Family-Child Resources

3995 E. Market Street
York, PA 17402
Ph: 717-757-1227
Fax: 717-757-1353
Website: www.f-cr.com

Occupational Therapy
for children

Occupational
Therapy
for children

PAT NUSE PRATT, M.O.T., O.T.R./L., F.A.O.T.A.
Private Practive,
Cleveland, Georgia

ANNE STEVENS ALLEN, M.A., O.T.R.
Formerly, Assistant Director,
School of Allied Medical Professions,
The Ohio State University, Columbus, Ohio

SECOND EDITION

with 233 illustrations
Illustrations by Jody Fulks, M.S., Medical Illustrator

The C. V. Mosby Company
ST. LOUIS • BALTIMORE • TORONTO   1989

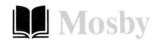

Editor: Richard A. Weimer
Editorial assistant: Adrianne H. Cochran
Project manager: Patricia Gayle May
Manuscript editor: Penny Susan Rudolph
Book design: Gail Morey Hudson
Cover design: The Archbault Group
Publisher: Thomas A. Manning

SECOND EDITION

The C.V. Mosby Company
11830 Westline Industrial Drive, St. Louis, Missouri 63146

Library of Congress Cataloging in Publication Data

Occupational therapy for children.

  Includes bibliographies.
  1. Occupational therapy for children.   I. Pratt,
Pat Nuse.   II. Allen, Anne S.
RJ53.025022   1989   615.8′5152′088054   88-25794
ISBN 0-8016-2466-5

C/VH/VH   9   8   7   6   5   4   3

Contributors

ANNE STEVENS ALLEN, M.A., O.T.R.

Formerly, School of Allied Medical Professions, The Ohio State University, Columbus, Ohio

PEGGY BARNSTORFF, M.O.T., O.T.R.

Pediatric Therapy Associates, Fort Collins, Colorado

JULIE CRITES BISSELL, M.A., O.T.R.

Occupational Therapy and Physical Therapy Services, Anaheim City School District, Anaheim, California

JANICE POSATERY BURKE, M.A., O.T.R./L., F.A.O.T.A.

Thomas Jefferson University, Philadelphia, Pennsylvania; Private Practice, Huntingdon Valley, Pennsylvania

DIANA P. BURNELL, Ph.D., O.T.R.

Private Practice and Consultation, Saratoga, California

RICARDO C. CARRASCO, M.Ed., O.T.R./L.

Occupational Therapy Department, Medical College of Georgia, Augusta, Georgia

FLORENCE CLARK, Ph.D., O.T.R., F.A.O.T.A.

Occupational Therapy Department, University of Southern California, Downey, California

IDA LOU COLEY, O.T.R.

Formerly, Children's Hospital at Stanford, Palo Alto, California

ANNE F. CRONIN, M.A., O.T.R.

Department of Occupational Therapy, University of Florida, Gainesville, Florida

FROMA JACOBSON CUMMINGS, O.T.R.

Upward Foundation, Phoenix, Arizona

CHRISTINE BOSONETTO DOANE, M.S., O.T.R./L.

Clinical Services, American Rehabilitation Services Atlanta, Georgia.

CHARLOTTE E. EXNER, M.S., O.T.R., F.A.O.T.A.

Towson State University, Towson, Maryland

LINDA A. FLOREY, M.A., O.T.R., F.A.O.T.A.

Rehabilitation Services, Children's Division, UCLA/Neuropsychiatric Institute, University of California, Los Angeles, California

JANET H. JOHNSON, M.S., O.T.R.

Colerain School, Columbus, Ohio

KATALIN I. KORANYI, M.D.

Department of Pediatrics, The Ohio State University, Columbus, Ohio

ZOE MAILLOUX, M.A., O.T.R.

Occupational Therapy Department, University of Southern California, Downey, California

M. JEANETTE MARTIN, M.Ed., O.T.R./L., F.A.A.M.D., F.A.O.T.A.

Georgia Retardation Center, Atlanta, Georgia

MARY A. McILROY, M.D.

Department of Pediatrics, The Ohio State University, Columbus, Ohio

MARTHA S. MOERSCH, M.Ed., O.T.R., F.A.O.T.A.

Formerly, Institute for the Study of Mental Retardation and Related Disabilities, University of Michigan, Ann Arbor, Michigan

ALISA PALMERI, O.T.R.

University of Connecticut Health Center, Farmington, Connecticut

DIANE PARHAM, M.A., O.T.R.

Occupational Therapy Department, University of Southern California, Downey, California

NANCY J. POWELL, Ph.D., O.T.R.

College of Pharmacy and Allied Health Professions, Wayne State University, Detroit, Michigan

PAT NUSE PRATT, M.O.T., O.T.R./L., F.A.O.T.A.

Private Practice, Cleveland, Georgia

SUSAN A. PROCTER, O.T.R.

Rehabilitation Engineering Center, Children's Hospital at Stanford, Palo Alto, California

CHARLOTTE BRASIC ROYEEN, Ph.D., O.T.R., F.A.O.T.A.

Office of Special Education Programs, U.S. Department of Education, Washington, D.C.

KAREN E. SCHANZENBACHER, M.S., O.T.R.

State University of New York at Buffalo, Buffalo, New York

JUDITH PELLETIER SEHNAL, M.S., O.T.R.

Easter Seal Rehabilitation Center
Waterbury, Connecticut

SUSAN DENEGAN SHORTRIDGE, M.H.S., O.T.R.

Developmental Health Care Services, Inc., Gainesville, Florida

BETTY SNOW, M.A., O.T.R.

Occupational Therapy Education Coordinator, Los Angeles County, California Children's Services, Los Angeles, California

LINDA C. STEPHENS, M.S., O.T.R./L., F.A.O.T.A.

The Adaptive Learning Center, Atlanta, Georgia

SUSAN K. TAUBER, M.Ed., O.T.R./L.

The Adaptive Learning Center, Atlanta, Georgia

Foreword

Children are a nation's richest resource. How a nation treats its childen is a measure of its civility. The authors of this comprehensive textbook have provided a vehicle for occupational therapists to improve and maintain the health of the nation's children and to assist them in achieving their optimal potential in growth and development. The concepts expressed in this book will facilitate learning for students and practitioners and promote high-quality health care for all children: from the presumably well to those who are ill, disabled, and dysfunctional; from birth through adolescence; and through the developmental stages that are critical to their chronological development.

The authors have addressed theory and practice in ways that provide basic understanding for the student who is developing entry-level professional competency and stimulation and challenge for the advanced student and experienced therapist. Occupational therapy practice in pediatrics encompasses case identification, screening, evaluation, treatment or intervention, re-evaluation, follow-through, and health maintenance. The settings in which the therapist practices include neonatal units in general hospitals; community preschools; elementary, junior, and senior high schools; neighborhood health centers; high-density housing developments; training schools and halfway houses for delinquent children and youth; special service agencies for adolescents; public health departments; and the home.

The authors have taken into account the reader's need to be aware of developmental principles and theories; the developmental process through adolescence; general pediatric health care; and the areas of illness, disability, and dysfunction that occur with infants, children, and adolescents, whether congenital or acquired. The authors have therefore provided the reader with tools, procedures, and techniques for identifying and assessing pediatric clients. They discuss the clinical reasoning process that assists readers in developing or sharpening the skill to analyze and synthesize data from evaluation and to plan and implement appropriate strategies for direct and indirect intervention. Direct and indirect intervention strategies are presented for working with children and significant others such as parents, teachers, siblings, and caretakers. The occupational performance frame of reference has served the authors well in the organization of many of their evaluation and treatment formulations.

Occupational Therapy for Children provides a state-of-the-art conceptualization of pediatric occupational therapy practice. In addition to the extensive literature synthesis, the contributors to this volume have shared their commitment as pediatric practitioners to the health care of the nation's children.

This book is a long-awaited contribution to the literature in the field of occupational therapy. It will surely advance the level of pediatric occupational therapy practice and the professionalism of the discipline.

Lela A. Llorens, Ph.D., O.T.R., F.A.O.T.A.

Professor, Chair, and Graduate Coordinator, Department of Occupational Therapy, San Jose State University, San Jose, California

Preface to second edition

As we developed the first edition of *Occupational Therapy for Children,* one of our objectives was to produce a text that would be of high enough quality and usefulness to warrant a second edition. We realized that, despite the very best efforts of the contributors, reviewers, editors, and publishers, there would be weak areas in the text. Also, due to the continually evolving nature of a practice profession, we knew that many areas of pediatric occupational therapy theory and technology were in transition, and that a significant portion of our content would soon require updating.

Since the publication of the first edition, we have maintained a file of suggestions, corrections, and comments received from helpful occupational therapy educators, practitioners, and students. In addition, we conducted a survey of faculty in a random sample of professional level occupational therapy curricula. We thank the respondents for their critiques, and hope that we have used their suggestions responsibly.

Accordingly, a number of changes have been made in this edition to update and improve the breadth of content, to increase the number of photographs and illustrations, and to improve the mechanics of using the text. In response to our own and others' concerns, and to keep pace with changes in the field, we have added chapters on program planning and evaluation, the development and treatment of hand function and dysfunction, independent living, early intervention, and private practice in pediatric occupational therapy. All of the continuing chapters have been updated, and our authors have expanded content on occupational behavior theory, neuromotor development, issues of parent involvement in the therapy process, activity adaptations, approaches to treating the learning disabled child, and ongoing changes in the legislative and practical aspects of working in public schools. The chapters on treatment of children with cerebral palsy and emotional and behavior disorders have been completely rewritten, with more emphasis on practice. Each chapter in this edition of *Occupational Therapy for Children* includes a set of study questions following the chapter summary. These are designed to be used by the student to examine his or her understanding of any specific diagnostic problem presented in the chapter. Some of the questions test knowledge and comprehension. Others test the student's ability to predict the possible impact of these diseases and conditions on a child's developmental progress and functional abilities. This new study aid will guide integration, analysis, and application of content. The authors hope that learning will be enhanced.

One of our disappointments with the first edition was the discontinuity caused by the test forms in the assessment chapters. Consequently, this edition presents most test forms as a group at the end of each chapter in which they are discussed, thereby allowing more continuity in the flow of the narrative text. Similarly, the assessment tools that were originally located in the appendixes have been moved to the ends of the chapters to which they pertain, with the exception of Coley's self-care assessment. This has been continued as an appendix, due to space considerations.

We hope these changes will improve the utility of the book, and welcome feedback. At this time, we do wish to reaffirm our intent to have *Occupational Therapy for Children* serve as a basic student text and general reference for practitioners. We do not and cannot provide in-depth information in the different specialty areas of practice: each of these merits a monograph or text of its own, and in fact many such resources are available to experienced therapists. Further, the cost of a volume that covered the state-of-the-art in all specialty areas would be prohibitive. We do believe that, added to the academic and clinical education required by the "Essentials," careful study of this text and thoughtful application of its content will enable an occupational therapist to plan and provide competent services to children. This is the guiding purpose for the development and revision of *Occupational Therapy for Children,* and our hope for its users.

The editors and contributors gratefully acknowledge the continued support, encouragement, and assistance of colleagues and loved ones.

Pat Nuse Pratt
Anne Stevens Allen

Preface to first edition

This book is about the practice of occupational therapy with children. To provide a sound basis for discussion of practice methods and modalities, we have included the most pertinent information about developmental theory, learning theory, and pediatric medicine. However, this book is not intended to take the place of good textbooks on development, pediatric medicine, health care delivery systems, or educational methods. We hope it will serve as a detailed collection of current and time-honored theory and practice in pediatric occupational therapy, as well as a guide to practice trends for the future.

We believe that each child has basic developmental needs and matures through a common developmental process. Yet we also recognize that each child is different and proceeds according to an individual timetable through this process. Many of the differences result from the nature of each child's play opportunities and experiences, as well as from the environments in which each child grows. The differences are also a result of each child's individual biological endowment and of the forces that may positively or negatively affect the growing child from embryo to adulthood.

The primary role of the occupational therapist in pediatrics is to help children play, grow, and develop many of the skills that will enable them to enjoy a satisfying adult life. Occupational therapists do this through the knowledgeable selection and use of everyday activities to evaluate and enhance children's development and competence.

We would like to introduce the reader to children, and to occupational therapy practice with them, through a process that is similar in sequence to a student's academic and clinical experiences. *Part I* introduces the general roles and functions of occupational therapy in pediatrics. This is followed by a survey of the different types of service facilities in which pediatric practitioners most frequently work. It will be noted that the trend is toward practice in education-oriented settings and that even medically-oriented practice is most often found in outpatient settings. This does not imply that inpatient, hospital-based practice is out-moded or unnecessary. It does reflect significant improvements in pediatric medical and surgical practices that now enable the majority of "problem children" to become medically stable enough to live at home, with due regard to funding constraints.

Part I concludes with a discussion of the persons who are important to the child and to the pediatric occupational therapist. It begins with the family and includes professional and technical members of the health care and educational teams.

Part II provides a compilation of the knowledge base for pediatric occupational therapy. This begins with a review of basic developmental principles and theories. The overview of major theories of child development provides a foundation for the discussion of pediatric occupational therapy. These theories are next integrated into a concise description of the developmental process from the prenatal period through adolescence.

Two chapters in this section provide basic information about child health care and the diseases and disabilities that cause problems for the children who are treated by occupational therapists. We have tried to select a broad variety of diagnostic problems and to provide timely information about cause, classification, course and prognosis, and general management. Implications for occupational therapy intervention will help to carry the focus of information from the pathological to the practical.

Part III uses the knowledge base to define the occupational therapy process. This section includes discussion of the parameters of occupational therapy intervention and broadly defines the generic modalities of practice, including occupational activities; human and object relationships; tools, materials, and equipment for activities; and special adaptation techniques. The generic processes of the discipline, activity analysis and activity adaptation, are presented as a framework for occupational therapy programming with children. A sequence for occupational therapy intervention provides a model for planning individual programs for children seen in treatment. We include a number of sample worksheets for organization and analysis of assessment information and program ideas are included throughout the text. This section also includes information about different instructional approaches that can be used with children, as well as contraindications related to particular methods. Collaborative programs and relationships with parents are necessary to develop play, self-maintenance, and school work skills to an optimal level. Guidelines for such interactive programs are presented in general and specific form.

A therapist's first encounter with a child will typically involve assessment of current function. *Part IV* presents information about the variety of assessment methods and instruments available to the pediatric occupational therapist. These range from methods of observation to the specialized procedures used to develop highly detailed understanding of a child's strengths and limitations. Causes of problems are also identified.

There is a growing concern among the members of the profession that occupational therapists often perform exhaustive evaluations that leave little time or resources for the actual treatment program that is to produce change. This book will emphasize assessment tools that use age-appropriate, familiar activities, and we hope that this will bridge the gap from testing to treatment. There are multitudes of tests available that have been designed to be administered to children, and each therapist will find occasion to develop new evaluation materials. However, we believe that the formal evaluation of children should be kept to the minimum necessary to obtain good information and retain the child's interest. Often as much accurate information can be obtained by watching a child play catch with a shadow for 5 minutes as by administering a 3-hour battery of tests. Therapists need to know what to look for and what they are seeing. This knowledge comes from study of child development and activity analysis.

Part V provides comprehensive information about practice methods and modalities that are used in all occupational therapy programming with children. These chapters in Part V present the major domains of activity. We believe that these domains of play, self-maintenance, and school work should be the beginning and end of each child's program if they are to be described as occupational therapy. The chapters will give detailed information about age-appropriate steps and modifications of basic activities for children. A wide variety of adaptive techniques and devices are presented that will enable children to explore and control their environments more independently.

A final word is pertinent to the content on school work activities in *Part V.* This section relates to a child's basic readiness and capacities for school work and preadult development. Most of this preparation will come through therapy experiences in play and self-maintenance activities. However, when a child has

specific problems identified during the school-age years, the therapist will need to develop additional programming to ensure the child's adequacy in the school environment. More relevant material will be found in Part VI in discussion of occupational therapy services in educational settings.

The chapters in *Part VI* are meant to provide a foundation for study in the specialty areas of pediatric practice. Although no chapter is exhaustive in discussing its topic, therapists should be able to begin working with special populations in a more confident manner as they seek additional resources to obtain specialist competence. Our finding is that most therapists tend to see two or three special populations of children most often as their interests and experience progress.

As in the chapter on diagnostic problems (Chapter 6), we have tried to present information about a broad variety of specialized practices. In addition to tying information into content presented in Parts I through V, each chapter presents the theories, assessment instruments, and treatment modalities essential to its focus. Part VI includes a chapter about the special characteristics of practice in the public school systems because this is where the greatest proportion of pediatric occupational therapy is now practiced. However, the methods and modalities discussed throughout Parts IV and V have been developed through both educationally- and medically-oriented practice environments and should not be considered extraneous material for the school therapist.

The contributing authors for this book may be recognized as experienced clinical educators who like to write. We looked for the former characteristic in selection of authors to ensure the timeliness and usefulness of practice information. Of course, without the latter quality it would be impossible to complete the book.

As female members of the occupational therapy profession, we and our contributing authors have made conscientious efforts to avoid terminology that might be considered sexist. Whenever possible, we have referred to children in plural form and used clinical examples of both female and male children. However, it is sometimes impossible to present descriptive material in readable style without the use of gender-related pronouns and possessives. In such instances, it is necessary to abide by the general policy of our publishing company to use the universal masculine forms. Please be aware that unless these forms are used in relation to a specific clinical or gender-related example, they are intended to describe characteristics and actions of both female and male children.

The primary purpose of this book is to serve as a basic text for the occupational therapy student who is involved in academic and fieldwork study in pediatrics. We hope it will serve as a continuing resource to that student long after graduation and certification and that it will also provide a basic reference for the experienced practitioner. Our own experiences as students and practitioners of occupational therapy have caused us to wish for, look for, and finally develop such a resource.

No book of this scope can be produced without the assistance and encouragement of many people. We would like to acknowledge the initiating contributions of Don Ladig and Ida Lou Coley, who conceptualized this comprehensive textbook and gave us the idea for its elaboration and production. Rose Hartsook helped establish an outline for the prodigious chapter on diagnostic problems, and Richard D. Sarkin, M.D. reviewed its content. His willingness to share information and resources and his enthusiasm for occupational therapy education were major factors in the completion of that chapter.

Elnora Gilfoyle, Lela Llorens, and Nancy Prendergast read pages and pages of manuscript, giving valuable and insightful comments that improved both content and presentation. Ann Wade, Karen Feltham, Ruth Humphry, and Debbie Russo assisted with the preparation of the chapter on cerebral palsy, as did the staff of the Franklin County Program, Forest Park School, Columbus, Georgia. A succession of therapists at the Colerain School developed several of the assessment instruments used in Chapters 9, 10, and 11: Kathy Campbell, Vera Demeter, Leni Heller, Marilyn Fetters, Janet Johnson, Mary Stover, and Marilee Wilde. Their development and refinement over the years of most useful instruments demonstrate one of the salutary components of occupational therapy practice today. Julie Garvin assisted with the sensory-integration section of Chapter 3; Carol Leaman and Carol Johnson generously provided assessment tools and guidance. We are indebted to the students of Herndon Elementary School, Atlanta, Georgia, for the photographs in Chapters 14 and 24. In addition, the faculty of the occupational therapy program at Ohio State University gave the kind of support that only friends of long standing and kind disposition can give. To all these colleagues who saw a need for this kind of book and contributed so generously to its development, we extend profound appreciation.

A special kind of acknowledgment must be made to Rosa Kasper whose constant grace, good humor, and editorial wisdom were the catalysts that kept the authors and editors working. David Clark and John Allen tolerated the kind of neglect that is induced by projects of this magnitude. Their understanding and nurture were necessary ingredients. And Scott and Stacy Clark modeled, posed, and assisted in many ways so that we could observe and write about what really happens.

Pat Nuse Clark
Anne Stevens Allen

Contents

PART
I

INTRODUCTION

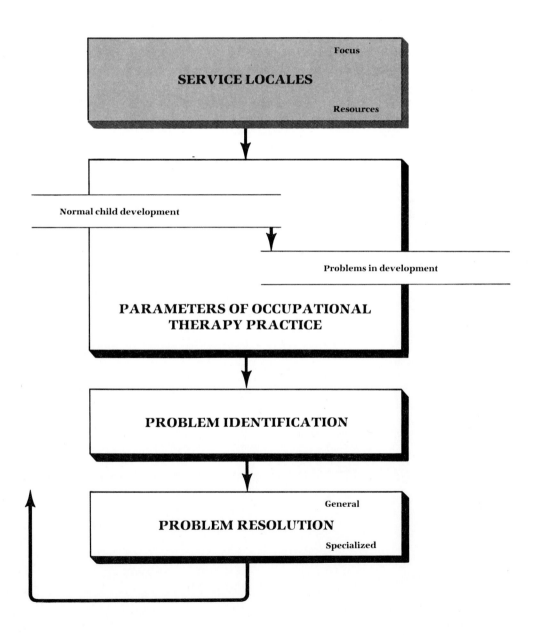

1

The role of occupational therapy in pediatrics

PAT NUSE PRATT
ANNE STEVENS ALLEN

ORGANIZING PRINCIPLES

In 1947 McNary[4] identified the following seven objectives of occupational therapy practice with children:

1. To offer diversional activity to the child when he is undergoing medical treatment,
2. To offer concentrated activity for development of motion of joints, strength of muscles, and coordination,
3. To provide specialized play to teach the elements of self-care,
4. To overcome fears and develop confidence through performance,
5. To encourage normal development in spite of physical, emotional, or intellectual handicap,
6. To provide socializing factors for those who need them and
7. To increase parental understanding of the child's problems through his performance (p. 20).

Thoughtful consideration of the general purposes of current pediatric occupational therapy practice reveals no substantive change in objectives. Certainly, the language of the profession has become more formal and specialized, as have the structure and content of practice. In the early programs the bulk of the occupational therapist's time was spent in actual treatment, namely, teaching children self-care and doing play and recreational activities with them. In contrast, today's therapist may devote longer hours to administrative and supervisory activities and conduct a more formal, comprehensive assessment before initiation of treatment.

The greatest changes in structure and content of occupational therapy practice have resulted from two forces: (1) the overwhelming transformation of contemporary living caused by twentieth century technology and (2) the resultant, concurrent growth and spe-cialization of the educational process. Adequate discussion of these two forces is beyond the purpose of this text. However, these forces have produced the following six change factors that are pertinent to occupational therapy:

1. The increased life expectancy of children with severe health problems.
2. The expanding scope and variety of publicly supported programs for children.
3. The burgeoning of knowledge in the human sciences, particularly in psychology, the neurosciences, and child development.
4. The impact of modern technology on both diagnostic and treatment aspects of children's programs.
5. The impact of regulatory mechanisms on organization, administration, and documentation of services.
6. The sophistication of methodology for clinical research and its application in occupational therapy.

The purpose of this book is to describe the structure and content of contemporary occupational therapy practice with children and to develop an understanding of the purpose of practice. It is therefore necessary to examine the knowledge that has accrued to the profession, including that resulting from the six change factors described in the preceding paragraph:

1. The current knowledge related to the causes, course, and prognosis of the problems that affect children who are seen by occupational therapists.
2. The focus and variety of settings, agencies, facilities, and service providers pertinent to occupational therapy practice.

3. The principles and processes of child development.
4. The assessment-diagnostic and treatment modalities that have been influenced by the application of research and other technology to occupational therapy practice.
5. The pertinent information related to compliance with regulatory mechanisms governing occupational therapy programs for children

It is premature to present a detailed discussion of the structure of occupational therapy practice before examining the knowledge that provides its foundation. However, it will be useful here to present an overall framework that guides, determines, and describes pediatric occupational therapy practice (Figure 1-1). This text essentially duplicates the framework in Figure 1-1 with the exception of the first two chapters, which are introductory and describe service locales, providers, and relationships. In practice, however, one component may never be clearly isolated from the others. It is necessary to have a basic familiarity with the people and places of a child's environments to discuss the child's development and problems in a knowledgeable manner. More detailed information about the dynamics of specialized service settings and mechanisms in relation to occupational therapy practices will be presented later in this book.

BASIC METHODS OF SERVICE DELIVERY

Chapman and Chapman[1] outlined a three-dimensional model of health care services that was based

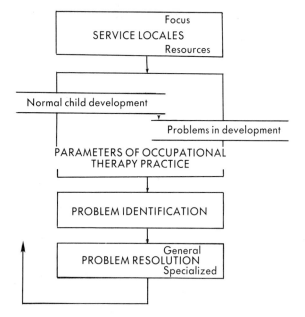

Figure 1-1 Organizing framework for comprehensive pediatric occupational therapy.

on the individual client's right to a healthful, productive life. They categorized services as:
1. Life-saving—directed toward prevention of imminent death.
2. Life-sustaining—directed toward health maintenance and prevention of disability.
3. Life-enhancing—directed toward maintenance, restoration, and development of the individual's sense of well-being, social productivity, and self-satisfaction.

It is clear that occupational therapy services are broadly directed toward the life-sustaining and life-enhancing dimensions of health care as described by Chapman and Chapman. In essence, occupational therapy treatment can be said to maintain and enhance the quality of an individual's life. This is an especially important outcome of health services for children with problems, because the biggest part of their lives lies ahead of them. Without life-sustaining and life-enhancing services, such as those delivered by occupational therapists, the future of many children would be less meaningful, less productive, and less satisfying.

A child is likely to receive occupational therapy services at various times during the course of a health problem or handicapping condition. These services may be provided by one or more therapists working through a variety of health care or educational agencies. Occupational therapy services may also differ in method according to the child's status and the agency's objectives. This concept of multiphasic service delivery through a variable course of time, place, and method of intervention constitutes a *continuum of service.*

This chapter will introduce the general methods and settings of occupational therapy services in pediatrics. Discussion of the changes in service over the course of time according to the progression of a child's health status and age will be incorporated into subsequent chapters on pediatric problems and treatment. The service methods described here are a modification of the model developed through the American Occupational Therapy Association (AOTA).[2]

Direct service

Direct service is the most basic method used to provide occupational therapy. This term implies a direct relationship between the child (service recipient) and the therapist (service provider). Usually direct service also denotes face-to-face, hands-on contact between recipient and provider. The usual sequence in direct service is assessment, treatment, and follow-up.

ASSESSMENT

Assessment is an evaluation process that is based on facts (data collected through different formal and informal objective measures of the child's performance) and sound clinical judgment. The latter is the subjective and interpretive component of assessment, and it is the end product of the therapist's individual experiences, namely, the therapist's training, practice, and theoretical frame of reference.

The initial phase of assessment is known as *screening.* In occupational therapy, screening usually includes observing the child in a natural activity situation and gathering baseline background information about the child. Screening permits the therapist to determine the need for more comprehensive and precise evaluation and subsequent occupational therapy treatment. Occasionally the therapist will decide that occupational therapy intervention is unnecessary or that such services are contraindicated until a later date.

Assessment is a continuing process as the therapist continually thinks through interactions and activity experiences with the child. However, at designated intervals the assessment becomes more structured and is thus recorded. This allows the therapist to:

1. Identify present performance
2. Define problems
3. Identify potential performance
4. Develop program objectives and modalities
5. Record and report progress to document change

TREATMENT

Treatment consists of a carefully selected program of change-enhancing activities that are administered by the therapist. The child's response to the activity is guided by the therapist, who is also responsible for changes and outcome of the treatment program. (The terms *treatment, therapy,* and *program* are often used interchangeably.) The structure and ramifications of treatment are complex and will be explored throughout this book.

FOLLOW-UP

When the child has obtained the optimal benefits from treatment or has shown no significant change over time (plateaued), therapy is discontinued. The child is assigned to follow-up status. This means that the child is rechecked by the therapist at fixed intervals. Follow-up appointments for children are generally scheduled every 3 to 6 months. This is usually more frequent than follow-up for adults because of the impact of the continuing developmental process on the child's functional level and needs. Frequent follow-up visits allow the therapist to monitor a child's progress and reinstitute therapy in a timely manner when needed.

Eventually the child will be discharged. Parents should always be advised of available resources for future therapy and related needs.

Outreach services

Outreach services are provided by occupational therapists to children who are under the primary care of other agencies. Often these agencies may already employ an occupational therapist. However, special children have special needs, and occasionally more experienced or specialized therapy services are indicated that are beyond the expertise of the agency therapist.

Outreach services usually follow the same assessment and treatment planning sequence as direct service with one important difference. After the assessment has been completed, the visiting therapist develops a *model program* for the child or children. This model program is then demonstrated and described in detail to the agency therapist. The goal is to increase the expertise of the local agency therapist who will continue and carry out the treatment at the agency. The outcome of treatment is a shared responsibility of both visiting and local therapists.

Outreach services are used most frequently to provide specialized services to rural areas. Typically the visiting therapist is employed at an urban, university-affiliated children's center and works with a local therapist whose practice and experience are more general (Figure 1-2).

Indirect service

Indirect service implies that the therapist does not engage in face-to-face, hands-on contact with the child.

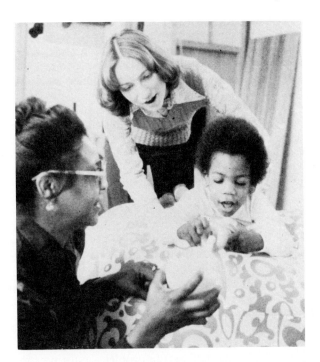

Figure 1-2   A visiting occupational therapist works with local staff to bring specialized skills to a small community hospital.

From Worley JS, "Occupational Therapy" in INTRODUCTION TO HEALTH PROFESSIONS, ed 3, The CV Mosby Co. With permission.

The concept can be misleading, because usually there is at least one direct contact with the service recipient, and often additional contacts are made at regular intervals. The essence of indirect service is that the bulk of treatment is administered by other direct service providers and based on recommendations made by the occupational therapist. The occupational therapist may or may not be held responsible for the outcome of treatment.

Therapists who work in large agencies with many potential clients, such as school systems, often use *monitoring* as the primary method of service delivery. The therapist directly assesses the child and develops a treatment program. Other direct care staff are then trained by the therapist to carry out program activities on a daily basis. The therapist rechecks the child and the consistency of the program and updates activities and assessment at regular intervals. Using a monitoring system, the therapist is responsible for the outcome of the program.

The responsibility for outcome shifts to the direct care providers in a *consultation* arrangement. The therapist may directly assess individual children and recommend program methods. Or the therapist may not evaluate directly but instead will interview staff members to obtain information about clients and agency procedures. The therapist then discusses and writes down broad recommendations for changes that could facilitate improved services for clients of the agency. The consultation process has its own formal structure and is usually of short duration. The therapist has no direct authority to enforce recommended changes but relies on an ability to influence the behavior of staff members.

In practice, most experienced therapists use a combination of direct, outreach, and indirect service methods to provide appropriate occupational therapy services to children. The emphasis on one method of service delivery over another is influenced by the type of agency in which the therapist is employed.

SERVICE SETTINGS

Almost one third of all practicing occupational therapists work in the field of pediatrics by providing services to newborns, toddlers, preschoolers, and kindergartners through adolescents. This clientele receives health services in numerous settings, depending on the age of the child, the severity and cause of the problem, and, to some extent, the parents' ability or willingness to pay for services.

Some children with severe problems must be cared for in custodial situations, while others with similar problems may live at home and go to public schools. Maintaining regular school programs for handicapped children among their normal peers is called *mainstreaming* and is mandated by federal law (p. 8.) Indeed, federal or local regulations affect all facets of pe-

diatric services. Concern is growing that payment schedules might become the determining factor in availability of services.

In all settings the occupational therapist attempts to help children adapt to their physical and emotional surroundings, to assure children the most normal development possible, to assist parents in learning how to understand and deal with their child's needs, and to offer opportunities for daily stabilizing diversion for children under stress.

Neonatal units

Specialized units for the care of newborns at risk are part of the nurseries in teaching hospitals and in specialty hospitals with high obstetrical case loads. These units serve newborns in need of special care, especially those whose survival is in doubt and those who appear to be well but are at risk of serious illness. These newborns are isolated in a sterile, protective environment and handled through sealed apertures in the sides of their bassinets. They are under 24-hour observation because of the rapidity with which life-threatening crises can occur. Nurses, physicians, respiratory therapists, developmental therapists, and other specialized personnel are involved in their care.

The determination of which newborns are to be placed in such units depends on institutional criteria, such as minimal weights, disease categories, or condition of the mother. The components of service are (1) direct observation of the newborn by nursing and medical personnel, (2) physiological and biochemical monitoring by electronic equipment and laboratory personnel, (3) diagnostic and therapeutic procedures, and (4) support of maximal mother-child contact.[3]

In the neonatal setting, developmental therapists, who are often occupational therapists, are involved in these therapeutic procedures by giving sensory stimulation to infants deprived of normal stimulation by the enforced isolation of the unit. These infants are frequently restrained to prevent interference with the tubes and other biomedical devices necessarily attached to them. Sensory stimulation is provided to counteract the negative developmental effects of this isolation and restraint. Splinting is sometimes used to maintain the infant in a safer functional position.

Public health departments and well-baby clinics

Public health departments are financed by city and county governments and offer certain clinical services to residents of the city and region. These services include communicable disease testing, immunization programs, and home health services. Mothers who have no family physician are encouraged to have their infants checked in the well-baby clinic, which is frequently operated under the county's maternal and child health funds, and to participate in the immunization program.

Occupational therapists working in well-baby clinics have the opportunity to develop infant stimulation programs and to teach the mothers about developmental play. This can often mean the difference between a neglected child who fails to develop socially and emotionally and a thriving, happy youngster.

Home health services

Home health services are offered to homebound persons of all ages. These services include bedside nursing, homemaking assistance, hot meal programs, and programs of occupational, physical, and speech therapies.

Home health services provide occupational therapy to children of all diagnoses who cannot be taken to central agencies or schools. Occupational therapy services to homebound children include programs for orthopedic and developmental disabilities. The goals are primarily rehabilitative in nature. Maintenance of health and function, assisting the child to develop in the home environment, and teaching family how to assist or care for the child are also goals of home health services.

Physicians' offices

Most children receive primary health care through the offices of private physicians. Detailed description of their services may be found in Chapter 5.

Occasionally physicians will arrange for therapists to provide assessment and treatment in their offices. Usually such arrangements are made with therapists in private practice. Such an arrangement is convenient for parents because it reduces the need to travel from office to office for services.

Community health centers

Community health centers offer a variety of services to clients from a localized area. The centers usually develop in response to specific needs and as a result of considerable community effort. They are funded in the following ways: by united appeals campaigns, by sliding-scale fee-for-service arrangements, by private endowments, by grants from governmental agencies, and by other sources tapped by enterprising citizens.

The health programs in these centers reflect the community's need for emergency services and general health care. Emphasis is usually on prevention.

Occupational therapy in community health is a diverse practice and often reflects the interests or specialties of the therapists on the staff, for the service potential far exceeds the ability of the center to develop needed programs. Pediatric occupational therapists in community health screen for developmental delay, teach play skills to parents and children, and provide specialized therapy programs for handicapped children.

Health maintenance organizations (HMOs)

Health maintenance organizations (HMOs) are a relatively new type of health agency that provide continuous, coordinated health services to members. These members enroll individually and prepay their medical expenses with a fixed monthly payment. Under such a system it is to the benefit of the HMO to keep health and medical costs low. One of the ways this is done is to prevent illness and maintain health.

There are two types of HMO. One provides care in a centrally located building with a group of physicians under contract to or employed by the HMO. The other type contracts with community-based physicians to give care in their own offices to HMO members. Occupational therapists seeking to practice in HMO settings find the first type, the so-called group staff HMO, more supportive of their services. Within the central location, occupational therapy programs answering pediatric needs can be developed. The therapist's role in such an agency would include consultation as well as direct service with a great deal of emphasis placed on preventive programs, such as screening for the early detection of developmental problems.

General and children's hospitals

General hospitals are found in small communities and in large cities and constitute the largest classification of hospitals. They accept patients of all ages and diagnoses, but they usually refer complex cases to appropriate specialty hospitals. They serve as the health and emergency center for their surrounding communities.

The occupational therapist in a general hospital provides many services because of the variety of problems and the relatively short stay of most patients. General hospitals require occupational therapists to serve in many capacities, for instance, (1) evaluating patients for physical function and developing therapeutic programs for them and (2) providing cardiac programs, burn care, and stroke rehabilitation. Similar functional services are provided for the pediatric unit but with additional emphasis on diversional programs and play therapy because of the emotional needs of children separated from their families.

Children's hospitals limit their patient services to the pediatric patient and therefore can usually offer a wider variety of pediatric occupational therapy than can the general hospital with its broader range of needs. In the children's hospital, probably as in no other setting, the seven objectives listed by McNary[4]

(p. 2) can each be realized in the same setting. A wide variety of pediatric diagnoses gives rise to a wide variety of treatment objectives. Length of stay is longer in the children's hospital than in the general hospital, making emotional and developmental support mandatory. Also found in children's hospitals are functional programs for the development of muscle strength, joint motion, and coordination for the orthopedically and neurologically handicapped child; socializing and developmental programs for all children, but especially for those with long hospital stays; and programs that build confidence and positive self-images in children who have experienced either psychological or physical trauma.

As with any program involving children, a second dimension of treating the child is working with the parent. Occupational therapists will teach parents the same skills the child learns and also teach them how to help the child.

Rehabilitation centers

Rehabilitation is defined as a return to the level of function enjoyed before the onset of the disease or injury that has interrupted the client's life. Children who have never attained any degree of independence and who must learn self-care and other basic living skills for the first time are said to undergo *habilitation*. Agencies that provide habilitative and rehabilitative services are called *rehabilitation centers* and are usually financed by private resources, such as insurance companies, union funds, and united appeals agencies. Payment for services often comes from the state division of rehabilitation services when adults are being served. Children's services are reimbursed by a variety of governmental agencies, both state and federal.

Rehabilitation centers provide the child with a broad range of concentrated corrective programs designed to restore function and advance independence. In addition to medical services, rehabilitation centers provide social and psychological services; occupational, physical, and speech therapies; tutors or classroom teachers; vocational counseling and prevocational testing; orthotic and prosthetic consultation; and other needed services, either in the center or by referral.

As in the children's hospital, the full range of occupational therapy objectives is applicable. Occupational therapists evaluate the children and design treatment programs that promote developmental skills, enhance independence and self-confidence, and develop physical function and coordination. The therapist functions as part of an interdisciplinary team, not only in treatment but also in decision making and problem solving.

Residential programs

Residential programs for the care of handicapped children usually serve the most seriously handicapped population and are usually operated by the state government. Institutions for the profoundly retarded, for the blind, and for the deaf are funded by the states, and the quality of their programs depends on the tax structure and philosophy of the incumbent administration.

Client evaluation, training in adaptive skills, and sensory integrative therapy are the primary concerns of the staff occupational therapists. Because of the residential nature of the institution, diversional programming is also within the purview of occupational therapy planning and of high importance for the stimulation, skill development, and self-confidence of the residents.

Institutions that are primarily custodial may offer little to attract a staff of occupational therapists. Occupational therapy is at its best in residential programs when it is closely allied to an educational program with teachers, occupational therapists, physical and speech therapists, and psychologists working together as a team.

Day training centers

Day training centers serve a population of educable mentally retarded and severely physically handicapped persons as an entry point to sheltered or assisted work. Adaptive skills and work skills are taught in these centers, usually to adolescents and young adults. Infants and younger children who are not able to attend public school are also clients of the day training centers. Referral can be made by schools, by the division of vocational rehabilitation, and by other agencies.

Clients go to the day training center on regular schedules three to five times a week. An educational rather than clinical atmosphere is maintained. Occupational therapy programs include evaluation and training in self-care, homemaking, and prevocational skills, including emotional and social skills that are required vocationally. Subcontracted work, such as simple assembly tasks, is sometimes available to be used primarily in client evaluation or training for future assisted placement. Occupational therapists will frequently analyze available jobs in the community to determine their appropriateness for specific clients and to suggest modifications that would enable clients to be successful on the job.

Schools

Occupational therapy services have long been established in specialized schools for handicapped children. Supported by funds from national agencies, service clubs, and other community organizations, both occupational therapy and physical therapy were made available primarily in private schools but also in public schools when the local system was large enough to accommodate a special school for children with special needs.

This imbalance was changed in 1975 through Public

Law 94-142. This bill mandated education for all handicapped children within public school systems through programs designed to meet the individual needs of these children. Transportation to the school, special teachers, and occupational, physical, and speech therapies were construed as education-related services necessary to meet these needs, and they were therefore provided by law.

Occupational therapy in the public schools has one primary aim—to improve the handicapped student's ability to participate in the special education program. Secondary aims are to consult with parents and teachers, enabling them to understand the needs of the individual child and to assist the child in attaining and applying adaptive skills to classroom and home situations.

Occupational therapists have different roles in private schools, depending on the mission of the particular schools. Those schools that are established to serve children of one handicap group, such as the mentally retarded or the deaf, will often have a staff of therapists to provide services similar to those described previously. These services can also be extended to the prevocational area through prevocational tests, work methods adaptation, job evaluation, and assisted placement.

Private schools are maintained by two primary sources: (1) full tuition and (2) combinations of tuition and charitable endowments. Their programs are less affected by government regulations, so the programmatic quality of these schools varies according to the philosophy of their proprietors and the demands of their clientele. Thus, they range from being excellent educational and training programs to being mere custodial care centers.

Preschool programs

Preschools are set up in churches and other central locations to provide socialization and environmental stimulation for children younger than kindergarten age. The Head Start program, established under the Economic Opportunity Act of 1964, is an example of such a program developed by public initiative and federal funds. Its purpose was to prepare disadvantaged children for elementary school programs. Individual grants were made to cities and localities to initiate programs at public locations. Services were later extended to children above the poverty level whose parents were required to pay according to their ability.

Private preschool programs are frequently sponsored by a church or other institution having space available. They depend on parental assitance, partial tuition, and subsidized overhead charges for support. There also are entrepreneurial preschools run for profit in private homes or commercial locations that depend totally on student tuition for support.

Occupational therapy in preschool settings is often practiced on a consultant basis and is entirely developmental in nature. Screening for developmental delay and evaluation of age-appropriate social and coordinative skills comprise the majority of the assessment in preschool occupational therapy. Developmental and sensory integrative techniques are used in treatment, either at the school or by referral to therapists in private practice.

Private practice

Pediatric occupational therapists in private practice frequently work as consultants to several agencies, preschools, or pediatricians. They may refer children for treatment to other practicing therapists, to staff Certified Occupational Therapy Assistants (COTAs), or to outpatient clinics. Consultants may also combine practice with their consultancies and see patients either at the patient's home or at their own offices.

Consultant, therapist, developmental specialist, prevocational evaluator—all these are roles filled by the occupational therapist in private practice. Services may be reimbursed by individual fees or a combination of patient fees and retainers paid by the employing agencies.

SUMMARY

The organizing principles of occupational therapy have their roots in McNary's original seven objectives.[4] Twentieth century technology and educational specialization produced six change factors that have influenced the practice of occupational therapy. The methods of service delivery and their locales have responded to these factors. At present, occupational therapists may practice in a variety of different settings and give direct, outreach, or indirect services.

REFERENCES

1. Chapman JE, and Chapman HH: Behavior and health care: a humanistic helping process, St. Louis, 1975, The CV Mosby Co.
2. Gilfoyle EM, and Hayes C, editors: Training: occupational therapy educational management in schools (TOTEMS), Rockville, Md, 1980, American Occupational Therapy Association, Inc (Supported by Grant #G007801499 US Department of Education, Office of Special Education and Rehabilitative Services, Vol I to IV.)
3. Korones SB: High-risk newborn infants, ed 3, St Louis, 1981, The CV Mosby Co.
4. McNary H: The scope of occupational therapy. In Willard HS, and Spackman CS: Occupational therapy, Philadelphia, 1947, JB Lippincott Co.

2

Relationships with other service providers

ANNE STEVENS ALLEN

Children with illnesses and emotional, physical, or mental deficiencies must be treated as "whole persons" within their environments. This is a truism not only in occupational therapy with its long history of concern for the wholeness of the patient, but increasingly in the other helping professions where technological specializations have often divided patient care into units defined by body systems or malfunctioning parts.

It has been suggested that society's present concern for the whole person has generated a need for interprofessional collaboration. Various specialists must learn to work together as one functioning unit to ensure respect for the patient as a whole person and to treat the person as one complex organism rather than treat only separate parts of that person.[1]

Collaborating groups of concerned, helping professionals are usually referred to as teams, and an extensive literature has developed that deals with the formation of teams and their ability to function effectively. Occupational therapists serve on many interprofessional teams and therefore work with many other helping persons. Not all such persons have the training in small group dynamics and interpersonal skills that is part of occupational therapy education. Most occupational therapists find that this part of their education (originally planned for patient interfaces) transfers most helpfully into professional interfaces. Careful attention should be paid to recognition of roles, clear communications, and shared decisions. These are effective tools for establishing relationships with the other persons involved in the care of children—medical and educational personnel and parents. This chapter will discuss the occupational therapist's relationship with medical and educational teams. For an interesting description of how teams develop to meet the specific needs of different patient populations while staying within the limits of realistic staffing for the agency, see Chapter 19.

THE MEDICAL TEAM

The medical team is made up of a variety of persons who are trained in different specialties and who each have different backgrounds, different values, and sometimes different goals. These specialists work together in varying configurations, depending on the needs of the patient. Sometimes the team is made up of a physician and nurse only; sometimes it encompasses the full spectrum of service providers—physician, nurse, social worker, occupational and physical therapists, speech pathologists, and so on. An important aspect of the health team is its ever-changing nature.

Baldwin,[2] one of the leading researchers in team evaluation, has compared teams to traffic on the Los Angeles freeway:

As with teams, cars (read team members) get on and off for different reasons, at different times, at different places, for different destinations, and with different speeds and sizes (read power and prestige).

Occupational therapists must be aware of the potential contributions of each specialist to the well-being of patients and must be able to adapt to the changing team members with their different "destinations . . . speeds and sizes."

Some occupational therapists have a very close relationship with other members of the medical team, while others practice more separately. A therapist on the staff of a children's rehabilitation unit might interact with the majority of the team members several times a day. A therapist in private practice might not make these contacts more than once a week. In both cases, however, and in situations between these two extremes, interprofessional relationships should be collaborative and understanding.

Good team relationships resolve the problems of overlapping roles among the professions. Informed professionals are aware of the areas of overlap and build cooperative relationships. Horwitz[5] suggests that these relationships can allow practitioners to work at their advanced skill levels for longer periods of time than can the practitioner who does not have access to team support and consultation.

Occupational therapists are trained in skills that sometimes overlap with those of physical therapists, social workers, psychologists, teachers, child developmentalists, and orthotists, to name a few. It is natural to desire autonomy, but this can be counterproductive in professional practice. Keeping open lines of communication; recognizing the skills, overlapping or specific, of other professions; and using those skills to complement one's own are hallmarks of professional competence.

It is the responsibility of each professional to interpret his or her role to others. An occupational therapist can never assume that members of other professions are knowledgeable about the role of occupational therapy in health services for children. A nurse who has experienced occupational therapy as a behaviorally oriented therapy in a clinic for adolescents will be hard pressed to understand the sensory integrative approach used in a school program. A physician who is accustomed to working with child developmentalists in one neonatal nursery must be introduced to the occupational therapist's overlapping expertise in a different neonatal department.

Occupational therapists must become experts at explaining their own functions, because their treatment goals are so often hidden within an apparently recreational activity. Group activities especially must be identified with specific treatment goals to make the practice credible and desirable.

Physicians

Although occupational therapists can practice without physicians' referrals, in pediatric services the pediatrician is not only a significant source of referrals but also a source of information about the patient and joint planning for the patient. The pediatrician is a medical specialist, having completed medical school and several years of specialized study and practice in children's diseases. Specialists in family practice have a similar length of medical preparation, but they work more broadly with conditions affecting the entire human life span and more intensively with family interactions. Both specialties are considered primary care, for the reason that children may go initially to a pediatrician or to a family care specialist for checkups or when ill. These physicians' offices, therefore, serve as ports of entry to the medical system. Physicians refer patients to other specialties as the need is perceived.

Consulting physicians are usually specialists to whom the child has been referred by the primary care physicians; they include orthopedists, ophthalmologists, neurologists, cardiologists, physiatrists, psychiatrists, and pulmonary specialists. It is not uncommon for a seriously ill child or one with multiple handicaps to have several consulting physicians, some of whom must be integral members of the treatment team; others can be more peripheral.

In reference to Baldwin's analogy,[2] the consultants represent the large, fast cars on the freeway, entering quickly and moving on. Occupational therapists should be prepared to relate to them by explaining occupational therapy services and establishing or modifying treatment goals to meet the particular condition. In working with all professional colleagues, these explanations should start with the benefits a particular patient can receive from occupational therapy and the goals to be set and worked toward. From here one can go on to generalities and from generalities to basic theory if the colleague expresses interest. But it is usually desirable to establish interprofessional dialogue by using specific cases.

Nurses

Nurses often serve a coordinating function in the delivery of patient services and can be directly responsible for referrals to occupational therapy and for making it physically possible for the child to go to treatment sessions. It is therefore wise for occupational therapists to acquaint themselves with the nursing staff, make clear to all nurses the role of occupational therapy, and work closely with them in coordinating programs. It is frequently difficult for a nurse who is caring for several patients to allow exceptions to the necessary floor routine for a patient who needs leniency for specific routines prescribed by occupational therapy. Whether a child is allowed to practice feeding skills during the very busy breakfast hour in an institution might very well depend on the relationship between the therapist and the nursing staff.

Nursing was the first of the many undergraduate health professions now in practice, and it has the largest number of practitioners. Student nurses can prepare for the certifying examination and become registered nurses through one of the following routes:

1. Hospital schools that are associated with teaching hospitals, which give classes and practical experience in a program usually 3 years in length. A diploma is awarded.
2. Community or technical colleges that give classes and laboratory experience and arrange for clinical practice with local hospitals. These programs are 2 years in length and award the associate of arts degree.

3. Four-year colleges and universities that offer undergraduate education along with nursing classes and laboratory experience. Clinical practice is arranged with suitable hospitals. The bachelor of science degree is awarded.

Registered nurses can specialize as pediatric nurses through on-the-job training and experience by acquiring specific pediatric nursing skills that other nurses who take general duty jobs do not attain because they transfer from service to service. There is also a classification known as pediatric nurse practitioner, which indicates that the nurse has completed advanced education, usually at the master's degree level, and has acquired advanced skills, particularly in physical assessment. These nurses can establish their own practices within a community but will generally establish a close working relationship with a specific physician or group of physicians.

Licensed practical nurses (LPNs) complete training programs 12 to 16 months in length, usually after high school, and sit for examinations in the state where they will practice. These nurses give bedside care and work under the supervision of registered nurses. Nursing aides are trained in high school vocational programs or on-the-job programs in hospitals. They assist both registered and practical nurses.

The different levels of nurse education make it difficult for newcomers in the health services field to make knowledgeable expectations of nursing staffs. In general, higher levels of education produce nurses with greater theoretical knowledge and therefore higher ability to plan programs, evaluate patients and systems, and make changes; the more technically trained nurses develop high skills in bedside care and the techniques of nursing. As with all generalizations, individual exceptions abound.

Physical therapists

Occupational and physical therapists work closely together in outpatient clinics, hospitals, special schools, public schools, crippled children's agencies, and private practice. Known together as the rehabilitation therapies, occupational therapy and physical therapy have, for the most part, many common goals in patient treatment. But their primary treatment modalities are vastly different. Their goals do overlap, however, and when this happens, the roles of the two professions begin to blur. It is to the advantage of those in both professions to observe the technical differences in one another's practices, even though a good case can be made for eliminating arbitrary boundaries with individual patients, particularly children. Where occupational therapists work with activities and stress adaptability, physical therapists work with physical modalities—for example, heat, ultrasound, mechanics, and water—and stress mobility. These are the foci of their educational programs and the thrust of their practices.

Because of their common treatment goals, working relations between the two professions are highly collaborative in most instances. Because of the vagaries of human nature and the economy, the two professions sometimes find themselves competing for patients. When this happens, it must be recognized, and steps must be taken to plan jointly for the good of the patient.

An example of role blurring between occupational therapy and physical therapy can be seen in the treatment goal of establishing trunk stability. The physical therapist must work toward this goal as a prerequisite to sitting and walking; the occupational therapist works toward the same goal as a prerequisite to sitting and using arms for feeding or other activities. Often the exercises that the physical therapist uses in working toward this goal with children look very similar to the activities the occupational therapist uses.

Physical therapy at present is essentially an undergraduate health profession, as is occupational therapy, terminating in the bachelor of science degree. However, physical therapy is officially moving toward establishing all basic education programs at the post-baccalaureate level. Both professions require extensive clinical experience before certification. Whereas occupational therapists can, and do, frequently work without physician referrals, physical therapists do not, a situation that tends to press the physical therapist into the medical model and the occupational therapist into the educational model. It is probably because of their similarities and in spite of their differences that the two professions achieve high degrees of the collaboration and cooperation that Beckhard[3] cites as the essence of health team success.

Speech and hearing specialists

Speech and hearing specialists receive their education at the master's or doctoral level and have studied such topics as speech and hearing disorders, the development of language, the physics of speech, theories and measurements of hearing, and phonetics. Depending on their area of specialization, they are referred to as speech and hearing therapists, speech pathologists and audiologists, logopedists, or phoniatrists.[4] They work only with the body systems having to do with verbal communication (talking and listening), but they see many of the same patients that occupational therapists see. These are primarily the children and youth who are developmentally delayed and children and adults who have suffered brain damage from cerebral vascular accidents, head trauma of various origins, and neurological conditions such as Parkinson's disease and multiple sclerosis.

Occupational therapists in schools for the deaf interact with the entire spectrum of these specialists in verbal communication. In hospitals, schools, and clinics they tend to work mostly with speech pathologists because of the common interest in the developmentally delayed and brain-damaged patients. Frequently occupational therapists will collaborate by incorporating procedures initiated by the speech pathologist into their own treatment time, for example, using pictures to stimulate proper word sounds as part of educational activities with developmentally delayed children. This is an example of combined treatment time made possible through careful planning by the two professionals. It works to the advantage of the patient both in economy and in reinforcement.

Social workers

Social workers are employed by hospitals, clinics, state and local agencies, and sometimes school systems to assist clients and families in their attempts to adjust financially, socially, and psychologically to the problems besetting them. Occupational therapists have frequent meetings with social workers as they each try to help the patient adjust to handicaps of illness, injury, family loss, and vocational stress. While occupational therapists work through activities, social workers employ counseling sessions and assistive negotiations with financial and social agencies.

There are several levels of social work practice, each capable of different contributions to the care of the client. The following levels were established by the National Association of Social Workers, Inc., and published in Standards for Social Services Manpower[6]:

Social service aide No educational requirements, on-the-job training.

Social service technician Completion of a 2-year community college education with an associate of arts or bachelor's degree from another field. This level is sometimes called mental health technician.

Social worker A baccalaureate degree from an accredited program.

Graduate social worker A master's degree from an accredited graduate school of social work.

Certified social worker Certification by the Academy of Certified Social Workers (ACSW) as being capable of the autonomous practice of social work.

Social work fellow Completion of a doctoral degree or substantial practice in a field of specialization following certification by ACSW.

Social workers recognize that social stresses arise from physical and mental illness, and they plan for services to the client that will minimize social dysfunction. Knowledge of agencies and how they operate, of how interagency referrals can be accomplished to the benefit of the client and family, and of cultural and ethnic differences that must be countered or planned for are all part of what the social workers bring to the health team.

Social workers frequently can assist the occupational therapist by finding resources for needed adapted equipment, by helping patients accept or psychologically adjust to various aspects of disabling conditions, and by facilitating interagency communications.

Prosthetists and orthotists

In the field of pediatrics, prosthetists are the persons who make and fit artificial limbs. Orthotists make and fit permanent splints and braces. Each specialist works closely with the prescribing orthopedist, physiatrist, or pediatrician to ensure the child's benefit and comfort. They also work closely with the occupational therapist who teaches the child to use the device in the way most effective for that individual.

Occupational therapists have a special relationship with orthotists because fabricating splints and orthotic devices has long been a part of occupational therapy practice. Occupational therapists' knowledge of anatomy, expertise with tools and materials, and dedication to increasing function produced some of the earliest orthotic devices within hospitals and rehabilitation clinics. In some areas, practice is now divided by body part—occupational therapists fabricate orthoses for the upper limbs and face and the lower limbs and trunk are the province of the orthotist. Service is usually provided by the most accessible qualified person.

Prosthetists and orthotists were at one time apprentice kinds of specialties where the necessary skills were acquired through on-the-job training. Standards were established in the late 1970s, and a national certifying examination was developed. Current requirements to sit for the examination include graduation from an accredited program and 1 year of experience.

Child developmentalists

Persons educated in the area of child development have a wide variety of skills and interests. They hold degrees at the bachelor's, master's, and doctoral levels and represent a broad range of special interests and skills: human development, family relationships, child evaluation, infant guidance and care, nursery school, and group care services. Occupational therapists meet these specialists primarily in the infant stimulation, child assessment, and play therapy programs. Depending on interest, level of education, and type of institution, there may be overlap with the occupational therapy program. It is to everyone's benefit to keep the lines of communication open and to discuss common treatment goals and methods.

Technical personnel

Hospitalized children may be alarmed at the array of technical personnel who jab them, prod them, stick things into them, aerate and ventilate them, and perform other incomprehensible and frightening procedures. During planned play periods, which are relatively nonthreatening situations, occupational therapists can often provide comforting interpretations of such treatments and procedures for the child. Cooperation in arranging treatment schedules with laboratory and x-ray personnel, respiratory therapists, and technicians who operate such diagnostic equipment as the electrocardiograph and electroencephalograph can work to the benefit of everyone's schedule by producing a relaxed, unfrightened child at treatment time.

THE EDUCATIONAL TEAM

The educational team is responsible for preparing children with the knowledge and skills essential for productive living in a complex technological society. Occupational therapists have varying degrees of interface with educators, depending in great part on whether occupational therapy is given at the child's home, in a hospital, clinic, private office, or school building. The occupational therapist must be aware of the child's educational achievements and objectives, whether therapy is seen as a separate, medically oriented treatment or as an integral part of the educational curriculum. Gaining this awareness requires communication and often a good measure of cooperation with the educational team. In school settings the occupational therapist is considered one of the educational team members. The following section will describe other members of this team: professional teachers, teachers' aides, other professionals, and support personnel.

Teachers

The teaching profession is made up of persons with specific expertise: kindergarten and elementary school teachers, secondary school teachers, special education teachers, guidance counselors, art and music teachers, teachers of industrial arts, home economics teachers, vocational education and automobile driving instructors, coaches and physical education teachers, and administrators. Whatever the specialization of the teacher, all teachers have in common the basic tenets of the profession and the requirements of their particular state regarding certification.

All states require certification for public school teachers, and many require it for teachers in private and parochial schools. The minimal requirement for certification is the bachelor's degree, with the infrequent exception of nursery and kindergarten teachers whose minimal requirement in some states is the associate of arts degree. Many states require teachers to work toward and achieve master's degrees within specified periods of time after employment. The education profession has thus mandated the continuing education that all professions encourage as an essential of continuing professional viability. Guidance counselors and teachers in special education are required to have teaching certificates as well as further qualifications in their special areas.

Occupational therapists often work closely with special education teachers because of their shared interest in handicapped children. These teachers have advanced skills in teaching children who are blind, deaf, emotionally disturbed, mentally retarded, and physically handicapped. They seek the expertise of the occupational therapist in planning for the child's classroom participation through the use of assistive devices, handling techniques, positive self-image and so forth.

The guidance counselor can supplement the prevocational work of the occupational therapist by supplying career information, selected testing services, and counseling with students about vocational, academic, and technical opportunities. The prevocational work that occupational therapists do with handicapped children should be carefully described and demonstrated to the guidance counselor to develop cooperative, effective services for the child. Refer to Chapter 29 for a thorough presentation of occupational therapy in the school system.

Therapists working outside the school system in clinics or other agencies usually familiarize themselves with the educational program of the particular patient as an aid to selecting appropriate and stimulating therapeutic activities. Teachers can be directly approached for conferences concerning the child.

Teachers' aides are trained to assist the professional teacher in the classroom in ways that give the teacher more time to do what he or she is primarily hired to do—teach. Aides will grade papers, monitor hallways, help children with outdoor clothing, and, in general, assist in any classroom or area of the school program. They are sometimes paid employees of the school system; other times they are volunteers. Because of the assistive nature of their job, aides are often directly involved with helping children adjust to the classroom or to feeding themselves or to doing other self-maintenance activities. Occupational therapists should ensure that the aides as well as the teachers are familiar with prescribed routines and equipment.

Other professionals

Others who also join the educational team as needed are speech and language teachers, audiologists, psychologists, and occupational and physical therapists. (See p. 12 for a discussion of physical therapy.)

Speech and language teachers have duties that differ from those of the special educators who are specifically trained to teach academic subjects to the deaf. The speech and language teachers teach communication processes and language skills to all needful children, including the deaf, and are qualified in the area of speech and hearing sciences. Similarly, audiologists evaluate the hearing ability of school children and recommend hearing aids or other treatments to improve hearing. More is written about speech and hearing personnel on p. 12.

Psychologists relate to the educational team in two ways: (1) as school psychologists hired by the school system and (2) as consulting or clinical psychologists used on a fee-for-service basis by the individual child and family. Licensure requirements vary from state to state, but in general, psychologists may be prepared at the master's or doctoral levels. They will perform services according to their level of qualifications and experience. Most psychologists who serve school systems are prepared to make psychological evaluations, give treatment, and interpret test results.

Support personnel

Bus drivers, maintenance workers, and dietary personnel contribute services to the educational program in their contracted areas and in ways that are not so apparent. The bus driver can have a great influence on the child with a mobility problem, and the dietary worker can influence the child with a feeding problem. All levels of personnel can contribute substantially to the therapeutic and educational programs if the therapists and teachers communicate goals, elicit suggestions, and instruct them in the use of assistive devices and techniques.

Administrators

The last decade has produced many regulations for health services and educational programs. Federal, state, and local laws have been enacted that regulate the finances, standards, and environments of most health and educational programs for children. Some laws limit the scope of services and others mandate extensions of existing services. All of these regulations must be applied and enforced by administrators who are thereby put into the position of setting parameters for the professional programs within their institutions. Their administrative skills and their knowledge of the capabilities of the professions within their departments affect the quality and nature of services delivered.

Administrators come from varied backgrounds. Some are promoted from within the professions whose programs they administer; therefore, they have intimate knowledge of the programs but varying degrees of administrative skill. Others are brought from such backgrounds as public health, business management, educational administration, or hospital administration. These persons have important expertise in the management of personnel, space, and finances but less knowledge of the professional services they administer. It is

important, therefore, for the administrators and the service professionals to work together so that administrative goals and service goals are clearly defined and compatible.

The effect of government regulations is felt throughout most service departments—as the variety of services offered and the quality of those services increases, documentation needs increase, generating more paperwork. It has been estimated that almost half of an occupational therapist's work is made up of paperwork required by government regulations. Everyone gains, therefore, from efficiently designed institutional procedures for complying with the many external demands on service personnel.

SUMMARY

Occupational therapists work with many professionals during their service to children. In health and educational institutions, as well as in the community at large, children are best served if the many persons involved in their treatment communicate and collaborate in goal setting and planning. A variety of professional and technical specialties have been introduced in this chapter to acquaint the reader with the level of knowledge and skills of their colleagues in the helping professions.

REFERENCES

1. Allen AS, Casto RM, and Janata MM: Interprofessional practice. In Allen AS, editor: New options, new dilemmas: an interprofessional approach to life or death decisions, Lexington, Mass, 1986, DC Heath and Co.
2. Baldwin DC, Jr: Some conceptual and methodological issues in team research. In Bachman JE, editor: Interdisciplinary health care: proceedings of the third annual Interdisciplinary Team Care Conference, Kalamazoo, 1982, Center for Human Services, Western Michigan University.
3. Beckhard R: Organizational issues in the team delivery of comprehensive health care, Millbank Mem Fund Q 50:287, July 1972.
4. Black JW: Speech and hearing science. In Allen AS, editor: Introduction to health professions, ed 3, St Louis, 1980, The CV Mosby Co.
5. Horwitz J: Interprofessional teamwork, Soc Worker 38:5, 1970.
6. Standards for social services manpower, Washington, DC, 1973, The National Association of Social Workers, Inc.

SUGGESTED READINGS

Allen AS, editor: Introduction to Health Professions, ed 3, St Louis, 1980, The CV Mosby Co.
Ducanis A, and Golin A: The interdisciplinary health care team, Germantown, Md, 1979, Aspen Systems Corp.
Kane RA: Interprofessional teamwork, Manpower monograph No. 8, Syracuse, NY, 1975, Syracuse University School of Social Work.
Lawson D: Education careers, New York, 1977, Franklin Watts.

PART
II

KNOWLEDGE BASE

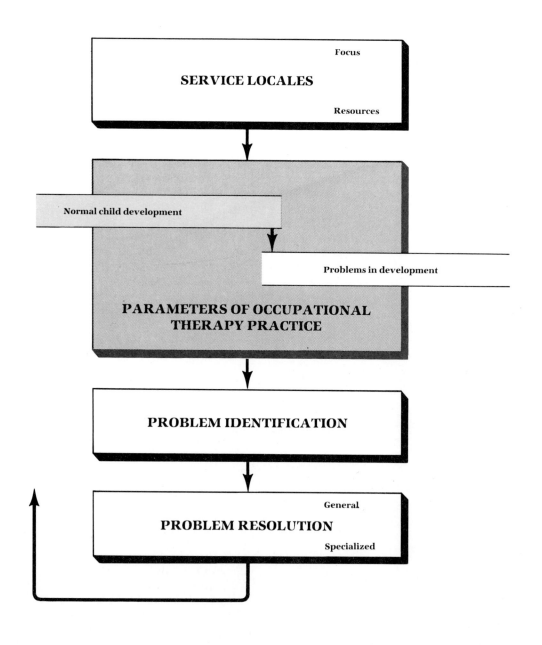

3

Developmental principles and theories

PAT NUSE PRATT
LINDA A. FLOREY
FLORENCE CLARK

In the course of studying child development, it is not uncommon to find ourselves reviewing our own life histories by watching children in public and comparing and contrasting events and behaviors with the theoretical models. These mental exercises are inescapable and appropriate. In fact, this retrospective-observational method gave impetus to the earliest concepts of human development in the past centuries.

In this century, however, developmental concepts have been tested by varying and increasingly sophisticated research methodologies. The end result is a vast amount of information available to occupational therapists and to other providers of children's services. It becomes a formidable tast to sort through the literature and determine the most salient theories and findings. This task is further confounded by the continued emergence of new findings, methodologies of child study, and even changing political climates that can call into question, dilute, and even refute long-standing theories.

With these constraints in mind, it is the purpose of this chapter to present a number of durable concepts and theories that can provide a foundation for occupational therapy practice with children. Some recent trends in the study of child and human development will also be considered, since these may well affect the direction of theory development and related practice methods. Chapter 4 will follow this theoretical content with a descriptive narration of the child development sequence. Chapters 3 and 4 should be used as a starting point in the study of child development. The references and recommended journals that follow this chapter should prove useful for the future study and updating of current knowledge.

BASIC PRINCIPLES OF DEVELOPMENT
Maturation and experience

At the core of most developmental theories is an explanation of the interplay between (1) human biological capacity and maturation and (2) the influence of the environment on the behavioral experiences of the individual. In fact, theories tend to be distinguished from each other by the specific weighting of these two factors or by an investigator's emphasis on a particular aspect of human biological function or environment. For example, B.F. Skinner highly values the influence of the environment on human development, whereas Sigmund Freud emphasized biological determinants of behavior. In effect, theorists generally agree that human development is both a process and the product of biological maturation and environmental experiences. *Development* may be defined as the sequential changes in the function of the individual or species. This should be differentiated from the concept of *growth,* which refers to those maturational changes that are physically measurable.

Parameters of development

There are three general parameters of development: biological, psychological, and social. Each parameter has subcategories that will be differentiated later in this section. *Biological development* is primarily related to enzyme systems that stimulate complex metabolic changes. There are two subcategories of *psychological development* that generally refer to those functions we attribute to interactive brain processes: the cognitive and affective (or emotional). In the infant, cognitive psychological function tends to be dominated by neurological maturation and behavioral motivations for survival. As the child develops, cognitive activity is measured by communication skills and the handling of abstract material. Affective development is characterized by the establishment of bonds of feeling and meaning with human and nonhuman objects in the child's environment. *Social development* provides the child with skills to live in a community of others and is a product of both the child's biological capacity to learn and the direct influence of the societal environment on the child's maturation. Learning may be equated with acculturation, that is, the acquisition, internalization, and use of skills necessary to function in society.

The parameters of development affect one another. For example, the ancient Chinese custom of footbinding was socially derived. It was believed that upper class women should have small feet. However, the practice prevented full development of the bones of the foot. And, because foot-binding limited the mobility of these women, it tended to restrict opportunities for emotional attachments. Another example is that when a person is depressed, there is a subsequent decrease in activity. Social experiences become limited, as well as the opportunity for physical exercise. A long-term result of depression can be a decrease in muscle tone, strength, and bulk. All social behavior is mediated by the basic biological capacities and psychological needs of the individual and the species and by the changing factors of the environment that impinge on an individual or group.

Dimensions of development

Development is an ongoing process that can be studied in two dimensions: longitudinal and cross-sectional. *Longitudinal development* refers to the chronological sequence of changes throughout the life span: year to year, stage to stage.[24] Investigators of longitudinal development tend to formalize their concepts in stage theories. These theories, such as Erikson's, identify functionally related processes and milestones over the course of time. In contrast, *cross-sectional development* examines discreet areas of function that occur simultaneously at any point in the individual's life.[29] Brazelton,[2] for example, is known for his intensive investigation that focuses on simultaneous development of infant maturation and behavior (Chapters 6 and 18).

Gradients of growth

There are several universal concepts of the directions, or gradients, of growth that have strong implications for treatment. The first principle is that *ontogeny recapitulates phylogeny,* that is, the growth of the individual mirrors the maturational development of the species. This is particularly important to the understanding of the sequential maturation of biological functions. Second, there is *cephalocaudal progression* of maturation. For example, the purposeful control of motor activity begins with movements of the head (cephalo) and develops gradually in descending order to the caudal (or tail) region of the body. There is a concurrent *proximodistal* gradient of growth from the midline of the body out to the fingers and toes. The change from mass to specific action, as movement becomes more discriminative and refined, is termed *differentiation.* Finally, there is increasing acceptance of the concept that the maturation of systems and functions proceeds toward the *integration,* rather than fragmentation, of the individual.[20,40]

Stress and adaptation

It is generally agreed that the behavior of living organisms is directed toward maintaining a state of *homeostasis,* or *equilibrium,* that is, a life-maintaining balance of all systems, parts, and forces intrinsic and extrinsic to the individual. *Stress* may be defined as an internal or external force that threatens homeostatic balance. *Adaptation* is the general term for the mechanisms used by the individual to restore homeostasis. The adaptive mechanisms may be physiological or behavioral, used with and without conscious control. The standard example of an unconscious adaptive mechanism is the response of the autonomic nervous system to prepare the body to deal with emergency situations. Similarly, when the child encounters an unfamiliar object, an adaptive pattern may be seen as the child first stands back and then bursts forward to seize the object, as if holding it will restore the sense of equilibrium.

Stress is now generally accepted as having both positive and negative values. The positive result of stress is the initiation of more discriminative, and therefore more mature and adaptive, behavioral responses. This result assumes that the individual has the physiological capacities and maturity to purposefully deal with a stressful situation and learn from it. The negative influence of stress is most likely to occur when stress is multidimensional or beyond the physiological capabilities of the individual, or when it is continuous to the point that the individual is unable to experience intermittent sensations of equilibrium. Such distress situations eliminate the discriminative learning aspects of adaptation that ordinarily promote development and allow the person to experience a sense of achievement.

Most theories of interest to occupational therapists attempt to explain the processes a child uses to adapt to stress, either of a particular type or at different stages. Very often theorists will link the healthy resolution of stressful situations to critical periods or events. The term *critical periods* refers to certain times in an individual's life when a particular type of development or learning can take place most readily or spontaneously.[30] For example, sometime during the sixth year of life, the child's visual and auditory functions, language and social development, and curiosity are at an optimal level for learning to read. This does not mean that the child cannot learn to read 1 year earlier or 10 years later. It simply means that this is developmentally the most opportune period, a time when the overall maturational *readiness* of the individual to engage in a new type of learning or experience is at its peak. Other examples of critical periods will be found in this chapter in discussion of various theories and in the developmental sequence presented in Chapter 4.

In contrast, the concept of *critical events* implies more rigid expectations. Critical events may be defined as certain situations that must take place within a given time period or else successful mastery of subsequent developmental tasks will be incomplete. Freud's psychopathological concepts of oral and anal fixation are examples of critical events hypotheses.[30]

It may be hypothesized that theorists who propose critical periods are more inclined to be environmentalists. In contrast, critical events theorists tend to place greater emphasis on biological factors in development. Although such a distinction is not invariant, it is useful as a guide.

General classifications of developmental theories

There may seem to be as many classification systems for theories as there are theories of child development. This section will review several classification systems that should be familiar to occupational therapists because of their relation to practice and research in services for children. Already introduced in this chapter were *stage theories,* which take a longitudinal view of development. The counterparts to these are known as *process theories,* which examine in detail the many variables influencing a particular type or stage of behavior.[29] Many of the elaborate stage theories, such as those developed by Freud and Piaget, demonstrate considerable depth at the process level.

Theories may also be classified broadly by their implicit view of the control of the developmental process. For example, there are *deterministic* and *nondeterministic* theories. The former indicates that the outcome of the developmental process is beyond the control of the individual. Examples of deterministic theory are found in the works of Freud and Skinner. The differences between their theories demonstrate that a determinist may see a human being as a responder to either the environment or to biological nature. In contrast, the nondeterminist view maintains that the individual can rise above biological and environmental destinies. Theorists Carl Rogers and Abraham Maslow were proponents of this view.[31]

Closely allied to the deterministic and nondeterministic perspectives are the preformational and epigenetic classifications. However, these models are associ-

ated with specific developmental influences. The *preformational model* was most popular in the last century and has been revived recently by the sociobiological theorists. This model proposes that a human being (or any species) is a product of biological-genetic determinants of behavior and that human functions will develop in a fairly uniform sequence regardless of environmental influences. The *epigenetic model* was favored by theorist Erikson who gave priority to environmental forces. This model proposes that growth and development are continuously shaped by the individual's ongoing experiences and interactions with the environment.[29]

Finally, theories may be classified according to the psychological school of thought that they represent (Table 3-1). The most commonly identified approaches are the psychoanalytic, humanistic, cognitive, behavioristic, and eclectic. In brief, *psychoanalytic theory* proposes that development and behavior are largely inner directed, generally resulting from the will of the unconscious. *Humanistic theory* is generally concerned with the self-actualization process, and the individual is viewed as a purposeful creature of plans, strategies, and choices.[29] A *cognitive theory* concerns the conscious, rational thought of the individual undergoing maturation and how this affects the individual's behavioral repertoire. *Behavioristic theory* is characterized by attention to the environmental stimuli and reinforcements that shape the individual's behavior over time. An *eclectic theory* tends to have a more humanistic view of the individual, but this approach is descriptively or methodologically influenced by one or more of the other schools of thought. Eclectic models appear to be more prevalent among theories of practice and are well represented by the occupational therapy theories described later in this chapter. Table 3-1 illustrates the classification of selected theories according to school of thought.

Although the developmental models that follow will be grossly classified as stage or process theories, each one also reflects some of the thinking represented by the systems of classification discussed in this section. Although it may seem academic now, these varied terms and definitions will most certainly resurface in the therapist's continued study of child development. Perhaps even more important is the fact that the philosophies they represent will be encountered among colleagues in practice settings. Therefore therapists must be familiar with the implied methodologies and approaches to treatment that each classification engenders.

STAGE THEORIES
The psychosexual theory of Freud

Discussion of Freud's theory in this chapter will emphasize his model of personality development. Freud proposed that personality arises from the biological, in-

Table 3-1   Classification of selected developmental theories

Focus of study	School of thought				
	Internal processes				External controls
	Psychoanalytic	Humanistic	Eclectic	Cognitive	Behavioristic
Stage theories			Gesell Havighurst		
					Kohlberg
	Erikson				
— — — — — — — — — Freud — —		— Reilly — —	— Llorens Gilfoyle and— Grady	— — Piaget — —	— — — — —
		Maslow			
					Sociobiology
			Interactionism Ayres		
					Skinner
		Rogers			Information processing
Process theories				Hemispheric specialization	

NOTE: This classification assumes that the focus of study in theories falls along a continuum of developmental stages and elaboration of processes. As discussed in the text, theoretical schools of thought tend to be differentiated according to their view of the control of behavior from internal processes to external forces.

stinctual energy of the individual and that this energy is differentiated through typical environmental experiences at different ages.

The age-related stages that Freud proposed have proved to be the most durable components of his work and have been applied with success to many populations beyond those originally studied (Table 3-2). It should be remembered that most of Freud's patients were upper middle income Viennese women of the Victorian era. Most of his theory was developed through painstaking analysis of the case histories of his patients. He worked with very few children. Therefore the bulk of his data related to childhood was collected from retrospective accounts by use of free association techniques to draw out details of the past hidden in the realms of the unconscious of his adult patients.

Freud was a physician who beame interested in neurological disorders, particularly those with no apparent organic base (the hysterical conversions). In keeping with his medical background, Freud assumed that there was a biological determinant for all behavior. Interestingly, the problems that he encountered most often among his patients are now seen to be reflections of a cultural era that repressed human sexuality. Of course, it is easier for us to identify the heavy environmental influence in the psychopathology that he studied because we are representatives of a different time.

With this background in mind, we can examine the development of the personality according to Freudian psychosexual theory. Structurally the three components of the personality are the id, the ego, and the superego. Each of these parts is engaged in interactive processes with the others, usually characterized by some conflict. Freud longitudinally identified five stages

of functional development. Remember that although Freud gave priority to the biological basis of behavior, he also recognized that the outcomes of each personality component and stage were influenced by environment.

STRUCTURE OF THE PERSONALITY

The initial, motivating part of the child's personality at birth is called the *id*. It represents the psychic energy of the child, the impetus for all behavior. The sole purpose of the id is to rid the person of tension by seeking out pleasurable sensations and avoiding pain. This purpose is called the *pleasure principle*. The id does not think; it only wishes and reacts. If all needs of the id were met, the infant would remain helpless.

Freud wrote that the id is able to conjure up mental images of the sensations that repeatedly give it pleasure. Therefore a hungry infant develops mental images of food through repeated satisfaction of the hunger needs. As the infant develops these images, he is able to use the *primary process* of the id, which is the calling up of mental images to satisfy a perceived need in the absence of the real object. The id does not know the difference between the real or the mental image. Satisfying use of either source is called *wish fulfillment.*

The id contains both the life and death instincts of the individual. The *life instincts* include hunger, thirst, and sex drives that ensure the survival of the individual and the species. The source of energy for these drives is called the *libido.* The opposing drives, the *death instincts,* are usually subordinate to life instincts but manifest themselves throughout life in the form of destructive energies and aggressive behaviors.

Table 3-2   Contrasted sequences of selected stage theories

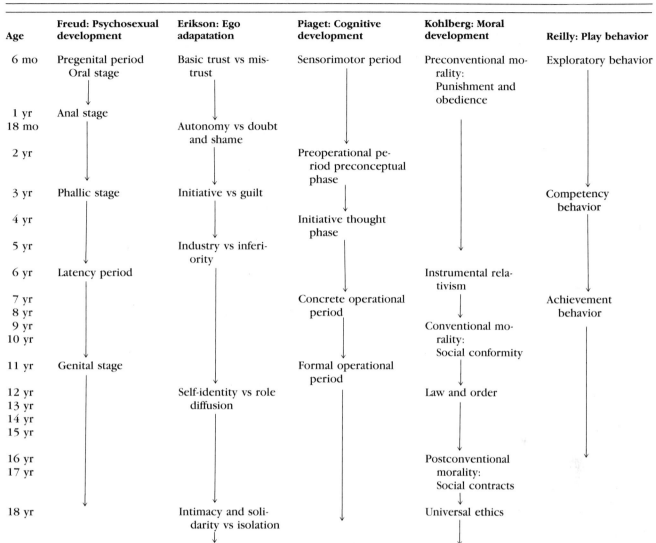

Age	Freud: Psychosexual development	Erikson: Ego adapatation	Piaget: Cognitive development	Kohlberg: Moral development	Reilly: Play behavior
6 mo	Pregenital period Oral stage	Basic trust vs mistrust	Sensorimotor period	Preconventional morality: Punishment and obedience	Exploratory behavior
1 yr	Anal stage				
18 mo		Autonomy vs doubt and shame			
2 yr			Preoperational period preconceptual phase		
3 yr	Phallic stage	Initiative vs guilt			Competency behavior
4 yr			Initiative thought phase		
5 yr		Industry vs inferiority			
6 yr	Latency period			Instrumental relativism	
7 yr			Concrete operational period		Achievement behavior
8 yr					
9 yr					
10 yr				Conventional morality: Social conformity	
11 yr	Genital stage		Formal operational period		
12 yr		Self-identity vs role diffusion		Law and order	
13 yr					
14 yr					
15 yr					
16 yr				Postconventional morality: Social contracts	
17 yr					
18 yr		Intimacy and solidarity vs isolation		Universal ethics	

The *ego* is the part of the personality that starts to develop after birth as the infant comes into contact with the mediating influences of the environment. At present we can consider it as the part of the personality that moderates the id's wishes according to environmental constraints.

The ego operates according to the *reality principle.* Nye[31] stated that the ego "attempts to differentiate between what is desired (by the id) and what is actually available (in the environment)" (p. 13). The *secondary process* used by the ego is called *reality testing.* This involves formulating a plan to obtain the desired object and then trying the plan out to see if it works.

The ego modifies libidinal energy through the *displacement process.* This is the transference of energy into alternative actions. The displacement of libidinal energy through a socially acceptable behavior is called *sublimation.* Freud believed that the world's progress toward civilization was dependent on sublimations. For example, if you are hungry and have a visitor, you do not satisfy the libidinal urges of the id by disappearing into the kitchen and eating alone. Instead, because of the mediating influence of the ego, you share the food with your guest.

The third part of the personality is the *superego.* This is the moral component of the personality that reflects the learned values of the culture. Freud believed that the child's parents have the greatest influence on the development of the superego. Operational constructs are the ego-ideal and the conscience. The *ego-ideal* is the child's conception of what other people expect in terms of good behavior. The *conscience* represents what is thought to be bad behavior. The superego uses feelings of pride to reward the moral actions of the ego and guilt to punish bad behaviors. Like the id, the superego is not objective. It responds to mental images as well as to personal actions. Only the ego is realistic as it balances the innate needs of the id with the environmentally molded demands of the superego.

LEVELS OF CONSCIOUSNESS

Freud is best known for his systematic study and organization of concepts related to the unconscious. He constructed a topographical model consisting of the conscious, the preconscious (meaning readily accessible to the conscious), and the unconscious levels. The content of the unconscious realm of the mind is considered to be available at the conscious level with great difficulty. Although only parts of the ego and the superego exist at the unconscious level, all of the id is unconscious. Only small aspects of the ego and the superego are at the conscious level at any one time. The major parts of these two components are stored in the preconscious mind and are called on as needed. Figure 3-1 depicts the relationship between Freud's concepts of personality and topography.

The ego acts as a gatekeeper to the unconscious, channeling through those needs of the id that can be met through socially acceptable ways. Libidinal urges that are in conflict with society (and its mirror the superego) are held back or sidetracked through *defense mechanisms.* There are a variety of defense mechanisms that may collectively be defined as irrational thinking that allow the ego to protect itself from anxiety when rational, adaptive processes are insufficient.

THE PSYCHOSEXUAL STAGES OF DEVELOPMENT

Freud postulated that the impetus for development at different stages of life is centered on obtaining pleasurable sensation in the erogenous zones. Each of his stages is named for the erogenous zone that presumably provided the greatest source of pleasure and con-

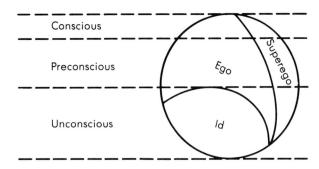

Figure 3-1 An integration of the structural and topographical models of the personality.

From Nye RD: Three psychologies: perspectives from Freud, Skinner, and Rogers, ed 2, Monterey, Calif, 1981, Brooks/Cole Publishing Co.

tact between the child and environment at that age (Table 3-2).

The *oral stage* is centered around the mouth and lips. Pleasure is derived through sucking, chewing, and feeding. The infant is dominated by the id toward meeting survival needs. The infant develops bonds of loving feelings with parents through their association with oral gratification.

The *anal stage* describes the second and third years of life. Pleasurable sensations are obtained through elimination activities of the anal and perineal sphincter muscles. The most important activity of the anal stage is toilet training. This provides the ego with its first great test of delaying sensory gratification in the face of social pressure.

The *phallic stage,* which covers the period from about 3 to 6 years, was the most controversial part of Freud's theory because of its stress on the child's incestuous feelings toward his or her parents. The centers of sensation here are the external genitalia. Pleasurable activities include masturbation and fantasizing. The latter is an example of the use of mental images to satisfy the libidinal urges of the id. The most important (and criticized) concept is the development of the *Oedipus and Electra* complexes. In essence, Freud hypothesized that children of this age have sexual drives toward parents of the opposite sex and aggressive drives toward parents of the same sex. This conflict signals the emergence of the superego, which in effect punishes the child for such fantasies. The ego responds to this anxiety-producing situation by suppressing the libidinal urges of the id and promoting identification with the parent of the same sex. Through reality testing the ego has realized that it cannot compete with the larger, stronger adult for the affections of the opposite sex parent. So it directs its energies toward becoming more like the larger, stronger, same sex parent.

The oral, anal, and phallic stages were collectively considered the *pregenital period.* Freud believed that the personality was essentially formed through this period. The child develops the ability to survive, to form emotional bonds, to delay gratification, to channel energy into socially acceptable behaviors, and to assume a sex role identity.

The *latency period,* which occurs during the elementary school years, is a time of quiescence and recovery from the turbulent conflicts of the phallic stage. It is essentially devoid of any psychosexual activity. The child shifts his interest from the self to the outside world and increases the quantity of social skills. Because Freud believed that the personality was already formed (through the pregenital period), he did not expect any qualitative changes in social skills to occur thereafter. In other words, although the child might learn to do many more things, the manner in which situations are approached will remain unchanged.

The *genital stage* is characteristic of the teen years, as hormonal changes reawaken the sexual drives of the individual. However, through the socialization process (sublimation and identification) the ego has learned to channel these drives appropriately. The youth seeks heterosexual relationships involving mutual gratification. This emergence of altruistic concerns is characteristic of the adolescent in other areas of life as well. If the ego is successful with sublimation and identification, a healthy adult is the result.

• • •

This discussion is limited to a very small portion of Freud's theory. He believed that the mark of the healthy adult is the ability to direct one's energies into love and work. Freud was deterministic in his view that physiological drives give impetus to all behavior. He was also essentially pessimistic about human nature, believing that these drives cause a continual conflict between the individual and civilization. The processes of sublimation and identification were central to controlling drives for the preservation of society.

Although Freud's theory is considered by many to be outdated, it still provides a foundation for subsequent developmental concepts. In addition, many of his concepts are still used in mental health facilities, particularly for diagnostic and analytical purposes. Application of his concepts appears to be more prevalent in private facilities. Freud was a prodigious writer, and many translations of his detailed work are still readily available for those who are interested in exploring his concepts further.[10,14,15,31]

The ego psychology of Erikson

It is almost inevitable to find the theory of Erik Erikson following that of Freud. Erikson began his study of psychology under Freud, and his theory reflects this affiliation. Erikson considered himself a psychoanalyst, even though he is viewed as the father of ego psychology and a pioneer of the humanistic school of thought.

Erikson took a more optimistic view of human nature and became intrigued with the functions of the ego in response to the environment. Whereas Freud saw the id as the most important aspect of the personality, Erikson gave priority to the adaptive response of the ego in the development of the individual. Much of Erikson's theory crystallized through his studies of the lives of famous people, such as Gandhi and Luther, as he sought to identify what characteristics allow people to go on living in the face of adversity. In addition, he conducted considerable treatment and study with children, including cross-cultural comparisons. He believed that play afforded the best opportunity for observations of adaptive and maladaptive responses of the ego.

Erikson divided the life span into the *eight stages of man.* Each stage is represented by a *personal-social crisis* that gives impetus to ego growth. Erikson accepted Freud's concept of the id as the prime motivator; however, he believed that the ego provided conti-

nuity to development. One of Erikson's most important assumptions was that society constitutes itself to provide opportunities for ego growth and identity. As we shall see, the tasks of adulthood direct the individual's attention to facilitating the development of the next generation. All crises recur throughout life, but these particular stages are the critical periods in which crises are best resolved to promote successful living. Erikson viewed development as an autotherapeutic process, that is, the successful resolution of a crisis repairs the wounds of its conflicts and gives the individual a sense of achievement. Erikson prefaced each stage with "a sense of" to refer to the continuing sense of mastery and achievement (Table 3-2). Each stage also results in the acquisition of an abstract personality quality, such as hope or wisdom.

BASIC TRUST VS MISTRUST

The infant from birth to about 18 months must develop psychological trust, the eagerness to approach new experiences without paralyzing fear. Trust develops through the care-giving attentions of the parents, particularly the mother. The initial sense of trust comes from the infant's realization that survival needs will be met and that she can exist in a state of comfort. The most difficult task for the infant is to maintain this trust in the absence of the mother. Erikson believed that the parents must provide gradual opportunities for separation that do not provoke excessive anxiety. *Hope* is the acquired characteristic of this stage.

AUTONOMY VS DOUBT AND SHAME

Autonomy vs doubt and shame is the stage of the 2- to 4-year-old toddler. It is characterized by holding on and letting go and is exemplified by the crisis that occurs through the toilet training process. Erikson specified the relationship of autonomy to the child's increasing control over his body. This permits independent movement into the outer world. Parents must provide opportunities for the child to make choices and develop a sense of self-controlled *will.*

INITIATIVE VS GUILT

The newly autonomous preschooler has mastered basic motor skills and must now build a repertoire of social skills to deal with the outer world. Central to this is the achievement of gender (sex) role identity. Erikson's view of the Oedipus and Electra situations closely parallels that of Freud's, but Erikson's view is more broadly concerned with the child's imitation of the variety of role behaviors. Through imitation the child learns to assume responsibility for himself within the confines of his still limited environment and develops a sense of *purpose.*

INDUSTRY VS INFERIORITY

The elementary school child experiences a period of slow, steady growth. The need for security is transferred from the family to the peer group as the child attempts to master the activities of her age. The peer group is used as a standard of performance against which the child can measure her own skill. The abstract objective of this period is the realization of *competence.*

SELF-IDENTITY VS ROLE DIFFUSION

Erikson studied the period of adolescence in great detail, and the scope of his theoretical formulations for this age is therefore much broader than Freud's. The masterful school child is suddenly shaken by the physiological changes of puberty and must struggle to regain control over his body, identity, and future. During adolescence the prolonged childhood draws to a close, and society asks the adolescent to make choices about adult roles. The teenager experiments with patterns of identity until a sense of continuity and control over the ego is regained and a perspective of the future is acquired. In spite of the often turbulent conflicts between adolescents and their elders, Erikson felt that the actions of both were directed to the same end of helping youth clarify their roles as members of society. Through resolution of the identity crisis the individual gains a sense of *fidelity,* the continuity of the past with the future.

INTIMACY AND SOLIDARITY VS ISOLATION

Earlier relationships have helped the young adult define himself or herself. Now the adult seeks to share that identity through the intimate relationships of marriage and family life. In concert with Freud's view, Erikson saw healthy adulthood as a time of love and work. The abstract capacity derived through this period is *love.*

GENERATIVITY VS SELF-ABSORPTION

The crisis of middle adulthood is to develop the feeling that one's life is meaningful and productive. The person must find a sense of security in the usefulness of his or her chosen personal, social, and economic roles for the continuity and preservation of society. *Caring* is the abstract phenomenon realized during this time of life.

INTEGRITY VS DESPAIR

The stage of integrity *vs* despair is continuous and largely dependent on a successful sense of generativity. It represents the appraisal of self-worth as the individual faces the physical, economic, and personal losses of old age. It is essentially a case of "it was a very good year" versus "if only." The objective of this stage is the achievement of *wisdom* and the ability to share a satisfying and encouraging philosophy of life with the younger generation.

• • •

It is interesting to note that Erikson began his adult life as an artist, a background that manifested itself in his books through the detailed "life space" portraits he presented in his reports of clinical cases and biographical analyses. His artist's eye as well as his interest in history and anthropology allowed his written work to acquire an insight into and an emphasis on environmental influences, which are lacking in Freud's theories. These factors, as well as the cross-cultural durability of his theories, make Erikson's works especially useful for occupational therapists.[7,15,30]

The cognitive theory of Piaget

Jean Piaget's concept of the child as a little scientist is remarkably reflective of his own youth. By age 10 he had published his first paper in a biology journal, and at 22 he had completed his doctoral dissertation on mollusks. He attended university at the time that Freud, Adler, and Jung were receiving recognition in Europe, and consequently he was influenced to study a good deal of philosophy and psychology. The academic atmosphere in early twentieth century Europe was very stimulating for the study of human nature, and it produced a number of great theorists such as Piaget, Erikson, and Maslow.

By training, Piaget was a zoologist. By vocation, he became a psychologist. His particular interest was in the genesis and theory of knowledge (genetic epistemology). Piaget's first employment was to assist Binet in the standardization of intelligence tests. What interested Piaget most was not the correct responses made by children during testing, but rather the consistency of patterns of incorrect responses at different ages. This interest led him to a research career investigating children's thought patterns. The experimental approach that he developed is called *methode clinique.* This method involved (1) presenting children with familiar objects, such as blocks, pieces of paper, and glasses of water; (2) constructing problem-solving situations with the objects; and (3) asking children to solve the problem *(actions)* and to explain how they had done this *(experience).* The importance of his method lies in the concern for the processes used by the children regardless of the correctness of their problem solving. Although his initial investigations were conducted with his own children, Piaget's studies have since been replicated with several thousand children.

Piaget's work developed a very elaborate theory of the process of cognition as it matures over the span of life from infancy to adolescence. It is necessary to first examine Piaget's major constructs relating to this process in order to understand the sequence of cognitive development periods.

MAJOR CONSTRUCTS

Piaget accepted the biological basis of behavior, but he was more concerned with the developmental *adaptation* of the individual in response to ongoing environmental experiences. He wrote[32] that "the theory of knowledge is . . . essentially a theory of adaptation of thoughts to reality (resulting from) an inextricable interaction between the subject and objects" (p. 24). He examined adaptation through the child's relationships with human and nonhuman *objects, time, and space.* He said that the child organizes his experiences into *mental schemes* (schemata, concepts) through use of mental operations. *Operations* may be defined as the cognitive methods used by the child to organize his schemes and experiences and to direct his actions. The totality of operational schemes available to the child at a given time constitutes the *adapted intelligence,* or cognitive competence, of the child.

The child's quest is for *equilibrium,* a balance between what he knows and can act on and what the environment provides for him. But the child is constantly faced with novel situations and stimuli and in fact would not learn and develop without disequilibrium. Two processes are used by the child to organize novel experiences (and restore equilibrium). *Assimilation* means that the child takes a new situation and bends it to match one of his existing schemes. This may result in some distortion of reality, but it is typically the first cognitive method we all use to confront new situations. For example, a young child who sees a furry, small, four-legged animal tends to call it a *dog.* However, if the child's mother is available and corrects the child with the information that the animal is a cat, the child must then use the process of *accommodation.* That is, the child develops a new scheme in response to the reality of the situation. Assimilation tends to result in generalization whereas accomodation improves discrimination. Both are important to the child's development, because although discrimination promotes cognitive maturity, generalization is necessary for organization and continuity.

SEQUENCE OF COGNITIVE PERIODS

Piaget also believed that there was an invariant, hierarchical development of cognition that proceeds from the simple to the complex, from the concrete to abstract, and from personal to worldly concerns. At first, thought is *egocentric,* that is, the child relates all experiences to himself. Through cognitive maturation, thought becomes decentered and *relativistic,* that is, relationships between time, objects, and space assume an importance independent of the child's own experiences. Piaget specified four maturational levels, or periods, of cognitive function: (1) sensorimotor, (2) preoperational, (3) concrete operational, and (4) formal operational.

THE SENSORIMOTOR PERIOD

The child from birth to about age 2 responds to and learns about his environment directly through his sensations and motor responses. The emphasis is on sensory, movement, and manipulative experiences with objects. This period is characterized by the most ego-

centric thought. Although it is the shortest time period of mental development, it is proportionally the most active.

Piaget differentiated six stages of sensorimotor activity. The *reflexive stage* occurs during the first month. The child's schemes begin in simple biological reflexes that are primitive, general, and related to survival. Piaget felt that the sucking and palmar reflexes, which modify to promote oral and manipulative exploration, are the most critical to early mental development. The baby assimilates sensory experiences, such as the taste of food, with the kinesthetic sensations derived from the reflexive movements of sucking. Through repetition, the child becomes more proficient in the use of reflexes to satisfy basic needs. There is no differentiation between self and object or between sensation and action.

The next sensorimotor stage, occurring in the second through the fourth months, is called *primary circular reactions.* The child repeats reflexive sensory motor patterns merely for the sake of pleasurable repetition. There is still no separation between sensation and action. Essentially the child is establishing primitive habit patterns as the precursors of voluntary movements that are associated with specific sensations.

The third stage, *secondary circular reactions,* evolves during the fifth through eighth months of life. At this time the child begins to show true voluntary movement patterns based on a coordination of vision and hand function. In effect, the child reaches for and grasps everything that is seen. When the action is rewarded by a pleasurable secondary sensation, such as the sound of a bell inside a toy, the infant will repeat the action. The child is beginning to have a primitive awareness of cause and effect.

The fourth stage of *coordination of secondary schemata* completes the baby's first year. This marks exciting changes in the child's operations as the child begins to direct movements in response to stimuli that cannot be seen. The child can respond to and then look for a sound and then look for an object that disappears from view. This marks the emergence of *object permanence,* the awareness that something or someone has continuity beyond the child's direct experience with it. In turn, object permanence signals the beginning of decentered thought.

This phenomenon has implications in affective-emotional development as well. The baby now realizes that when the mother leaves the room, she does not cease to exist. The baby can begin to listen for sounds of his mother in a nearby room and gradually realizes that he can use sound stimuli to find the missing mother (since locomotor development is also progressing rapidly at this age). As shown in Erikson's theory, this awareness is critical to the child's progress toward independence.

The fifth sensorimotor stage, which lasts until about 18 months, is called *tertiary circular reactions.* The child's mental behavior is characterized by searches for new schemes. This development parallels a motor stage when the child is suddenly able to walk and crawl about freely, and parents are hard pressed to keep their youngsters from getting into everything. Although it happens by chance, one of the most important results of this stage is the beginning of *tool use.* The child discovers that he can get more food into his mouth with a spoon or that a distant pull toy can be obtained by pulling on the attached string that previously had no function for him. Prehension patterns become more refined and precise in the process.

The sixth stage of sensorimotor activity, the transitional stage, is marked by *inventions of new means through mental combinations.* It generally occurs during the last 6 months of the second year. This stage is mentally demonstrated through insight and physically characterized by purposeful tool use. The child is looking for alternate means to solve problems. These changes are in large part aided by the child's increasing motor proficiency in speech production and by an expanding receptive vocabulary. The child can now begin to label or symbolically represent mental schemes. Whereas during the previous stages all schemes were represented as sensorimotor experiences, the child is now beginning to represent concepts without direct manipulation.

THE PREOPERATIONAL PERIOD

With the emergence of language and symbolic representation of schemes, the child's cognitive patterns undergo significant changes. Through acquisition of verbal schemes, the child is able to expand his conceptual repertoire more rapidly. In addition, symbolic representation allows the child to organize what he knows and to call on a scheme at will. During the time from 2 to 7 years of age, children learn to systematically manipulate their environments through development of the organizing operations called classification, seriation, and conservation.

Classification is the organization of objects according to similarities and differences. At first, children classify according to one common stimulus characteristic, such as color. Two-year-old children can be seen making little stacks of blocks with each stack a different color. When they have mastered classification according to one common characteristic, children begin to notice other shared characteristics as well as discrete differences. Classification becomes multidimensional. The dog and cat of the example given earlier for assimilation and accommodation become classified as pets. Classifications may be made according to sensory characteristics, spatial arrangements, and readily observable cause and effect relationships.

Seriation is the relationship of one object, or classification of objects, to another. As with classification, this operation is initially exercised at a unidimensional level. Proximity of objects tends to afford the earliest

stimulus for seriation. However, as the child matures and vocabulary increases, he can rank-order objects in terms of size, weight, color intensity, and other sensory characteristics.

Conservation is the end product of the preoperational period. It permits the child to recognize the continuities of an object or class of objects in spite of apparent change. A typical Piagetian example would be to show the child a ball of clay. The clay is flattened or rolled out in front of the child who is then asked if the amount is the same. A child who is still unable to conserve sees that the physical appearance is different and would say that the amount is not the same.

The most primitive kind of conservation is by the number of objects (in different spatial arrangements). Later the child begins to conserve mass (as in the clay example), area, length, and volume. The ability to conserve is critical to learning to read and do math, for the child must learn to recognize the sameness of sounds and values in letters and numbers regardless of their arrangements.

The preoperational period is divided into two distinct phases. The 2- to 4-year-old child is considered *preconceptual.* The chief task here is for the child to expand her vocabulary and thus increase the quantity of symbolic representations. Typically classification is the primary operation that develops at this time, although the child is also learning verbal concepts that will promote use of seriation and conservation. Play provides the arena for learning, and the child spends considerable time in verbal play.

The *intuitive thought phase,* from about age 4 to 7, provides the child with substantially more social-environmental contacts. The child uses a tremendous amount of imitation by copying whatever is seen and repeating whatever is heard. Children happily relate all the family secrets in great detail. The child answers questions and solves problems intuitively, not really knowing how conclusions were reached. Seriation and conservation develop during this phase as the child is able to deal with multiple characteristics of objects. Through classification and seriation the child begins to use inductive reasoning to relate parts to the whole. This marks the transition to concrete operations.

THE CONCRETE OPERATIONAL PERIOD

The concrete operational period, which covers the life span from about age 7 to 11, is important for the acquisition of reversibility, spatial concepts, and rules. During this time the child is still stimulus and experience bound; he can only think about things that are at least available for sensory manipulation.

Reversibility is an extension of conservation and allows the child to develop more spatial awareness. Children learn that they cannot only add 2 numbers, but that they can also subtract. They gain an understanding that the constant features of an object, such as the conservation of the clay mass, permit it to be returned to its previous state.

Rules are not new to the concrete operational child, but understanding of rules becomes more realistic and complete, and therefore the child is able to apply them. There are rules of causation that prescribe general cause and effect; rules of attribution, related to social causation, such as custom to outcome or event to event; and moral rules for right, wrong, and situational appropriateness. Mature understanding and application of rules continue to evolve through the formal operations period. For example, the preoperational child knows that he should not hit another child because "Mommy says not to." In the concrete operational period the child will refrain from hitting because "It is wrong." At the formal operational level, the adolescent can explain that hitting is a form of violence that has an impact on society and that it is justified only under certain conditions.

Classification, seriation, conversation, reversing, and rule use allow the child to develop systematic ways of organizing parts to wholes and determining parts of wholes. The child begins to make combinations and elementary permutations (combinations of combinations). The use of concrete operations constitutes *empirico-inductive thinking,* that is, the child is able to solve problems by use of information that is concretely available to him.

THE FORMAL OPERATIONAL PERIOD

The formal operational period, which is the final cognitive period, begins at about 11 years of age and continues through the teen years. It signals the transition to mature thinking. The adolescent begins to think about things that are beyond his experience and manipulative control, and he can begin to use mental, language-based manipulation. A typical characteristic is the developing ability to organize one's time and to relate one's schedule to other people's schedules. The adolescent's thoughts are generally relativistic, that is, he sees relationships of object to object or event to event as having importance regardless of direct personal experiences. An interest in world events and social problems is manifest. The youth internalizes abstract values.

The ability to perform mental manipulations demonstrates the teenager's proficiencies with permutations and the laws of probability. Because of these, the adolescent is able to conceptualize possibilities. Plans can be made and tried out mentally and changed according to mental judgments regarding the soundness of the plan. This ability to analyze problems and to plan possibilities is called *hypothetico-deductive thinking* and is used by adults in most situations that can be dealt with on a cognitive rather than an emotional basis.

Piaget believed that this sequence of development leads to the cognitive maturity of adulthood. The rep-

resentative of this is a person with values, goals, plans, and an understanding of one's purpose in society. Piaget and Inhelder[33] stated that maturation of cognition is dependent on:

1. Organic growth, especially the maturation of the nervous system and endocrine glands. . .
2. Experience in the actions performed upon objects. . .
3. Social interaction and transmission and
4. A balance of opportunities for both assimilation and accommodation (p. 154)

Knowledge of Piaget's theory is critical to occupational therapists who plan programs for children. Regardless of the psychosocial or neurological approaches used in treatment, the therapist in an activity-based situation is interacting with a thinking child. The selection and structure of an activity in accordance with the operational skills and concepts of the child are essential. This can be particularly tricky whan a child is in transition from one period to the next. Because most of Piaget's work on children's cognition has been translated from the original French, which has different grammatical structure and often offers no readily available English terminology, his work is often difficult to read. However, a number of Piaget's colleagues[33] have described his theory for the English-speaking reader. Other authors have contributed significant works.[29,30,32]

Other stage theories
KOHLBERG: STAGES OF MORAL DEVELOPMENT

Lawrence Kohlberg[23] was interested in the relationship between Piaget's concepts of cognitive development and the acquisition of moral value schemes. He designed a series of fascinating experiments that presented moral dilemmas to children and young adults of different ages (Figure 3-1). Like Piaget, he did not make judgments about the correctness of children's choices, but instead he collected data about the concepts used by the children to make moral decisions. He described three discrete levels of moral development, each having two complementary stages.

The first level is called *preconventional morality.* Obedience is the limit to morality until about 8 years of age. Choices are governed by egocentric concerns. The first stage, *punishment and obedience,* is based on the child's desire to avoid punishment from the larger, parental authority figures. The second stage, *instrumental relativism,* is slightly decentered. Decisions are based on personal needs and occasionally on the needs of others when they can be of help to the individual. In other words, you scratch my back, I'll scratch yours.

Conventional morality, the second level of moral development, emerges around 9 or 10 years of age (late concrete operations) and is characterized by social conformity. Its appearance indicates some internalization of rules of social causation. The third stage, *social conformity,* demonstrates behavior that is pleasing to others. It is easy to see how this follows the patterns of instrumental relativism. This is the age when children become very serious about their responsibilities to help with classroom chores. Concern with *law and order* marks the fourth stage. Moral behavior is very rule bound in response to emerging notions of social order and fairness. A typical behavior of this stage is concern with cheating and other infractions of honor codes.

The third level of moral development, *postconventional morality,* is marked by relativistic thinking. There is an effort to define moral principles (rather than obedience) that are flexible for different situations. This is characteristic of the older adolescent with mature formal operations who can consider many variables and possibilities. In the fifth stage, *social contracts,* the young adult makes moral decisions based on social values, with an awareness of the legal implications. A typical example of social contracts thinking is demonstrated by the conscientious objector who registers to provide humanitarian services as an alternative to serving in the army. Kohlberg believes that only a small percentage of individuals attain the sixth stage of moral thinking, *universal ethics.* This stage is represented by the great humanitarian who demonstrates a life commitment to preserving the rights and dignity of man, such as Martin Luther King, Jr.

It is interesting to note that Kohlberg's stages lag behind those of Piaget in a chronological sense. This would indicate that levels of cognition must be fairly mature before an individual can use the higher level operative methods to reexamine abstract issues of morality and obedience. Just as adults tend to use concrete and formal operations flexibly according to the merits of a situation, they also use variable stage moral thinking in dealing with everyday situations. It appears that when a situation is novel and does not readily lend itself to assimilative use of moral schemes, the individual tends to direct a higher level of moral thinking toward the situation.[20,23,40]

MASLOW: HUMANISTIC PSYCHOLOGY

Abraham Maslow[15] is generally considered the father of humanistic psychology in the United States. He, like Piaget and Erikson, was profoundly influenced by European philosophical trends during the Age of Enlightenment. He outlined a *hierarchy of basic human needs* that are believed to appear in the following longitudinal sequence.

The *physiological needs,* such as food, water, rest, air, and warmth, are necessary to basic survival. The next level is characterized by the need for *safety,* broadly defined as the need for both physical and physiological security. The need for *love and belonging* promotes the individual's search for affection, emotional support, and group affiliation. The need for a sense of *self-esteem,* which is defined as the ability to regard one's self as competent and of value to society, is evidenced as persons grow. The need for *self-actualization,* which represents the highest level, is attained through achievement of personal goals.

Maslow proposed that each of these needs serve as motivators to achieve a higher level of human potential. There is a progression of development that begins with the satisfaction of biological, egocentric needs, proceeds through needs for social group affiliation, and culminates in the use of intellectual capacities to affect the broader community of the individual.

If the lower level needs are not met, the individual is not able to direct his energies toward higher levels. For example, if a girl and her boyfriend have just broken up, it is difficult for either of them to concentrate on their studies. Instead they turn to friends (group affiliation) to reestablish feelings of love and belonging.[15,20]

GESELL: DEVELOPMENTAL SCHEDULES

Arnold Gesell[22] was a physician whose work gave impetus to the medical specialty of pediatrics. Through his practice, Gesell accumulated data on children's performance of everyday activities, and he was the first to put a timetable on development through a series of developmental schedules. Most of the items on standard developmental evaluations in use today are based on Gesell's findings. The origins of these developmental behaviors are often taken for granted, and Gesell has received little recognition outside of the health care field.

Most of Gesell's work concerns what to look for, how to find it, and at what ages. It would be impossible to list here all of the ages and items that were identified, but a few key definitions should be useful.

Gesell used the term *behavior* to collectively define all kinds of reactions to stimuli, voluntary or involuntary. In contrast, a *behavior pattern* is considered a discreet, voluntarily repeatable response of the neuromotor system to a specific stimulus situation. The developmental schedules help chart key categories of behavior patterns that are critical to determining the progress of the child. *Motor behavior* is directed toward postural control and locomotion. *Adaptive behavior* patterns are used to manipulate the environment. *Language behaviors* include vocabulary, articulation, and social communication skills. The *personal-social behaviors* are learned controls of bodily functions, such as hygiene and grooming. *Maturity stages* are chronological periods of development in which certain behavior patterns characteristically appear for the first time.

Adaptation is the coordination of physical maturation with the skill demands of the environment. In his studies Gesell found that this was not a smooth process. Typically, behaviors become less adaptive when the child is in a period of rapid physical growth. When the growth spurt subsides, the child is able to concentrate on coordinating his body in the practice of socially acceptable behavior patterns. This cycle of alternating periods of positive and negative adaptation is called *reciprocal interweaving.*[22]

HAVIGHURST: DEVELOPMENTAL TASKS

Robert Havighurst, a renowned American educator, proposed that a person must learn specific groups of skills at different ages to meet social expectations. The acquisition of a particular group of skills enables a person to perform adequately the age-appropriate roles of player, student, worker, or retired person. Havighurst believed that it was the ability of the person to learn, rather than merely respond to situations, that differentiated man from animals.

Havighurst believed that each developmental task had biological, psychological, and sociological bases. Similarly, he proposed that the achievement of each task could be facilitated or inhibited by these three forces. The concept of *sensitive periods* was described as the time at which biological, psychological, and sociological conditions were most appropriate to the achievement of a developmental task. These particularly sensitive times often provided a "teachable moment" when the child or adult is most apt to integrate all previous learning to master the skills of a new developmental task with social guidance. Therefore Havighurst analyzed each task in terms of its biological, psychological, and sociological bases, as well as its educational implications.

Havighurst's *Developmental Tasks and Education*[18] is easy to read and interesting in its discussions of the cultural variations and programmatic implications of the following tasks:

1. Tasks of infancy and childhood
   a. Learning to walk
   b. Learning to take solid food
   c. Learning to talk
   d. Learning to control the elimination of body wastes
   e. Learning sex differences and sexual modesty
   f. Achieving physiological stability
   g. Forming simple concepts of social and physical reality
   h. Learning to relate oneself emotionally to parents, siblings, and other people
   i. Learning to distinguish right and wrong and developing a conscience
2. Tasks of middle childhood
   a. Learning physical skills necessary for ordinary games
   b. Building wholesome attitudes toward oneself as a growing organism
   c. Learning to get along with age-mates
   d. Developing fundamental skills in reading, writing, and calculating
   e. Developing concepts necessary for everyday living
   f. Developing a conscience, morality, and a scale of values
   g. Developing attitudes toward social groups and institutions
3. Tasks of adolescence
   a. Achieving new and more mature relations with age-mates of both sexes
   b. Achieving a masculine or feminine social role
   c. Accepting one's physique and using the body effectively
   d. Achieving emotional independence of parents and other adults
   e. Preparing for marriage and family life
   f. Preparing for an economic career
   g. Acquiring a set of values and an ethical system to guide behavior—developing an ideology
   h. Desiring and achieving socially responsible behavior
4. Tasks of early adulthood
   a. Selecting a mate
   b. Learning to live with a marriage partner
   c. Starting a family
   d. Rearing children
   e. Managing a home
   f. Getting started in an occupation
   g. Taking on civic responsibility
   h. Finding a congenial social group
5. Tasks of middle adulthood
   a. Assisting adolescents to become responsible and happy adults.
   b. Achieving adult civic and social responsibility
   c. Reaching and maintaining satisfactory performance in one's occupational career
   d. Developing adult leisure-time activities
   e. Relating oneself to one's spouse as a person
   f. Accepting and adjusting to the physiological changes of middle age
   g. Adjusting to aging parents
6. Tasks of later maturity
   a. Adjusting to decreasing physical strength and health
   b. Adjusting to retirement and reduced income
   c. Adjusting to the death of a spouse
   d. Establishing an explicit affiliation with one's age group
   e. Adopting and adapting to social roles in a flexible way
   f. Establishing satisfactory physical living arrangements

It is appropriate to conclude this section on stage theories with Havighurst's sequence. Essentially Havighurst's work[18] is a compilation of concepts developed and studied by the previously discussed theorists. The tasks given are self-explanatory and very useful to the therapist to get a quick overview of the social expectations for patients at a particular time of life.

PROCESS THEORIES

This section on process theories is generally limited to Skinner's theory of operant conditioning and Rogers' humanistic theory of the self. This approach was chosen because most of the other process theories are variations of the work of these two men or of the theorists presented in the section on stage theories. Skinner's approach is behavioristic and superficially contrasts sharply with Rogers' ideas. However, it should be recognized at the start that Skinner and Rogers are equally concerned with the individual's opportunity to achieve maximal potential. The difference between the two lies in the school of thought that gives each man his methodological orientation. Skinner's view of man is considerably less mechanistic than that of other behaviorists.

Skinner's theory of radical behaviorism

B.F. Skinner is considered a radical behaviorist, not because he is at the extreme of behaviorism, but because he leans toward the opposite pole. He acknowledges the importance of genetic endowment; he accepts feelings, thoughts, and other "inner events" as behaviors; and he is concerned with self-knowledge and creativity as cultural essentials. In addition, as will be shown, he believes that the initiation of behaviors involves a voluntary element rather than merely a set of uncontrolled responses to environmental stimuli. In these aspects his thinking is radically different from the traditional school of behaviorist thought. It is precisely these differences that make his theory useful to occupational therapists. It must be added, however, that Skinner is strictly a behaviorist in methodology and insists on identification of behaviors that are measurable. However, the range of behaviors that he sees as being measurable is fairly broad.

The components of Skinner's work that are presented here constitute a theory of behavioral development and learning. Skinner believes that all human behavior is shaped by the environment and that bits of behavior may be randomly emitted in response to an environmental stimulus. That is, the organism tries out a behavior that has worked before. Or, an involuntary, reflexive response is elicited by the environmental stimulus. The bit of behavior is then reinforced in some way by the environmental consequences that follow it. Bits of behavior include genetic traits that have proved useful to the species in a given environment and that have been passed on through generations. This sequence of (1) stimulus situation, (2) behavioral response, and (3) environmental consequence constitutes a *contingency of behavior.* It is the mechanism through which the environment shapes behavior.

Skinner clearly states that the environment selects those behaviors that it will reinforce and ignores or punishes those behaviors that are not adaptive. For ex-ample, a young child encounters a dog for the first time. Reaching into his behavioral repertoire, the child emits a reaching-and-touching behavior. If the dog responds by nuzzling, licking the child, and providing the child with a generally pleasant sensory experience, it may be said that the child has been positively reinforced (rewarded) by the environmental consequences. The environmental consequences, or *reinforcements,* of a bit of behavior may be defined as controls that strengthen, weaken, or maintain that particular behavior. If the child comes to associate reaching and touching as a means to obtain a pleasant reaction from dogs, he would tend to repeat that behavior under similar stimulus situations. Thus his behavior would be strengthened and maintained as long as it was generally effective in obtaining positive reinforcement. If, on another occasion the child pets the dog and the dog runs away, the reaching-and-touching behavior might be weakened. In the first instance the behavior was reinforced by the environment. In the latter situation reinforcement was absent, that is, not given and therefore negative. If the dog ran away often enough, it is probable that the child's reaching-and-touching behavior with dogs would be extinguished.

The third type of environmental control, called aversive control, punishment, or a *punitive contingency,* is recognized and defined by Skinner. However, he specifically advocates against its use, because its effects on behavior are unpredictable and generally do not promote adaptation. Punishment has been a common form of behavioral control throughout the ages and is generally expected to eliminate behaviors. If the child reached and petted the dog and was bitten, that would be a form of punishment. If this resulted in avoidance of all future dog encounters, as sometimes happens in this situation, the contingency would be maladaptive. The child still has not learned the most effective behavior to use when approaching strange dogs.

The above example of the child and the dog is also useful for discussion of Skinner's concept of *contingencies of survival.* Certain genetic characteristics, such as having adequate vision to see the dog, a musculoskeletal system that produces a stroking movement, and a neurological system that permits one to approach animals calmly, have proved useful to the survival of the species. These characteristics have enabled humans to domesticate animals through the ages for assistance with food production, transportation, and physical safety. In contrast, the species that did not have these characteristics were forced to rely on their own bodies for sustenance, travel, and security. This has not always proved effective, as witnessed by the great number of species that have become extinct.

To recapitulate, Skinner believes that all behavior is a result of the environmental control of the individual, the culture, and the species. He specified that man, the species, and the culture are part of the environment and therefore control as much as they are controlled. Skinner[36] points out that most of man's environment is man-made and that

Man has changed himself greatly as a person in the same period of time by changing the world in which he lives . . . .Man has "controlled his own destiny". . .the man that man has made is a product of the culture man has devised. He has emerged from two quite different processes of evolution: the biological evolution responsible for man the species and the cultural evolution carried out by that species (p. 198).

What Skinner rejects is the traditional concept of *autonomous man* who functions with no controls. Skinner provides a number of behavioral explanations for the concepts typically used to support the idea of autonomous man. For example, *aggression* is often said to be part of human nature. Skinner would say that this behavior resulted from contingencies of survival. He also points out that aggressive behaviors are strengthened and maintained by here-and-now contingencies of reinforcement. For example, we tell children that it is wrong to hit another child, but then we encourage them to stand up for their rights or to be tough in sports activities. To use Skinner's example, if a man attacks another man and gets the other man's possessions, the attacker is positively reinforced by the goods he has acquired.[36]

A traditionally humanistic concept is the capacity for *self-awareness.* Skinner says this is largely dependent on language, which has been acquired and shaped by the verbal community. Small children do not verbally describe their feelings as a spontaneous behavior. Instead, they learn to describe their feelings because they are questioned regarding these. Even a simple How are you? helps to shape this behavior. The problem with self-awareness, according to Skinner, is its accessibility. A person's verbal bahavior may be incongruent with his nonverbal behavior, so it is more difficult to analyze and control it precisely.

Another characteristic capacity of man that has been described as uniquely human is the ability to *think.* Skinner acknowledges that the ability to think is a complex process with a foundation in the genetic endowment of the species (and therefore evolved through contingencies of survival). A behavioral explanation of thinking is that the culture teaches people to make fine discriminations, to solve problems, and to follow rules, including rules for finding rules. For example, children are taught very early to go to a police officer for help, even if they have had no direct contact with such a person. They can be shown a police officer on television or in a book and be reasonably accurate in subsequent real-life situations that require them to identify this person. Skinner suggests that when a person recalls a concept, it is because something in the present situation elicits a response, in a weakened or altered form, that was acquired on another similar occasion.

Self-identity is readily explained in behavioral terms as a "repertoire of behavior appropriate to a given set of contingencies" (p. 189).[36] Skinner says there are a variety of "selfs" that develop according to the specific contingencies of the varied environments of a person's life. Problems arise when an environment changes and becomes inconsistent with prior contingency patterns. For example, children use one set of behaviors with their families and another set with friends. The first few times that they are in a blended situation with family and friends they are unsure of the environmental consequences and try out both sets of behaviors in a haphazard fashion. Typically, parents will respond by complaining that their child was influenced by the poor behavior of the neighbor's children.

For the purposes of this discussion, the final aspects of human nature to be considered are related to the ability to manipulate the environment. Traditionally, *manipulative ability* has been considered one of the hallmarks of the view of man as autonomous. Skinner explains this characteristic simply as a result of contingencies of survival. Manipulative ability improved man's chances for survival when man emitted eye-hand behaviors that changed the environment. Because these behaviors over time had such a strong impact on the survival of the species, the ability to produce them came to be highly valued. In behavioral terms, manipulative behaviors were increasingly accompanied by positive social-cultural reinforcements. In fact, cultures eventually began to systematically train its members to use manipulative techniques that improved their capacity to change the environment.

The concept of environmental manipulation is coupled with the notion of *industry.* Industry may be defined as the person's rate of emitting behaviors that change the environment. Because such behaviors are highly valued by society, it provides satisfying rewards for higher rates of emitting such behaviors.

A word of caution is in order when reading the works of Skinner. They must be read carefully from start to finish, because he uses logical arguments, and scanning will not provide an accurate picture of radical behaviorism.[31,37-39]

Rogers' self theory

Like Maslow, Carl Rogers believed that people have an inborn need for self-actualization. Rogers took a positive view of human nature that was both deterministic (driven by the actualizing tendency) and epigenetic. Central to Rogers' theory is the individual's *inner experiencing,* that is, how one perceives oneself, one's relationships, and one's environment. Rogers acknowledged the instrumental influence of the environment in the development of the self, but he believed that the individual has the capacity to choose responses to the environment that will maintain a sense of personal control.

Many of Rogers' ideas were developed through his clinical practice and academic career in psychology. He also studied for the ministry, and although he did not complete this course, it provides some explanation for the direction of his thinking. One of his characteristic research methods was the use of the Q-sort. Patients were given cards printed with statements of feelings and personal attributes and then asked to divide the cards into two stacks representing the perceived self and the ideal self. This procedure was repeated at various times throughout the course of therapy to measure changes in the discrepancy between the perceived and the ideal selves.

Rogers is best known for his formulation of *client-centered therapy.* Like Erikson, he believed that each individual has, and must find within himself orherself the resources for growth, adaptation, and self-actualization. Client-centered therapy was designed to elicit these resources, and the therapist takes a nondirective role that encourages the client to say what he or she really feels and wants to do. The *nondirective approach* is readily applied in occupational therapy, when the therapist urges the child to "show me what you can do" and "tell me what you think." This approach has been described by Knickerbocker.[21]

Concepts of the developmental process. Rogers conceptualized the infant as being essentially a clean slate for the development of the self. The totality of sensations constitutes reality. Like and dislikes are clearly demonstrated in response to pleasant and aversive stimuli.

The child grows to want the pleasurable sensations experienced through love and acceptance of *significant others.* Initially these significant others are the child's father and mother. This need for positive regard forces the child to examine what he does that pleases and displeases his parents. He learns to view himself through others' eyes and to suppress feelings and other inner experiences. This is believed to occur because the child receives *conditional positive regard* from the parents; love and acceptance are given under certain conditions according to the child's actions.

Through growth and increased contacts with the outer world, the child slowly loses sight of himself. Externally derived values and feelings of self-worth are internalized. This alienation of the self from the natural organismic (innate) experience is called the *basic estrangement* of humans. The degree to which this prevents the individual from following the self-actualizing tendency is dependent on the amount of *unconditional positive regard* the person receives from significant others.

Rogers' developmental goal for an individual was for the individual to become a fully functioning person. In essence, this is an individual with an existential approach to life who deals with each new situation based on its own merits and on the individual's own true feelings about the situation. Such persons are able to use reality testing to improve the quality of life, rather than to put up with a constrained existence. Rogers[34] provided the following description:

> He is able to experience all of his feelings and is afraid of none . . . he is his own sifter of evidence, but is open to evidence from all sources; he is completely engaged in the process of being and becoming himself, and thus discovers that he is soundly and realistically social . . . He is a fully functioning organism, and because of the awareness of himself which flows freely in and through his experiences, he is a fully functioning person (p. 288).

This discussion of Rogers' theory is to some extent limited by the content of his writing. In contrast to the behavioral tradition of Skinner's work, which is largely-descriptive, Rogers' work[35] is primarily prescriptive for clinical psychology, education, and other socializing institutions. The works of Knickerbocker[21] and Nye[31] are also noteworthy.

CURRENT TRENDS IN DEVELOPMENTAL THEORY

Current investigators of child development appear to be more concerned with process than were the earlier theorists who have been described thus far. It may be hypothesized that stage theories have been fairly well defined to this point and are generally accepted for the basic structure that is provided. A review of the literature in child development in recent years reveals four areas of study that have begun to influence the thinking and practice of occupational therapists: (1) hemispheric specialization, (2) sociobiology, (3) interactionism, and (4) information processing. These terms are from the literature and, though not necessarily parallel, seem to be commonly accepted.

Hemispheric specialization

In the late 1960s it became an accepted practice to "split" the brains of individuals with intractable epilepsy. In simple terms, portions of the interhemispheral connections were surgically cut to reduce the spread and intensity of electrical activity caused by seizures. Although such surgery had been practiced earlier with animals, the use of the techniques with humans provided scientists with a unique opportunity to examine the functions of the brain's two hemispheres.

Earlier it had been believed that the hemispheres were basically similar in function, even though one hemisphere would become dominant in control of fine movements. If the left hemisphere became dominant, then the person would be right-handed. The opposite would hold true if the person was right hemisphere dominant. Dominance was generally believed to be controlled by heredity. In addition, it was clinically well established that individuals who had survived cerebral vascular accidents showed definite signs of hemispheric function asymmetry. After experiencing a lesion in the right hemisphere, patients typically had visual-spatial and affective impairment. In contrast, those individuals whose cerebral vascular accidents had occurred in the left hemisphere demonstrated deficits in language production and motor planning. However, there was no information available from intact human brains to corroborate these findings.

However, researchers have since developed a number of techniques that are used to examine separate functions of the cerebral hemispheres, as demonstrated by those individuals on whom interhemispheric commissurotomies have been performed. Replicated results over the years from such investigators as Sperry, Gazzaniga, Kimura, and Geschwind[11] clearly indicate that there are differences in hemispheric functions. It appears that the right cerebral hemisphere plays a greater role in our perception and association of visual and auditory stimuli that are nonverbal. For example, recognition of music, art, and faces appears to be subject to adequate function of the right hemisphere. In contrast, the left cerebral hemisphere is more critical to perception and association of verbal and other symbolic material. Differences are both anatomical and physiological.

In addition to intraindividual differences, there also appear to be interindividual differences. It is now believed that left hemisphere functions are more highly specialized in women and that right hemisphere functions are more highly developed in men. Although researchers warn that socialization may exaggerate these differences to a greater degree, this neurophysiological gender difference tends to account for the greater proficiency of women in language-related subjects and the gravitation of men toward math and visual-spatial subjects such as engineering.

Similarly, learning styles and interests are derived, at least initially, from the influence of an individual's more highly developed hemisphere. The right dominant child will perform better in traditional educational programs that emphasize verbal skills. In contrast, the left dominant individual reaches a higher level of achievement when engaged in multi-sensory, experiential learning.

Persons with dominant right hemispheres may be more interested in art, architecture, and engineering, whereas persons with dominant left hemispheres would gravitate more toward teaching, sales, and writing.[11,20]

Findings on hemispheric specialization and other related data from the neurosciences are effecting an increasing number of changes in health care and educational programs. Service providers, including occupational therapists, are more routinely identifying hemisphere-related learning styles and planning program activities accordingly. The impact of hemispheric specialization is particularly notable in treatment of individuals with known or suspected brain damage, in art programs for children, and in services for learning disabled adolescents. Continuing data from the neurosciences can be expected to support the devlopment of increasingly sophisticated approaches to human service delivery.

Sociobiology

The concepts and speculations generated by sociobiology are even more controversial. Sociobiology is defined as "the application of evolutionary principles to the social behavior of animals. . .and human beings as well" (p. 1).[5] This discipline proposes that much of the behavior of human beings that has heretofore been considered socially derived, and therefore environmentally derived, is actually genetically transmitted. Researchers have sought to identify universal behaviors among species and relate the development of those behaviors through natural selection. They propose that each species develops a unique behavioral repertoire over time through the natural selection of those characteristics that are most adaptive for the species. Their concern is not with the different cultural patterns that are used to refine the behaviors, but rather with the species-specific behaviors that are the bases of the cultural patterns. Barash[5] pointed out that although there are thousands of language patterns used by different humans, the capacity to speak, develop, and learn a language and communicate with others is biologically derived and shared by the entire species. Again, the critical difference that the sociobiologists make is that these capacites are genetically, rather than socially, transmitted.

The concepts of sociobiology have been rejected by some social scientists on the grounds that the theory does not account for individual differences and that it has an aura of determinism that could conceivably be used to support discriminative practices.[41] Selected review of the literature in sociobiology indicates that individual differences are not overlooked but are deemphasized.[39,42]

In contrast, Thomas[41] noted that sociobiological concepts provide considerable explanation for the growing evidence of the complexity of infant behavior. The human capacities for reflexive responses, sensory perception, speech, and learning are recognized as biologically determined. What has been questioned until recently is how well developed these capacities are at birth.

Interactionism

The concept of interactionism, as defined by Thomas,[41] includes several components. These include the inborn complexity of infant behavior, the plasticity of the human development, and the variable effects of the child's temperament. Simply stated, interactionism postulates that the child is an active social being who contributes to continuity and change in his developmental environment.

As was alluded to earlier, research data now indicate that infants have definite behavioral patterns at birth, including preferential attention to a variety of auditory, visual, tactile, and gustatory stimuli. Active learning, as evidenced by the rapid manifestation and replication of neurodevelopmental reflexes, begins immediately after birth. Imitative behaviors appear within 2 weeks. These behaviors are now defined as being social rather than reflexive.[41] Whereas it was formerly emphasized that infants learned to respond differentially to their mothers' behaviors, researchers now speak in terms of mothers' increasingly differentiated responses to infants' behaviors.[1]

Similarly, it is becoming clearer that the residual effects of early or traumatic experiences are not as permanent as previously thought. Numerous studies of children from varied early environments who later had the opportunity for enriching experiences have led investigators to conclude that the human capacity for change is as important in child development as is the capacity for steady, continuous maturation. Considerable research is now directed toward understanding the influence of multiple attachments at different stages of life.[41] Equally relevant is information about a child's capacity to recover from traumatic experiences, such as separation from parents through divorce or death, as the child develops. Again, the influence of multiple attachments is considered critical, particularly in relation to the need for adequate gender role models.[49] It appears that a child's adaptive development is best facilitated by a balanced combination of continuity and change, rather than overemphasis on either mode.

Finally, interactionism is concerned with the influence of the child's temperament. As a logical extension to the awareness of the strength of the infant's cognitive behaviors and learning, researchers have begun to look at the way the growing child's temperament affects the behaviors and attitudes of others, as well as how the child's temperament affects her response to others. For example, the child who is perceived as "not caring about schoolwork" may be ignored by teachers. If this perception is accurate, such lack of attention may not be as negative an influence on the child as was formerly believed. However, if the child's attitude is a reflection of fear of failure with schoolwork, then neglect by the teachers could be even more threatening to the child. A long-term study by Thomas[41] indicates that there are clear-cut patterns of consistency of temperament over time, and that these patterns in turn contribute to variations in development.

Cognition and learning

In addition to the concern with physiological and social foundations of behavior, recent study in child development has been directed toward the examination of cognitive behaviors and learning. Although Piagetian theory had been generally well accepted as an explanation of the developmental maturation of a child's thought content, it left gaps in the understanding of how cognition and learning take place. Researchers have relied heavily on combining concepts from information processing and social learning theories to develop a more sophisticated explanation of the two phenomena.

The early development of *information processing* theory has been attributed to Klahr and Wallace.[9] In essence, information processing is actually a conceptual model of how the brain operates from the information it receives. The development of computer technology has provided researchers with terminology for the processes that are involved in cognition.

Information processing uses a simple input-operations-output model. The input includes any sensory stimuli that are received through the sensory organs and transmitted to the central nervous system. Therefore input is dependent on attention, curiosity, exploration, sensory awareness, and sensory recognition. The operations (or cognitive functions) include storage in long- and short-term memory, concept formation, association, sorting, and retrieval strategies. These operations are subject to physiological variations such as age, level of consciousness, and general well-being. The output of cognition is represented by thought or action as the individual makes a choice, moves, or speaks. Output is modified by concurrent operations related to affect and attention.[29]

The information processing model has been widely adopted in psychology and education, and occupational therapists need to be familiar with its relevance to sensory integrative function (Chapter 23). It is a useful tool for both research and program design because of its simplicity and well-defined terminology.

One application of the information processing model is shown in Kaluger and Kaluger's[20] conceptualization of the learning process. Using model components studied by the early social learning theorists, Kaluger and Kaluger propose that *learning* is the cognitive process through which the individual gathers information and is able to knowledgeably select the appropriate behavior(s) to reach a desired goal.

The information processing model for learning (Figure 3-2) shows the three main process components and two universal bases involved. The learning processes provide input to the individual. Learning methods are the operational components. Learning outcomes, or outputs, include specific knowledge and behaviors. Motivation to achieve a goal is essential to the initiation and continuity of learning, as is the development of a repertoire of knowledge and cognitive abilities.

Kaluger and Kaluger remind us that learning is an active process and will not occur if the goal is not meaningful to the child or if the knowledge and con-

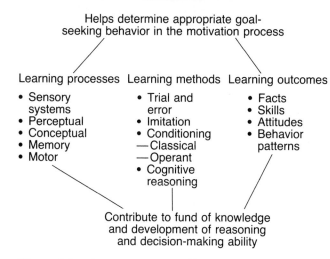

LEARNING

Helps determine appropriate goal-
seeking behavior in the motivation process

Learning processes   Learning methods   Learning outcomes

- Sensory
  systems
- Perceptual
- Conceptual
- Memory
- Motor

- Trial and
  error
- Imitation
- Conditioning
  —Classical
  —Operant
- Cognitive
  reasoning

- Facts
- Skills
- Attitudes
- Behavior
  patterns

Contribute to fund of knowledge
and development of reasoning
and decision-making ability

Figure 3-2   Component parts of learning process that influence quality of goal-seeking behavior.

From Kaluger GA, and Kaluger MF: Human development: the span of life, ed 3, St Louis, 1984, The CV Mosby Co.

ceptual skills to be attained through the learning situation have no personal relevance. Perhaps it is a sign of maturity when the accumulation of knowledge for its own sake is a goal.

To summarize, the trend toward identification of universal sequences of development that dominated child study through the 1960s has given way to concern with the processes of development and function that underlie such sequences. There appears to be an increasing tendency to examine how the broad range of social, biological, and psychological influences affect different areas of behavior. This trend is reflected in the theoretical frameworks that have developed in pediatric occupational therapy practice. The frameworks that are presented here have been derived from occupational therapists' studies of the various theories of child development. What differentiates the occupational therapists' theories is their concern with integration of these developmental theories to provide an explanation of the process of occupation in purposeful activity.

MAJOR THEORETICAL APPROACHES TO PEDIATRIC OCCUPATIONAL THERAPY
Reilly: an explanation of play

LINDA A. FLOREY

Children engaged in play spend endless hours in doing things and concentrating on things that for all intents and purposes have no observable value except to the children themselves. What children seem to gain from their involvement in play is an experiential know-how that they use to solve daily living situations. The play of childhood seems to provide individuals with strategies for coping with the unknowns of the here and now and for future life experiences.

Mary Reilly's major focus has been to formulate a theoretical explanation of play that gives substance to clinical impressions that play (1) has an organizing effect on human behavior and (2) is a critical base for adult competence. Reilly proposed that the ultimate service play provides is to give meaning to the complexities of society. She stated[34] that "human adaptation falters when meaning cannot be derived from environmental interactions" (p. 15). The central question Reilly raised is how play enables meaning to be attributed to the events of everyday life.

Reilly speculated that the very obvious and commonplace nature of play does not lend itself to rigorous scientific investigation as a discrete phenomenon. Discussion of the values and functions of play is interspersed among many theories of human behavior; however, play had rarely received prominence as a major construct. Instead, play had been approached through the back door in major theories of evolution, psychology, sociology, philosophy, biology, and anthropology. Although a theory might discuss play, it was generally discussed as a vehicle for the development of some other construct.

Reilly was convinced that play figured importantly in attempts to evoke competency in disabled individuals. Therefore she concentrated on (1) the explanatory framework by which play phenomena are examined, (2) the learning system through which the play process is explained, and (3) the play progression through which the changes in the outcome of the play process can be viewed.[34]

THE EXPLANATORY FRAMEWORK

Our knowledge of play is drawn from biology, psychology, sociology, and anthropology. Anyone attempting to examine or explain play must acknowledge this multidimensional nature of the phenomena. Reilly stated[34] that "existing theories about behavior are limited in their ability to explain multiple dimensions and integrating mechanisms." (p. 118). She addressed the question that what is needed is an interdisciplinary approach to explanation. The vehicle she selected for interdisciplinary examination of play is general systems theory.

*General systems theory** addresses the complexity of phenomena, identifies the limits to which theoretical models explain the actions of a phenomenon, and pro-

*Discussion of general systems theory here is limited to Reilly's interpretation as presented in reference.[34] Similarly, her interpretation is used for discussion of concepts attributed to Vickers, Berlyne, Buhler, White, and McClelland. Primary references for these authors may be found in Reilly's book.

vides relationships between the various models. For example, the theoretical model that explains temperature control in the body is not the appropriate model to explain human cognition, and vice versa.

Key concepts within general systems theory are (1) the nature of systems and (2) hierarchy. The nature of systems addresses the relationships of parts to wholes, structure to function, and exchange and array of energy. Systems are described with respect to the degree of complexity in the organization of behavior. Hierarchy specifies the levels of complexity and the rules by which such complexity is ordered. The whole of a system is composed of many parts, or subsystems. Hierarchy specifies the ordering of subsystems according to the complexity of each one.

The overall function of a hierarchy is to process change from simple to complex and from lower to higher forms of behavior. It implies a sense of order both in the immediate time frame and also within larger time frames. A hierarchy is composed of stages in which older and simpler forms of behavior are transformed into newer, more complex forms. The first level of a hierarchy is the initial and most simple part of a system. Each succeeding level is more complex than the preceding levels. The higher levels direct the lower ones, although there must be stability at the lower levels for the higher levels to provide any direction.

By use of a general systems framework, Reilly saw play as one system that is part of the larger system of behavior. Within play there are subsystems that are arranged in a hierarchical manner. Play is a subsystem of the imagination system of learning. The subsystems within play are exploratory, competency, and achievement behaviors.

A PLAY SYSTEM OF LEARNING

Reilly speculated that the outcomes of play are learning to symbolize and learning meanings. The play-learning process cannot be conceptualized as a fixed connection between stimulus and response under high-need states. She believed that the traditional, behaviorally oriented learning theories are too simplistic to explain the complex nature of play. Instead, she drew on the appreciative system of learning to support her concepts.

The appreciative system of learning was developed by Geoffrey Vickers, a British lawyer and public administrator. He believed that the task of learning was to find a way to look at and examine the many choices presented by a complex society. Reilly believed that the appreciative system provides a way to interpret and give meaning to information. Learning is "a product of the interaction of external facts of reality with internal values" (p. 131).[34] The tendency of *symbols* (or schemata) to link with values is the key to the learning process and enables the individual to derive meanings. The overall product of the appreciative system is judgment.

Reilly believed that a play system of learning operates in a fashion similar to the appreciative system. However, the assumptions made and the ultimate purposes differ. The appreciative system assumes that a symbol formation process is already in operation. The play system does not hold such a conviction, but instead it asks how the symbol formation and classifying processes of the mind are formed. The appreciative system is designed to explain how reality is evaluated, whereas the play system of learning explains how reality is explored and how the exploratory process teaches meaning.

Reilly viewed the *imagination* as being central to symbol formation. Symbols require meaning within one's imagination. Symbols translate sensation into meaning as they name and describe aspects of reality and provide a shorthand representation of the individual's experiences. By storing meaning and codifying experiences, symbols establish a ground plan for communication. Because symbols speak for reality, the imagination is considered a language domain.

The three subsystems of the imagination that process information into meaning are (1) the myth subsystem, (2) the dream subsystem, and (3) the play subsystem. Each subsystem serves different functions and uses different symbols for expression. The *myth subsystem* uses word symbols to represent reality. This component serves the thinking behavior of human beings, and the ultimate product is the logic of reality. The *dream subsystem* uses visual imagery to represent reality. It serves the feeling behavior of humans. The product of this subsystem is the organization of feelings for social relationships. The *play subsystem* uses rules of action to represent reality. It serves the doing behavior of humans and addresses the technology of reality. The *rule* as a symbol seeks to learn, "What is this?" and "What can be done with this?" The product of the play subsystem is *skill* configuration. Rules provide a code through which the results of actions are stored. The yield of the code is skill.

All three subsystems serve the imagination system of learning, but the rule as a symbol is most relevant to understanding play. Reilly stated[34] that "the symbol of the rule is a product of the built-in characteristic of a nervous system that asks 'What is this?'" (p. 140). Reilly drew on the work of psychologist Berlyne to explain the roles of curiosity and conflict in the rule symbolization process. *Curiosity* is a drive triggered by the external stimuli of novelty, uncertainty, degree of conflict, and complexity of incoming information. These stimuli all entail conflict, and by virtue of the conflict they generate, they serve to increase the arousal of the organism. Excessive arousal is relieved by specific exploration. Exploratory responses resolve conflict by favoring one response over another, by providing additional information, or by allowing time to work out a new response to the stimulus pattern.

Reilly believed that play is energized by curiosity, and that, as a consequence, reality is explored to obtain the rules of how objects, people, and events work. The rule as a symbol generates meaning in the course of exploratory action. The rule comes to represent the strategies for knowing (or learning) how to do something with objects, people, and events within the boundaries of time, space, and purpose. Reilly stated [34] that "complex organizations of rules learned specifically from action of experience give rise to the skill configurations upon which the competency of man and the technology of his society are founded" (p. 145).

PLAY PROGRESSION

In the play system of learning, skill configurations are acquired, combined, and recombined into different products over time. Reilly hypothesized a progression of play behavior through three hierarchical stages: (1) exploratory behavior, (2) competency behavior, and (3) achievement behavior (Table 3-1). Each stage expresses a higher level of excitement and requires a greater degree of control. Although curiosity is the underlying force that drives the system, each stage is documented by its own motivational force.

Exploratory behavior in play is usually seen in early childhood or when an event is very new or different. Reilly proposed that exploratory play is motivated by *functional pleasure*, a concept described by Buhler. Because anxiety and pressure from unmet basic needs inhibit exploratory behavior, functional pleasure occurs only when major needs have been satisfied. In this stage children tease and test reality as their imaginations search for rules of how things work and do not work. Exploratory play produces schemata for understanding what something is and what can be done with it. For this to occur, the environment must be perceived as secure. The hallmark of this stage is the search to attribute meaning to motions, objects, and people. If the environment permits, feelings of hope and trust are generated.

Competency behavior is characterized by the need to deal with the environment and the need to be influenced by the environment through feedback mechanisms. Reilly proposed that this stage is motivated by the *efficacy drive,* as described by White. Children learn what effects they can have on the environment and what effects the environment can have on them. Through sensory, social, and other forms of feedback, children learn the results of their interactions and continually attempt to monitor their actions to achieve results. This is when the "do it myself" attitude reigns and children repeat activities over and over again to achieve a goal. Competency behaviors provide schemata, or understanding strategies, by which tasks can be mastered. The hallmark of this stage is persistence, which leads to task mastery and feelings of self-confidence and self-reliance.

Achievement behavior incorporates the learnings of the two previous stages. The nature of achievement was drawn by Reilly from the work of McClelland. The *achievement motive* that McClelland proposed is

guided by sets of expectations that are developed through anticipated or past achievement satisfactions or dissatisfactions. Expectations are formed out of universal experiences with problem solving, such as learning to walk, talk, read, or sew. These expectations involve competition with a standard of excellence. Although standards of excellence can be self-related, they are generally set by someone other than the child. Achievement behavior becomes more extrinsically guided as standards are linked to external requirements for pass, fail, good, and bad. Achievement behavior produces schemata for understanding how one's efforts measure up (or compare) in the public domain. This stage is characterized by competition, which has elements of risk and outright danger. Courage is the hallmark of this stage, and feelings of skillful mastery in a puzzling environment are generated.

• • •

In conclusion, Reilly believed that, in play, individuals acquire different kinds of rules that give meaning to environmental transactions. The rules of sensory motor action provide children with skills necessary to learn the rules of role behavior. In turn, the rules of role behavior equip children with the skills to learn the rules of cooperation and competition. Thus the early manipulation of objects and people and engagement in arts, crafts, and games yields the risk-taking behaviors seen in craftsmanship and sportsmanship. The results of engagement in these risk-taking behaviors are seen as necessary preconditions for engagement in adult workmanship. Reilly saw the play of childhood as the precursor to adult competency. The engagement of disabled individuals in arts, crafts, or games enables them to work and play through the exploratory, competency, and achievement processes by which competency is evoked.

Llorens: facilitating growth and development

Lela Llorens' work[24-28] has been broadly influenced by the developmental theorists who were discussed in prior sections of this chapter. Unlike the other occupational therapy theoretical frames of reference presented here, Llorens' model is designed to apply to adults as well. (It should be noted that the other three theorists are also broadly concerned with a life span approach to occupational therapy; however, their theories as presented here are limited to pediatric practice.)

In her 1969 Eleanor Clark Slagle Lecture, Llorens[24] proposed that occupational therapists focus on physical, social, and psychological parameters of human life tasks and relationships. Within this context the therapist looks at individual functions and their integration, both during specific periods of life (horizontal development) and over the course of time (longitudinal development). The therapist's role is conceptualized as that of a change agent, facilitating the growth and development of the individual.

The premises of Llorens' theoretical framework, are the following:*

1. That the human organism develops horizontally in the areas of neurophysiological, physical, psychosocial, psychodynamic growth and in the development of social language, daily living and sociocultural skills at specific periods of time;

2. That the human organism develops longitudinally in each of these areas in a continuous process as he ages;

3. That mastery of particular skills, abilities, and relationships in each of the areas of neurophysiological, physical, psychosocial, and psychodynamic development, social language, daily living and sociocultural skills, both horizontally and longitudinally, is necessary to the achievement of satisfactory coping behavior and adaptive relationships;

4. That such mastery is usually achieved naturally in the course of development;

5. That the fundamental endowment of the individual and the stimulation of experiences received within the environment of the family come together to interact in such a way as to promote positive early growth and development in both the horizontal and longitudinal planes;

6. That later the influences of extended family, community, social and civic groups assist in the growth process;

7. That physical or psychological trauma related to disease, injury, environmental insufficiencies, or interpersonal vulnerability can interrupt the growth and development process;

8. That such growth interruption will cause a gap in the developmental cycle resulting in a disparity between expected coping behavior and adaptive facility and the necessary skills and abilities to achieve the same;

9. That occupational therapy through the skilled application of activities and relationships can provide growth and development links to assist in closing the gap between expectation and ability by increasing skills, abilities, and relationships in the neurophysiological, physical, psychosocial, psychodynamic, social language, daily living and sociocultural spheres of development as indicated both horizontally and longitudinally;

10. That occupational therapy through the skilled application of activities and relationships can provide growth experiences to prevent the development of potential maladaptation related to insufficient nurturance in neurophysiological, physical, psychosocial, psychodynamic, social language, daily living, and sociocultural spheres of development, both horizontally and longitudinally.

With these 10 statements, Llorens sought to identify factors of development that would guide occupational therapy practice. The skills, abilities, and relationships that are critical to the child's development become the tools of the occupational therapist. As part of the Slagle Lectureship she constructed a life span model of developmental theories and activities. In later work she more specifically defined the critical activities to em-

phasize their importance as occupational therapy media. The activity categories include the following[26]:

1. *Sensory activities.* These activities provide sensory stimulation to the developing individual and are generally initiated by the self or significant others. These activities are enjoyed for their sensory pleasure and include rolling, tossing in the air, swinging, and being cuddled.

2. *Developmental activities.* The specific object of developmental activities is the learning and acquisition of skills. Most developmental activities involve object manipulation. These activities tend to be specifically age-related, although most result in skills that will be upgraded in performance of activities appropriate to a later age. Developmental activities are enjoyed, because they provide a sense of mastery and include arts, crafts, creative and dramatic play, and school readiness activities.

3. *Symbolic activities.* These activities are specifically related to gratification of basic needs and expression of feelings. Although the time to learn different symbolic activities may be age-related, performance of the activities generally will continue in a similar form throughout the life span. Symbolic activities include eating, collecting, and leading groups.

4. *Daily life tasks.* These tasks are a reflection of cultural expectations in day-to-day life. Whereas eating is symbolic and universal, the techniques used by the individual to feed himself or herself are culturally determined. Daily life tasks include other routine, age-related activities such as using transportation, working, and cleaning house.

5. *Interpersonal relationships.* Llorens has continually stressed the need to consider human interactions as both developmental and occupational therapy activities. The nature and quality of interpersonal relationships change throughout the life span, and mastery of the skills required for interaction is critical to adequate engagement in the other types of activities. Such relationships include the one-to-one dyad, parallel cooperative work, and nurturing.

Using this theoretical framework, Llorens has designed and described a systematic approach to the occupational therapy process that addresses both the horizontal and longitudinal dimensions of development. Through analysis of the developmental tasks, life roles, and expectations of the individual, and through analysis of the potential effects of stress, trauma, and disease, the therapist is able to identify service needs. Llorens conceived occupational therapy as a problem-solving process that uses a balance of artful caring and consideration with knowledge of the human sciences.[26]

In 1981, Llorens[27] explored the meaning of activity within the occupational therapy process. She suggested that the actions of the therapist involve the use of purposeful activity for organized, controlled stimulation of adaptive role behaviors of the patient. Llorens hypothesized that direct and indirect stimulation of the cen-

---

*From Llorens LA: 1969 Eleanor Clark Slagle Lecture: facilitating growth and development: the promise of occupational therapy, Am J Occup Ther 24:93, 1970.

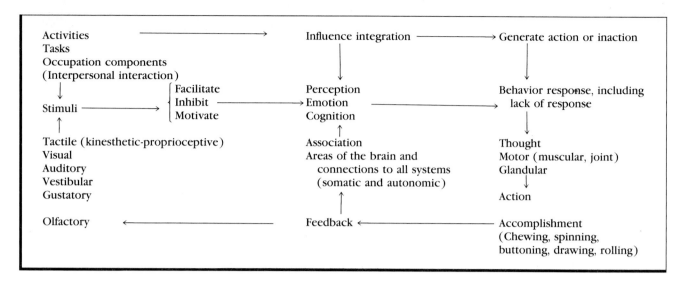

Figure 3-3 Sensory processing model for analysis of activities, tasks, and occupations.

From Llorens LA: Activity analysis: agreement among factors in a sensory processing model, Am J Occup Ther 40:104, 1986.

tral nervous system can be controlled by the therapist through the activity process (Figure 3-3). Activities must be analyzed and selected for their normalizing relation to the physical, psychological, and social components of individual task performance and to the totality of life role requirements.

Recently, Llorens reported on a study that investigated the application of model components in activity analysis. A nonrandom sample of 80 occupational therapy students used the model to analyze their own participation in five representative tasks. In addition to the components labelled in Figure 3-3, students considered 13 factors that were descriptive of the intersensory processes of perception, emotion, and cognition. Results of the study indicate that the components of this model, which applies neurobehavioral concepts to the occupational therapy process, provide a useful framework for activity analysis.[28]

Because so much of Llorens' work before and since her Slagle Lectureship has dealt specifically with the practice of occupational therapy, it is beyond the scope of this chapter to provide a complete review. Numerous references to her work appear throughout the assessment and treatment chapters.[24-28]

Gilfoyle and Grady: spatiotemporal adaptation

The theory of spatiotemporal adaptation formulated by Elnora Gilfoyle and Ann Grady is particularly useful as a "normal" development background for understanding the developmental disabilities. In addition to combining concepts from the work of Piaget, Gesell, and Erikson, their approach draws from the clinical theories of Ayres and the Bobaths (see also Chapters 20 and 23).

Gilfoyle and Grady have used the term *spatiotemporal* to connote adaptation as a process of interactions between the individual and an environment of time and space (Figure 3-4). Adaptation from primitive fetal reflexes to higher levels of function takes place through the maturation of the nervous system. Of primary importance to the adaptive response is *sensory-motor-sensory (SMS)* process of receiving, integrating, and acting on environmental input. The inborn genetic differences of the child, coupled with environmental variations, produce the unique self-system of the child. Reflex behaviors give way to posture and movement strategies, and these in turn are organized into purposeful behaviors, activities, and skills through the individual's successful experiences with the environment.

There are four components to the adaptation process. *Assimilation* is the sensory reception of stimuli from within and outside the body. The motor response of the body to stimulation is called *accommodation.* The organized process of relating a specific stimulus situation with a discrete motor response is *association.* Through repetition of this SMS pattern, the child is able to apply the process of *differentiation.* This means that the child is able to discriminate between the essential and nonproductive elements of his motor response in the given stimulus situation and can thereafter refine the accommodative pattern.

The SMS process of spatiotemporal adaptation is viewed as a spiralling continuum (Figure 3-4). Development makes up the continuous part of the process,

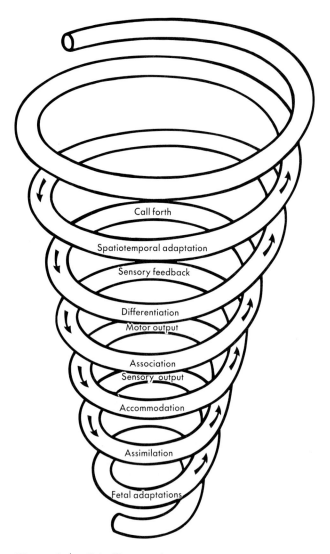

Figure 3-4   Spiralling continuum.

From Gilfoyle EM, Grady AP, and Moore JC: Children adapt, Thorofare, NJ, 1980, Slack, Inc.

and the interaction between older, undifferentiated SMS behaviors and newer discriminative behaviors promotes the spiralling effect. The following three principles[13] govern the direction of the spiralling continuum:

1. The child's adaptation process with new experiences is dependent upon the past acquired behaviors.
2. With the integration of past experiences with new experiences, the past behaviors are modified in some manner and result in higher level behavior.
3. The integration of higher level behaviors influences and increases the maturity of lower level behaviors (p. 50).

In effect, behavioral maturation and refinement in one activity tend to promote growth in other areas. The totality of functional development reaches higher levels.

Gilfoyle and Grady have defined a sequence for the development of purposeful activity that is useful to occupational therapy practice. In brief, this begins with a primitive phase during which the child visually explores the environment and becomes aware of her hands. Through the transitional phase, which occurs roughly from the fifth through the ninth month, visually guided development of grasp and release leads to the ability to explore objects. During this time also the infant's locomotor development is significant. With achievement of each milestone toward an upright posture, the function of the infant's hands can be directed less toward maintaining postural stability and more toward exploring objects in the environment. The mature phase of development of purposeful activity begins with the acquisition of fine prehension and progresses through the refined manipulative skill that allows the child to control objects. Gilfoyle and Grady believe that each child develops a set of prehension skills that are both unique to the individual and universally characteristic of the species.

The positive effects of stress discussed in the beginning of this chapter are detailed by Gilfoyle and Grady and are seen as a challenge to adaptation. However, they differentiate the concept of *spatiotemporal stress,* which means that the adaptive demands of a stimulus situation exceed the functional capacities of the child. In this case, rather than establishing new behavioral patterns, the child "calls up" lower level behaviors to adapt to the new situation. As a temporary measure, this provides the child with the opportunity to "get his bearings" and through association and differentiation of old and new, to determine what elements of the lower level behaviors offer some chance of acting on the new situation. This is a normal process. However, if the spatiotemporal stress continues without respite, either as a result of environmental causes or of an impairment of the SMS integration process, developmental deviation can occur. Then the child experiences *spatiotemporal distress.*

The preceding discussion may be clarified by a review of the theoretical premises of spatiotemporal adaptation, as described by Gilfoyle and Grady*:

1. Development is a function of nervous system maturation which occurs through a process of adaptation.
2. Adaptation is dependent upon attention to and active participation with purposeful events of the environment. Without active participation, the nervous system is deprived of certain forms of sensation (sensory feedback) which, in turn, affects maturation.
3. Purposeful events (behaviors and activities) provide meaningful experiences for enhancement of maturation by directing a higher level adaptive response.
4. Higher level responses result from integration with and modification of acquired, lower level functions, thus adaption

---

*From Gilfoyle EM, Grady AP, and Moore JC: Children adapt, Thorofare, NJ, 1980, Slack, Inc, p 208.

of higher level functions is dependent upon a certain degree of association/differentiation of specific components of lower level performance.

5. Adaptation spirals through primitive, transitional, and mature phases of development occurring at the same time within different body segments. The concurrent development of phases considers the adaptation of posture and movement strategies to purposeful behaviors and activities and the linking of behaviors and activities for adaptation to skill

6. Environmental experiences may present situations of spatiotemporal stress. With stress, the system calls forth past acquired strategies, behaviors, and activities to act upon the demands of the environment and maintain the system's homeostasis.

7. Spatiotemporal distress provokes dysfunction when the adaptation process is interrupted or incomplete resulting in maladaptation. With dysfunction a child repeats purposeless lower level performances. Repetition of purposeless performances results in regression and ultimately leads to developmental disability.

These premises provide a rationale for Gilfoyle and Grady's approach to treatment. They give considerable weight to the possibility of establishing new SMS pathways in a young nervous system (see Ayres' theory in the following section). This is achieved through a purposeful activity program that promotes spatiotemporal adaptation through active (as opposed to passive) SMS experiences. They differentiate purposeful activity as that which is initiated and directed toward interaction with objects and events in the environment. (This contrasts with the body-centered actions that Gilfoyle and Grady describe as purposeful behaviors.) The therapist's primary role is to structure the environment with stimulus situations that will challenge the child to act through purposeful activity and avoid spatiotemporal distress.[12,13]

Ayres: sensory integration

FLORENCE CLARK

As formulated by A. Jean Ayres, sensory integration theory provides a broad developmental perspective about how the brain develops the capacity to perceive, learn, and organize behavior. Ayres defines *sensory integration* as the organization of sensory input in the brain for the emitting of adaptive responses. Developed through 20 years of research, the theory stands as an elaborate description of how sensory integration develops, how it is enhanced, and how it results in more complex responses. As a developmental theory it has logically evolved from occupational therapy because of the discipline's concern with sensory processing and adaptive responses as foundations of purposeful activity. The uniqueness of sensory integration rests on the depth in which it addresses the neurobiological foundations of behavior.

Ayres' background in occupational therapy and edu-

cational psychology has been supplemented by postdoctoral study at the Brain Research Institute of the University of California in Los Angeles. Her early interest in perceptual disorders arose from clinical experiences as an occupational therapist. At that time her caseload of patients included individuals with overt brain damage secondary to cerebral vascular accident (CVA) and cerebral palsy. Gradually her interest extended to the apparently similar perceptual problems of children who seemed to have no upper motor neuron damage and yet were rather loosely called "brain damaged." Largely because of the accessibility and availability of categorical grant funding, most of Ayres' clinical research (through which the theory has been validated) was conducted with children who had perceptual or learning disabilities. Because of this research her theory is commonly identified with learning disability. It must be reemphasized, however, that sensory integration theory has its roots in the study of normal neurobehavioral development. Attention to sensory integrative function is emphasized throughout this text as an integral part of occupational therapy practice. Ayres believed that sensory integrative theory and treatment is applicable to a wide variety of neurological disorders in children, including mental retardation, autism, and aphasia. In 1979 Ayres published *Sensory Integration and the Child*[4] with hopes that it would correct the bias of overidentification of the theory with learning disorders.

There are many facets to sensory integration theory, not all of which are pertinent to this chapter. What will be emphasized here are Ayres' proposals about the development of the child's capacity to learn, perceive, and organize behavior. Chapter 23 discusses the research and formulations of the theory related to treatment of children with learning disabilities. Many portions of Chapter 23 apply to children with other neurological handicaps. Other discussions of sensory integrative function as it relates to occupational therapy practice are found throughout the chapters on assessment and programming.

The key concepts in sensory integration theory are derived from basic research on the vertebrate brain. Therefore, comprehension of the theory, as detailed in Ayres' works,[3,4] depends on extensive reading of the neurobiological literature and on solid preparation in neuroanatomy and neurophysiology.

THE IMPORTANCE OF SENSORY INTEGRATION

Sensory integration involves the organization of sensations from two or more sensory modalities (such as the tactile and vestibular modalities) for the purpose of emission of adaptive responses. Essentially the theory depicts streams of electrical impulses from a variety of sensory receptors converging in the central nervous system. The net effect is that this multitude of information must be localized, sorted, ordered, and organized so that it becomes meaningful. Collectively the hypothesized neural process that performs these operations is called sensory integration. Because it occurs in the brain, the process is not directly observable. However, some of its posited outcomes, like behavioral organization and adaptive responses, may be observed. *Perception*, or the ability to attach meaning to sensation, is described by Ayres as one other result of sensory integration.

When sensory integrative function is effective, the adaptive responses that are emitted are defined as successful, goal-directed, purposeful responses to some environmental challenge. A child is considered to have emitted an adaptive response when his actions are appropriate and successfully meet environmental demands. The complexity of adaptive responses varies. For example, at one end of the continuum the child might emit the simple response of being able to hold on and stay put on a stationary swing. The opposite end of the continuum could be the child's complex response of standing on a swing as it rapidly moves while at the same time throwing beanbags at a target. In sensory integration theory the efficiency of adaptive responses and the efficacy of sensory integrative function are mutually dependent.

Ayres placed great emphasis on the importance of adequate sensory integration as a foundation for normal learning and emotional behavior. She believed that learning occurs in the brain and that learning disorders reflect some irregularity in brain function. Ayres proposed that abstract, complex operations such as reading, auditory-language processing, and visual processing depend on intersensory processing of tactile, vestibular, and proprioceptive stimuli, particularly at the brain stem level. She reasoned that higher cognitive functions that are related to academic learning can be enhanced through better integration of the somatosensory systems when irregularities in those systems can be diagnosed.

Ayres' theory does not place equal emphasis on all the sensory systems. Although initially the visual system was emphasized, subsequent research suggests the importance of tactile, vestibular, and proprioceptive stimuli integration as a primary foundation for auditory and visual processing and for the acquisition of language and academic skills. Therefore the tactile and vestibular systems are conceptualized as unifying sensory systems. These systems are believed to provide the sensory input that forms the basic relationship of the individual to gravity and the environment. Ayres believed that vestibular input may prime the nervous system for adaptive function. If the vestibular system is not functioning efficiently, interpretation of other sensations may be distorted.

To support the theoretical postulates that sensory integration underlies behavioral and emotional adaptation, Ayres cited studies by Harlow.[16,17] Harlow's findings indicated that tactile stimulation provides a foundation for emotional attachment to a mother figure. In his studies Harlow discovered that monkeys who were raised with terry cloth surrogate mothers that could be touched, clung to, and hugged showed better adjustment than monkeys who were raised with surrogate mothers made of wire. Contact with the wire mothers did not provide supportive tactile experiences.

Vestibular stimulation and adequate integration of vestibular stimuli are also considered critical to emotional adjustment. Ayres pointed out that all living things must relate to the earth's gravitational pull. Ayres[3] described gravity as "the most constant universal force in our lives" (p. 40). Children are viewed as being endowed with a strong drive to master the force of gravity, which culminates in the assumption of an upright posture and accounts for the appeal of activities that challenge gravity, such as skiing or riding a roller coaster. Efficient integration and modulation of vestibular stimuli are considered by Ayres to be essential for mastery over the earth's gravitational pull. When gravity is experienced as a threat, and a reluctance to move results, children may demonstrate personality disorders associated with the fear of movement. Ayres hypothesized that these children have irregularities in the modulation of vestibular input.

NEURAL STRUCTURES AND RELATIONSHIPS

In her theoretical presentations, Ayres emphasized only those neural structures that are thought to play a major role in sensory integration. These structures include the spinal cord, the reticular formation, the thalamus, and the vestibular nuclei of the brain stem, the cerebellum, and the cerebral hemispheres.

The spinal cord contains many tracts that carry sensations to the brain, and it relays motor messages from the brain to the cranial and peripheral nerves. While some sensory integration is believed to occur within the spinal cord, Ayres proposed that most of the processing is at higher levels of the nervous system.

Ayres postulated that the structures of the brain stem have the greatest role in sensory integration. The reticular formation is composed of neurons that have the capacity to receive multisensory input (convergent neurons). This structure therefore plays a major role in the integration of stimuli from several senses and from the two body sides and in the regulation of attentional mechanisms. The thalamus and the vestibular nuclei of the brain stem are other structures that contribute greatly to sensory integration processes.

The cerebellum is another structure believed to play a crucial role in sensory integration. Ayres described it as a processor of all types of sensations, particularly those related to the force of gravity and to movement. Finally, the cerebral hemispheres, particularly the cortices, are depicted as the regions that integrate and form associations between all types of sensation. The unique integration that occurs in the cortical association areas is the comparison of present sensory messages to stored past experiences.

The interrelationships among these structures are illustrated when a child feels and observes a puzzle piece. Touch sensations are detected in receptors of the peripheral nerves of the hand, while visual sensations are received in the retinas of the eyes. Via the spinal cord and cranial nerves, these sensations eventually reach the brain stem where attention, localization, and organization begin. In the cerebral cortex details are processed, and the new visual and tactile sensations are associated with past experience. The cumulative effect of neural processing at the various levels leads to a meaningful motor response that is directed by the cerebral cortex and modulated through the cerebellum. This process results in the child's accurate placement of the puzzle piece into the form board.

This example illustrates an important principle of sensory integration theory: higher cortical processes are dependent on adequate organization of sensation in the brain stem. Another principle related to the adequacy of cortical functions is called *lateralization.* In sensory integration theory this is defined as the tendency of specific processes to be handled more efficiently by one side of the brain than the other. The establishment of hemispheric lateralization is viewed as dependent on effective sensory integration, especially of stimuli from the two body sides, at the brain stem level. Ayres posited that when the whole body and all of the sensory systems are working in concert and when sensations are efficiently organized at respective levels of the nervous system, adaptation, learning, and emotional satisfaction are natural outcomes.

THE DEVELOPMENT OF SENSORY INTEGRATION

Ayres' writings[3,4] supply a detailed account of how the child's nervous system develops capacities for sensory integration. The immature nervous systems of newborns have few interconnections between neurons, and they lack appreciable myelination in the cerebral cortices. Consequently, infant behavior is generally stereotypic and regulated by lower neural centers that lack the restraining and modulating influences of the higher brain structures. As the infant interacts with the world, neural interconnections are formed through the increased branching of dendrites (arborization). Sensory stimulation of appropriate kinds and amounts is deemed critical to the development of interconnections at the neural synapses and to the infant's capacity to perceive and adapt to the environment. In the central nervous system the neural flow can be inhibited or facilitated via the interactions of neurotransmitters at the synaptic connections. The result is modulation of sensory reception so that the child can selectively attend to relevant stimuli. Feedback provides the child with continual information about the results of actions and influences ongoing sensory integration. Gradually organization of vestibular sensations helps the infant adapt to the earth's gravitational pull through the

achievement of an upright posture. At about 2 years of age the child learns to climb and, through integration of tactile and proprioceptive sensations, she forms a sensory picture of how body parts are related. Sensory integration of visual and somatosensory stimuli is enhanced as the child gains mastery over tool use during the third through seventh years.

In Ayres' theory the status of sensory integration in a child is viewed as a product of genetic endowment and environmental experiences. Within the normal population individual differences will exist in the ability to organize sensation for use. Ayres[3,4] identified the following four principles of brain development that relate to the achievement of each child's maximal potential for sensory integration:

1. *The brain innately seeks out those sensations that will be organizing.* Children are designed to receive pleasure from activities that help to organize their brains. In sensory integration theory it is proposed that neural organization will be optimally promoted if children are encouraged to express this inner drive. The child's choices of play activities are believed to be motivated by this inner drive to seek organizing sensations. Play activities are therefore regarded as critical to brain development.

2. *The brain must interpret sensory stimuli before it can respond adaptively to those stimuli.* This principle implies that presentation of meaningful amounts and kinds of sensory stimulation will further the developing child's capacity to adapt to environmental demands. For example, rocking a newborn baby will promote better neural processing as long as the frequency and duration of rocking are appropriate to the baby's organizational capacities. This principle proposes that infants and children should be afforded opportunities to receive stimuli from movement, sight, sound, and touch.

3. *Ontogenetic brain development of the individual is enhanced by many of the same factors that promoted phylogenetic brain development across the species through evolution.* Evolutionary theory suggests that brain development of species occurred in response to environmental demands. The neural processing will be enhanced if growing children are provided with opportunities to successfully adapt to environmental challenges.

4. *As the brain evolved, higher and newer structures like the cerebral cortex remained dependent on adequate functioning of older structures.* The newer structures can process more complex information, but they do so with the benefit of sensory integration that occurs at lower levels of the nervous system. This principle suggests that it is appropriate to emphasize the importance of brain stem sensory integration as a foundation for efficient cortical function.

Principles of sensory integration theory that apply more directly to treatment are described in Chapter 23 and detailed in Ayres' writings.[3,4] It must be emphasized, however, that this theory is continually evolving and is modified in accordance with results of continual research conducted and published by Ayres and other investigators. Therefore serious study of sensory integration theory requires attention to relevant journal articles.

DISCUSSION

Sensory integration theory has transformed many aspects of pediatric occupational therapy. Although Ayres' thinking was broadly influenced by Piaget's description of the sensorimotor stage and by Rood and the Bobaths (Chapter 20) who addressed the relationship of sensory stimuli to motor responses, her sensory integration theory included many new ideas. A critical, differential concept of Ayres' theory is the shift of emphasis from the motor response to its foundations in neural processing. This focus has resulted in a new way of perceiving the sensory-motor dimension of child development.

SUMMARY

Each child who is seen in occupational therapy is in the midst of a dynamic process of growth, maturation, and adaptation. Therefore knowledge of the human development process is critical to the foundation of occupational therapy theory and practice. This chapter has reviewed basic principles of growth and development, as well as selected systems for classification of theories. Stage theories, which examine longitudinal aspects of development, and process theories, which look in detail at one facet of development, make up the most basic classification system.

The best accepted stage theories were developed through the work of Freud, Erikson, and Piaget. Each of these men formulated a series of recognizable stages that correspond to the usual development of one area of human function. Freud's work related to the biologically based psychosexual development of the child as the foundation of emotional and social behavior. Erikson followed much of Freud's thinking but placed greater emphasis on the role of the environment as the moderator of individual adaptation. Piaget concentrated on the cognitive development of the child and formulated a series of periods that are differentiated by the child's use of progressively more elaborate mental operations. He also emphasized the role of environmental experiences as determinants of cognitive and adaptive development.

Other stage theories that are particularly useful to occupational therapy practice include Kohlberg's stages of moral development, Maslow's hierarchy of human needs, Gesell's schedules of adaptive behavioral development, and Havighurst's model of developmental tasks for each major age of human life. Each of these models helps to expand concepts of Freud, Erikson, and Piaget, especially as they apply to age-related activities.

The work of Skinner and Rogers accounts for the most durable process theories. Skinner emphasized the role of the environment in shaping the behavior of the individual and the species. Rogers also recognized the role of the environment but emphasized the importance of a healthy self-concept as a foundation for successful adaptation.

Current trends in developmental theory tend to emphasize process. Scientists are examining the relationship between specialized brain hemisphere functions and human behavior. In addition, they are looking to sociobiology to help differentiate between those human capacities that are derived through the species and those that are environmentally shaped. Current research indicates that many of the social, adaptive, and emotional characteristics of children that were earlier thought to be environmentally shaped may have a greater foundation in inborn capacities. Finally, followers of Skinner's behavioral approach and other learning theorists have turned to information processing theory to examine the cognitive functions of the child.

Developmental theories are only useful to occupational therapists if they can be operationalized for practice. This chapter has presented reviews of the theoretical frameworks of Reilly, Llorens, Gilfoyle and Grady, and Ayres. Each of these occupational therapists integrated their studies of developmental theory to formulate an approach to occupational therapy practice in pediatrics. Reilly concentrated on play as the fundamental occupation of the developing child through which the skills that underlie adult competence are shaped. Llorens integrated the developmental theories to propose a model of occupational therapy practice that is related to horizontal and longitudinal aspects of development in the child's life. Gilfoyle and Grady examined the spiralling development of sensory and motor functions of the child as the foundation for purposeful human activity. Ayres studied the role of the brain and its sensory integrative processes that organize and direct observable behavior. No single framework for occupational therapy practice is all inclusive; each must be considered in relation to the others and applied according to the needs of individual children. A derived conceptual model of practice that integrates concepts of the developmental and occupational therapy theories found here is presented in Chapter 7.

STUDY QUESTIONS

Observe children in home, play, and school environments; record behaviors noted in a 20 minute period.
   What developmental concepts and theories are illustrated?
   What concepts and theories seem to be contradicted?
   How and why?

REFERENCES

1. Ainsworth MDS: Infant-mother attachment, Am Psychol 34:932, Oct 1979.
2. Als H, and Brazelton TB: A new model of assessing the behavioral

organization in pre-term and full-term infants: two case studies, J Am Acad Child Psychiatry 20:239, 1981.

3. Ayres AJ: Sensory integration and learning disorders, Los Angeles, 1972, Western Psychological Services.

4. Ayres AJ: Sensory integration and the child, Los Angeles, 1979, Western Psychological Services.

5. Barash D: The whispering within, New York, 1979, Harper & Row, Publishers, Inc.

6. Clark PN: Human development through occupation: theoretical frameworks for contemporary occupational therapy practice, part 1, Am J Occup Ther 33:505, 1979.

7. Erikson EH: Childhood and society, ed 2, New York, 1963, WW Norton & Co, Inc.

8. Flavell JH: Cognitive development, Englewood Cliffs, NJ, 1977, Prentice-Hall, Inc.

9. Forman GE, and Sigel LE: Cognitive development: a life-span view, Monterey, Calif, 1979, Brooks/Cole Publishing Co.

10. Freud S: An autobiographical study. Translated by Strachey J, New York, 1952, Norton Library.

11. Geschwind N: Specializations of the human brain. In Scientific American: the brain, San Francisco, 1979, WH Freeman & Co Publishers.

12. Gilfoyle EM, and Grady AP: Posture and movement. In Hopkins HL, and Smith HD: Willard and Spackman's occupational therapy, ed 5, Philadelphia, 1978, JB Lippincott Co.

13. Gilfoyle EM, Grady AP, and Moore JC: Children adapt, Thorofare, NJ, 1980, Slack, Inc.

14. Hall CS: A primer of Freudian psychology, New York, 1964, Mentor Books.

15. Hall CS, and Lindzey G: Theories of personality, ed 3, New York, 1978, John Wiley & Sons, Inc.

16. Harlow HF: The nature of love, Am Psychol 13:673, 1958.

17. Harlow HF: Love in infant monkeys, Sci Am 200:68, 1959.

18. Havighurst RJ: Developmental tasks and education, ed 3, New York, 1972, David McKay Co Inc.

19. Hetherington EM: Divorce: a child's perspective, Am Psychol 34:851, Oct 1979.

20. Kaluger G, and Kaluger MF: Human development: the span of life, ed 3, St Louis, 1984, The CV Mosby Co.

21. Knickerbocker BM: A holistic approach to the treatment of learning disorders, Thorofare, NJ, 1980, Slack, Inc.

22. Knoblock H, and Pasamanick D, editors: Gesell and Amatruda's developmental diagnosis, ed 3, New York, 1975, Harper & Row, Publishers, Inc.

23. Kohlberg L: Stage and sequence: the cognitive developmental approach to socialization. In Groslin D: Handbook of socialization theory and research, Chicago, 1969, Rand McNally & Co.

24. Llorens LA: 1969 Eleanor Clark Slagle Lecture: facilitating growth and development: the promise of occupational therapy, Am J Occup Ther 24:1, 1970.

25. Llorens LA: The effects of stress on growth and development, Am J Occup Ther 28:82, 1974.

26. Llorens LA: Application of developmental theory for health and rehabilitation, Rockville, Md, 1976, American Occupational Therapy Association, Inc.

27. Llorens LA: On the meaning of activity in occupational therapy, Journal of the New Zealand Association of Occupational Therapy 32:3, 1981.

28. Llorens LA: Activity analysis: agreement among factors in a sensory processing model. Am J Occup Ther 40:103, 1986.

29. McDavid JW, and Garwood SG: Understanding children: promoting human growth, Lexington, Mass, 1978, DC Health & Co.

30. Maier HW: Three theories of child development: the contributions of Erik H Erikson, Jean Piaget, and Robert R Sears, and their applications, rev ed, New York, 1969, Harper & Row, Publishers, Inc.

31. Nye RD: Three psychologies: perspectives from Freud, Skinner, and Rogers, ed 2, Monterey, Calif, 1981, Brooks/Cole Publishing Co.

32. Piaget J: Psychology and epistomology: towards a theory of knowledge. Translated by Rosin A, New York, 1971, The Viking Press.

33. Piaget J, and Inhelder B: The psychology of the child. Translated by Weaver H, New York, 1969, Basic Books, Inc, Publishers.

34. Reilly M: Play as exploratory learning: studies of curiosity behavior, Beverly Hills, Calif, 1974, Sage Publications, Inc.

35. Rogers CR: Freedom to learn, Columbus, Ohio, 1969, Merrill Publishing Co.

36. Skinner BF: Beyond freedom and dignity, New York, 1971, Bantam Books, Inc.

37. Skinner BF: About behaviorism, New York, 1974, Vintage Books.

38. Skinner BF: Walden two, ed 2, New York, 1976, Macmillan Publishing Co.

39. Smith JM: The concepts of sociobiology. In Stent GS, editor: Morality as a biological phenomenon, Berkeley, Calif, 1978, University of California Press.

40. Sprinthall RC, and Sprinthall NA: Educational psychology: a developmental approach, ed 3, Reading, Mass, 1981, Addison-Wesley Publishing Co, Inc.

41. Thomas A: Current trends in developmental theory, Am J Orthopsychiatry 51:580, 1981.

42. Wilson EO: Introduction: what is sociobiology? In Gregory M, Silvers A, and Sutch D, editors: Sociobiology and human nature, San Francisco, Calif, 1978, Jossey-Bass, Inc, Publishers.

RECOMMENDED JOURNALS

American Journal of Occupational Therapy
American Journal of Orthopsychiatry
American Psychologist
Annual Review of Psychology
Child Development
Developmental Medicine and Child Neurology
Developmental Review
Journal of Educational Psychology
Infant Development and Behavior
Merrill-Palmer Quarterly
Monographs of the Society for Research in Child Development
Occupational Therapy Journal of Research
Physical and Occupational Therapy in Pediatrics
Scientific American

4

The developmental process: prenatal to adolescence

SUSAN DENEGAN SHORTRIDGE

Development is a continuous process. It proceeds stage by stage in an orderly sequence, despite individual variations. Both biological and psychological development adhere to these rules. Llorens[45] emphasizes the importance of "master of particular skills, abilities, and relationships . . . for successful achievement of satisfactory relationships." According to DiLeo[15] development is:

> . . . a continuum. It advances upward and forward, not in a linear fashion, but more like a spiral, with its downward as well as upward cycle, yet always a bit more upward and a bit less downward, each stage representing a level of maturity whose features are qualitatively different yet derived from and dependent upon earlier stages (p. 3).

Childhood is indeed the magic time in the life span when development blossoms. From the moment of conception through the adolescent years the child passes through many facets of developmental growth. These facets include the physiological, sensorimotor, cognitive, and social-emotional domains.

Periods of growth show great variation; however, for the purpose of clarity, the division of growth periods and their approximate age ranges follow:

Growth period	Approximate age
Prenatal	From 0 to 280 days
Ovum	From 0 to 14 days
Embryo	From 14 days to 8 weeks
Fetus	From 8 weeks to birth
Birth	Average 280 days
Neonate	First 4 weeks after birth
Infancy	First year of life
Early childhood	From 1 to 6 years
Middle childhood	From 6 to 12 years
Adolescence	From 12 to 18 years

PRENATAL PERIOD

Preparation for childbirth begins both biologically and psychologically in the mother before the delivery date. The 280 days following the last menstrual cycle affords ample time to adjust to the developing child.

Biologically the mother's body has been making changes and adjustments in anticipation of the delivery. During the first trimester of pregnancy the adaptive reactions of the uterus greatly influence the developing fetus. Abdominal distention begins to occur because of hyperplasia of smooth muscle fibers, especially in the vicinity of the implantation sites. The preparation of the muscular layer of the uterus is extremely important, because it will open the cervix, help push the baby out, and form ligatures to cut off the blood supplying the lining of the uterus. This hypertrophy continues to keep pace with the growth of the fetus and is largely caused by the increased production of estrogen.

Psychologically pregnancy brings forth sensations that a woman has not known before. The "mystery of birth" becomes less of a fantasy when fatigue, nausea, tenderness of the breasts, or frequent urination occur to remind the woman of her changed state. As pregnancy advances the perception of fetal movement, or quickening, directs the woman's focus even more strongly toward her body and the birth of her child. Before the birth event three distinct phases of development occur in utero. These are the germinal stage, the embryonic stage, and the fetal stage.

The first prenatal stage, which is the period of the ovum, or the *germinal stage,* lasts approximately 2 weeks. This period is initiated from the moment of fertilization to implantation in the uterus. The major emphasis during this period is in the change from a fertilized egg to a complex structure that will consist of 800 billion cells at birth. The structural changes that occur during cell differentiation are seen in the change from a zygote to a blastocyst. The blastocyst is a free-floating sphere that remains in the uterus for approximately 2 days. During this time cells cluster to one side of the blastocyst to form the embryonic disk from which the fetus will develop. The remaining cells form distinct layers. The upper layer, called the *ectoderm,* will become the infant's epidermis and its derivatives, that is, the sensory organs, brain, and spinal cord. The lower layer, the *endoderm,* will later form the digestive system, as well as the liver, pancreas, and salivary glands, and the respiratory system. The *mesoderm,* or middle layer, differentiates into the dermis, muscles, skeleton, and excretory and circulatory systems. The outer cells of the blastocyst, called the *trophoblast,* give rise to the protective and nutritive membranes of the intrauterine environment: the placenta, umbilical cord, and amniotic sac. Once this cell mass is fully implanted in the uterus it is called an embryo.

The second stage of prenatal development, the *embryonic stage,* is swift and lasts from 2 to 8 weeks. Although of short duration, this prenatal period is characterized by rapid growth. The fourth week shows an embryo with a beating heart. Between the fourth and the eighth week the eyes, ears, nose, and mouth become more clearly recognizable, signifying cephalocaudal development. By the end of the first 8 weeks after conception, 95% of the body parts have appeared through the continued process of differentiation. At the end of this prenatal period the embryo is recognizable as a tiny human.

The third prenatal period, the *fetal stage,* lasts from the end of the second month until birth. The appearance of the first bone cells at 8 weeks signals the name change from embryo to fetus. This is the longest of the prenatal stages. At this developmental period almost all of the structures and systems found in the newborn have developed, and many are already functional. These structures are primitive and must be developed further before they can be considered completely functional. This is perhaps most clearly seen in the primitive movements of the fetus.

A light touch to the mouth area of an embryo will cause the entire body to convulse, but spontaneous movement does not occur until later (p. 27).[2]

These primitive movements continue to refine over the next 7 months. Milani-Comparetti and Giodoni[50] characterized the period from 7 months' gestation to birth in terms of fetal competencies for readiness to be born. These include *fetal locomotion,* which allows the fetus to move around the fetal chamber to find the correct presentation for physiological birth, and *fetal propulsion,* which is the active movement of the fetus involving an extension pattern of thrusting. To understand the tremendous growth and development that occur

during this fetal stage, each event should be assessed separately (Table 4-1).

Prenatal influences

The interaction of heredity and environment strongly influences the prenatal period (Table 4-1). An ideal environment for the fetus is one that includes an adequate supply of oxygen and nutrients via the functional placenta and umbilical cord, as well as freedom from disease organisms, toxic chemicals, abnormal genes or chromosomes, and maternal stress. Inherited abnormalities make up only a small proportion of birth defects.

About 20 percent of known birth defects can be traced primarily to hereditary factors. Genetic traits in one or both parents cause a disease or abnormal condition in the child. Another 20 percent or so of birth defects are due to something in the environment of the baby that affects it while it is developing inside the mother. (The remaining 60 percent are caused by the interaction of hereditary and environmental factors.)[7]

Pregnancy is influenced not only by alcohol, coffee, smoking, and stress of the mother, but also by numerous environmental influences outside the woman's control.

Because of rapid growth during the embryonic period, the unborn child is most vulnerable to environmental insults and disruptions. The effects of many of these prenatal influences depend on the relative stage of development, that is, the point in the developmental sequence when the change in the prenatal environment occurs. Sensitive periods are times during which a particular influence or stimulus from another part of the environment evokes a specific response.

CHILDBIRTH
Labor

At approximately 40 weeks the uterus begins to undergo rhythmical contractions that ultimately lead to the birth of the child. This sequence of events is referred to as labor or parturition.

Labor consists of three stages. The first stage, which entails the major portion of the duration of labor, is dilation of the cervix. The rhythmical contractions signaling pain begin to push the fetus downward while the muscle fibers surrounding the cervical opening are pulled upward by the upper segment of the uterus. The further stretching of the cervix may cause the amniotic sac to burst and release its flow of "waters." These muscular processes of the first stage of labor are involuntary. The maternal abdominal muscles should remain relaxed to allow the uterus to rise during contraction. This rise assists in positioning the fetal head toward the cervix, and it promotes normal dilation. Relaxation resulting from the absence of fear hastens relaxation of

Table 4-1 Prenatal development during the fetal stage

Stage	Physical development	Motor development
Third month	Length = 3 inches Weight = 1 ounce Eyelids fused Fingers and toes well formed Fingernails growing Sex differentiation*	Kicks, makes fist, turns head, but movement not recognizable by mother
Fourth month	Length = 6 inches Weight = 6 ounces Most rapid growth*	Sucking Pushing with limbs Quickening noted by mother
Fifth month	Length = 12 inches Weight = 1 pound	Sleeps and wakes
Sixth month	Length = 14 inches Weight = 2 pounds Red, wrinkled skin Eyes unfused Taste buds form	Grasp reflex present Slight, irregular breathing Hiccup
Seventh month	Viable* Growth slows	
Eighth and ninth months	Wrinkled skin fills out with fat Weight = ½ pound a week All intrauterine development completed*	Startle reflex present Responds to light and sound Motor action limited because of increasingly tight fit of uterus

Adapted from Annis LF: The child before birth, London, 1978, Cornell University Press.
*Most important characteristic of time period.

the muscle fibers surrounding the cervix and is one of the purposes of childbirth education classes.

Delivery of the infant through the cervical canal and vagina marks the second stage of labor. The physical act of "bearing down" complements the uterine contractions. It is during this stage of delivery that conscious control of breathing and relaxation can facilitate the natural birth process. The birth canal has a tremendous ability to stretch, and, since the bones of the fetus' skull have not yet fused together, the head serves as a pliable instrument for widening the cervix and the vagina. This second phase of labor begins with head-first passage of the fetus into the birth canal. The head-first birth presentation is seen in approximately 95% of the labors; the remaining 5% involve deviation from the cephalocaudal position and are termed malpresentations.[63]

The third stage of delivery consists of expelling the amniotic sac, the placenta, and membranes that are all referred to as the afterbirth.

INFANCY
Physiological development

The neonate comes into the world looking more like a wrinkled old person than a Gerber baby. Typically the physical appearance of the neonate is characterized by reddish skin covered by vernix caseosa. The vernix caseosa is an oily protection against infection that dries in a few days' time. The head appears larger than the body and is usually elongated and bumpy as a result of molding during birth. In addition, the flat, broad nose that is formed of cartilage is often temporarily pushed out of shape by the birth process. Acrocyanosis, caused by sluggish peripheral circulation and mottling in response to cold, may also be present. The neonate's eyelids are usually puffy, making the eyes appear small. The eyes, smoky blue for the first month or two, change gradually to their permanent color. Hair may be abundant or scanty. Often the permanent hair color is different from that at birth. The external breasts and genitals of both males and females may look enlarged. This appearance is temporary and is caused by female hormones that passed to the baby before birth.

The average weight of the neonate is 7 pounds 2 ounces. During the first few days of life most neonates lose 5% to 10% of their body weight because of passage of meconium and urine, as well as delays in feeding. This weight shift is usually regained by 10 days of age. The average length of the neonate is between 19 and 22 inches.

Following birth the full-term neonate must make profound adjustments to his new life. The once totally dependent neonate emerges into a new environment as a separate entity who must now be responsible for respiration, circulation of the blood, digestion, and temperature regulation.

The traditional cry at birth signals a message to the mother that the baby has arrived and is inspiring air for the first time. Breathing is irregular, rapid, and shallow, involving the abdomen more than the chest. During the first few days after birth the neonate experiences periods of coughing and sneezing. This serves to clear the mucus and amniotic fluid from his airways.

The onset of breathing also marks a significant change in the neonate's circulatory system. A change in the vascular resistance alters the blood flow that once passed via the placenta. Closure of a valve between the right and left atrium *(foramen ovale)* and a vessel that leads from the aorta to the pulmonary artery *(ductus arteriosus)* occurs within the first 10 days of life. In addition, the lungs continue to expand.

Before birth the placenta provided nourishment as well as oxygen for the fetus. After birth the neonate must obtain nourishment from the mother in an external environment. The initial move toward feeding behavior is complemented by hunger contractions, rooting, sucking, and swallowing mechanisms that are present at birth and stimulate physiological maturation.

The neonate's temperature regulation system also gradually changes. Within the uterus the infant's skin was maintained at a constant temperature. The neonate's subcutaneous fat layer is inadequate for insulation, and the large skin surface area contributes to heat loss. Swaddling and heat lamps are frequently used to maintain temperature.

Sensorimotor development

From the moment of birth the neonate shows specific behavioral stages. Wolff[80] was able to separate and identify six newborn behavioral stages: regular sleep, irregular sleep, drowsiness, alert inactivity, waking activity, and crying. These stages have distinct conditions and specific properties. The neonate's response to stimulation depends on this state and on the stimulus.

The neonate's motor responses contribute to his organization of the world and to his survival within its boundaries. The neonate's gross motor activity is developed from movement patterns that began in the intrauterine environment and from the maturation of reflex behavior that is primarily controlled from the spinal and brain stem level (Table 4-2).

The neonate is capable of more than reflex behavior. He demonstrates orientation, attention, and habituation to visual, auditory, and tactile stimuli.

Following the first month of life the neonate is identified as an infant. At this time of life, motor responses in head control, sitting, rolling, and locomotion continue to develop from simple to complex skills (Table 4-2). At 4 weeks the infant's head position is dominated by the tonic neck reflexes. Head lag is noted in the pull to sitting position; however, the infant is able

to lift his head long enough to turn it while he is on his stomach (prone position) to attain a more comfortable cheek-resting posture. By 16 weeks the infant is able to lift his head at a 45-degree angle to the supporting surface. Visual stimulation and an increased ability to deal with gravity allow the infant to attain a more erect head posture. The infant's progression continues so that he is able to support himself propped on his forearms, and, finally, he is able to support himself by extending his arms and resting on the palms of his hands. This developmental sequence of head control is assisted by the emerging righting reactions and the disappearance of the tonic labyrinthine and asymmetrical tonic neck reflexes. The Landau reflex allows the infant to extend his trunk and extremities as he attains pivot prone postures.

Following head control, the infant is able to roll. He first develops the ability to roll from his back (supine position) to his side, then from his stomach to his side, and then from his stomach to his back. The neonatal neck righting reflex allows the trunk to follow the head. By 7 months the infant is able to roll voluntarily from stomach to back, and back to stomach.

The neonate of 4 weeks of age sits with a rounded back and a head that is erect only momentarily. In the infant, however, more muscle extension exists, and the infant's ability to control her head and trunk result in a more upright sitting posture. The 7-month-old can sit with back support provided by a chair or pillow or with arms propped forward in a tripod posture. By 10 months the infant can sit erect and unsupported for several minutes and soon progresses from a sitting to prone posture. By 12 months the infant can sit, rotate, and pivot without losing her balance and attain a creeping position from sitting.

Parents' eager anticipation of their infant's first steps often causes them to regard the spontaneous stepping seen at birth as an advanced motor skill of their "unique offspring." These reflexive stepping movements are visible shortly after birth; however, the complex coordination necessary for walking does not occur until 9 to 15 months of age. Before walking the infant becomes mobile in many ways.

Creeping refers to four-point mobility with only the hands and knees on the floor. This reciprocal limb motion demonstrates integration of many of the primitive reflexes before engagement in the more complex voluntary process of ambulation. With creeping and crawling come increased trunk flexibility and rotation. The emergence of equilibrium and protective reactions assists the 10- to 12-month-old infant in creeping as fast as others can walk.

The ability to stand is influenced by the emergence of postural stability. When her weight bearing is secure, a 7-month-old girl bounces in delight of her new skill and practices the freedom of movement from flexion to extension. She begins to prepare for the upright posture by first attaining a kneel-standing posture, then

Table 4-2   Sequences in Motor Development

Gestation		Birth	1 month	2 months	3 months	4 months	5 months	6 months	7 months	8 months	9 months	10 months	12 months	18 months
28 weeks	35 weeks													

PRIMITIVE REACTIONS

Rooting
  Enables infant to find nipple; allows active contraction of neck muscles
Suck-swallow
  Enables attainment of nourishment
Moro
  Breaks up flexion posture to permit extension of trunk and extremities
Traction-grasp
  Allows reflexive momentary grasp
Crossed extension
  Used later with positive support to maintain balance on one leg; integration needed for reciprocal movements
Flexor withdrawal
  Serves as protective response to noxious stimuli
Plantar grasp
  Integration needed for standing
Neonatal neck and body righting
  Allows logrolling from supine to sidelying
Neonatal positive support
  Allows weightbearing in upright position
Proprioceptive placing (LE)
  Allows foot to be placed flat on surface; primitive form of ambulation
Proprioceptive placing (UE)
  Needed for supporting body weight on forearms and extended arms
Spontaneous stepping
  Precursor to mature walking
Tonic labyrinthine
  First manifestations of gravitational influences to head orientation
Asymmetric tonic neck (ATNR)
  Enhances supportive framework of voluntary motion
Symmetric tonic neck
  Promotes four point kneeling by breaking up extensor pattern
Palmar grasp
  Allows infant to reach out for toy with full palmar grasp

GROSS MOTOR DEVELOPMENT

	Stage 1	Stage 2	Stage 3	Stage 4	Stage 5	Stage 6
Head control	Supine - TNRs dominate; Prone - Rotates head to rest on cheek	TNRs integrate; head in midposition; Lifts head in midposition from prone on elbows	Infant lifts head in supine; Prone on hands, tries to pivot	Gets on hands and knees to creep		Completed
Sitting	Marked or complete head lag in pull-to-sit; Momentary head righting in sitting, rounded back	Slight head lag in pull-to-sit; Head erect, set forward in sitting; Lumbar curvature	Sits erect momentarily; Sits propped	Sits with good control, no support; Goes from sitting to prone	Sits erect, pivots in sitting position; Goes from sitting to creeping	Seats self in small chair
Rolling	Partially rolls supine to sidelying	Rolls prone to side	Rolls from supine to prone, prone to supine	Completed		
Locomotion			Sustains most of weight standing; Bounces actively	Creeps on hands and knees, pulls up to feet, stands and lowers while holding on, stands supported with hands held	Pulls to feet while holding railing, Cruises sideways, Walks with one hand held	Walks alone; Runs stiffly; Walks upstairs with one hand held; climbs into adult chair

HAND FUNCTION

	Stage 1	Stage 2	Stage 3	Stage 4	Stage 5	Stage 6
	Reflex, automatic hand grasp (See Palmar grasp); Ocular fixation, beginning eye-hand coordination; Reaching, scratching, but unable to secure object; Ulnar-palmar grasp	Palmar grasp	Radial-palmar grasp; Radial raking at a string	Radial-digital grasp; Crude release	Pincer grasp; By 15 months, builds tower of two 1-inch cubes	Builds tower of three to four 1-inch cubes

Adapted from: Barnes ML, and others: The neurophysiological basis for patient treatment, Morgantown, WVa, 1978, Stokesville Publishing Co. Gessell A, and Amatruda CS: Developmental Diagnosis, ed 2, New York, 1954, Harper & Brothers.

progressing to a half kneel, and finally to full standing. A 10-month-old boy practices rising and lowering postures by supporting himself on furniture. At this time the infant becomes interested in objects denied him. This interest stimulates an even stronger desire to stand when the objects are moved out of reach. The development of cruising at 12 months of age helps the infant coordinate his high center of gravity and short legs.

The infant's first efforts of unsupported forward movement are often seen in short, erratic steps, unnecessary lifting of the legs, and uncontrollable excitement. By 12 months most infants can walk with help. By 18 months they are able to move throughout their world with the help of a relatively immature balance system, a high protective guard of the upper extremities, and a wide-based gait. When hurried, the infant may regress to the initial creeping pattern. However, with maturational changes in the infant's body proportions and the development of strength and coordination, walking becomes the primary means of mobility. Walking brings forth new avenues of exploration and a sense of autonomy. The parent must now protect this moving, explorative infant more than previously.

The infant's hands provide a means to reach out to the world and discover it. As in all development, sequences of motor development do not occur independent of each other. The development of mobility and hand function occurs simultaneously, each progressing chronologically toward maturation (Table 4-2).

The grasping reflex is present at birth and allows the infant to have automatic contact with anything placed in his palm. The first 12 weeks involve contacting objects more with the eyes than with the hands. Infants look, stare, and grope at objects within their visual fields. By the fourth month infants develop more voluntary control over their activities. The first voluntary, physical, prehensile activity is swiping at objects. By 5 months reaching toward an object develops, although the grasping skill is limited to a precarious ulnar-palmar grasp in which the fifth and fourth fingers press the object against the palm. Infants can be observed alternating between looking at their hands and looking at the object (Figure 4-1). Palmar grasp follows as all four fingers hold the object against the palm. Subsequent sequences are: radial-palmar grasp, second and third fingers hold object against palm; radial-digital grasp, object is secured by thumb, index and middle fingers; and pincer grasp, object is secured by tips of thumb and index finger.

In conjunction with the development of sitting, the infant starts to coordinate all the preceding manipulatory skills for grasping activities. The infant still notes the visual and tactile components of manipulation in the visual and oral inspection of most objects.

The presence of associated movements results in voluntary movement in one limb accompanied by involuntary movement in the other until 5 to 6 years. Voluntary grasp precedes voluntary release, which

does not occur until 10 months, and this complements the development of the flexors before development of the extensors. For a detailed discussion of arm-hand function, see Chapter 13.

Cognitive development

The cognitive development of the infant, as described through Piaget's sensorimotor period, has already been discussed in detail in Chapter 3. The cognitive process in this period is first initiated through reflexive reactions to stimuli and later becomes more purposive as the infant accidentally discovers behaviors that affect the environment. The infant's attention is gradually directed away from his own body as he becomes aware of the results of his activity. This process proceeds to experimentation as the infant tries to produce new events. Through this change the infant's cognitive repertoire that develops includes schemata for the actions of his own body and the concept that objects in the environment are influenced by his body's actions. The infant does not yet understand the effects of other persons on objects.

Although most cognitive development is expressed through sensorimotor exploration, infants are also involved with the development of communication. Prelinguistic speech is a central theme and proceeds through distinct stages. Lennenberg[43] identified seven stages of prespeech that progress from undifferentiated crying to expressive jargon (Table 4-3).

Physiological maturation is central to the development of expressive speech. The pseudocry and cooing are made possible by changes in the infant's vocal equipment. The larynx, which contains the vocal cords, changes as the child grows, allowing the infant to produce a greater variety of sounds. Because the ability to produce different sounds is evidenced in crying, lack of crying ability in the infant may indicate brain damage.

Social-emotional development

The infant's emotional transition from the protective, neutral womb is dramatically changed at the moment of birth. The sense of basic trust or mistrust becomes a primary theme in the child's affective development. The primary concern of the infant is to maintain body functions of the cardiovascular, respiratory, and gastrointestinal systems. As the infant matures the focus then moves to increasing competence in interacting with the environment through his body functions. According to Erikson,[19] "the first demonstration of social trust in the baby is in the ease of his feeding, the depth of sleep, the relaxation of his bowels." Erikson also included the quality of maternal relationships:

. . . the amount of trust derived from earliest infantile experience does not seem to depend on absolute quantities of food or demonstration of love, but rather on the quality of the maternal relationship. Mothers create a sense of trust in

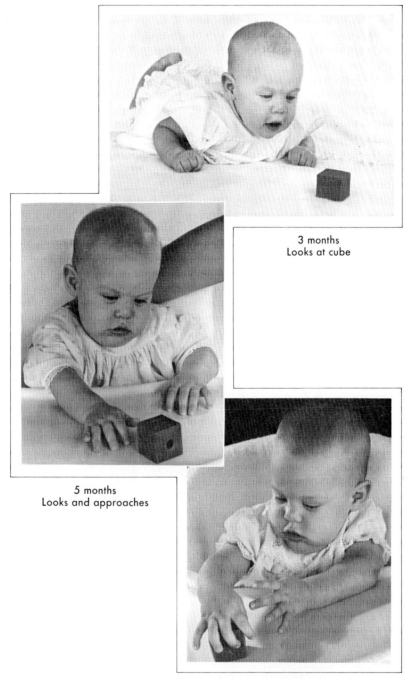

3 months
Looks at cube

5 months
Looks and approaches

6 months
Looks and crudely grasps with whole hand

Figure 4-1   Developmental progression of prehensile behavior.   *Continued.*

From Ingalls AJ, and Salerno MC: Maternal and child health nursing, ed 3, St Louis, 1983, The CV Mosby Co.

their children by that kind of administration which in its quality combines sensitive care of the baby's individual needs and a firm sense of personal trustworthiness within the trusted framework of their culture's life style (p. 249).[19]

The basic trust relationship is one that has varying degrees of involvement. Rubin and others[59] believed that feelings of maternal love are not endowed but acquired over time within experiences between two people. This is seen in the progression of contact between mother and infant—first from the mother's fingertips, then with her hands, and lastly with her whole arms as an extension of her body. Klaus and others[40] discussed

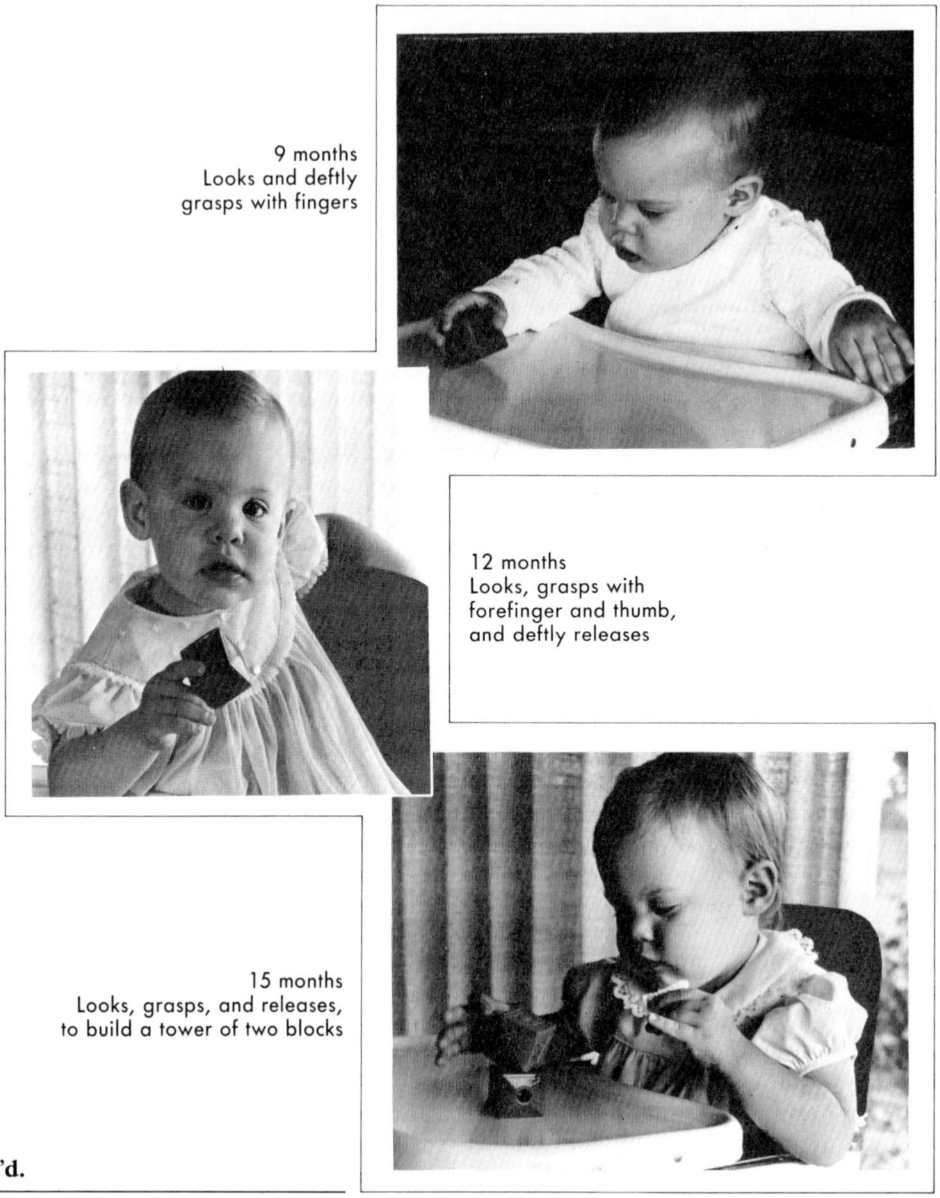

9 months
Looks and deftly
grasps with fingers

12 months
Looks, grasps with
forefinger and thumb,
and deftly releases

15 months
Looks, grasps, and releases,
to build a tower of two blocks

Figure 4-1, cont'd.

the importance of the en face position and stressed the importance of this early eye-to-eye contact between mother and infant in the attachment process.

The importance of the quality of maternal relationships was demonstrated earlier by Harlow and Zimmerman[31] in their studies of infant attachment relationships among rhesus monkeys. Their research demonstrated that it was not the mere provision of nutrients, but rather the close body contact that was essential to the attachment process.

Ainsworth[1] discussed the attachment process in terms of four stages of attachment. These include undiscriminating social responses (2 to 3 months), discriminating social responses (4 to 6 months), active initiative in seeking proximity and contact (7 months), and goal-corrected partnership or the ability to alter mother's plans to fit better the child's own. Precursors of attachment affect the first two stages of the development of attachment and include both reflexive and early sensorimotor behaviors such as rooting-sucking, looking, listening, smiling, vocalizing, crying, grasping, and clinging.

The role of the father must not be overlooked in the attachment process. Greenberg and Morris[29] identified strong evidence of paternal feelings and involvement with the neonate by new fathers. The father-neonate bond was characterized by engrossment, suggesting that fathers develop feelings of preoccupation, absorp-

Table 4-3 Stages of speech preceding the real word

Stage	Speech development
1	Undifferentiated crying: reflexive, produced by expiration of breath
2	Differentiated crying: varied patterns and intensities; pitches signal hunger, sleep, anger, or pain
3	Cooing: chance movement of vocal cords produces simple sounds; first sounds are vowels; first consonant is *h* (6 weeks)
4	Babbling: repetition of simple vowel and consonant sounds (3 to 4 months)
5	Lallation: accidental repetition of what has been heard (6 to 12 months)
6	Echolalia: conscious imitation of sounds (9 to 10 months)
7	Expressive jargon: meaningful utterances that sound like sentences with pauses, inflections, and rhythms (2 years)

Adapted from Lennenberg EH: Biological functions of language, New York, 1967, John Wiley & Sons, Inc.

Figure 4-2 Activities of daily living

Dressing
2 years: Puts on shoes, socks, and shorts. Takes off shoes and socks.
3 years: Dresses and undresses fully; needs help with buttons, back and front, left or right shoe.
4 years: Can manage buttons completely.
5 years: Can dress completely and often tie shoelaces, but cannot do tie.
Feeding
2 years: Has learned chewing and swallowing and can use a spoon well enough to feed self without accidentally inverting it.
3 years: Can feed self with little or no spilling. Can pour out from a jug into cup if not heavy. Feeding skills are now learned and become part and parcel of social skills in accordance with family standards of table manners.
Toilet training
2 years: By this age will tell mother he is "wet" and indicate that he wants to go "potty." Generally clean and almost dry by day.
2½ years: Dry at night if "lifted" late in the evening. (Variation is common, and boys tend to be later than girls.)

Adapted from Gesell A, and Amatruda CS: Developmental diagnosis, ed 2, New York, 1954, Harper & Brothers.

tion, and interest in their neonate within the first 3 days after birth.

EARLY CHILDHOOD
Physiological development

Preschoolers are much more mobile than infants. They have completed the transition from quadrupedal to bipedal motor skills. In addition, the preschool period is marked by its own special emergents: the development of autonomy, the beginning of expressive language, and sphincter control. The growth rate of the preschooler is less dramatic than that of the infant. The child at this age is still top heavy with a large cranium and small lower jaw, similar to the cupids in Renaissance paintings. The abdomen sticks out, since a relatively short trunk must accommodate the internal organs. The posture may appear lordotic.

Physiological differences from the mature adult are noted in the characteristic shape, position, and structure of the middle ear. The eustachian tube, which is shorter, more horizontal, and wider than that of the adult, allows free passage to invading organisms and thus increased susceptibility to ear infections in the younger child. The digestive tract also shows lack of full maturation. The shape of the stomach is straight and has less than half the capacity of the average adult stomach. This structural disparity results in frequent stomach upsets in the preschooler.

The special senses demonstrate noteworthy differences as well. The taste buds are more numerous and are located on the side of the cheeks and the throat as well as on the tongue. Because of the immaturity of the macula of the retina, the young child is farsighted.

Significant physiological changes occur in the physiological pathways necessary for sphincter control. Thus the preschooler is capable of entering and successfully completing toilet training. This is evidenced in the change from bulky diapers to training pants.

Sensorimotor development

Preschoolers are amazingly competent individuals. They initially walk with a wide stance and body sway because of their short stature; however, as they physically mature, the preschoolers' repertoire of motor activity steadily advances. The preschoolers' motor development is observed primarily in refinement. Coordination and the ability to voluntarily control movement increase significantly with each yearly advancement.

The 3-year-old who is able to stand on one foot eventually progresses into the 5-year-old who can skip on both feet. The child-directed activity is evidenced in small muscle coordination and activities of daily living (Figure 4-2).

Cognitive development

Symbolic representations of the preschooler, particularly in language, are the hallmarks of what Piaget termed the preoperational stage of cognitive development from 2 to 7 years.[55] The child is now able to represent people, objects, and places through the use of words as symbols. Symbols used by children have personal reference for them. The inability to comprehend a general language meaning used in the adult world is demonstrated in a lack of mutually agreed on verbal framework and emphasizes the preconceptual content of the preschooler's speech.

The child's egocentrism, or the belief that everyone perceives and interprets the world in exactly the same way, inhibits the development of such desirable behavior as acceptance of another person's point of view. Preschoolers relish their interactions with the environment through imaginative play; however, they are still not able to share or adhere to "fair play."

Children in the preoperational period still have difficulty distinguishing mental, physical, and social reality. They act as though they are the center of the universe. This is displayed in artificialism, animism, centration, and irreversibility.

This cognitive period is divided into two parts: (1) the preconceptual stage, ages 2 to 4 and (2) the intuitive stage, ages 5 to 7. The ability of the child to handle multiple characteristics marks the preconceptual stage. Children's reasoning skills are simple. Their experiences are not broad enough to allow them to understand the relationships between representatives of a class and the class itself. Between the ages of 4 and 7 years, children appear to cope intuitively with the physical world, but they continue to be dominated by egocentrism and illogical reasoning. They approach logical thinking but are constantly distracted by the surface appearance of things.

Psychosocial development

Erikson[19] defined the early psychosocial phase of early childhood as autonomy vs shame and doubt. Autonomy dominates the early part of the preschooler's psychosocial development from 2 to 4 years. The preschooler is adamant about making his or her own decisions. The development of trust in the environment and the improvement in language bring forth control over self and the corresponding strengthening of the preschooler's autonomous nature.

The discovery of the body and how to control it promotes independence in feeding, dressing, and toileting. The success in doing things for himself instills a sense of confidence and self-control in the preschooler.

The negative side of autonomy is a sense of shame or doubt. If the child fails continuously and is labeled messy, inadequate, or bad, shame and self-doubt are learned. Shaming may lead to "secret determination to try to get away with things, unseen."[19] In Erikson's words:

This stage, therefore, becomes decisive for the ratio of love and hate, cooperation and willfulness, freedom of self-expression and its suppression. From a sense of self control without loss of self esteem comes a lasting sense of good will and pride; from a sense of loss of control and of foreign over control comes a lasting propensity for doubt and shame (p. 254).[19]

Erikson described the latter part of the psychosocial period as initiative vs guilt. Children aged 4 or 5 explore beyond themselves. They seek new experiences for the pleasure of knowing, understanding, and getting projects started. The child's world entails real and imaginary people and things. If the child's seeking activities are successful, effective, and meet with parental approval, a sense of initiative is developed. This provides a foundation for learning to deal with people and things in a constructive way and provides a method for looking for new solutions, answers, and reasons. As parental voices are internalized via the superego, children may experience guilt. Severe criticism or punishment may teach children to feel guilty. Children need a balance between the initiative to carry out activities and the sense of responsibility for their own actions.

Peer play becomes an important avenue for the preschooler's social development. The preschooler is now able to combine motor, language, and cognitive abilities to become an active participant. Play is essential to the child's continued development in these areas. Although adult-child relationships represent different social interactions, early home experiences are said to influence later peer relations. Evidence supports the fact that children whose attachments to their mothers are rated as secure tend to be more responsive to other children in nursery school.[52]

Preschool play has a large sensorimotor component, although intellectual growth has progressed beyond this period. Exploration is an important facet of preschoolers' developing initiative; consequently, they are observed manipulating and sensing all aspects of their world of toys.

Play progresses from simple to complex interactions. To separate play from other activities, Garvey[24] proposed that any activity be defined as play if it (1) was engaged in simply for pleasure, (2) had no purpose other than the activity itself, (3) was something the player chose to do, (4) required the player to be "actively engaged" in it, and (5) was related to other areas of the player's life, that is, furthered the individual's cognitive and social development, enhanced creativity, or improved problem-solving abilities. Parten[54] observed the interactions of nursery school children who ranged in age from 2 to 5 years. *Solitary play* was identified in the younger child who tended to play alone, and social interaction was likely to consist of looking at someone else. *Parallel play* was engaged in by those children who were involved in similar activities but who displayed little direct communication. *Associative play* involved shared materials and conversational exchanges but not necessarily play toward a single goal. *Cooperative play* was identified as engagement in a single activity with a commonly accepted set of rules. Much of the past research generated in the area of preschool play has been confirmed in later literature. Recent studies indicate that middle-class preschoolers engage in more associative and cooperative play than lower-class preschoolers.[59]

The development of autonomy provides a foundation for the preschooler's imagination. Now the young child not only explores the world through his senses, but he uses thinking and reasoning to imagine future situations. Play includes fantasy and motor activities that are complemented by words, rhymes, or noises. The power of symbolic thought enables the child to go beyond the immediate perception of objects and react to them in a manner that can be wishful rather than real.

The preschooler's progression to games with rules requires a stronger component of social skills.[56] The child must now conform to established guidelines, and the rule now replaces the symbol. The game presents a real-life situation during which the preschooler tests his newfound social graces. Chapters 3 and 15 discuss play as an essential component of development for all children.

MIDDLE CHILDHOOD
Physiological development

With the continued development of initiative, the school-aged child is seen playing throughout neighborhoods and schoolyards. The middle, or school-age, years, as they are sometimes referred to, stress the relative tranquility between the turmoil of autonomous growth of the preschool years and the identity crisis of the adolescent years.[66] Striking physical differences are noted in growth patterns. Physical development is characterized by slow but steady advances in height and weight that will continue until puberty. The basic pattern of body build, which shows such great variation, also affects motor skills. Problems sometimes arise because the school-aged child wants to copy new things done by friends, but physical limitations prevent success.[8] A wide span of abilities is thus seen: the child may be one who is selected first for participation in sports, or he may be left sitting on the sidelines only to watch. The period of slow growth ends with the onset of the pubescent growth spurt. Although this is generally associated with adolescents, some school-aged children have already entered this phase of development. Growth increases at about age 9 in girls and age 11 in boys. These physical growth differences result in the disparity of height between the sexes. The older elementary school female child is larger than her male counterparts, whereas the younger female child does not show as much variation.

The facial features of the school-aged child have changed by becoming more distinct and individual. The successive losses of baby teeth and the appearance of permanent teeth distinguish the changing face to a greater degree. At almost any time children can display gaps in their smiles, a loose tooth, or a tooth just erupting. The 6-year-old is clearly identified by this toothless grin, while his 8-year-old counterpart is recognized by the front teeth that loom disproportionately large in his smile.

Organ systems show continued maturation, specifically in the development of keener vision. The digestive system shows added maturity with fewer upsets and longer food retention. Ears are less likely to become infected than they were during the preschool period. The growth of the lower part of the face changes the position of the eustachian tube by making it longer, narrower, and more slanted. It is now harder for disease organisms to invade, and troublesome ear infections are fewer.

Sensorimotor development

Gross motor development during the elementary school years continues to focus on refinement of previously acquired skills. With this refinement, hours of repetition of activity to attain mastery of common interests are seen. Motor capabilities are very diverse for this age group. The skills of the average 8- to 9-year-old include swinging a hammer well, sawing, using garden tools, sewing, knitting, drawing in good proportion, writing or printing accurately and neatly, cutting fingernails, riding bicycles, scaling fences, swimming, diving, roller skating, ice skating, jumping rope, and playing baseball, football, and jacks.[26,66]

Research indicates that children who master a physical skill tend to think better of themselves.[48] Not only does self-esteem improve, but children who have attained mastery of a skill enjoy greater acceptance by other children.[11,53]

It is not uncommon for a child this age to plead for the opportunity to become involved in an activity and then abandon it because of lack of skill or interest. School-aged children's high activity levels provide them with the opportunity to develop strength, coordination, agility, flexibility, and balance. Assessment of readiness is important for parents to consider during the child's quest for increased involvement because of the relative expense of participation and the need to enhance the child's sense of industry rather than inferiority.

Cognitive development

The cognitive period of concrete operations (7 to 11 years) gives the child an opportunity to grasp concepts and relationships in the physical world.[55] He understands space and time and can think in terms of future and past. The middle school child uses reasoning as a primary basis for conceptualizing the world. Older children are now able to weigh several pertinent factors at one time, but their thinking is limited in flexibility. They are still not able to see abstracts, but they deal with concrete objects. The period of concrete operations is highlighted by the addition of two mental operations: reversibility and decentration. Reversibility now enables the school-aged child to try out different courses of action mentally, rather than relying on sensorimotor aspects of the situation. In addition, this mental process results in quicker problem-solving capabilities. The child is also able to decenter or pay attention to more than one physical characteristic at a time. These add to the systematic, logical, concrete thinking of the school-aged child. This is seen most clearly in the child's recognition of constancy and his beginning understanding of conservation.

Social-emotional development

During the middle years the child is busy with basic school subjects, perfecting motor skills, and participating in activities with like-sex peer groups. The time of industry vs inferiority is highlighted by building new skills and refining old ones. Middle school children focus on meeting challenges in themselves as well as those presented by the environment. Industry, meaning to build, is evidenced in the child's exploration of the inner workings of things and not just physical appearance. According to Erikson,[19]

The inner stage seems set for "entrance into life," except that life must first be school life, whether school is field or jungle or classroom. . . He now learns to win recognition by producing things. . . He has experienced a sense of finality. There is no workable future within the womb of his family and thus becomes ready to apply himself to given skills and tasks. . . He develops a sense of industry—i.e., he adjusts himself to the inorganic laws of the tool world (p. 258).

Comparison with peers is increasingly important during this time. A negative evaluation of one's self compared to others or an inability to attain mastery of industrial achievements can result in a sense of inferiority.

The school-aged child is beginning the quest for independence of identity. School-aged children are less egocentric and able to view themselves more objectively. Children at this age have a definite subculture that includes magical rituals and gangs and is exclusively limited to children. This separate subculture is quick to criticize the different sizes and shapes of its members, and it is common for membership to entail a nickname related to these differences as a rite of passage.[66]

Rejection by the child's peers may result from lack of conformity in dressing or physical appearance. Data suggest that social skills are also important determi-

nants of peer acceptance. Children who rarely praised their peers, who had difficulty communicating, and who did not know how to initiate a new friendship were found to be unlikely candidates as friends.[28]

Middle school children may aspire to be teenagers, emulating teenage dress and current slang; however, questions of masculinity and femininity are prominent. Boys associate with boys, and girls associate with girls, each sex pursuing its own separate interests and identities with little communication in between.

Age becomes psychologically important to the middle school child. Both boys and girls tend to associate primarily with peers of the same age. It is not uncommon to add halves or "almost" to age description. The middle school child who is aged 7½ or almost 8 may also declare proudly following schools' end that he is in the next school sequence despite a summer's waiting period.[66]

During this age children begin to turn their backs on adults and unite to form a society of children. Values from peers become significantly more important than those of adults. One of the major functions of the peer group involves changing the child's attitudes. The peer group may strengthen existing attitudes, weaken those in conflict with peer group values, or establish new ones.[32] Data indicate that children between 7 and 10 years are highly compliant; they shift consistently in the direction of the peer consensus.[4] Children tend to be less compliant as they approach the adolescent age group.

This society of school-aged children dominates neighborhood streets and backyards with their refreshment stands, bicycle races, clubhouses, and endless explorations of woods, trash cans, and rain-swept streets. Large numbers of school-aged children are seen congregating in group activity, which includes such popular games as hide-and-seek, tag, hopscotch, swing the statue, red light—green light, blindman's bluff, dodgeball, and red rover. Many of the middle school child's games are accompanied by ritualistic chants. The words are often empty of any literal meaning; however, the sense of participation in group ways aids in this repetition.[66]

The child's progression from structured ritualistic games to participation in competitive games with a score is seen in his perception of rules. Piaget identified stages of moral development including rules.[56] Early in the child's thinking (age 4 to 7), rules are viewed as absolute, sacred, and untouchable. Later, children (aged 7 to 10) recognize that rules come from somewhere and they accept what these rule-maker authorities say. Finally, late in the elementary school years (age 10 to 11) children cast aside their belief in the absolute infallibility of rules because they have gained the knowledge that man is the creator of such rules. Children now no longer accept adult authority, rules, or society without questioning them.

ADOLESCENCE
Physiological development

Adolescents are surely identified by the unique circles with which they symbolically identify. However, no formal rite of passage exists for the adolescent in the United States. Various cultural expectations within our society complicate this adolescent time period. States differ in laws concerning when one can leave school, drive a car, or marry without parental consent.

There is great discussion regarding distinction between physical maturation and culturally defined roles. *Pubescence* refers to the period of time encompassing the physical changes that lead to puberty. These include the physiological growth of reproductive functions and maturation of primary sex organs resulting in secondary sex characteristics. Pubescence lasts an average of 2 years and ends in puberty. According to Ausubel[3] the normal sequence of development during pubescence is as follows:

Girls	Boys
Initial enlargement of breasts	Beginning growth of testes
Straight, pigmented pubic hair	Straight, pigmented pubic hair
Kinky, pigmented, pubic hair	Early voice change
Age of maximal growth	First ejaculation of semen
Menarche	Kinky pubic hair
Growth of axillary hair	Age of maximal growth
	Growth of axillary hair
	Marked voice changes
	Development of the beard

In the male these characteristics include the regular production of sperm by the testes, the development of the penis, growth of pubic and axillary hair, and marked voice changes. The deepening of the voice in the male is a result of the growth of the larynx in ventrodorsal diameter.[8] Female secondary sex characteristics become obvious in the emergence of breasts, a change in bodily proportions, as well as the onset of menstrual periods and the hormonal reactions that accompany them. *Puberty* is the resolution of all morphological and physiological changes in the growing boy or girl while the gonads mature. The adult state refers to sexual maturation and the ability to reproduce.

The adolescent growth spurt is perhaps the most outstanding physical change that occurs and signifies a time when the velocity of growth doubles. Even to those who live with the adolescent, the growth spurt appears to occur almost overnight. This phenomenon is partially a result of the fact that during the full year that surrounds the point at which peak height growth is measured children usually grow between 2.5 and 4.5 inches. The growth of 5 to 6 inches in a year is not rare. The average age onset of the adolescent growth spurt is approximately 14½ years for boys and 12½ for girls. Much of the growth occurs in the long bones of the legs and arms and is stimulated by the increased output of sex hormones (testosterone in the male and estrogen in the female).

Males and females react differently to their newfound height. Tall females may require reassurance to foster a positive body concept, while tall males are more likely to be pleased with this rapid addition of height. Shorter males are apt to need reassurance, since the timing of the adolescent growth spurt is controlled primarily by genetics.[8]

The process of sexual maturation brings forth many complex social and emotional problems. It is a period of relative sexual maturity in contrast to relative immaturity of social and mental development, and the result of these newfound hormonal changes is confusing. Personal appearance becomes a source of conflict. There is greater emphasis on the good looks of physical attractiveness and physique than at any other time. The culture's current definition of attractiveness serves as the established norm for bodily proportions and facial features. Adolescent girls tend to be more interested in and concerned about their physical appearance than boys. The adolescent may gaze continually in the mirror, comparing his or her own appearance to the ideal seen in magazines or on television. Marked deviations from idealized norms and cultural stereotypes of masculinity and femininity may adversely influence the adolescent's self-concept and treatment by others.[17] With experience and maturation, some changes in this overwhelming concern about appearance may be expected.

Cognitive development

The development of formal operational thought is a highlight of adolescence. Complex material can now be conceptualized without reliance on concrete schemata. The ability to imagine an infinite variety of options establishes the presence of hypothetical reasoning. The addition of reasoning permits mature understanding of such subjects as mathematics and philosophy. The adolescent's ability to think about his or her own thinking signifies complex mental operations. The mature teenager can now consider all possible relationships that might exist and evaluate these relationships one by one to eliminate the falsity and arrive at the truth. Additional discussion of adolescent cognitive development is found in Chapter 3.

Social-emotional development

Erikson[19] emphasized the role of identity is the adolescent's psychosocial development. During this period society begins to ask the youth to define his or her own role and career aspirations. Erikson believed that to solve one's identity crisis, one must be committed to a role, which in turn means showing commitment to an ideology. The adolescent must define a personal ideology and confirm beliefs, values, and ideals. This commitment, or fidelity, should coincide with prerequisites for the adolescent's desired occupation. The acting out of behaviors, experimentation with new roles, fantasy, self-doubts, and rebellion are seen as the adolescent attempts to establish a firm identity and role that will be most suited to him or her. If a youth fails to integrate a central identity or cannot resolve conflicts between roles and a value system, ego diffusion is the result.

Elaborating on Erikson's theory, Marcia and Freidman[47] evaluated adolescents' levels of crisis and commitment in relationship to occupational choice, religion, and political ideology. They described four identity statuses. These identity statuses were modes of dealing with the identity issue characteristic of adolescents. Those classified by these modes were defined in terms of the presence or absence of a decision-making period (crisis) and the extent of personal investment (commitment) in two areas: occupation and ideology.

Identity achievers are individuals who have shown a commitment to an occupation and to an ideology. They have experienced a decision-making period. *Foreclosures* are adolescents who have never experienced a crisis. They are committed to occupational and ideological positions but have adopted identities that have been parentally chosen with little or no question. *Identity diffusions* are young people who have no set occupational or ideological direction. They may or may not have experienced crisis, but their defining characteristic is their lack of concern regarding lack of commitment. *Moratoriums* are individuals who are currently in crisis. They have a vague commitment to an occupation or ideology but are in a state of search.

The establishment of ego identity, including occupational identity, is often complex and potentially confusing for the adolescent. Even at the age of 25, one young adult in four is still uncertain what vocation he or she should choose. Decisions concerning occupations interact with other choices in development so that when commitment to the occupational choice is firm, the individual has to some extent fitted himself or herself for it.

There exist a multitude of theories of vocational choice and development. Ginzberg[27] presents a developmental theory proposing movement through three primary psychological periods: a fantasy period, a tentative period, and a realistic period.

Super and others[69] present an extensive psychological theory of vocational choice and development. Super differentiates between the adolescent's self-concept and vocational self-concept. The adolescent must translate his self-concept into occupational terms to develop the vocational self-concept. He identifies five vocational behaviors; although ages are typical of the age range, these developmental tasks are not rigidly defined (see Chapter 16).

Tiedman and O'Hara[73] proposed a theory of vocational development by using Erikson's stages of general personality development as a basis. The emphasis of ego identity is closely intertwined with career development.

Since the central theme of adolescence focuses on identity, the adolescent is in conflict between the emerging responsibility of being an adult and the past classification of being a child. By relieving the pressure of adult society's expectations, the peer group serves as a support system for the young person who is trying to make this transition from childhood to adulthood. As adolescents are faced with this pressure, aggressive rebellion may result. This rebellion is often displayed in increased social contact outside of the home. A desire to escape from the demands of parents and community and to retreat to an environment where one's views are appreciated is seen in group attachment.[66] The heightened importance of the peer group increases the adolescent's desire to conform to the values, customs, and fads of the peer culture. This culture often proclaims its differences through symbolism in manners of dress, language, or food fads.

Although the rise of peer attachment introduces an important source of social control into the life of the young person, both peers and parents are important. Data suggest that, depending on the meaning and context of the social relationship, parents *or* peers may be more important. Sorenson found that 88% of the young people surveyed had considerable respect for their parents as individuals, while 48% desired more parental support of their own political and social opinions.[90] These differences in opinion tended to be on finer points of policy rather than on the overall issue. Lerner and Knapp[44] assessed the comparability of parents' and adolescents' attitudes toward societal issues. Their results indicate that although both groups were able to successfully assess the attitudes of each other, "there was a tendency for parents to minimize discrepancies between themselves and their children and a tendency for adolescents to magnify such discrepancies" (p. 35).

SUMMARY

An overview of growth and development, from conception through adolescence, clearly identifies that children are complex individuals. The overt characteristics of physiological, sensorimotor, cognitive, and social-emotional domains are variable for each child. All children, however, must mature through an identifiable developmental sequence to achieve their maximal potential.

STUDY QUESTIONS
1. What are the major developmental characteristics during the three prenatal periods?
2. Describe the sequence of sensorimotor development that

culminates in the infant's having the ability to use both hands to manipulate objects.

3. How does the process of early childhood development facilitate the pre-schooler's achievement and sense of autonomy?
4. Relate the social-emotional development of the adolescent to physical maturation.
5. What characteristics of adolescent development contribute to involvement in activities such as student government or basketball?

REFERENCES AND SELECTED READINGS

1. Ainsworth MDS: The development of infant-mother attachment. In Caldwell BM, editor: Review of child development, vol 3, Chicago, 1973, University of Chicago Press.
2. Annis LF: The child before birth, London, 1978, Cornell University Press.
3. Ausubel DP: Theory and problems of adolescent development, ed 2, New York, 1977, Grune & Stratton, Inc.
4. Berenda RW: The influence of the group on the judgments of children; an experimental investigation, New York, 1950, King's Crown Press.
5. Bevling CM, and Jacobson CB: Link between LSD and birth defects reported, JAMA 221:1447, 1970.
6. Bibba M, and others: Follow-up study of male and female offspring of DES-exposed mothers, Obstet Gynecol 49(1):1, 1977.
7. Birth defects, Pub No 59-93, White Plains, NY, The National Foundation—March of Dimes.
8. Brophy JE: Child development and socialization, Chicago, 1977, Science Research Associates, Inc.
9. Campbell S: Fetal growth. In Beard RW, and Nathanillsz PW, editors: Fetal physiology and medicine, London, 1976, Holt-Saunders, Ltd.
10. Carr DH: Chromosome studies in selected spontaneous abortions: conception after oral contraceptives, Can Med Assoc J 103:343, 1970.
11. Clarke HH, and Greene WH: Relationship between personal-social measures applied to 10-year-old boys, Res Q 34:288, 1963.
12. Coffey VP, and Jessop JW: Maternal influenza and congenital deformities: a prospective study, Lancet 2:935, 1959.
13. Corner GW: Congenital malformations—the problem and the task. In Morris F, editor: Congenital malformations, Papers and discussions presented at the first International Conference on Congenital Malformation, Philadelphia, 1961, JB Lippincott Co.
14. Davids A, and others: Anxiety, pregnancy and childbirth abnormalities, J Consult Clin Psychol 25:74, 1961.
15. DiLeo JH: Child development: analysis and synthesis, New York, 1977, Brunner/Mazel Inc.
16. Drillien CM, and Wilkerson EM: Emotional stress and mongoloid births, Dev Med Child Neurol 6:140, 1964.
17. Dwyer J, and Mayer J: Variations in physical appearance during adolescence. Part 2. Girls, Postgrad Med J 42:1967.
18. Ebbs JN, and others: Influence of prenatal diet on mother and child, J Nutr 22:515, 1941.
19. Erikson EH: Childhood and society, ed 2, New York, 1963, WW Norton & Co, Inc.
20. Erikson EH: Insight and responsibility, New York, 1964, WW Norton & Co, Inc.
21. Foster JA: Physical status and development of the neonate. In Tudor M, editor: Child development, New York, 1981, McGraw-Hill Book Co.
22. Frazier TM, and others: Cigarette smoking: a prospective study, Obstet Gynecol 81:988, 1961.
23. Fricker H, and Segal S: Narcotic addiction, pregnancy and the newborn, Am J Dis Child 132:360, 1978.
24. Garvey C: Some properties of social play, Merrill-Palmer Q. 20:163, 1977.
25. Gesell A, and Amatruda CS: Developmental diagnosis, ed 2, New York, 1954, Harper & Brothers.
26. Gesell A, and others: The child from five to ten, rev ed, New York, 1977, Harper & Row, Publishers Inc.
27. Ginzberg E: Toward a theory of occupational choice: a restatement, Voc Guide Q 20:169, 1972.
28. Gottman J, and others: Social interaction, social competence, and friendship in children, Child Dev 46:709, 1975.
29. Greenberg M, and Morris N: Engrossment: the newborn's impact upon the father, Am J Orthopsychiatry 44(4):520:1974.
30. Hanson JW, and others: Fetal alcohol syndrome: experience with 41 patients, JAMA 235:1458, 1976.
31. Harlow HF, and Zimmerman PR: Affectional responses in the infant monkey, Science 130:421, 1959.
32. Hartop WW: Peer interaction and social organization, In Mussen PH, editor: Carmichael's manual of child psychology, ed 3, vol 2, New York, 1970, John Wiley & Sons, Inc.
33. Herbst AL, and others: Adenocarcinoma of the vagina, N Engl J Med 284(16):878, 1971.
34. Horrocks JE, and Weinberg SA: Psychological needs and their development during adolescence, J Psychol 74:51, 1970.
35. Jacobsen C: Association between LSD in pregnancy and fetal defects. In Brazelton TB, editor: Effects of prenatal drugs on the behavior of the neonate, Am J Psychiatry 126(9):95, 1970.
36. Janerich DW, and others: Oral contraceptives and congenital limb-reduction defects, N Engl J Med 291:697, 1974.
37. Jones KL, and others: Pattern of malformation in offspring of chronic alcoholic mothers, Lancet 1:1267, 1973.
38. Kaminski M, and others: Rev. Epidemiol Sante Publique 24:27, 1976. (English translation by Little RE, and Schnizel A: Alc Clin Exp Rep 2:155, 1978.)
39. Karelitz S, and others: Infants' vocalizations and their significance. In Bowman P, and Manters H, editors: Mental retardation: proceedings of the international medical conferences, New York, 1960, Grune & Stratton, Inc.
40. Klaus MH, and others: Human maternal behavior at the first contact with her young, Pediatrics 46(2):187, 1970.
41. Kolodny RC, and others: Depression of plasma testosterone levels after chronic intensive marijuana use, N Engl J Med 290:872, 1974.
42. Landesman-Dwyer S, and Emanuel I: Smoking during pregnancy, Teratology 19:119, 1979.
43. Lennenberg EH: Biological functions of language, New York, 1967, John Wiley & Sons, Inc.
44. Lerner RM, and Knapp JR: Actual and perceived intrafamilial attitudes of late adolescents and their parents, J Youth Adolesc 4:17, 1974.
45. Llorens LA: Application of a developmental theory for health and rehabilitation, Rockville Md, 1978, American Occupational Therapy Association.
46. Marcia JE: Development and validation of ego-identity states, J Pers 1:118, 1967.
47. Marcia JE, and Freidman ML: Ego identity status in college women, J Pers 38(2):249, 1970.
48. McGowen RW, and others: Effects of a competitive endurance training program on self concept and peer approval, J Psychol 86:57, 1974.
49. Metcaff J: Association of fetal growth with maternal nutrition. In

Falkner F, and Tanner JM, editors: Human growth. Part 1. Principles of prenatal growth, New York, 1978, Plenum Publishing Corp.

50. Milani-Comparetti A: Pattern analysis of normal and abnormal development: the fetus, the newborn, and the child. In Seaton DS, editor: Development of movement in infancy, Chapel Hill, NC, 1981, Division of Physical Therapy, The University of North Carolina.

51. Montagu M, and Ashley F: Prenatal influences, Springfield, Ill, 1962, Charles C Thomas, Publisher.

52. Moore SB: Correlates of peer acceptance in nursery school children, Young Child 22:281, 1967.

53. Nelson DO: Leadership in sports, Res Q 37:268, 1966.

54. Parten MB: Social participation among preschool children, J Abnorm Psychol Soc Psychol 27:243, 1932.

55. Piaget J: The origins of intelligence in children. Translated by Cook M, New York, 1952, International Universities Press, Inc.

56. Piaget J: The moral judgment of the child, New York, 1955, Macmillan Publishing Co, Inc.

57. Rhodes AJ: Virus infections and congenital malformations. In Morris, F, editor: Congenital malformations, Papers and discussions presented at the first International Conference on Congenital Malformations, Philadelphia, 1961, JB Lippincott Co.

58. Rothman KJ, and Louik C: Oral contraceptives and birth defects, N Engl J Med 229(10):522, 1978.

59. Rubin KH, and others: Free play behaviors in middle and lower class preschoolers: Parten and Piaget revisited, Child Dev 47:414, 1976.

60. Rugh R, and Shettles LB: From conception to birth: the drama of life's beginnings, New York, 1971, Harper & Row, Publishers Inc.

61. Schonfeld WA: Primary and secondary sexual characteristics: study of their development in males from birth through maturity with biometric study of penis and testes, Am J Dis Child 65:535, 1943.

62. Schulman CA: Sleep patterns in newborn infants as a function of suspected neurological impairment of maternal heroin addiction, Unpublished paper presented to the meeting of the Society for Research in Child Development, Santa Maria, Calif 1969.

63. Seeds JW, and others: Malpresentations, Clin Obstet Gynecol 25(1):145, 1982.

64. Shelesynak MC: Decidualization: the decidua and the deciduoma, Perspect Biol Med 5:503, 1962.

65. Sherman A, and others: Cervical-vaginal adenosis after in utero exposure to synthetic estrogen, Obstet Gynecol 44(4):531, 1974.

66. Stone JL, and Church J: Childhood and adolescence. A psychology of the growing person, ed 3, New York, 1973, Random House, Inc.

67. Stott DH: Abnormal mothering as a cause of mental abnormality, J Child Psychol 3:79, 1962.

68. Strauss M, and others: Behavior of narcotics—addicted newborns, Child Dev 46:887, 1975.

69. Super DE, and others: Career development: self-concept theory, New York, 1963, College Entrance Examination Board.

70. Sutton-Smith B, and others: Development of sex differences in play choices during preadolescence, Child Dev 34:119, 1963.

71. Swann C: Rubella in pregnancy as an aetiological factor in congenital malformations, stillbirth, miscarriage and abortion, Br J Obstet Gynecol 56:341, 591, 1948.

72. Tanner JM: Physical growth. In Mussen PH, editor: Carmichael's manual of child psychology, ed 3, vol 1, New York, 1970, John Wiley & Sons, Inc.

73. Tiedman DV, and O'Hara RP: Career development: choice and adjustment, New York, 1963, College Entrance Examination Board.

74. Uchida IA, and others: Maternal radiation and chromosomal aberrations, Lancet 2:1045, 1968.

75. US Congress, Senate, Congress of the Judiciary, Subcommittee to investigate the administration of the Internal Security Act and the internal security laws of the Committee on the Judiciary; Marijuana-hashish epidemic and its impact on the United States security, Washington, DC, 1974, second session of the 93rd Congress (hearing).

76. US Food and Drug Administration: Caffeine and birth defects—tempest in a coffee pot? Pediatr Alert 5(19):73, 1980.

77. Versuhalmy J: Infants with low birth weight born before their mothers started to smoke cigarettes, Am J Obstet Gynecol 112:277, 1972.

78. Watson EH, and Lowrey GH: Growth and development of children, ed 5, Chicago, 1967, Year Book Medical Publishers, Inc.

79. Weathersbee PS: Heavy coffee intake, miscarriage linked, Muncie Evening Press, p. 19, Oct 1975.

80. Wolff P: The causes, controls and organization of behavior in the neonate Psychol Issues (Monogr. 17) 1:entire issue, 1966.

81. Yamazaki JN, and others: Outcome of pregnancy in women exposed to the atomic bomb in Nagasaki, Am J Dis Child 97:448, 1954.

5

General pediatric health care

MARY A. McILROY
KATALIN I. KORANYI

DELIVERY OF HEALTH CARE SERVICES
General aspects

Quality pediatric health care strives toward one primary objective: to enable each individual to pursue childhood and enter adulthood at his or her optimal state, physically, intellectually, and emotionally. Occupational therapists share this objective. In striving toward this goal, occupational therapists must collaborate with parents, physicians, and other resource personnel and therefore understand the various components of pediatric health care and their effective use.

Children receive pediatric health care in various settings, including private offices of pediatricians and family physicians, hospital or community clinics, health department stations, and hospital emergency rooms. Despite differences in locations, staffing, costs, and other amenities, each program offering pediatric care should share the common aim just stated.

Health care needs of children vary over time. The vast majority of the physician's effort in pediatrics is involved in the delivery of health promotion services and acute episodic care. Smaller amounts of time are given to rehabilitation, the coordination of home health care, and the establishment of educational programs. This chapter will present a description of each of these types of care and detail more thoroughly the most important aspects of preventive care and acute episodic care.

Health promotion

Prevention of illness, screening for disease, and monitoring health through well child checks are accepted goals of pediatrics and are essential in standard practice. Health promotion extends beyond prevention and maintenance and attempts to teach patients and families the importance of healthy life-styles.

Health promotion is a long-term process through which patients and families are assisted in accepting the responsibility for health care. It encourages them to take an active role in determining their own health, rather than relying on curative medicine in the future. The development of a mutually satisfying physician-patient-family relationship is important for the success of this process. A constructive relationship allows for better care during acute problems and crises, whether physical or psychosocial, and permits more effective counseling and teaching at routine visits (Figure 5-1). An effective relationship should also help patients and parents develop self-esteem and self-help skills to deal with routine daily problems. The desired result of such efforts in health promotion is to have patients and families establish lifetime goals and patterns that will be beneficial to good health and that will encourage appropriate use of health services.

Preventive and screening services, which are vital parts of pediatric health care and health promotion, will be discussed in detail later in this chapter. The aim of such services is the prevention of mortality and the minimization of morbidity from the many illnesses that afflict children. Early intervention is a necessary part of preventing mortality and morbidity and requires caregivers who are skilled in effective interviewing and the detection of problems. Routine checkups with thorough physical examinations may aid in the early identification of physical problems. Opening the lines of communication about behavior, development, school performance, sex education, and family relationships will assist in early diagnosis and treatment of many of the most common problems in childhood. Parents are often reluctant to begin the discussion about a child's behavior and, in fact, may not recognize a developing pattern of difficulty unless physicians use a developmental approach to health promotion. By using basic

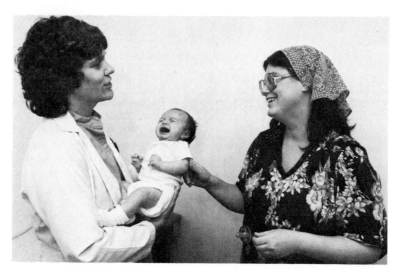

Figure 5-1 Effective and constructive physician-family relationships permit better care and counseling and help parents develop self-confidence in dealing with problems.

knowledge of the stages of development in childhood, the physician can question parents about the most common problems occurring in the child's age group. If the answers indicate that abnormalities exist, treatment programs can be instituted. Often the discussion indicates that the parents need education and understanding of the normal childhood stages, and this aspect of early intervention may prevent potential psychosocial morbidity.

Acute episodic care

Many visits to pediatric health caregivers are for diagnosis and treatment of acute problems, such as infections, minor trauma, or other physical complaints. Upper respiratory tract diseases, otitis media, and diarrheal illnesses account for a large proportion of these visits. In general, acute illnesses are most common between 6 months and 4 years of age. A small peak is often seen in the first 2 years of school, but otherwise the frequency decreases with increasing age. Data from the *National Health Survey,*[7] collected by household interview, indicate the children under age 6 have about 3.8 acute illnesses each year, while children aged 6 to 16 have 2.8 acute illnesses.

Many of the acute illnesses of childhood are mild and self-limited, yet they account for a large part of the demand for physician's time. Patients with acute illnesses seek care from private offices, community clinics, urgent care centers, and hospital clinics and emergency rooms. The use of scattered services interrupts continuity of care, but it frequently occurs. The education of children and families to deal with minor symptoms by themselves and to use health care services wisely may have great impact on the cost and delivery of health care.

Habilitation and rehabilitation

Children with handicaps have various needs that can best be met through comprehensive care programs. The physician often serves as a coordinator for the various agents of the child's program. More importantly, the physician should be an advocate for the handicapped patient so that the child and family can live more comfortably with long-term disabilities. Children with handicaps need a great variety of experiences that are appropriate for their ages. The physician assists the family in ensuring that the appropriate programs and opportunities for learning, social interaction, and physical habilitation are provided for the child. Encouraging the family to help the handicapped child lead a fulfilling life, where self-discipline rather than overindulgence prevails, is an important aspect of chronic care (Chapter 8).

The physician serves as a referral source for specialists and services available in the community, such as occupational and physical therapists, psychologists, relief caretakers, public health nurses, special schools, and special education classes. The physician also serves as an advisor for decisions about the child's education and residence plans, such as mainstreaming a child with special needs into a regular classroom or placing a previously institutionalized child into alternative living arrangements.

Unfortunately, some children with handicapping conditions do not have a primary care physician directing their overall care. These children may be seen by multiple subspecialists, each dealing effectively, but specifically, with isolated aspects of a child's problems. Despite many visits to these specialists, the patient's general health care, developmental needs, behavioral changes, and family relationships may be overlooked or ignored.

Many reasons exist to explain the lack of follow-up care by the primary physician. Some patients may not recognize the need for such services or may expect that the physician subspecialists or other health care personnel will tell them when to see the general physician. They may resent the involvement of so many subspecialists, who indeed may be superficial in their relationships with the family and may offer differing opinions about a concern. Patients may feel the primary care physician has relinquished caring for them by virtue of referrals to subspecialists who manage some aspects of the child's care. Financial constraints and transportation problems are among other stated reasons for lack of continuity with the primary physician.

The impact may be great in situations in which handicapped children are not cared for by a primary care physician. Even such important aspects of health promotion as immunizations and screening tests may be neglected because subspecialists don't perform or monitor such procedures. Developmental, behavioral and psychosocial issues may be poorly dealt with, if discussed at all. Parents are often unsure to whom they should direct their questioning. If they seek answers about behavioral or emotional issues from a subspecialist who is untrained in that area, their concerns may be ignored or minimized. The parents may view this lack of discussion or action by the subspecialist as an indication that the matter is insignificant and of no concern. Or they may feel they were foolish to mention the issue and then may be reluctant to raise other concerns later.

Occupational therapists can play a beneficial role for their patients by identifying children who are not receiving primary care and then assisting those families in finding a primary physician. If a previous relationship with a primary care provider was satisfactory for the family, then it may be sufficient to suggest the family seek input from that physician regarding general health issues. Because of temperament, interest or training, some physicians are better suited than others to provide ongoing care to handicapped children and their families. If a family's previous experience with a primary care physician was unsatisfactory, they can be encouraged to seek care from another primary physician who has been recognized by other community professionals and families for providing good care to handicapped children.

Home health care

Continuing health care in the home for a high-risk child, such as a low birth weight infant, a child who fails to thrive, or a child with multiple handicaps, may be provided by visiting public health nurses. They serve as a liaison between the family and the physician or medical facility.

In addition, homemaker services are available to help families who cannot provide adequate care to a child because of various problems such as maternal illness or insufficient knowledge in child care or homemaking.

Educational programs

Education of children and families constitutes a large part of the pediatrician's efforts. There is little research showing how this is most effectively accomplished. In providing routine care the pediatrician has an excellent opportunity to discuss various health problems, preventive care, anticipatory guidance, and child safety. In addition, teaching materials (videotapes, pamphlets) can be made available in patient waiting areas. Individuals responsible for the care of children can offer group discussion programs regarding health care through organizations such as schools, parents' groups, and churches. Occupational therapists may be called on to participate in this role in community education. Informing the general public regarding important health issues, such as immunizations, health hazards, and safety, can be done through the news media.

PREVENTIVE PEDIATRICS
General aspects

One important part of health promotion, as mentioned previously, is preventive care. Three aspects of preventive care can be identified. First is the prevention of specific childhood illnesses through immunizations. Second is the attempt to prevent disability from asymptomatic diseases by use of screening tests. Early detection of asymptomatic diseases, such as hypothyroidism and phenylketonuria, permits treatment before the disease impairs its victim. Screening of development is also essential because the prevention or minimization of developmental delays and dysfunctions is an important segment of general pediatric health care.

A third aspect of service in preventive care is the promotion of good health through the teaching of healthy life habits and counseling concerning proper diet, exercise, and accident prevention, among other things.

In addition, preventive care is provided in other ways. Physicians try to detect and treat symptomatic diseases as early as possible to prevent secondary complications or sequelae. Habilitative and rehabilitative services are sought to prevent physical and emotional dysfunction from chronic disabling diseases. Both of these aspects are discussed in other chapters of this book.

Well child care

Regularly scheduled health supervision visits for children are important for the assessment of general health, growth, and development. They permit effective administration of immunizations and allow for important screening tests to be performed. These practices will be discussed later in this chapter.

Routine visits also allow for anticipatory guidance in preparing parents for both the certainties and uncertainties of the future.[1,2] (For a more detailed discussion of this topic, see Suggested Readings: Cataldo; Green and Haggerty; and Behrman and Vaughan.) For example, when a baby is 2 to 3 months old parents should be informed that the ability to roll over will be developing in the following 2 or 3 months. This knowledge prepares the parent so that the infant is not left unguarded on a surface where he might roll off the edge and fall to the floor. Similarly, since most infants undergo a decrease in appetite at around 1 year of age, parents need to be aware of this change so that they avoid unnecessary conflicts concerning feeding. Uncertainties, for example, a child's reaction at times of stress or crisis, should also be discussed to aid the parent in being prepared to handle such situations.

At these visits the physician can assess the mental and emotional well-being of the patient and the family unit. Although this is not strictly preventive care, it does allow for, if necessary, the early intervention for problems such as behavior abnormalities, discipline difficulties, parental anxieties about normal variations, and toilet training.[1,2,6] These problems, although not causing physical illnesses, lead to psychosocial morbidity, which may have effects throughout an individual's life.[11]

Health care visits for preventive services must be sufficient in number and frequency to meet the individual needs of the child. Determining the optimal number of visits or procedures for all children or parents is impossible. But guidelines and recommendations have been published by the American Academy of Pediatrics[5] "for the care of well children who receive competent parenting, who have not manifested any important health problems and who are growing and developing satisfactorily."

Clearly, many circumstances or conditions may indicate a need for additional visits, and the physician will determine the need and pattern. More frequent visits are indicated for children with low birth weight or with congenital problems that cause no serious difficulties but result in parental anxiety. Also at risk and generally requiring increased professional contact are families with a previous child with an abnormality, those who have lost a child, adoptive or foster parents, and parents who are found to be in greater need of education and guidance, such as teenage mothers.

The current American Academy of Pediatrics' recommendations[5] reflect this emphasis on meeting individual needs. They suggest that each health supervision visit should include initial or interval history, measurements of growth, physical examination, sensory screening and developmental appraisal as indicated by age, immunizations and diagnostic tests according to age, discussion of findings, and counseling that concerns problems or anticipatory guidance.

The timing of health supervision visits in the first 2 years has previously been scheduled around the immunization needs of the child, rather than out of concern for the developmental needs of the child and parents. The need for immunizations at certain ages still holds true, but the intervals can be more flexible in an attempt to avoid rigid adherence to providing well child care at specific ages. This attitude also allows for completing a health supervision visit with a visit initiated by a minor acute problem whenever possible.

Six well child visits are recommended as a minimum in the first year, generally at 4 weeks, 2 months, 4 months, 6 months, 9 months, and 12 months. In the second year three health supervision appointments are encouraged at 15 months, 18 months, and 24 months. Each of these visits is important for documenting satisfactory growth and development, discussing dietary and feeding practices, and assessing parental needs for guidance or reassurance. Immunizations are also necessary at the 2-, 4-, 6-, 15-, 18-, and 24-month visits. The immunization schedule will be discussed later.

Beyond 2 years of age the need for routine health promotion visits is generally diminished, but it will vary according to the health of the particular child and the family conditions. Yearly visits are encouraged from 3 to 6 years of age (Figure 5-2). The American Academy of Pediatrics[5] recommends six routine visits in alternate years for school-aged children 8 to 18 years of age. For the older child and adolescent these visits serve a much different purpose. Very few abnormal conditions will be discovered in asymptomatic children in these groups. Although documentation of normality and the updating of immunizations is important, more pertinent topics for these visits include be-

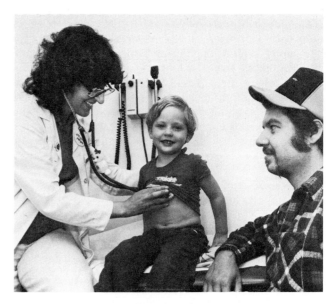

Figure 5-2 Routine visits for healthy children document normalcy and allow for discussions of parental concerns about behavior, development, peer relationships, and school performance.

havioral concerns, school performance, family and peer relationships, psychomotor development, and sexual development. With adolescents, counseling about drug and alcohol use and about sexual behavior is valuable. (For further reading on this subject, see Suggested Readings: Daniel; Felice and Friedman; and Mercer.)

Screening tests and procedures

Screening procedures are one of the major thrusts of health promotion and are a part of all the routine visits described previously. Various tests are performed at different visits according to age and will be discussed individually in this section. The purpose of the screening tests is to identify illnesses or abnormalities in specific functions that are more likely to respond to corrective treatment while being asymptomatic and that may be more difficult to correct after symptoms are evident or when secondary problems appear. Extremely important, then, to the success of screening for disease is the assurance that programs exist for the treatment of children with abnormalities identified through screening.

Some screening procedures detect diseases that are asymptomatic in early infancy but will lead to damage if left untreated. For example, infants with hypothyroidism appear normal at birth. Over the first few months, characteristic physical signs may occur, but they may be subtle. Mental retardation will occur unless treatment with thyroid replacement is instituted within the first 2 months. A screening test to detect hypothyroidism at birth is now in use in many areas and is valuable in preventing this avoidable retardation.

Developmental screening may help identify treatable diseases and is beneficial for recognizing delays so that appropriate counseling of parents and attempts at remediation can occur. Early therapeutic intervention for the primary developmental problem often leads to a more successful outcome. In addition, the occurrence of secondary developmental difficulties may be prevented by early recognition and treatment programs. Especially responsive to early attempts at correction are those developmental delays and dysfunctions that result from a patient's major health and environmental problems, such as burns, diabetes, or neglect.

The prevention of secondary problems is important. Aiding a child to develop appropriate adaptive maneuvers or mechanisms to compensate for a primary disability may prevent a later need for extensive rehabilitation.

Most physicians recommend some caution in the use and application of screening tests results. The importance of appropriate identificaton of a child at risk and the provision of needed services has already been stated. But evidence has shown that children who are labeled as having problems or as being at risk for developing problems have an increased chance of later dysfunction. This effect seems to be related to a child's change in self-image and his expectations as a result of being labeled abnormal.

Occupational therapists should be cognizant of such effects and should be extremely careful in discussing with parents and patients the results of developmental testing and their implications. Significant discrepancies must be communicated to the primary physician, and questions of etiological factors and prognosis should be referred back to the physician for discussion with the family.

MONITORING GROWTH

Growth parameters of height, weight, and head circumference aid in screening infants and children for problems that result in abnormal growth. Abnormalities can be either insufficient rate of growth or excessive rate of growth, and either variation may be seen in height, weight, and head circumference. In fact, knowing whether there is an abnormality in only one parameter or in two or all three measurements is important because that knowledge will often suggest different etiological explanations.

Measurements of weight and height (supine length in infants) should be recorded accurately at every visit to the physician or caregiver. Head circumference (Figure 5-3) is most valuable during the first 3 years when the rate of head growth is the greatest. It is generally not recorded beyond that age. Standard curves or growth charts are available and delineate the percentile ranking of any measurement according to age (Figure 5-4). The data obtained from the patient should be plotted on such a graph at each visit. This process provides a visual display of the data and quickly alerts the physician to abnormalities that otherwise might be overlooked.

Single measurements provide little valuable informa-

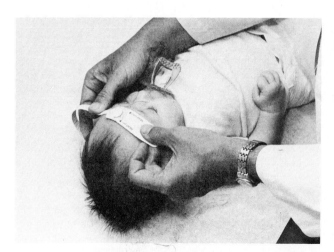

Figure 5-3 Occipitofrontal head circumference measures the largest diameter of an infant's head and is vital to detect insufficient or excessive head growth.

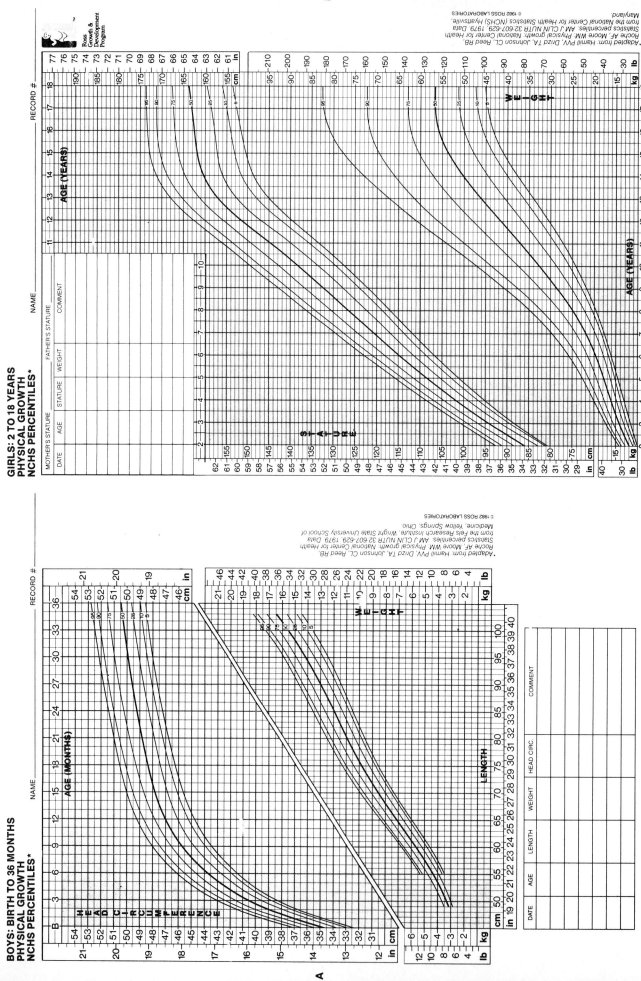

Figure 5-4 **A,** Standard growth curve for plotting lengths and weights of infant boys from birth to 36 months. **B,** Standard growth curve for plotting heights and weights of girls from age 2 to 18 years. *Adapted from Hamil, PVV, and others: Am J Clin Nutr 32:607, 1979.*

tion in most cases, unless they deviate markedly from normal or demonstrate a significant discrepancy between simultaneously obtained percentiles for height, weight, and head circumference. For example, if the baby's length and weight at a single examination are at the 50th percentile, but the head circumference is less than the 10th percentile, abnormalities of the skull or central nervous system should be suspected. The subsequent measurement and recording of growth parameters at each visit allow comparison over time, and a change of two or more percentile lines (for example, from 50th to 10th) signifies a need for explanation.

Among the most common abnormal settings is one in which an infant or toddler shows significantly less weight gain than expected while continuing to grow normally in length and head circumference. Generally this picture reflects a nutritional basis for the inadequate growth. The physician must then try to delineate whether there exists a problem in acquiring adequate intake, in losing excessive quantities of calories, or in using food delivered to the body. Insufficient intake may result from poor feeding practices, maternal ignorance or neglect, poverty, or birth defects, such as cleft palate, which may hinder the mechanics of feeding. Excessive loss of calories may be caused by recurrent vomiting or losses in stool from diarrhea or malabsorption. Improper utilization of food may be seen in metabolic disorders such as diabetes, glycogen storage diseases, or cystic fibrosis.

Other patterns of abnormalities should indicate different concerns. Lack of adequate growth in length or height may be seen in metabolic derangements such as renal disease, hypothyroidism, or hypopituitarism. Early excessive growth in height may signify precocious puberty. In severe central nervous system disorders with brain damage, growth curves will often show markedly low values in height, weight, and head circumference. An infant whose head growth is more rapid than expected will show a change toward higher percentiles or may have a head circumference greater than the 95th percentile for his age and would likely be evaluated for hydrocephalus.

Accurate and repeated measurements of height, weight, and head circumference are an exceptionally good screening tool for detection of many illnesses and problems. Routine use of these statistics may aid the physician in early detection of diseases, and it also provides other health personnel involved in a patient's care some objective data that may be reassuring with regard to the patient's general health or that may arouse concern, resulting in consultation with or referral back to the physician.

SENSORY EVALUATION

Sensory screening for vision and hearing is mandatory to detect major defects early, to enable development to progress as normally as possible, and to permit maximal rehabilitation before school age for those in whom normal development has been altered.

Children's eyes must be examined for screening purposes in early infancy, before beginning school, and at intervals during the school years. Examination of the infant's eyes should be done several times during the first 6 months. At birth this may consist of only a determination of light perception (blinking in avoidance when a bright light is presented) and visualization of a red reflex by funduscopy. By 3 or 4 months of age the infant should be able to follow a light 180 degrees and therefore demonstrate both visual perception of the light and conjugate movements of the eyes. The eyes should be assessed for alignment by checking to see if light reflects from the same location in both eyes when the patient looks at the light. Further screening procedures can also be done to detect intermittent changes in alignment. This testing is performed by interrupting a patient's conjugate gaze at an object by using a thumb or other block in front of one eye (Figure 5-5). The examiner observes for deviation of that eye away from the object of gaze. Such deviation is readily detected as the interrupted eye moves back into conjugate alignment when vision is no longer blocked.

Visual acuity and muscle alignment should be screened between 3 to 5 years of age and again at other visits during the school years. Acuity can be checked by using standard eye charts or small projection machines. Because this screening is simple and requires minimal equipment, schools and communities will often provide large screening programs. Children with abnormalities of acuity or alignment should be referred for appropriate and thorough evaluation by their physician.

Hearing and language are informally assessed at each visit as the physician interacts with the patient or observes patient-parent communications. The newborn

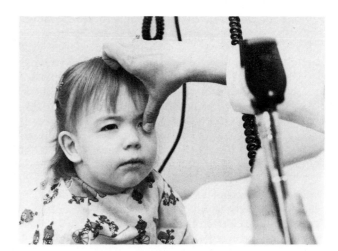

Figure 5-5 Screening for intermittent abnormalities in ocular alignment is performed by blocking the vision of one eye and then observing for correction of alignment to return the eye to conjugate gaze when vision is no longer blocked.

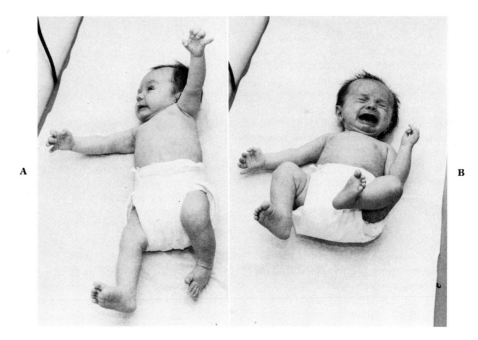

Figure 5-6   The Moro reflex is a normal neurological response in early infancy, often elicited by loud noises or a sudden change in position. **A,** The initial phase involves stiffened extension of arms and legs. **B,** The second phase is flexion and abduction of extremities and, often, crying.

or young infant should respond to a loud noise or clap with blinking of the eyes or a Moro response (Figure 5-6). Normal hearing is demonstrated in 6- to 9-month-olds by their attempts to locate a familiar sound. A bell or rattle can be used to produce sound, and older infants should turn their heads to locate it. The older infant should also be making babbling sounds. At 12 months hearing is indicated by the following of simple directions and the use of two or three meaningful words. Vocabulary continues to expand and the complexity of language increases so that by 3 years of age the child should be able to speak in simple sentences.

Screening of hearing should be done again before the beginning of school so that any loss that might impair classroom work can be dealt with before academic problems are created. Many communities and schools provide hearing screening programs to be certain this service is provided to all children, not just to those who seek professional health care.

Abnormalities in vision or hearing, if detected by occupational therapists in the course of patient evaluation or therapy, should most certainly be communicated to the referring physician to assure that adequate evaluation has been or will be done.

DEVELOPMENTAL ASSESSMENT

Developmental appraisal should occur at every contact between patient and caregiver and is an important aspect of each visit. Initially, simple observation of the infant's motor and social development suffices. As the infant develops, more motor and social skills become obvious, and language and cognitive abilities appear. These capabilities become progressively more complex with age, and the physician must not only observe but also interact with the patient to determine developmental level. Through informal assessment the physician should identify the infant or chid likely to benefit from more formal evaluation, whether performed in the office situation or in a referral system by occupational therapists or other trained personnel.

For screening purposes, the Denver Developmental Screening Test[4] is widely used. It allows establishment of a baseline for an infant's development and can be used repeatedly up to age 6 to help measure progress. It is a brief sampling of abilities and is limited in items tested at very early ages, but it can provide an estimation of a child's developmental course. Concerns noted by informal evaluation or deficiencies noted on the Denver Developmental Screening Test assessment should receive more extensive evaluation by personnel trained in standardized developmental appraisals. The occupational therapist often serves as a resource for evaluation and therapy of noted delays, and the therapist can assist in the establishment of home programs, occupational therapy sessions, or referrals to community programs. In this role the occupational therapist can support the physician-patient relationship and enhance the care given to the child and family.

METABOLIC SCREENING

Several specific screening tests are used routinely in pediatric health supervision. In many states neonates are screened by blood tests for the presence of metabolic diseases such as phenylketonuria, hypothyroidism, or galactosemia. The benefits of early detection of these diseases, which will be discussed in the next chapter, are obvious, since in many cases early treatment can prevent or minimize mental retardation or other pathological consequences of the disease.

HEMATOLOGY TESTING

Hemoglobin or hematocrit testing is a valuable screen for anemia and is usually performed in infants at 9 to 12 months of age. Nutritional anemia from iron deficiency is common at this age among disadvantaged populations. Treatment with iron preparations is fairly simple and will prevent the complications of anemia. Parents of anemic patients also need counseling about proper diet and nutrition for children. The American Academy of Pediatrics[5] suggests hemoglobin or hematocrit testing again at 2 to 4 years of age, during late childhood, and in adolescence. Sickle-cell testing should be done at 9 to 12 months in all black infants. Identification of sickle-cell disease or trait cannot change its presence. However, recognition of the existence of this inherited abnormality can result in effective education of patients and families so that early therapy is received when illness or complications occur and so that genetic counseling concerns are addressed. Also at 9 to 12 months of age, a lead level should be meaured if indicated, especially in infants living in older homes in inner city areas. The presence of lead overload should be diagnosed so that any necessary treatment is provided and recurrence is prevented.

TUBERCULOSIS SCREENING

Recommendations concerning the use of routine tuberculosis screening tests have changed. The risk of tuberculosis infection is extremely low for most children in the United States. For this reason, nonselective testing of children is not believed to be an efficient public health practice. The American Academy of Pediatrics Committee on Infectious Diseases considers acceptable[9] the following two options: no routine testing or testing three times—in infancy (12 to 15 months), preschool (4 to 6 years), and adolescence (14 to 16 years). For children at high risk of acquiring tuberculosis, annual tuberculosis skin testing is still recommended.

URINE TESTING

The benefit of routine urinalysis and urine culture in healthy children is controversial. During preschool and early school years urine cultures of asymptomatic girls may yield positive results in 1% to 2%. But it is unclear what relationship this finding has to the develop-

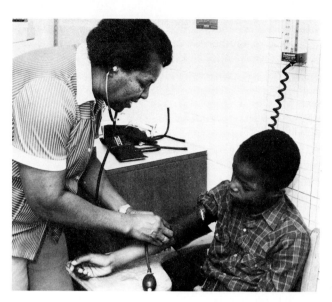

Figure 5-7 Blood pressure screening should be performed in all children over 3 years old.

ment of chronic renal disease and whether treatment of asymptomatic bacteriuria prevents such complications.

BLOOD PRESSURE SCREENING

Blood pressure screening is recommended[5,10] for all children 3 years of age and older (Figure 5-7). Previously most childhood hypertension was thought to be secondary to renal disease, metabolic abnormalities, or other pathological causes, and extensive evaluation was warranted. Essential or primary hypertension is becoming increasingly recognized in children, although debate still exists as to what blood pressure levels actually constitute hypertension and at what point treatment is indicated.[10] Prevention of the adult complications of hypertension (heart disease, stroke) seems to be a logical aim and might be aided by the detection of elevated blood pressure during childhood and by effective therapy, where appropriate.

Immunizations

Prevention of childhood illnesses and their morbidity and mortality is one of the proven benefits of pediatric health supervision. Death and disability from poliomyelitis and measles are almost unknown today. Tetanus occurs uncommonly, and deaths and brain damage from pertussis have decreased remarkably.

Immunizations against diphtheria, tetanus, pertussis, poliomyelitis, measles, mumps, rubella and haemophilus influenzae type b infections are given routinely during infancy and early childhood. Recommended schedules have been established to provide early and effective protection from these diseases. Table 5-1 dis-

Table 5-1 Recommended[9] immunizations and ages for their administration

Recommended age	Vaccines(s)
2 months	DTP*, OPV†
4 months	DTP, OPV
6 months	DTP
15 months	MMR‡
18 months	DTP, OPV
24 months	HBPV§
4-6 years	DTP, OPV
14-16 years	Td‖

Adapted from Report of the Committee on Infectious Diseases, Elk Grove Village, Ill, 1986, American Academy of Pediatrics.
*DTP, Diphtheria and tetanus toxoids with pertussis vaccine.
†OPV, Oral attenuated poliovirus vaccine.
‡MMR, Live measles, mumps, and rubella viruses in a combined vaccine.
§HBPV, Haemophilus b polysaccharide vaccine.
‖Td, Adult tetanus toxoid (full dose) and diphtheria toxoid (reduced dose) in combination.

plays the schedule as currently recommended.[9]

Known risks and side effects do occur from these immunizations, but the vast majority are very mild (fever, irritability, soreness at the site) and are to be expected. Severe reactions to pertussis vaccine are rare, and even rarer are documented cases of vaccine-related poliomyelitis. The details of these complications have been well described in other texts.[3,8,9] Despite these risks, it is a matter of major concern for the public and individual health and welfare that children receive the recommended immunizations.

Nutrition

Nutrition counseling has accrued added significance as people begin to realize that good health is a result of good health practices, not just good medical care. The converse is also true: bad health is not a result of poor medical care, but it may develop from unhealthy lifestyle practices.

Health promotion for children includes the encouragement of better feeding habits and sound nutrition. The trend toward breastfeeding is increasing and should be supported by individuals responsible for child health care. Nutritious and complex infant formulas are available when babies are not nursed, and they are recommended in preference to whole cow's milk or skim milk. Cow's milk products are a potential cause of microscopic blood loss from the gastrointestinal tract. Cow's milk has insufficient iron to meet an infant's needs, and it has higher sodium and renal solute content than human milk or commercial formulas.

Introduction of solid foods should be delayed until 6 to 7 months of age. Recent changes in prepared infant foods have markedly decreased the content of salt and sugar, both of which had been added for adult tastes. In addition, attention must be given to supplementation of the diet with vitamins, iron, or fluoride when conditions warrant.

The importance of nutrition extends far beyond the feeding of infants. As pediatric practice moves more into the role of health promotion, increased attention is being given to prevention of illnesses in adulthood. Heart disease, stroke, and cancer cause the majority of deaths in American adults. Many of the habits that contribute to adult morbidity from these problems begin in childhood.

The prevention of obesity in adulthood can probably be aided by the discouragement of obesity in childhood. Advice to parents is important to change the idea that a happy baby has to be a fat baby and to encourage proper nutrition (but not overnutrition) throughout childhood.

Sodium intake is felt to play a role in adult hypertension. It is unclear if control of sodium intake in infancy and childhood will contribute to decreasing the incidence of hypertension. While the answer to that question is being sought, prudent eating practices might include the avoidance of excessive salt.

Obesity and salt intake have been mentioned as contributors to heart disease. Lack of exercise also contributes, and continuing exercise programs should be encouraged by those who provide health care to children.

Smoking is associated with the development of lung cancer, and the use of alcohol and drugs contributes to the number of accidental deaths. The prevention of such problems through education of children and families has not been sufficiently researched to determine effectiveness, but such programs deserve a trial. The aim of health promotion in pediatrics is to keep an individual healthy throughout his or her entire life, not just during childhood.

ACUTE EPISODIC CARE
General considerations in outpatient care of sick children

Ambulatory care services provide for both emergency and nonemergency care of sick children. In recent years there has been a growth of ambulatory services for children. This increase has resulted from several factors, such as the rising cost of inpatient care and the recent advances in diagnostic and therapeutic procedures by which children can now be treated in an outpatient setting.

Acute care cannot be scheduled in advance, so health care facilities must be prepared for urgent calls. Ideally the same physician or group of physicians will provide acute and ongoing care for the child. If the child has been examined periodically at the same office or clinic, it is assumed that a complete personal and family history is available, thus the physician can concentrate on the acute visit. If the child is being seen for the first time by the physician, a brief history regarding factors that may influence the present illness (for example, allergies, chronic illness) must be obtained. A follow-up appointment for a complete history and examination can be arranged. For those children who usually receive only episodic or crisis care, it is important to provide preventive health care during the visit for the acute illness. If a child does not have an established source of continuing health care, it is important to emphasize and encourage the benefits of such service.

The emotional aspects of an illness also deserve consideration. Children seldom understand illness. They often view sickness as a punishment for bad behavior. The physician needs to keep in mind the various ages and levels of understanding of children and direct all explanations in a way that is meaningful to the patient. The child deserves simple but honest explanations regarding the illness, procedures, and expected degree of discomfort. Parents may worsen the situation because they often feel guilty, anxious, and tired, and they may ventilate their frustrations on the child or the health care personnel.

The hospitalized child

Many children are hospitalized at least once during childhood. Because of the emotional stress for the child and the family and the significant expense, hospital admissions should occur only when diagnostic and treatment procedures cannot be performed on an ambulatory basis.

If it is at all possible, the family should be prepared for the hospital admission so that potential problems can be addressed before they arise and anxieties can be diminished. When children are admitted to the hospital, they often feel that they are being punished; they feel abandoned by their parents and they are afraid. In many hospitals preadmission visits are arranged for the child and the parents to develop a sense of familiarity with the setting, the procedures, and the personnel. Showing one child a patient who is happily eating ice cream after a tonsillectomy could allay that child's fears regarding his own surgery. In addition to the hospital tours, materials such as coloring books, pamphlets, or videotapes can be made available to families.

A child should be allowed to express his fears, whether real or fantasized. Preparation at home and in the hospital by playing out fears (for example, giving a shot to the doll) and by role-playing games (for example, as doctor or nurse) may provide insight to the child's fantasies and help alleviate some of the fear. In case of an emergency admission many of the preparations cannot take place, and the event is often confusing and hectic. Nevertheless, the physician and the nurse should try to answer questions of the parents and the child.

Children should be admitted to a pediatric unit and, if possible, matched with children of similar ages. A realistic and fair statement as to the estimated length of the hospitalization is important. All personnel need to be aware that children are not little adults and that they have special needs. Before any kind of procedure the physician should talk with the patient and explain what will be done and why it is necessary. For children terms such as *mend a break, fix up,* or *make well* are preferred over more threatening and confusing medical terms. When it benefits the patient, a support person (parent, nurse, or occupational therapist) should be permitted to accompany the child for procedures, such as radiographs, venipuncture, and even minor surgical procedures.

Care should be taken that children do not witness very agitated or very sick patients; tubes, machines, and bandages can be frightening to them. In the event a child is exposed to a very ill or dying patient, he deserves a sensitive and careful explanation.

Parental attitudes help to allay a child's fears, so parents and hospital personnel need to cooperate and understand each other. The child may view the hospitalization as a rejection or lack of love by his parents. The parents and hospital personnel need to become aware of possible changes in the behavior of a child during or after hospitalization, such as regressive behavior, increased clinging, antagonism, or agressiveness. Parents should be encouraged to bring to the hospital some familiar object (for example, a favorite toy or blanket) that suggests a tie to the security of home. Frequent visits by parents should be encouraged.

Pediatric units should have age-appropriate playrooms or recreational areas for the children. School-aged children staying for an extended period of time (over 2 weeks) should continue their education through homework or hospital-based teachers. Whenever it is possible, hospitalized children should be allowed to get out of their rooms, go to other hospital areas, or receive passes to leave the hospital for a few hours.

Childhood morbidity

Morbidity is much more difficult to measure than mortality. Most childhood illnesses are minor traumatic injuries and acute infectious diseases that leave no sequelae. However, a portion of these problems will lead to chronic conditions or result in psychosocial difficulties.

The incidence of various illnesses has changed tremendously over the past decades. Diseases that were once prevalent, such as poliomyelitis, measles, tuberculosis, and diphtheria, have disappeared as the leading causes of mortality and morbidity. After the age of 1 year, accidents (in particular, motor vehicle accidents) are the leading cause of mortality in childhood. The second cause before 4 years of age is congenital malformations, while malignancies are the second cause of mortality from 4 to 18 years of age.

The *new morbidity* is a term frequently used now.

In pediatric health care this refers to the recently noted increase in care provided for behavior problems, school difficulties, and family social problems. This has occurred because the incidence of severe illness in childhood has decreased as a result of better technology, the prevention of many childhood diseases, and improved treatment of illness. Childhood health care personnel must keep pace with changing causes of morbidity and mortality, and their efforts must be directed toward prevention and treatment of these problems.

SUMMARY

Occupational therapists are called on to direct or participate in efforts to facilitate a child's development of age-appropriate abilities and to help that child respond to the environment with whatever adaptations are necessary. It is important, therefore, that significant health concerns be identified and properly addressed before treatment is initiated or whenever they appear during the course of therapy.

When appropriate pediatric health care services are effectively delivered, as described in this chapter, the child in need of occupational therapy should be readily identifiable. The careful monitoring of physical, mental, and psychosocial development through the use of routine health promotion visits and screening procedures will provide the physician with the necessary understanding of the child's primary developmental problem and level of abilities and aid recognition of other health problems. Such background information is of great importance for the occupational therapist designing treatment plans, along with determinations of whether the problems are temporary or permanent, what the expected outcomes and prognoses are, and what influence any health problems may have on both the child's development and therapy. Obvious, then, is the need for maintaining effective communications between occupational therapists and the primary physician to meet the changing needs of the child.

STUDY QUESTIONS

1. Identify three problems that may occur when a handicapped child is being cared for only by subspecialists. Describe how an occupational therapist might address with the family the need for ongoing health supervision with a primary care physician.
2. Identify the parameters of growth that should be monitored in children and discuss why these aspects should be carefully recorded and evaluated.
3. Describe how the parents and the health care professional can prepare a child emotionally for an elective hospital admission.
4. Name five illnesses that can be prevented by adequate childhood immunization.

REFERENCES

1. Chamberlin RW: Prevention of behavioral problems in young children, Pediatr Clin North Am 29:239, April 1982.
2. Christopherson ER: Incorporating behavioral pediatrics into primary care, Pediatr Clin North Am 29:261, April 1982.
3. Feigin RD, and Cherry JD: Textbook of pediatric infectious diseases, Philadelphia, 1981, WB Saunders Co.
4. Frankenburg WK, and Dodds JB: The Denver Developmental Screening Test, J Pediatr 71:181, 1967.
5. Guidelines for health supervision of children and youth, News and comment, May 1982, American Academy of Pediatrics.
6. Metz JR and others: A pediatric screening examination for psychosocial problems, Pediatrics 58:595, 1976.
7. National health survey, Series 10, No 141, Washington, DC, 1981, US Department of Health and Human Services.
8. Recommendation of the Immunization Practices Advisory Committee, Morb Mort Week Rep, Center for Disease Control 34(27): entire issue, 1985.
9. Report of the Committee on Infectious Diseases, ed 20, Elk Grove Village, Ill, 1986, American Academy of Pediatrics.
10. Report of the Second Task Force on Blood Pressure Control in Children — 1986, Pediatrics, 79:1, 1987.
11. Starfield B: Behavioral pediatrics and primary health care, Pediatr Clin North Am 29:377, April 1982.

SUGGESTED READINGS

Behrman RE, and Vaughan VC, editors: Nelson textbook of pediatrics, ed 12, Philadelphia 1983, WB Saunders Co.

Cataldo MF: The scientific basis for a behavioral approach to pediatrics, Pediatr Clin North Am 29:415, April 1982.

Daniel WA, Jr: Adolescents in health and disease, St Louis, 1977, The CV Mosby Co.

Feldman KW: Prevention of childhood accidents: recent progress, Pediatr Rev 2:75, Sept 1980.

Felice ME, and Friedman SB: Behavioral considerations in the health care of adolescents, Pediatr Clin North Am 29:399, April 1982.

Green M, and Haggerty RJ, editors: Ambulatory pediatrics III, Philadelphia, 1984, WB Saunders Co.

Hospital care of children and youth, Evanston, Ill 1978, American Academy of Pediatrics.

Mercer RT: Perspectives on adolescent health care, Philadelphia, 1979, JB Lippincott Co.

North AF, Jr, and others: Screening in child health care, Pediatrics 54:608, 1974.

Paulson JA: Patient education, Pediatr Clin North Am 28:627, Aug 1981.

Rudolph AM, editor: Pediatrics, ed 17, Norwalk, Conn, 1982, Appleton-Century-Crofts.

6

Diagnostic problems in pediatrics

KAREN E. SCHANZENBACHER

This chapter provides occupational therapists with specific information regarding diagnostic problems commonly encountered in their pediatric populations. An overview is provided for each problem, consisting of the etiology, symptoms, complications, diagnostic and treatment procedures, and the prognosis. Discussions related to prevention, new trends and issues, and implications for occupational therapy are also included. The information in this chapter serves as the basis for subsequent chapters that describe specific services occupational therapists provide for children with various diagnostic problems.

PRENATAL PROBLEMS

A normal, healthy baby is the wish of every prospective parent. While that wish is realized in the vast majority of pregnancies, a small percentage present risk factors that jeopardize the developing fetus. These pregnancies necessitate the use of specific diagnostic and intervention strategies that are designed to eliminate or minimize the effects of these factors. If prevention is not possible and birth defects are inevitable, the prospective parents are at least provided with a chance to begin to make the difficult decisions and adjustments surrounding that knowledge.

This section deals with complications surrounding the prenatal period of development. It discusses types of birth defects and their causes, the detection and monitoring of high-risk pregnancies, fetal diagnostic and intervention procedures, and the implications for occupational therapy.

BIRTH DEFECTS

Approximately 5% of all children have major birth defects and many others have minor variations of physical development.[50] These birth defects may be caused by genetic abnormalities, infections, unusual mechani-

cal forces, toxic agents, poor maternal health and nutrition, or a combination of these factors. The March of Dimes defines a birth defect as "an abnormality of structure, function, or body metabolism which often results in physical or mental handicap, shortens life, or is fatal."[22]

Chromosomal abnormalities

Humans normally have 23 pairs of chromosomes in each cell of the body. Smaller or larger numbers of chromosomes cause specific problems.

Excess chromosomal material is evidenced in the trisomy syndromes. The most common trisomy syndrome is trisomy 21, or Down syndrome, which is characterized by one additional chromosome 21. This syndrome, found in approximately 1 in 660 neonates, causes very specific mental and physical problems. While a wide range of physical characteristics may be associated with Down syndrome, a few are common to the majority of the children. Most of the children have a short and stocky stature with a protruding abdomen. Their heads are often small and flattened at the back, with upward slanting eyes that have abnormal epicanthal folds. Other common facial features include: low set ears, a flat nose, and often the mouth is held slightly open with the tip of the tongue protruding. Extremities are shorter than normal and fingers and toes are usually broad and short. The palms of the hands usually have a single crease known as the "simian" crease.

These children have delays in attaining specific motor milestones, weak muscle tone (hypotonia), gait difficulties, and fine and gross motor dexterity problems. They sometimes have difficulty performing unplanned motor movements (dyspraxia).[87]

Related health problems often include: cardiovascular abnormalities, obesity, increased respiratory and other infections due to immune system inefficiency, gastrointestinal problems, and an apparent increase in the risk of leukemia.[50,53] One problem that is potentially dangerous to the child is the atlanto-axial dislocation. This condition results in a tendency for dislocation to occur between the first and second cervical vertebrae. If this dislocation were severe enough it could do spinal cord damage. If this dislocation is found through x-rays, surgery may be performed and precautions given to the family about roughhouse play or participation in activities that put stress on this joint.

Trisomy 18 is seen much less often, affecting only 1 in 3,500 infants.[50] The additional chromosome 18 causes a number of malformations, including: a weak cry and small mouth, decreased skeletal tissue, fused toes (syndactyly), hand problems, and pelvic abnormalities. As many of these babies have feeding problems in addition to problems caused by the malformations, survival rate is only about 10%. Those babies who do survive are usually severely mentally retarded.

Babies born with trisomy 13 are very rare—only 1 in 15,000 births.[50] Characteristics include: poor brain development, cleft lip and palate, skin defects on the scalp, heel deformities, and often, extra fingers and toes that may be fused. The survival rate for these babies is less than 20% and those who do survive have many problems including severe mental retardation, seizures, and failure to thrive.[50]

A decrease in the number of chromosomes (45 or less) also causes problems. Many of the fetuses who have this type of genetic abnormality die early in gestation. One exception to this statement is children born with Turner's syndrome. This syndrome is found in approximately 1 in 5,000 females (only), and is caused by one missing sex chromosome. These babies may be born with webbing of the neck, congenital edema of the extremities, and may have cardiac problems. Small stature, obesity, and underdeveloped ovaries that cause infertility and absence of secondary sexual characteristics are symptoms that must be dealt with in the school-aged child and adolescent with Turner's syndrome. Most of these children do not have mental retardation, which certainly improves their functional prognoses.[50]

There are many other chromosomal abnormalities caused by a missing portion of an individual chromosome (deletion) or by a portion of a chromosome breaking off and reattaching to another chromosome (translocation). The incidence of these events is much more rare than any of the chromosomal problems discussed so far. Also, because the amount of chromosomal material that is missing or duplicated is so variable, the resulting conditions are expressed very differently. Problems common in these types of conditions are mental retardation, abnormal brain development, and facial abnormalities.

Genetic abnormalities

Genetic diseases are inherited abnormalities caused by abnormal genes that have had a negative effect on development. There are four different patterns of gene inheritance. The first, autosomal dominant inheritance, indicates that an abnormal gene is present on one of the non-sex chromosomes. Usually this gene has been directly passed from one of the parents to the child. On rare occasions the gene is not present in either the mother or father and it is then known as a new or "fresh" mutation. There is no carrier state; if the gene is present the baby will have the abnormal characteristics. An example of an autosomal dominant illness is von Recklinghausen's disease (neurofibromatosis), which results in multiple subcutaneous and connective tissue tumors and causes neurologic impairments.

The second pattern, autosomal recessive inheritance, indicates that an abnormal gene must be in a paired condition as it is less potent. This condition exists, as with the first pattern, on non-sex chromosomes. Commonly, both parents are carriers but have no symptoms of the illness. Examples of common autosomal recessive illnesses are cystic fibrosis, phenylketonuria, and diabetes. Many of the inherited diseases and illnesses have this pattern of inheritance and in many instances the carrier states can be detected using various diagnostic procedures.

A third inheritance pattern is x-linked inheritance. In this case the abnormal gene sits on the female sex chromosome, the x chromosome. Because this gene is recessive, in females the normal gene on the second sex chromosome prevents expression of the disease. However, males who inherit the abnormal gene on their mother's x chromosome will be affected. Duchenne type muscular dystrophy and hemophilia (factor VIII deficiency) are examples of diseases inherited through this pattern.

The last type of pattern is the polygenic or multifactorial inheritance. As the name implies, many genes are needed from both parents before the problem will occur in the child. Some congenital heart problems, cleft lip and palate, and meningomyelocele (neural tube defects) are examples of polygenic inheritance problems.

Toxic agents

Other birth defects are caused by adverse changes that take place within the fetal environment. Substances and factors that negatively affect the developing fetus are called *teratogens.* Drugs, radiation, chemicals, and industrial wastes are the most common teratogens known to affect fetal development. Table 6-1 lists some common teratogens and their possible effects on the developing fetus. It is important to remember that a number of factors determine whether a teratogen will affect the fetus. The dosage, the gestational stage of the infant, and the specific sensitivity of the developing organs at the time of exposure to the teratogen are all factors that contribute to the outcome.[136]

One of the most serious examples of a fetal syndrome caused by maternal exposure to a teratogen is fetal alcohol syndrome (FAS). FAS is a specific pattern

Table 6-1 Effects of common teratogens on developing fetus

Substance or factor	Effect on fetus
Drugs	
Alcohol	Intrauterine growth retardation; mental deficiency; stillbirth. Babies born to chronic alcoholics may have fetal alcohol syndrome or withdrawal symptoms.
Aspirin	In large amounts may be fatal or cause hemorrhagic manifestations.
Cortisone	Possible relation to cleft palate.
Caffeine	Increased incidence of miscarriage; limb and skeletal malformations.
Dilantin	Fetal hydantoin syndrome (growth and mental deficiency; abnormalities of the face; anomalies of the hands).
Heroin, codeine, morphine	Hyperirritability; shrill cry; vomiting and withdrawal symptoms; decreased alertness and responsiveness to visual and auditory stimuli. Can be fatal.
LSD	Spontaneous abortions; chromosomal changes; suspected anomalies.
Lead	Spontaneous abortion; intrauterine growth retardation; congenital anomalies; anemia. Can be fatal.
Tetracycline	Stains teeth, inhibits bone growth.
Thalidomide	Phocomelia; hearing loss; cardiac anomalies. Can be fatal.
Tobacco	Intrauterine growth retardation.
Tranquilizers	All may cause withdrawal symptoms during the neonatal period.
Hormones	
Diethylstilbestrol (DES)	Cancer of reproductive system in females (20 years later); reproductive anomalies in males.
Chemicals and industrial wastes	
Methylmercury	Congenital abnormalities; growth retardation. Can cause abortions.
Pesticides (some types)	Congenital anomalies
Social factors	
Maternal stress	Increased fetal anomalies; premature labor; mongoloid birth.
Poor nutrition	Prematurity; toxemia, anemia, intrauterine growth retardation; lower levels of intellectual performance.
Radiation	Congenital anomalies; growth retardation; chromosomal damage; mental deficiency; stillbirth.

Adapted from Klaus MH, and Farnaroff AA: Care of the high-risk neonate, Philadelphia, 1979, WB Saunders Co; and Schuster CS, and Ashburn SS: The process of human development: a holistic approach, Boston, 1980, Little, Brown & Co; and Shortridge SD, unpublished material.

of altered growth structure and function seen in babies of alcoholic women.[76] FAS is the third leading cause of birth defects and mental retardation and has been reported to occur in 1 in 600 to 1,000 live births in the United States.[52] It occurs in approximately 30% to 45% of infants born to chronic, heavy daily drinkers and in approximately 11% of babies born to mothers who drink moderately.

Alcohol, like other teratogens, causes a spectrum of defects that vary from severe physical and mental problems that are readily detectable at birth to more subtle learning problems that may not be detected until school age.[76] The principal features of FAS include: prenatal and postnatal growth deficiencies with weight and head circumference being most affected; typical craniofacial features including ptosis, a long philtrum, short palpebral fissures, maxillary hypoplasia, and a thin vermilion of the upper lip; musculoskeletal problems that include congenital dislocations, foot positional defects, cervical spinal abnormalities, specific joint alterations, flexion contractures at the elbows, and tapering of the terminal phalanges.[76,126] Many of these craniofacial and skeletal defects are secondary to the effect of the alcohol on brain development.[52,76]

Also a result of alcohol's effect on brain development is the impaired intellectual performance displayed by these children. This can range from learning disabilities to profound mental retardation with an average IQ of 63 reported.[76] Functionally, these children often have speech problems, otitis media causing hearing and auditory perceptual problems, poor attention spans, and fine motor dysfunction demonstrated by weak grasp and poor eye-hand coordination.[76,149]

Children with Alcohol Related Birth Defects (ARBD) usually have decreased intellectual capacities, disturbances in sleep and behavior patterns, lack of motor coordination, and any of the physical anomalies described under FAS.[52] The nature and extent of fetal injuries produced by alcohol depends on a number of factors including: the amount of alcohol consumed per day; the time during the pregnancy that the alcohol was taken; whether food was eaten near the time of alcohol consumption; whether other substance abuse occurred during the pregnancy; and the general health of the mother.[52]

The prognosis for FAS children varies with the extent and severity of the various malformations and growth deficiencies. Two other important factors to consider are the severity of the maternal alcoholism and the quality and stability of the home environment.[76]

Hypothetically, FAS could be completely preventable if the public were educated to the deleterious effects of alcohol on unborn babies and changed its behavior accordingly. It seems that the best that can be hoped for is a reduction in the number of babies born with FAS and ARBD. It is recommended that ingestion of alcohol during pregnancy be limited to an occasional small drink.

Maternal and paternal health

The general health and nutrition of the mother, and also the father in certain instances, can either enhance or limit the ability of the mother-to-be to conceive or maintain the pregnancy. For example, exposure of the father to certain chemicals, maternal underweight (under 120 pounds) or overweight (over 180), age of the parents, drug and substance abuse, and abnormalities of maternal or paternal genital tracts are but a few of the factors that might affect conception. In addition to these physical factors, a multitude of psychosocial and socioeconomic factors can affect conception.[50]

Once conception has taken place, the intact mental and physical well-being of the fetus is critically linked to the well-being of the mother. Chronic health problems or chronic diseases can also cause spontaneous abortions, fetal malformations, premature births, fetal growth problems, or can present other problems to the mother or the fetus. Diabetes, high blood pressure, severe anemia, transplacental or ascending infections, heart disease, cancer, toxemia, and various surgical procedures are examples of conditions that can present these kinds of problems.

Chronic stress is also believed to have the potential to cause birth defects, because it reduces the blood flow to the uterus, thus limiting the amount of nutrients and oxygen to the fetus. In addition, stress causes the release of hormones, such as cortisone, that in turn can have a teratogenic effect on the fetus.[148,151]

Maternal nutrition

Maternal nutrition is important before conception as well as throughout the pregnancy. Maternal malnutrition during periods of fetal growth may be very detrimental to the health of the baby. For example, a reduction in protein and caloric intake between 26 and 32 weeks of gestation can permanently reduce the number of brain cells.[137] Continued poor maternal diet is believed to result in low birth weight, neuromuscular disorders, and, later in life, learning disabilities.[22]

Maternal infections

The fetus may be infected by a variety of organisms. Some of the infections are passed from the mother to the fetus during pregnancy (transplacental infections) while others are present in the vagina and are passed to the baby at birth (ascending infections). These infections invade the fetus at a time when it has a very limited capacity to ward off disease and, in the case of transplacental infections, at a time when they can have a profound effect on growth and development or the formation of tissues and organs.[50]

The most common of these infections are often referred to as the STORCH infections. Each of these illnesses presents a different set of characteristics and each is caused by a specific virus or infection. Table 6-2 summarizes these five infections, classifies them by type of infection, and summarizes their effect on the fetus.

A serious illness, not included in the STORCH acronym, is gonorrhea. With gonorrhea, the baby is exposed to the bacteria at the time of birth (ascending infection). The bacteria that penetrates the anterior cell

Table 6-2 Intrauterine infections (STORCH)

Name	Cause	Type*	Effects
Syphilis	Parabacterial infection	A	Large liver and spleen; jaundice; anemia; rash; rhinorrhea
Toxoplasmosis	Parasitic infection	T	Deafness; blindness; mental retardation; seizures; pneumonia; large liver and spleen
Rubella	Virus	T	Meningitis; hearing loss; cataracts; cardiac problems; mental retardation; retinal defects
Cytomegalovirus	Virus	T	Hearing loss; in severe form problems are similar to rubella
Herpes	Virus	A	Localized form: lethargy, rash, respiratory distress, jaundice, enlarged liver and spleen. Generalized form: attacks CNS causing MR, seizures and other problems

*A - ascending
 T - transplacental

layer of the eye can result in a purulent infection. If untreated the eye infection can progress to meningitis or other systemic infections. To prevent this possibility, all states require administration of a solution containing silver nitrate, or a topical antibiotic, to neonates' eyes immediately after birth. As a result of this treatment, gonorrhea has been reduced greatly in neonates.

Identifying the high-risk pregnancy

Early identification of the high-risk pregnancy is of utmost importance to ensure the best results for the greatest number of mothers and infants.[96] This requires the establishment of a network of professionals, paraprofessionals, and lay people concerned with prenatal and postnatal care. Counselors, teachers, therapists, social workers, nurses, and others who come in contact with pregnant women should provide education and counseling geared toward the prevention of the high-risk pregnancy and toward the early referral of any pregnancies that may be at risk. Organizations and agencies concerned with public education should be identified and their activities encouraged. Finally, for those pregnancies that will require special diagnostic and intervention strategies, a highly trained and well-equipped obstetrical care team must be available.[96]

Several studies[65,72,103] have described assessment systems that help distinguish the high-risk patient from the low-risk patient. These systems provide uniform record-keeping of specific factors that have been identified as determinants of perinatal morbidity and mortality. These factors include maternal age, socioeconomic status, race, nutritional status, past medical and obstetrical histories, and current medical and pregnancy problems.[72] The assessments are designed to systematically gather data during the first pregnancy care visit, the third trimester, early in labor, later in labor, and during the postnatal period.[96] Once the high-risk pregnancy is identified, specific diagnostic and intervention strategies may be initiated.

Evaluation of the fetus

Various biochemical, hormonal, and physical approaches now allow many fetal complications to be diagnosed. The approaches discussed here are the ones most often encountered by occupational therapists in reviewing both research literature and the charts and records of their patients. Included are the following procedures: ultrasonography, amniocentesis, fetoscopy, and selected laboratory procedures.

Ultrasonography has replaced radiography as the preferred method of measuring fetal development, because it is believed to be a safer procedure.[154] With ultrasonography, short pulses of low-intensity, high-frequency ultrasound waves are transmitted through the woman's abdomen to the uterus and the fetus.[29] These signals are reflected back from tissue mass, cre-

ating a two-dimensional picture of the fetus, placenta, uterine wall, and amniotic fluid. Types of problems commonly diagnosed from this procedure include multiple pregnancy complications, fetal structural abnormalities, uterine and placental problems, and intrauterine growth problems.

Ultrasonography can also help determine the gestational age of the fetus, sex of the fetus, head shape and size, and bone development. Ultrasound has come under some criticism for its greatly expanded use with non-risk pregnancies. Concern is raised that the effects of exposing the unborn child to high frequency sound is still unknown.[119] The National Institutes of Health suggest that this technique be used if there is vaginal bleeding, ectopic pregnancy, suspected congenital problems, and to guide the needle during amniocentesis.[119]

A second procedure commonly used in fetal assessment is amniocentesis. In this procedure a needle is inserted through the abdominal and uterine walls and into the amniotic sac where approximately 1 ounce of amniotic fluid is withdrawn.[15] Analysis of the fluid and the discarded fetal cells contained in the fluid allows the detection of specific chromosomal abnormalities, inborn errors of metabolism, and fetal malformations (Figure 6-1).

For example, if a concentration of the compound alpha-fetoprotein (AFP) is found in the amniotic fluid, spina bifida may be present. Tay-Sachs disease, thalassemia, and Down syndrome may also be detected by evaluating the fetal cells. As the gender or sex of the fetus may also be determined by amniocentesis, parents concerned with the possibility that their baby may be born with a sex-linked disorder, such as muscular dystrophy or hemophilia, may be helped in their difficult decision-making process.

The risks associated with amniocentesis are consid-

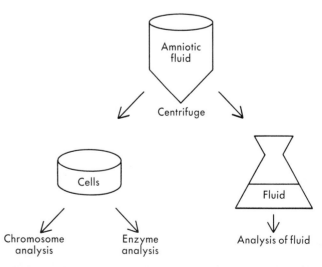

Figure 6-1 Analysis of amniotic fluid.

ered very small, although instances of miscarriages, infections in the mother, increased respiratory difficulties and pneumonia, and needle punctures of the fetus have been reported.[105] While it would seem that the benefits of the procedure far outweigh the risks, only a small percentage of at-risk mothers take advantage of the procedure.[15] Reasons for this phenomenon have been the high cost, fear of the procedure, fear of the associated risks, lack of knowledge that the procedure exists, and inaccessibility to the procedure.[15]

The National Institutes of Health recommend amniocentesis in the following situations: when the mother is 35 years of age or older; if there is a history of chromosomal abnormalities; if there is a reason to suggest a birth defect; or if the mother, or any ex-wife of the husband, has had a miscarriage.[119]

Fetoscopy is another diagnostic procedure that is being used to a greater extent. In this procedure a small tube is inserted through the mother's abdominal wall and into the amniotic fluid. A fiberoptic light source on the end of the tube, or fetoscope, allows the physician to detect congenital malformations. In addition, a syringe may be used to take placental blood samples that can be used to detect such blood diseases as sickle-cell anemia.[112]

A new technique, chorionic villus sampling (CVS), is growing in use. This diagnostic technique involves inserting a tube through the vagina and suctioning a sample of microscopic uterine cells that are destined to help form the placenta. Analysis of these cells can determine certain genetic abnormalities. As this procedure can be done 60 days earlier than amniocentesis and as the results come back from the laboratory in 2 to 4 days as opposed to 2 to 3 weeks, the benefits for counseling and decision making are great. Proponents of this procedure predict it will replace amniocentesis within 5 years if the incidence of spontaneous abortions following the procedure can be lowered.[119]

Many high-risk pregnancies require the continued monitoring of various biochemical and hormonal factors through the use of specific laboratory techniques. For example, during a diabetic pregnancy, blood glucose concentrations must be constantly monitored to ensure that they stay within acceptable ranges. Other laboratory tests may be used to determine fetal pulmonary maturity. This factor is important to the physician in determining the optimal time of delivery, because it is now known that the risk of intrauterine death often increases approaching term in the diabetic pregnancy.[137] These procedures are believed to have helped reduce perinatal mortality in the diabetic pregnancy.[104]

It is anticipated that in the next decade many of these techniques will be refined and many new procedures developed. As a result, even more conditions and risk factors will be diagnosed prenatally, thus making that wish for a healthy baby a reality for more prospective parents than ever before.

Treatment of the fetus

Although most of the techniques now being used in fetal treatment have been developed within the last decade, the risks, benefits, and long-term impact of these techniques on all aspects of development are still largely unknown. Some of the risks that have been identified include infections, premature rupture of membranes, premature labor, puncture of fetal organs and blood vessels, and damage to the fetus, risks that often do not become critical until later in the pregnancy.

One of the first successful intrauterine procedures was the blood transfusion. In this procedure blood is directly administered to the fetus in cases of severe anemia as a result of blood incompatibility. Another technique, now commonly used, is the infusion of various drugs directly into the amniotic fluid where the fetus later ingests the drug. This procedure has been used to correct vitamin deficiencies, thyroid malfunctions, and heart rate irregularities.[71]

A procedure that is still in the experimental stages is the draining of excess fluid from fetal structures into the amniotic fluid. For instance, the treatment of fetal hydrocephalus consists of inserting a prenatal brain shunt into the enlarged ventricle in the brain and draining the excess cerebral spinal fluid into the amniotic fluid. A similar procedure is used in cases of hydronephrosis, a condition that results in urine backing up into the abdomen because of a urinary blockage.

Perhaps the most sophisticated procedure attempted so far is extrauterine surgery. The uterus is opened, then the fetus is exposed for surgery and returned to the uterus for the remainder of the pregnancy. This procedure has been attempted only a few times to date and is still considered highly experimental.[71] While fetal surgery may eventually save hundreds of babies a year from lives of disability, in the near future many medical problems still must be solved.

Fetal treatment also presents many moral and ethical questions. For example, is the therapy warranted? Which fetuses should be treated? What is the optimal period of intervention? Should the multiply handicapped child be treated? Can an obstetrician be sued for not diagnosing a fetal problem? Is it the parent's decision to decide if a procedure can or cannot be used on their child? When and under what conditions are abortions to be performed? The answers to these and countless other questions will unfold as the state of the art and science of perinatology is refined and expanded and as its procedures and policies are scrutinized by society.

Implications for occupational therapy

The role of the occupational therapist in prenatal care is still emerging and therefore must be hypothesized to some extent. Obviously the occupational therapist will not be directly involved in the medical procedures themselves, but as the focus of intensive care nurseries expands to include prevention and parent education, the occupational therapist will have a great deal to offer.

In the area of prevention an occupational therapist might be involved with the community task force charged with establishing and monitoring the prenatal network that is so necessary for high-quality care for the mother and fetus. Also, an occupational therapist would be helpful in working with the handicapped population in attempts to reduce some of the high-risk factors associated with pregnancies among that population.

Another role of the occupational therapist could be to share information at prenatal classes for prospective parents. Topics that occupational therapists might be asked to present include early infant stimulation, selection of infant toys, prenatal sensory or motor development, and activities to foster bonding and attachment.

Finally, the occupational therapist may become involved with the prospective parents of a handicapped baby. Who better than an occupational therapist could answer questions about the possible effects of a particular disability on the child's development or on specific tasks of daily functioning? These and other roles will emerge as techniques advance and new needs are discovered in this exciting new arena of practice.

PERINATAL COMPLICATIONS

The period just before, during, and immediately after birth is known as the perinatal period. Many factors can affect the birth process and also that critical period immediately after birth when the neonate must make so many biophysical adjustments to extrauterine life.

This section discusses major problems found in the perinatal period, describes medical procedures used with neonates in distress, overviews some of the neonatal assessments, and discusses implications for occupational therapy.

Complications surrounding the birth process

Labor and delivery are a very critical time in the pregnancy. Some of the factors that negatively affect these processes are maternal in origin, while others are caused by infant complications.

Many of the maternal illnesses that were discussed as presenting high-risk factors during the prenatal period of the pregnancy may also lead to the development of problems at this time of the pregnancy. For example, the diabetic pregnancy not only presents the prenatal complications already discussed, but it also in-

volves complications in this period, such as toxemia, large babies, and babies who may be hypoglycemic after birth because of the excess insulin their bodies have produced.[83] Another example is the mother with a bacterial or viral infection, such as syphilis or gonorrhea, at the time of birth. While these diseases will no longer produce malformations, they may be transmitted to an immune-deficient neonate and cause serious and sometimes fatal results.[15]

A potentially dangerous maternal illness is toxemia, or preeclampsia. This syndrome consists of high blood pressure and edema in the lower extremities, and protein may be detected in the urine. If untreated, the mother may progress to eclampsia, which is often characterized by seizures, severe headaches, nausea, elevated pulse rate and temperature, and coma. Premature births, low birth weight babies, and even death have been attributed to these conditions.[70]

Other maternal complications may be related to placental problems or physical structural problems of the uterus or the pelvis. For example, placental problems can endanger the fetus by causing prematurity or by interfering with fetal blood circulation. Abruptio placentae is a condition in which the placenta prematurely separates from the uterine wall. In placenta previa the placenta lies over the cervical opening, and when labor begins, the cervix dilates and the placenta tears. Physical problems include uterine fibroid tumors that may hinder fetal growth, problems with premature dilation of the cervix, or a pelvis too small to allow passage of the fetal head.

The two most common infant factors affecting labor and delivery are birth defects and multiple pregnancies. Malformations of critical body organs are present in some birth defects. These may cause serious medical problems, some of which are incompatible with survival. Other birth defects may cause problems because of their unique characteristics. For example, babies born with hydrocephalus, or spina bifida myelomeningocele, or osteogenesis imperfecta may each have unique problems during the birth process.

Multiple births also have the potential to pose complications during this process. These complications include premature births, prolapsed cord, toxemia in the mother, and difficult deliveries as a result of unusual positioning of one or more of the fetuses.[15,136]

Medical management during labor and delivery

Many of these maternal and infant factors affect the oxygen supply to the fetus. Because there is a direct correlation between fetal oxygen level and fetal heart rate, heart rate is carefully monitored throughout the labor and delivery process. For instance, the normal range of fetal heart beats is 120 to 160 per minute. If this drops to below 100 beats per minute, it could indicate that the fetus is not getting enough oxygen and that immediate emergency medical care is required.[136]

Fetal heart rate may be monitored externally or internally. External monitoring is done by holding a stethoscope against the mother's abdomen and counting the number of beats per minute. Another method consists of attaching an electronic microphone to the mother's abdomen that continually monitors fetal heart rate and uterine contractions. Internal monitoring may be accomplished by inserting an electrode into the vagina and attaching it directly to the presenting part of the fetus.

The cesarean section may be performed as a lifesaving technique in many of the situations mentioned. This procedure consists of administering a general anesthetic to the mother and surgically removing the baby through an incision in the mother's abdomen. While the cesarean section must be performed to save the lives of babies, it does create some potential risks to both the mother and the baby. As the procedure is considered major surgery, the mother is subjected to potential hazards from the general anesthetic, the possibility of infection, and postoperative pain and discomfort. Babies delivered by cesarean section are more likely to develop respiratory distress, because they are born with fluid in their lungs. Normally, this fluid is expelled from the lungs during the first stages of labor.[136] They are also often more lethargic because of the effect of the anesthetic.[58]

Complications in the first weeks

In the first minutes and hours after birth, major changes should take place that allow the neonate to breathe, blood to circulate to all parts of the body, nutrition to be absorbed, and temperature to be regulated. But in some neonates these changes do not take place automatically nor early enough and the resultant problems must be treated. Especially vulnerable are the premature and the postmature neonates.

The premature neonate is defined as a baby born anytime before the 36th week of gestation or, in other words, more than 1 month before the anticipated due date. Because of aggressive obstetrical management and advances in techniques and equipment, more and more of these premature babies are surviving. Today, neonates who weigh as little as 750 g (1.6 pounds) and who are as young as 24 to 27 weeks' gestational age are surviving.

These preemies do not look like full-term babies, but more like fetuses, especially if they are very premature. Specific characteristics vary with gestational age, but they often have paper-thin skin that is brittle and red in color, and they may lack skin creases if they are younger than 32 weeks of gestational age. They may also have decreased tone and joint mobility and the babies younger than 34 weeks may lack ear cartilage and breast buds.[81,90]

The postmature, or postterm, neonate is usually defined as a baby born after 42 weeks of gestation. These neonates may possess the following physical characteristics: a long, thin body; thick scalp hair; and dry cracked skin resulting from the loss of the vernix caseosa. In addition, they may show signs of recent weight loss if the placenta was no longer able to provide all the nutrition needed causing stored fat to be used as a food source.[50]

Respiratory problems are common in neonates and can be dangerous. Some of these problems are acute in nature and others are considered chronic lung diseases. Respiratory distress problems may be caused by many things such as the aspiration of amniotic fluid or meconium; malformations or tumors of the respiratory organs; neurological diseases; central nervous system damage; drugs; air trapped in the chest or pericardium (sac surrounding the chest); and pulmonary hemorrhages.[50,81]

One of the acute respiratory problems often found in any neonate, especially preterm babies, is *hyaline membrane disease*. This disease is caused by a deficiency of surfactant, the chemical that prevents the alveoli from collapsing during expiration. As this chemical is not produced until about the 34th to the 36th week of gestation, many preemies are born with this deficiency. As the air sacs collapse, oxygen absorption and carbon dioxide elimination is hindered and the babies need at least supplemental oxygen and frequently need more intensive mechanical ventilation support. After 3 to 4 days of treatment, most infants begin to recover as surfactant begins to be produced by the baby's body or when an artificial substitute is administered. Some infants will develop chronic lung problems following hyaline membrane disease.

Chronic lung disease implies a long-term need for supplemental oxygen. The chronic lung disease often seen in neonatal centers is *bronchopulmonary dysplasia* (BPD). Initially, these neonates would have had some type of acute respiratory problem that precipitated the prolonged use of mechanical ventilation and other types of necessary, but perhaps traumatic, interventions. Due to the ventilation, airways begin to thicken, excess mucous forms, and alveolar growth is retarded. As a result, babies who develop BPD are often susceptible to respiratory infections and other respiratory problems until they are 5 and 6 years old. Problems, such as bronchopulmonary dysplasia, that are a result of the techniques used to save neonates' lives, are called iatrogenic disorders; Table 6-3 lists some of the more common ones.

Today's artificial respirators are sophisticated and allow careful control of the oxygen mixtures. In addition, they are designed to maintain a constant pressure on the alveoli, thus keeping them open in the absence of surfactant. This is known as *positive end-expiratory pressure* (PEEP), which has significantly lowered the

Table 6-3 Examples of iatrogenic conditions and disorders common in premature neonates

Intervention or procedure	Resulting disease or complication
Blood transfusions and intravenous procedures	Infections
Prolonged intravenous feeding	Liver damage, clots in the kidneys, feeding difficulties
Prolonged artificial ventilation	Bronchopulmonary dysplasia

rate of fetal death and overall risk of severe developmental delays.[54,67]

Three major cardiovascular changes must take place at birth. The foramen ovale, the hole between the right and left atria, must close. Also the ductus arteriosus and ductus venosus must close to allow blood to flow to the lungs and to the liver, respectively. Many complications can arise when these changes do not occur. One of the most common conditions found in premature newborns with respiratory distress syndrome is *patent ductus arteriosus* (PDA). In this condition the ductus arteriosus does not constrict, and this can lead to eventual heart failure and inadequate oxygenation of the brain. Treatment includes the administration of the drug *indomethacin,* which often triggers closure of the arterial wall. Surgery follows if the drug does not work.[64,92]

Another cardiovascular complication that may occur during the perinatal period is intracranial hemorrhage. This may occur prenatally, during the birth process, or postnatally. The site and the extent of the bleeding affect the prognosis. For example, extracranial bleeding, or cephalohematomas, are usually considered minor and usually cause no permanent damage. On the other hand, subdural, subarachnoid, and intraventricular hemorrhages are much more serious and, depending on the extent of damage, may cause seizures, brain damage, cerebral palsy and even death.[157]

Biochemical complications affect the premature neonate as well as the full-term neonate. One of the most common biochemical problems is jaundice, or icterus. This condition is characterized by a yellow discoloration of the skin and eyes as a result of an increase in the bilirubin level. Bilirubin is a by-product of the normal process that discards dead blood cells. When the bilirubin level rises slightly—a relatively common event in neonates—treatment may consist of simply placing the neonate under fluorescent lights. This speeds up the elimination of the bilirubin.

Hyperbilirubinemia (increased blood level of bilirubin) poses a serious threat to newborns. The most common cause of hyperbilirubinemia is Rh incompatibility. In the past this syndrome, called *kernicterus,* caused many fetuses to die in utero, and those who survived suffered brain damage, cerebral palsy, a high-frequency hearing loss, discoloration of the teeth, and sometimes paralysis of the upward gaze.[111]

Today the drug *RhoGAM,* which is a gamma globulin, is injected into Rh-negative women after the birth or miscarriage of each newborn. It blocks the formation of antibodies in the mother's circulation, and subsequent Rh-positive newborns will be born without problems. This treatment has resulted in the virtual disappearance of kernicterus.[15]

Two other biochemical complications are hypoglycemia and hypothermia. Hypoglycemia, or low blood glucose level, can cause the newborn to be jittery, appear lethargic, vomit, and have seizures or apnea spells. Giving the newborn sugar intravenously usually prevents permanent damage. The premature newborn is very susceptible to loss of heat, or *hypothermia.* There are two major reasons for this: (1) an inability to regulate temperature and (2) a reduced amount of fatty tissue to act as insulation.

Immaturity of the central nervous system may also cause complications. For example, some neonates have spells in which they have irregular respiratory patterns. If these hesitations last longer than 20 seconds, if the baby becomes cyanotic, or if the heart rate slows during these breathing irregularities, the term *apnea* is applied to the symptoms. An immature nervous system often does not send strong enough peripheral signals about the stretch and pressure feedback from the chest and lungs nor does it have the central organizational abilities to coordinate the respiratory cycle.

Another example of a condition often found in an immature nervous system is *sudden infant death syndrome* (SIDS). While the exact cause and site of involvement are not as yet confirmed, the brain stem is believed to be involved, and sensory processing has been found to be slower in some infants. Equipment such as rocker beds have proved helpful to stimulate some infants to breathe, as have certain medications such as caffeine and aminophylline.[85] If the spells continue, it may be helpful to have an apnea monitor that sounds an alarm if the infant stops breathing. In addition, many physicians are recommending that the parents of infants with histories of apnea participate in cardiopulmonary resuscitation (CPR) courses.

In addition to apnea and sudden infant death syndrome, an immature central nervous system may cause sucking and swallowing problems that hinder nutritional intake. Some newborns may have to be fed intravenously by a gastrostomy tube, which is inserted through the abdomen into the stomach, or by a nasogastric tube, which is inserted up the nose and down the esophagus to the stomach. *Hyperalimentation* is the term used for the administration of intravenous solution that contains sufficient glucose, vitamins, amino acids, and electrolytes to meet the nutritional needs of these neonates.[152]

A variety of hearing and visual problems continues to be found in neonates in spite of the tremendous technical and medical advances that have been made to date. One of the earliest visual deficits reported was *retrolental fibroplasia* (RLF). During the 1940s and 1950s, many babies became blind as a result of a detached retina that is now known to be caused by a combination of increased blood oxygen levels with elevated blood carbon dioxide levels. Today, RLF is more often referred to as *retinopathy of prematurity* (ROP) and is still seen within this population. Unfortunately, it is not yet possible to predict which premature babies will develop this condition and which will not, as not all premature babies who have required lengthy periods of time on supplemental oxygen have developed this problem. While aggressive monitoring of blood oxygen levels has lessened the role oxygen plays in causing this condition, other preventive factors and potential causative factors must be researched since some studies actually indicate a rise in the number of babies being born with this problem.

In addition to ROP, neonates may be born with, or develop shortly after birth, a number of visual abnormalities. Included in this category would be eyes that are missing, misformed, or missing the iris; cataracts; glaucoma; and tumors. Other visual impairments that have been reported are myopia, strabismus, and visual tracking delays.[50]

The incidence of hearing impairments among special care nursery neonates is much greater than among normal neonates. Possible causes of these hearing losses are congenital factors, intrauterine infections (rubella, CMV), anoxia and asphyxia, intracranial hemorrhages, hyperbilirubinemia, and abnormalities of the hearing structures and organs themselves.[50] Many nurseries screen their neonates for early hearing losses using the brainstem-evoked technique, an electrophysical test that measures peripheral and brainstem auditory acuity.

Many of these neonates also demonstrate neuromotor delays, behaviors or patterns not found in the normal full term baby. Because occupational therapists are very involved in helping to describe these problems and in helping to minimize the effects of these conditions, they are discussed in detail in Chapter 18.

An intestinal disorder called *necrotizing enterocolitis* (NEC) is thought to be caused by some type of infection. It is a serious intestinal disorder, occurring at about 2 weeks of age, in which the bowel stops functioning and may rupture. Antibiotics usually help solve the problem but surgery may have to be performed to remove or repair a section of the colon. In these neonates, unlike in adults, the colon often regenerates.

Generalized bacterial infection, or sepsis, is a serious concern in all nurseries. Neonates are susceptible to infection because of their incomplete defense or immune systems. Newborns may contract infections in the nursery from staff and visitors, from medical procedures such as blood transfusions, or from the insertion of tubes for feeding and respiratory support. Early diagnosis is essential, because the infection can spread rapidly through the newborn's body. Blood cultures are taken to identify the specific organism, and antibodies are given intravenously. Usually the newborn's condition improves within 2 or 3 days with this treatment.

Problems of neonates who are small or large for gestational age

The small for gestational age (SGA) neonate is often defined as a newborn whose birth weight is below the 10th percentile for gestational age as measured by standardized growth charts.[90] The majority of small for gestational age newborns are born at or near term but are small for their age. These newborns may suffer from a number of medical problems, including congenital anomalies; difficulty with thermal regulation, polycythemia, or hypoglycemia; and pulmonary problems such as aspiration syndrome, pneumomediastinum, and pneumothorax.[150]

The growth for small for gestational age infants varies, depending on the duration of the intrauterine problems that caused the stunting.[150] Some studies indicate that if the child's growth and development have not caught up to normal curves by 3 years of age, the child will remain smaller than normal throughout life.[59] It has been stated that the small for gestational age infant has a higher incidence of developmental disabilities when compared to average infants.[59,136]

The large for gestational age (LGA) neonate is often defined as the neonate whose birth weight is above the 90th percentile on the growth charts. Medical problems of these neonates include hypoglycemia; birth injuries resulting from prolonged or difficult labor or birth; and orthopedic problems resulting from the restricted room in utero.

Assessment of the neonate

At birth a neonate's neuromuscular, cardiovascular, and respiratory systems must be appraised to determine how well the neonate has responded to the birth process and extrauterine life. The Apgar scoring system provides this information by rating the neonate's color, heart rate, reflex irritability, muscle tone, and respiratory effort.[9]

Assessment of a neonate's gestational age is very important, especially in planning for the needs of the premature neonate. Clinical assessment of gestational age is based on the knowledge of various postures, reflexes, and external body characteristics at specific fetal ages.[7,10,18,159]

The three most commonly used clinical assessments for determining gestational age are (1) the Dubowitz and Dubowitz Clinical Assessment of Gestational Age,[47]

(2) the Lubchenco Clinical Estimate of Gestational Age,[90] and (3) the Newborn Maturity Rating and Classification. One of these assessments is usually given at birth and again during the first few days of life if low scores were noted in specific areas or if variations occurred between the results and other approaches to determine gestational age. All the assessments are used to evaluate neuromuscular signs as well as condition of skin, lanugo, breasts, plantar creases, ears, and genitalia.

A thorough physical examination is usually done after the newborn is 24 hours old, because it is after that time that problems such as seizures, intestinal obstructions, jaundice, apnea, hematomas, and other conditions become identifiable.[129] The physical condition and appearance of the following body structures are part of the examination: skin, head, eyes, nose, mouth, neck, thorax, lungs, heart, abdomen, genitalia, anus, trunk and spine, and extremities. In addition, general appearance, reflex presence and integration, tone, and quality of movement are observed.[129]

Many examinations also assess the social and interactive abilities of the neonate. The abilities to locate and orient to sensory stimuli, to react to environmental conditions, and to interact with caregivers are important factors in growth and development and in the bonding and attachment process.

The Brazelton Neonatal Behavioral Assessment Scale (BNBAS) is one of the most commonly used measures of social-interactive responses in the neonate.[25] This scale is designed to look at both the neurological and interactional functioning of a neonate during the first month of life.

Other assessments that explore various aspects of the caretaker-child interactional processes are the Mother-Infant Play Interaction Scale[153]; the Maternal Attachment Assessment[12]; and the Neonatal Perception Inventories.[28] Assessments that specifically look at child abuse factors include the Perinatal Screening for Child Abuse Potential[66]; the Index of Suspicion[108]; and the Child Abuse Potential Inventory.[100]

Follow-up testing

Professionals in most health care, medical, and educational settings agree that the biophysical, cognitive, and psychosocial progress of the types of neonates discussed should be monitored throughout the infant and preschool years to detect any developmental delays. A variety of tests have been designed to accomplish this goal. Some of the most often used tests are the Denver Developmental Screening Test (DDST)[59]; the Bayley Scales of Infant Development (BSID)[12]; the Revised Gesell-Amatruda Developmental Scales[82]; the Gesell Preschool Test[6]; the Miller Assessment for Preschoolers[98]; the Erhardt Developmental Prehension Assessment[51]; and the Brigance Inventories.[26] In addition to these traditional developmental skills, functional skills such as self-care, feeding, and mobility; and cognitive skills such as organizational abilities, general knowledge and comprehension, pre-reading and pre-math skills, and speech and language skills must be monitored. Other skills such as coloring, printing, cutting, manipulating objects, and play performance are also critical to the child's successful role performance. Specific assessments that can be used to evaluate these latter skills as well as specific roles and functions of the occupational therapist working with infants and preschoolers are discussed in Chapters 10, 11, 16, and 19.

Implications for occupational therapy

The first goal of the neonatal intensive care nursery is to ensure the physical survival of the neonate. But once the medical problems have been overcome or at least stabilized, it is time to address other equally important factors that relate to the quality of life of both the neonate and the parents. For example, the environmental stimulation must be examined, caregiver-infant interaction must be nurtured, and the sensorimotor abilities, psychosocial skills, and functional skills of the neonate must be assessed.

An occupational therapist knowledgeable in the assessment and treatment of these factors can be a tremendous asset to the interdisciplinary team used in most neonatal units. In addition, occupational therapists have much to offer during follow-up evaluations geared toward monitoring the growth, development, and functional skills of high-risk neonates and neonates with diagnosed problems (Chapter 18).

MUSCULOSKELETAL PROBLEMS

This section will discuss the components of the musculoskeletal system, their reactions to disorders and injuries, and selected musculoskeletal problems of particular interest to occupational therapists.

Components and functions of the musculoskeletal system

The musculoskeletal system consists of the following six major components:[131]

1. Bones that provide a framework for the body; serve as levers for the skeletal muscles; protect body organs; produce platelets, erythrocytes, and leukocytes; and store calcium, magnesium, phosphorus, and sodium
2. Joints that allow for segmentation of the skeletal system and help facilitate movement
3. Articular cartilage that provides a cushioning effect and allows free movement
4. Skeletal muscles that provide active motion and the maintenance of posture
5. Ligaments that facilitate or limit motion and provide support

6. Tendons that also facilitate or limit motion and provide support

Musculoskeletal reactions to disorders and injuries

When subjected to abnormal conditions, bone tissue will either die or continue to live by making some type of adaptation. An increase or decrease in the amount of bone tissue deposited may take place; there may be an increase or decrease in bone resorption; or a combination of these two circumstances may occur.[121] If these reactions occur in just one bone, it is called a *localized reaction;* but if many bones are affected, it is referred to as a *generalized reaction.*

In children and adolescents, the epiphyseal plates are particularly vulnerable to injury or growth disturbances, for example, decreased blood supply, pressure from fluid or tissue buildup, and injury to the plate itself. As a result of these abnormal conditions, growth may be stopped entirely or restricted to one part of the plate and not another. The result of pressure and abnormal twisting forces can be the rotation of the bone toward the source of the pressure.

The various components of a synovial joint are shown in Figure 6-2. These parts may also react to abnormal conditions. For instance, articular cartilage has little power to regenerate itself; therefore, under abnormal conditions it often degenerates and the peripheral edges begin to thicken and eventually ossify.[131] Often the synovial membrane reacts by producing an excessive amount of fluid, by thickening, or by forming adhesions to the articular cartilage. The joint capsule and surrounding ligaments react by either stretching, which causes joint instability, or becoming tighter, which can impair the range of motion of the joint.

Finally, adverse conditions can affect any or all of the components of the skeletal muscle motor unit. When this occurs, the skeletal muscle may react by degenerating, contracting or shortening, becoming weaker and smaller (atrophy), becoming larger (hypertrophy), or regenerating.[131]

Selected musculoskeletal disorders and conditions

EPIPHYSEAL PLATE DISORDERS

Fractures of the unossified epiphyses in children and adolescents account for about 15% of all childhood fractures.[131] Figure 6-3 depicts the Salter-Harris classification system for these injuries. This system is based on two factors: the relationship of the fracture or separation to the growing cells of the epiphyseal plate and (2) the mechanism of injury.[131] The prognosis for growth disturbances worsens with each type; therefore Type V is the most serious.[60] Although some epiphyseal fractures are complicated, causing growth disturbances, Salter states that approximately 85% of these disorders do not cause permanent growth disturbances.[131]

The clinical picture for a child with a fracture of an epiphyseal plate includes pain and swelling. X-ray films are taken of both the injured extremity and the normal extremity to compare the two and help with the diagnosis. Immobilization or decreased weight bearing are usually the only treatments that need to be taken, and with time the fracture heals. More serious fractures, with accompanying deformities, are discussed later in this chapter.

As mentioned earlier, prolonged twisting forces may cause changes in epiphyseal plate growth, causing the long bones to twist in the direction of the abnormal force. These are known as *internal, external,* or *combinational torsional deformities.* For example, "toeing out" is very common in young children. This deformity

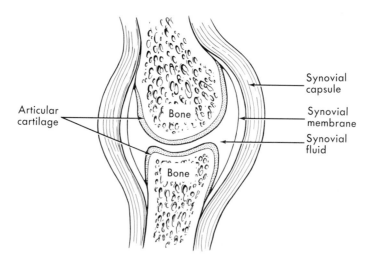

Figure 6-2 Components of a typical synovial joint.

is characterized by externally rotated feet and knees and by limited internal rotation of the femur. It is often seen in infants who habitually sleep in the prone position with their legs externally rotated, and this causes external femoral torsion. Conversely, children who spend a great deal of time sitting on the floor with knees in front, feet out to the side, and femora internally rotated (the "television position" or "W-sitting"), may begin to "toe in," resulting from the internal femoral tension.

Bow legs, or *genu varum,* is an example of a deformity caused by combinational torsional forces, that is, prolonged internal torsion to the tibia and external torsion to the femur. This deformity is often present at birth because of prenatal posturing, but it usually corrects itself unless compounded by specific neuromus-

cular problems or unusual sleeping and sitting postures that continue to apply the abnormal torsions.

Marfan's syndrome, also called arachnodactyly or hyperchondroplasia, is a disorder that causes excessive growth in all the epiphyseal plates. It is considered a hereditary condition with an unknown cause. Symptoms include increased height and decreased weight for chronological age, excessive length of the extremities, scoliosis, depressed sternum, stooped shoulders, flat feet, and excessive joint flexibility. Additional problems may occur, such as dislocation of the optic lens[131,152] and heart disease that includes dilation of the aorta. Medical treatment includes surgical intervention for any skeletal deformities that interfere with function.

Chondrodystrophia, also called chondrodystrophy

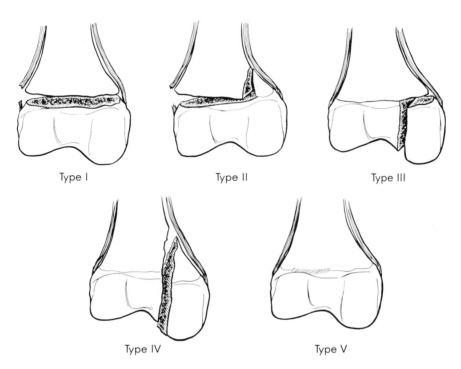

Figure 6-3 Salter-Harris classifications of epiphyseal plate injuries.

TYPE	INJURY AND GROWTH EFFECTS	MECHANISM
I	Complete separation of epiphysis along plate; growing cells remain with plate	Shearing force
II	Complete separation of epiphysis with fracture (fx) into metaphysis; growth cells remain with plate	Bending and shearing forces
III	Incomplete separation along epiphyseal plate, fx through epiphysis. No damage to growth cells	Intraarticular
IV	Fx through epiphysis, plate, and into metaphysis	Intraarticular
V	No separation or fx but epiphysis and plate have received severe blow sufficient to interrupt growth	Crushing force through epiphysis

or achondroplasia, has the opposite effect of Marfan's syndrome by stunting epiphyseal plate growth and causing dwarfism. This disorder is transmitted by an autosomal dominant gene and is characterized by very short limbs, a small face (head size is average because of normal growth of the cranial bones), and decreased height that seldom exceeds 4 feet. Skeletal abnormalities such as lumbar lordosis, coxa vara, and cubitus varus may also be present. To improve both function and appearance, orthopedic surgery is often performed.[131]

DISORDERS CAUSED BY DEPOSITION OR RESORPTION IMBALANCES

Osteogenesis imperfecta, also called brittle bones or fragilitas ossium, offers an example of a disorder characterized by decreased bone deposition. It is a congenital type of osteoporosis that is transmitted by an autosomal dominant gene. The result is a serious disorder in which fractures can result from very minor traumatic situations. The severity of the disorder varies greatly depending on the time of onset (Table 6-4). Multiple fractures or repeated fractures to the same bone may cause a limb to become misshapen and eventually muscularly underdeveloped because of the long periods of immobilization and disuse. Prevention must be attempted through, at least, the use of padded arm and leg protectors and, in severe cases, long leg braces and crutches.[131] To provide internal support and to correct deformities that may develop, surgical procedures using metal rods and segmental osteotomies may be helpful.

Osteopetrosis, or marble bones or Albers-Schönberg's disease, is an autosomal recessive disorder that is characterized by a great increase in the amount of bone that results from defective resorption.[89,131] Gradually the bones become dense and the hemopoietic marrow spaces are infiltrated with bony deposits, causing aplastic anemia. Other local complications may include pathological fractures of the neck of the femur, nerve deafness or blindness as the nerve foramina begin to close because of bony encroachment, and enlargement of the liver and spleen. In severe cases hydrocephalus and mental retardation may be present. Prognosis is poor, and many children die in childhood. Treatment includes the administration of steroids and aggressive treatment of the anemia.

DISORDERS CAUSED BY INFECTION

Osteomyelitis is an inflammation of the bone marrow that may be caused by puncture wounds, infection adjacent to the bone, or microorganisms that travel in the blood.[123] Initially the organisms settle in the distal end of the metaphysis, and as the disease progresses the infection spreads throughout the bone and outward to the periosteum. Initial symptoms include pain, tenderness, and unwillingness to use or bear weight on the involved limb. These symptoms are followed by a fever, soft tissue swelling, and often anorexia.[160]

Treatment must be initiated as soon as possible, because prolonged infection may cause bone destruction, pathological fractures, septic arthritis, and eventually growth disturbances.[131] Diagnosis is usually made based on clinical signs, and confirmation is made from specimen aspiration test results, blood cell counts, and positive radiographic evidence.[123,131] Initial treatment usually consists of oral or intravenous antibiotic therapy for at least 3 weeks with bed rest and immobility of the affected body part. If improvement is not seen, surgery is done, which includes drilling into the bone to remove the pus and damaged tissue and putting in place drainage tubes and intravenous tubes that are used to infuse the site with a saline and antibiotic solution.[131] Following these procedures, splinting of the extremity or traction helps to prevent the spread of infection, reduces pain, and prevents contractures.[2] Relapses can lead to chronic osteomyelitis that may involve continued discharge of pus from a sinus over the infected area, pain, or the formation of an abscess cavity in the bone itself. Bed rest and antibiotics may clear the problem, or surgical procedures may have to be repeated. Chronic untreated osteomyelitis presents serious medical problems that can be minimized by early detection and prolonged antibiotic therapy.[2,123,131]

Another disorder that is spread by infection is *tuberculosis.* On occasion tuberculosis of the bone (tuberculous osteomyelitis) occurs as an isolated lesion, but it usually forms from infection at a primary lesion in another part of the body or from an adjoining joint.[2] The most common sites for tuberculosis of the bone are the long bones, synovial joints, and vertebrae.

The joints most often affected are the hip and the knee. Symptoms include pain, muscle spasm, reduced joint motion, and muscle atrophy. Initially swelling of the soft tissue around the joint is noted. Then the synovial membrane changes, and articular cartilage necrosis occurs. Finally the adjacent bones may begin to collapse.[131]

Tuberculosis of the spine, or Pott's disease, usually begins with pain, tenderness, and muscle spasms in the

---

Table 6-4 Effect of onset of osteogenesis imperfecta

Fetal type	Most severe	Fractures occur in utero and during birth. Mortality is high.
Infantile type	Moderately severe	Many fractures occur in early childhood. Severe limb deformities and growth disturbances occur also.
Juvenile type	Least severe	Fractures begin in late childhood. By puberty bones often begin to harden and fewer fractures occur.

back. As the disease progresses, the anterior sections of the vertebral bodies begin to collapse, causing the spine to tilt anteriorly.[2] Infection may spread to adjacent disks and vertebrae or to the spinal cord. Pott's paraplegia may be a direct result of spinal cord involvement or a result of pressure on the cord.

The treatment for bone tuberculosis includes the use of antituberculous drugs, rest, a nutritious diet, immobilization of the infected joint or limb, surgical drainage, and, on occasion, arthrodesis or bony fusion.[2,123]

DISORDERS OF THE JOINTS

A major cause of physical disability in children under the age of 16 is *juvenile rheumatoid arthritis* (JRA). It is estimated that approximately 250,000 children in the United States suffer from some form of this disease.[2] This disease usually begins between the ages of 2 and 4 years of age and is more common in girls.[131]

The exact cause of juvenile rheumatoid arthritis is unknown, but the following factors are believed to play undefined roles in its cause: genetics, emotional trauma, histocompatibility antigens, viruses, and antigen-antibody immune complexes.[2]

Juvenile rheumatoid arthritis is usually described as taking three different forms: (1) pauciarticular, (2) polyarticular, and (3) systemic, or Still's disease. The pauciarticular form usually affects only a few joints. Involvement is often asymmetrical, and there are few or no systemic manifestations. The joints most often affected are the knee, hip, ankle, and elbow. Many times overgrowth in the long bones surrounding the inflamed joint causes gait problems and flexion contractures. Many children suffering from pauciarticular juvenile rheumatoid arthritis develop iridocyclitis, an inflamed condition of the iris and ciliary body of the eye that can lead to blindness if early treatment is not begun.[2,131]

In the polyarticular form, onset is often abrupt and painful with symmetrical involvement of the wrist, hands, feet, knees, ankles, and sometimes the cervical area of the spine. Other symptoms include a low-grade fever, malaise, anorexia, listlessness, and irritability.[131]

Systemic juvenile rheumatoid arthritis, or Still's disease, consists of polyarticular symptomatology plus involvement in other organs such as the spleen and lymph nodes.[2] Signs and symptoms include a high fever, rash, anorexia, enlargement of the liver and spleen, and an elevated white blood cell count.[131] Epiphyseal plates adjacent to an affected joint may initially show an acceleration of growth but later may be destroyed, causing local growth retardation.

The prognosis for juvenile rheumatoid arthritis varies, depending on a number of factors, but it is important to remember that the largest percentage of children (the pauciarticular type) often recover completely within 1 to 2 years. Only about 15% of all children with the disease will have permanent disabilities.[131]

Medical management primarily centers on the use of the following therapeutic drugs (in order of preference): salicylates; nonsteroidal, antiinflammatory analgesic drugs; gold salt injections; and adrenocorticosteroids.[131] Surgical repair and reconstruction are seldom recommended for children. Other forms of treatment may include splinting, active and passive range of motion of the joints, and monitoring each joint to maintain maximal function and prevent deformity.[123,131]

In summary, children with JRA may be in pain at times, may show signs of fatigue, and may have reduced range of motion in one or more joints. As a result, they may have difficulty performing activities of daily living and certain school tasks. Adaptive equipment such as pen and pencil grips, dressing aids, and built-up handles on utensils or other adaptations to feeding equipment often improve functioning and reduce fatigue and stress on joints. Seating needs must be monitored to help reduce fatigue and prevent undue pressure on joints as well.[16]

A disease that is a form of polyarthritis is *ankylosing spondylitis,* or Strümpell-Marie disease. The time of onset is usually 18 to 30 years of age, and it occurs predominately in young men.[2] This disease is characterized by a progessive bony ankylosing of the spine, beginning in the sacroiliac region and progressing upward to the cervical region. Eventually the spine becomes one rigid mass of bone. The proximal joints of the extremities are also often affected.

Treatment methods for this disease include the administration of salicylates or phenylbutazone, activity to maintain function, radiation therapy for relief of pain, and surgical procedures such as spinal osteotomy, interposition arthroplasty, and resection arthroplasty.[2,131] It should be remembered that no treatment halts the disease, but all methods must be used to limit immobility and prevent fusion of the spine.[2]

A severe orthopedic problem that is seen at birth is *arthrogryposis multiplex congenita,* or amyoplasia congenita. It is characterized by stiff, spindly, deformed joints in the extremities that are caused by either defectively formed (hypoplasia) or absent (aplasia) muscle groups or, on occasion, secondary to a defect in the anterior horn cells of the spinal cord.[131] Common clinical deformities include clubfoot, hip dislocation, flexion or extension deformity of the knee, flexion deformities of fingers and wrists, extension deformities of the elbows, and adduction deformities of the shoulder.[57]

Treatment presents an orthopedic challenge that may include casting, splinting, surgery on bones and soft tissue, and daily passive stretching of the joints.[131]

DISORDERS OF THE SPINE

The most common congenital abnormality of the spine is *spina bifida,* in which the laminae of one or more of the vertebrae are incompletely closed during the fourth week of prenatal development. This defect

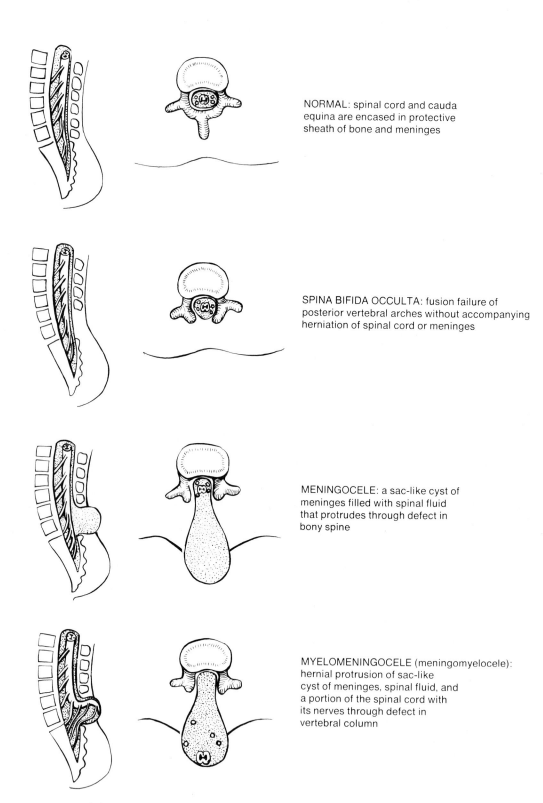

NORMAL: spinal cord and cauda equina are encased in protective sheath of bone and meninges

SPINA BIFIDA OCCULTA: fusion failure of posterior vertebral arches without accompanying herniation of spinal cord or meninges

MENINGOCELE: a sac-like cyst of meninges filled with spinal fluid that protrudes through defect in bony spine

MYELOMENINGOCELE (meningomyelocele): hernial protrusion of sac-like cyst of meninges, spinal fluid, and a portion of the spinal cord with its nerves through defect in vertebral column

Figure 6-4 Three forms of spina bifida.

From Whaley L, and Wong D: Nursing care of infants and children, ed 2, St Louis, 1983, The CV Mosby Co.

may be seen at any spinal level but most often occurs in the lumbosacral region.

The degree of impairment depends on the level and degree of spinal cord involvement. This continuum of impairment ranges from no functional impairment, to mild muscle imbalances and sensory losses, to paraplegia, and even to death in severe cases.[131]

The three types of spina bifida are illustrated in Figure 6-4. The mildest form is spina bifida occulta. Many times in this form of spina bifida there are no external manifestations visible, or the skin overlying the defect may be dimpled, pigmented, or covered with hair. Internally the spinal cord may be divided by a bony spur or congenital neoplasm, or there may simply be a slight bony malformation of one or more vertebrae.[95]

Spina bifida with meningocele is characterized by a sac, or meningocele, visible above the bony defect. This sac is covered with skin and subcutaneous tissue, contains cerebral spinal fluid, and while the meninges extend into the sac, the spinal cord remains confined to the spinal canal.

Spina bifida with myelomeningocele is the most severe form of the disorder. In this form the sac may be covered with only a thin layer of skin or the meninges, and the spinal cord or nerve roots protrude into the meningocele.

Complications with this form of spina bifida include meningitis and hydrocephalus. Infection is easily contracted because of environmental exposure of the meninges and spinal cord. Hydrocephalus is a common secondary complication that may be caused by either a developmental defect in the brain, such as aqueduct stenosis, or by the lower portion of the brain (and part of the cerebellum) slipping through the foramen ovale, a condition known as *Arnold-Chiari syndrome.*[15,131]

The medical management of the spina bifida child depends on the degree of involvement, but ideally the sac should be removed as soon as possible. Additional surgery may include the implantation of a shunt to relieve excessive ventricular pressure. Orthopedic intervention may include bracing, crutches, casting, and orthopedic shoes.[123,131] Other medical procedures may involve controlling urinary and bowel continence and infections and preventing renal deterioration.[123,140]

The rehabilitation goals for these children include the attainment of the highest level of physical functioning possible and the achievement of maximal independence in all areas of daily functioning. Counseling; the long-term monitoring of physical, cognitive, and psychosocial functioning; special education; and vocational training may be implemented to achieve these goals.

Congenital scoliosis is another relatively common spinal abnormality. The condition is usually characterized by two lateral spinal curves, the severity of which is variable. In mild cases the curvature may be inconspicuous to external observation, and if a healthy spine exists above and below the curvature, further progres-

sion is unlikely.[131] If the curvature is more severe or if the condition exists with other abnormalities such as absent or fused ribs or multiple hemivertebrae, early surgical treatment must be done to prevent permanent deformities and subsequent growth complications.[131]

DISORDERS OF THE UPPER EXTREMITIES

The most common congenital abnormalities of the hands are (1) excess number of fingers (polydactyly) and (2) webbing of the fingers (syndactyly). In *polydactyly* a variety of things may occur: the existence of one or more complete extra digits, or the duplication of just a portion of a finger or thumb. The decision to surgically remove a digit or portion of a digit is based on radiographic information, functional assessment, and cosmetic considerations.[131]

Webbing of the fingers may exist between two adjacent fingers or may involve three or four fingers. Usually the webbing extends along the proximal portion of the fingers, but occasionally it may extend the length of the fingers. Bones and joints may be involved in addition to the soft tissue. Typical reconstructive surgery involves surgical separation of the digits and skin grafts.[131]

Relatively rare abnormalities of the upper extremities include hypoplasia or aplasia of the radius; dislocation of the head of the radius; hypoplasia of the clavicles; and a congenital high scapula (Sprengel's deformity). In each of these problems surgical interventions will be attempted if function and cosmetic appearance can be improved.

Congenital amputations of the upper extremities may be as minor as a missing finger or part of a hand, or as major as the absence of one or both of the extremities. During the prenatal period, for varying reasons, the soft tissue and overlying skin in a small area of the limb fail to grow in circumference, thus forming what are called *congenital annular constricting bands.*[131] If the constriction is shallow, no deformity may occur, or the distal portion of the extremity may enlarge because of edema. But if the constriction is severe, the extremity may be amputated below the constriction.[131]

Types of limb deficiencies include *amelia,* which is the absence of an arm; *phocomelia,* which refers to a limb that is missing the proximal part; *paraxial deficiency,* which consists of a normal upper part of the limb with either the radial part of the arm and attached fingers undeveloped or the ulnar part of the arm and attached fingers undeveloped; and *transverse hemimelia,* in which a part of a forearm or hand or part or all of the fingers are missing.[124]

Treatment of children with severe congenital amputations consists of fitting them with prostheses as early as 6 months of age. This helps to prevent the formation of habits that might interfere with adapting to the prostheses and also allows the child to interact with the environment through age-appropriate bimanual activities.[131,145] Treatment may also include early referral to an amputee clinic. An interdisciplinary team can work with the child on preprosthetic activities as well as help the family adjust to the child's deficiency.

DISORDERS OF THE LOWER EXTREMITIES

Congenital abnormalities of the feet include polydactyly, syndactyly, and assorted adduction (varus) and abduction (valgus) deformities of one or more toes. The treatment of these conditions is very similar to that described for the hands.

The most important abnormality of the foot is *clubfoot,* or talipes equinovarus. The incidence of clubfoot is high (2 per 1,000 live births), with boys being affected twice as often as girls.[2,131] The condition is often bilateral with major clinical features that include forefoot adduction and supination, heel varus, equinus through the ankle, and medial deviation of the foot in relationship to the knee.[2,131] Underdevelopment of the muscles in the lower legs may also be noted.

The exact cause or causes of clubfoot are unclear, but during fetal development something adversely affects the development of the muscles on the medial and posterior aspects of the legs, causing them to be shorter than normal.[2,131] These contractions in turn lead to the bone and joint problems.

Complete correction of clubfoot is very difficult to attain. Many times the deformity will be corrected in infancy only to recur during periods of rapid growth.[131] Initial treatment consists of manually correcting the deformity with gentle pressure and then using one of the following methods for holding the foot in the correct position: casting, metal splints of the Denis Browne type, adhesive strapping, and special boots.[2] Gradually the amount of time the child spends in the piece of equipment is decreased until the child is only in it at night. If progress has not been noted in 2 to 3 months, soft tissue operations such as tendon lengthenings, tendon transfers, and capsulotomies may be performed. Salter[131] states that these early operations can greatly decrease recurrence of the problem.

In older children and in neglected cases or recurrent cases, treatment may have to be geared toward the creation of a plantigrade foot so that the child can walk on the sole of his foot.[2] The soft tissue surgeries mentioned earlier may be used, as well as bony operations such as arthrodesis of joints, osteotomies, and the insertion of a bone wedge on the medial side of the calcaneus to correct the line of weight bearing.[2]

Hypoplasias of the fibula, tibia, and femur are rare but serious congenital abnormalities. Often when the fibula is affected, a built-up foot and brace may help to compensate for the leg length discrepancy. Hypoplasia of the tibia is often unsuccessfully resolved by reconstructive surgery; therefore, amputation is performed at the knee, and the child is subsequently fitted with a prosthesis.

Cogenital problems of the knee include hyperextension of the knee, called genu recurvatum, and dislocation of the patella. Genu recurvatum is usually corrected with plaster casts, and dislocation of the patella may require reconstructive soft tissue operations.[131]

Congenital dislocation of the hip is almost as common as clubfoot (1.5 per 1,000 live births) and is also often bilateral, but, unlike clubfoot, many more girls than boys are affected.[131] The causes of congenital hip dislocation (head out of socket) and subluxation (head partially out of socket) are both genetic and environmental. For example, hip laxity may be genetically inherited or may be a result of a hormonal secretion of the uterus.[2] Environmental factors include birth complications from uterine pressure or poor presenting positions. Also, the unstable hip may be dislocated or subluxed by sudden, passive extension or by positioning that maintains the legs extended and adducted.[2,131]

Early diagnosis of this abnormality is critical, because delay can cause serious and permanent disabilities. Three clinical observations that may be used in diagnosing congenital hip dislocation are the Ortolani test, Galeazzi's sign, and Trendelenburg's sign.

The Ortolani test consists of flexing the infant's knees and hips and then alternately adducting and pressing the femur downward and then abducting and lifting the femur. If the hip is unstable, it will dislocate when it is adducted but will reduce back into the socket as it is abducted.[131] The evaluator will feel and often hear a "click" as this happens. Galeazzi's sign consists of one knee being lower than the other when the child is placed in the supine position on a table with knees flexed to 90 degrees. This results from the dislocated femur lying posteriorly to the acetabulum.[131] Trendelenburg's sign consists of the hips dropping to the opposite side of the dislocation and the trunk shifting toward the dislocated hip when the child is asked to stand on the foot of the affected side.

If treatment is begun within the first few weeks of life, normal development of the hip can nearly always be assured. The longer it goes unresolved, the poorer the prognosis.[2] Specific treatment techniques vary according to the age of the patient when treatment is initiated, but generally the techniques, ranging from those used on the younger child to those used on the older child, include stabilizing the hip in an abducted and flexed position to facilitate femoral and acetabular development. This may be accomplished with splints, traction, the hip spica plaster cast, or the pillow splint.[2,131] If these methods do not correct the problem, a number of surgical procedures may be used to correct bony and soft tissue problems.[2] In severe cases arthrodesis or total replacement arthroplasty may be performed.[2] Again, it should be emphasized that every infant should be examined for this deformity in the first weeks of life to prevent the complications this defect can cause.

Congenital amputations of the lower extremities are not as prevalent as those in the upper extremities.[2,131] They are just as serious when they do occur.

Terminology and management strategies are the same as described with the upper extremity amputee.

Implications for occupational therapy

Occupational therapists have worked with children with assorted musculoskeletal problems for many years. Specific treatment goals will vary, depending on the condition and the needs of each child. In general, occupational therapy goals will include assisting with the physical habilitation or rehabilitation of the child; monitoring and fostering development; and working on various self-care, play and leisure, and work skills that the child needs to perform his roles at home, in school, and in the community (Chapter 24).

NEUROMUSCULAR CONDITIONS

This section discusses various diseases and conditions that are of interest to occupational therapists because they primarily interfere with the ability of children to engage in motor interactions with their environment. The site of the damage may be the brain, the anterior horn cells, the peripheral nerves, the neuromuscular junction, or the muscle itself. These diagnostic problems are collectively referred to as neuromuscular conditions.

Selected neuromuscular diseases and conditions

THE MUSCLES

The muscle cells are thought to be the primary site of disease in the muscular dystrophies. All forms of muscular dystrophy are the result of specific genetic defects that cause biochemical and structural changes in the surface and internal membranes of the muscle cells. These changes cause a progressive degeneration and weakness of various muscle groups.[101]

A somewhat debated type of muscular dystrophy is *congenital muscular dystrophy* (CMD). While the literature dates back to the mid-1960s, it does not appear to provide definitive data on incidence, essential features, or long-term follow-up.[86]

The disease is transmitted by autosomal recessive inheritance. Essential features reported in various studies include hypotonia and multiple joint contractures from birth, general muscle weakness and atrophy, and normal intelligence.[86] Associated problems include clubfoot, torticollis, diaphragmatic involvement, congenital heart defects, and spinal defects.[45,86] Often little to no progression of the disease is seen after childhood, and some functional improvement may be seen around this time.[86]

Diagnosis is made from the presence of high serum levels of the muscle enzyme creatine kinase; by electromyography analysis; and by examination of muscle tissue taken during biopsy. Clinical examination often reveals a "floppy" child with muscle weakness in the face, neck, trunk, and limbs; decreased muscle mass; and absent deep tendon reflexes.[86]

Two other forms of muscular dystrophy are *limb-girdle* and *facioscapulohumeral*. In *limb-girdle muscular dystrophy* the initial muscles affected are the proximal muscles of the pelvic and shoulder girdles. Onset may begin anywhere from the first to the third decade of life, with progression being either slow or moderately rapid. Its hereditary pattern is autosomal recessive like the congenital form.

Facioscapulohumeral muscular dystrophy is autosomal dominant, and onset usually occurs in early adolescence. Although severity varies greatly from patient to patient, involvement is primarily in the face, upper arms, and scapular region, as the name implies. Clinical manifestations include a slope to the shoulders, decreased ability to raise arms above shoulder height, and decreased mobility in the facial muscles that gives a "masked" appearance.[101]

The most common and the most severe form of muscular dystrophy is called *Duchenne's dystrophy*. It is inherited in a sex-linked recessive manner, affects males, and has an incidence of 0.2 per 1,000 live births.[15]

Symptoms usually begin between the second and sixth years of life. Parents describe their child as having difficulty climbing stairs and rising from a sitting or lying position. The child stumbles and falls excessively and tires easily.[101] A distinctive characteristic of this form is the enlargement of calf muscles and sometimes of forearm and thigh muscles, giving the appearance of strong, healthy muscles (Figure 6-5). However, this en-

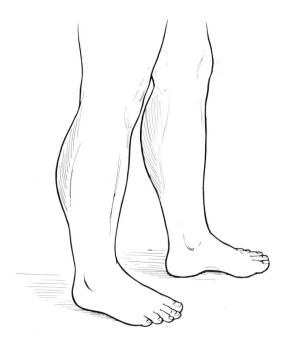

Figure 6-5   Enlarged calf muscles in Duchenne's muscular dystrophy.

largement is caused by extensive fibrosis and proliferation of adipose tissue, which, when combined with the other pathological changes in the muscle tissue, actually causes muscle weakness. This phenomenon is referred to as pseudo-hypertrophy of muscles.

Involvement begins in the proximal musculature of the pelvic girdle, proceeds to the shoulder girdle, and finally affects all muscle groups. As leg and pelvic muscles weaken, the child will often use his arms to "crawl" up his thighs into a standing position from a kneeling position. This is known as Gower's sign and is diagnostically very significant (Figure 6-6). Mobility is one of the first functions to be lost, and wheelchair dependence is common by 9 years of age. Gradually the simplest activities of daily living become difficult and then impossible. In the advanced stages of the disease, lordosis and kyphosis are common, as are contractures at various joints. Death, usually as a result of infection, respiratory problems, or cardiovascular complications, often occurs before the early twenties.[97,98,101]

At this time there is no treatment that will arrest or reverse the dystrophic process, but antibiotic therapy and other advances in dealing with pulmonary complications have helped to extend life expectancy.[101] Also, the use of orthopedic devices and adaptive equipment and activity can increase mobility, minimize contrac-

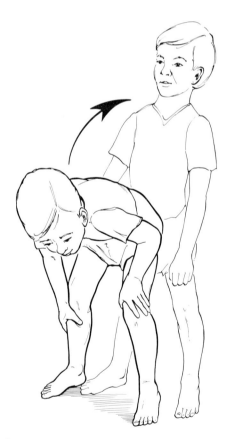

Figure 6-6   Child with Gower's sign.

tures, delay spinal curvatures, and maximize independence in daily activities and thus in role functioning.

The term "dystrophy" is usually reserved for certain genetically determined disorders such as those just described. All other disorders of muscles are usually called "myopathies."[115] Congenital myopathies are rare in infants; however, when they occur they are usually caused by autosomal dominant patterns of inheritance but may also be caused by prolonged treatment with certain drugs such as steroids.[19,115] Clinically, the children present similarly to the dystrophies with proximal muscle weakness of the face, neck, and limbs.[19,115] Congenital dislocation of the hip, scoliosis, seizures, and reduced cognitive skills may also be present.[115] Diagnosis is made by muscle biopsy. Unlike the dystrophies, progression of the condition is slow to nonexistent, making the prognosis much better.

THE NEUROMUSCULAR JUNCTION

An example of a disease that affects the neuromuscular junction occasionally in children is *myasthenia gravis.*[99] When this disease enters the body, antibodies are produced that block or greatly reduce the neurotransmitter acetylcholine from being released into the synaptic gap, thus impairing nerve impulses and causing impairment of movement.[15]

Symptoms include drooping of the eyelids, and general muscle weakness that usually worsens as the day progresses.[15] Treatment includes a medication called neostigmine that prevents the breakdown of acetylcholine. With medication and proper rest, these children can lead relatively normal lives.

THE PERIPHERAL NERVES

Guillain-Barré syndrome, an acute polyneuropathy, is caused by a virus that infects the peripheral nerve roots. For some reason the body interprets these infected roots as foreign bodies and begins to destroy them: a phenomenon known as an autoimmune response. This disease is normally rare (1 per 100,000 live births), but in 1976 the incidence rose sharply as a complication of the swine flu vaccination program.[15]

Clinical symptoms usually begin with an upper respiratory infection, progress to muscle weakness and paralysis in the lower extremities, and then involve the upper extremities and diaphragm.[15] However, the nerve fibers often regenerate over a period of months, and normal functioning usually returns.[48]

THE ANTERIOR HORN CELLS

Poliomyelitis is a viral disease that affects the anterior horn cells of the spinal cord. In less severe forms of the disease, symptoms may last a few days or weeks and consist of flu-like symptoms with no clinically detectable neurological deficit.[15,123] The paralytic form of polio, on the other hand, progresses quickly to meningitis and muscle weakness, followed by some degree of paralysis.[15] Often, for example, the anterior horn cells of the cervical and lumbar regions are involved, causing quadriplegia and interfering with innervation to the diaphragm and intercostal muscles, thus hampering or completely eliminating the person's ability to breathe independently.[15]

Before 1955 thousands of infants and children contracted poliomyelitis each year, but for the last decade less than 50 cases have been reported in the United States.[123] The reason for this is the highly successful oral polio immunization program recommended for infants between 2 and 4 months of age (Chapter 5).

THE BRAIN

Cerebral palsy is a disorder of movement and posture expressed through variable impairments in the coordination of muscle action and of sensation caused by a nonprogressive brain lesion that may have occurred in utero, around the time of birth, or after birth.[17,24]

Factors already discussed may cause the lesion or lesions leading to cerebral palsy, but the ones most often described are prematurity, intracranial hemorrhage, neonatal anoxia, poor maternal prenatal conditions, hyperbilirubinemia, multiple pregnancy, and malformations of the central nervous system.[32,134] In addition, cases of genetically determined lesions that cause specific types of cerebral palsy have been reported. These cases have been attributed to an autosomal dominant pattern of inheritance and have been traced through several generations of the families.[40] Lesions that develop in the infant period are often caused by trauma, neoplastic factors, intracranial hemorrhages, central nervous system infections, toxicity, or complications surrounding conditions and diseases such as uncontrolled hydrocephalus or sickle-cell anemia.[73,109]

The incidence of cerebral palsy was reported to be 7 per 1,000 live births in 1956,[113] but a survey of more recent studies indicates a range of 0.6 to 2.4 per 1,000 live births.[68] Reasons for this apparent reduction in the overall number of cases include improved obstetrical care, technological advances in prenatal and neonatal care, and improved management of maternal infections and diseases such as rubella, diabetes, and Rh incompatibility.[61,68] For example, the incidence of athetosis has dropped because of improved treatment and prevention of hyperbilirubinemia,[61] and spastic diplegia has been reported to be declining in incidence because of advances in neonatal care.[68]

Injury to the brain often results in disorders other than motor impairments. The specific type of associated condition that develops depends on a variety of factors including the location of the damage in the brain; the severity or extent of the damage; and the time of development that the damage occurred.[15,32] It is important to remember that each child with cerebral palsy will have a unique set of problems including one or more of the following conditions.

A wide continuum of problems with the visual system may include impaired vision, blindness, limitations in eye movements and eye tracking, squinting, strabismus, eye muscle weaknesses, and eye incoordination.[15,32,73] In addition, children with cerebral palsy may have visual perception problems that can interfere with school progress. It is estimated that 40% to 50% of cerebral palsy children have visual defects of some type.[15,73]

Auditory disturbances include hearing (acuity) problems that can range from slight hearing loss to total deafness. Auditory perceptual problems and agnosia are also common.[15,73] An estimated 25% of children with cerebral palsy have some type of auditory disturbance.[73]

Sensory integration disorders are estimated to occur in approximately 14% of these children; they include various vestibular, tactile, and motor planning problems.[73] All types of speech and feeding disturbances may be found in this population. Inadequate coordination of facial, neck, tongue, lip, and respiratory muscles as well as inadequate swallowing mechanisms all contribute to these problems. Excessive (high) tone or inadequate (low) tone can also be a major contributing factor. Speech disturbances occur in approximately 25% of this population.[73]

Delays are also seen in cognitive development with approximately 50% to 75% of these children having below average intelligence.[15,73] This would include all types of mental retardation from mild to profound.

Seizure disorders are estimated to occur in 25% to 35% of the cases and range in intensity from petit mals to grand mals. They are more likely to occur in children with spastic cerebral palsy than with other forms.

Lastly, these children must be monitored for signs of behavioral problems and psychosocial delays that can become serious problems if not found early and corrected. Evaluation of these areas should be an integral part of the total assessment and treatment regimen for these special children.

A comprehensive medical assessment is necessary with cerebral palsy because of its multiple problems. The physician usually bases the diagnosis on abnormal delays in development that have been observed during physical examinations and on what the parents have reported over a period of months or years. Types of problems that should alert the physician that something may be wrong include: the retention of primitive reflexes, variable tone, hyperresponsive tendon reflexes, asymmetry in the use of extremities, clonus, poor sucking or tongue control, and involuntary movements.[15,123] Another clue might be a large discrepancy between motor and intellectual areas of development.[15]

Medical management of cerebral palsy may encompass pharmacological, orthopedic, and neurosurgical approaches. Many medications have been used in an attempt to help alleviate the motor problems associated with cerebral palsy. For example, dantrolene (Dantrium) and diazepam (Valium), have been reported to reduce spasticity and tone in some children.[15,123] Another medication, levodopa, is believed to have possible benefits with athetoid children.[123]

Orthopedic procedures range from bracing and splinting to orthopedic surgery. Batshaw[15] states that bracing and splinting may be used to maintain range of motion, prevent contractures, improve functioning, and prevent or delay orthopedic surgery. Bracing and splinting may also be used as an integral part of postoperative treatment.

Various surgical procedures may be employed with these children. Some of these procedures are designed to increase range of motion through the release, lengthening, or transfer of affected muscles.[15] For example, a hamstring release might benefit walking, or a transfer of hip adductors might help the child to sit. Surgery may also be needed to correct hip dislocation by releasing the hip adductors and severing their nerve connections.

Although prognosis varies for each type of cerebral palsy, most children with cerebral palsy will live to adulthood, but their life expectancy is less than that of the normal population.[15] Functional prognosis varies greatly from type to type, with hemiplegia and spastic diplegia having a better prognosis than the more severe, rigid types.

Chapter 20 provides detailed information on the specific types or classifications of cerebral palsy, overviews the specific motor and postural problems these children have, and addresses the specific roles and functions of the occupational therapist with these children.

Seizures are another example of a group of neuromuscular conditions whose center of dysfunction is in the brain. A seizure may be defined as a temporary, involuntary change of consciousness, behavior, motor activity, sensation, or automatic functioning. A seizure starts with an excessive rate and hypersynchrony of discharges from a group of cerebral neurons that spreads to the adjoining cells.

Some seizures may be directly attributed to the factor or factors that trigger the seizure. For example, acute factors often described are hypoglycemia, fever, trauma, hemorrhages, tumors, infections, and anoxia.[15,123] Other seizures may be attributed to previous scarring and structural damage or to hormonal changes.[123] Many seizures, especially in children, have no discernible underlying disease and are therefore idiopathic in nature.

Many authors classify seizures by their clinical characteristics or symptoms. With this form of categorization there are four major types of seizures: (1) grand mal seizures that account for 40% to 50% of the total incidence, (2) petit mal seizures that occur 12% to 15% of the time, (3) focal or psychomotor seizures that occur 5% of the time, and (4) mixed-type seizures that account for the remainder of time.[123]

A child having a grand mal seizure may have an aura, or sensation that the seizure is about to begin. This is usually followed by a loss of consciousness during which the body becomes rigid or tonic, and then rhythmical clonic contractions of all the extremities occur. Incontinence is frequent. The seizure may last for 5 minutes followed by a postictal period that may last from 1 to 2 hours in which the child is drowsy or in a deep sleep.[15,123]

Petit mal seizures are characterized by a momentary loss of awareness and no motor activity except eye blinking or rolling. There is no aura, the seizures usually last only 5 to 10 seconds, and there is no postictal period. One important factor to remember with this type of seizure is that they are frequently mistaken for "daydreaming." Petit mal seizures are common in children and in early adolescents, but they are seldom seen after the age of 15.[123]

Psychomotor seizures, or temporal lobe seizures, may consist of tonic-clonic movements, but they also show automatic reactions such as lip smacking, chewing, and buttoning and unbuttoning clothing. In addition, the individual may appear to be confused and disorganized, and he may have sensory experiences such as smelling and tasting items not in the environment and hearing sounds of various types.[15,123]

Minor motor seizures include those found in infancy. The most common type of seizure in infancy is the febrile seizure. This is often a single, brief episode that is precipitated by fever and usually is unassociated with either prior or residual neurological signs or with an abnormal electroencephalogram (EEG).[123]

Two other mild forms of seizures are (1) myoclonic seizures that consist of contractions by single or small groups of muscles and (2) akinetic seizures in which the primary problem is a loss of muscle tone.[15]

A child who has a seizure must undergo a thorough evaluation so that the factors causing the seizure can be determined. A family history, medical history, and developmental history must be completed, as well as an electroencephalogram to help determine the type of seizure.

Anticonvulsive medications are administered in an attempt to control the seizures. In theory these medications increase the intensity required to trigger the seizure or eliminate the recruitment of surrounding cells. Batshaw[15] and Roberts[123] have described some of the common side effects from these anticonvulsive medications: cataracts, weight gain, high blood pressure, pathological fractures, drowsiness, hair loss or gain, nausea, liver damage, vomiting, gum enlargement, hyperactivity, anorexia, and lymphoma-like syndrome. Commonly prescribed medications include: valproic acid (Depakene), phenytoin (Dilantin), phenobarbital, ethosuximide (Zarontin), and carbamazepine (Tegretol).

Implications for occupational therapy

The services provided by occupational therapists to children with neuromuscular problems are steeped in years of tradition. Roles are well established and usually understood and accepted by parents and other professionals. With some of these children the first concern is to provide them with normal sensory and motor experiences. Another important goal is to position and support them so that they may begin to develop specific skills. In other children the focus may be on other aspects of daily functioning, such as selecting leisure activities or learning to drive or selecting activities that will foster vocational development (Chapters 20 and 24).

DEVELOPMENTAL DISABILITIES

This section addresses other developmental disabilities found in childhood, namely, autism, learning disabilities, and mental retardation. In general, the developmental disabilities are characterized by prenatal, perinatal, or early childhood onset, and each disability has the potential to affect all areas of the child's development and to impair the child's performance of many functional tasks and skills.

Autism

Autism is one of the most devastating of the chronic developmental disabilities because of the unusual combinations of sensorimotor and behavioral characteristics displayed by these children.

The National Society for Autistic Children estimates that approximately 5 autistic children are born per 10,000 live births and that four times as many boys as girls are afflicted with the disorder.[11] Autistic children are found in families of all racial, ethnic, intellectual, and socioeconomic backgrounds.[110]

The disorder is complicated by the fact that it often coexists with other problems such as mental retardation, seizure disorders, and a number of diseases associated with organic brain damage. The fact that a large percentage of autistic children also suffer from cognitive deficiencies has been a controversial but relatively accepted issue. For example, Ornitz[110] explains that the cognitive deficiencies exhibited by autistic children are just as real as in mentally retarded children and that 75% of the autistic children can be expected to perform at a retarded level throughout their lives. DeMyer and others[43] state that 70% of these children have IQ scores lower than 35. The National Society for Autistic Children estimates that 60% of all austistic children have IQ scores below 50; 20% have IQ scores between 50 and 70; and 20% have scores of 70 or more.[11]

As mentioned earlier, autism is often seen in conjunction with conditions that are associated with brain damage, including phenylketonuria, congenital rubella, Addison's disease, celiac disease, retrolental fibroplasia, cerebral lipidosis, and infantile spasms.[41,84,121] Seizure disorders also occur in high incidence in autistic children. Both psychomotor and grand mal seizures have been reported in the autistic population.[41,84]

In the almost 40 years since Leo Kanner[27] first identified 11 children as having "extreme autistic aloneness," many theories have been suggested for autism. At first it was hypothesized that the parents' inability to provide appropriate nurture because of their extreme personality types and traits or because of their psychopathies caused the child to withdraw socially and become autistic.[21,36] Next came the theorists who proposed that various hereditary and biological factors were present but that the parents were still at least partially responsible for causing the syndrome.[116] These theorists were followed by ones who focused on the "psychological" problem of the child. During this period autistic children were described under the term *childhood schizophrenia*.[20,61] Today there is general agreement among most researchers that the syndrome of autism is caused by organic brain pathology. However, at this time the location of the exact affected site or sites in the central nervous system is not certain, nor are the factors that cause this organic pathology known.

The behavioral characteristics of autism are usually manifested before 30 months of age and may be categorized into five subclusters.[110] Disturbances in relating to persons and things affect the autistic child's ability to establish meaningful relationships with people and inanimate objects. While abnormalities in this area vary with age and degree of severity, they directly involve interactions that require initiative or reciprocal behavior from the child. Specific behaviors that are observed are poor or deviant eye contact, delayed or total lack of a social smile, apparent aversion to physical contact, delayed or absent anticipatory response to being picked up, and an apparent preference for being alone.[94,110] Disturbances in relating to inanimate objects are often observed during the play of autistic children. Many times a toy or an object is not used in the manner that it was intended but instead is twirled, spun, flicked, tapped, or in other ways manipulated, arranged or rearranged. In addition, the autistic child's use of play materials is often rigid and inflexible; these children seldom demonstrate cooperative and imaginative play.[162]

Disturbances in communication may be thought of as being on a continuum from severe to mild. At the severe end of the continuum appears a complete lack of speech, or mutism. At the other end of the continuum normal language accompanied by only slight articulation or tonal deficits may be seen. Many other communication problems have been described at points along the continuum. For instance, much of the speech of autistic children is repetitive, or echolalic, in nature. Classic echolalia consists of parrotlike repetitions of phrases immediately after the child has been exposed to them, while delayed or deferred echolalia consists of the repetition of phrases at a later time. Echolalic speech occurs out of social context and appears to have little or no communicative value. Other types of speech and language problems include syntax problems, atonal and arrhythmic speech, pronoun reversals, and a lack of inflection and emotion during communication.[118]

Onset can occur at either of two times, as described in the literature: at birth and anytime up to the age of 30 months. But regardless of the time of onset, most autistic children display disturbances of their developmental rate. Specifically, they will show deviations and discontinuities in the normal sequence of motor, language, and social milestones.[55,56] For example, an autistic child may demonstrate the ability to perform one task precociously, such as sitting up, but another motor task, such as pulling to the standing position, may be delayed well past the normal time. Or the child may walk on time but not learn to run until many years later.

Disturbances of motility are considered to be indicative of central nervous system dysfunction in autistic children.[42,120] Deviant motility may involve the arms, hands, trunk, lower extremities, or entire body. Motor patterns in the upper extremities are very common and include wiggling and flicking of fingers, alternating flexion and extension of the fingers, and alternating pronation and supination of the forearm.[120] Other motility patterns often seen include head rolling and banging, body rocking and swaying, lunging and darting movements, toe walking, dystonia of the extremities, involuntary synergies of the head and proximal segments of the limbs, and an inability to perform two motor acts at the same time.[32,42]

Disturbances of sensory processing and perception have been reported in autistic children for almost 20 years. Eric Schopler[135] in 1965 first described the abnormal responses of autistic children to various visual, vestibular, and auditory stimuli. Since then many research studies have attempted to unearth and describe these various dysfunctions by using techniques such as film microanalysis, electronystagmography, sensory-evoked potentials, and many less technical methods.[34]

A. Jean Ayres[13] describes two types of sensory processing problems in autistic children. The first deals with the registration of, or orientation to, sensory input. It appears that in autistic children the neurophysiological processes that decide what sensory stimuli will be brought to their attention are working correctly sometimes but not at others.[13] Therefore they react normally to sensory stimuli one minute, and the next minute (hour or day) they may overreact or underreact to the same stimuli.

The second sensory processing disturbance described by Ayres involves the control or modulation of a stimulus once it has entered the system.[13] Again, the autistic child is believed to be capable of exerting control at times but not at other times, resulting in a child who processes tactile information normally at times and who at other times appears to be the victim of uncontrolled overstimulation—the tactilely defensive child.

While most autistic children have normal life expectancies, the functional prognosis has not been good to date. In 1967 Rutter and Lockyer[130] reported in follow-up studies of autistic children that fewer than 2% were functioning effectively and holding a job in the community; 50% were institutionalized; and the remainder were at home functioning at various levels but needing considerable help from the family. In 1980 Cerreto[30] predicted that about 20% of the autistic children should be capable of making a good social adjustment and able to lead an independent life and work; another 20% will need help in adjusting to life and work; and 60% will remain severely handicapped and be unable to live independently. These prognostic figures may be accurate indicators of the overall potential of these children, or they may simply reflect the state of the art today in diagnosing and treating these children's special problems.

As no one method of treatment has yet proved to be totally effective in treating autism, an interdisciplinary approach is usually selected. The role of the physician on the interdisciplinary team is to make appropriate referrals, offer support to the parents, monitor the child's progress, and often prescribe medications. The medications used with these children are varied: sedatives, stimulants, major and minor tranquilizers, antihistamines, antidepressants, and psychotomimetics.[110] It is felt that these medications work best when used in conjunction with attempts at corrective socialization and special education.[110]

Learning disabilities

Many different labels are used synonymously with the term *learning disabilities*. Some of the more common labels that have been applied are the following:

Minimal brain dysfunction (MBD)
Minimal brain injured (MBI)
Minimal cerebral dysfunction (MCD)
Slow learner
Educationally handicapped
Educationally maladjusted
Special learning disorder
Neurologically handicapped
Neurologically impaired
Perceptually handicapped
Specific language disorder
Dyslexia
Hyperactive child
Attention deficit

Why so many labels? First of all, these terms reflect the jargon of the large number of professionals from both the educational and health fields who have become involved with these children. Also reflected in these terms are the demands, preferences, and restrictions of parental and political groups and agencies.

Defining learning disabilities has been as difficult as labeling the condition. Many "official" definitions are available, but the following definition taken from Public Law 94-142, the Education for All Handicapped Children Act,[158] has been the most influential:

A disorder in one of the more basic psychological processes involved in understanding or in using language, spoken or written, which may manifest itself in an imperfect ability to listen, think, speak, read, write or do mathematical calculations.

The learning disabled child has average or above average intelligence, has adequate sensory acuity (is not blind or deaf), and has been provided with appropriate learning opportunities. In spite of all these positive features, there is a significant discrepancy between the child's academic potential and the child's educational performance.

While different studies and agencies report varying incidence figures, the figure most often given is approximately 10% of the school population. As with autism, more boys than girls are affected, in this instance a 4:1 ratio.[15]

A child with learning disabilities may display any number of the behaviors listed under the following eight categories:[35]

Disorders of motor function include both motor skills and motor activity level. Motor skills dysfunctions may range from clumsiness, to poor performance in gross or fine motor skills, to problems planning new tasks (dyspraxia), to reflex and equilibrium problems, to sensorimotor problems in a number of areas. Occasionally tics, grimaces, and choreoathetoid movements in the hands may be seen. The child may be described as always being in motion (hyperactive) or being slow and lethargic (hypoactive).

Educational disorders can occur in one or more academic subjects. Related educational skills that are often described as being dysfunctional in a learning disabled child are copying from the blackboard, printing and cursive writing, the organization of time and materials, understanding written and oral directions, symbolic confusion (reversals of letters, and so on), cutting, coloring and pasting, and keeping place on the page.

Disorders of attention and concentration include short attention span and other attentional deficits, restlessness, impulsivity, and motor and verbal perseveration.

Characteristics included under *disorders of thinking and memory* are poor ability for abstract reasoning, difficulty with concept formation, and poor short- and long-term memory.

Difficulties with speech and communication may include difficulty shifting topics of conversation and difficulty with "small talk," the sequencing of words, sentences or sounds, slurred words, and articulation errors. Chapter 22 details the various communication disorders found in learning disabled and other types of children.

Auditory difficulties associated with learning disabled children often stem from auditory perceptual and auditory memory problems and not acuity (hearing) problems. Children with these types of problems are often the ones who cannot remember the oral directions just given to them (auditory memory), cannot sound words out or blend sounds into words (phonemic synthesis), cannot block out background noise (speech-in-noise), and who cannot remember the sequencing of sounds, words, or numbers (auditory sequencing). These types of problems often affect school performance and should be explored by an audiologist familiar with the specific instruments and programs that are available to assess and to treat these auditory perceptual (central auditory processing) problems. The high incidence of allergies and ear infections in learning disabled children puts them at risk for auditory perceptual problems.[79,163]

Learning disabled children often have various *sensory integrative and perceptual disorders.* Because the base of support (good tone and cocontraction, integrated reflexes, functional postural and equilibrium reactions, and adequate processing and modulation of sensory output) is weak in many of these children, they are not adequately prepared for various laterality and directionality concepts and tasks that require visual perception skills. Their specific sensory integration problems will be discussed in Chapter 23.

Last but not least, learning disabled children may demonstrate *psychosocial problems* such as throwing temper tantrums or demonstrating antisocial behavior. Their social competencies may be delayed based not only on their ages but also on their intelligence. Many of these children are sensitive and decidedly at risk for poor self-esteem and self-concept problems, because they have the intelligence to know when they are being teased and to know the frustration of being good at some things and not at others.

It appears that a number of factors can cause learning disabilities. In some cases, heredity appears to be a possibility, allergies are another factor, sensory integrative dysfunctions have been found in others, and all the prenatal, perinatal, and early childhood factors that have been mentioned earlier are potential contributors.

The role of the physician in the management of learning disabilities is similar to that with autistic children: referrals are made when special evaluations and services are needed, the child's progress is monitored, parental support and guidance are provided, and, on occasion medications are prescribed to control agitation and hyperactivity.

The prognosis for learning disabled children is the best of all the developmental disabilities. Although most will retain some degree of learning disability as adults, the vast majority will be contributing members of society.[74] As with all disorders, prognosis will be affected by the severity of the disability. Therefore the milder learning disabled persons should not be limited in their life and career skills. But those with severe learning disabilities may need vocational planning and counseling and minor adaptations to ensure as high a level of social, emotional, and vocational functioning as possible.

Mental retardation

The following definition for mental retardation is from Public Law 94-142, the Education for All Handicapped Children Act[158]:

. . . significant subaverage general intellectual functioning existing concurrently with deficits in adaptive behavior and manifested during the developmental period, which adversely affects a child's educational performance.

This means that to be labeled mentally retarded an individual must score 2 or more standard deviations below the mean on a standardized IQ test, the individual must be impaired in the ability to adapt to the environment, and the cause of the mental retardation must have occurred prenatally to age 18 years.

Four degrees of severity are usually given: *mild, moderate, severe,* and *profound.* Figure 6-7 shows the bimodal distribution of intelligence. It also shows the levels of severity as they relate to this distribution. Mildly, or educable, mentally retarded children have an IQ range of 55 to 69. Characteristics include the ability to learn academic skills at the third to seventh grade level and the usual achievement of social and vocational skills adequate to minimal self-support (67% are employed and 80% are married).[123]

Moderately, or trainable, mentally retarded children have an IQ range of 40 to 54. This group is unlikely to progress past the second grade level in academics; they can usually handle routine daily functions and do unskilled or semiskilled work in sheltered workshop conditions. Some type of group home or supervised hous-

ing situation is usually the best placement for these individuals.

Severely retarded children have an IQ range of 25 to 39. These individuals can usually learn to communicate, they can be trained in elemental health habits, and they require supervision to accomplish most tasks.

Profoundly retarded children have IQs below 25. These children need nursing care for basic survival skills. Usually they have minimal capacity for sensorimotor or self-care functioning.

It has been estimated that there are over 300 causes of mental retardation.[53] These causes are usually categorized under the following headings: acquired conditions (toxins, trauma, infection, prematurity); chromosomal problems; multiple congenital anomaly syndromes; central nervous system malformations; neurocutaneous syndromes; and metabolic and endocrine disorders.

Many prenatal, perinatal, and postnatal factors can cause a child to be diagnosed as being mentally retarded. Descriptions of some of the clinical types of mental retardation commonly seen by occupational therapists follow. The trisomy syndromes, as discussed under the birth defects section of this chapter, constitute some of the most common clinical types of mental retardation. Two other quite common clinical types of mental retardation are microcephaly and hydrocephaly. *Microcephalic* children have abnormally small heads, usually resulting from genetic factors or from prenatal factors such as the umbilical cord being wrapped around the head. Because brain weight is also lessened, these children are usually mildly to profoundly retarded.[53] *Hydrocephaly* is caused by a buildup of cerebrospinal fluid in the cerebral ventricles. As the fluid increases, pressure is exerted on the brain and eventually the sections of the skull begin to spread apart, enlarging the diameter of the

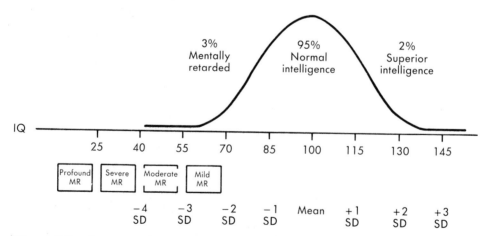

Figure 6-7　Criteria for determining the four degrees of severity in mental retardation.

head. Unchecked, the condition is fatal. However, shunts are now used to remove the excess cerebrospinal fluid from the ventricles, thus minimizing the damage.

Two metabolic disorders also have the potential to cause mental retardation if left undetected and untreated. *Galactosemia* is a recessive, inherited metabolic disorder that prevents the child from converting lactose, a sugar in milk, into glucose, the sugar that can be absorbed and metabolized. Large amounts of lactose in the blood, over a period of time, can cause damage leading to mental retardation.[15,53] *Phenylketonuria* (PKU) is a disorder in which a defective enzyme system prevents phenylalanine, a normal constituent of proteins, from converting to tyrosine.[53] Large accumulations of phenylalanine in the blood can also cause mental retardation. The incidence of galactosemia and PKU has dropped tremendously due to infant screening procedures and early intervention.

Approximately 80% of retarded children have additional problems.[123] For example, it is estimated that approximately 50% have speech problems, 50% have ambulation problems, 20% have seizures, 25% have visual problems, and 40% have chronic conditions such as heart disease, diabetes, anemia, obesity, and dental problems.[123]

The physician's role begins with a history that focuses on gestation, neonatal events, illnesses, and developmental progress.[123] During the physical examination all major and minor abnormalities must be identified to detect the possibility of a syndrome.[123] In addition, laboratory tests such as chromosomal analysis, metabolic tests, and EEGs may be ordered. Referrals for psychological, education, developmental, and speech and hearing evaluation may be made and then interpreted for the parents. Services must be determined, and parents, siblings, and other family members must be given support and advice.

Today the emphasis in the field of mental retardation is toward deinstitutionalization, normalization, and providing mentally retarded individuals with every opportunity to be able to reach their maximal level of functioning in the least restrictive environment.

Implications for occupational therapy

Occupational therapists have been working with mentally retarded and autistic children for many years. What has changed is the expanded number of settings for therapy. Not long ago, mentally regarded children, no matter what their level of functioning, were institutionalized because that is where the services were offered. The same situation was true for autistic children. Today there is a varied continuum of program options available to these children. These options are offered not only by institutions but also by private developmental centers, public and private schools, governmental agencies, and parent and professional groups.

The most recent developmental disability to be of concern to occupational therapists is learning disability. Today a substantial percentage of occupational therapists work with learning disabled children in school-based practice (Chapters 21, 23, and 27).

RESPIRATORY PROBLEMS

This section discusses three major chronic respiratory conditions found in children. In addition, it discusses otitis media, which, while located in the ear, often accompanies upper respiratory infections, colds, and allergic conditions.

Selected diseases and conditions
CYSTIC FIBROSIS

Cystic fibrosis (CF) is an autosomal recessive inherited disorder in which the mucus secreted by various exocrine glands becomes abnormally thick and sticky.[115] Exactly what causes these changes is unknown. Cystic fibrosis is found almost exclusively in Caucasians and has an incidence of approximately 1 in 2,000 live births.[15]

Chronic pulmonary disease is the most serious complication of cystic fibrosis.[123] A chronic cough, wheezing, lower respiratory infections, abscesses and cysts, hemoptysis, and recurrent pneumothorax are all examples of the serious pulmonary complications that develop in cystic fibrosis. Other complications often related to cystic fibrosis are: clubbing of the fingers resulting from hypoxemia, nasal polyps, and enlargement of the right side of the heart (right ventricular hypertrophy), which may eventually cause heart failure.[44]

Pancreatic insufficiency causes characteristic foul smelling and greasy stools. Associated problems include malabsorption; clinical diabetes; deficiencies of vitamins A, E, and K; and gastrointestinal obstruction.[123]

In the liver, bile ducts often become blocked, resulting in destruction of cells behind the blocked ducts. While this is a serious problem, a positive point is that children's livers are often capable of regeneration.

In the female reproductive system the ovaries are not affected, and the child does not become infertile, but problems are commonly found with the cervical mucous glands. In the male the testes are not affected, but sterility does occur often because sperm cannot travel through the vas deferens.

Also in cystic fibrosis the sodium absorption inhibiting factor is affected, which causes excessive amounts of sodium chloride to be secreted from the sweat glands onto the skin. This phenomenon provides important diagnostic information that is often gathered in two vastly different but important ways. First, mothers often detect that their children taste salty when they kiss them. This alerts the physician who will perform the simple diagnostic test known as the "sweat test." In this test an electrode is placed on the skin, causing the child to sweat at the contact site. A sample of the sweat is taken. If excessive levels of sodium chloride are detected, the diagnosis is made.[123]

Medical management consists of vigorous antibiotic, enzyme, and vitamin therapy and sound nutritional counseling. In an effort to keep the lungs as free as possible, the following physical or respiratory therapy techniques may be employed: mist tent therapy, intermittent positive pressure breathing, aerosol therapy, and postural drainage techniques.[123]

One of the promising procedures for the future is the heart-lung transplant. Today, this procedure is used only with the chronic CF patients who are in a life-threatening situation. However, as the heart-lung transplant is perfected it is expected to be used more frequently.

The prognosis for cystic fibrosis is not good. Some of these children die in infancy, while others may do relatively well until adolescence, when there is some evidence that girls do more poorly than boys.[91,146] The life spans of children with cystic fibrosis are slowly lengthening as a result of improved maintenance techniques; however, many CF children still die before they are 20 years old.

OTITIS MEDIA

Otitis media is one of the most common infections in children. Approximately 30% of all children in the age range of 6 to 36 months show evidence of middle ear problems.[80] In otitis media the eustachian tube usually becomes blocked and fluid forms in the middle ear. One of the following organisms is usually found: pneumococcus, hemophilus influenzae, or streptococcus. Milder cases of otitis media may go undetected. However, the following symptoms often accompany this condition: pain, a sense of fullness in the ear, a low-grade fever, vertigo, nausea, and loss of balance.[102,123]

Investigators studying the long-term effects of otitis media have suggested possible language and cognitive delays,[163] hearing loss,[79] and central auditory processing problems.[79,163] Of special interest to occupational therapists is the possible relationship between otitis media and vestibular disorders. Although further research is necessary to verify this relationship, initial data warrant considering vestibular dysfunctions as possible contributors to some of the developmental delays found in children with otitis media.[133]

The goal of medical treatment is to eradicate the organisms, clear the fluids, and prevent chronic serous otitis media.[23] This is accomplished by the administration of antibiotics such as penicillin, ampicillin, amoxicillin, or sulfonamides.[23] The insertion of tym-

panostomy tubes may be necessary in more chronic cases of otitis media.

ASTHMA

Asthma is characterized by bronchial hyperreactivity that causes airway constriction in the lower respiratory tract and reported bouts of wheezing. Roberts[123] reported that approximately 5% of the boys and 3% of the girls under 15 years age suffer from hay fever or asthma.

Many factors can cause the wheezing. If it is evoked by external factors, such as dust, it is called *extrinsic asthma*, and if it is evoked by internal stimuli, such as infection, it is called *intrinsic asthma*. In many instances a multifactorial etiology exists, which consists of environmental sensitivity and familial predisposition.

Status asthmaticus is a serious asthmatic condition in which normal outpatient assistance does not improve the condition and emergency medical intervention is needed.

Treatment for asthma may include environmental control measures, skin testing, immunotherapy for allergies, emotional support, and usually a combination of two classes of pharmacological agents: methylxanthine and beta-adrenergic agonists.[31]

TUBERCULOSIS OF THE LUNGS

Tuberculosis of the lungs is one of the oldest diseases reported to be found in humans. It is an infectious disease caused when the tubercle bacillus is inhaled into the lungs. Symptoms include fatigue, a persistent cough, hemoptysis, and chest pain.[152] Lesions occur in one or more lobes of the lungs. It is not uncommon for individual lesions to heal by calcification, thus allowing the disease to go into an inactive or arrested stage.[152]

A number of different tuberculin tests may be performed that indicate whether an individual has ever been infected or exposed to tubercle bacillus. However, these tests do not reveal whether the infection is currently active or inactive. These tests consist of applying tuberculin to the skin directly or intradermally and then watching for a local inflammatory reaction within 48 to 72 hours or 48 to 96 hours, depending on the test administered. Diagnosis may also be done through the examination of sputum samples and through chest x-ray films.

Treatment consists of chemotherapy using medications such as ethambutol, isoniazid (INH), para-aminosalicylic acid (PAS), or streptomycin.[123] Bed rest and nutritional counseling may also be recommended. In advanced cases various surgical procedures may be required.

While tuberculosis is not as prevalent as it was 20 years ago, it is still found in certain parts of the country and is more prevalent among certain populations, such as American Indians.

Implications for occupational therapy

Occupational therapy involvement with children with respiratory problems may occur at two different levels. At the secondary level the occupational therapist must be aware of complications, signs, and symptoms and possibly adjust some treatment methods. This situation would occur in those cases where the respiratory situation was secondary and probably an acute problem to the patient's major handicapped condition. Many days of treatment are missed because of respiratory illnesses.

On a primary level of involvement the occupational therapist might be directly involved in the treatment of the respiratory condition or disease. This might involve the implementation of activities to improve respiratory output, help with energy conservation, or direct concern with deficit self-care, play, and leisure activities or work tasks.

CONGENITAL CARDIAC DEFECTS

This section discusses the major cardiovascular conditions found in the neonatal and early childhood periods of life. Congenital heart defects are second only to problems concerned with prematurity when the leading causes of death in pediatric hospitals are determined.[81]

Patent ductus arteriosus (PDA) was discussed earlier in the perinatal section of this chapter. The other major types of congenital heart conditions will be described here. They are atrial septal defects, ventricular septal defects, tetralogy of Fallot, and transposition of the great vessels. In addition, rheumatic fever will be discussed, because it is one of the most serious cardiac illnesses found in children.

Atrial septal defects

When an opening in the septum between the right and left atrial chambers occurs, it is called an atrial septal defect (ASD) (Figure 6-8). This opening may be of any size and can occur anywhere along the septum. As a result, when the left atrium contracts, blood is sent into the right atrium. This is called a left-to-right shunt and causes more blood than normal to be sent to the lungs, resulting in "wet lungs," a condition that makes the lungs more susceptible to upper respiratory infections. This also causes the right atrium, and especially the right ventricle, to work much harder, and it can eventually cause heart failure in the older child. Other symptoms include poor exercise tolerance and the appearance of being thin and small for age. Information for diagnosis is gathered from listening to the characteristics of the murmur, evaluating chest x-ray films and electrocardiograms, and administering heart catheterization.

Surgical procedures are not routinely done until the

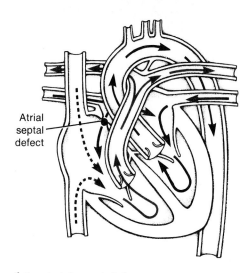

Figure 6-8 Atrial septal defect.

From Whaley L, and Wong D: Nursing care of infants and children, ed 2, St. Louis, 1983, The CV Mosby Co.

child is 4 or 5 years of age. Until that time, the child is closely watched for complications, especially signs of heart failure.

Ventricular septal defects

Ventricular septal defects (VSD) are the most common type of congenital cardiac malformations and are often more serious than atrial septal defects.[123] This type of defect consists of a hole or opening in the muscular or membranous portions of the ventricular septum (Figure 6-9).

Etiological factors are often idiopathic, but congenital infections, various teratogenic agents, and genetic predisposition may also contribute to the cause.[49]

In these defects the blood flows from the left ventricle to the right ventricle, a left-to-right shunt, and as in an atrial septal defect, an increased amount of blood is pumped to the lungs. The defect is considered more serious if the opening is in the membranous section of the septum, because the size of the hole is not, at least somewhat, diminished during contraction as happens in openings in the muscular part of the septum.

Symptoms associated with this defect include feeding problems, shortness of breath and increased perspiration, fatigue during physical activity, increased incidences of respiratory infections, and delayed growth.

As in atrial septal defects, the diagnosis is based on the murmur, chest x-ray film results, electrocardiograms, and heart catheterization. In these defects improvement often occurs after 6 months of age, and over 50% of the cases correct themselves by the age of 5 years.[38] However, if the extent of damage is great, or if the hole does not repair itself, surgical procedures to

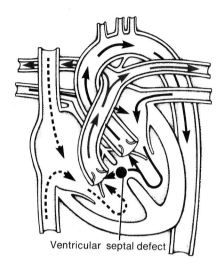

Figure 6-9 Ventricular septal defect.

From Whaley L, and Wong D: Nursing care of infants and children, ed 2, St Louis, 1983, The CV Mosby Co.

close the defect may need to be undertaken early in the child's life.

Careful monitoring of these children must occur to prevent the life-threatening situation known as Eisenmenger's complex. In this situation pulmonary vascular obstruction has occurred as a result of prolonged exposure to increased blood flow and high pressure. Eventually the heart is no longer capable of pumping against the increased pulmonary pressure, and blood pools in the right ventricle. This poses a medical emergency, requiring immediate surgical intervention.

The prognosis for infants with ventricular septal defects continues to improve as both surgical techniques and management of heart failure progress.[123]

Tetralogy of Fallot

As the name implies, there are four different problems associated with tetralogy of Fallot: (1) pulmonary valve or artery stenosis plus (2) ventricular septal defect present prenatally causing (3) a right ventricular hypertrophy, and (4) overriding of the ventricular septum by the aorta[123] (Figure 6-10).

The etiological factors are probably similar to those described under ventricular septal defects, but it is felt that they must occur in the early weeks of fetal development when the right ventricle is at a critical stage.[78]

Physiologically the unoxygenated blood that is returning from the body cannot easily exit to the lungs because of the pulmonary stenosis. Instead, it takes two paths of least resistance: the defect, creating a right-to-left shunt, and the aorta.

Symptoms include central cyanosis, coagulation defects, clubbing of fingers and toes, feeding difficulties, failure to thrive, dyspnea, and "tet" spells during which the child suddenly squats to his knees. It is believed

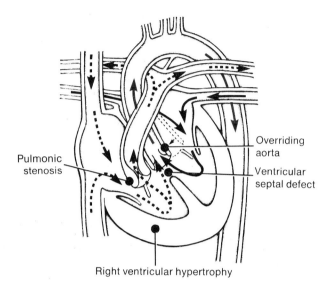

Figure 6-10 Tetralogy of Fallot.

From Whaley L, and Wong D: Nursing care of infants and children, ed 2, St Louis, 1983, The CV Mosby Co.

that this squatting action raises systemic vascular resistance and decreases the shunting.[78]

Diagnosis is usually based on cyanosis; analysis of the heart murmur; right ventricular hypertrophy and right axis deviation demonstrated on the electrocardiogram; a chest x-ray film revealing the characteristic "boot-shaped heart"; and echocardiography demonstrating the overriding aorta.[78,123]

Management consists of medication to reduce the frequency and severity of the "tet" spells.[123] Surgery is ideally delayed as long as possible. In severe cases a temporary shunt may be put in to bypass the stenosis. Later, "total correction" surgery is done in which the pulmonary outflow obstruction is removed, the VSD is closed, and the aorta may be enlarged.

As with VSD, prognosis is improving as techniques and maintenance improve. Operative mortality has been reduced to 20%,[123] but surgery is still a dangerous and complicated procedure.

Transposition of the great vessels

Transposition of the great vessels involves the anatomical transfer of the great arteries. Severity depends on the amount of mixing between the two sides of circulation.[81] This can be accomplished by coexisting congenital cardiac defects, such as a VSD, or a pulmonary stenosis, or congenital transposition of the ventricles, called *corrected transposition*.[123] The severity of the symptoms varies, but cyanosis, congestive heart failure, and respiratory distress are common.

Diagnosis may be helped by the use of echocardiography, which can help identify the transposition, and by heart catheterization.

Treatment techniques include enlarging the foramen ovale by inserting a catheter with a balloon tip through the foramen ovale and into the left atrium. Next the catheter is pulled back through the foramen ovale to enlarge it, thus increasing the flow of oxygenated blood to the right atrium.[123] Another procedure involves excising the atrial septum and inserting a patch that redirects the blood flow. A third technique that is very new involves severing the great vessels at their bases and reattaching them to the proper ventricles.[123]

Rheumatic fever

Acute rheumatic fever occurs from 2 to 4 weeks after an acute infection of streptococcal pharyngitis. The incidence of rheumatic fever has been greatly reduced in the past century but should still be considered a potentially dangerous condition.

School-aged children are most frequently affected, especially following a streptococcal pharyngitis epidemic. Rheumatic fever usually begins with one of the following serious symptoms: carditis, polyarthritis, or chorea.[123]

As there is no laboratory test specific for diagnosing rheumatic fever, a combination of factors from the following diagnostic criteria must be substantiated:[47]

Minor criteria	Major criteria
Clinical	Carditis
Arthralgia	Polyarthritis
Fever	Erythema marginatum
History of infection in recent weeks	Chorea
	Subcutaneous nodules
Lab	
Increased erythrocyte sedimentation rate	
Presence of C-reactive protein (CRP)	

Treatment consists of prescribing bed rest plus administering antibodies (usually penicillin) and antiinflammatory agents. Most patients will take penicillin from the time of diagnosis until approximately 15 to 20 years of age as a preventive measure to prevent recurrence. It appears that a high percentage of children who experienced carditis during the first phase of rheumatic fever will experience future heart problems.[123]

Implications for occupational therapy

As in the case of respiratory conditions, the involvement of occupational therapy in congenital cardiac defects may be direct or indirect. For example, congenital heart defects are often found as secondary diagnoses in handicapped children. Children with Down syndrome or other types of mental retardation and multiply handicapped children may have histories of congenital heart problems. In these cases occupational

therapists must be aware of the associated signs, symptoms, treatment procedures, and medications to watch for complications and for the effect of these conditions on the child's functioning.

Direct involvement might include participation on a pediatric rehabilitation team. In this instance, the occupational therapist would be concerned with physical restoration as well as the monitoring of various developmental and functional skills.

HEMATOLOGICAL PROBLEMS
Selected diseases and disorders

The following selected blood diseases and disorders found in children are reviewed in this section: iron deficiency anemia, sickle-cell anemia, hemophilia, idiopathic thrombocytopenic purpura, Tay-Sachs disease, thalassemia, and acquired immune deficiency syndrome (AIDS).

IRON DEFICIENCY ANEMIA

Iron deficiency anemia is the most frequent blood condition in infancy and childhood. Iron is an essential part of the hemoglobin module and when it is deficient, problems may occur. Children with this condition are most often asymptomatic, but may be pale in appearance, irritable, listless, and may have some growth delays and feeding difficulties. The primary cause of iron deficiency anemia is dietary. The diagnosis is usually made easily with office screening procedures that are routinely conducted because of the high incidence of this condition within the pediatric population.

In the young child, treatment consists of giving the child iron-enriched cereals and formulas. Breast milk contains easily absorbed iron while whole milk has insufficient iron and must be supplemented. The older child should be given a diet rich in foods containing a high amount of iron such as liver, beans, peas, and whole grain cereals.

SICKLE-CELL ANEMIA

Sickle-cell anemia is a hereditary, chronic form of anemia in which abnormal sickle, or crescent-shaped, erythrocytes are present that contain an abnormal type of hemoglobin called Hemoglobin S.[142] In the United States most cases occur in black Americans, of whom 1 in 10 are carriers of the trait, and 1 in every 400 to 600 black neonates have the disease.[122] Sickle-cell is rare in Caucasians but can be found in people of Hispanic, Middle Eastern, and Mediterranean ancestry.

It is now possible to determine this condition in the newborn. A few states already require sickle-cell screening for all neonates and more states are considering this course of action.

The clinical course of children with sickle-cell anemia is interspersed with episodes of severe worsening called *sickle-cell crises* that can be grouped into four types.[142] *Aplastic* and *hyperhemolytic* crises are characterized by imbalances in the production and premature destruction of red blood cells. These may cause the hemoglobin to decrease by 50%, necessitating immediate transfusions. *Sequestrian crises* consist of the sudden and rapid enlargement of the spleen. This type of sickle-cell anemia traps much of the blood volume and can possibly cause shock or death. Painful, or *vaso-occlusive crises* are characterized by pain in the hands, feet, toes, and abdomen.

Sickle-cell anemia affects other organs as well. Lungs may become infected, and hypoxemia is common; liver and kidney involvement causes urine problems and hematuria; cerebrovascular accidents may occur; the legs develop ulcers; and spleen damage can leave the child defenseless against major infections.[142]

Medical management is limited to the treatment of symptoms: transfusions, antibiotic therapy, and making the child comfortable. Recently the use of penicillin has been reported to reduce the risk of life-threatening infections. Overall prognosis is poor, since this is a disease that is both physically painful and potentially emotionally crippling.[123]

HEMOPHILIA

The hemophilias are characterized by greatly prolonged coagulation time (clotting) that results in abnormal bleeding. They are sex-linked hereditary disorders and occur almost exclusively in males.[142]

There are two major types. Hemophilia A, or classic hemophilia, is caused by a deficiency of a factor in plasma necessary for blood coagulation. This factor has been called factor VIII, antihemophilic globulin, and antihemophilic factor.[152] Hemophilia B (Christmas disease) results from a deficiency of clotting factor IX.

Symptoms are not usually noticeable or bothersome until near the end of the first year of life, then soft tissue hemorrhages begin to occur. The intracranial hemorrhage is one of the most dreaded and serious complications of hemophilia. Bleeding into joints (hemarthrosis) can cause severe musculoskeletal problems that can lead to joint deterioration if untreated. The following procedures can be used to protect the joints: blood can be drained from a joint; chemical agents can be injected into the joint; and a specific preventive range of motion activities can be initiated. Surgical procedures, such as joint replacements or synovectomies contain some element of risk for hemophiliac patients.[122]

Soft tissue hemorrhages and hemarthroses are treated at home by replacing the missing factor to a level that will again control the bleeding. This is called *replacement therapy,* and most children can be trained to administer their own infusions.

The prognosis is steadily improving for this disease. Life expectancy used to be 20 to 30 years; it has now lengthened to 52 years.

IDIOPATHIC THROMBOCYTOPENIC PURPURA

The central problem in idiopathic thrombocytopenic purpura (ITP) is the fact that the blood plate-lets are being destroyed faster than they can be produced. Simply stated, patients with this disease develop antibodies that destroy their own platelets.

About one half of the children with idiopathic thrombocytopenic purpura have had an infectious illness within 6 weeks of the diagnosis. These cases have a better prognosis, with 90% recovering.[152] Symptoms include bleeding from the mouth and skin when injured, intracranial hemorrhage, increased clotting time, and hemorrhages in internal organs.[93] Treatment with corticosteroids may help, but these agents have long-range side effects. Platelet transfusions and splenectomy are used as emergency procedures.

While most patients recover to the point that they may not demonstrate symptoms, their bodies often continue to destroy platelets but at a level that is matched by increased bone marrow production.[123]

TAY-SACHS DISEASE

Tay-Sachs disease is a degenerative nervous system disorder caused by the absence of an enzyme usually found in the blood called hexosaminidase A. This enzyme converts GM_2 ganglioside, a product of nerve cell metabolism, into a nontoxic substance. As this is not happening in Tay-Sachs disease, the toxic substance builds up in the brain and other body organs and leads to brain damage.

This disorder is common in Jewish persons whose ancestry can be traced to the Mediterranean region.[15] Today nearly 1 out of every 10 American Jews carry the Tay-Sachs gene.[15] As Tay-Sachs is an autosomal recessive trait, both parents must be carriers of the abnormal gene for the disease to be passed to the child.

Children with Tay-Sachs disease appear healthy at birth and seem to develop normally until about 6 months of age at which time they begin to deteriorate.[15] Within the next 3 to 5 years the children lose motor functioning, become profoundly mentally retarded, become blind and deaf, and often suffer seizures.[15] Death occurs usually no later than 5 years of age.

Carriers of Tay-Sachs disease can be detected by a simple blood test. In addition, through amniocentesis, the disease can be detected in the fetus by examining the amniotic fluid for the presence of hexosaminidase A. These tests, in addition to the relatively small and well-defined population in which the disease is primarily found, make Tay-Sachs disease hypothetically a preventable condition.[123]

Prevention becomes even more important when it is remembered that there is no cure. Treatment procedures can only make the child as comfortable as possible until death occurs. Research efforts are focusing on a number of treatment approaches that may someday offer help for these children. For example, the search continues for a substance that could substitute for the hexosaminidase A or for a procedure to graft healthy cells into Tay-Sachs patients so that the transplanted cells could produce hexosaminidase A. Research is also progressing on gene transplantation from normal into defective cells. Until an effective treatment is found, the best strategy is prevention through genetic counseling.

THALASSEMIA

Thalassemia is one of the most common inherited hematological diseases. It is an autosomal recessive trait affecting primarily those of Greek or Italian descent.[15]

In this disease the red blood cells are characteristically misshapen and lack normal amounts of hemoglobin. A blood test can determine if an individual carries the abnormal gene. In addition, this condition can also be detected prenatally through the use of amniocentesis.

This disease has a mild to severe continuum. As in Tay-Sachs disease, the children appear healthy at birth but during the first year or two they become pale and listless, develop poor appetites, and have frequent infections; their bones become thin and brittle; and facial bones take on a characteristic look.[15] As the condition worsens, the spleen, liver, and other organs enlarge. Many children require surgery to remove the spleen, and they require many blood transfusions. There is no cure for the disease at this time. As with Tay-Sachs disease, the hope lies in prevention and research.

ACQUIRED IMMUNE DEFICIENCY SYNDROME

A relatively new and very serious disease that is being transmitted to children is *acquired immune deficiency syndrome* (AIDS). AIDS is a disease that infects and damages cells of the immune system, thus making the child vulnerable to life-threatening illnesses that do not affect children with normal immunity. The virus that causes AIDS and AIDS-related complex (ARC) has had several different names including human T-lymphotrophic virus (HTLV), lymphadenopathy-associated virus (LAV), and most recently human immunodeficiency virus (HIV).

T-4 lymphocytes are the type of white blood cells primarily affected by the AIDS virus. This type of lymphocyte is primarily made up of helper cells and inducer cells which, when diminished, lessen the body's abilities to carry out normal immune responses. Once the AIDS virus has infected some cells it has the ability to lie dormant for weeks to years while the infected person remains healthy and apparently free of symptoms.

Some persons infected with AIDS develop AIDS-related complex (ARC), which includes symptoms such as swollen glands, fever, chills, diarrhea, weight loss, fatigue, dizziness, night sweats, dry cough, unexplained bleeding from any body opening or from growths on the skin or mucous membranes, and signs of unexplained confusion and disorientation.[4,107,141] It is not known at this time what percentage of persons with ARC will develop AIDS.

Persons with the AIDS disease itself have symptoms similar to those with ARC. In addition, they often develop other problems such as rare, fatal diseases. For example, the HIV virus may attack the central nervous system causing severe motor problems such as ataxia and paraplegia. Many AIDS patients develop bacterial infections as well as a parasitic infection of the lungs called *Pneumocystic carinii pneumonia* (PCP).[4,107,141] This infection is almost never seen outside of patients with immune disorders. PCP shows a good response to antibiotic treatment but the patient often must stay on the antibiotics for long periods of time to prevent relapses.[4] Herpes simplex and cytomegalovirus are two other serious viruses commonly found in AIDS patients.

Certain types of cancers are also found in persons with AIDS. A rare skin cancer, Kaposi's sarcoma, causes purplish nodules and patches to appear on the skin and inside the mouth, nose, or eyelids. Additional problems develop in the gut and lungs.[4,141] Other types of cancers in AIDS patients include: lymphomas, carcinomas of the lung, and an unusual type of cancer of the rectum.[1,8]

Most children contract AIDS from their infected mothers before or during the birth process. In one case AIDS was probably caused by infected breast milk[2,8] and a few cases of infection through transfusion of blood or blood products were reported prior to the screening now done on all blood products.[2,8] The specific symptomatology found in infants and children with AIDS varies slightly from the adult form. Symptoms usually begin to appear at about 5 months of age; however, cases have been reported with children as young as 1 month and as old as 21 months.[128] Most of the infants appear chronically ill with failure to thrive, infections, hepatosplenomegaly, and diarrhea.[2,8,107,138] Other common symptoms include persistent oral infections, pneumonia (PCP), otitis media, and rashes. It appears that, unlike adults, children rarely develop Kaposi sarcoma.[139]

Medical treatment of AIDS in children is complicated by the multiplicity and severity of the problems. A variety of drugs are used to fight the various infections. Monthly administration of gammaglobulin has appeared to help improve immunologic test results and decrease the incidence of bacterial and viral infections in some children.[10] Also, intravenous alimentation may be needed to correct nutritional problems.[139]

The prognosis for children with AIDS appears poor at this time. The course of the syndrome is rapid; many children die within 2 years of onset.

Implications for occupational therapy

Advances in the medical treatment of hematological diseases, conditions, and disorders have helped to reduce the long-term biological effects. This fact has changed the overall role of occupational therapy with this population.

Fewer of the children require orthopedic equipment such as splints and adaptive equipment. Careful monitoring can be done of the child's biophysical development in general; in particular, the range of motion in joints, strength, asymmetrical changes, and pain can be monitored. Families may need help in selecting appropriate play and leisure activities that facilitate maximal activity levels in the child.

An exception to this positive trend is AIDS. The incidence of AIDS is projected to escalate within the coming years presenting a challenge of great proportions to all health care and medical personnel. Much work must be done to determine what assessments will be most effective in determining the specific problems of these children and their families. Next, treatment techniques will have to be validated for this population. Last, but certainly not least, occupational therapists working with these children will have to confront and overcome their own fears and misconceptions about death and dying and about this disease itself, at least in these early years of research into its etiology and control.

NEOPLASTIC DISORDERS

Cancer, somehow, seems even more insidious when it attacks children. This section will discuss some of the major cancers of children and young adults.

Acute lymphoblastic leukemia

Leukemia is the most common neoplastic disease of childhood, occurring in 3 to 4 children per 100,000, with a peak incidence between 2 to 6 years. The cause is unknown, but changes in gene structure, viruses, and various environmental teratogens are all being studied as possible etiological factors.

Acute lymphoblastic leukemia (ALL) is characterized by the uncontrolled multiplication of immature white blood cells, which prevents the bone marrow from producing normal blood cells.[123] Symptoms include loss of weight; night sweats; chronic fatigue; paleness; a high fever; repeated infections; purpura; and enlarged lymph nodes, spleen, and liver. Diagnosis is usually made by examining a specimen of bone marrow for lymphoblasts. Blood counts are also taken.

The goal of medical management is the achievement of complete "cure" by inducing remission, eliminating cells in "sanctuaries" like the central nervous system, and maintaining the remission.[123] Specifically, treatment is conducted in three phases. The first phase is called *induction therapy* and is designed to rid the bone marrow and the rest of the body of the leukemia cells. The second phase is called *central nervous system prophylaxis* and is aimed at killing cells in the brain and spinal cord. The third phase of treatment is called *maintenance therapy* in which chemotherapy is administered to treat small deposits of cells that remain after remission.[114]

Prognosis is much improved over previous years, with the majority of patients going into remission for at least 5 years. Many go long periods of time with no recurrent signs.[123]

Wilms' tumor

Wilms' tumor is the most common abdominal neoplasm in children, with an incidence of 1 in 10,000 to 15,000 live births. Peak incidence is at 3¼ years.[123]

Sonography may help to distinguish a tumor from a fluid-filled cyst. If a tumor is found to exist, surgery should be performed as soon as possible. This is followed by radiation and a chemotherapeutic regimen.[123]

Prognosis is now favorable for recovery, with even the most involved level of cases having a 50% cure rate.[123]

Hodgkin's disease in children

The highest peak of incidence of Hodgkin's disease in children is between 5 and 8 years, with a second peak in the mid-teens. Cause is unknown, but a viral agent is suspected.

The presenting problem is often an enlarged but painless cervical node. Other symptoms include fever, chills, night sweats, and weight loss.[100,152]

A histological examination of the node reveals the presence of Reed-Sternberg cells if Hodgkin's disease is present. A clinical examination may detect an enlarged liver and spleen. Diagnosis is based on the extent of the disease, as is prognosis. Treatment consists of radiotherapy and chemotherapy.

Implications for occupational therapy

While the prognosis for many childhood cancers is good, even the most hopeful situation is a crisis for the child and the family. Many times the diagnostic and treatment procedures have side effects that are physically and psychologically devastating.

If the child's condition is terminal, the situation is even more difficult. In our culture death is not only unexpected in childhood but it is also considered an unnatural event. Occupational therapy has a significant role to play with a child who is dying, the family, and significant others in the child's life (Chapter 28).

ENDOCRINE DISORDERS AND CONDITIONS

The hormones secreted by the endocrine glands enter the bloodstream and travel to a second site where they have a specific effect on a body organ or another gland. In children the endocrine glands have an effect on metabolism, growth, sexual maturity, and stress control. This section provides an overview of the endocrine conditions and disorders commonly seen in children.

Type I diabetes

Type I diabetes* (juvenile diabetes, growth onset diabetes mellitus, or insulin-dependent diabetes) is a chronic metabolic disorder resulting from an extremely low level of insulin production or no production at all. This type of diabetes is found in children and young adults. A large number of children seem to develop the disorder at 10 or 11 years of age.

The exact cause of Type I diabetes is unknown. It appears, however, that genetic predisposition plays a role, as does infection. One hypothesis is that the beta cells of the pancreas are damaged as a result of virus infections. It has been noted that newly diagnosed cases of Type I diabetes rise as the number of cases of viral infections rise at various times of the year.

Early symptoms include increased voiding, increased thirst, and dehydration. Later symptoms include acidosis, vomiting, hyperventilation, and eventually coma.

The general goals of treatment are to ensure satisfactory growth, ensure emotional development, help the child acquire some degree of normal life, resolve the symptoms, prevent ketoacidosis, and prevent long-term sequelae, such as renal and cardiac damage and eye disease.[46,158] The achievement of these goals is very difficult because it depends on maintaining a delicate balance between so many factors: exercise, nutritional intake, hormones, emotions, and many other internal and external influences on blood sugar levels.

Effect on growth and metabolism

Following stimulation by the hypothalamus, the pituitary gland secretes the thyroid-stimulating hormone (TSH) into the bloodstream. This hormone stimulates the thyroid gland to produce thyroxine, a hormone that affects body growth, metabolism, and brain growth. If the thyroid gland secretes too little thyroxine, brain development may be hampered during the critical prenatal and infant periods of life. Later in development body growth may decrease or stop, and the child may develop dry skin, become constipated, and show a decreased heart rate.

To prevent, or at least minimize, the effects of thyroid deficiency, early diagnosis is critical. Today many states have mandated screening for this deficiency during the first few days of life. Once the

deficiency is found, the children are given daily dosages of thyroxine for as long as they continue to show a deficiency.

On the other hand, an overproduction of thyroxine can cause sleeplessness, diarrhea, and a slight tremor in the upper extremities and increase in appetite with no weight gain. Growth is usually not affected in this condition. Treatment consists of the administration of a medication that blocks the production of thyroxine. In extreme cases surgery may be used to remove part or all of the thyroid gland, thus reducing the production of thyroxine. The child can then be given correct dosages of thyroxine on a daily basis.

Also influencing the growth of the child is a growth hormone that is produced in the pituitary gland. If this hormone is deficient or absent, growth is slowed or stopped and deviations appear on growth charts. Treatment consists of injections of a similar hormone taken directly from human cadavers or from pigs, as the hormone cannot yet be synthesized. In fact, this hormone is in such scarcity that dissemination is controlled by the National Pituitary Center, and children who qualify for the program are treated only until they reach a height of 5 feet, 6 inches.

Effect on sexual maturity

The hypothalamus stimulates the pituitary gland, which in turn stimulates the testes to produce testosterone and the ovaries to produce estrogen. Both these hormones accelerate growth of the bones, assist in the fusion of the growth plate, and contribute to the development of secondary sex characteristics. These hormones can be deficient or excessive. A balance can be achieved through medication and hormone administration.

Reaction to stress

Another example of an endocrine gland is the adrenal gland. The same cycle begins with the hypothalamus stimulating the pituitary gland, which in turn stimulates the adrenal gland to secrete dopamine, norepinephrine, and epinephrine.[123] These agents affect other organs as well by providing negative feedback to the pituitary gland to stop the secretion of the adrenocorticotropic hormone. The purpose of this particular cycle is to help the body deal with stressful situations.

Implications for occupational therapy

Advances in medical treatment have reduced the need for most of these children to receive occupational therapy. But therapists must be familiar with signs and symptoms, treatment techniques, and possible side effects of these techniques in case a child has or develops any conditions as secondary problems during therapy for other problems.

*This type is insulin-dependent diabetes, which differs from Type II diabetes, or non-insulin-dependent diabetes.

GASTROINTESTINAL AND RENAL CONDITIONS

This section discusses the major disorders and diseases of the gastrointestinal and renal systems in children.

Crohn's disease

Crohn's disease is a chronic, inflammatory disorder of the intestinal tract that is accompanied by the formation of granulomas, fistulas, abscesses, and perianal disease. Pain and bloody diarrhea are also present. The cause is unknown.[123]

Treatment consists of anti-inflammatory agents, steroids, a bowel management program, and psychological support.[123] Surgery does not reverse the damage, but 80% of all patients face surgery at one time or other. Recurrence is virtually assured.[39]

Renal failure

Acute renal failure (ARF) of the kidney may be a result of trauma, toxins, temporary obstruction, or decreased blood flow to the kidney. Treatment for the underlying cause and temporary dialysis should eliminate the problem.

Chronic renal failure (CRF) is a permanent, progressive reduction in renal function. Renal diseases, such as focal glomerular sclerosis and membranoproliferative nephritis, or systemic disorders, such as systemic lupus erythematosus and vasculitis, may cause chronic renal failure.[123]

The uremic syndrome refers to the group of symptoms caused by reduced renal functioning and compensatory behaviors. It includes acidosis, dermatological changes, gastrointestinal problems, changes in the eyes, cardiac problems, neurological changes, and bleeding.[3]

Treatment centers on dialysis and transplantation. The much publicized problem with transplantation is finding a donor in time. The irony is that the technique has been perfected to the point that 75% of the kidneys transplanted into children function well for at least 3 to 5 years.[123]

Biliary atresia and neonatal hepatitis

Biliary atresia appears soon after birth and usually involves a restriction of the bile duct, not a complete closure as the name implies. It is now believed that there is a relationship between this condition and neonatal hepatitis. It is believed that some insult or pathogen produces a self-limiting disease in some infants (neonatal hepatitis) and a potentially fatal disease in others (biliary atresia).[123]

Most cases of both diseases are idiopathic but various viral, chemical, and genetic pathogens have been proposed and are being investigated.[123] The incidence of both diseases is about 1 in 10,000 births.[123]

Clinically, infants with these two diseases are very similar. These infants are usually healthy at birth but develop hyperbilirubinemia. Their livers and spleens are enlarged, urine is dark yellow, and if biliary obstruction is serious the stools may be acholic.[123] In addition, hepatic cirrhosis and encephalopathy are present.[123,147]

It is very difficult to differentiate between these two diseases. A variety of lab tests, a liver biopsy, and exploratory laparotomy may all help identify which problem the infant has.[123,147] Children believed to have neonatal hepatitis receive supportive management for hepatic insufficiency.[123] Prognosis for neonatal hepatitis is good, with approximately 50% showing full recovery and another 30% recovering with slight liver damage.[123]

Biliary atresia patients usually face surgery if their condition is serious. New surgical procedures such as portoenterostomy retards the progressive loss of liver function.[147] In some cases, patent bile ducts can be anastomosed to the intestine through surgery.[123] While the prognosis is improving with the new procedures, some end-stage biliary atresia patients will need a liver transplant.[147]

Hepatitis

Older children may contract hepatitis from a variety of infections. There are two major types of hepatitis, hepatitis A and hepatitis B. Hepatitis A is a more acute illness with symptoms in young children including fever, fatigue, listlessness, and diminished appetite. In the adolescent, these symptoms may be more severe, accompanied by jaundice and joint pain. Hepatitis B is more severe with symptoms often lasting for months.

For patients with acute hepatitis, bed rest and nutritional restrictions are usually prescribed. Patients with severe involvement may be hospitalized. Complete recovery occurs in 80% to 90% of these patients; however, 3% to 5% will develop chronic active hepatitis and will be "carriers" of hepatitis B surface antigen.

Work continues on how best to manage hepatitis carriers and how to protect persons working and living with all hepatitis patients. Immune serum globulin, administered shortly after exposure to both types of hepatitis, is effective in protecting against the disease. Vaccines to prevent hepatitis are still being developed.[123]

Implications for occupational therapy

Children with these disorders and diseases are usually very ill—some critically. But as progress is made in medical management, such as transplants, the focus is shifting to other problems the children may have on a more long-range basis. As life expectancy increases, investigators are beginning to look at such issues as motor and mental developmental delays in these children.[147] Where occupational therapists once saw these children in acute hospital settings, they will be seeing them in follow-up preschool clinics and eventually in school-based settings.

TRAUMATIC INJURIES

Hundreds of thousands of children are seriously injured and thousands more die each year as a result of accidents. The four leading types of fatal accidents are motor vehicle accidents, drownings, burns, and poisonings.[123] Other accidents, while not fatal, cause injuries that may leave the children with life-long physical or emotional scars. This section discusses specific types of traumatic injuries that often require the evaluation and treatment services of occupational therapists.

Head trauma

Head injuries during childhood constitute a major medical and public health problem. Approximately 4,000 children per year die from head injuries in the United States. Three to four times that number are seriously injured and must endure prolonged hospitalizations and life-long complications of some degree.

The vast majority of these cases are caused by motor vehicle accidents involving cars, bicycles, or motorcycles. Other cases are caused by self-inflicted injuries such as falls, and still others are caused by assault or penetrating wounds, such as gunshots.

Head traumas are often classified as closed or open. A closed head trauma indicates a blow to the head that has not caused an open or penetrating wound. An open head trauma denotes a penetration or laceration. Open wounds often require additional treatment, such as debridement, removal of bone fragments or other foreign bodies, surgical repair of blood vessesl, closure of the wound, and tetanus prophylaxis.

Damage to nervous system tissue may occur at the time of impact or penetration. However, secondary damage may occur resulting from brain swelling, intracranial pressure, hematomas, emboli, and hypoxic brain conditions.[75,117] It is these secondary causes of nervous system damage that must be prevented or at least minimized through early medical intervention.

Two distinct clinical patterns in unconscious children with head injuries are described.[117] In the first type the child goes into unconsciousness or coma immediately after the trauma. In the second type, known as the pediatric concussion syndrome, the child may become unconscious right after the injury but then become lucid before showing further signs of involvement. These may include drowsiness, vomiting, loss of consciousness, and even more serious indicators such as Babinsky's sign, decerebrate posturing, and even brain death.[117] The pediatric concussion syndrome may resolve at any stage of its continuum or complete its full course.

Once the child's condition is stabilized, his level of consciousness is determined. One scale that is often used is the Glasgow Coma Scale.[75] This system ranks children according to their ability to elicit sounds or words; their responses to tendon reflex testing and motor responsiveness in general; and their ability to voluntarily or involuntarily open their eyes.[117] Next, a neurological assessment of brain stem reflexes is conducted. Additional diagnostic procedures may involve computerized tomography (CT scan), electroencephalography (EEG), angiography, and radiography to determine the extent and location of fractures.

Treatment includes the close monitoring and control of cerebral circulation and of intracranial pressure through the use of sophisticated devices and control systems. When intracranial pressure cannot be controlled by use of traditional means, a large dose of barbiturate, such as phenobarbital, may be administered. If this attempt fails to control the pressure, lowering of the body temperature may help. Withdrawal from the latter two forms of treatment is difficult and may cause sleep disturbances, behavioral problems, apnea and some decreased intellectual functioning.

The prognosis for children who receive the type of treatment described is good. The majority of children with head trauma make a good recovery or are only moderately handicapped and are able to return to a regular school setting.[117] The milder effects include auditory and visual perceptual deficits, body image problems, difficulties with some minor gross and fine motor skills, a slowing of response, and moderate problems with some types of academic performance.[15,117]

Children who have shown decerebrate posturing, flaccidity, scores of less than 5 on the Glasgow Coma Scale, or prolonged coma are considered to have a guarded prognosis.[117] These children often require rehabilitation for ambulation, motor skills, self-help skills, language and cognitive skills, plus the previously mentioned problems.[27] In addition, some children will demonstrate severe emotional disturbances that will require professional help.[27]

Burns

Every year burn accidents cause the death of approximately 1,800 children and result in serious medical conditions in 1,500 other children.[123]

In addition to these serious medical problems from burns, thousands of other children suffer burns of a milder nature. Smith and O'Neill did a retrospective study of children admitted to a regional burn unit and found that, in the under 10-year-old population, scalds from hot beverages and foods and scalds caused by hot water in the bathtub caused 74% of all burns.[144] In the 10- to 16-year-old group, burns caused by flammable materials (matches, chemicals, gasoline, etc.) were responsible for the majority of burns.[144] In both age ranges only about 7% of the burns were attributed to house fires.[144]

Among the serious burns, smoke inhalation, respiratory failure, hypovolemic shock, renal failure, and post-traumatic infection are the major factors associated with death.[123] The severity of the burn injury is determined by the depth, exact location, and extent of body surface affected.

Clark[33] described the aims of burn treatment: prevention of infection and burn shock, early skin coverage, correction of cosmetic damage, restoration of function, and integration back into the environment. As burned tissue provides a fertile bed for infection, many types of intervention procedures must be used to minimize the possibility of sepsis. Environmental bacteria must be minimized. Surface bacteria must be reduced by using medicated ointments, administering antibiotics, removing dead tissue early, and covering the areas with skin grafts.[33] Burn shock is prevented by administering various intravenous solutions that help replace lost body fluids. Nutrition may be maintained through tube feedings, oral feedings, and intravenous feedings if indicated.[156]

Deformities, contractures, and loss of motion must be prevented by early intervention. Exercise programs, splinting, proper positioning, pressure garments, and reconstructive surgery are all methods used to limit the long-term effects of burn injuries. A child who faces a long hospital stay will need to have academic assistance to prevent any educational delays. The family and the child may need counseling in adjusting to any disfigurements or any limiting physical conditions. Without this help the emotional handicap may be as great as the physical one.[161]

Musculoskeletal injuries resulting from trauma

Fractures are extremely common in children. As prenatal and perinatal fractures and those of the epiphyseal plate were discussed earlier in this chapter, this section will describe fractures caused by traumatic injuries occurring in the early childhood and adolescent years.

Most childhood and adolescent fractures occur in normal play, sports, and recreational situations, but thousands of children are injured each year in traffic accidents.

Fractures may be classified in many ways. An open fracture refers to the fact that there is an open wound or penetration caused by an object outside the body or caused by the bone penetrating from within the body. A closed fracture indicates that no penetration has occurred. Open fractures present added complications because the wound must be closed in addition to treating the fracture. The risks of infection and soft tissue and nerve damage are higher with the open fracture and complications are more common.

Traumatic fractures are often complicated by the fact that bones are displaced and malaligned. If not corrected, this can cause permanent deformities in the child or adolescent. Figure 6-11 shows some of the most common deformities that can be caused by a serious fracture.

Children's ligaments are stronger than the associated epiphyseal plates. Therefore, when stress is applied, it is more common to find a fracture than a damaged ligament. However, when severe tension is applied to muscles, nerves, and tendons, damage can occur. Treatment is usually aimed at protecting the damaged part from stretching during the healing process.[132] The child must begin to exercise as soon as possible to prevent decreased joint motion and muscle power loss. Surgical repair may also be needed.

Treatment of childhood and adolescent fractures rarely requires open reduction (surgery) and the injured bone simply needs to be immobilized and protected so that the natural healing process can take place. However, if serious malalignments and displacements (especially rotational malalignment and lateral angulation) do not self-correct, if serious epiphyseal plate damage has occurred, or if any other problems are causing the bone not to heal correctly, open reduction to correct the problems will be necessary.[60,131]

Peripheral nerve injuries

Infants and children occasionally suffer traumatic injuries, perinatally and postnatally, that temporarily or permanently cause peripheral nerve injuries. For example, breech deliveries with after-coming arms can cause brachial plexus lesions.[115] These babies might demonstrate weakness or wasting of the small muscles of the hands and sensory diminution in the areas of the hand and arm served by this plexus.[115]

In older children, compressions, severe joint injuries, fractures, nerve lesions or infiltrations, excessive exercising of a specific body part, and tumors often cause damage to the brachial or lumbosacral plexus as well as to the median, ulnar, and the common peroneal nerves. When these nerves are injured, sensory diminution, motor weakness or wasting, and pain are common symptoms.[115]

Diagnosis is made using a combination of techniques such as family and medical histories, nerve conduction studies, observations of sensory and motor involvements, muscle biopsies, EMGs, and in more serious accidents, surgical exploration.

Specific treatment depends on the extent, progression, location, and especially the cause of the nerve damage. In general, treatment techniques include rest, splinting, nerve and local anesthetic injections, and surgical intervention to relieve nerve compression.[115]

Implications for occupational therapy

Children with head trauma, severe burns, and serious fractures or peripheral nerve damage will all require extended occupational therapy intervention of

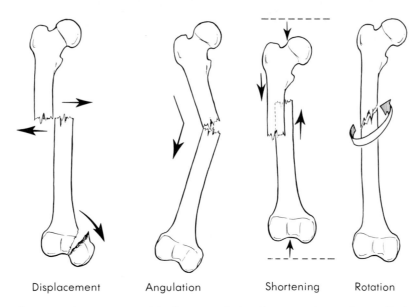

Displacement   Angulation   Shortening   Rotation

Figure 6-11 Deformities caused by fractures. **A,** Displacement; **B,** angulation; **C,** shortening and overriding; **D,** rotational.

some type. The information contained in Chapters 13, 24, and 25 will detail the types of problems that occupational therapists may be able to address. As medical advances increase the survival rates among children with these diseases and conditions, treatment goals will change to incorporate the monitoring of various components of growth and development and the various skills these children will need to live functional, productive, and happy lives.

SUMMARY

This chapter has presented an overview of specific diagnostic problems commonly encountered by occupational therapists in a variety of pediatric settings. In most instances, the various diagnostic problems presented here will be supplemented with additional information in subsequent chapters. References cited throughout the chapter will lead the student to more detailed information on the various topics discussed.

STUDY QUESTIONS
Select one specific disease, disorder, or condition.
1. List four major symptoms.
2. Will this disease, disorder, or condition worsen? If yes, what additional symptoms or problems will develop?
3. What is the cause of this disease, disorder, or condition? Could it have been prevented? How?
4. How is it diagnosed?
5. List two medical treatment techniques.
6. How will the symptoms listed in question 1 affect the child's developmental progress:
   a. Physical development
   b. Psychosocial development
   c. Cognitive development

7. Predict how symptoms and problems associated with this disease, disorder, or condition might affect the child's functioning in the following areas:
   a. Play/leisure
   b. Self-maintenance activities
   c. Work within preschool, school, or vocational readiness settings.

REFERENCES AND SELECTED READINGS

1. Acquired immune deficiency syndrome: 100 questions and answers, Albany, 1986, New York State Department of Health.
2. Adams JC: Outline of orthopedics, ed 9, New York, 1981, Churchill Livingstone, Inc.
3. AIDS and children, Washington, DC, 1986, American Red Cross and US Public Health Service.
4. AIDS: The facts, Washington, DC, 1986, American Red Cross.
5. Alfrey A: Chronic renal failure: manifestations and pathogenesis. In Schrier RW, editor: Renal and electrolyte disorders, Boston, 1976, Little, Brown & Co.
6. Ames LB, Gillespie C, Haines J, et al: Gesell preschool test manual, Flemington, NJ, 1984, Programs for education.
7. Amiel-Tison C: Neurological evaluation of the maturity of newborn infants, Arch Dis Child 43:89, 1968.
8. Ammann AJ, Cowan MJ, and Wara DW: Acquired immunodeficiency in an infant: possible transmission by means of blood products, Lancet 1:956, 1983.
9. Apgar V: A proposal for a new method of evaluation of the newborn infant, Curr Res Anesth Analg 32:260, 1953.
10. Apgar V, and James LS: Further observations on the newborn scoring system, Am J Dis Child 104:419, 1962.
11. Autism fact sheet, Washington, DC, 1980, The National Society for Autistic Children.
12. Avant K: A maternal attachment strategy. In Humenick SS, editor: Assessment strategies in the health care of young children and childbearing families, Norwalk, Conn, 1982, Appleton-Century-Crofts.

13. Ayres AJ: Sensory integration and the child, Los Angeles, 1980, Western Psychological Services.
14. Ballard JL, Kazmaier K, and Driver MA: Simplified assessment of gestational age, Pediatr Res 11:374, 1973.
15. Batshaw ML, and Perret YM: Children with handicaps: a medical primer, Baltimore, 1981, Paul H Brookes Publishing Co.
16. Battersby C: Pupils with juvenile arthritis, Australian Occ Ther Journal, 31(1), 1984.
17. Bax MCO: Terminology and classification of cerebral palsy, Developmental Medicine and Child Neurology 6:295, 1964.
18. Bayley N: The Bayley Scales of Infant Development, New York, 1969, The Psychological Corp.
19. Beary JF, Christian LL, and Johansin NA: Manual of Rheumatology and Outpatient Orthopedic Disorders, ed 2, Boston, 1987, Little Brown & Co.
20. Bender L: Schizophrenia in childhood: its recognition, description and treatment, Am J Orthopsychiatry 26:499, 1956.
21. Bettelheim BJ: A mechanical boy, Sci Am 200:117, 1959.
22. Birth defects: tragedy and hope, White Plains, NY, 1981, The National Foundation—March of Dimes.
23. Bluestone CD, and Shurin PA: Middle ear disease in children: pathogenesis, diagnosis, and management, Pediatr Clin North Am 21:379, 1974.
24. Bobath K: A Neurophysiological Basis for the Treatment of Cerebral Palsy, Philadelphia, 1980, JB Lippincott Co.
25. Brazelton TB: Neonatal behavioral assessment scale, Philadelphia, 1973, JB Lippincott Co.
26. Brigance A: Brigance Inventories, North Billerica, Mass, 1981, Curriculum Associates.
27. Brink JD, and Woo-Sam J: Physical recovery after severe closed head trauma in children and adolescents, J Pediatr 97(5):721, 1980.
28. Broussard ER: Psychosocial disorders in children: early assessment of infants at risk, Contin Educ Fam Physician 44:42, 1978.
29. Campbell S: Fetal growth. In Beard R, and Nathaniels P, editors: Fetal physiology and medicine: the basis of perinatology, Philadelphia, 1976, WB Saunders Co.
30. Cerreto M: The diagnosis of childhood autism, Galveston, Spring 1980, The School Health Newsletter, The University of Texas Medical Branch.
31. Chai H, and Newcomb R: Pharmacologic management of childhood asthma, Am J Dis Child 125:757, 1973.
32. Churchill J, and others: The etiology of cerebral palsy in premature infants, New York, 1971, American Academy for Cerebral Palsy.
33. Clark AM: Burns in childhood, World J Surg 2:175, 1978.
34. Clark F: Research on the neuropathophysiology of autism and its implications for OT, Occup Ther J Res 30:3, 1983.
35. Clements SD: Minimal brain dysfunction in children: terminology and identification, NINDB Monograph No 3, Washington, DC, 1966, US Department of Health, Education and Welfare.
36. Clerk G: Reflections on the role of mother in the development of language in the schizophrenic child, Can Psychiatr Assoc J 6:252, 1961.
37. Colbert EC, and Koegel RR: Toe walking in childhood schizophrenia, J Pediatr 53:219, 1958.
38. Collins G, and others: Ventricular septal defect: clinical and hemodynamic changes in the first five years of life, Am Heart J 84:695, 1972.
39. Cooke W: Survey of results of treatment of Crohn's disease, Clin Gastroenterol 1:521, 1972.
40. Cooper W, German J, and Lame E: Genetic implications of cerebral palsy, J Bone Joint Surg 47:1673, 1965.
41. Creak EM: Childhood psychosis: a review of 100 cases, Br J Psychiatry 109:84, 1963.
42. Damasio AR, and Maurer RG: A neurological model for childhood autism, Arch Gen Psychiatry 35:777, 1978.
43. DeMyer M, and others: Prognosis in autism: a follow-up study, J Autism Child Schizophr 3:199, 1973.
44. di Sant' Agnese PA, and David PB: Research in cystic fibrosis, J Pediatr 8:711, 1976.
45. Donner M, Rapola J, and Somer H: Congenital musuclar dystrophy: a clinico-pathological and follow-up study of 15 patients, Neuropaediatrie 6:239, 1975.
46. Drash A: The control of diabetes mellitus. Is it achievable? Is it desirable? J Pediatr 88:1074, 1976.
47. Dubowitz LMS, and Dubowitz V: Gestational age of the newborn; a clinical manual, Reading, Mass, 1977, Addison-Wesley Publishing Co, Inc.
48. Eisen A, and Humphreys P: The Guillian Barré syndrome, Arch Neurol 30:438, 1974.
49. Engle MA: Ventricular septal defects: status report for the seventies, Cardiovasc Clin 4(3):282, 1972.
50. Ensher GL, and Clark DA: Newborns at Risk: Medical Care and Psychoeducational Intervention, Rockville, Md, 1986, Aspen Publishers, Inc.
51. Erhardt RP: Erhardt Developmental Prehension Test, Laurel, Md, 1982, RAMSCO Publishing Co.
52. Fetal Alcohol Syndrome, Task Force Report to the Governor, Albany, 1979, State of New York.
53. Fils DH: The developmental disabilities handbook, Los Angeles, 1978, Western Psychological Services.
54. Fisch, RD, and others: Physical and mental status at 4 years of age of survivors of the respiratory distress syndrome, J Pediatr 86:497, 1975.
55. Fish B: Involvement of the CNS in infants with schizophrenia, Arch Neurol 2:115, 1960.
56. Fish B: Longitudinal observations of biological deviations in a schizophrenic infant, Am J Psychiatry 116:25, 1959.
57. Fishbein J: Birth defects, Philadelphia, 1963, JB Lippincott Co.
58. Fisher D, and Paton J: The effect of maternal anesthetic and analgesic drugs on the fetus and newborn, Clin Obstet Gynecol 17:275, 1974.
59. Fitzhardinge P, and Steven E: The small-for-date infant. I. Later growth patterns, Pediatrics 49:671, 1972.
60. Fleisher G, and Ludwig S: Textbook of Pediatric Emergency Medicine, Baltimore, 1983, Williams and Wilkins.
61. Franco S, and Andrews B: Reduction of cerebral palsy by neonatal intensive care, Pediatr Clin North Am 24:639, 1977.
62. Frankenburg WK, and Dodds J: Manual: Denver Developmental Screening Test, Denver, University of Colorado Medical Center.
63. Friedland GH, Satzman BR, Rogers MF, et al: Lack of transmission of HTLV-III/LAV infection to household contacts of patients with AIDS or AIDS-related complex with oral candidiasis, N Eng J Med 314(6):344, 1986.
64. Friedman WF: Medical management of ductus arteriosus, Prenatal Care 77:18, 1977.
65. Goodwin J, Dunne J, and Thomas B: Antepartum identification of the fetus at risk, Can Med J 101:458, 1969.
66. Gray JD, and others: Prediction and prevention of child abuse and neglect, Child Abuse Neglect Int J 1:45, 1977.
67. Gregory GA, and others: Treatment of the idiopathic respiratory distress syndrome with continuous positive airway pressure, N Engl J Med 284:1333, 1971.
68. Hagberg B, Hagberg G, and Olow I: The changing panorama of

cerebral palsy in Sweden 1954-1970. I. Analysis of general changes, Acta Paediatr Scand 64:187, 1975.

69. Havelkova M: Follow-up study of seventy-one children diagnosed as psychotic in preschool age, Am J Orthopsychiatry 38:846, 1968.

70. Hellman L, and Pritchard J, editors: Williams' obstetrics, New York, 1975, Appleton-Century-Crofts.

71. Henig RM: Saving babies before birth, The New York Times Magazine, vol 18, Feb 1982.

72. Hobel C, and others: Prenatal and intrapartum high risk screening: prediction of the high risk neonate, Am J Obstet Gynecol 117:1, 1973.

73. Hopkins HL, and Smith HD: Willard and Spackman's occupational therapy, ed 6, Philadelphia, 1983, JB Lippincott Co.

74. Ingram TS, Mason AW, and Blackburn I: A retrospective study of 82 children with reading disability, Dev Med Child Neurol 12:271, 1970.

75. Jennett B, and Teasdale G: Management of head injuries, Philadelphia, 1981, FA Davis Co.

76. Jones KL: Fetal alcohol syndrome, Pediatrics in Review, vol 18(4)122, Oct 1986.

77. Kanner L: Autistic disturbances in affective contact, Nervous Child 2:217, 1943.

78. Karp R, and Kirklin J: Tetralogy of Fallot, Ann Thorac Surg 10:370, 1970.

79. Katz J: The effects of conductive hearing loss on auditory function, ASAA, 20(10), 879, 1978.

80. Kessner DM, Snow CK, and Singer J: Assessment of medical care in children, Contrasts in health status, Washington, DC, 1973, Natl Academy of Science, vol 13.

81. Klaus MH, and Fanaroff AA: Care of the high-risk neonate, Philadelphia, 1979, WB Saunders Co.

82. Knoblock H, Stevens F, and Malore A: Manual of developmental diagnosis, ed 3, Philadelphia, 1980, Harper and Row, Publishers Inc.

83. Koivisto M, Blanco-Sequeiros M, and Krause V: Neonatal symptomatic and asymptomatic hypoglycaemia: a follow-up study of 151 children, Dev Med Child Neurol 14:603, 1972.

84. Kolvin J: Psychoses in childhood: a comparative study. In Rutter M, editor: Infantile autism: concepts, characteristics and treatment, London, 1971, Churchill Livingstone.

85. Korner AF, and others: Reduction of sleep apnea and bradycardia in preterm infants on oscillating water beds: a controlled polygraphic study, Pediatrics 61:528, 1978.

86. Lazaro RP, Fenichel GM, and Kilroy AW: Congenital muscular dystrophy: case reports and reappraisal, Muscle Nerve 2:349, 1979.

87. Lemeshow S: The handbook of clinical types in mental retardation, Boston, 1982, Allyn and Bacon, Inc.

88. Lewis J, Spero J, and Hasiba V: Death in hemophiliacs, JAMA 236:1238, 1976.

89. Livingstone C: Outline of orthopedics, ed 9, New York, 1981, Churchill Livingstone.

90. Lubchenco LO: Assessment of gestational age and development at birth, Pediatr Clin North Am 17(1):125, 1970.

91. Mangos J, and Talamo R, editors: Cystic fibrosis: projections into the future, New York, 1976, Grune & Stratton, Inc.

92. McCarthy JS, Zies LG, and Gelband H: Age-dependent closure of the patent ductus arteriosus by indomethacin, Pediatrics 62:706, 1978.

93. McClure P: Idiopathic thrombocytopenic purpura in children: diagnosis and management, Pediatr Clin North Am 55:68, 1975.

94. McConnell OL: Control of eye contact in an autistic child, J Child Psychiatry 8:249, 1967.

95. Menelaus MB: The orthopaedic management of spina bifida cystica, London, 1971, E & S Livingstone.

96. Merkatz IR, and Fanaroff AA: Antenatal and intrapartum care of the high-risk infant. In Klaus MH, and Fanaroff AA, editors: Care of the high-risk neonate, Philadelphia, 1979, WB Saunders Co.

97. Miller G, Tunnecliffe M, and Douglas P: IQ, prognosis, and development in muscular dystrophy, Brain and Development, 7:7, 1985.

98. Miller LJ: Miller assessment for preschoolers, Englewoods, Col 1982, Knowledge in Development Foundation.

99. Millichap JG, and Dodge RR: Diagnosis and treatment of myasthenia gravis in infancy, childhood, and adolescence, Neurology 10:1009, 1960.

100. Milner JS, and Wimberly RC: An inventory for the identification of child abusers, J Clin Psychol 25(1):95, 1975.

101. Muscular dystrophy fact sheet, New York, 1980, Muscular Dystrophy Association.

102. Nager G: Pathology of acute and chronic otitis media and their complications. In Gerwing K, editor: Otitis media and complications, Springfield, Ill 1972, 103, Charles C Thomas.

103. Nesbitt R, and Aubry R: High-risk obstetrics. II. Value of semi-objective grading system in identifying the vulnerable group, Am J Obstet Gynecol 103:972, 1969.

104. New M, and Fiser R, editors: Diabetes and other endocrine disorders during pregnancy and in the newborn, Prog Clin Biol Res 10:13, 1976.

105. NICHD National Registry: Midtrimester amniocentesis for prenatal diagnosis: safety and accuracy, JAMA 236:1471, 1976.

106. Norris D, and others: Hodgkin's disease in childhood, Cancer 36:2109, 1973.

107. Oleske J, Minnefor A, and Cooper R: Immune deficiency syndrome in children, JAMA 249 (17):2345, 1983.

108. Olsen RJ: Index of suspicion: screening for child abusers, Am J Nurs 1:108, 1976.

109. O'Reilly D, and Walentynowicz J: Etiological factors in cerebral palsy: an historical review, Dev Med Child Neurol 23:8, 1981.

110. Ornitz E: Childhood autism: a review of the clinical and experimental literature, Calif Med 118:21, 1973.

111. Oski FA, and Naiman JL: Hematologic problems in the newborn, Philadelphia, 1972, WB Saunders Co.

112. Patrick JE, Perry TB, and Kinch RA: Fetoscopy and fetal blood sampling: a percutaneous approach, Am J Obstet Gynecol 119:539, 1974.

113. Perlstein M, and Barnett H: Nature and recognition of cerebral palsy in infancy, JAMA 148:1389, 1952.

114. Pinkel D: Treatment of acute leukemia, Pediatr Clin North Am 23:117, 1976.

115. Pryse-Phillips W, and Murray TJ: Essential neurology, ed 2, Garden City, NY, 1982, Medical Examination Pub Co.

116. Rank B: Intensive study and treatment of preschool children who show marked personality deviations or "atypical development" and their parents. In Caplan, G, editor: Emotional problems in early childhood, New York, 1955, Basic Books Inc, Publishers.

117. Raphaely RC, and others: Management of severe pediatric head trauma, Pediatr Clin North Am 27(3):715, 1980.

118. Ricks DM, and Wing L: Language, communication and the use of symbols in normal and autistic children, J Autism Child Schizophr 5:215, 1975.

119. Riukin J: Prenatal previews, American Health, p 13, Jan-Feb, 1987.

120. Ritvo E, Ornitz E, and LaFranchi S: Frequency of repetitive behavior in early infantile autism and its variants, Arch Gen Psychiatry 19:341, 1968.

121. Ritvo E, and others: Correlation of psychiatric diagnoses and EEG findings, Am J Psychiatry 126:37, 1970.

122. Rizza CR, and Mathews JM: Management of the haemophilic child, Arch Dis Child 47:451, 1972.

123. Roberts KB: Manual of clinical problems in pediatrics, Boston, 1979, Little, Brown & Co.

124. Robertson E: Rehabilitation of arm amputees and limb-deficient children, London, 1978, Cassell, Ltd.

125. Rogers MF, Thomas PA, and Starcher ET: Acquired immune syndrome in children: report of the Center for Disease Control national surveillance, 1982 to 1985, Pediatrics 79(6):1008, 1987.

126. Rosset HL: A clinical perspective of the fetal alcohol syndrome, Alcoholism: clinical and experimental research, 4(2), p 119, 1980.

127. Rubinstein A, Sicklick M, and Gupta A: Acquired immunodeficiency with reversed T4/T8 ratios in infants born to promiscuous and drug-addicted mothers, JAMA 249 (17):2350, 1983.

128. Rubinstein A, Schooling for children with acquired immunodeficiency syndrome, J of Peds, 109 (2):242, 1986.

129. Rudolph AJ, and Kenny JD: Anticipation, recognition, and transitional care of the high-risk infant. In Klaus MH, and Fanaroff AA, editors: Care of the high-risk neonate, Philadelphia, 1979, WB Saunders Co.

130. Rutter M, and Lockyer L: A 5 to 15 year follow-up study of infantile psychosis. II. Social and behavioral outcome, Br J Psychiatry 113:1183, 1967.

131. Salter RB: Textbook of disorders and injuries of the musculoskeletal system, ed 2, Baltimore, 1983, Williams & Wilkins.

132. Salter RB, and Field P: The effects of continuous compression on living articular cartilage: an experimental investigation, J Bone Joint Surg 42A:31, 1960.

133. Schaaf RC: The frequency of vestibular disorders in developmentally delayed preschoolers with otitis media, Am J of Occ Ther, vol 39(2):247, 1985.

134. Scherzer AL, and Tscharnuter I: Early Diagnosis and treatment in cerebral palsy: a primer on infant developmental problems, New York, 1982, Marcel Dekker, Inc.

135. Schopler E: Early infantile autism and receptive processes, Arch Gen Psychiatry 113:1183, 1965.

136. Schuster CS, and Ashburn SS: The process of human development: a holistic approach, Boston, 1980, Little, Brown & Co.

137. Schwartz R, Field G, and Kyle G: Timing of delivery in the pregnant diabetic patient, Obstet Gynecol 34:787, 1969.

138. Scott, GB, Buck BE, and Letterman JG: Acquired immunodeficiency syndrome in infants, N Eng J Med 310 (2): 76, 1984.

139. Shannon KM, and Ammann AJ: Acquired immune deficiency syndrome in childhood, J of Peds 106 (2) 332, 1985.

140. Sharrard WJ, and Zachary RB: A controlled trial of immediate and delayed closure of spina bifida cystica, Arch Dis Child 38:18, Feb 1963.

141. Sherman LM: Cancer and AIDS. In Tigges KN, and Marcil WM, editors: Terminal and life threatening illness: an occupational behavior perspective, Slack, Inc. (In press.)

142. Sickle-cell anemia fact sheet, White Plains, NY, 1981, The National Foundation-March of Dimes.

143. Smith DW: Recognizable patterns of human malformation, ed 3, Philadelphia, 1982, WB Saunders Co.

144. Smith RW, and O'Neill TJ: An analysis into childhood burns, Burns, vol 11(2):117, 1984.

145. Spencer EA: Functional restoration—amputations and prosthetic replacement. In Hopkins HL, and Smith HD, editors: Occupational therapy, ed 6, Philadelphia, 1983, JB Lippincott Co.

146. Stern R, and others: Course of cystic fibrosis in 95 patients, J Pediatr 89:406, 1976.

147. Stewart SM, Vary R, Waller DA, et al: Mental and motor development correlates in patients with end-stage biliary atresia awaiting live transplantation, Pediatrics, vol 79(6), June 1987.

148. Stott DH: The child's hazards in utero. In Howells JG, editor: Modern perspectives in international child psychiatry, New York, 1971, Brunner/Mazel, Inc.

149. Streissguth AP, Clarren SK, and Jones KL: Natural history of the fetal alcohol syndrome: A 10 year follow-up of 11 patients, Lancet 2:89, 1985.

150. Sweet AY: Classification of the low-birth-weight infant. In Klaus MH, and Fanaroff AA, editors: Care of the high-risk neonate, Philadelphia, 1979, WB Saunders Co.

151. Synder C, Eyres SJ, and Barnard E: New findings about mothers' antenatal expectations and their relationship to infant development, Am J Matern Child Nurs 4:354, 1979.

152. Thomas CL: Taber's cyclopedic medical dictionary. Philadelphia, 1981, FA Davis Co.

153. Thompson E, and others: The mother-infant play interaction scale, Austin, TX, 1980, The University of Texas School of Nursing.

154. Thompson H: Evaluation of the obstetric and gynecologic patient by the use of diagnostic ultrasound, Clin Obstet Gynecol 17:1, 1974.

155. Thompson R: Juvenile onset diabetes, Can Med Assoc J 114:783, 1976.

156. Trunkey D, and Parks S: Burns in children, Curr Prob Pediatr 6(3):3, 1976.

157. Tsiantos A, and others: Intracranial hemorrhage in the prematurely born infant, J Pediatr 85:854, 1974.

158. US Office of Education: Education for all Handicapped Children Act, Public Law 94-142, Fed Reg 42:42478, 1977.

159. Usher R, McLean F, and Scott KE: Judgment of fetal age: clinical significance of gestational age and an objective method for its assessment, Pediatr Clin North Am 13:835, 1966.

160. Weldvogel F, Medoff C, and Swartz M: Osteomyelitis: a review of clinical features, therapeutic considerations and unusual aspects, N Engl J Med 282:198, 1970.

161. Wilkins TJ, and Campbell JL: Psychosocial concerns in the paediatric burn unit, Burns 7:208.

162. Wing L, and others: Symbolic play in the severely mentally retarded and in autistic children, J Child Psychol Psychiatry 18:167, 1977.

163. Zinkus PW, Gottlieb ML, and Shapiro M: Developmental psychoeducational sequelae of chronic otitis media, Amer Jour Dis Child, 132:1100, 1978.

PART III

BASIC PRINCIPLES OF OCCUPATIONAL THERAPY INTERVENTION

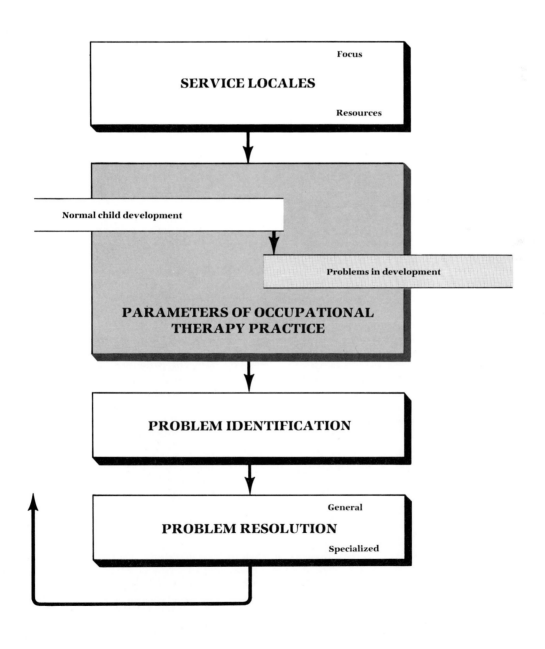

7

Occupational therapy in pediatrics

PAT NUSE PRATT

The four theoretical approaches to pediatric occupational therapy reviewed in Chapter 3 share a humanistic view of the child (and the species) as an adaptive creator. An integration of the constructs of these and other theories and models of occupational therapy proposes an approach to practice that has been called "human development through occupation."[3,4] This chapter presents the philosophy of practice developed for this approach and discusses generic processes and modalities of occupational therapy. These concepts have been expanded and modified somewhat from their original presentation so that their ideas can be applied more directly to pediatric practice. In addition, a description of the sequence and basic components of occupational therapy in pediatrics is presented.

A PHILOSOPHY OF PRACTICE
View of man

Human adaptation is distinguished by the child's capacity to purposefully affect his own world of self, culture, and environment. The unique richness of this creative function is the product of two biological characteristics: (1) the ability of the human brain to formulate and symbolize concepts and (2) the ability of the human hands to translate concepts into action. The child's awareness of these abilities, through successive and successful interactions with the environment, promotes the will for purposeful activities.[7,9]

Purposeful activities are broadly defined as the goal-directed use of a person's body systems, time, energy, interests, and attention in environmental interactions.[10,17,23] The child spends most of his time occupied in certain types of purposeful activities that support performance of chosen personal, social, and occupational roles.[1] Occupational roles and the supportive *occupational activities* are distinguished from other kinds of purposeful activities by two characteristics: (1) the use of hands and tools to explore and manipu-

late the environment and (2) the direct or indirect relationship of occupational activities to cultural continuity. There is a recognized sequence to the emergence and primary engagement of the human in such occupational activities.[18] This includes the development and use of:

1. *Self-maintenance,* including self-care, sleep, rest, recreation, and other activities directed toward the preservation of the self and the species and preparation for work and play.[19,24]
2. *Play* as the anticipator and facilitator of subsequent goal-directed activities. Play includes sensorimotor exploration; symbolic activities such as art and drama; crafts; and games. The behaviors and skills acquired through playful exploration of the self, culture, and environment serve as the learning bridge to adult competence and creative achievement.[25]
3. *Work* as the economic function of humans in their world and the healthy state of man the achiever.[24,25] Work includes the educational and prevocational activities of the child in addition to the vocational and home management activities of the adult (Figure 7-1).

View of health

The child's maturing ability to direct and affect his or her purpose in life may be seen as a primary indication of general well-being, or health. Humans maintain health through engagement in a flexible balance of work, play, and self-maintenance activities, which develop and change throughout the life span.[19,24] The infant's work of learning is blended into playful sensorimotor exploration of the environment. As the child ages, the structure of his learning becomes more formalized through school, family, peer group, and community activities. The infant's involvement in self-maintenance activities is superficially passive until one con-

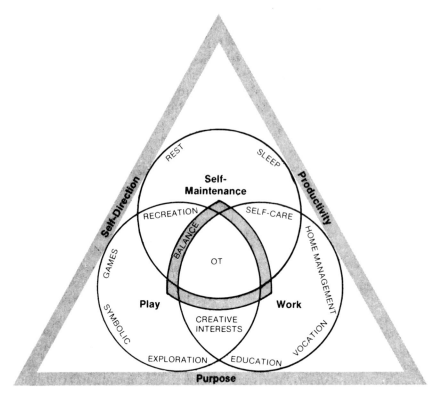

Figure 7-1 Conceptual model for the philosophy of practice: occupational activities and occupational therapy.

From Clark PN: Am J Occup Ther 33:578, Sept 1979.

siders the role of his crying behaviors in his daily routine. Again, with maturation the child gradually assumes more direct responsibilities for various self-care tasks.

In a healthy state the individual is able to adapt and achieve a satisfying life and is able to function adequately in chosen personal, social, and occupational roles.[22] *Role performance* involves the use of pertinent purposeful activities, including the various skills, habits, rules, tasks, and relationships acquired through the acculturation of the individual.[2,7,17]

The healthy performance of an individual is influenced by four major factors. First, the child's basic *biological endowment*, which includes the various body systems, functions, and genetic capacities, provides her with the potential to develop and learn a variety of skilled activities. Second, there is a hierarchical *maturation* of these basic endowments as the child grows and accommodates to changing environments, assimilating new experiences and learning. Together these two physiological processes provide a foundation of sensory, integrative, motor, and cognitive functions that permit the development of adaptive skills. The interaction between the individual and culture, physical space, and other environmental elements becomes increasingly complex throughout the life span. Therefore

human performance must change and adapt as it is influenced by the third factor of *cultural, spatial, and temporal requirements.* The child must learn to effect a satisfying balance between meeting internal needs and adapting his behavior to external influences. The emergent, socialized *personal needs* change in concert with the three other performance factors, becoming the fourth determinant of one's "normal" performance. The human capacities that develop through the interaction between these internal and external forces provide a foundation of emotional and social functions (Figure 7-2).

Throughout life the individual encounters physiological, social, and psychological problems that may or may not impede performance of various roles and role activities. Analysis of the effect of such problems on socially adequate, personally satisfying performance and critical elements of development is both qualitative and quantitative.[16] Several questions arise. Is the individual capable of resolving the problem, adapting to it, or coping with it independently? With children in particular one needs to consider whether the coping process in itself is a hazard to the developmental progression. Is the nature of the problem such that it threatens to delay, disrupt, or impair functions, life role skills, or both? If the problem is sufficient to cause a dysfunction

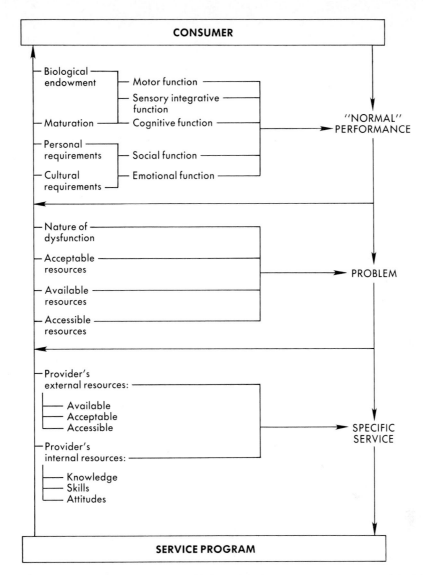

Figure 7-2 Conceptual model for the philosophy of practice: a continuum of health and dysfunction.

Adapted from Clark PN: Am J Occup Ther 33:579, Sept 1979.

in the individual's performance and balance of daily tasks and roles, what resources are available, acceptable, and accessible to the child and family (Figure 7-2)? For example, a learning disabled child might have parents who both work, and therefore he needs to receive occupational therapy services through the school. However, he may not meet the eligibility requirements for that school's therapy services if his schoolwork is not 2 years below age level. If he lives in a county where there are no clinical occupational therapy services for children, and his parents cannot change their work schedules, life-style, and standard of living, he will probably go without occupational therapy treatment.

View of the profession

It is the heritage and concern of occupational therapy that awareness of the child's special needs for both purpose and balance in life activities be applied to health service delivery.[7,24] Occupational therapy is viewed as an applied health service that is concerned with the quality and satisfaction of daily living from birth to death, as evidenced through occupational role performance.[16] The scope and delivery of such a service may be as complex and varied as the nature of human occupation.

It is the belief of the discipline that "man, through use of his hands, as they are energized by mind and will, can influence the state of his own health" (p. 2).[23] It is the mandate of occupational therapists to provide services that support the child's achievement of health through engagement in purposeful activities. Inherent in this mandate is a second: that occupational therapy services must be relevant to the time, cultures, and environments that are meaningful to the child. Accordingly, service programs must be designed and carried out that use goal-directed, meaningful, and age-appropriate activities to influence the quality of human development and life adaptation.

The core of occupational therapy service delivery is the therapist's use of the activity analysis and adaptation processes. Both analysis and adaptation of the activity are determined by the functional components and developmentally antecedent skills required to perform it. The intervention process will require attention to the enhancement and integration of sensory-integrative, motor, cognitive, emotional, and social functions *as these relate to* performance of daily occupational activities. The outcome of occupational therapy service delivery is always determined by the child's mastery of tasks and relationships necessary to actively engage in play, self-maintenance, school, and prevocational activities.[16] Regardless of the complexity of services to enhance functional components of behavior, if the program does not follow through to ensure an optimal level of performance in required everyday activities, it is not occupational therapy.

The occupational therapist may work with children of varied age and diagnostic groups in a broad spectrum of health care, educational, and social service settings. Services provided include assessment of the child's performance of play, self-maintenance, educational, and prevocational tasks and the design, execution, and evaluation of individualized, goal-directed programs. The goals of occupational therapy intervention are always related to the following.[15]

1. The *development and maintenance* of functions and skills necessary for performance of the desired or required occupational activities
2. *Prevention* of inadequate development, deterioration, or loss of those functions necessary to engage in play, educational, prevocational, and the various self-maintenance activities
3. *Remediation,* or rehabilitation, of dysfunction that impairs acceptable performance of daily occupational activities
4. *Facilitation* of the child's adaptive capacity to influence his or her own life and health status
5. *Collaboration,* communication, and cooperation in the planning and achievement of goals with the child and significant others in the child's life, including family and other service providers.

BASIC PRINCIPLES OF PRACTICE

In essence, the practice of occupational therapy must be directly related to each child's overall mastery of age-appropriate occupational role requirements

(that is, player or student) and must also support the achievement of goals and balance in the broader scope of personal and social roles (that is, son-daughter or boy-girl). Therefore the therapist must be familiar with the human development process, its functional and skill components, and its sequence, and the therapist must relate these to the needs of the child within a continuum of health and dysfunction.

The constructs of "human development through occupation" suggest that there are processes and modalities that are generic to occupational therapy services. The processes are activity analysis and activity adaptation. The modalities include occupational activities, relationships, special activity adaptation techniques, and the tools, materials, and equipment of the activity process.

Analysis and adaptation of generic modalities

Occupational activities are selected from the age-appropriate play, work, and self-maintenance categories described earlier. The therapist analyzes the activity by considering the functional content and quality required to perform the activity and the antecedent developmental skills that are needed. The activity is also analyzed to determine if it is meaningful to the age-related role requirements of the child. For example, if the child will be attending school, will the activity be required of the child there, or will it at least promote the child's performance of similar activities in the school setting?

Once the activity is selected, the therapist can structure it and make use of the other generic modalities. From the study of Freud, Piaget, and Erikson the therapist is aware of the motivational utility of the child's *relationships* with human and nonhuman objects. This characteristic of human behavior can be used to stimulate the child to active participation in the activity process. For example, a favorite toy can be used to stimulate the infant toward achievement of a new motor function. Or the therapist can urge the child to complete a craft project as a gift for a parent or favorite relative. When working with young children (Chapter 8), it has proven to be most effective to make direct use of infants' relationships with their mothers by training the mothers to carry out treatment programs.

The activity itself can be modified by use of special *adaptation techniques* that can include such a method as changing the position of the child's body or working surface. The therapist may use some special physical techniques, such as direct sensory stimulation, to enable the child to perform better in the chosen activity. The activity process itself may be modified by breaking tasks down into components by use of a simple-to-complex, step-by-step progression of skill development. Another method is to alter expectations for independent performance of the activity in view of the functional limitations of the child. For example, the therapist may scoop food onto a spoon for the child but expect the child to bring the spoon to his mouth independently.

The therapist may also teach the child to use compensatory methods. In essence, this means teaching the child to substitute the use of a well-developed function for a function that is either temporarily inadequate or poorly developed. For example, if a child has broken an arm but wants to remain independent in self-care, the therapist can teach the child to use one-handed techniques in the varied activities.

The *tools, materials,* and *equipment* of the activity are in themselves important modalities and are often the easiest part of the process to adapt. Adaptations can be made according to the developmental sequence of activity performance. Typically, small children can control a ball better with both hands before they can throw with one hand. Therefore the person helping the child learn to do this activity might start out with bilateral throwing of a large ball and progress to a smaller ball as the child gains control of the movement.

There is also a large variety of tools and materials that are collectively known as *adaptive equipment.* This equipment runs the gamut from bent-handle spoons to electronic door openers (and beyond) and often opens up a new world of independent performance for the child. However, adaptation of materials does not necessarily require special devices. Often a simple substitution, such as Play-doh for plastic clay, may make the activity more achievable for a child. It is clear that in addition to having a good knowledge of developmentally appropriate activities, the therapist must also be able to approach activity performance in a flexible way.

The process of breaking an activity into steps to facilitate performance of the necessary skills is also used to enable the child to learn what to do. The teaching skills of the therapist are important, and the therapist must learn a variety of teaching techniques to deal with a varied pediatric population.[3,4,6,13,20]

This preliminary discussion of activity analysis and adaptation may be clarified further by Figure 7-3. This form allows the therapist to analyze the activity according to the components stressed earlier, and it provides information that can be used to adapt the activity to the needs of a child. For example, if the therapist finds that a child lacks the developmentally antecedent skills to perform an activity independently, then a program of the earlier occurring activities would be in order first. Analysis of essential and variable functions permits the therapist to identify activity adaptations that can be tailored to a specific child's functional capacity.

A SEQUENTIAL MODEL OF THE OCCUPATIONAL THERAPY PROCESS

As was previously mentioned, activity analysis and adaptation are generic processes of occupational therapy. A number of categories of occupational therapy modalities were introduced and briefly discussed in relation to the generic processes. These modalities may be used both to assess and to enhance the development and skill performance of the child throughout the occupational therapy intervention process. Figure 7-2, which demonstrates the continuum of normal performance and dysfunction, also represents the sequence of events that leads the child to occupational therapy services.

Figure 7-3 Model for activity analysis in pediatric occupational therapy

1. Description of the activity.
2. Properties of the activity.
   a. Tools, materials, techniques, and equipment used in the activity.
   b. Steps in the activity process.
   c. Relationship to occupational role development and performance.
   d. Human and object relationships inherent in the activity process.
3. Performance requirements of the activity.
   a. Developmentally antecedent skills.
   b. Component functions used in the activity process.

Function	*Essentials*	*Variables-adaptables*
Sensory integrative		
Motor		
Cognitive		
Emotional		
Social		

The two major components of the service process are (1) assessment and (2) program development and evaluation. The latter may be considered *treatment,* and the terms are often used interchangeably. However, this book will use program development and evaluation more frequently for several reasons. First, this terminology is more widely accepted in the educational and social service agencies that are the major employers of pediatric occupational therapists. In addition, it will serve as a reminder of the program evaluation requisite. Together the two components form a continuum of problem identification and problem resolution. Assessment is the problem identification component of practice, whereas program development and evaluation are concerned with problem resolution. These two components are not mutually exclusive. Much valuable information for assessment purposes is evidenced during programming, and often assessment activities become the foundation of the child's program. In addition, each component has several distinct phases, which are shown in Figure 7-4 and will be discussed in detail here.

Assessment

Assessment is an evaluative process that is based on facts (data collected through different formal and informal objective measures of children's functions and performance) and sound clinical judgment. The latter is the subjective and interpretive component of assessment, and it is the product of the individual therapist's experience that includes training, practice, and theoretical frame of reference. The importance of clinical judgment should not be underestimated. It is the critical difference between a collection of data and meaningful assessment.[16]

Assessment is a continuing process as the therapist constantly thinks through interactions and activity experiences with the child. However, at initial contact and at designated intervals throughout intervention, assessment becomes more structured in formal reports. This allows the therapist to:

1. Identify present performance
2. Define problems
3. Identify potential performance
4. Develop program objectives and modalities
5. Record and report progress to document change

The initial contact between the therapist and the child serves as a general performance *screening.* It is necessary to determine whether the child appears to have problems in play, self-maintenance, educational or prevocational activity performance. Also, at this time it may be useful to refer the child to other disciplines and resources for more effective problem identification. The therapist must determine if occupational therapy will help or hinder. Sometimes it may be more efficient to delay the start of occupational therapy until after another service provider has worked with the child. Or the problem may be minor or situational and merely require some timely discussion with the parents and available follow-up as needed.

BASIC METHODS OF ASSESSMENT

Decisions regarding intervention are usually based on data from a variety of resources and the therapist's general problem analysis. Several basic methods are used to collect pertinent information about a child. First, the therapist will *observe* the child, preferably within an uncontrived activity performance situation. For example, the child might be seen in a hospital playroom or in a classroom. Skilled observation requires that the therapist carefully use all senses and record data objectively. An increasingly popular method of observation is to record the child's activity on videotape, which can then be analyzed later with less loss of information.

Whenever possible, the therapist will conduct short *interviews,* with the child, significant others (family and associates), and other members of the service delivery team. The components of a good interview were described by Gillette[11] as being carefully structured, open-ended questions; unbiased observing, listening, and feedback; and objective recording of data.

Next, a *performance-based screening test* may be administered to the child to identify his developmental level, as well as his general performance capacities and weaknesses. The use of a standardized developmental evaluation is highly recommended, because it will provide a normative baseline for continued assessment and descriptive information for program planning.

Standardized tests are recommended for this part of screening because of the way they are constructed, administered, scored, and interpreted. A standardized test is constructed for use with a specific population of people who share some common characteristics. The population could be as specific as a group of multiply handicapped preschool children or as broad a population as 8-year-old children. When the test is constructed, it is repeatedly administered to a sample of this population until it is refined enough to make predictions about that population.

GENERAL PROBLEM ANALYSIS

General problem analysis is a thought process (adapted from Llorens[16]) that is used by the therapist to guide initial planning for individuals and groups. The process is based on the therapist's knowledge of child development and pathological processes. First, the therapist will identify the critical elements of development and role performance for the age of a given child. Next, the problem is defined and described. This would include prediction of the course and outcome of the problem, other service providers and procedures that are commonly associated with that problem, and special considerations and precautions involved in management of the problem by the therapist and others.

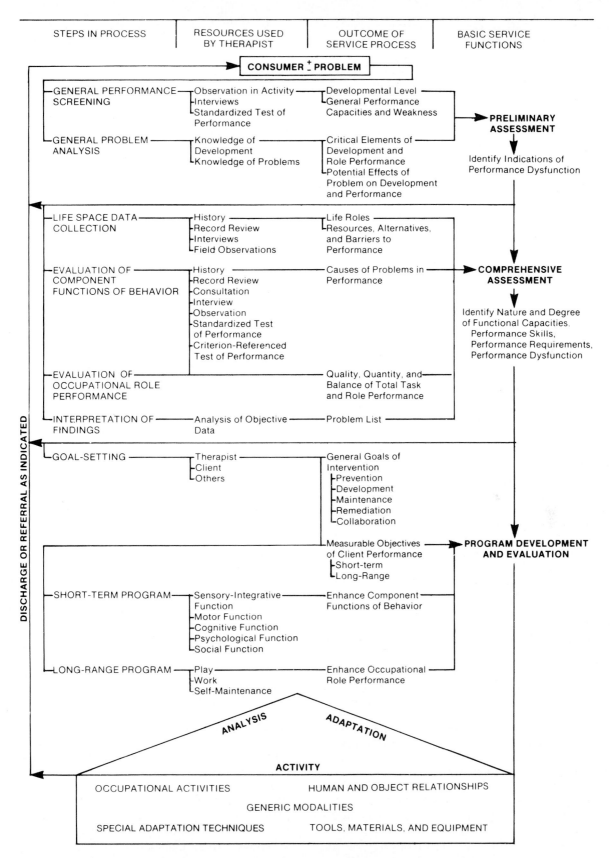

Figure 7-4   Sequential model of the occupational therapy process.

From Clark PN: Am J Occup Ther 33:583, Sept 1979.

Next, the therapist will consider what the effects of the problem, as described, might be on attaining and maintaining the critical developmental task and performance requirements of that age. This estimation is a global process, but it requires the use of activity analysis and the consideration of how the component functions of behavior might be affected. The result of this analysis is the identification of potential areas of performance dysfunction that need to be assessed by the therapist and that later will serve as the focus of program development. The occupational therapist then evaluates data collected during screening in relation to the potential effects on occupation role performance predicted by the general problem analysis.

It should be reinforced here that general problem analysis is a thought process, a way of approaching *planning* for a new client or developing a service program for a group who share similar presenting problems. It is useful for occupational therapy students to practice using this method in written form until they become attuned to using the thought process. In addition, a written version of general problem analysis is valuable as a prospectus for a new service program. It will indicate the rationale for occupational therapy intervention, specific foci of the service programs, and space, staff, material, and equipment needs. A sample of a general problem analysis is shown in Figure 7-5. Although the information about general problem analysis is presented here after screening, this thought process begins as soon as the therapist is notified of a new referral.

COMPREHENSIVE ASSESSMENT

The preliminary part of the assessment process, or screening, can help the therapist begin to determine what the child needs to be able to do that he or she cannot do to satisfy self, family, and society. Results of general performance screening guide the design of further evaluation as the therapist seeks to identify more precisely the nature and degree of a child's functional capacities and skills, as well as program goals. Comprehensive assessment includes the following:

1. *Life space data collection.*[5] Through history-taking, interviews, and field observations the therapist defines the child's life roles and environmental and cultural performance requirements. External resources, alternatives, and barriers to performance are clarified.

2. *Evaluation of component functions of behavior.* Formal and informal measures of functional capacity are used to determine why a child has problems doing every day activities. The therapist, guided by general problem analysis and screening results, assesses sensory-integrative, cognitive, social, motor, and emotional functions. Specific evaluation of one functional area may be more indepth than others, depending on the presenting problems.

Information about functional capacities may be collected by the therapist through observation, inter-views, and administration of standardized and criterion-referenced tests. Standardized tests were discussed in detail in the section on screening. *Criterion-referenced* tests are nonquantifiable measures of performance. They may be commercially produced or therapist made. Behavioral statements about functions or descriptions of a skill are collected from various legitimate resources and listed. For example, if a therapist wanted to evaluate a young child's emotional functions and used Erikson as a reference, a criterion-referenced test might include "Does not cry when mother leaves room."

Data may also be collected from other service providers through the use of record review and consultation. Information is taken from charts, reports, team meetings, and individual discussions. The use of assessment findings from other sources helps to limit duplication of services to a child who may already be overwhelmed by professional attention. Interpretation of the assembled data will provide a picture of the child's capacities and deficits in the five component functions (Figure 7-4).

3. *Evaluation of occupational role and activity performance.* Concurrently, the therapist also measures the child's ability to perform specific activities required in daily self-maintenance, play, educational, and prevocational roles. The variety of assessment methods used remains the same but with focus on total task performance. Evaluations of performance in these activities will be both qualitative and quantitative and will also identify the appropriateness of balance between the different categories of occupational activities. For example, does the child take so long to put on a shirt independently that he frequently misses the bus for school? Would it be feasible to use some adaptive equipment or limited assistance from the mother so that he can benefit from school opportunities and still maintain a sense of independence? Considerations of this type guide the transition from assessment to program planning.

Program development and evaluation

Through the assessment process the therapist has identified child-specific performance dysfunctions and problems, that is, what areas and types of activity performance require occupational therapy intervention and why. Often a prioritized list of problems is constructed, either individually by the therapist or jointly with team members.

Program goals and objectives can be developed with the child and family through the consideration of the assembled data and the availability of occupational therapy and other services. *Program goals* describe long-term expectations of treatment and will be consistent with the general goals of occupational therapy, as described earlier and shown in Figure 7-5. *Objectives* can be conceptualized as the short-term accomplish-

FIGURE 7-5　General problem analysis

Client: Johnnie Jones
Age: 6
Sex: Male
Life and occupational roles: Boy, son, playmate, brother, student
Problem: Juvenile rheumatoid arthritis
Meaningful others: Parents, siblings, peers, teachers, other relatives, adults in the neighborhood.
Critical elements of development and role performance at this period of life: Learning academic skills; improving motor and perceptual skills; learning to get along with peers; learning social and sexual roles; developing an independent self-concept; moving into the community; developing concrete operations.
Common definition and description of presenting problem: A systemic disease with inflammation of the joint capsule; involves one or more joints; intermittent low-grade fever; pain, swelling, redness, and stiffness. Requires rest, periods of immobilization, medical and nursing care, laboratory procedures, chemotherapy.
Potential disruptions to performance:
　Sensory-integrative: General decrease in sensory stimulation, especially tactile and kinesthetic; vision may be impaired by fever and medications.
　Motor: Decreased muscle strength, speed, flexibility, precision, and impulsion. Decreased practice and refinement of motor patterns.
　Cognitive: Delay of academic learning; interference and effect on perceptual-motor experiences; possible delay on transition to concrete operations because of diminished activities.
　Emotional: Less opportunity for reaching out; forced into dependency; regression may occur; sexual identity could be disrupted.
　Social: Separated from meaningful others, especially peer group; decreased competitive and cooperative interaction experiences; decreased social language development.
　Developmental tasks: All tasks are affected by decreased opportunity, especially physical, academic, and peer group skills.
　Occupational role performance: Limited mobility affects skill development and maintenance in all areas. Subject to dependence in self-care and in initiating activities in other realms.
Areas indicated for occupational therapy assessment: Age-related task performance; evaluation of sensory, motor, and emotional functions. Information on other functions could be obtained from teachers, physician, nurses, parents, social worker, or psychologist.
Suggested procedures: Observation, standardized developmental evaluation for age, interviews with child and parents regarding occupational role and activity history; assessment of play and self-maintenance skills; range of motion and functional muscle strength tests; tests of visual perception and sensory awareness; possibly a projective activity battery. Check on family and developmental history; intellectual assessment and school performance; peer interaction if in a children's unit.
Possible goals for occupational therapy intervention:
　Direct: Maintain developmental-performance skills, especially play, self-care, and socialization; maintain healthy self-concept; prevent loss of joint motion; prevent excessive dependency.
　Indirect: Support bedside academic program; facilitate home management, including parent-child relationships; support medical regimen through the monitoring of performance response to medications and through the use of graded activity program and adherence to medical precautions.
Possible program modalities: Board games at bedside with two or three children; resting splints as necesary to protect joints and maintain range of motion; gross motor play on inflatables; adapted diet to facilitate self-care in feeding; adapted dressing techniques as necessary; reading, story-telling, and dramatic play.

Adapted from Llorens LA: Application of a developmental theory for health and rehabilitation, Rockville, Md, 1976, American Occupational Therapy Association, Inc.

ments that will enable the child to achieve long-term goals.

Next, a therapy program is designed to meet those objectives, based on the therapist's use of the activity analysis process with generic modalities. Fidler[8] stated that occupational therapists select activities that duplicate, simulate, or represent the natural activities of the child's required repertoire. As discussed earlier, pro-

gram activities may be adapted to facilitate independent activity performance.

SHORT-TERM PROGRAM

Most frequently the initial, short-term goals and program will be directed toward improving basic capacities in the five component functions. This practice is supported by the theoretical frameworks presented in

Chapter 3. It is proposed that most programs should begin with attention to the physiological components (sensory-integrative, motor, and cognitive functions.) Research reports support the effectiveness of this approach in early programming.[2,14,21] In pediatric occupational therapy, play activities provide the most appropriate modalities for development of component functions. The use of play as a therapeutic modality will be discussed in detail in Chapter 15.

LONG-TERM PROGRAM

The long-term objectives and program are concerned with promoting acceptable performance in required occupational role activities. Therefore the therapist works with the child to develop skills in specific play, self-maintenance, and academic and work readiness activities.

At different intervals throughout the process of intervention, the therapist will retest and reassess the performance status of the child to determine program effectiveness. Goals and objectives must maintain relevance to the changing needs of the child. It is particularly important for the therapist to keep in touch with the family and significant others to ensure continuity and consistency of the program with environmental demands. Moving to a new house or entering a new school can have profound implications for program changes. A two-dimensional review of the intervention process (Figure 7-4) may be used to check relationships between and within components of assessment data, program goals and objectives and program modalities.

DISCHARGE, REFERRAL, AND FOLLOW-UP

It should be remembered that at any time through the sequence of occupational therapy intervention, services may be discontinued. Occasionally this is because of circumstances beyond the therapist's control, such as acute illness or family relocation. However, termination is generally subject to tacit agreement by all parties involved. Because of growth patterns, children tend to reach plateaus of performance, and continued therapy during these times often becomes unproductive. In such instances it is useful to institute "vacation from therapy" periods. This pattern of discharge should be accompanied by a specific follow-up date as well as an open door for parents' contacts before that.

At other times therapy may be discontinued because of a life change of the child that necessitates delivery of occupational therapy through another agency. An example of this is when a child enters a school system that provides direct therapy services. In this case contacts need to be made early with the accepting agency therapist to ensure program continuity and to prepare the child for the changes. Very often children do become attached to their therapists, but they seem to respond nicely when changes are explained in terms of "growing up." Again, an open-door policy with the family should exist, but with the understanding that future contacts will be handled cooperatively with the new therapist.

The preceding cases relate to children whose problems require long-term occupational therapy services. The therapist will also see a number of children whose problems require only short periods of intervention. In this instance therapy is terminated with the expectation that the child can accomplish necessary tasks of the moment and should have little or no difficulty with future developmental requirements. Any problems that are foreseen are carefully discussed with the parents, and the child, if possible. Referrals to other agencies or services are made to ensure adequate supports for remaining or unforeseen problems. As usual, there exists an open-door policy, and the therapist will usually schedule a follow-up appointment within the next 6 months.

STANDARDS OF PRACTICE

The American Occupational Therapy Association (AOTA), through its Commission on Practice, has developed standards of practice in different specialty areas. Included among these are standards for developmental disabilities and school system services. The sequential model of practice presented in this section is in accord with AOTA recommendations, and each may help clarify the other.

SUMMARY

The developmental theories used by occupational therapists and the "human development through occupation" model suggest that the therapist is concerned with development, integration, adaptation, competence, and initiative in task performance. Therefore therapy is directed toward providing opportunities to enhance the child's preparedness to deal with the activity performance requirements of daily living. The tools of the occupational therapist are the activities of daily living in the broadest sense.[15] The processes of activity analysis and adaptation are the core functions of the occupational therapist. These functions are used throughout an intervention process that identifies and resolves children's problems through assessment, program development, and evaluation.

STUDY QUESTIONS

1. What are the three major types of occupational activities and what common characteristics do they share?
2. What are the generic modalities of occupational therapy? Give an example of each.
3. Using the model for activity analysis shown in Figure 7-3, analyze:
   a. Playing with a kaleidoscope
   b. Playing with Tinkertoys
   c. Playing gin rummy
4. Using the general problem analysis format shown in Figure 7-5, prepare an intervention plan for:

a. Susan, aged 8 months, with a diagnosis of Down syndrome
b. Fred, aged 8 years, with a diagnosis of childhood autism
c. Annie, aged 16 years, diagnosed with sickle-cell anemia

REFERENCES

1. Bertrand AL: Social organization: a general systems and role theory perspective, Philadelphia, 1972, FA Davis Co.
2. Carlsen PN: Comparison of two occupational therapy approaches for treating the young cerebral-palsied child, Am J Occup Ther 29:267, 1975.
3. Clark PN: Human development through occupation: theoretical frameworks in comtemporary occupational therapy practice, part 1, Am J Occup Ther 33:505, 1979.
4. Clark PN: Human development through occupation: a philosophy and conceptual model for practice, part 2, Am J Occup Ther 33:577, 1979.
5. A curriculum guide for occupational therapy educators, Rockville, Md, 1974, American Occupational Therapy Association, Inc.
6. Cynkin S: Toward health through activities, Boston, 1979, Little, Brown & Co.
7. Fidler GS, and Fidler JW: Doing and becoming: purposeful action and self-actualization, Am J Occup Ther 32:305, 1978.
8. Fidler GS: Personal communication, 1975.
9. Florey LL: Intrinsic motivation: the dynamics of occupational therapy theory, Am J Occup Ther 25:319, 1971.
10. Gilfoyle EM, Grady AP, and Moore JC: Children adapt, Thorofare, NJ, 1981, Slack, Inc.
11. Gillette NP: Occupational therapy and mental health. In Willard HS, and Spackman CS, editors: Occupational therapy, ed 4, Philadelphia, 1971, JB Lippincott Co.
12. Heard C: Occupational role acquisition: a perspective on the chronically disabled, Am J Occup Ther 31:243, 1977.
13. Hopkins HL, and Smith HD: Willard and Spackman's occupational therapy, ed 5, Philadelphia, 1978, JB Lippincott Co.
14. King LJ: A sensory-integrative approach to schizophrenia, Am J Occup Ther 28:529, 1974.
15. Lansing SG, and Carlsen PN: Occupational therapy. In Valletutti P, and Christoplos F, editors: Interdisciplinary approaches to human service delivery, Baltimore, 1977, University Park Press.
16. Llorens LA: Application of a developmental theory for health and rehabilitation, Rockville, Md, 1976, American Occupational Therapy Association, Inc.
17. Llorens LA:1969 Eleanor Clark Slagle Lecture: Facilitating growth and development: the promise of occupational therapy, Am J Occup Ther 24:93, 1970.
18. Matsusuyu J: Occupational behavior: a perspective on work and play, Am J Occup Ther 25:291, 1971.
19. Meyer A: The philosophy of occupational therapy, Am J Occup Ther 31:639, 1977.
20. Mosey AC: Occupational therapy: configuration of a profession, New York, 1981, Raven Press.
21. Norton Y: Neurodevelopmental and sensory integration for the profoundly retarded multiply-handicapped child, Am J Occup Ther 29:93, 1975.
22. Pelligrino E: Preventive health care and the allied health professions. In Hamburg, J, editor: Review of allied health education, Lexington, 1973, University of Kentucky Press.
23. Reilly M: 1961 Eleanor Clark Slagle Lecture: Occupational therapy can be one of the great ideas in 20th century medicine, Am J Occup Ther 16:1, 1962.
24. Reilly M: A psychiatric occupational therapy program as a teaching model, Am J Occup Ther 20:61, 1966.
25. Reilly M: Play as exploratory learning: studies in curiosity behavior, Los Angeles, 1974, Sage Publications, Inc.

8

Parent and family involvement

MARTHA S. MOERSCH

This chapter focuses on the current equal emphasis in practice and the literature on parents *and* families as important determinants of treatment success. This change has become increasingly apparent over the past 20 years, evidenced by the requirement of an individualized family service plan in Public Law 99-457 and by the Education of the Handicapped Act Amendments of 1986.

OCCUPATIONAL THERAPY LITERATURE ON PARENT INVOLVEMENT

Occupational therapists have always been aware of the important role that parents play in helping to carry out treatment plans for children, but the occupational therapy literature has not reflected this awareness to the extent that literature of other disciplines has.

Differences between the first and fifth editions of Willard and Spackman's traditional textbook of occupational therapy[109] indicate that therapists are increasing the documentation of their involvement with parents. In their 1947 edition, Willard and Spackman[109] mentioned parents three times. By 1978, in the fifth edition, Tiffany[95] noted that it was highly desirable that the occupational therapist be involved in parent counseling or family treatment. It was also noted that therapists in acute pediatric settings could expect to spend "50 percent of their time working with adults under stress—the patients' families" (p. 428)[45] and that the entire family of the child with cerebral palsy should be active members of the treatment team.[57] Parents were discussed at length in the chapter on blindness and deafness: Wade[104] showed empathy for parents and recognized that good relationships with them were necessary to ensure maximal benefits to the blind or deaf child.

Knickerbocker,[62] writing in 1965, appears to be the first occupational therapist to write about the art and philosophy of involving parents. Many of her suggestions are almost identical to the current literature on

appropriate ways to involve parents. These include the following: ask for suggestions from parents; recognize the value of parents' contributions; do not isolate the child from the parents when treating the child; build on parents' strengths; direct actions toward maintaining a cohesive family unit; make sure that parents know why as well as how to carry out their child's program; help parents develop appropriate perspectives of the capabilities and deficiencies of their child; and structure the therapy program with the goal of developing more effective parent-child relationships.

In 1969 Vulpe[102] reported a home program that provided successful experiences for parents by teaching them to use concrete activities related to their child's developmental patterns. Since the early seventies, occupational therapists have published increasing amounts of material about parents and therapists working together.*

Research studies of aspects of parental involvement have been scarce in occupational therapy. However, there are some related investigations: Petersen[84] studied stress and identified resources for reducing stress in mothers of handicapped children. A pilot study by Johnson and Deitz[60] found that the mothers of physically handicapped preschool children "spent significantly more time engaged in physical child care activities than did the mothers of normal preschoolers" (p. 578). Sparling and Rogers[91] authored a preliminary report (suggesting minor revisions) on the pilot study of Feeding Interaction Report—Scale and Treatment (FIRST), an instrument that assesses oral motor and interactive behaviors of children at risk for developmental disabilities. Howard[56] used the Preschool Play Scale to compare developmental play ages, and found that physically abused children had lower developmental play ages than nonabused children.

---

*References 2-4, 11, 16, 20, 22, 23, 29, 31, 32, 44, 49, 61-63, 66, 67, 72, 75, 76, 78, 80, 86, 101-104.

THERAPIST-FAMILY RELATIONSHIPS
The child

As the therapist develops and maintains a relationship with parents, the parents must sense that the therapist always has the child's welfare as top priority. Otherwise, there is no basis for a therapist/parent relationship. This concept may be difficult to keep in mind during the sometimes stressful process of developing a rapport with parents. The following behaviors should be incorporated in interactions with children and parents:

- The therapist should acknowledge the child as an active participant. "Show mommy how you can close your lips on the spoon." Refrain from talking to parents of a 4- or 5-year-old as if the child were not present.
- Children should be included in the decision-making process whenever possible. It is better for the child to hear what takes place in the parent-therapist conference than to develop anxiety, fear, and fantasy about what is being said.[15]
- Children should be given appropriate explanations of the goals of their occupational therapy programs.
- Children need role models to help them develop self-esteem, someone to note or foster their accomplishments. Parents can observe therapists and be made aware of how families can contribute.
- Therapists should show respect for the child as a person. Featherstone,[30] both a professional educator and a parent of a handicapped child, notes that a professional "offers parents a chance to savor the ordinary but delicious pleasure of parental pride and delight" (p. 183) when he treats the handicapped child as any other child.

The parents
GENERAL CONSIDERATIONS

The therapist should see that at least part of the initial visit of the child and his parents is spent discussing what occupational therapy is and what it can be expected to do for children. It is important that both parents be present for as much of the initial evaluation as possible. If only one parent is present, it will be necessary for this parent to explain findings and recommendations to the other parent and thereby risk being put in the position of having to defend the program. Even when both parents are present, they should also be given written reports.

GUIDELINES FOR HOME PROGRAMS

The nature of a child's growth and development and the occupational therapist's goal to help children attain their maximal potential levels of growth and development require home programs to be included in occupational therapy treatment. The following guidelines will assist therapists in developing home treatment programs to be carried out by parents and families.

- Develop the home program following the initial meetings with the child and parents. These meetings are for orientation, interview, comprehensive evaluation, parent informing, and treatment planning.
- Visit the child's home for some of the initial meetings, if possible.
- Give parents written reports of all findings and plans as they are developed.
- Determine treatment objectives jointly with parents, as well as appropriate activities to meet the objectives. Specify which portions of treatment will take place at home.
- Write objectives in areas of the child's strengths and weaknesses. This assures parents of some success.
- Demonstrate the treatment activities and explain their rationale; teach the parents to perform the activities, observe their practice, correct their mistakes, and make necessary adaptations; answer parents' questions you have answers for and be honest about questions you do not have answers for; and provide emotional support to the parents.
- Encourage parents to join you in frequent problem-solving sessions.
- Monitor parents' program implementation and make appropriate adaptations and changes in conjunction with the parents.
- Reevaluate and write new objectives at frequent intervals (3- to 6-month intervals recommended).
- Vary activities to maintain continued interest of both child and parents and for generalization of learning.

Occupational therapists have discussed home programs in numerous publications.* Program suggestions appear throughout the discussions of practice in this text.

MOTIVATING PARENTS

Therapists often ask how to motivate parents to carry out treatment programs. Three ways are (1) be sure the program works for the child, (2) be sure the parent will achieve some success, and (3) be sure the program includes areas of major concern to the parents.

Parent motivation is usually increased by setting up treatment activities that can be carried out in the daily routine of the family, such as gross motor activities during bath and diapering times, rough and tumble play with a parent or sibling, or fine motor manipulation board games that other family members enjoy.

Parents are usually more motivated if they have had a part in planning the program. The therapist should make reasonable requests of the parents. It is not necessary that the treatment program be done in the same way or at the same time each day. However, for some-

---

*References 4, 23, 49, 61-63, 66, 72, 75, 86, 102, 103.

parents a very structured program seems to be more motivating.[72] A parent who is overwhelmed by the constant problems brought on by a handicapped child and has experienced feelings of helplessness may welcome a home program that is written precisely and includes a section for recording comments by the parent.

It is also worthwhile to think of motivating parents for themselves, to increase their feelings of worth and accomplishment. This effort at motivation might take place during clinical activities but can be focused on the parent as on the child. One definition of motivate is "to stimualte active interest in (some study) through appeal to associated interests." Observe the parents for indications of interests or abilities which can be praised or at least recognized with a positive approach.

Offer parents opportunities to assist other parents, take part in a teaching session, assist in making decisions, or exercise autonomy in some way. But be sure opportunities are offered in a way that parents recognize they can choose to say no. Programs that give parents opportunities to meet on a one-to-one basis to provide emotional support and resource information are excellent vehicles for developing parent motivation, especially in rural areas where families feel isolated.

FOSTERING PARENT-THERAPIST INTERACTIONS

Therapists must be objective in evaluating their own actions as they try to work out positive relationships with parents. Knickerbocker[62] suggested that therapists who assume major treatment responsibility for the child may "imply that the parents' responsibility ends at the clinic door" (p. 129). Therapists should guard against assuming authoritarian roles that seem to put them in superior positions because this can interfere with therapist-parent communication and make it more difficult for parents to assume their responsibilities. Therapists should be alert to possibilities that they may "mother" or "father" the child as a way of fulfilling their own needs for parental roles; in so doing they "may tend to usurp the rightful responsibilities of the child's own parents" (p. 130).[62]

Anderson and Hinojosa[3] presented findings from their experience and from the literature related to establishing professional partnerships with parents of handicapped children. They gave numerous examples of basic principles for working with parents but stressed that systematic methods were not usually effective because of the individual needs and differences in parents. They concluded that "The occupational therapist's time spent with parents may be more important and therapeutic than time spent in direct treatment of the child" (p. 460).

The following suggestions, paraphrased from Roos[85] are ways of building productive work relationships between parents and professionals.

- Parents should be accepted as team members, considered as colleagues, and have their contributions treated with respect.
- Parents and professionals should recognize and discuss their preconceived notions or negative expectations of each other.
- Professionals should accept parents "where they are."
- Professionals should share relevant information with parents.
- Professionals should maintain good commmunication with a minimum of professional jargon.
- Professionals should select methods and techniques; parents, and children if appropriate, should make the final selection of goals and objectives.
- Parents and professionals need mutual support and encouragement from each other.
- Parents and professionals should never compete with each other or undermine each other's efforts with the child.

SPECIAL CIRCUMSTANCES OF PARENTS

The pediatric occupational therapist is likely to find that a variety of circumstances exist among parents.

Marital problems affect many parents of handicapped children because marital problems affect a high percentage of the population as a whole and because there is the added stress of caring for a disabled child.[30,108]

Single parents head many families with handicapped children. Problems that may arise are not necessarily related to singleness itself, but to the lack of another adult who can provide support.[6] Bronfenbrenner[10] noted that one of the five factors that determine the effectiveness of early intervention programs for children is the "presence in the home of another adult besides the principal caretaker" (p 18).

Therapists will encounter *those other than biological parents in the parental role,* such as adoptive parents, stepparents, foster parents, guardians, grandparents, siblings, other relatives, agency representatives, and friends. The occupational therapist's relationship with surrogate parents will usually be the same as with biological parents, and the suggestions of Roos[85] will usually apply to anyone in the parental role. However, the person who is legally designated as responsible in the child's state of residence, including the handicapped person, must sign all legal documents.

Parents with handicapping conditions are likely to be among the parents of children that therapists treat. *Children of Handicapped Parents*[94] includes chapters on parenthood in a variety of handicapped persons, from both clinical and research perspectives. This resource includes discussion of problems faced by parents with emotional problems, mental retardation, physical disabilities, diabetes, and deafness. A major purpose of the book is to point out that very little information is available on such parents and to urge that research studies be conducted from the viewpoint of both legal and public policy issues. There are concerns for the rights of disabled persons to have children and concerns for children's rights to grow up in positive environments. Policies are being made without benefit of knowledge and will continue to be so made until further research has occurred.[94]

Bingham[8] was diagnosed as having multiple sclerosis at the age of 27. Over 20 years later, she wrote *One Step More, Lord!* This book recounts her life as a wife, mother of two, and active participant in religious and community activities both for her own benefit and on behalf of her husband and children. Her story exemplifies experiences encountered by parents who have long-term illnesses.

Mentally retarded parents are sometimes found among parents of handicapped children. Such parents can usually manage to maintain themselves and their families in at least a marginal manner, but they may need help in crises.

Dickerson, Eastman, and Saffer[25] developed *Child Care Training for Adults with Mental Retardation, Vol 1, Infants,* which includes training units on holding, dressing, feeding, diapering, bathing, and playing with infants. The authors believe that "all adults who live in the community should have the opportunity to learn how to interact with infants and children in a caring and safe manner" (p. 1). They constructed a training program so that mentally retarded adults could "develop competency in their interactions with children, become trustworthy sitters for other parents' children, and be better prepared for parenting their own children" (p. 1).

Parents who abuse and neglect children are found throughout society.[17,29,108] Major focus in the 1960s was on physical abuse, sexual abuse was the focus in the 1970s, and Garbarino, Guttmann, and Seeley[34] expect psychological maltreatment to become well known in the 1980s and 1990s. Garbarino, Guttmann, and Seeley[34] wrote *The Psychologically Battered Child* for professionals and students who work with children. Unlike physical abuse and neglect and sexual exploitation, psychological abuse is not easily described or recognized. Also, psychological abuse or maltreatment takes on different aspects depending on the age of the child. The book considers the psychological maltreatment categories of terrorizing, isolating, ignoring, rejecting, and corrupting as they occur in the development periods of infancy, early childhood, school age, and adolescence. Case histories are used to illustrate the categories within developmental periods as well as the implications for identification, assessment, and intervention. Major emphasis is on parent-child relations in the home. The book's extensive reference list covers all three areas of child abuse. Other resources include instruments, key organizations, and state chapters of the National Committee for Prevention of Child Abuse.

Therapists should also be aware of possible problems among parents at low economic or educational levels who have other ill or dependent family members or who make frequent geographical moves and must therefore locate new community resources and emotional support systems.

Siblings

Through discussions with parents or through their own observations, therapists can determine the need of siblings to know and understand the handicapped child's condition, to know the implications of the handicapping condition as it relates to them, and to know the future expectations related to the handicapped child. There are numerous publications on siblings.*

Seligman[88] reviewed research findings on siblings and concluded that "whether normal siblings are not affected, are helped, or harmed by the presence of a handicapped brother or sister is unanswerable" (p. 170).

Grandparents

Parents may report that they have more difficulty coping with the concerns and questions of their parents than they do with those of their nonhandicapped children. This is not unexpected, since grandparents have concerns for both the beloved grandchild and their own beloved child. Parents may also report more difficulties with grandparents who live far away.

However, parents usually report positive aspects of involvement of the grandparents in the care of a handicapped child. The grandparents provide emotional support, sitter or respite care, financial assistance, and attention to the other children in the family so that the parents are able to spend more time with the handicapped child. Therapists are likely to have relationships with grandparents that can facilitate the child's therapy. Grandparents are good sources of information about the child, because many children willingly cooperate with grandparents. Grandparents often have more time than working parents to play with or teach the child, and they contribute in many ways to a normal family life for the child.

Grandparents can also contribute to friction within a family, as when a husband or wife may be forced to take sides for or against inlaws or each other.[15] Moersch[77] described possible problems in households made up of children, parents, and grandparents. When fathers are unable to accompany mothers to clinic visits of the child, the grandmother often goes along to help. This may result in increasing the competency and effectiveness of the mother and grandmother and strengthening their alliance. By contrast, the father becomes less competent and effective. Extreme examples have shown that grandparents, especially the grandmother, assume the parental role in opposition to one or both parents and the child becomes uncertain as to who the real mother or father is. In such families, children who are already prone to learning or emotional

---

*References, 1, 11, 15, 84, 88, 108.

problems seem to suffer from living with too many adults who expose them to different and contradictory expectations of behavior. Other factors negatively affecting the child are parents and grandparents who act as individuals rather than family units in managing the children.

Northcott,[82] who worked with young deaf children for many years, cautioned professionals in programs for young handicapped children to be aware of the special situation of the single parent and the parent in a multigeneration family under one roof.

Others: relatives, neighbors, friends, the public

Therapists do not usually have active relationships beyond the immediate family of the child. However, the child's welfare can be affected if the parents have difficulties maintaining a normally functioning environment. To educate relatives, neighbors, friends, or other persons who seem likely to interfere with family relationships, the therapist can make use of the ongoing efforts of schools, churches, the press, movies, television, the government, and others to influence attitudes toward people with handicapping conditions. These efforts can provide information and influence public policy. It is hoped they can also suggest positive alternative actions to family associates.[7]

THE THERAPIST'S PREPARATION TO RELATE TO FAMILY MEMBERS

A group of 30 pediatric occupational therapy leaders determined that the highest priority for pediatric content in curriculum for training pediatric occupational therapists was working with parents and families.[83] Increasing numbers of universities are developing academic courses about working with parents and families; instructors sometimes assign students to spend time with families of handicapped children. Clinical placements of occupational therapy students may provide opportunities for some students to work with parents in pediatric acute care hospitals and other programs that emphasize parent involvement. But when and where do most therapists get sufficient practice in working with parents to feel comfortable in doing so? Probably only when they begin working in a program in which parent involvement is an integral part of the structure. Early intervention programs for handicapped or high-risk infants have been good sources for learning to work with parents, especially those programs that include home visits. Home visits bring about intimate associations with families who have to add the care of a handicapped child to their normal responsibilities. Here the home visitor becomes a "participant in both the joys and sorrows of the families, including critical illnesses and death as well as the successful attainment of program objectives" (p. 41).[77]

Although reading should not be emphasized over active participation, there are many publications on working with parents and families.*

NATURE OF PARENT INVOLVEMENT
Infant and preschool years

Literature on parent involvement since the mid-1960s pertains overwhelmingly to the infant and preschool years. This is explained in part by the focus of medical and educational research on young children, belief in the importance of the family setting for early learning, availability of funds, expectations of parents to care for their young children, and recognition by professionals of the personal satisfaction and career opportunities in working with infants and preschool children.

Anderson[2] reviewed pediatric research findings as a basis for selecting sensory assessment and treatment methods for a neonatal intensive care unit. Concern was expressed for the possible negative effects of early sensory experiences on the "delicate reciprocal reinforcement system between parent and infant" (p. 22) and on later parent-child interactions.

Parents and therapists with limited experience in high-risk neonatal care will benefit from Lucas's[67] account of her home and family accommodations when her 2-month-old, 4 pound daughter was released from the neonatal intensive care unit. From her background as an occupational therapist, Lucas was able to provide appropriate care with many adaptations.

McCollum[70] studied gaze patterns in mother and infant interactions in play and instructional situations. Such studies provide information for "understanding caregiver-infant interactions as well as for designing interventions that take these patterns into account" (p. 517).

For ways in which parents of preschool children may become involved in their children's treatment/education, see Chapter 19. An operational preschool program that builds parental involvement is described.

The majority of early preschool programs[41,43,48,107] were for disadvantaged children and were aimed at improving cognitive and social levels of the children. Handicapped children were added as the result of the movement toward ensuring the rights of all people and because of the influence of parent groups. Medical advances in neonatal care, studies of parent-infant bonding, and general feelings of "the earlier the better" reduced the age level of special programs to birth, and the parent involvement literature increased even more.

Childhood years

State and national mandatory special education laws reflect the concept of parents' rights in legislative and

---

*References 15, 30, 38, 47, 70, 71, 76, 96, 97.

educational practices. The laws at both state and federal levels continue to change and parents and therapists must monitor these changes.

As parents and therapists work together with the school-aged child, they may be interested in *Teaching Students with Learning and Behavior Problems.*[105] Although the book notes that it applies to both clinical and classroom settings, it is clearly for teachers of children with mild to moderate learning impairment and behavior impairment. It is recommended as one of the best recent publications on teaching these children. A parent interested in being well prepared for Individualized Education Plan meetings would find much material in this book as to what occurs in up-to-date schools. The content includes information on social interactions and behavior, teaching competencies, structuring the learning environment, microcomputers, cognitive training, and other topics of possible interest to therapists working in school systems.

The school-aged child who is handicapped becomes increasingly different from the normal school-aged child. The handicapped child has difficulties developing peer relationships and requires more assistance from his or her parents, becoming even more dependent on them. The parent-child relationship suffers because of the parents' anxiety and expectations that are higher than the child can meet.[3]

Adolescent years

The nature of parent involvement in the lives of all children changes drastically when the children reach adolescence. It appears that adolescence is such a critical time that whether the child is ill or handicapped seems secondary in importance. At the same time, the presence of a handicapping condition increases the possibility that the child will not acquire the basic survival skills so important in adult life.[18]

Parents of children with all levels of handicapping conditions are well aware of the changes that occur when the children reach adolescence. Parents of a severely retarded son were surprised at the abrupt changes that came with puberty after they had assumed that a mentally slow child would also show slow physical development. They found instead that there was a difference between having a retarded child and having a retarded teenager.[73] One intellectually bright but severely physically handicapped person considered that the success of her life was a result of her parents' repeated advisements throughout her early years that she could be anything she wanted to be.[12] It is especially hard for parents of mildly handicapped children of adolescent age to strike a balance between their love and concern for their children and their children's need to acquire the "skills and competencies necessary to function independently of parents, to become gainfully employed, and to assume adult responsibilities" (p. 1.)[69]

Some special educators believe that both parents and professionals should have a thorough understanding of all that adolescence implies,[18] that "emotional development and the self-concept of a mildly handicapped adolescent may be of paramount importance" (p. 52),[69] and that the period of secondary education often brings about increased family stress, socialization problems, and interpersonal conflict.[69] Most of the interactions of professionals and parents of mildly handicapped adolescents will take place in the secondary educational environment, and the parent involvement will of necessity be less visible and less active. Professionals must realize how important it is that there be candid discussion between themselves and parents with understanding on the part of both.[69] Persons filling parent counseling roles must be aware of the special problems of the secondary school because of the number of personnel involved and the "impersonal structure of the school" (p. 124).[69]

The *Exceptional Education Quarterly* devoted an entire issue to the subject of mildly handicapped adolescents. Entitled "Special Education for Adolescents and Young Adults,"[21] it presented such topics as educational options, career preparations, work-oriented curriculums vs academic education, and the similarities between learning disabled and low-achieving secondary school students. It also dealt with emotional factors, such as the depression and suicide potential and the vulnerability of partially blind and hard-of-hearing adolescents to psychiatric disturbance, and the need for sex education for handicapped persons. The importance of social skills, the impact of mandatory minimal competency testing, and the greater prevalence of learning disabled persons among officially delinquent youth were discussed. This issue is an exceptionally informative resource for both professionals and parents.

Perceptually handicapped adolescents often have difficulty feeling loved, develop inadequate self-concepts, then become more and more depressed, and finally go on to have severe emotional and behavior problems. These children must feel "genuinely, unconditionally loved, . . . and they need more affection . . . " (p. 128).[13]

Preparation for adulthood

Parents, and persons working with them, have major concerns as to what will happen when disabled children grow up. Moving beyond adolescence brings about many changes for the soon-to-be adults and their families—changes that require careful planning on the part of families and others. Recognition of these concerns brought about publication of *The Right to Grow Up: An Introduction to Adults with Developmental Disabilities.*[92] The authors discuss various aspects of the transition period as well as mature and elderly years, including living arrangements, vocational training and work opportunities, sexuality, marriage and parenthood, recreation and leisure, participation in religious activities, independent living, and self-advocacy. They also focus on primary needs of all persons for acceptance, appreciation, and respect. Both parents and therapists will find in the book much information that applies to persons with all types of special needs.

As commissioner of the Administration on Developmental Disabilities, Elder[28] noted that a major shortcoming of our governmental system is that "young adults with developmental disabilities, graduating from the public education system have extremely limited options" (p. 53) and stressed the need for a continuum of services in this transition period.

Harris[46] believes that parents should begin consideration and discussion of the moral and legal aspects of parenting a handicapped adult before childhood is over because parents' views of the future will affect how they rear and educate their child. He urges professionals to introduce considerations of long-term parental responsibilities into their relationships with parents of young children.

The *Adult Transition Model*[55] was developed to bridge the gap between public schools and postschool community agencies and to promote the goals of productivity, independence, and integration into the community as measures of success and quality of life. The workbook format includes sections on administration, staff education, student training, and parent education. The parent education section provides detailed information and sample forms as well as emphasizing the importance of involving, increasing awareness, alleviating concerns and fears, and helping parents.

Hobbs[51] urged development of public policies to help young people with chronic illness and disabilities make the transition to adulthood. There must be recognition on the part of both parents and professionals that young people must be allowed, and encouraged to become adults.

Mental retardation

The literature on parent involvement has been greatly influenced by the problems associated with mental retardation (see references). Both early and contemporary programs for high-risk children have had prevention of mental retardation as a major purpose. Since preschool programs for handicapped children became widespread, many of the children served are mentally retarded, such as those with Down syndrome or those who were multiply handicapped with various degrees of mental retardation as one of the handicaps.

Chronic illness

The 5 year project, Public Policies Affecting Chronically Ill Children and Their Families, conducted at the Vanderbilt Institute for Public Policy and directed by Nicholas Hobbs served to bring chronic illness to the attention of the public in the early 1980s as did President Kennedy's interest in mental retardation in the early 1960s. The study considered diabetes, severe asthma, leukemia, cystic fibrosis, sickle-cell anemia, and similar medical conditions as the chronic illnesses that before the late 1950s and early 1960s usually resulted in early deaths of the affected children. These children live well into adulthood due to developments in the basic sciences and in medical care. New problems and new demands have followed the scientific and medical progress: the years of financial and emotional burdens for the families, leading to the conclusion that "The time has come for policy makers to turn their attentions to children who have chronic illnesses, to their families, and to supporting effective programs for them" (p. xviii).[50]

The project has been highly publicized beginning with an interim report in 1983, later published in *Rehabilitation Literature*,[53] followed by a formal report[51] and an accompanying resource book.[52] *Strengthening Families*[50] is a related book that focuses on *all* children and, like the reports, makes "existing knowledge available to policy makers" (p. 7). The project and resulting reports have had significant impact and should have momentous consequences.

Campbell, a psychiatrist,[13] gives insight into the effects of chronic illness on children, writing that chronically ill children become resentful and defiant because of "(1) substitution of medical procedures as a manifestation of love . . . . and (2) poor limit-setting and lack of behavioral control by the parents" (p. 130). If not controlled, the children will manipulate and control the parents and will use the "outright threat of purposely succumbing to the illness" (p. 130).

Other disability areas

Literature on parent involvement with learning disabilities,* physical disabilities,† sensory deficits,‡ emotional problems,§ and autism[42,87,106] is available but to a lesser degree than that which is related to mental retardation and chronic illness.

Children at risk

As occupational therapists expand their areas of practice to include facilitation of growth and development in well children who are at risk for developmental problems, they see parent involvement as a major vehicle for implementation of their programs.

Finn[31] described a community intervention and prevention model for children, parents, and schoolpersonnel in an inner-city area. Parents were helped to learn

---

*References 4, 13, 18, 21, 32, 63, 89, 105.
†References 23, 44, 54, 62, 86.
‡References 23, 46, 49, 75, 86, 104.
§References 4, 23, 29, 31

about mothering skills, elements of children's developmental processes, toy construction from household items, and other positive parent-child interactions in both group and home visit situations. The program emphasized the parents as decision makers regarding their children, the provision of basic emotional support for parents, and preserving and respecting the values and life-styles of the parents.

Gillette[35] set up an art workshop for the mothers of preschool children who were identified by the school as exhibiting less than optimal mothering behaviors toward their children. The mothers who were selected had difficulties in one or more of the areas of "discipline; intimacy; giving (in other than material ways); allowing freedom of expression, especially when it was 'messy'; permitting the development of autonomy in the child; and denying the existence of certain personal needs which resulted in a sense of depletion and frustration in the mother herself" (p. 128).[35] The preschool children themselves were "considered to be poor educational, emotional, or behavioral risks for the community" (p. 127).[35] Results of the program led to the assumption "that an increase in [the mother's] own sense of personal value can lead to more mature behavior in regard to other persons" (p. 129).[35] It was not possible to identify specific changes in the mothering behavior at the time of reporting. The program itself is an example of how occupational therapists can take part in parent involvement with the intent of benefiting children.

Llorens[66] included a brief description of a program for teenage mothers as one example of her use of objective setting to establish an occupational therapy program within an inner-city community. The mothers were helped through an education-consultation process to increase their own interpersonal growth and development as one means of preventing ineterpersonal difficulties within the mother-infant relationship.

In 1978 Morris[80] suggested parent education in well baby care as a new role for the occupational therapist. She reported that pediatric clinics were ideal locations for parent education programs for teaching mothers the mental health aspects of child care, how to support their child's cognitive development, and alternative ways of interacting with their child.

Ellsworth[29] described a parent education program that was designed to counteract the increasing incidence and severity of child abuse and neglect among children of Army families, as well as the alarming prevalence of parents ill prepared to rear socially and emotionally healthy children. The program, developed and directed by an occupational therapist and an Army health nurse, followed a 10-week seminar and group counseling format for parents, accompanied by developmental assessment and play therapy sessions for their children. Provisions were made for appropriate follow-up treatment for the children and counseling for the parents.

ISSUES OF PARENT INVOLVEMENT
Parents as individuals

A notable aspect of the parent involvement literature of the 1980s is the focus on parents as individuals, as having the right to lives of their own, apart from being parents of handicapped children.

Parents Speak Out, published in 1978, was one of the earliest of the "tell it like it is" books and was written by persons who were both professionals and parents of disabled children.[98] *Before and After Zachariah: a family story about a different kind of courage* is a similar book written by a mother of a handicapped child.[64] *Parents Speak Out: Then and Now,* published in 1985, contains the original chapters of the 1978 book as well as updated accounts by the authors; the preface notes that the editors plan to revise the book every 5 or 6 years with updates so that readers can follow life cycles of families.[100] These books are highly recommended for parents, professionals, and students.

Parents as individuals need "self-nourishment"; privacy; time to attend to marital relationships; social contact with the outside world; interesting occupations, hobbies, and recreation; and freedom from or help with coping with unusual stresses that are exacerbated by the presence of a disabled child, such as poor physical health, emotional problems, financial difficulties, and stigma.[74,79,84]

Play and parent-family involvement

It is appropriate to link play and parent involvement in a book on how occupational therapy can help children play, grow, learn, and develop skills that will enable them to enjoy satisfying adult lives. Various types of play, from infant stimulation to educational games for teenagers, take place within the family environment. Helpful examples are given in *Teaching With Toys: Making Your Own Educational Toys* for children up to age 3 and *Growing With Games: Making Your Own Educational Games* for children aged 3 to 6.[36,37] The two books were written for parents and children who enjoy playing together; they were also written to enhance learning for children with learning disabilities.

Occupational therapists have used the normal day-to-day interactions of mothers and children to determine how mothers can provide sensory stimulation to their infants,[20] how mothers can be helped to understand sensory integrative problems of their children,[4] and how mothers can make their children's everyday environments more positive.[32] Day[20] found that in a 4- to 6-week-old infant, playing was second only to feeding in providing the greatest amount of stimulation. On a per minute basis, playing provided more stimulation than any other activity, and playing was an important provider of all types of stimulation. Ayres[4] described how parents can involve their children in sensory integrative activities in the form of play to encourage adap-

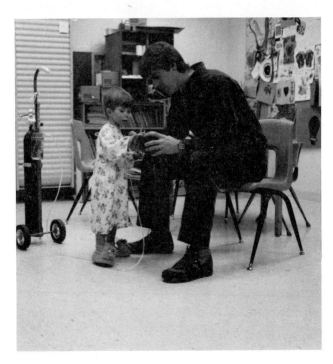

Figure 8-1 In addition to giving loving support to their hospitalized children, parents can often act as co-therapists or teachers.

tive responses and to enhance the children's self-esteem. Gordon and Lally[41] used play activities in their classic studies of disadvantaged mothers and their children. Later, the play activities were published for the use of other parents.[39,40]

Many of the intervention programs[41,43,107] in the 1960s and early 1970s for high-risk children made extensive use of home visitors. One of the major duties of the home visitor was to demonstrate play activities to the parents and to encourage parents to play with their children. There are many books on play and games for children of all ages.

Parent as teacher or therapist

The topic of parents as teachers or therapists arises often in descriptions of programs for individuals or groups of children with handicaps. For the most part, the situation is either casually accepted or upheld as being desirable, beneficial, and expedient.*

Positive reports of parents acting as teachers come from persons well known in early programs for children at risk, such as Weikart[107] and Gordon and Lally.[41] Subsequently, others such as Shearer and Shearer,[90] Vulpe,[102,103] and Baker[5] developed programs in which parents were teachers for retarded children and others. Morris[80] wrote that "The parent

can serve as an effective teacher when given training and experience in learning alternative ways of interacting with the child" (p. 75).

Shapero and Forbes[89] reviewed parent involvement in programs for learning disabled children and reported that a hands-off policy for parents as teachers was evident throughout the 1960s, but the policy changed completely by the early 1970s. It appears that parents as teachers can positively affect the academic performance of learning disabled children.

Another term to describe parents in the teaching role is *cotherapist,* which was used by Schopler[87] in a statewide program for autistic children in North Carolina. Parents carry out individualized home programs and also help out in the classrooms. *Provider of informal therapy* is the term used to describe "the introduction of therapeutically useful actions into the daily care and handling program" (p. 383),[54] especially for children with cerebral palsy (Figure 8-1).

In 1970 Moersch established the major feature of an early intervention program that was incorporated into the Early Intervention Project for Handicapped Infants and Young Children[78] in 1973. Parents were to be supported as the major treatment providers for their handicapped children. *Major treatment provider* could be looked on as a general term, since staff members were from various disciplines. The term was selected after thoughtful consideration of the intended philosophy of the program, namely, that such young handicapped children need care throughout their waking hours. Spe-

---

*References 5, 9, 14, 71, 90, 102, 103, 107.

cialized therapy programs two or three times a week are not sufficient.

The term *treatment* was selected because of its current usage by interdisciplinary teams to denote purposefully and thoughtfully planned management. The parent's treatment would include what all parents do to care for their babies—parent oriented activities instead of teacher-therapist oriented.

With the terminology established, it then became the responsibility of the project staff to develop treatment plans to fit into routine child care. The physical therapist determined what the child needed under the rubric of physical therapy, what part of the physical therapy could be done as exercises by the parents, and how the parents could incorporate the exercises into diapering, dressing, bathing, and playing with the child. The occupational therapist, speech therapist, psychologist, and special educator made similar discipline-related decisions. Parents became aware of the importance of establishing communication, naming items around the house, or singing to the child, but would never stop everything to have a period of speech therapy.

The Early Intervention Project made a point of not calling the parents "teachers" or "therapists." The outcome was that many of the activities of occupational, physical, and speech therapists; special educators; and psychologists were translated into normal child care activities and carried out by people called "parents"[78,86] (Figure 8-1).

There are those who oppose putting parents in the position of teachers or therapists on the grounds that this practice can diminish their roles as mothers or fathers. Tyler and Kogan[101] reviewed findings from studies reported in 1972 and 1974 of parent-child interactions with young children with cerebral palsy. They found that both mother and child showed more negative behaviors when the mother was performing therapy than when mother and child were playing. There was progressive reduction of warm and positive behaviors in both mother and child over a 2-year period. They suggested that teaching mothers to be therapists could be an intrusion into the parent role, and they recommended that parents be guided toward healthy interactions with their children. A subsequent study was undertaken in which mothers were provided behavioral instruction to help them develop warm and positive behaviors toward their children. The positive effect of mothers in the second study emphasized that the "mother's role as an attentive audience and in enjoying the child's play can be important components" (p. 155)[101] in mother-child interactions.[99]

Turnbull and Turnbull,[99] both professionals and parents of a handicapped child, urge that more study be done on parents as teachers and on the consequences of this practice for the parent-child relationship and for the child's self-image. They caution about the "possible implicit message to the chid: 'You need to get well— you are unacceptable as you are' " (p. 120).

A parent[59] notes, "It appears that in some cases professionals become more and more reliant on parents. Most parents feel that their main role is as a home care-giver. They are not and should not have to be teachers, case workers, therapists, and program developers" (p. 3).

Whether one speaks of the parent as teacher, therapist, co-therapist, or treatment provider, the important point is whether the professional feels comfortable helping the parent to assume the role and whether the parent feels comfortable in doing so. In *Helping Your Exceptional Baby,* Cunningham and Sloper[19] used the following low-key way of introducing the helping process to parents:

> Teaching is the art of getting someone to learn. Learning has taken place when someone can do something [he] could not do before. So anything that helps someone learn something new can be called teaching. Seen like this, we are all teachers. We all help each other and our children learn (p. 101).

Parent as advocate

The establishment in 1950 of the Association for Retarded Children (later changed to the Association for Retarded Citizens) and other parent groups is generally noted as the beginning of parent advocacy. Parent involvement does not necessarily have an active connotation, but parent advocacy requires the watchful and active participation of parents in securing services for their children.[69]

Staff members of the Early Intervention Project worked to help parents become advocates for their own and for all handicapped children.[11,78] Two of the parents described a successful parent advocate situation in their own words[58]:

> We have found it necessary to advocate for Laura with regard to the school bus. We needed to be sure that a seat appropriate to her size and type of handicap was provided for her. Since she was not sitting independently when she first began to ride the bus, we had to request an infant safety seat. As she has grown and developed, we've made sure that the appropriate safety changes have been made. . . . We feel that advocating in school for our child is not just a privilege but a responsibility that we are obligated to fulfill in order to ensure the best possible education for our daughter (p. 28, 29).

Markel and Greenbaum[68] saw the need for parents to take more assertive roles, including advocacy, and compiled in workbook format *Parents Are to be Seen and Heard: Assertiveness in Educational Planning for Handicapped Children.* This book used actual situations reported by parents and is helpful for parent group meetings, workshops, and individual parents.

Parent Counseling

When a telephone caller asks, "Will you talk with a mother about feeding her cerebral palsied child?" what pediatric occupational therapist would say no? If the same therapist was asked whether he or she is qualified as a counselor, what would the answer be?

What qualifies someone for counseling? Buscaglia[12] said that it depends on the questioner's definition of counseling and that "there appears to be little agreement concerning what counseling really is or should be. What is viewed as a *given assumption* or *common sense* to a traditional psychotherapist may be seen as a vague, meaningless opinion to a behaviorist" (p. 43). Buscaglia challenged

Medical doctors, psychologists, counselors, educators, physical and occupational therapists, social workers, psychiatrists, and all those in the helping professions, to become more cognizant of the desperate need the disabled person and the family have for good, sound, reality-based guidance (p. 5).

Many occupational therapists are reluctant to call themselves counselors. However, in reality they often find themselves in counseling roles with patients, clients, students, and others. As is true with counselors from any discipline, occupational therapists must be aware of the limitations of their knowledge and expertise and must decide when the needs of the person being counseled go beyond their expertise. At this point the occupational therapist has the same professional obligation as does any other counselor; to refer the person to a counselor with the appropriate expertise. Within these constraints, occupational therapists can still provide a great deal of beneficial counseling to the parents of handicapped, ill, and at-risk children.

The reading parent

Therapists can often help parents gain understanding of their own situations through reading literary works that deal with the human condition. In *The Uses of Bibliotherapy in Counseling Families Confronted with Handicaps,* Mullins[81] describes how professional workers can make use of literature in both formal and informal ways for helping families and children. Reading materials should be made available to parents who wish to use them. Therapists should be sensitive to the reluctance of parents of young handicapped children to read technical books that discuss disabilities in great detail and that are accompanied by photographs of persons of all ages and in all stages of the disability.

Many books on handicapped children* have lists of resources and readings for parents. From such lists, parents and therapists can identify books and articles on play and stimulation activities, sex education, growth and development, adaptive equipment, child abuse, attitudes toward people with handicaps, terminal illness and death, managing behavior problems, baby sitting and respite care, sibling reactions, the fu-

---

*References 7, 11, 47, 69, 81, 93.

ture of the handicapped child, and many types of handicapping conditions.

REACTIONS AGAINST PARENT INVOLVEMENT

It would be dishonest to imply that all parents are in favor of being involved in training and educating their handicapped children. Parent involvement appears to develop more naturally among parents of infants, since parents naturally assume that they will provide care for their infants. Such assumptions do not necessarily apply to older children.

Meyer,[73] in describing the life of her 18-year-old severely retarded son, said that she "would have been very grateful for any therapeutic help when he was an infant, but there was none available at that time" (p. 110). When her child was finally accepted into a program, she was grateful that the program "did not encourage parental involvement in other than typical school functions. I had spent twenty-four hours a day for six years with my child . . .; relief from constant child management allowed me the luxury of contributing [as a volunteer in community social and health agencies] and increased my own feelings of worth" (p. 110).

Turnbull and Turnbull[99] commented on the amount of time involved in educational matters. They feel that parent involvement and advocacy keep some parents so busy that they are thereby excluded from their own mainstream experiences with parents of nonhandicapped children. They question the emphasis on benefit to the child and suggest that parent involvement should also benefit the parents by "reducing stress, increasing family coping, and improving relationships within the family (parent and sibling) and with the handicapped child" (p. 116).[99]

The Turnbulls[99] felt strongly about the current emphasis on parents under Public Law 94-142, in which the "concept of parent participation pervades the requirements [of the law and] extends the right and arguably the duty to parents of handicapped children to assume the role of educational decision maker" (p. 115). Some parents have neither the desire nor the capabilities to assume this responsibility; furthermore, opportunities for actual decision making are much more limited than the law implies. Turnbull and Turnbull suggested that programs "tolerate a range of parent involvement choices and options, matched to the needs and interests of the parents" (p. 120).[99]

Jenkins[59] speaks of a "growing tendency toward professional dependency on parents that transcends most parental capacities and serves to escalate normal complexities in the family environment" (p. 3). Based on a British study, McConkey[71] concluded: "We have to accept that some parents will wish to opt out of whatever type of involvement we offer, either through force of circumstances (overcrowding of homes, social or marital problems, emotional and physical exhaustion) or from a desire to lead a life of their own" (p. 26).

It is obvious that many parents have concerns similar to those expressed above. A local Association for Retarded Citizens, in an editorial,[27] asked that its members have "ongoing discussion about establishing some balance between the desirability of and need for parental input and the concern that service providers might lean on parents too heavily" (p. 3).

Parents as managers

As an answer to the reactions against parent involvement, it is proposed that parents serve as managers of their handicapped child, not *case managers* but *managers.* Case manager is an institutionalized role that receives its authority and direction from an agency; case managers serve useful purposes for clients and agencies. Various persons have proposed that parents be case managers for their handicapped children, and in some agencies parents do fill this role, with authority and direction coming from the agency.

As *manager* of a handicapped child, authority and direction come from the family itself. Some of the attributes of this manager have been suggested.

- "You (the parent) can help the most . . . . (A)lthough you will want to take the advice of the pediatrician, family doctor, or specialist, remember that the baby is *your* baby and the day to day decisions are *yours*" (p. xii).[96]
- "Parents are the logical choice for (managers as) chief coordinators and evaluators of service, . . . (with) a sense of control over events in their own lives and their child's life. Parents, by experiencing this sense of potency, may act with greater confidence and purposefulness when confronted with choices or situations not to their liking" (p. 279).[65]
- "Each family (manager) must sort through advice, take what is helpful, and discard the rest. Advice givers, as helpful as they are, come and go on a daily, weekly, or monthly basis. Families must ultimately take responsibility for solving as many of their own problems as possible" (p. 12).[38]
- "Gradually I began to feel that I wasn't so out of control, that I did have some power . . . you *can* learn things and make wise decisions as you gain confidence and experience. Parents have to realize that they can have this power (as managers)" (p. 5).[47]
- ". . . whether (parents) will become (managers) directly relate(s) to how much power they feel they have and how well they can sort through what is best for themselves and for their child . . . . (Y)ou (the parent) can decide where your child will go, just the way parents of normal children do" (p. 6).[47]
- "(Parents) have capacities for creative problem solving and coping which professionals can respect, promote, and encourage" (p. 34).[47]
- "I remember (Beckie's mother's) stories of shuttling Beckie from one expert to another . . . only to emerge with the realization that she was Beckie's expert. The teachers, therapists, and miscellaneous professionals had their areas of expertise, but she alone knew the whole story. She was Beckie's primary helper, monitor, coordinator, observer, record-keeper, decision-maker, (and manager)" (p. 155).[1]

The following are three examples of parents who have served as managers for their children.

As Temple Grandin[42] recounted her life as an autistic person, now a Ph.D. candidate and world famous design and construction expert, the strong, supporting role of her mother was uppermost in her mind. Her mother prepared her for kindergarten, told her how much fun school and learning new things would be, and discussed Temple's problems extensively with the teachers; helped Temple achieve above grade level reading ability and raised her self-esteem by serving her "grown-up" tea; found the right medical, educational, and social resources for her; and wrote many supportive letters to Temple. She effectively *managed* Temple's interactions with those persons who were important in helping her to grow up.

The mother of a young teen-aged son with learning disabilities described how she was *managing* her son's care and activities. The discussion took place during a conference on learning disabilities that she attended. She familiarized herself with the many medical, educational, and social needs of her son and with resources for meeting these needs. She worked as an individual for her son's benefit and with other parents for the benefit of all handicapped children. She monitored the school placements of her son and felt that P.L. 94-142 enabled her to do this. She determined and met criteria for each move from a segregated special education class to a regular class. She seemed especially pleased that she had finally secured a place for him on the soccer team, as well as the support of the coach and team members.

On January 24, 1987, the *Sarasota Herald-Tribune* carried a feature story on the family of Gail and John Graves and their five children that demonstrates how an active family with a handicapped member can demand the utmost of a parent as *manager.* The three middle children, girls aged 10, 12, and 14, are pursuing acting careers in current roles ranging from television commercials and "Saturday Night Live" productions to plays at Lincoln Center and the children's chorus at the Metropolitan Opera. Their acting interests determine where the mother and five children live, which is now in New York City. A 19-year-old-son is on leave of absence from school because of severe leg and back problems and is an outpatient at a New York hospital for special surgery. A 17-year-old daughter, Kelly, has

Down syndrome; she attends the Kennedy School for Handicapped Children and requires special treatment, education, and attention. Her mother reports that Kelly is doing very well and that all family members work with her. The three actresses attend a professional school for young actors next door to their apartment in the morning and travel from acting, singing, dancing, and music lessons to auditions in the afternoon. John Graves lives in Sarasota where his federal litigation practice either forces or allows him to travel most of the time and gets him to New York City often.

SUMMARY

As occupational therapists become more active in programming for infants and for children whose disabilities require long-term or lifetime attention of parents or other adults, the topic of parent involvement in therapy programs becomes increasingly important. Since the beginning of the 1970s, public opinion and philosophy, legislation, and governmental regulations have created a climate of child care that makes it necessary for individual or agency service providers to involve parents. Because of the thoughtful and constructive comments from parents and professionals and, perhaps, the belligerent comments of others, agencies at all levels are examining the roles that parents have been forced into and are now inclined to allow parents more options.

Knowledge and understanding of what is involved in the parenting of disabled children remain of uppermost importance to those persons planning to work with disabled children and their families. Application of this knowledge and understanding is in transition.

A welcome trend can be seen in this chapter—that of research on parents and families of handicapped children. It is in its early stages but a beginning has been made. Those ready to begin research studies will find numerous areas of need already identified.*

STUDY QUESTIONS

1. Think of three situations that might disrupt the working relationships between parents and professionals. List possible ways to resolve these situations. Discuss your ideas with other students or colleagues.
2. At a new early intervention program for handicapped children from birth through age 3, a staff meeting has been called to discuss how parents will be involved. Assume the roles of three staff members, describe a different way of involving parents for each of the three members, and give reasons for and against each way.

*References 9, 14, 26, 33, 38, 47, 50, 51, 52, 88.

REFERENCES

1. Ackerman J: Update: preparing for separation. In Turnbull RH, and Turnbull AP, editors: Parents speak out: then and now, Columbus, 1985, Charles E Merrill Publishing Co.

2. Anderson J: Sensory intervention with the preterm infant in the neonatal intensive care unit, Am J Occup Ther 40:19, 1986.
3. Anderson J, and Hinojosa J: Parents and therapists in a professional partnership, Am J Occup Ther 38:452, 1984.
4. Ayres AJ: Sensory integration and the child, Los Angeles, 1979, Western Psychological Services.
5. Baker BL: Support systems for the parent as therapist. In Mittler, P, editor: Research to practice in mental retardation: care and intervention, vol 1, Baltimore, 1977, University Park Press.
6. Baker BL, Clark DB, and Yasuda PM: Predictors of success in parent training. In Mittler, P, editor: Frontiers of knowledge in mental retardation: social, educational, and behavioral aspects, vol 1, Baltimore, 1981, University Park Press.
7. Baskin BH, and Harris K: More notes from a different drummer: a guide to juvenile fiction portraying the disabled, New York, 1984, RR Bowker Co.
8. Bingham O, with Bingham RE: One step more, Lord!, Nashville, TN, 1984, Broadman Press.
9. Blancher J, editor: Severely handicapped young children and their families: research in review, Orlando, 1984, Academic Press, Inc.
10. Bronfenbrenner U: Who needs parent education? Position paper prepared for the Working Conference on Parent Education, Flint, MI, 1977, sponsored by the Charles Stewart Mott Foundation.
11. Brown SL, and Moersch MS, editors: Parents on the team, Ann Arbor, 1978, The University of Michigan Press.
12. Buscaglia L: The disabled and their parents: a counseling challenge, Thorofare, NJ, 1975, Charles B Slack, Inc.
13. Campbell DR: How to *really* love your child, Bergenfield, NJ, 1977, New American Library.
14. Campbell P, editor: Special needs report, 1: (1), 1986.
15. Chinn PC, Winn J, and Walters RH: Two-way talking with parents of special children, St. Louis, 1978, The CV Mosby Co.
16. Cohn MS, and Caffey KJ: Handi-sitters: how to sit for the handicapped, 1812 Mapleleaf Boulevard, Oldsmar, Fla, 1979, Handi-Sitters.
17. Colman W: Occupational therapy and child abuse, Am J Occup Ther 29:412, 1975.
18. Cruickshank WM, Morse WC, and Johns JS: Learning disabilities: the struggle from adolescence toward adulthood, Syracuse, 1980, Syracuse University Press.
19. Cunningham C, and Sloper P: Helping your exceptional baby, New York, 1980, Pantheon Books, Inc.
20. Day S: Mother-infant activities as providers of sensory stimulation, Am J Occup Ther 36:579, 1982.
21. Deshler DD, editor: Special education for adolescents and young adults, Except Educ Q 1(2):entire issue, 1980.
22. D'Eugenio DB: But he doesn't fit in the car seat anymore. In Brown SL, and Moersch MS, editors: Parents on the team, Ann Arbor, 1978, The University of Michigan Press.
23. D'Eugenio DB, and Moersch MS, editors: Developmental programming for infants and young children, vol 4, 5, Ann Arbor, 1981, The University of Michigan Press.
24. Dickerson MU, and Brown SL: A search for a family. In Brown SL, and Moersch MS, editors: Parents on the team, Ann Arbor, 1978, The University of Michigan Press.
25. Dickerson MU, Eastman MI, and Saffer AM: Child care training for adults with mental retardation, vol 1, Infants, Downsview, Ontario, 1984, National Institute on Mental Retardation Publications.
26. Dokecki PR, and Zaner RM, editors: Ethics of dealing with per-

sons with severe handicaps: toward a research agenda, Baltimore, 1986, Paul H Brookes Publishing Co.

27. Editorial, Washtenaw Association for Retarded Citizens, ARC Outlook, June-July 1986.

28. Elder JK: Priorities of the administration on developmental disabilities for fy 84, Ment Retard 22:53, 1984.

29. Ellsworth PD: Parent education: a definite approach to the problem of child abuse and neglect. In US Army Health Services Command Publication: Current trends in ambulatory patient care, Fort Sam Houston, Texas, Washington, 1978, US Government Printing Office.

30. Featherstone H: A difference in the family: life with a disabled child, New York, 1980, Basic Books, Inc, Publishers.

31. Finn JL: The children's developmental workshop. In Llorens LA, editor: Consultation in the community, Dubuque, IA, 1973, Kendall/Hunt Publishing Co.

32. Friedman B: A program for parents of children with sensory integrative dysfunction, Am J Occup Ther 36:586, 1982.

33. Gallagher JJ, and Vietze PM: Families of handicapped persons: research, programs, and policy issues, Baltimore, 1986, Paul H Brookes Publishing co.

34. Garbarino J, Guttmann E, and Seeley JW: The psychologically battered child, San Francisco, 1986, Jossey-Bass Publishers.

35. Gillette NP: Occupational therapy belongs to the community. In Llorens LA, editor: Consultation in the community, Dubuque, IA, 1973, Kendall/Hunt Publishing Co.

36. Goldberg S: Growing with games: making your own educational games, Ann Arbor, 1985, The University of Michigan Press.

37. Goldberg S: Teaching with toys: making your own educational toys, Ann Arbor, 1981, The University of Michigan Press.

38. Goldfarb LA, and others: Meeting the challenge of disability or chronic illness: a family guide, Baltimore, 1986, Paul H Brookes Publishing Co.

39. Gordon IJ: Baby learning through baby play: a parent's guide for the first two years, New York, 1970, St. Martin's Press, Inc.

40. Gordon IJ, Guinagh B, and Jester RE: Child learning through child play; learning activities for two and three year olds, New York, 1972, St. Martin's Press, Inc.

41. Gordon IJ, and Lally JR: Intellectual stimulation for infants and toddlers, Gainesville, Fla, 1967, Institute for Development of Human Resources.

42. Grandin T, and Scariano MM: Emergence: labelled autistic, Novato, Ca, 1986, Arena Press.

43. Gray SW: Home-based programs for mothers of young children. In Mittler P, editor: Research to practice in mental retardation: care and intervention, vol 1, Baltimore, 1977, University Park Press.

44. Griswold PA: Play together, parents and babies, New York, 1972, United Cerebral Palsy, Inc.

45. Hamant C: Pediatrics. In Hopkins HL, and Smith HD, editors: Willard and Spackman's occupational therapy, ed 5, Philadelphia, 1978, JB Lippincott Co.

46. Harris GA: Fairy tales, beatlemania, and a handicapped child. In Turnbull RH, and Turnbull AP, editors: Parents speak out: then and now, Columbus, 1985, Charles E Merrill Publishing Co.

47. Healy A, Keesee PD, and Smith BS: Early services for children with special needs: transactions for family support, Iowa City, 1985, The University of Iowa.

48. Heber R, and Garber H: The Milwaukee project: a study of the use of family intervention to prevent cultural-familial mental retardation. In Friedlander B, and Sterritt G, editors: Exceptional infant. Vol 3: assessment and intervention, New York, 1975, Brunner/Mazel, Inc.

49. Hill L: Working with blind pre-schoolers, Am J Occup Ther 31:417, 1977.

50. Hobbs N, and others: Strengthening families, San Francisco, 1984, Jossey-Bass Publishers.

51. Hobbs N, Perrin JM, and Ireys HT: Chronically ill children and their families, San Francisco, 1985, Jossey-Bass Publishers.

52. Hobbs N, and Perrin JM, editors: Issues in the care of children with chronic ilness: a sourcebook on problems, services, and policies, San Francisco, 1985, Jossey-Bass Publishers.

53. Hobbs N, and others: Chronically ill children in America, Rehab Lit 45:206, 1984.

54. Holt KS: Neurological and neuromuscular disorders. In Gabel S, and Erickson, MT, editors: Child development and developmental disabilities, Boston, 1980, Little, Brown & Co.

55. Horton B, Maddox M, and Edgar E: Adult transition model: planning for postschool services, Seattle, 1984, University of Washington.

56. Howard AC: Developmental play ages of physically abused and nonabused children, Am J Occup Ther 40:691, 1986.

57. Howison MV, Perella JA, and Gordon D: Cerebral palsy. In Hopkins HL, and Smith HD, editors: Willard and Spackman's occupational therapy, ed 5, Philadelphia, 1978, JB Lippincott Co.

58. Jaworowski S, and Jaworowski R: A baby goes to "school." In Brown SL, and Moersch MS, editors: Parents on the team, Ann Arbor, 1978, The University of Michigan Press.

59. Jenkins C: Open letter, Washtenaw Assoc for Retarded Citizens, ARC Outlook, June-July 1986.

60. Johnson CB, and Deitz JC: Time use of mothers with preschool children: a pilot study, Am J Occup Ther 39:578, 1985.

61. Kinnealey M: Service programs in the university affiliated programs. In Llorens LA, editor: Consultation in the community, Dubuque, Iowa, 1973, Kendall/Hunt Publishing Co.

62. Knickerbocker BM: A parent-oriented occupational therapy program for the multiply handicapped child. In West WL, editor: Occupational therapy for the multiply handicapped child, Chicago, 1965, Board of Trustees of the University of Illinois.

63. Knickerbocker BM: A holistic approach to treatment of learning disorders, Thorofare, NJ, 1980, Charles B Slack, Inc.

64. Kupfer F: Before and after Zachariah: a family story about a different kind of courage, New York, 1982, Delacorte Press.

65. Laborde PR, and Seligman M: Individual counseling with parents of handicapped children: rationale and strategies. In Seligman M, editor: The family with a handicapped child: understanding and treatment, New York, 1983, Grune and Stratton, Inc.

66. Llorens LA: Problem-solving the role of occupational therapy in a new environment. In Llorens LA, editor: Consultation in the community, Dubuque, Iowa, 1973, Kendall/Hunt Publishing Co.

67. Lucas G: Accommodating the premature infant at home, Occup Ther Forum, Eastern Edition, 2(1):1, 1987.

68. Markel GP, and Greenbaum J: Parents are to be seen and heard: assertiveness in educational planning for handicapped children, San Luis Obispo, Calif, 1979, Impact Publishers.

69. Marsh GE, II, and Price BJ: Methods for teaching the mildly handicapped adolescent, St. Louis, 1980, The CV Mosby Co.

70. McCollum JA: Looking patterns of mentally retarded and nonretarded infants in play and instructional interactions, Am J Men Def 91:516, 1987.

71. McConkey R: Working with parents: a practical guide for teachers and therapists, Cambridge, Mass, 1985, Brookline Books.

72. McKibbin EH: An interdisciplinary program for retarded children and their families, Am J Occup Ther 26:125, 1972.

73. Meyer JY: One of the family. In Brown SL, and Moersch MS, editors: Parents on the team, Ann Arbor, 1978, The University of Michigan Press.

74. Meyerson RC: Family and parent group therapy. In Seligman M, editor: The family with a handicapped child: understanding and treatment, New York, 1983, Grune & Stratton, Inc.

75. Moersch MS: Training the deaf-blind child, Am J Occup Ther 31:425, 1977.

76. Moersch MS: History and rationale for parent involvement. In Brown SL, and Moersch MS, editors: Parents on the team, Ann Arbor, 1978, The University of Michigan Press.

77. Moersch MS: The handicapped child in a trigenerational family, Paper presented at American Occupational Therapy Association Conference, Detroit, April 25, 1979.

78. Moersch MS, and Wilson TY, editors: Early intervention project for handicapped infants and young children, final report, Ann Arbor, 1976, Institute for the Study of Mental Retardation and Related Disabilities (ERIC Document #ED 132804).

79. Moroney RM: Family care: toward a responsive society. In Dokecki RR, and Zaner RM, editors: Ethics of dealing with persons with severe handicaps: toward a research agenda, Baltimore, 1986, Paul H Brookes Publishing Co.

80. Morris AG: Parent education in well-baby care: a new role for the occupational therapist, Am J Occup Ther 32:75, 1978.

81. Mullins JB: The uses of bibliotherapy in counseling families confronted with handicaps. In Seligman M, editor: The family with a handicapped child: understanding and treatment, New York, 1983, Grune and Stratton, Inc.

82. Northcott WL: Developing parent participation. In Lillie DL, editor: Parent programs in child development centers, Chapel Hill, 1972, The University of North Carolina Press.

83. Pediatric Occupational Therapy: Challenges for the future: Proceedings of the Maternal and Child Health/Boston University Occupational Therapy Symposium (edited by Henderson A, Lawlor M, and Pehoski C), May 1986, Medford, Mass.

84. Petersen, P: The therapist as a family resource, AOTA Dev Dis Special Interest Section Newsletter, 7(4):1, 1984.

85. Roos P: Parents of mentally retarded children—misunderstood and mistreated. In Turnbull AP, and Turnbull HR III, editors: Parents speak out: views from the other side of the two-way mirror, Columbus, 1978, Charles E Merrill Publishing Co.

86. Schafer DS, and Moersch MS, editors: Developmental programming for infants and young children, vol 1, 2, 3, rev ed, Ann Arbor, 1981, The University of Michigan Press.

87. Schopler E: Treatment of autistic children: historical perspective. In Mittler P, editor: Research to practice in mental retardation: care and intervention, vol 1, Baltimore, 1977, University Park Press.

88. Seligman M: Siblings of handicapped persons. In Seligman M, editor: The family with a handicapped child: understanding and treatment, New York, 1983, Grune & Stratton, Inc.

89. Shapero S, and Forbes CR: A review of involvement programs for parents of learning disabled children, J Learn Disabil 14:499, 1981.

90. Shearer MS, and Shearer DE: Parent involvement. In Jordan JB, and others, editors: Early childhood education for exceptional children, Reston, VA, 1977, Council on Exceptional Children.

91. Sparling JW, and Rogers JC: Feeding assessment: development of a biopsychosocial instrument, Occup Ther J Res, 5:4, 1985.

92. Summers JA, editor: The right to grow up: an introduction to adults with developmental disabilities, Baltimore, 1986, Paul H Brookes Publishing Co.

93. Thain WS, Casto G, and Peterson A: Normal and handicapped children: a growth and development primer for parents and professionals, Littleton, Mass, 1980, PSG Publishing Company, Inc.

94. Thurman SK, editor: Children of handicapped parents: research and clinical perspectives, Orlando, 1985, Academic Press, Inc.

95. Tiffany EG, Psychiatry and mental health. In Hopkins, HL, and Smith HD, editors: Willard and Spackman's occupational therapy, ed 5, Philadelphia, 1978, JB Lippincott Co.

96. Tingey-Michaelis C: Handicapped infants and children: a handbook for parents and professionals, Baltimore, 1983, University Park Press.

97. Turnbull AP: Moving from being a professional to being a parent: a startling experience. In Turnbull AP, and Turnbull HR, editors: Parents speak out: views from the other side of the two-way mirror, Columbus, Ohio, 1978, Charles E Merrill Publishing Co.

98. Turnbull AP, and Turnbull HR III, editors: Parents speak out: views from the other side of the two-way mirror, Columbus, Ohio, 1978, Charles E Merrill Publishing Co.

99. Turnbull AP, and Turnbull HR III: Parent involvement in the education of handicapped children: a critique, Ment Retard 20:115, 1982.

100. Turnbull HR, and Turnbull AP, editors: Parents speak out: then and now, Columbus, 1985, Charles E Merrill Publishing Company.

101. Tyler NB, and Kogan KL: Reduction of stress between mothers and their handicapped children, Am J Occup Ther 31:151, 1977.

102. Vulpe SG: Home care and management of the mentally retarded child, Toronto, 1969, National Institute on Mental Retardation.

103. Vulpe SG: Vulpe Assessment Battery: developmental assessment, performance analysis, individualized programming for the atypical child, ed 2, Toronto, 1977, National Institute on Mental Retardation.

104. Wade AS: Occupational therapy for problems with special senses: blindness and deafness. In Hopkins HL, and Smith HD, editors: Willard and Spackman's occupational therapy, ed 5, Philadelphia, 1978, JB Lippincott Co.

105. Wallace G, and Kauffman J: Teaching students with learning and behavior problems, ed 3, Columbus, Ohio, 1986, Charles E Merrill Publishing Co.

106. Warren F: Update: call them liars who would say, "all is well." In Turnbull RH, and Turnbull AP, editors: Parents speak out: then and now, Columbus, Ohio, 1985, Charles E Merrill Publishing Co.

107. Weikart DP: Designing parenting education programs, Paper presented at the Working Conference on Parent Education, Flint, Mich, 1977, Charles Stewart Mott Foundation.

108. White R: The special child: a parents' guide to mental disabilities, Boston, 1978, Little, Brown & Co.

109. Willard HS, and Spackman CS: Occupational therapy, Philadelphia, 1947, JB Lippincott Co.

PART
IV

PRINCIPLES AND TECHNIQUES OF OCCUPATIONAL THERAPY ASSESSMENT IN PEDIATRICS

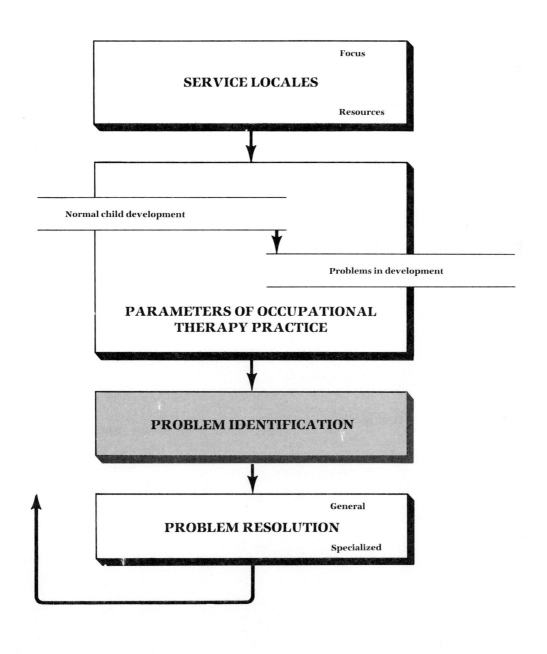

9

Basic methods of assessment and screening

PAT NUSE PRATT
IDA LOU COLEY
ANNE STEVENS ALLEN
KAREN E. SCHANZENBACHER

BASIC METHODS

This chapter focuses on the use of a variety of basic methods to screen children to determine the need for occupational therapy services. Guiding questions for clinical observation of the child will provide a foundation for any other screening or formal evaluation. In addition, this chapter discusses a number of commonly used standardized and criterion-referenced screening instruments that are often used by occupational therapists in pediatric settings. Information on basic methods used for assessment was presented in Chapter 7. It might be useful to review that section before proceeding further.

A questioning mind is critical to the assessment process. It is an asset to know what questions to ask of oneself and others. Questions are formulated and answers often found through the study of normal development, principles of structure and function, and the behavioral sciences.

Among the most valuable skills a therapist can possess are the abilities to observe, to be flexible and spontaneous, and to be creative with play and other activities that foster intrinsic motivation in children. Supporting these clinical attributes are foundation skills that are solidly grounded: a sense of organization and problem-solving strategies for developing the child's potential in daily life activities.

To begin, the importance of taking a broad view is emphasized. The therapist must look at the total child interacting within multiple environments. The child should not be considered merely in terms of an "oral-motor problem" or "dressing problem." Life systems are too closely intertwined. The task of the therapist is to make a thorough search: unravel and discover *why* the child can do some things and not others in his daily life routine.

Looking at the total child: clinical observations of basic skills

The following information will provide a foundation for and direction to the therapist's search for what a child can or cannot do.[3] Assessment begins by focusing attention on the child at rest in supine and prone positions. Movement is minimal, but signs of head control and the child's use of his head for orientation may be noted. The broad task is to view postural tone throughout the body and to survey structural components, carefully considering the inhibitors of activity performance. These may include stress, static postures, contractures of muscle tissue, tightening of skin, fusion of joints, structural deformities, and atrophy of muscles. Conditions that contribute to discomfort and pain, such as swelling, inflammation, and tenderness, can also affect mobility. Observations of the child at rest permit the therapist to develop a baseline picture from which to evaluate subsequent movement and its quality. Philosophically, and in practice, movement and independence in activity performance are linked together, each contributing to the other.

THE CHILD AT REST: SUPINE POSITION

Postural components. The therapist should ask the following. What is the child's prevailing posture? Does flexion or extension predominate, or is the body-position asymmetrical? Is the child bound by prevailing postures, or can he easily initiate volitional movement? What is the quality and type of postural tone: hypertonic, hypotonic, fluctuating, or appropriate to the age of the child? Does the child appear to rest comfortably in this position (Figure 9-1, *A*)?

Stabilization and control of the head. Can the child turn his head to the side without moving his arms or legs? Can he follow an object visually without head movement? Is the child's head in midline? Does he demonstrate neck extension or shoulder retraction?

Structural components of body systems. Are the child's shoulders level? Is his rib cage symmetrical? What is its shape? Is the pelvis level? Are there discrepancies in arm or leg length? Are there obvious joint contractures in the elbows, wrists, fingers, hips, knees, or ankles? Are there deformities or joint subluxation at the shoulder, wrist, metacarpophalangeal joints of the fingers, hips, knees? Are the joints enlarged or reddened? Are there nodules around the joints? What is the appearance of muscle tissue: tense, flaccid, atrophied, or hypertrophied? What is the appearance of the child's skin: dry, moist, tight, loose, warm, or cold? What is its color?

THE CHILD AT REST: PRONE POSITION

Stabilization and control of the head, trunk, and shoulders. Postural components of the prone position are examined as with the supine position. In addition, the therapist will consider any changes in the child's head control in the prone position. Can the child extend his neck so that his head is free in space? Can neck extension be maintained without bobbing his head? Are the child's arms caught under his body or are they used appropriately to support upper body weight on his elbows or in an extended position? Where are the child's elbows in relation to his shoulders, and are his hands open or fisted? Is the child's head in a normal position in space (Figure 9-1, *B*)?

Structural components of body systems. Are the child's scapulae symmetrical? Is the child's spine relatively straight, or is there evidence of lordosis, kyphosis, or scoliosis? Are the buttocks elevated by tightness at the hips or spinal deformity? Are there obvious joint contractures at the elbows, hips, knees, or ankles?

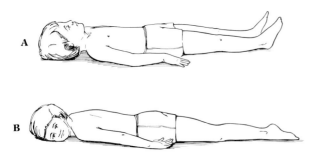

Figure 9-1 Normal resting postures. **A,** Supine. **B,** Prone.

ROLLING

The body is engineered for flexibility so that individuals can move freely, easily, and in most instances without conscious effort. However, patterns of movement are learned through practice and repetition and are gradually refined. During observation, note the child's use of his head, shoulders, and hips, as well as his ability to rotate along the body axes. Abnormal patterns and asymmetry may interfere with mobility. Factors related to body structure may require adaptation.

Where does the child initiate movement for the roll: from the head, shoulder and arm, trunk, hip and leg, or combinations of these? Does he become asymmetrical and lose control? Is rolling accomplished more readily to the right or left side? Are movements exaggerated with head thrust backwards or back extended? Does the child demonstrate log or segmental rolling, or has the child developed an adaptive pattern to accomplish this activity?

ACHIEVING THE SITTING POSITION

As infants gain stability of the neck and shoulders, acquire increased extensor tone for trunk stability, and are able to break through mass patterns of flexion and extension, they develop the ability to flex at the hips and elevate the upper body in space. They come to grips with the forces of gravity and are helped to maintain sitting position by postural reactions, guided by visual and vestibular processes, that keep the body upright in space. Can the child bring his head forward and lift it from a resting surface? How does the child "come to" sitting: with ventral push-off, dorsal push and partial rotation, or symmetrical push-off from the supine position (Figure 9-2)? Does the child roll to the side and push up sideways? Do the hips and knees flex when sitting is achieved? Do the child's legs need to be stabilized before sitting can be achieved? If the child cannot come to the sitting position alone, what is the position of his head when he is pulled to sitting? Is there head lag? Is the back rounded? Is there resistance at the hips?

SITTING

Sitting is normally an effortless task. The individual is not aware of the mechanisms at work that orient his head in space nor the work of his extensor muscles to keep his head erect. Trunk stability, or the balance of the vertebral column, depends largely on the posterior trunk musculature, the abdominal and intercostal muscles. As one sits, the trunk balances on the pelvis, which is a narrow sitting base unless the legs are extended and spread. The body, with its numerous movable parts, is a series of structural segments, one placed on top of the other. Maximal stability is assured when the centers of gravity of the segments lie in a vertical line centered over the base of support. In the body structure, when one segment is unaligned, there is usually a compensatory disalignment of another segment

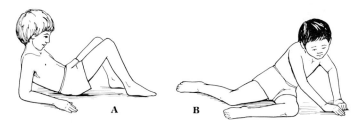

Figure 9-2 Coming to sit. **A**, Symmetrical. **B**, Ventral push.

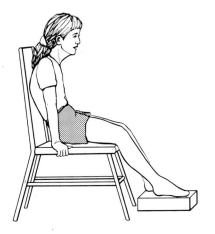

Figure 9-3 Insufficient hip flexion in sitting results in rounded spine and forward thrust of head.

to maintain a balanced position of the body as a whole (Figure 9-3).

The important functional areas to observe as the child sits are head and trunk alignment, the sitting base, and the amount of support required and provided by the arms. What is the position of the child's head? Is control maintained effortlessly in a stationary position or during free rotation? What does the child's back look like: is it rounded, symmetrical, or asymmetrical? What is the position of the hips? Are they extended or comfortably flexed? Is the child's weight distributed evenly over a narrow or wide sitting base? Can the child sit with her legs extended for a reasonable period of time? Is the child comfortable in the sitting position, or is he insecure?

Where are the child's arms, and does she use her hands as props? If so, how is her weight-bearing on the arms achieved: forward, right or left side, or backward propping? Is protective extension active and functional with elbows extended, or does the child tend to flop over on bent elbows? Are her hands open or fisted?

If a child can sit unsupported, can she lean forward and then recover balance? Can the child pivot her trunk while sitting to reach for objects that are not at midline? Are her hands free for manipulative play, or are they held insecurely close to the body? Is the

child's head up with her eyes alert? Is the child comfortable in this position, or is there evidence of postural insecurity?

REACHING

Reaching multiplies the demands for postural security. Observe that as the child extends his arms outward from his body the center of gravity rises and his balance is less stable. Movement of the arms requires the child to make quick shifts in position to maintain balance. The maturation of postural stability to the point of maintained upright positioning permits development of the amazing process of human hand use. Obviously, this cannot occur while the child must use all of his energy to maintain body position against the forces of gravity.

If the arms and hands are to do something, cocontraction is required at the proximal joints and at the midline to stabilize and maximize the forces exerted by the moving muscles. To reach all body parts, including those at the periphery, the child must actively move his scapulae and shoulders in all planes. The elbow joint calibrates the reaching parameters toward the head and feet. Combinations of range at the shoulder, elbow, and wrist bring the child's hand, with its valuable prehensile qualities, in contact with superior body surfaces. Flexibility of the spine and range of motion at the hips and knees permit the child to reach all the way to his toes.

Can the child bring her hands together at midline? Can she bring one or both hands to her mouth, behind her head, and to the small of her back; pronate and supinate her hand and forearm; reach straight overhead and out to the side without loss of trunk stability; and bend over at the waist, touch her toes, and return to an upright sitting position without loss of control and balance? Does the child reach equally well with each side and with both arms together? What seems to interfere with her function?

HAND USE

As the child performs fine motor tasks with his hands, the rest of his body tends to be quiet, as if providing a silent framework for intricate movement. This is an important message from nature that should be recalled by the therapist when working with the child on eating skills or the fine manipulations required for fastening clothing. Postural stability is a critical prerequisite to human hand use.

Grasping involves complex movements. The long flexors and extensors of the hand pass over several joints, potentially affecting movement in multiple locations. The tenodesis action of the wrist is an example of such phenomena. Fine prehension includes rotation and abduction of the thumb for opposition to the volar finger pads. Similarly, slight flexion of the fingers at the metacartpophalangeal and interphalangeal joints is needed to position the fingertips for prehension. Various degrees of movement between pronation and supination place the hand in angular planes during performance of such manual skills as writing, eating, playing, and cleansing after a bowel movement.

The therapist should observe to see if the child can oppose all fingers to the thumb (Figure 9-4, *A*). Are such movements awkward or fluid? Are they performed in digital sequence or arbitrarily? Can the child straighten his fingers with his wrist in a neutral position? Can his fingers be fully extended from a fisted position? Is extension of the child's fingers exaggerated when he reaches for an object?

What is the position of the child's wrist during grasping? (Figure 9-4, *B*). Is the child's grasp on objects forced? What is the position of the forearm during grasping: pronated, supinated, or in midposition? Is the thumb used in an immature scissors pattern, or is mature pincer function evident? (Figure 9-4, *C*). What is the quality of muscle tone, strength, and coordination?

Are fine tremors noted in the hand? Does the child drop objects easily, or does she have difficulty releasing objects?

Clinical observations: the child interacting with the environment

The focus thus far has been on the components of motor function, such as balance, stability, muscle strength, synergy, coordination, and range of motion. These indispensable elements of movement and static postures are required for activity engagement. This view has been directed toward seeing the "entire body" in space. Now it is appropriate to look at the "whole child."

The questions to be asked are the following: How does the child respond to stimuli in the environment? What is the child's style of interaction with inanimate and animate objects? What attracts the child's attention and what intrigues, motivates, distracts, or disorganizes him? How does interaction with the environment affect the "doing" of the child? The search continues to find the child's unique combination of abilities that promote function and to sift out those elements that interfere with function.

THE CHILD'S USE OF SENSORY MODALITIES

Does the child show preferential use of a sensory modality? For example, an individual may rely on sight, hearing, or touch in his interactions with people and objects. Does the child look selectively and have visual

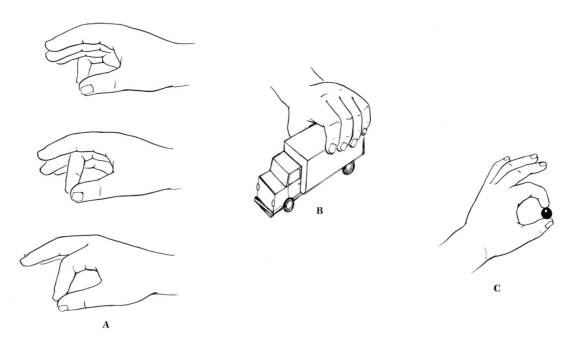

Figure 9-4 Normal prehension patterns. **A,** Checking opposition, thumb to fingers. **B,** Gross grasp with wrist extended. **C,** Pincer grasp, tip prehension.

interest in people, in people's activities and interactions, in objects, and in furnishings? Does the child attend to sound and explore objects that have a distinctive smell? Are heights and balancing activities avoided or approached eagerly? Does the child tend to touch and manipulate objects before proceeding with a task?

THE CHILD'S MOTOR RESPONSES

Does the child organize and carry out motor tasks in logical sequence, or does his motor planning appear impaired? Is it necessary to demonstrate a task or put a child passively though task patterns, or does the child initiate a new activity independently? Are the child's movements impulsive, controlled, or restrained?

COGNITIVE STYLE

The therapist will need to analyze problems of task performance in light of all observed chracteristics. Sometimes motor ability is adequate to the task, but performance may be immature or impaired because of cognitive factors. How does the child approach a task: impulsively, automatically, analytically, or by using trial-and-error methods? How does the child respond to verbal direction? How many steps of a task can the child remember and process at a time? Is thinking concrete or abstract, and does the child show any awareness of and judgment related to safety factors?

SOCIAL RESPONSES AND COMMUNICATION

Intricately interwoven with engagement in activity is the child's participation in the larger activity of a social world. As skill in object manipulation increases, the activity itself requires less concentration, and the child looks out to compare his performance against that of others. Or, the child recognizes that others around him are doing things that may or may not relate to him. The child's social interaction is commensurate with his ability to communicate by using verbal and nonverbal processes.

Does the child demonstrate eye contact during interactions with other persons? How much does she pay attention to others, whether engaged in an activity or not? Does the child seem to prefer to play alone, alongside others, or in cooperative interaction? Does the child appear to perceive social feedback related to herself or others?

Does the child rely predominantly on speech to express himself, or does he use manual and facial expressions as well? Does he use automatic phrases? Does the child show indications of perseveration of ideas, word searching, or blocking? Does the child initiate conversation with elaboration of ideas, or does he merely answer questions with brief phrases?

Although specific behaviors can be observed the reality is that behaviors occur within the context of the total environment. Therapists are also processing global interactions and integrating all that is seen into composite impressions of function. It is advisable to carefully consider the setting within which one gathers those impressions. The clinical setting is always artificial, and therefore limits the scope of evaluation and problem-solving. It does not represent the natural arenas of the child. In a sense, one is seeing the child in isolation, removed from the familiar surroundings of daily life: home, school, and playground.

THE CHILD AT HOME

At the child's home the therapist has the opportunity to view the child's characteristic adaptation in its fullest dimension. This is the most significant environment, because it contains those persons who can contribute most to the quality of the child's life.

There are many things to consider in this environment that directly or indirectly affect the child's development of function. These include the type of neighborhood; rural, urban, or suburban location; the terrain; and climatic factors. The therapist should explore the house and yard, noting the presence of stairs and other barriers to mobility. The interior of the house is important, including space for mobility aids and other adaptive equipment, storage areas, and how the family feels about changing the home environment to make it easier for the child to function. The therapist needs to know how busy the family life is and how the family manages daily schedules. The primary caregiver's skills and attitudes must be assessed to identify how much assistance is given to the child, how it is given, how responsibility is shared by other family members, and what the stresses of caretaking are. The availability of extended family help and respite care should be explored. Therapists need to determine how well the family will be able to follow through with therapy goals, including what realistic expectations can be established. The family's understanding of their child's potential and limitations, and their attitudes toward fostering maximal independence will be important to the outcome of occupational therapy intervention. The therapist needs to clearly identify what help the family is seeking, what they want to change, and where they want to begin.

THE CHILD AT SCHOOL AND PLAY

Success in school depends in large part on how comfortable the child feels in the environment and how well the environment is structured to permit the child to use her abilities, gain satisfaction, and receive recognition. Teachers, bus drivers, classmates, and other persons with whom the child comes in contact and who understand the disability can give valuable support for increasing independence by encouraging efforts. School represents a major part of the child's life and is critical to preparation for adulthood.

When therapists observe a school environment, they are bound by tradition and tend to look at practicalities to begin identifying and then solving problems. They will want to know if the child can sit at a desk or if some other arrangement will be necessary. Will the teacher's body and voice, as well as the blackboard, be readily accessible to the child? Will the child be able to reach for and put away books without assistance? How will toileting and eating be managed, as well as mobility within the school classroom, hallways, and grounds? What are the time constraints for mobility? What arrangements are needed regarding use and maintenance of wheelchairs and other adaptive equipment? Where will these items be stored? Who will assist the child with these? Do school personnel understand when to assist and when to insist on independent performance? These are important considerations that require the collective help of the child, parents, school staff, classmates, and therapists.

There are other issues to consider as well that are related to peer acceptance and the child's integration into the social fabric of the school. Factors to note include whether the child seems to be different from peers in the classroom. For example, is the child dressed like the others in the class? Does the child's disability affect others in the room to the point of overt or covert reactions? Are the students and teacher comfortable with a child who may be different? How well does the child communicate with others? Since gaining acceptance from peers is a gradual process in all situations and for all human beings, the child may require help in relating, in making appropriate social overtures, and in being able to help others become at ease in his presence.

Observation in a play setting provides unique insight into the way a child interacts in her own world. Does the child play alone or with peers? Does the child initiate play, go along with peer group activities, or participate only in play situations that are structured by adults? Does the child prefer to play indoors or out? What are the age-level interests reflected in play? Are regressive or higher levels of function used? What social play and cognitive patterns are evidenced? Is the child's participation in play active or passive?

One of the special values obtained through such observation is a picture of the child's personally-directed, comfortable use of capacities, functions, and skills. The therapist needs to remember that among all children ranges of engagement in play can vary from minute to minute, activity to activity, and group to group. Because of this situational variability, multiple unobtrusive observations of play are recommended, with supplementary interviewing of parents and others, before final decisions are made about the child's status as a player. (See Chapter 15 for additional information about assessment of play behaviors.)

Through the basic process of clinical observation of the child at rest, in a variety of functional postures, in familiar environments, and at play, the therapist records impressions and evolving questions. One of the recurring questions should be: Does this child already have the resources to achieve a satisfying level of independence, or will occupational therapy services make a critical difference in the quality of this child's life? As the therapist reviews his or her notes of observation, the need for more information generates the use of other forms of screening. Figure 9-5 provides a checklist to guide the observations described to this point.

Interviewing

Various types of interview formats are used to obtain information about children. Interviews are often conducted by the therapist with both parents, sometimes supplemented with data obtained through questionnaires.

There are several basic forms of interviewing. The most structured type is guided by an outline of questions. The interviewer asks the questions as specified on the outline, and the respondent provides answers that are linked by the constraints of the outline. The interviewer discourages discussion of extraneous material. This is called the *limited or structured response interview.*

A *semistructured interview* uses a basic outline of questions that have been developed to elicit thoughful responses from the person. Although the interviewer will be careful to ensure collection of basic data, the questions have an open-ended quality that allows additional useful information to be obtained. In other words, the therapist who uses a semistructured format does so to prevent overlooking important information about a child that might not fit into frequently used categories. For example, a question might be worded, "How does your child play with brothers and sisters?" Clearly, such questions are designed to elicit descriptive information rather than yes-no responses.

A third type of interview is designed to obtain *free responses.* Open-ended questions are used to help the respondent examine and report on the meaning of experiences and perceptions. This method is frequently used in nondirective therapy and in assessment for mental health programs. The free response method differs from the semistructured interview in that the interviewer has fewer preconceived expectations about the nature of the information to be revealed.

INTERVIEWING SKILLS

To obtain useful information through an interview, the therapist must have command of the subject matter to be discussed. When an interview elicits information that is outside the therapist's expertise, appropriate referral for problem resolution is indicated. The therapist must be able to analyze and conceptualize content obtained through interviews into a meaningful whole (gestalt). Simple completion of interview forms without this follow-up step of integrating details into the overall assessment of the child is a waste of everyone's

Figure 9-5 Checklist for initial observations

BASIC SKILLS

A. Resources for and inhibitors of activity performance
B. Rest: Supine
 1. Prevailing posture
 2. Quality and type of tone
 3. Head stabilization and control
 4. Visual function
 5. Musculoskeletal symmetries
 6. Appearance of joints
 7. Muscle bulk
 8. Skin
C. Rest: Prone
 1. Head stabilization and control
 2. Neck stabilization and control
 3. Position and control of shoulders and arms
 4. Hand position and appearance
 5. Skeletal symmetries
 6. Spine
 7. Hip position
 8. Joints
D. Rolling
 1. Rotational patterns used
 2. Head, shoulder, and hip positions
 3. Musculoskeletal symmetries
 4. Lateral differences
E. Coming to Sitting
 1. Head stabilization
 2. Patterns used
 3. Trunk and spine stabilization and control
 4. Leg stabilization and control
F. Sitting
 1. Head and trunk alignment
 2. Spine
 3. Hips
 4. Weight-bearing pattern
 5. Leg positions
 6. Postural security
 7. Use and position of arms
 8. Ability to maintain position during hand use
G. Reaching
 1. Bilateral hand and arm pattern
 2. Trunk stability
 3. Quality of movements
 4. Lateral differences
 5. Inhibitors of function
H. Hand Use
 1. Opposition
 2. Quality of finger and thumb movements
 3. Tenodesis effect
 4. Wrist and forearm influences
 5. Prehension patterns used
 6. Muscle tone
 7. Release patterns

ENVIRONMENTAL INTERACTIONS

A. Use of Sensory Modalities
 1. Response to environment
 2. Preferred sensory modalities
 3. Attentional levels
 4. Exploratory behaviors
B. Motor Responses
 1. Initiative
 2. Motor planning and sequencing
 3. Motor control
C. Cognitive Style
 1. Problem-solving strategies
 2. Response to direction
 3. Memory
 4. Abstract function
 5. Awareness of safety functions and judgment
D. Social Responses and Communication
 1. Visual contacts
 2. Communication patterns
 3. Social interaction and responsiveness
E. Home Environment
 1. Neighborhood description and demographics
 2. Home and property description
 3. Caregiver needs and skills
 4. Family attitudes, life-styles, and schedules
 5. Inhibitors of function
F. School Environment
 1. Physical description and requirements
 2. Caregiver description, needs, requirements, and skills
 3. Special needs of the child
 4. Peer descriptions and relationships
 5. Communication abilities and patterns
G. Play Environment
 1. Description and requirements
 2. Social interaction
 3. Individual and group interests
 4. Level and quality of participation and engagement

time. It may be noted that the expertise of the professional level occupational therapist (OTR) is rarely needed for the administration of the limited response interview. Instead, the therapist's skills are better used in semistructured and free response formats. Within these formats the therapist's knowledge is used to develop and explore new ideas that surface during an interview. Responses to one question may be seized on to develop new questions or to obtain more considered information.

The skilled therapist becomes expert in gaining the participation of the respondent. This may be done in a number of ways. First, the purpose and focus of the interview are clearly explained. The therapist develops a comfortable atmosphere that permits the respondent to reply openly. The therapist frequently reviews assembled information with the respondent to ensure accurate understanding of what has been said. The therapist listens attentively and without bias, making a conscious effort to allow for feedback. The therapist is aware of shifts in conversation, recurrent references, and inconsistencies and gaps and explores concealed meanings. Finally, the occupational therapist considers the effect of the physical setting, the hour of the day, and other external influences on the interview process.

USE OF HISTORIES FOR SCREENING

Many occupational therapists have developed interview formats to obtain histories of skill development, activity participation, and life-space data. Two are included here. The *developmental history* (Figure 9-6) was constructed to obtain initial intake information as well as background data on developmental milestones and parental expectations of occupational therapy. It serves as a representative semistructured interview and

---

Figure 9-6   Developmental history

Child's name:_____   Birthdate:_____ Age:_____
  Mother's name:_____   Father's name:_____
  Home address:_____
  Home phone no.:_____   Business phone no.:_____
  Prenatal history: Please describe the pregnancy:
Birth: Weight:_____ Height:_____   Duration of pregnancy:_____
  Type of delivery:_____
  Complications at birth?_____
  Treatment received by baby or mother?_____
Postnatal history: Please list and describe any important injuries or illnesses, including ear and chest infections. At
  what ages did these occur?
  _____
  _____

Milestones: At what age did your child:
Turn head side to side?_____   Sit alone?_____
Lift head while lying on tummy?_____   Crawl-creep?_____
Roll over?_____   Pull to standing?_____
Cruise, walk with support?_____ Walk alone?_____ Run?_____
Climb stairs?_____ Walk down stairs?_____ Swallow?_____
Chew?_____ Drink from cup?_____ Feed self with spoon?_____
Babble?_____ Say words?_____ Speak in phrases?_____
Speak in sentences?_____ Play with children?_____
Have you noticed any differences compared to your other children?
_____
_____

Do you have any family/living problems which you think might affect your child's development or therapy?
_____
_____

What does this child like?
_____
_____

Dislike?
_____
_____

has been used in face-to-face discussion with parents. It can also be given in questionnaire form to parents to complete at home where they may have more complete records available.

Takata's play history was also developed for use with an interview or questionnaire. It examines the child's play history by obtaining information about his preferred forms of play and play context. In addition, this form is used to obtain information about current play content and skills of the child. From the data collected the therapist develops a description of the child as a player and a prescription for necessary play experiences that will be provided through occupational therapy intervention[9] (Figure 9-7).

SCREENING INSTRUMENTS

A veritable supermarket of screening instruments is available commercially. Most screening tests are performance based and therefore examine the child's skills

in activity situations. Screening tests may focus on self-care activities, object manipulation skills, social skill development, language and cognition, or a combination of these areas. Such combination tests are considered adaptive development tests.

The screening instruments used by occupational therapists in pediatrics are usually criterion-referenced. The majority of commercially available or published tests have a standard or recommended administrative procedure. Those that are true *standardized tests* should always include standard administrative, scoring, and interpretive procedures that are based on normative data and acceptable test development and evaluation procedures.

Standardized tests

There is a prescribed way to administer a standardized test that is to be followed by anyone who uses the test. There are also prescribed ways to score the test

---

Please describe your child's problems.

_____

What would you like us to help you and your child do?

_____

What other therapy and/or special education programs has your child had? Now receiving?

_____

Please indicate with a plus (+) the items that you feel are strengths in this child and please use a minus (−) to identify those factors that you feel are weaknesses in this child.

_____response to smells and tastes   _____response to touch
_____response to visual stimuli   _____response to movement
_____response to sounds   _____response to eating
_____ability to manage physical/motor requirements of play/school activities.
_____ability to manage thinking requirements of play/school activities.
_____self-feeding _____dressing _____toileting
_____grooming _____gross-motor coordination
_____fine-hand coordination _____general activity level
_____attention span _____social skills _____motivation
_____response to family _____response to other children
Does your child use glasses, hearing aid, braces, wheelchair, or other special equipment for daily activities?

_____

Are there any allergies, seizures, or other medical problems we should know about?

_____

Is there anything else you would like us to know at this time that you feel can help us provide better services for your child?_____

Do we have your permission to take photographs of your child for evaluation and student training purposes?
_____Yes   _____No
May we obtain copies of your child's records from your child's physician or other agencies? Please list:_____

_____

Signature:_____ Date:_____

Figure 9-7 Takata's play history

---

(1) *General information*
   Name: Birthdate: Sex:
   Date: Informant(s):
   Presenting problem:
(2) *Previous play experiences*
   A. Solitary play
   B. Play with others:
      mother father sisters brothers playmates
      other family members   pets
   C. Play with toys and materials (earliest prefer-
      ences)
   D. Gross physical play
   E. Pretend and make-believe play
   F. Sports and games: group collaboration
      group competition
   G. Creative interests: arts   crafts
   H. Hobbies, collections, other leisure-time activ-
      ities
   I. Recreation social activities
(3) *Actual play examination*
   A. With what does the child play?
      toys   materials   pets
   B. How does the child play with toys and other
      materials?
   C. What type of play is avoided or liked least?
   D. With whom does the child play?
      self parents brothers sisters peers others
   E. How does the child play with others?
   F. What body postures does the child use during
      play?
   G. How long does the child play with ob-
      jects?   With people?
   H. Where does the child play?
      Home: indoors   outdoors
      Community: park school church other areas
   I. When does the child play?
      Daily schedule for weekday and weekend?
(4) *Play description*
(5) *Play prescription*

From Takata N: Play as a prescription. In Reilly M, editor: Play as exploratory learning: studies of curiosity behavior, Beverly Hills, Calif,
1974, Sage Publications, Inc.

and to interpret the scores. Usually raw scores are obtained from the number of test items passed by the
child. These raw scores may be transformed into meaningful data through the use of tables that accompany a
test kit. With use of the tables, raw scores are interpreted as developmental age levels, skill quotients, or
standard scores. Standard scores are derived through
analysis of the raw scores of the population of subjects
who were tested during the test construction phase.
These calculated scores indicate an individual's relative
standing within the performance variations for that
population. If the test has been administered and
scored properly, and if the test is valid and reliable,
then these interpretive scores (age levels, quotients, or
standard scores) may be assumed to indicate the individual's capacities or weaknesses.

Before a standardized test is released for public use,
it will be subjected to analysis for validity and reliability. The *validity* of a test indicates whether it measures
the skill or function it was designed to measure. There
are several kinds of validity. Logical validity is demonstrated when the test items are directly and obviously
examples of the process to be measured. Content validity refers to the relative weighting of test items as they
are used to measure a quality. For example, when predicting motor ability, is the value given for raising
one's head while in the prone position equal to the
value of rolling from the supine position to the side?
How many items would be needed to adequately assess
the motor skills of an infant? The third, most important
type of validity is called construct validity. Through
correlations of scores obtained by the sample population on the new test and other recognized tests of the
same phenomena, the test developer can determine if
the test has predictive value.

The *reliability* data for a standardized test indicate
the strength of its predictive value. Normally there are
two measures of reliability, each having a different
function. Test-retest reliability (also called stability) is
determined by administering the test two or more
times to each child in the sample within a fairly short
time period. The objective is for the children's individual scores to remain fairly consistent in each administration. In addition, the test should be measured for interrater reliability. Typically, two or more testers will
administer the test to each child in a sample. The goal
here is to have score consistency regardless of who administers the test. If either reliability measure is weak,
the test developer must reexamine the standardized
administration and scoring methods and refine the test
until more consistent (stable) findings are obtained.[8]

The process of test development and its necessary
constraints merit attention. It is generally agreed that
the variability of human characteristics and behaviors
makes the development of "the perfect test" an elusive
dream. The standardization of a test requires the participation of human subjects. Given individuals' commitment to freedom of choice, it is always difficult to find
adequate samples of subjects to take a test in its development stage, especially when the sample aims to represent every conceivable segment of minorities and
majorities of the total population distribution. When
children are to be tested, this task is compounded because of parental considerations regarding the privacy
of their own lives and sensitivity about the exploitation
of their children. Therefore test developers who are
able to obtain a sizable sample of children (N =
>1,000) have accomplished an admirable feat. When
they have been able to obtain a sample of subjects that
somewhat approximates a regional population distribution according to age, race, sex, and socioeconomic
factors, this is even more appreciable. Finally, in the
rare cases when fairly representative samples are ob-

tained in different regions of the country, there is evidence of herculean effort on the part of the test developers that may take a decade or more to achieve.

Therefore, although therapists are well advised to check out carefully the reliability, validity, and normative data of standardized tests, consideration of the constraints of test development should be weighed against negative criticism. Obviously some tests will be poorly constructed, standardized, and evaluated. However, many tests that have flaws in these areas may still be useful and represent application of the highest standards of test development within a constrained situation. As long as the therapist is aware of the limitation of a test, it may be used knowledgeably.

Criterion-referenced tests

As discussed in Chapter 7, criterion-referenced tests are nonquantifiable measures of performance. Typically, performance is judged by arbitrary ratings that vary in precision. More precise ratings can sometimes be determined by frequency of behavioral occurrence, such as "never," "1 to 3 times out of 10," "4 to 7 times out of 10," and so on. However, a frequency rating may not always be useful for program planning; therefore, descriptive terms are often used. For the example given, there might be such descriptors as "in presence of therapist," "in presence of other children," or "in any situation." Both sets of descriptors are examples of quasi-ordinal scales, which use ranked levels of performance that have no weighted equivalence. Although not often subjected to the rigors of standardized test construction and usually without reliability data, criterion-referenced tests usually have sufficient logical validity to provide useful information. An example of a well-constructed criterion-referenced test is the Early Intervention Development Profile (Chapter 11).

In addition to commercially available tests, other criterion-referenced instruments may be found in the literature and in local clinical facilities. Many of these tests have been so well researched by knowledgeable therapists that they are equally, if not more, useful for specific clinical needs. The key to working with such *"therapist-made"* tests is in the clarity of description for administration of test items. In addition, referencing of resources used to develop the test is important for future generations of therapists who adopt its use at the same or different facilities. It is satisfying to note an increasing trend in the collection and publication of validity and reliability data for "therapist-made" tests that are reported in the professional literature. These practices can be applied as well to tests that are developed by local occupational therapy staff, as discussed by Royeen in Chapter 31.

The remaining purpose of this chapter is to describe and discuss several representative screening instruments that can be used in a variety of occupational therapy settings for children. The screening instruments presented in this chapter are generally directed

Figure 9-8   Test analysis format

Title and authors:

What the test proposes to measure:

Population for whom the test was developed:

Test format
  A. Type of instrument
  B. Test content
  C. Administration
  D. Scoring
  E. Interpretation
Include information about the basic type of instrument that is being used, for example, interview, criterion-referenced, or standardized test. Then briefly discuss basic administration guidelines that pertain to the entire test. For example, is information obtained by report of parents, or by presenting tasks to children? How is the test set up? Are there time limits for items in general? Include basic information about scoring and interpretation procedures.

Advantages of the test:

Disadvantages of the test:

Purchasing information:

References:

toward assessment of overall developmental status. Additional screening tests that are used to evaluate specific areas of function or task performance are discussed in Chapters 10 and 11. For purposes of organization, these are divided into commercial tests and therapist-made tests. A test analysis format has been developed (Figure 9-8). This chapter will present a completed analysis of the Denver Developmental Screening Test because it is the screening instrument most commonly used with children. Other screening methods that are discussed here or encountered in practice may be similarly analyzed. The model analysis provided here will organize additional study of tests through the primary test reference and evaluative information from other similar resources.

Commercial tests
APGAR SCORING SYSTEM

The technology of neonatology has grown tremendously (Chapter 16), and screening of the newborn is critical to timely application of life-sustaining and enhancing procedures. Cardiac, neurological, and respiratory systems must be appraised to determine how well a neonate has responded to the birth process and ex-

---

Figure 9-9   Test analysis: Denver Developmental Screening Test—Revised

---

Test measures: Screening of developmental accomplishments in four areas
1. Personal-social: Ability to get along with people and care for self
2. Fine-motor adaptive: Ability to see and use hands
3. Language: Hearing, comprehension, vocabulary, verbal expression
4. Gross motor: Postural and locomotive patterns
Test identifies delays in development in these areas.
Population: Children from birth to 6 years.
Test format: This is a standardized test involving:
1. Task performance of specific activities by child.
2. Parent interview using specific questions; pass by "Report" of "R." To be used only if child cannot be observed performing tasks.
A standard, purchased test kit, forms, and manual are used. The form can be reused at successive test periods, rather than a new one.
Administration:
1. Establish rapport with parent and child. Child may sit on parent's lap during testing time but should be able to reach test material easily.
2. Calculate child's age in years and months.
3. Highlight the appropriate age line on the DDST-R form from top to bottom. Include subtractions of time if the child was more than 2 weeks premature.
NOTE: *Steps two and three should be completed with care as correct interpretation of results depend on accuracy here.*
4. Although the order in which test items are given is flexible, the items must be administered in the manner specified in the manual. An easy procedure to follow is to give the child blocks to play with as questions regarding birthdate and prematurity are asked and the age line is drawn. Items in the personal-social sector that are not likely to be observed during the test and can be passed on parental report can then be asked while the child continues to explore the blocks and becomes comfortable with the examiner.
5. Frankenburg[7] recommends that each child be given the abbreviated version of the test to determine the need for administration of the entire screen. The abbreviated version of the test includes the three items in each of the four sectors that are immediately to the left of, but not touching, the child's age line, for a total of 12 items. Items passed are scored with a "P" at the right end of the bar.
6. If a child does not pass any one of the 12 items, the test developers recommend that the entire screen be administered.
7. Scoring: P = Pass.

Table 9-1   Apgar scoring system

Sign	Score 0	Score 1	Score 2
Heart rate	Absent	Slow (below 100)	Over 100
Respiratory effort	Absent	Slow, irregular, hypoventilation	Good, crying lustily
Muscle tone	Flaccid	Some flexion of extremities	Active motion, well flexed
Reflex irritability	No response	Cry, some motion	Vigorous cry
Color	Blue, pale	Body pink, hands and feet blue	Completely pink

Total score	Condition
0 to 3	Severe distress
4 to 6	Moderate difficulty
7 to 10	Absence of stress

From Apgar V: Curr Res Anes Analges 32:260, 1953; and Apgar V and others: JAMA 168:1985, 1958.

trauterine life. The Apgar Scoring System provides this information by rating the baby's color, heart rate, reflex irritability, muscle tone, and respiratory effort.[1] This test is not given by occupational therapists. However, information from the test is frequently used by thera-pists and others who treat high-risk, developmentally disabled, and medically unstable infants.

Scores for each of the five factors are computed 1 minute and again 5 minutes after birth. Each factor is rated on a scale of 0 to 2, and the sum of individual

---

Figure 9-9, cont'd.   Test analysis: Denver Developmental Screening Test—Revised

8. Delays: Items to left of age line that are failed. These are colored in on ends of bars for easy identification. Percentages indicate number of children at each age who have passed item. R = Parent interview accepted performance by report if cannot be observed. 23 = Footnote number = Instructions given on back of test form.

	25%	50%	75%	90%
R			///////////////	
23			///////////////	

9. Interpretation:
  Abnormal = a. 2 or more sectors with 2+ delays, or
            b. 1 sector with 2+ delays and 1 sector with 1+ delay and no passes intersecting the age line
  Questionable = a. 1 sector with 2+ delays or
            b. 1 sector with 1+ delay and no passes intersecting the age line
  Untestable = When refusals occur in numbers large enough to cause the test result to be questionable or abnormal if refusals were scored as failures.
  Normal = Anything else.
Advantages of test:
1. Speedy administration and scoring
2. Can be done by support staff with training and supervision
3. Validated against Bayley and Stanford-Binet tests
4. Large and good socioeconomic and ethnic distribution of standardization sample (N = more than 1,000)
5. Test-retest reliability: 90%-100%
6. Interrater reliability: 80%-95%
7. Validity: Positive 0.73 agreement on passes
          Negative 0.22 agreement on failures
Disadvantages: Cannot get clear-cut developmental level without abusing test. The test developers have stressed repeatedly that the DDST is to be used only for screening; they warn against using the test for diagnostic purposes.

---

scores is called the Apgar score. The closer the total is to 10, the better the condition of the neonate is considered to be. Scores equal to or less than 6 usually indicate the need for some type of intervention. Table 9-1 further details the Apgar Scoring System.

It is generally agreed that the Apgar score accomplishes its purpose: to provide delivery room personnel with important information that helps them plan the management of the neonate immediately after birth.[10] Attempts have also been made to determine the ability of the Apgar score to predict survival potential and to see if there is a correlation between the Apgar score and long-range intellectual, neuromuscular, and other specific disorders. These studies have produced a variety of conclusions. For example, one study found that the Apgar score was satisfactory for the prediction of survival of infants whose birth weight was over 1,000 grams but had poor prognostic value for infants weighing less than that.[2] A study by Drage and others[5] found that low birth weight infants who had unsatisfactory 5-minute Apgar scores had an increased percentage of neurological abnormalities at 1 year of age. But these same subjects at 4 years of age showed almost no neurological abnormalities, indicating that limitations may be short-lived.[4] No follow-up study of the school performance of these children was reported, although

such assessment seems warranted. These and other studies attempting to confirm or deny the predictive validity of the Apgar score are most interesting, but more research is needed.

DENVER DEVELOPMENTAL SCREENING TEST (DDST)

The Denver Developmental Screening Test[6,7] is widely used by pediatricians, occupational therapists, and many other child care personnel to screen for developmental delays. The test was developed in 1967 by Frankenburg and Dodds of the University of Colorado Medical Center and has generally well-accepted normative data. The test administration process and form were revised and reevaluated for reliability and findings reported by Frankenburg in 1981.[7]

Because this test is simple to administer, actual test administration is easily performed by well-trained assistant-level personnel. Therapists are cautioned to remember that this is a screening instrument. Its developers did not intend that it be used to establish clear-cut developmental levels of performance or be used for diagnostic purposes. They recommend the administration of comprehensive developmental and neurological evaluations for such purposes. The test analysis for the Denver Developmental Screening Test-Revised is

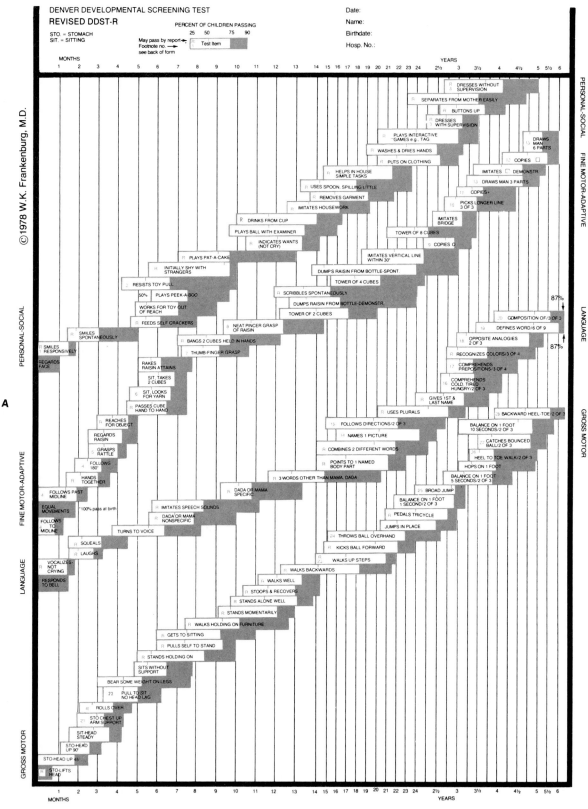

Figure 9-10 Denver Developmental Screening Test form. **A,** Front. Denver Developmental Screening Test form. **B,** Back, with directions from numbered items on testing form. From Frankenburg WK, Dodds JB, and Fandel AW: Denver Developmental Screening Test manual, ed 2, Denver, 1970, LADOCA Project & Publishing Foundation, Inc. Available from LADOCA Project & Publishing Foundation, Inc, E 51st St & Lincoln St, Denver, Colo 80216.

1. Try to get child to smile by smiling, talking or waving to him. Do not touch him.
2. When child is playing with toy, pull it away from him. Pass if he resists.
3. Child does not have to be able to tie shoes or button in the back.
4. Move yarn slowly in an arc from one side to the other, about 6" above child's face. Pass if eyes follow 90° to midline. (Past midline; 180°)
5. Pass if child grasps rattle when it is touched to the backs or tips of fingers.
6. Pass if child continues to look where yarn disappeared or tries to see where it went. Yarn should be dropped quickly from sight from tester's hand without arm movement.
7. Pass if child picks up raisin with any part of thumb and a finger.
8. Pass if child picks up raisin with the ends of thumb and index finger using an over hand approach.

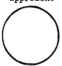   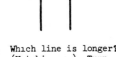

9. Pass any enclosed form. Fail continuous round motions.
10. Which line is longer? (Not bigger.) Turn paper upside down and repeat. (3/3 or 5/6)
11. Pass any crossing lines.
12. Have child copy first. If failed, demonstrate

When giving items 9, 11 and 12, do not name the forms. Do not demonstrate 9 and 11.

13. When scoring, each pair (2 arms, 2 legs, etc.) counts as one part.
14. Point to picture and have child name it. (No credit is given for sounds only.)

  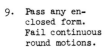 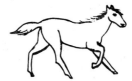   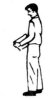

B

15. Tell child to: Give block to Mommie; put block on table; put block on floor. Pass 2 of 3. (Do not help child by pointing, moving head or eyes.)
16. Ask child: What do you do when you are cold? ..hungry? ..tired? Pass 2 of 3.
17. Tell child to: Put block on table; under table; in front of chair, behind chair. Pass 3 of 4. (Do not help child by pointing, moving head or eyes.)
18. Ask child: If fire is hot, ice is ?; Mother is a woman, Dad is a ?; a horse is big, a mouse is ?. Pass 2 of 3.
19. Ask child: What is a ball? ..lake? ..desk? ..house? ..banana? ..curtain? ..ceiling? ..hedge? ..pavement? Pass if defined in terms of use, shape, what it is made of or general category (such as banana is fruit, not just yellow). Pass 6 of 9.
20. Ask child: What is a spoon made of? ..a shoe made of? ..a door made of? (No other objects may be substituted.) Pass 3 of 3.
21. When placed on stomach, child lifts chest off table with support of forearms and/or hands.
22. When child is on back, grasp his hands and pull him to sitting. Pass if head does not hang back.
23. Child may use wall or rail only, not person. May not crawl.
24. Child must throw ball overhand 3 feet to within arm's reach of tester.
25. Child must perform standing broad jump over width of test sheet. (8-1/2 inches)
26. Tell child to walk forward, ⟨footprints⟩ heel within 1 inch of toe. Tester may demonstrate. Child must walk 4 consecutive steps, 2 out of 3 trials.
27. Bounce ball to child who should stand 3 feet away from tester. Child must catch ball with hands, not arms, 2 out of 3 trials.
28. Tell child to walk backward, ⟨footprints⟩ toe within 1 inch of heel. Tester may demonstrate. Child must walk 4 consecutive steps, 2 out of 3 trials.

DATE AND BEHAVIORAL OBSERVATIONS (how child feels at time of test, relation to tester, attention span, verbal behavior, self-confidence, etc,):

Figure 9-10, cont'd.   Denver Developmental Screening Test form.

shown in Figure 9-9, and a sample score sheet is shown in Figure 9-10. Awareness of the types of items used in this test is useful to the therapist because similar items are used on the more comprehensive developmental evaluations.

Therapist-made tests
CHECKLISTS

Very often therapists will develop checklists to assist with referrals and screening. Checklists are simple lists of factors or behaviors that the therapist considers important to note. For example, the checklist shown in Figure 9-5 is a useful tool to guide one's clinical observations according to the questioning process presented earlier in this chapter. Checklists do not constitute comprehensive evaluations. They are merely reminders to guide the direction of the screening or assessment.

A one-page checklist for referral to occupational therapy was developed by Carol Leaman, Fulton County Schools, Atlanta, Georgia (Figure 9-11). To help determine the need for occupational therapy ser-

---

Figure 9-11 Checklist of symptoms that may suggest a need for an occupational therapy referral

---

Guidelines:
1. Child is 9 years old or under
2. Child has many of the symptoms checked in Section I *plus* one of the other sections.

Section I
_____ Has trouble with cutting, tracing activities
_____ Has trouble pasting one piece of paper on another
_____ Has difficulty reading the writing on the blackboard
_____ Has difficulty copying from the blackboard
_____ Has difficulty spacing his letters as he writes them
_____ Reverses letters more often than his classmates
_____ Sometimes reads words backwards
_____ Does not have normal hand dominance; not skillful with either hand
_____ Sometimes gets right and left confused
_____ Hyperactive; distractible; poor attention span

Section IA (underreactive vestibular disorder)
_____ Has trouble holding head up while sitting
_____ Becomes tired easily
_____ When shifting body in chair, sometimes falls out of seat
_____ Stumbles and falls more frequently than others his age
_____ Sometimes makes no attempt to catch himself when falling
_____ Large movements are clumsy
_____ Has a hard time keeping his balance in games, in P.E., on equipment
_____ Is not really good at sports or does not enjoy them
_____ Throwing or catching a ball may be difficult
_____ Walks or runs into furniture, walls
_____ Oversteps or understeps obstacles
_____ Feels heavy or stiff when you try to help him position body
_____ Runs in the wrong direction when playing a team sport
_____ Often stands too close to other people
_____ Often bumps into people

Section IB (overreactive vestibular disorder)
_____ Does not stumble or fall, yet wants physical assistance
_____ Becomes anxious when feet leave the ground
_____ Has an unnatural fear of falling or of heights
_____ Does not have fun on the playground equipment or with moving toys
_____ Dislikes rough-housing, somersaults, rolling on the floor, jumping
_____ May avoid climbing, walking on a raised surface, over bumpy ground
_____ Is alarmed if suddenly pushed backward
_____ Is threatened when other people move him
_____ May not allow others to stand nearby when he is working
_____ Uses the stair banister more than other children

Section IC (developmental dyspraxia: a motor planning problem)
_____ Has not learned to do many self-help activities at age-appropriate level
_____ Has trouble putting on clothes, using buttons, zippers, and laces
_____ Does things in an inefficient way
_____ Appears weak, has low muscle tone
_____ Is accident-prone; has many little accidents (spilling milk)
_____ Needs more protection than other children
_____ Is more emotionally sensitive; feelings are easily hurt
_____ Cannot tolerate upsets in plans and expectations
_____ Complains more about minor physical injuries
_____ Bruises, bumps, and cuts seem to hurt more than they do in other children
_____ Is apt to be stubborn or uncooperative
_____ Wants things his way
_____ Has a shortage of skills; has to practice each skill over and over
_____ Once a skill is learned, it is performed well
_____ Has trouble with pencil control; is messy
_____ Is slow to learn new games or new motor skills

From Carol Leaman, OTR, Fulton County Schools, Atlanta, Ga.
Adapted from text of Ayres AJ: Sensory integration and the child, Los Angeles, 1979, Western Psychological Services, Inc.

---

vices of classroom students, the teachers can review items on the checklist to see if problem students demonstrate one or more of the behaviors indicated. Leaman has divided checklist items into four categories to assist the therapist in determining primary problem areas. Although this checklist was developed for elementary school children under 9 years of age, similar behavioral items can be developed to assist with referrals for other age groups and problems. In Leaman's checklist, section I relates to terminal behaviors. Sections IA through IC are used to identify clusters of behaviors for diagnostic purposes.

Another type of checklist was developed by therapists at the Colerain Elementary School in Columbus, Ohio. This Student Checklist (Figure 9-12) is used by therapists to organize initial data collection from

---

Figure 9-12 Student checklist

Name_____ Birthdate_____
Diagnosis:
Precautions:

Activities of daily living skills

Ambulation

Walks _____   Wheelchair _____
Independent _____ Walker _____   Independent _____ Dependent _____
Crutches _____ Cane _____   Assistance, long distances _____
Stairs: Independent _____ Dependent _____ Assistance _____
Comments:

Dressing

	Dependent	*Needs some assistance*	*Independent*
Coat	_____	_____	_____
Upper extremity	_____	_____	_____
Lower extremity	_____	_____	_____

Comments:

Feeding

Independent _____ Set up only _____ Minimal assistance _____ Dependent _____
Special utensils, equipment needed _____
Comments:

Toileting

	Yes	No	
Bathroom independence	_____	_____	Transfers: Independent _____
Urinary appliance _____	_____	_____	Assistance _____ Dependent _____
Diapers (independent)_____	_____	_____	
Braces (independent)_____	_____	_____	

Comments:

Communication

Verbal _____   Nonverbal _____
Clear _____ Articulation problems _____   Bliss symbols _____
                                                                     Other _____

Written communication	*Legible*	*Illegible*
Prints _____	_____	_____
Cursive _____	_____	_____
Types _____	_____	_____

Comments:

_____   _____
                 Therapist   Therapist

If you have any questions, concerns, or problems please feel free to contact us.

records and reports that is related to ambulation, self-care, and communication activities. Therapists can make note of reported independent and dependent performance, as well as assistive devices already in use by the student.

A developmental checklist (Figure 9-13) can be useful for screening large groups of children in an agency where therapist hours are limited. Three to five representative activities are given at each age level that generally indicate adequate performance of play, self-main-

Figure 9-13	Developmental checklist	

Neurological development to 5 years	1. Tonic neck reflex 2. TLR 3. Response to touch 4. Protective extension 5. Body righting
1 to 3 months	Lifts head Follows moving object
4 to 7 months	Transfers toy hand to hand Approaches mirror
8 to 12 months	Raises self to sitting position Finger-feeds self
13 to 18 months	Makes pencil marks Cooperates in dressing
19 to 24 months	Squats in play Identifies pictures by pointing Feeds self with spoon
25 to 36 months	Runs well Holds pencil with fingers Pulls on simple garment
37 to 48 months	Alternates feet going upstairs or rides tricycle Copies circle Feeds self well (spoon and fork)
49 to 60 months	Catches ball Copies crosses Distinguishes front, back of the clothes or *self* Acts out fantasies in play
5 to 7 years	Recites letters of alphabet Differentiates right from left Exhibits hand dominance Performs somersault Plays well with other children
7 to 10 years	Performs well in competition sports with other children Verbalizes plans for adult life Can read and write at grade level Can do math at grade level Independent in self-care
10 to 15 years	Prefers peer group activities Enjoys one hobby Travels independently Grade level academic performance (C− or better) Grade level athletic performance (C− or better)
15 to 20 years	Active interest in community-world affairs Preparation for adult occupational role Grade level academic performance Satisfactory peer relationships

tenance, and school work tasks. Therapists might ask the referring individuals to use the checklist as a guide for identifying children who are unable to meet the performance criteria in two or more items at each age level.

MAKE YOUR OWN TESTS

All of the screening instruments presented here, including commercial tests, were at one time drafted together out of need by one or two individuals with knowledge and ingenuity. Some were developed to the point of usefulness in one facility, while others have been modified and subjected to extensive item analysis and standardization procedures. Within that one facility, the therapist-made test may be more reliable than other tests that have been developed further for commercial use.

This point is made to emphasize the importance of the therapist's grounding in developmental processes and problems, and the ability to formulate questions that will provide answers to guide effective treatment. Often the therapist may find that parts, but not the wholes, of different tests are useful with a particular population of children. Such a finding is common among therapists who work with developmentally disabled children because of children's variable age level development in different skill areas. Rather than subjecting a child to lengthy evaluation by using all tests, it may be more practical and sensitive to develop a therapist-made test that integrates the critical items from a variety of appropriate tests. It is important for the therapist who does this to retain information on the test form about the sources of items used, as well as any variations made in the items for the new test format. Clearly the usefulness of any instrument depends on the experience, perceptiveness, and knowledge of the test administrator. It is advisable for therapists to be familiar with correct administrative procedures for test items before adapting them.

SUMMARY

This chapter has presented basic methods of clinical evaluation, including observation, interviewing, and history taking, as well as a number of standardized and criterion-referenced screening instruments for children. The test instruments discussed include both commercially available and therapist-made tests that are used to obtain information about developmental history and to identify problems in functional status and general performance competencies. This initial part of the occupational therapy assessment clarifies the need for more comprehensive evaluation and treatment. Considerable information can be obtained through careful observation of the child in relation to various activities and environments. This requires that the therapist use a questioning attitude based on and supported by knowledge of the human growth and development processes and human function.

STUDY QUESTIONS

1. Using the "Checklist for Initial Observations" (Figure 9-5) as a guide, observe three able-bodied children: an infant or toddler less than 2 years of age, a primary grade child, and a high school student. Compare differences and quality of performance of different age levels.

2. Using Takata's "Play History" (Figure 9-7), interview one or both of your parents. Ask them to describe you at an age you can remember. How do your memories of that time differ in relation to the content drawn from the play history?

3. Select a child or adolescent age level that interests you. Review related growth and development information from Chapters 3 and 4 and from other available references. Select six functions, skills, tasks, or activities that you believe are especially representative of the designated age to serve as a screening test. Administer the six test items to two able-bodied children. How does the children's performance compare? Administer the test to two more children: one with an acute condition and one with a chronic disability; compare their performance. Does your screening test discriminate differences?

REFERENCES

1. Apgar V: A proposal for a new method of evaluation of the newborn infant, Curr Res Anes Analges 32:260, 1953.

2. Apgar A, and James LS: Further observations on the newborn scoring system, Am J Dis Child 104:419, 1962.

3. Coley IL: Pediatric assessment of self-care activities, St Louis, 1976, The CV Mosby Co.

4. Drage JS, Berendes H, and Fisher PD: The apgar score at four years: psychological examination of performance. In Pan American Health Organization: Perinatal factors affecting human development, World Health Organization Scientific Publications 185:222, 1969.

5. Drage JS, et al: the Apgar score as an index of infant morbidity, Dev Med Child Neurol 8:141, 1966.

6. Frankenburg WK, Dodds JB, and Fandel AW: Denver Developmental Screening Test manual, ed 2, Denver, 1970, LADOCA Project and Publishing Foundation, Inc.

7. Frankenburg WK, et al: The newly abbreviated and revised Denver Developmental Screening Test, J Pediatr 99:995, 1981.

8. Hasselkus BR, and Safrit MJ: Measurement in occupational therapy, Am J Occup Ther 30:429, 1976.

9. Takata N: Play as prescription. In Reilly M, editor: Play as exploratory learning: studies in curiosity behavior, Beverly Hills, Calif, 1974, Sage Publications.

10. Taylor KM: The Apgar scoring system. In Humenick SS, editor: Analysis of current assessment strategies in the health care of young children and child-bearing families, Norwalk, Conn, 1982, Appleton-Century-Crofts.

10

Instruments to evaluate component functions of behavior

PAT NUSE PRATT
ANNE STEVENS ALLEN
RICARDO C. CARRASCO
FLORENCE CLARK
KAREN E. SCHANZENBACHER

Through the screening process and general problem analysis (Chapters 7 and 9) the therapist is able to identify deficits in the child's performance that indicate the need for occupational therapy services. Screenings typically raise more questions in the therapist's mind than answers. These questions guide the selection of formal evaluation measures. The therapist will want to determine why the child has problems doing everyday activities. To begin to find the causes of these problems, the therapist will evaluate the status of sensory integrative, motor, cognitive, social, and emotional functions. Depending on the presenting problems, specific evaluation of one functional area may be done in more depth than others.

Evaluation procedures used to determine functional states include interviews, observations, administration of standardized and criterion-referenced tests, and manipulation and palpation of the child's body parts by the therapist. Again, the variety of tools available through commercial resources, the literature, and colleagues is virtually limitless. However, for this chapter a representative sample of some of the more widely known evaluative procedures is presented. Test analyses are included for the Frostig Developmental Test of Visual Perception, the Developmental Test of Visual-Motor Integration, the Purdue Perceptual Motor Survey, and the Erhardt Developmental Prehension Assessment. A number of other tests will also be discussed.

As discussed previously, knowledgeable use of tests and other measurements is the occupational therapist's professional responsibility. Such use is based on careful study of test manuals and materials, adequate practice of test procedures prior to use in a clinical situation, and an awareness of the strengths and limitations of test purpose, procedures, and results. It is helpful to administer unfamiliar tests both to normal children and to a colleague for purposes of self-correction and comparison.

Until a therapist is experienced in the use of a particular test, she should administer the test as prescribed in the literature and only to individuals representative of the population for whom the test was developed. With experience and clinical judgment, the therapist can use a test with other individuals or groups of children, making modifications in procedure and interpretation as indicated. However, the findings of such modified use of a test should be reported accordingly and are best used for program planning rather than for diagnostic purposes.

TESTING MOTOR FUNCTION

Because the occupational therapist is greatly concerned with the manifestations of motor behaviors in activity performance, considerable emphasis is often placed on motor function tests. Therefore the variety and specificity of tests for motor function that have been developed for and by occupational therapists are greater than for other functional areas. It would be difficult to familiarize oneself with every test available that measures motor function. However, selections from the group of tests presented here should permit the therapist to develop a comprehensive assessment of the motor functions of most children.

Palpation

In addition to visual observation, one of the most basic methods of clinical assessment is *palpation.* This process may be conceived as a tactile-proprioceptive examination of surface and deeper body structures and their functions. Palpation is most frequently used by occupational therapists to assess skin texture and temperature, muscle bulk, tone and actions, joint integrity and restrictions, bony landmarks, and reflex/reaction patterns.

Palpation cannot be learned from a book, but rather through clinical instruction from an experienced therapist. However, guidelines can be presented here to enhance the clinical learning experience. Whaley and Wong[52] note that "a thorough knowledge of anatomy is essential in differentiating palpation of normal body structures from abnormal ones" (p. 169). Gentle pressure of the therapist's warm hands or fingers should be applied gradually to feel the structures in question. The nonpalpating hand is often used to stabilize or move the main body part, according to the needs of the examination. Fingertips (not nails) are best used when fine discrimination is needed; palmar surfaces of the fingers and hands are more useful in comparing size or function of two paired body parts. The back of the hand is highly sensitive for assessing skin texture and temperature.

Whaley and Wong[52] also recommend that the child be as relaxed as possible during palpation to provide the most accurate information and to strengthen the interpersonal relationship. They suggest such strategies as gentle rocking and storytelling, beginning with superficial and progressing to deeper palpations, and delaying palpation of painful areas until the end of the examination. In clinical occupational therapy practice, it is often helpful to allow the child to similarly palpate the therapist, either before or after a specific examination is made. This practice allows the child to understand better what specific action is needed, to feel more comfortable with the examination process, or simply to engage in a dramatic play experience with the therapist.

Tests for neurodevelopmental reactions and reflexes

A number of systems for testing the maturational patterns of the neuromotor system have been developed, including those by Fiorentino[20] and Milani-Comparetti.[39] To use any of these tests it is necessary to understand the general categories of neurodevelopmental reactions and be aware of the principles of reflex maturation and testing. Figure 10-1 provides an overview of critical information. (Reference to relevant sections of Chapter 4 is also useful.)

Bearing the infant's state in mind, despite the fact that reflex evaluation may be the procedure used most often with younger children, it is generally best to perform these tests at the close of a testing session. The responses of infants and young children to the different tests range from slightly irritated to openly resistive, and the procedure does little to establish rapport between the child and the therapist. Therefore it is better to present the child with enjoyable play activities early in the therapeutic relationship and save the reflex testing until the child shows a recognizable amount of positive responsiveness.

GENERAL PROCEDURES

In most neurodevelopmental tests the child is placed in a relatively static posture by the examiner. Postural tone and body symmetry are noted in the resting position. Then the examiner will touch or move the child, using a prescribed pattern of stimulus. The motor response that is elicited by the stimulus constitutes the reflex or reaction.

MILANI-COMPARETTI MOTOR DEVELOPMENT SCREENING TEST

The Milani-Comparetti Motor Development Screening Test[39] is a particularly useful system because the evaluation form clearly demonstrates time ranges for the emergence and disappearance of primitive and postural reactions. The reactions are tied to the development of locomotor patterns that begin in the supine position and progress to movement in upright walking. The instructions for test administration are clear, concise, and easy to follow. The protocol sheet provides a graphic record of the child's progress toward neuromotor maturity (Figure 10-8 at the end of this chapter). Therapists are referred to the administration manual for more detailed information about the development and use of this test.[31]

FIORENTINO REFLEX DEVELOPMENT SYSTEM

The Fiorentino Reflex Development System is widely used. It was developed by Mary Fiorentino,[20] an occupational therapist. It is organized according to postural patterns of apedal, quadrupedal, and bipedal locomotion, and the level of central nervous system control of the reflexive pattern. There are subcategories of different types of reactions that occur and recur at each level. There is a maturational component through different forms of similar reactions as the child matures, and primitive subcortical reflexes are replaced by higher reactions with more cortical control. The Fiorentino system is well documented elsewhere.[20,27]

AMIEL-TISON NEUROLOGICAL EVALUATION OF THE NEWBORN AND INFANT

This test was developed by Amiel-Tison[1] based on 20 years of practice with healthy and high-risk premature, full-term, and older infants at Baudelocque Hospi-

---

Figure 10-1 Neurodevelopmental reactions and reflexes

Definitions

1. *Attitudinal (postural) reflexes:* Those reactions that automatically provide for maintenance of the body in an upright position through changes of muscle tone in response to the position of the body or its parts.
2. *Equilibrium reactions:* Responsible for body adaptation in response to a change in the center of gravity. Results in head and trunk righting toward vertical body alignment, changes in extremities to balance weight shifts through extension and abduction, and also protects body balance.
3. *Labyrinthine:* Refers to the inner ear that contains vestibular sensory organs that are sensitive to progressive movements, acceleration or deceleration forward, turning movements, and to changes of direction in relation to gravity.
4. *Phasic reactions:* Movement reflexes that coordinate muscles of the limbs in patterns of either total flexion or total extension.
5. *Righting reactions:* Function to keep the upper part of the body upright and to maintain the head and trunk in their proper relationship. Stimuli go through the labyrinths and to tactile receptors in the trunk, neck, and ears.
6. *Optical righting reactions:* Considered separately because these are dependent on the occipital cortex of the cerebral hemispheres.
7. *Static or tonic reactions:* Changes in distribution of muscle tone throughout the body, either in response to a change in position of the head and body in space (stimulus through labyrinths) or in the head in relation to the body (stimulus through proprioceptors in the neck muscles).

Principles of reflex maturation and testing

1. Maturation of central nervous system control results in the appearance of more adaptive and discriminative reactions rather than totally different, new reactions.
2. Neuromotor development is continuous, although not all areas mature simultaneously or at the same rate.

3. A child experiences both dormant and regressive periods of neuromotor maturation.
4. Flexor tone predominates in the limbs of the newborn. This decreases in the arms by 3 to 5 months and in the legs by 4 to 5 months.
5. There is an important interrelationship between muscle tone and reflex development. Reactions that include extension components do not appear until flexor tone begins to diminish.
6. It is important to differentiate the stimuli used to elicit a specific reflex (for example, noxious, tactile, proprioceptive).
7. Close observation is important as the infant moves constantly into and out of reflex patterns.
8. Some reflexes can be observed only through spontaneous behavior and cannot be elicited through testing.
9. Some reflexes are imposable (can be elicited by testing) at one age and not another.
10. Confusion exists because various authors label the same reflex with different names, label different reflexes with the same names, and test the same reflex with different stimuli. These practices lead to conflicting conclusions regarding ages of onset, disappearance, and so on.
11. The infant's state of being is important during testing:
    a. Wakefulness: During sleep there is complete hypotonia. The infant should be observed both during the resting state (awake, but not engaged in activity) and during spontaneous activity. Be alert to any signs of postural asymmetry between the two sides of the body.
    b. Mood: Crying increases muscular tension.
    c. Health: Pathology influences reflexive behaviors.
    d. Satiation: Hypotonia occurs after nursing when the infant is satiated, while increased muscular tension resulting from crying occurs shortly before feeding.
    e. Age: Specific age is determined by period of gestation.

Adapted frtom Carol Johnson, University of Florida, Gainesville, Fla, 1973.

---

tal in Paris. Designed to measure active and passive muscle tone, the test also detects transient and permanent abnormalities in neurological development. The ranges of muscle tone development and limits of each test item are based on findings reported in the literature.

The test is used to assess neuromotor function of infants from 0 to 12 months, but should not be used with premature infants who have not attained 38 to 42 weeks' gestational age. The Amiel-Tyson test is intended to be used on a monthly basis to monitor history, sleep patterns and seizures, examination of the

skull, muscle tone, selected reflexes and reactions, spontaneous motor activities, resting postures, and classic neurological signs. The test is not standardized, but it does have inter-observer reliability information. Test forms are reproducible and procedures can easily be learned using a videotape.* The examination requires no special equipment and can be administered with the infant in an Isolette, a crib, or on an examining table.[1,38]

---

*Available through Case Western Reserve University Health Science Center, Cleveland, Ohio 44106.

Motor performance tests

MOVEMENT ASSESSMENT OF INFANTS (MAI)

The MAI was developed by Chandler and colleagues[15] at the Child Development and Mental Retardation Center of the University of Washington. The test is designed to provide a detailed, systematic appraisal primarily of motor performance during the first year of life. Quantified and descriptive data are elicited regarding muscle tone, primitive reflexes, automatic reactions, and volitional movement. The MAI can be used to identify motor dysfunction in infants up to 12 months and to establish a baseline for intervention. The test monitors development of infants and older children whose motor performance is at or below the 1 year level.

The test manual contains a 4-month profile, and an 8-month profile is being evaluated for its reliability and predictive validity.[26] The MAI can also be used for clinical research and is a valuable teaching tool for skillful observation of movement and motor development in normal and handicapped children. The test manual and forms are purchased and additional items can be readily found in the clinical setting.

NORTON'S BASIC MOTOR EVALUATION

Norton's Basic Motor Evaluation was designed to assess the quality of sensorimotor performance and to identify the predominating inborn reactions that are related to a child's deficits in sensorimotor function. Therefore this test battery examines both reflex reactions and purposeful movement patterns. The original format of the test was developed by Semans in 1965 for assessment of children with cerebral palsy. In the Semans version the child was placed in a position and asked to hold it. In contrast, Norton's adaptation[41] was designed for the child with a less severe handicap, and it requires that the child assume and hold the position after a verbal command is given. Demonstration and physical assistance are given only if the child appears to have difficulty following directions.

The therapist observes the child according to a number of criteria. These include the quality of movement (such as smoothness and balance), motor planning and body scheme, flexibility and bilateral symmetry, and comprehension and memory for instruction. The therapist analyzes patterns of pathological movement to determine problems in balance, coordination, perception, or behavior. Because this evaluation includes interesting activities, children appear to enjoy participation. The test provides a useful measure of the movement criteria mentioned if the therapist closely observes the child's performance. Use of a videotape to record the child's performance can be particularly helpful for analysis and follow-up. Although the test was designed for use with learning disabled children, it can readily be applied to other populations to obtain information about general motor function. (See Figure 10-12 at the end of this chapter.)

QUICK NEUROLOGICAL SCREENING TEST

The Quick Neurological Screening Test (QNST) was developed by Mutti, Sterling, and Spalding.[40] The test is used to help determine a child's maturity of motor development, skill in large and small muscle control, motor planning, sequencing and rhythm, spatial organization, visual and auditory perceptual skills, balance, and attention disorders. Although the QNST was originally intended for use with learning disabled children, it is also discriminative with adolescents and adults with learning problems. The test population age range is from 5 years to adulthood.

The QNST can be used as a screening tool but is not intended for diagnosis of neurological handicap, brain damage, or dysfunction. The test can be administered in about 20 minutes, and raw scores are converted to "high," "suspicious," or "normal" ratings using a table in the test manual.

BRUININKS-OSERETSKY MOTOR DEVELOPMENT SCALE

The Bruininks-Oseretsky Motor Development Scale is a standardized test of motor development that is administered individually to children 4½ to 14½ years of age. Gross and fine motor skills are evaluated according to performance on a group of 46 items that are divided into eight subtests. The fine motor subtests include upper limb coordination, response speed, visual-motor control, and upper limb speed and dexterity. Gross motor skills are measured on running speed and agility, balance, bilateral coordination, and strength subtests. Activities include gross motor and paper-and-pencil tasks, such as walking a balance beam and drawing a straight line between two points.

The entire battery can be administered in under an hour, and requires a large room. Using the manual enables the tester to convert raw scores to standard scores and approximate age equivalents. Test development and evaluation of the Bruininks-Oseretsky scale has been extensive. The tests discriminate well between nonhandicapped populations and learning disabled and mentally retarded children. Interrater reliability is excellent, probably because of the well-written and amply illustrated administration and scoring procedures. Test/retest reliability is generally good for the entire battery. Individual subtest stability at the higher ages in the range shows more variability. In general this is an excellent evaluation instrument to use with school-aged children who demonstrate motor problems without obvious physical handicap, if adequate space is available.[11]

Ziviani, Poulsen, and O'Brien[53] reported on a study that compared test scores for the Bruininks-Oseretsky with Southern California Sensory Integration Test (SCSIT) results of 49 learning disabled children. Results showed a significant correlation of Bruininks-Oseretsky scores with 14 out of 18 scores on the SCSIT, representing those Southern California tests that involve a gross or fine motor component. Although the sample was small, results suggest that the Bruininks-Oseretsky might be useful as a screening tool with learning disabled children to determine the need for administration of a complex sensory integration test battery. It should be remembered that this study was not done with tests from the newer Sensory Integration and Praxis Tests (SIPT). Although many tests of the SIPT are similar to those of the SCSIT, it cannot be assumed that the same correlation would be found between Bruininks-Oseretsky and SIPT scores until further research findings support such a correlation.

PURDUE PERCEPTUAL-MOTOR SURVEY

The Purdue Perceptual-Motor Survey is used to assess performance of a series of perceptual motor skills that are designed to detect errors in perceptual-motor development in children. Its purpose is to identify areas for remediation. The skills are grouped into five main areas: posture and balance, body image and differentiation, perceptual-motor match, ocular movements, and form perception. The test battery was designed by Roach and Kephart[45] at Purdue University in Indiana and was one of the earliest tests developed to evaluate this area of function. It is a performance-based test and is included in this section because clinical experience has shown that it is more useful to the occupational therapist for the assessment of motor functions than for sensory-integrative functions. The test analysis is found in Figure 10-2.

Evaluation of Hand Function

A number of hand function tests, both published and unpublished, have been developed for children. These are often differentiated from similar tests for adults because of linear changes in a child's hand function that occur from infancy through adolescence. Assessment of hand function includes measures of prehension development, strength and dexterity of prehension patterns, and coordination and skill development. As Exner discusses in Chapter 13, occupational therapists

---

Figure 10-2 Purdue Perceptual-Motor Survey

Test measures: The survey was designed to detect errors in perceptual motor development and to designate areas for remediation. It does not provide diagnostic information. It is a survey of perceptual motor skills that are grouped into five areas of posture and balance, body image and differentiation, perceptual-motor match, ocular pursuits, and form perception.

Population: It is recommended for children aged 6 to 10 years. The survey should not be used with children who have specific sensorimotor deficits such as blindness, paralysis, or known motor involvement. Results of tests administered to children with a measured IQ below 80 may be questionable.

Test format:

    Content: This is a performance-based test that requires a manual, rating sheet, and the following equipment: balance beam, 4-foot-long pole, small pillow, mat, chalkboard, chalk, penlight, paper and pencil, and a table and chair appropriate to the child's size.

    Administration: By use of the manual and equipment, 22 items plus 11 subitems are administered, and results are recorded in a scoring booklet. Common problems are listed for each task, and the examiner places a checkmark by each observed characteristic.

    Scoring: Ratings from 1 to 4 are assigned for the child's performance on each item. A 4 indicates adequate performance; a 1 indicates that the child had considerable difficulty with an item. Ratings for items are transferred to a summary sheet to allow for score comparisons among the five areas. A composite score of 65 or higher indicates that the child is achieving within normal limits.

Interpretation: The lack of information concerning interpretation of ratings has been a source of criticism. The examiner is instructed to check the profile on the summary sheet to estimate major areas of difficulty that will require programming. Therefore the survey is most useful to experienced clinicians who are able to extract diagnostic information through observation of the child during test administration.

Advantages: Administration can be accomplished in about 30 minutes and is relatively simple. The survey can be used as a screening device and as a valid indicator of the need for diagnostic testing. Results are very useful for program planning. Reliability correlations for this test are generally good.

Disadvantages: Norms were obtained from 200 children in grades 1 through 4 at one school in Indiana only. A clinical sample of 97 "nonachievers" was matched to children in the normative group to establish validity estimates. Ratings were also correlated with teacher estimates of pupil performance, but the coefficient was not strong. Interpretations of findings are not well discussed in the manual. Standardization norms are not clearly presented for each age range.

Purchasing information: From Roach EG, and Kephart NC: The Purdue Perceptual-Motor Survey, Columbus, Ohio, 1971, Merrill Publishing Co.

take a broad view of the components of hand function, because it is so intricately representative of the interaction between functional development and childhood performance.

MEASURES OF PREHENSION DEVELOPMENT

These tests are based on the maturational and experiential development of prehension patterns from gross arm movements to fine tip prehension. Illustrations of these patterns are found in Chapters 4 and 13. Through observation and activity analysis, the therapist can select representative developmental activities to assess the emergence and precision of hand use.

Two systems of prehension development testing are both valuable models of their type and also exceptionally useful in the clinical setting. *The Erhardt Developmental Prehension Assessment* (EDPA)[19] is a research-based instrument that is commercially available and deserves special attention. The EDPA was developed by Rhoda Erhardt, an occupational therapist, and includes test items that assess postural antecedents of prehensile patterns. Therefore it is as useful for assessing those children who have not yet developed isolated hand function as it is for those children who have. A test analysis is shown in Figure 10-3.

In 1971, Skerik, Weiss, and Flatt[48] and then Weiss and Flatt[51] described a developmental test of prehension patterns. It was originally developed through their

---

Figure 10-3   Erhardt Developmental Prehension Assessment

Test measures: Components and skills of hand function development. Test items were developed through extensive literature review. Three major sections, divided into 17 subsections, measure involuntary arm-hand patterns; the arms at rest; the asymmetrical tonic neck reflex; grasping reactions; placing responses; avoiding responses; voluntary movements; arm approach in prone and sitting positions; grasp and release of dowel, cube, and pellet; manipulation skills; crayon or pencil grasp; and drawing skills.

Population: Different sections of the test contain criterion-referenced behaviors that normally occur from birth to 6 years. Erhardt states that the 15-month level indicates prehensile maturity and would therefore be the baseline for measurement of older children.

Test format:

Content: This is a criterion-referenced test that uses a test booklet, the primary reference for scoring and interpretation, and a test kit of items specified by Erhardt but developed by the individual therapist.

Administration: Test items are presented in the sequence shown in the test booklet. Items are administered through observation of movement patterns and presentation of selected objects to the child. With older children, test administration may be expected to take up to 1 hour.

Scoring: As items are administered, the examiner makes notations in the test booklet according to prescribed symbols. Developmental age levels for each of the subtests are determined by the highest level pattern that is considered well integrated. Each of the subsections indicates which patterns should be considered permanent throughout life. Performance that indicates the need for intervention is also noted in scoring.

Interpretation: Approximate age levels for the three main areas of hand function (primarily involuntary hand-arm patterns, voluntary movements, and pre-writing skills) are synthesized from average

developmental levels in each pertinent subsection. Erhardt makes clear that the test is a clinical tool that is designed primarily to identify discrete areas for intervention. Therefore the derived developmental levels for each of the three areas would be considered less important than the descriptive information about hand function that is generated by the test.

Advantages: This test provides a detailed assessment of a broad range of motor skills and functions that contribute to the development of prehension. The gradings of the sequences of function are more highly developed than in any other test of prehension patterns available. It is therefore a highly useful tool to the occupational therapy clinician and researcher.

Disadvantages: The administration and scoring instructions for the test are in general poorly detailed. Use of the author's text assists the examiner to some extent with this problem through the detailed case examples that are given. More precise definitions for some of the objects to be used for test administration would be helpful. In the primary reference Erhardt discussed the interrater reliability study that was conducted. Two groups of eight therapists used the test booklet to score the videotaped performance of two handicapped children per group, and agreements were subjected to statistical analysis. Interrater correlations varied from fair to very good. Individual items were analyzed in light of the variable correlations, but the outcome of this process is not clear. It is unfortunate that interrater comparisons were not performed with the evaluations of normal children. Erhardt also stated that the test had been evaluated through clinical use by a number of therapists in several states. However, the results of this field testing have not been reported to date.

Purchasing information: From Erhardt RP: Developmental hand dysfunction: theory assessment treatment, Laurel, Md, 1982, RAMSCO Publishing Co.

work with children who had congenital hand anomalies. However, because the test uses everyday activities of children to assess hand function, it can be used with other children as well. An adapted version of the Skerik, Weiss, and Flatt evaluation is shown in Figure 10-4.

HAND STRENGTH AND DEXTERITY MEASURES

Until recently, normative data have not been made available for many of the standard measures of hand strength and dexterity that have been used with adults. It is rewarding to have such data now increasingly available, to monitor and document improvement in function.

Mathiowitz, et al[37] obtained dynamometer readings from 471 normal children aged 6 to 19 years. These data shown in Table 10-1 provide useful information about *grasp strengths* expected of children in this age range. Mathiowitz, et al stated that they used the standard measurement procedure recommended by the American Society of Hand Therapists (ASHT). This requires the child to be seated, with shoulder adducted and neutral, elbow flexed to 90 degrees, forearm in neutral, wrist with 0 to 30 degrees dorsiflexion and 0 to 15 degrees ulnar deviation. The dynamometer was set at the second slot. By report of the researchers,

theirs has been the first study of children's hand strength that consistently specified and applied the ASHT procedure; for that reason their norms are presented here. Mathiowitz, et al also collected data on pinch strength of the sample children, but encountered problems in applying a standard procedure for positioning hands and pinch meters.

The *Purdue Pegboard Test*[23] is another measure of hand function that has proved useful with adults for many years. It measures finger dexterity through timed tests of separate hand insertion of pegs, simultaneous insertion of pegs with both hands, and a bimanual peg, washer, and collar assembly task. The Purdue Pegboard Test is particularly useful in predicting employability of disabled individuals. Recent studies (Mathiowitz, et al[36] and Gardner and Broman[23]) have reported normative data on Purdue Pegboard performance of children and adolescents; their findings are shown in Table 10-2. This standardized test should be administered according to procedures described in the test manual in order to use the normative data.

MEASURES OF HAND SKILLS

Many of the developmental tests administered by occupational therapists include items that measure

---

Figure 10-4   Hand function evaluation

Score: 0 = Child cannot grasp object.
      1 = Child completes grasp in manner
         of his own adaptation.
      2 = Child uses mature grasp pattern.

Pattern-activity	*R-L*	*Comments*
Hook grip: MCP joints flexed. Carry a small suitcase.		
Hook grip: MCP joints extended. Carry a plastic pail with handle.		
Power grip: Thumb adducted. Use a toy hammer.		
Power grip: Thumb abducted. Hold a 1-inch dowel.		
Lateral pinch: Standard. Hold a key.		
Tip pinch: Standard. Insert tipped lace through 1-inch bead.		
Palmar pinch: Standard. Use a needle for sewing cards.		
Palmar pinch: Cylindrical. Hold an empty tin can.		
Palmar pinch: Spherical Hold a small rubber ball.		
Palmar pinch: Disk. Hold a plastic stacking ring.		
Pinch strength:		
Differences between active and passive range of motion in hand:		

Adapted from Skerik SK, Weiss MW, and Flatt AE: Am J Occup Ther 25:98, 1971.

Table 10-1   Average performance of normal subjects on grip stength (lb)

Age	Hand	MALES			FEMALES		
		Mean	SD	Range	Mean	SD	Range
6-7	R	32.5	4.8	21-42	28.6	4.4	20-39
	L	30.7	5.4	18-38	27.1	4.4	16-36
8-9	R	41.9	7.4	27-61	35.3	8.3	18-55
	L	39.0	9.3	19-63	33.0	6.9	16-49
10-11	R	53.9	9.7	35-79	49.7	8.1	37-82
	L	48.4	10.8	26-73	45.2	6.8	32-59
12-13	R	58.7	15.5	33-98	56.8	10.6	39-79
	L	55.4	16.9	22-107	50.9	11.9	25-76
14-15	R	77.3	15.4	49-108	58.1	12.3	30-93
	L	64.4	14.9	41-94	49.3	11.9	26-73
16-17	R	94-0	19.4	64-149	67.3	16.5	23-126
	L	78.5	19.1	41-123	56.9	14.0	23-87
18-19	R	108.0	24.6	64-172	71.6	12.3	46-90
	L	93.0	27.8	53-149	61.7	12.5	41-86

Adapted from Mathiowitz, et al: Grip and pinch strength: norms for 6 to 19 year olds. Am J Occup Ther 40(10):705, 1986. With permission.
Note: The mean scores for individuals, aged 14 to 19 years, may be slightly low (0 to 10 lb lower than they should be) due to instrument error detected after the study.

Table 10-2   Average performance of normal subjects on the Purdue Pegboard*

Age	N	Subtest	Mean†	SD	SE	Low	High
		MALES					
14-15	26	Right hand	49.5	4.0	.77	41	57
		Left hand	46.4	5.0	.97	33	56
		Both hands	39.5	5.1	1.01	26	47
		Assembly	119.7	18.4	3.61	78	162
16-17	32	Right hand	49.6	4.5	.80	42	60
		Left hand	47.8	4.9	.86	39	60
		Both hands	40.2	4.0	.70	31	47
		Assembly	119.8	18.2	3.22	85	164
18-19	29	Right hand	49.5	5.4	1.00	30	57
		Left hand	48.0	4.6	.86	37	56
		Both hands	40.4	4.3	.81	28	46
		Assembly	123.2	15.4	2.86	81	154
		FEMALES					
14-15	28	Right hand	51.6	4.8	.91	42	61
		Left hand	47.9	5.0	.95	40	61
		Both hands	40.3	3.6	.67	34	47
		Assembly	114.0	17.0	3.22	76	141
16-17	33	Right hand	52.6	4.4	.76	44	62
		Left hand	49.4	5.2	.90	38	58
		Both hands	42.4	4.3	.76	33	50
		Assembly	122.4	18.2	3.17	81	151
18-19	28	Right hand	54.8	5.8	1.09	44	65
		Left hand	51.1	4.1	.78	42	60
		Both hands	44.3	4.9	.92	34	53
		Assembly	134.5	16.4	3.10	107	179

Adapted from Mathiowitz, et al: The Purdue Pegboard: norms for 14- to 19-year olds. Am J Occup Ther 40(3):176, 1986. With persmission.
*Sum of three trials.
†For right, left, and both hands subtests, score equals number of pegs placed in 30 sec. For assembly subtest, score equals number of pegs, collars, and washers assembled in 60 sec.
SD, standard deviation. *SE,* standard error.

skilled hand use. Object manipulating, coloring, writing, cutting, and measurement skills are often included.

Evaluation of general motor function

Occupational therapists will also want to assess muscle strength, range of motion, and muscle tone of many children seen in practice. Methods for evaluation of these characteristics are well documented.[27,42] Assessment of muscle tone is discussed in Chapters 9 and 20. There are many other formats available through the sources mentioned. Figure 10-5 shows page one of a composite form that can be used to record this information. This format was developed as part of the initial evaluation process used by the occupational and physical therapy staff of Colerain Elementary School, Columbus, Ohio. The Colerain form is also used to record developmental locomotor skills, from head control to walking, as measured on the Milani-Comparetti Motor Development Screening Test, the Denver Developmental Screening Test and other developmental evaluations.

It should be noted that data related to the areas of muscle strength and range of motion are generally not measured or recorded in as much detail as might be used for adult clients. This is in part because there are few normative data on strength in children and in part because of the limited usefulness of such data. With children the emphasis of assessment tends to focus more on the end performance of motor function than on isolated measures of musculoskeletal movement axes. The primary exception to this rule would be with those children who are seen before and after surgery for traumatic musculoskeletal injuries. In such cases therapists will perform detailed assessment of joint movement and muscle strength preoperatively and postoperatively.

TESTING SENSORY INTEGRATIVE FUNCTIONS

What occupational therapists refer to as sensory integrative function has had numerous other labels. For the purposes of this book, the term *sensory integrative functions* will include the awareness, discrimination, and recognition of sensory stimuli from the environment and the central nervous system's use of this sensory information to direct motor behavior. The occupational therapist focuses on sensory integrative function as the individual's capacity to use his senses to guide movements in daily life activities. This is a broad concept, and it refers to thinking and planning as well as execution of the broad range of motor behaviors.

Many tests have been developed to assess visual perception (that is, visual sensory awareness, discrimination, recognition, and utilization). Fewer tests are available to assess sensory integrative processing of the other five senses. This has resulted in the occupational therapist's heavy reliance on the Southern California Sensory Integration Tests (SCSIT) and on therapist-made tests of the other sensory modality functions.

Tests of visual perception

THE MOTOR-FREE VISUAL PERCEPTION TEST

The Motor-Free Visual Perception Test was developed by Calarusso and Hammill[14] to provide a rapid measure of visual sensory processing that does not require hand movements on the part of the child. Children are shown a series of test plates that measure simple visual discrimination, visual form constancy, gestalt perception, visual matching, and visual memory. The child can give a verbal response if he is unable to point to the correct item. Obviously the test is used with great difficulty with children whose severe motor handicap affects communicative ability.

The test is fairly well standardized with an adequate normative sample, validity, and reliability data. The test can be administered in its entirety in less than 15 minutes. Scoring provides a perceptual age and perceptual quotient. Although such scores are useful for monitoring progress and communicating with other professionals, they should not be considered inviolate indications of the child's level of function. It is more pertinent to look at the child's performance in each of the five areas of the test to determine areas of weakness and the need for remedial activities.

DEVELOPMENTAL TEST OF VISUAL-MOTOR INTEGRATION (VMI)

The Developmental Test of Visual-Motor Integration was developed by Beery[6] to determine specific areas of difficulty in visual motor behavior, with an emphasis on visual perception and motor coordination during pencil reproduction of geometric forms. The test is widely used by educators and psychologists and has proved useful to occupational therapists who want a quick measure of a child's eye-hand coordination in a pencil-and-paper task. A test analysis is shown in Figure 10-6.

FROSTIG DEVELOPMENTAL TEST OF VISUAL PERCEPTION

Frostig and others[22] first published the Frostig Developmental Test of Visual Perception in 1964, and it has been widely used since. The test represents one of the earliest and most durable tests of visual perception. The test seeks to measure five skill areas that Frostig defined as eye-motor coordination, figure-ground perception, shape constancy, position in space, and spatial relationships. These areas were chosen because of their importance to school readiness. The test can be administered to individuals or groups, and it is therefore useful for occupational therapists who need to screen large numbers of children. Figure

---

Figure 10-5 Colerain Elementary School Occupational and Physical Therapy Screening Evaluation

Child's name _____
Birthdate _____   Date of evaluation _____
1. Area of involvement/diagnosis:

2. General information—previous program, family, medical:

3. Development skills—motor skills, residual reflexes:

4. Muscle tone:

5. Muscle strength:
   Upper extremity   *Lower extremity*
   R   L   R   L

6. Limits in ROM:
   Upper extremity   *Lower extremity*
   R   L   R   L

7. Appliances:

8. Ambulation/mobility and transfers:

Reprinted with permission from Columbus Public Schools and Colerain Elementary School, Columbus, Ohio.

Figure 10-6 Developmental test of visual-motor integration (VMI)

Test measures: The test is a measure of the child's ability in eye-hand coordination. The test correlates best with reading ability and is basically a tool for educational assessment.

Population: This test can be administered to children 2 to 15 years of age, but it was designed to be used primarily for children in preschool and in the early primary grades. The manual includes instructions for individual and group administration.

Test format:
   Content: This is a pencil-and-paper test that uses a test booklet with 24 geometric forms to be copied.
   Administration: The test may be administered to individuals or groups. Shapes are to be copied in the sequence presented in the booklet, without use of an eraser. It is best to provide the student with a pencil that has no eraser. Only one attempt is allowed for each form. The examiner begins by presenting the first form and, when certain that the child understands what is to be done, allows the child to proceed independently.
   Scoring: Raw scores are obtained by counting the total number of forms passed, up to three consecutive failures. The manual provides scoring criteria with extensive examples of correct and incorrect reproduction of forms.
   Interpretation: Raw scores are converted to perceptual age equivalents. Performance on items is to be used for program strategies. Beery presents a sequence of worksheet-type program recommendations that may be used to improve performance.

Advantages: The test can be administered quickly to groups and individuals and is best used as a screening device.

Disadvantages: The information obtained from test administration is limited by the nature of test items. Test development data are not contained in the administration manual for ready reference.

Purchasing information: From Beery KE: Developmental test of visual-motor integration: administration and scoring manual, Chicago, 1967, Follet Publishing Co.

10-9 on p. 186 provides detailed information about the Frostig test in a test analysis.[21,22]

Tests of auditory perception

Whenever possible, tests of auditory perception are best administered and interpreted by speech pathologists or audiologists, who have greater expertise in these areas. Occupational therapists can readily obtain and discuss relevant information with these professionals in preparation for program planning. However, when speech or hearing services are not available, occupational therapists may need to obtain information about such areas as auditory discrimination and memory. In such instances the following tests are useful.

ILLINOIS TEST OF PSYCHOLINGUISTIC ABILITIES (ITPA)

The Illinois Test of Psycholinguistic Abilities is a widely accepted test battery that is used to delineate areas of difficulty related to communication skills. It is well standardized, and norms are available for children aged 2 to 10 years. Kirk, McCarthy, and Kirk[30] developed the test to measure components of communication according to a psycholinguistic model. This model states that the three major processes involved are decoding (stimuli reception), association, and encoding (expressive behavior). The test measures 12 areas of these processes, including grammatical closure and sound blending. Of particular interest to occupational therapists are its subtests that assess the following auditory perceptual functions: auditory reception, auditory association, verbal expression, auditory closure, and auditory sequential memory. The Illinois Test of Psycholinguistic Abilities measures visual areas as well: visual reception, visual association, visual closure, and visual sequential memory. The entire test battery frequently takes several hours to administer and requires careful preparation on the part of the administrator. As with the Sensory Integration and Praxis Tests, it is recommended that therapists who plan to use this test practice its administration with a number of normal children before using it clinically.

In a review of literature related to the Illinois Test of Psycholinguistic Abilities, Clark[16] cautioned occupational therapists to be aware that its predictive validity is questionable for learning disabled students. Test stability varies from weak to good. Therefore researchers have recommended that the test not be used by itself but in conjunction with other standardized tests.

DICHOTIC LISTENING TESTS

The dichotic listening test, which was developed by Broadbent[9,10] and later refined by Kimura,[28] is used by occupational therapists and audiologists to assess the status of speech lateralization in children. These tests provide an index believed to represent the relative efficiency of the right versus the left cerebral hemisphere functions that process auditory input of various types. It should be noted that the derived index is not considered a perfect indicator of speech lateralization.[28]

The procedure involves simultaneous presentation through headphones of a pair of auditory stimuli that have been stereophonically taped in a manner that administers one of the pair to each ear. Single sets of two digits, words, or nonsense syllables are used most frequently. Following the presentation of each stimulus pair, the subject is asked to indicate what was heard. Typically, right-handed individuals demonstrate greater accuracy in reporting what they heard through the right ear. When this result occurs, the computed index suggests a right over left ear advantage in accuracy of auditory processing.[5]

According to Kimura,[29] right ear advantage is interpreted to suggest lateralization of language processing in the left hemisphere of the brain. The basis for this inference resides in the arrangement of the neuroanatomical pathway from the ears to the regions of the cerebral cortex that are specialized for auditory processing.[46] Kimura[29] believed that impulses that travel via contralateral pathways from the ears to the hemispheres are processed more readily than stimuli that are conveyed over ipsilateral pathways.

Occupational therapists have used the dichotic listening tests as part of an overall assessment of sensory integrative function in which status of cerebral lateralization is one consideration (Chapter 23). Ayres[4,5] and Koomar and Cermak[33] are recommended reading.

Somatosensory tests
DEGANGI-BERK TEST OF SENSORY INTEGRATION (TSI)

In 1979 DeGangi[17] of the Georgia University Child Development Center published a performance-based test of sensory integrative function for children aged 3 to 5. The original test was made up of 21 items that assessed postural control, reflex integration, bilateral motor integration, oculomotor control, and vestibular function. Normative data were obtained from 113 children who represented a mix of racial and socioeconomic characteristics.

Eventually the test was refined to 36 items[7,18] that related to three main categories of function. Postural control items require the child to perform activities that elicit stabilization of the neck, trunk, and upper extremities as well as muscle cocontraction of the neck and upper extremities. Bilateral motor coordination items involve the child in activities that measure components of laterality and integration of the two body sides, including trunk rotation, midline crossing, rapid unilateral and bilateral hand movements, and dissociation of trunk and arm movements. Reflex integration includes testing symmetrical and asymmetrical tonic neck reflexes in the quadruped positions and tests of associated reactions in the upper extremities. Items related to oculomotor and vestibular functions were subsumed into the other three areas of measurement.

Although a fairly small sample was used for standardization, item analysis and test validation procedures were generally rigorous, and the test is useful to occupational therapists. The TSI has strong domain and construct validity; interobserver reliability measures are generally acceptable. Different samples of children were selected to match the requirements of various psychometric studies.

Test administration is similar to Norton's Basic Motor Evaluation, but the emphasis is on relating scores to sensory integration development. Intervention can therefore be more specifically focused. The manual provides comprehensive information on grading and interpretation of scores in each item and for clusters related to the three areas addressed. DeGangi and Berk[18] noted variability of the discriminative value of different test items in relation to different levels of dysfunction. Most test materials and forms are packaged in a kit, and additional required items are commonly available in pediatric settings or toy shops. The entire test can be administered to preschool children in about half an hour, which is advantageous when considering the test tolerance of younger children.

THE SENSORY INTEGRATION AND PRAXIS TESTS

Developed by A. Jean Ayres and colleagues, the Sensory Integration and Praxis Tests (SIPT)[2] replace the Southern California Sensory Integration Tests (SCSIT)[3,4] for comprehensive assessment of related functions. Like the earlier test series, the SIPT is standardized for children 4 through 8 years of age; some visual perception tests are standardized for children through 10 years. The normative study for the SIPT drew children of various ethnic and socioeconomic levels from a representation of rural and urban areas throughout North America. Children were randomly selected from public and private schools, organizations, and children's centers that agreed to participate in the study. To implement the standardization project, over 100 normative examiners and faculty were trained. Selection of project staff was based on previous SCSIT certification, experience with clinical, research, or educational use of the SCSIT, potential access to agencies and normative subjects, as well as willingness and time availability.

The sequence of tests (Figure 10-10 at the end of this chapter) is specifically designed to identify patterns of function and dysfunction in sensory integration and praxis. Selection of test items was based on the use of similar items in other tests, logical validation by theory, clinical experience, and item analysis. Tests must be presented in the order given with no extraneous conversation. Talking should be limited to administrative procedures to control the amount and degree of environmental stimulation to the child. Unnecessary conversation on the tester's part generates additional stimulation for the child that can confound the test results. As a rule of thumb, it is helpful to tell the child in advance that you can only say certain things to him during the test, but look forward to having a long conversation afterward.

The prescribed sequence of test administration requires 2 to 3 hours with the child. The Southern California Postrotary Nystagmus Test (SCPNT), formerly a separate test, is now part of the SIPT battery. The SIPT materials, as well as computerized reports and interpretations, are now available through the publisher. SCSIT materials will be available for a limited period but eventually will be phased out.

The revision and additions to the SIPT were designed to address many earlier concerns regarding SCSIT validity, reliability, and normative data.[2,3,4] Figure 10-10 at the end of this chapter presents the functional correlates of the SIPT, arranged according to the sequence of test administration.

For competent administration and interpretation of the SIPT, the completion of related certification coursework through Sensory Integration International (SII) is recommended and may ultimately be required to purchase the tests. Qualifications for the certification on courses include previous coursework in the neurosciences and tests and measurements, as well as previous clinical experience. In the future, course participants may also be required to have completed a master's level study program.

CLINICAL OBSERVATIONS

One of the clinically valuable components of the SCSIT was observation of the child's performance in a group of neuromotor and oculomotor tests.[4] Many of these tests were drawn by Ayres from traditional neurological examination procedures. Although a standardized format for these procedures has not been published by Ayres, a number of interpretive forms were developed over the years by therapists who were certified in administration of the SCSIT. The modification of one such form is shown in Figure 10-11 found in the appendix to this chapter. This clinical observation process incorporates additional measures that have proved useful in clinical practice.

RESEARCH TRENDS

Ongoing research in occupational therapy is particularly active in the area of sensory integrative function. As discussed by Clark and colleagues in Chapter 23, the standardization project for the SIPT is one of many areas of endeavor. One ongoing project reported by Royeen[47] concerns the development of a self-report test of tactile defensiveness. This intriguing project had children use a modified Likert scale to report the degree to which a series of statements applied to them. Statements were written as attitudes and related to the children's feelings and responses to a range of tactile stimuli experiences and situations. In addition to the potential usefulness of the specific scale for identification of tactilely defensive children, the method of measurement deserves attention. Of particular interest would be the use of such self-report tests for assessment of cognitive, social, and emotional functions.

SENSORY AWARENESS TESTING

Tests for sensory awareness, such as those of tactile recognition (stereognosis) and dermatomal patterns, are occasionally used with children who have lower motor neuron problems. Methods for these tests have been described.[27,42] However, the therapist needs to remember that sensory testing must be adapted to the experiential and cognitive levels of the children to be tested. For example, very young children cannot be expected to discriminate between pennies and dimes, for which their only concept may be "money."

Tyler[49] reported on a sensory test that was specifically designed for use with children aged 2 to 4 years. Seven common play and self-care items were chosen for manual identification by the child. Criteria for item selection included familiarity to children, small size, availability, texture variation, and presence of the items in the young child's language repertoire. Tyler encouraged children to manipulate and verbally label items before testing, and eliminated items from individual test protocols if the child could not label them.

Tyler administered items as a "guessing game" to a normative sample of 98 children. Items were presented to seated children to feel with their hands behind their backs. Items were presented to the children in random order, first in one hand and then in another. If the child incorrectly labeled the object, the examiner encouraged the child to manipulate it, with his vision occluded, for additional time. Average time for test administration was 4 minutes.

An adapted format for Tyler's test is found in Figure 10-7. Tyler found the greatest variability of correct responses among the 2-year-olds, and hypothesized that the skills required for sterognosis develop during this period. The entire range of 2- to 4-year-olds had the most difficulty with identifying the button, possibly because of language inadequacy or because this item is similar to the penny.

TESTING COGNITIVE FUNCTIONS

Superficially it may appear that there are fewer tests of cognitive, social, and emotional functions. However, it should be remembered that it is difficult to obtain physical measures of function in these areas. Instead these functions must be inferred through evaluation of the child's maturing performance in developmental tasks. The child's performance is reflected against the therapist's study of human development and the therapist's familiarity with the variations that normal children exhibit in manifestation of theoretical constructs. Therefore, although several tests that have been designed to measure cognitive levels and psychosocial functions are presented here, most assessment of these areas will be done during the therapist's administration of developmental and performance evaluations that will be discussed in Chapter 11.

Collaboration with psychologists and educators

Cognitive development and function are often tested by teachers and clinical psychologists who are well trained in the administration of intelligence tests. Specialized training and even certification are necessary to administer and interpret many such instruments. Therefore the occupational therapist should consult with these professionals to determine if reports are available about a child's performance on the Wechsler Intelligence Scale (WISC-R), the Stanford-Binet, the Bender-Gestalt, the Wide Range Achievement Test (WRAT), or other similar tests. Careful review of these reports should provide the therapist with substantial information about the child's intellectual capabilities, as well as offer clues to the child's thinking and learning styles.

However, if such information about cognitive function is not available from psychologists or teachers, several commercial tests that are fairly valid and reliable can be easily administered by the occupational therapist without additional training. These include the Goodenough-Harris Drawing Test and the Wachs Analysis of Cognitive Structures.

Cognitive tests
GOODENOUGH-HARRIS DRAWING TEST

The Goodenough-Harris Drawing Test is relatively simple to administer, and because it uses drawing, children generally enjoy taking it. The test is based on the premise that children's drawings reflect the maturation of cognitive representations.[24]

The test may be administered on an individual basis or in groups. Normative information is provided for children age 3 to 15 years; however, Harris cautions that the sample of 3- and 4-year-olds was smaller, and therefore the test is less predictive for this age range. The child is asked to draw three pictures: a man, a woman, and a self-portrait. The test administrator will ask the child to explain each of the pictures, to clarify what each component of the drawings represents to the child. To score the test the therapist contrasts body part details included in the child's drawing with normative criteria. The test manual gives clear definitions and examples of scoring for the various body parts so that scoring is generally objective. Raw scores (for number of acceptable body parts) can be converted to standard scores, quality scores, and percentile rankings to yield an impression of the child's intellectual development.[25] It should be noted that the test manual does not contain information about the test development. The user is referred to Harris' formal text[24] for more detailed information about theoretical framework and standardization.

WACHS ANALYSIS OF COGNITIVE STRUCTURES (WACS)

Wachs, an optometrist, became interested in cognitive development and learning problems through his work with children who had visual-motor and perceptual disorders. In collaboration with Hans Furth, Wachs studied Piagetian theory and research methodology extensively. With this background, Wachs and Vaughan[50] developed a test that uses typical Piagetian tasks to evaluate cognitive development of children in the preoperational age range (3 to 6 years). The Wachs Analysis of Cognitive Structures is more complex to administer than the Goodenough-Harris Drawing Test, but the information it provides can be helpful to occupational therapists. The test also serves as a model for the construction of Piagetian tasks for evaluative purposes.

The Wachs Analysis of Cognitive Structures is com-

Figure 10-7 Stereognostic test for preschool children

Child's name: _____ Date of birth: _____
Test date: _____
Object   *Right-left Comments*
1. Two-inch diameter rub-
   ber ball
2. Five-inch plastic spoon
3. Two-inch metal car with
   movable wheels
4. Three-inch plush stuffed dog
5. One-inch toy plastic chair
6. U.S. penny
7. One-inch plastic button,
   two times as thick as
   penny, with four holes*
TOTAL SCORE: _____ RIGHT: _____ LEFT: _____
Scoring: 2 = Identifies correctly when object
             is first presented.
         1 = Gives incorrect label on first
             presentation, but then self-corrects
             after additional manipulation.
         0 = Unable to give correct
             known label.
Note: Omit any items from the test that the child
cannot label during the initial exploratory period.

From the American Occupational Therapy Association, Inc: Copyright 1972, vol 26, No 6, p 256, A stereognostic test for screening
tactile sensation, NB Tyler.
*Correct identification of the button may indicate the development
of finer discriminative abilities.

posed of 15 task clusters that relate to four cognitive abilities: manipulation of materials, visual representation, graphic representation, and manual identification. The test requires little verbal response from the child; instead it is a performance-based assessment of the child's use of body and sense thinking. The test demonstrates the development of cognitive schemes in each of the four areas. Raw scores are converted to standard scores and percentile rankings.

Internal consistency and interrater reliability of the test are excellent. The normative samples for this test were small. However, one of the special features of the test is that it was also administered experimentally to a number of "atypical" groups of children, including high-risk, Eskimo, Indian, retarded, African, and deaf children. The test manual provides considerable data that can be used by the therapist to interpret test results, and it makes note of cultural implications for treatment planning.

As with other tests mentioned earlier, it is advisable for the interested therapist to practice administration of the Wachs Analysis of Cognitive Structures with normal children before clinical use. Naturally, one should study the manual carefully and review pertinent information about Piagetian theory.

TESTING PSYCHOSOCIAL FUNCTIONS
Projective techniques

For many years occupational therapists have used projective techniques to assist in the assessment of emotional states of their patients. Unstructured art materials are presented to the clients with variable instructions from the therapist about how the media are to be used. The therapists record observations of the client with regard to task involvement, approach to the activity, attention span, motivation, and feelings expressed by the client during engagement in the activity. A number of projective batteries that are used with adult clients have been reported in the occupational therapy literature, but there is less information about the use of projective techniques with children. Typical activities that are used to elicit projective information include finger painting, drawing, clay sculpture, and mosaic tile arrangement. The most essential element to the process is the therapist's ability to encourage the client to discuss what he is thinking about and doing.

Llorens and Bernstein[34] reported on the use of finger painting as a projective medium for emotionally disturbed children. The unstructured and reversible nature of finger painting was found to allow one child to express a range of feelings about his family problems, as well as recognize changes in his own behavior through discussions with the therapist. In another publication related to programming for this population, Llorens and Rubin[35] suggested that behavioral observations during activity involvement be rated according to the adequacy of attention span, ability to concentrate, ability to follow verbal directions, degree of motor activity, relatedness to therapist, dependence-independence (of behavior), and affect and mood. Behavioral manifestations of these characteristics may be rated as inadequate, transitional, and adequate. It is recognized that assessment through projective techniques is more subjective and depends on the sound clinical expertise of the therapist. Essentially the use of projective techniques represents the use of activity analysis as an evaluation tool.

Data-based observation of behavior

One of the most frequently employed techniques for the identification and assessment of adaptive and maladaptive behaviors is the use of data-based observation. The occupational therapist or another professional begins the assessment with detailed note-taking on observed behaviors. *Target behaviors* that appear to interfere most with effective social adaptation and emotional adjustment are identified and ranked. From this list the therapist and program team can identify a few behaviors that are most suited to immediate intervention. It should be noted that the behaviors that are first targeted for change might not be the most maladaptive. Instead the behaviors chosen will generally be those that are believed to be most amenable to change within the current time frame.

The next step is for the therapist and other staff who will work to eliminate the target behaviors to obtain baseline *frequency rates* on the occurrence of said behaviors. Most facilities have a specific internal data collection sheet, or they use commercial forms for this purpose. Data are usually collected within fixed time intervals, such as 5-, 10-, or 30-minute periods. Often therapists will use a small mechanical counter so that they can "click off" behaviors as these occur without interrupting the task. At the end of the data base period the behavioral frequency is recorded. The staff members will review baseline data and establish objectives for behavior change. For example, if a child was observed pushing other children five times in a 10-minute period on the playground, the staff members might establish an immediate objective to reduce the frequency of pushing by 40%, that is, to three times in one 10-minute period in that location. A long-term goal might be to eliminate the behavior completely.

Thereafter at regular intervals the frequency of the behavior is measured and notes may be made by the therapist regarding any variations in the behaviors. One of the critical observational requirements throughout the process will be the therapist's identification of situations *(environmental contingencies)* that appear to stimulate or inhibit behavioral frequency. This type of assessment process is used throughout the course of treatment as data collection continues until there is closure on the target behaviors. It should be noted that the *treatment* itself will usually consist of a reward for performance of an adaptive behavior, such as asking another child to move out of the way. Or the child may be rewarded for not exhibiting the maladaptive behavior, that is, when he has not pushed. In this behavior modification approach it is considered inappropriate to punish the child for exhibiting the maladaptive behavior unless all other routes to behavior change have been exhausted without success.

Although the example just mentioned relates to psychosocial dysfunction, data-based observations can be used to record changes in all areas of concern to the occupational therapist. For example, the therapist might use this technique to record changes in standing tolerance, increased assistive use of a weak hand, or spontaneous interactions with other children. Data-based observation is a powerful tool for measurement of change. The most important elements are the identification of appropriate targets for observation and data collection, as well as recognition of environmental contingencies for behavior change. Again, the therapist's use of activity analysis is the key to successful application of this technique.

The Preschool Play Scale

In 1974, the Knox Play Scale[32] was published in a collection of studies on play. The scale was a framework for analysis of observed activities used to assess the social-emotional maturation of newborn through 6-year-old children through their play behaviors. Knox's scale was based primarily on Erikson's concepts of play and psychosocial development. A revision of the instrument, called the Preschool Play Scale, was reported by Bledsoe and Shepherd.[8] The revised scale is presented in detail in Chapter 11.

Piers-Harris Children's Self-Concept Scale

Subtitled "The Way I Feel About Myself," the Piers-Harris Children's Self-Concept Scale[43] is a self-report instrument designed to look at correlates of the self-concept of children in grades 3 through 12. The scale consists of 80 questions that may be answered in 15 to 30 minutes, depending on whether it is administered individually or to a group. Results may be reported in stanines, percentiles, or individual scores for each of the six factors measured: behavior, intellectual and school status, physical appearance and attributes, anxiety, popularity, and happiness and satisfaction. While this test was designed primarily as a research tool to look at the development of a child's self-concept, it is also useful in clinical and counseling settings and as a screening instrument to identify children in need of intervention.

Studies measuring the internal consistency and stability reported coefficients ranging from .71 to .93. Concurrent validity studies comparing the Piers-Harris to other self-concept, peer, and teacher rating methods are inconclusive, with correlations ranging from -0.64 to 0.68. Further information on reliability and validity studies are discussed in a research monograph.[44]

Burk's Behavior Rating Scales

The Burk's Behavior Rating Scales (BBRS) consist of the school age version[12] and the preschool and kindergarten edition.[13] The school age version is intended for use with children in grades 1 through 9 and the other edition was designed for children aged 3 to 6. Both tests use parent or teacher reports on checklists to identify particular behavior problems and patterns of problems shown by children.

Categories of behavior patterns include: excessive self-blame, excessive anxiety, excessive withdrawl, excessive dependency, poor ego strength, poor physical strength, poor coordination, poor intellectuality, poor academics, poor attention span, poor impulse control, and poor reality contact. Additional areas are: poor sense of identity, excessive sense of persecution, excessive aggressiveness, excessive resistance, and poor social conformity.

Both scales have acceptable standardization and validity information that are reported in the test manual. The manual includes test forms, which can also be ordered separately. Profile sheets are used to convert raw scores into "not significant," "significant," and "very significant" ratings. Separate parents' and teachers' guides are also provided. The guides define categories of dysfunctional behavior as well as possible causes and suggest ways to help children who exhibit maladaptive behavior. The manual also makes recommendations for intervention approaches at home and school.

SUMMARY

This chapter has focused on the presentation of a selected group of tests, some more widely known than others. These tests are used to evaluate different component functions of behavior: the motor, sensory integrative, cognitive, psychological (emotional), and social processes that enable children to do the things they do. Assessment of these functions is critical to the therapist's understanding of why children have problems in everyday activities. Findings from these tests allow the therapist to develop treatment programs that will improve functional processes to improve the child's task performance. Testing in these functional components accompanies comprehensive evaluation of the child's performance skills in play, self-maintenance, school work, and prevocational activities (Chapter 11).

STUDY QUESTIONS

Using the resources discussed in this chapter, select at least three appropriate test instruments or evaluation methods to use for your assessment of each of the following children and adolescents:

1. An 8-month-old boy with poor head control and other delayed motor milestones.
2. A 3-year-old girl who is withdrawn and ignores other children during play. Parents report that her preferred toys typically use auditory stimuli.
3. A 6-year-old boy whose first grade teacher is concerned about his poor handwriting and participation in classroom activities.
4. A 13-year-old boy who has been diagnosed with Duchenne's muscular dystrophy for 5 years and is now unable to stand without bilateral support.

Explain why each of the tests or procedures you have selected is appropriate. What information do you expect to obtain from administration?

REFERENCES

1. Amiel-Tison C, and Grenier A: Neurologic evaluation of the newborn and the infant, New York, 1983, Masson.
2. Ayres AJ: Sensory Integration and Praxis Tests: administrative directions for normative examiners, Los Angeles, 1984, Western Psychological Services.
3. Ayres AJ: Southern California Sensory Integration Tests: test manual, revised, Los Angeles, 1980, Western Psychological Services.
4. Ayres AJ: Interpreting the Southern California Sensory Integration Tests, Los Angeles, 1976, Western Psychological Services.
5. Ayres AJ: Dichotic listening performance in learning-disabled children, Am J Occup Ther 31:441, 1977.
6. Beery KE: Developmental Test of Visual-Motor Integration: administration and scoring manual, Chicago, 1967, Follette Publishing Company.
7. Berk R, and DeGangi G: DeGangi-Berk Test of Sensory Integration Manual, Los Angeles, 1983, Western Psychological Services.
8. Bledsoe NP, and Shepherd JT: A study of reliability and validity of a preschool play scale, Am J Occup Ther 36:783, 794, 1982.
9. Broadbent DE: Listening to one of two synchronous messages, Exp Psychol 44:51, 1952a.
10. Broadbent DE: Speaking and listening simultaneously, Exp Psychol 43:267, 1952b.
11. Bruininks RH: Bruininks-Oseretsky Test of Motor Proficiency: examiner's manual, Circle Pines, Minn, 1978, American Guidance Service.
12. Burks HF: Burk's Behavior Rating Scales Manual, Los Angeles, 1986, Western Psychological Services.
13. Burks HF: Burk's Behavior Rating Scales: preschool and kindergarten edition manual, Los Angeles, 1983, Western Psychological Services.
14. Calarusso RP, and Hammill DD: Motor-Free Visual Perception Test, Novato, Calif, 1972, Academic Therapy Publications.
15. Chandler L, Andrews M, and Swanson M: Movement assessment of infants, Rolling Bay, Wash, 1980, MAI, PO Box 4361, Rolling Bay, Washington, 98061.
16. Clark FA: The Illinois Test of Psycholinguistic Abilities: considerations of its use in occupational and physical therapy practice, Phys Occup Ther Pediatr 2:29, Winter 1982.
17. DeGangi G: Assessment of sensorimotor integration in preschool children, Washington, DC, 1979, Georgetown University Child Development Center.
18. DeGangi GA, and Berk RA: Psychometric analysis of the Test of Sensory Integration, Phys Occup Ther Pediatr 3:43, Summer 1983.
19. Erhardt RP: Developmental hand dysfunction: theory assessment treatment, Laurel, Md, 1982, RAMSCO Publishing Co.
20. Fiorentino MR: Reflex testing methods for evaluating CNS dysfunction, Springfield, Ill, 1972, Charles C Thomas, Publisher.
21. Frostig M, Maslow P, Lefever DW, and Whittlesey JRB: The Marianne Frostig Developmental Test of Visual Perception: 1963 standardization, Palo Alto, Calif, 1964, Consulting Psychologists Press.
22. Frostig M, Lefever DW, and Whittlesey JRB: Administration and scoring manual for the Marianne Frostig Developmental Test of Visual Perception, Palo Alto, Calif, 1966, Consulting Psychologists Press.
23. Gardner RA, and Broman M: The Purdue Pegboard: normative data on 1334 school children, J Clin Child Psych 1:156, 1979.
24. Harris DB: Goodenough-Harris Drawing Test: manual, New York, 1963, Harcourt Brace Jovanovich Inc.
25. Harris DB: Children's drawings as measures of intellectual maturity: a revision and extension of the Goodenough Draw-a-Man Test, New York, 1963, Harcourt Brace Jovanovich Inc.
26. Harris SR, et al: Predictive validity of the Movement Assessment of Infants, J Dev Behav Pediatr 5:336, 1984.
27. Hopkins HL, and Smith HD: Willard and Spackman's occupational therapy, ed 6, Philadephia, 1983, JB Lippincott Co.
28. Kimura D: Cerebral dominance and perception of verbal stimuli, Can Psychol 15:166, 1961.
29. Kimura D: Some effects of temporal lobe damage on auditory perception, Can Psychol 15:156, 1965.
30. Kirk SA, McCarthy JJ, and Kirk W: Illinois Test of Psycholinguistic Abilities, Urbana, Ill, 1968, University of Illinois Press.

31. Kliewer D, Bruce W, and Trembath J: The Milani-Comparetti motor development screening test: administration manual, Omaha, Nebr, 1977, Meyer Children's Rehabilitation Institute.

32. Knox SH: A play scale. In Reilly M, editor: Play as exploratory learning: studies of curiosity behavior, Beverly Hills, 1974, Sage Publications, p 247.

33. Koomar JA, and Cermak SA: Reliability of dichotic listening using two stimulus formats with normal and learning disabled children, Am J Occup Ther 35:456, 1981.

34. Llorens LL, and Bernstein SP: Finger painting with an obsessive-compulsive organically-damaged child, Am J Occup Ther 17:120, May-June, 1963.

35. Llorens LL, and Rubin EZ: Developing ego functions in disturbed children: occupational therapy in milieu, Detroit, 1967, Wayne State University Press.

36. Mathiowitz V, and others: The Purdue Pegboard: norms for 14- to 19-year olds, Am J Occup Ther 40:174, 1986a.

37. Mathiowitz V, Weimer D, and Federman S: Grip and pinch strength: norms for 6-19 year olds, Am J Occup Ther 40:705, 1986b.

38. McCarraher-Wetzel AP, and Wetzel RC: A review of the Amiel-Tison Neurological Evaluation of the Newborn and the Infant, Am J Occup Ther 38:585, 1984.

39. Milani-Comparetti A: Routine developmental examination in normal and retarded children, Dev Med Child Neurol 9:631, 766, 1967.

40. Mutti M, Sterling H, and Spalding N: Quick Neurological Screening Test, Navato, Calif, 1978, Academic Therapy Publications.

41. Norton Y: Minimal cerebral dysfunction, part II: modified treatment and evaluation of movement, Am J Occup Ther 26:186, May-June, 1972.

42. Pedretti LW: Occupational therapy: practice skills for physical dysfunction, ed 2, St Louis, 1985, The CV Mosby Co.

43. Piers E, and Harris D: Piers-Harris Children's Self Concept Scale, Nashville, Tenn, 1969, Counselor Recordings and Tests.

44. Piers E, and Harris D: Children's Self Concept Scale: Research monograph #1, Nashville, Tenn, 1977, Counselor Recordings and Tests.

45. Roach EG, and Kephart NC: The Purdue Perceptual-Motor Survey, Columbus, Ohio, 1971, Merrill Publishing Company.

46. Rosenzweig MR: Representations of two ears at the auditory cortex, Am J Physiol 167:147, 1951.

47. Royeen C: The development of a touch scale for measuring tactile defensiveness in children, Am J Occup Ther 40:414, 1986.

48. Skerik SK, Weiss MW, and Flatt AE: Functional evaluation of congenital hand anomalies, part I, Am J Occup Ther 25:98, March 1971.

49. Tyler NB: A sterognostic test for screening tactile sensation: thesis abstract, Am J Occup Ther 26:256, July-August, 1972.

50. Wachs H, and Vaughan LJ: Wachs Analysis of Cognitive Structures, Los Angeles, 1977, Western Psychological Services.

51. Weiss MW, and Flatt AE: Functional evaluaton of the congenitally anomalous hand, part II, Am J Occup Ther 25:139, April 1971.

52. Whaley L, and Wong D: Nursing care of infants and children, ed 2, St Louis, 1983, The CV Mosby Co.

53. Ziviani J, Poulsen A, and O'Brien A: Correlation of the Bruininks-Oseretsky Test of Motor Proficiency with the Southern California Sensory Integration Tests, Am J Occup Ther 36:519, 1982.

Appendix to Chapter 10

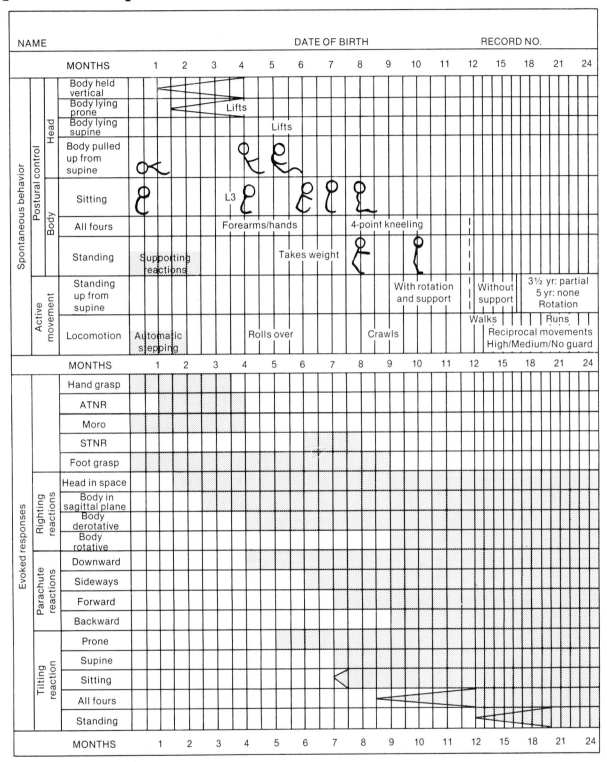

Figure 10-8   Milani-Comparetti Motor Development Screening Test.

From Milani-Comparetti A, and Gidoni E: Dev Med Child Neurol 9:631, 766, 1967.

Figure 10-9 Frostig Developmental Test of Visual Perception

Test measures: Frostig and associates postulated that what is usually referred to as visual perception actually consists of a number of different functions that develop relatively independently of each other. The test proposes to measure what the authors consider to be five fairly discrete areas that have particular relevance to school performance. These five abilities are:
1. Eye-hand coordination
2. Figure-ground perception
3. Perception of shape constancy
4. Perception of position in space
5. Perception of spatial relationships

Population: The Frostig test was developed for use as a screening device for preschool through first-grade children. Normative data for ages 4 to 8 are available. It is believed that any child over 10 years of age who does not score within the maximum age group for which any subtest is scaled may be presumed to have difficulty in the skill that subtest assesses.

Test format:

Content: This is a paper-and-pencil test that uses a protocol booklet, manual, and scoring materials. The booklet contains five subtests with several items in each test that are graded according to difficulty.

Administration: Normally individual administration should take no more than 45 minutes by following the manual, but there is great variability. Children who have learning disabilities frequently take longer or become too restless to complete the test at a single sitting. Group administration is possible if auxiliary personnel are available to monitor children and answer questions. Children with known problems should always be tested individually.

Scoring: Raw scores are determined for performance on each subtest. Scoring materials, such as overlays and lists of criteria, are included with test kits.

Interpretation: The raw scores are converted to perceptual age equivalents that serve as indicators of the age levels at which a child is believed to be functioning in abilities measured by each of the subtests. The perceptual age equivalents are then computed into scale scores that correlate the child's perceptual age to chronological age. In general, uniformly low scores suggest retardation rather than specific learning disability. A scatter of high and low scores suggests a disorder of visual perception. A perceptual quotient can be calculated in a manner similar to that for determining IQ. This may be converted to a percentile ranking by indicating how the child's performance compares to that achieved by the normative sample for his age group.

Advantages: The Frostig test is a good initial screening instrument, because it allows evaluation of a variety of behaviors in addition to evaluation of a variety of visual skills. These include test taking, following instructions, and the handling of the motor-planning tasks involved in writing. The test is simple to administer and grade because the manual has been written clearly. Adaptations of test administration are available for children who are deaf, do not speak English, are physically handicapped, or are emotionally disturbed.

Disadvantages: Standardization of the test was done with a somewhat small and primarily middle-income local population. Therefore findings with children of different socioeconomic or ethnic backgrounds should be viewed accordingly. Some of the subtests become less valid for the older child because of worksheet experience in school and because the child can use cognitive skills to second guess the items in spite of genuine visual perception problems. This is particularly true of the position in space and spatial relationships items.

Purchasing information: From Frostig M, and others: The Marianne Frostig Development Test of Visual Perception: 1963 standardization, Palo Alto, Calif, 1964, Consulting Psychologists Press.

References: Frostig M, Lefever DW, and Whittlesey JRB: Administration and scoring manual for the Marianne Frostig Developmental Test of Visual Perception, Palo Alto, Calif, 1966, Consulting Psychologists Press and Frostig M, and others: The Marianne Frostig Developmental Test of Visual Perception: 1963 Standardization, Palo Alto, Calif, 1966, Consulting Psychologists Press.

Figure 10-10   Definitions and functional correlates of the sensory integration and praxis tests

1. *Space Visualization:* This test demonstrates the child's ability to discriminate spatial elements of objects (geometric forms), including, in the more advanced items, mental manipulations (movements) of objects in space. Formboard puzzles are presented to the child in different positions, with variable visual coordinates. Space visualization is critical to daily tasks that require object assembly/construction. SIPT revisions include the protocol sheet and test instructions.

2. *Figure-ground discrimination:* This visual perceptual function allows the individual to concentrate on one stimulus against a field of many competing stimuli. The test items require the child to select a specific picture from a background of distracting pictures. Visual figure-ground discrimination enables the child to focus on words during reading.

3. *Standing and Walking Balance:* This test measures the child's ability to maintain balance with and without vision, on both feet or on one foot, on a dowel of the floor, heel to toe, and tandem walking. Standing and walking balance skills are necessary to maintain an upright posture in various gross and fine motor tasks.

4. *Design Copying:* This pencil and paper test measures a combination of visual perception of a geometric design and the capacity of the brain to direct the hand in duplicating that design. This combination allows the child to learn to write letters and numbers. This measure of graphic praxis is obtained by the recording and scoring of the child's approach to figure reproduction, simultaneously as the child is drawing the figure.

5. *Postural Praxis:* This test evaluates a child's ability to imitate positions or postures as demonstrated by the examiner. This test replaces the SCSIT Imitation of Postures test. Some old test items were deleted and new ones added. Timing and scoring criteria were revised.

6. *Bilateral Motor Coordination:* This measures smooth performance of executed movements of both hands or both feet together in smooth, rhythmic patterns. Both motor planning and integration of the two body sides are measured. Criteria includes timing, rhythm, and sequencing of movements patterns. Bilateral coordination is critical to smooth performance of gross motor activities such as bicycle riding or dancing, and fine motor activities such as supporting paper while writing.

7. *Praxis on Verbal Command:* This test measures the ability to motor plan body postures based on verbal directions without visual cues. It therefore measures auditory language processing as well as motor praxis. This process is critical to following directions for unfamiliar activities.

8. *Constructional Praxis:* This test measures a child's ability to relate objects to each other in space through "structures I and II." Structure I requires the child to construct a "building" after the examiner provides a demonstration. Structure II asks the child to reproduce a different block design from a visual model, without demonstration by the examiners. Measurement is according to accuracy and placement of design. Constructional praxis is important in motor planning a course of action for object assembly and three-dimensional design.

9. *Postrotary Nystagmus:* This test measures the duration and regularity of eye oscillations after spinning—a normal vestibulo-ocular reflex. This reaction is important to maintaining balance as well as coordinating eye function with body movements. The SIPT version includes revised directions for test administration language.

10. *Motor Accuracy:* This test measures the degree of changes in sensorimotor coordination in the arms and hands, guided by visual cues. The test emphasizes the motor aspect of tracing over a large pattern, and relates to activities such as cutting, writing, and performing sports activities.

11. *Sequencing Praxis:* This measures the ability to replicate a series of hand and finger movements after demonstration by the examiner. Emphasis is on the serial movements rather than rhythm and smoothness. Elements of visual, auditory, and kinesthetic memory are also tapped by the test.

12. *Oral Praxis:* This test measures the ability to motor plan and sequence oral positions and movements following the examiner's demonstration. Oral praxis is important in performing unfamiliar movements when eating, learning new sounds, and developing smooth articulation.

13. *Manual Form Perception:* The test has been significantly revised from the SCSIT to more effectively measure stereognostic function. This use of tactile functions is important in performing routine activities precisely, such as buttoning or counting money. Part I still requires the subject to identify the counterpart of a hand held object on a presented board. However, the stimulus blocks and visual shapes have been changed. Part II is new and requires the child to feel a shape with one hand and use the other hand to tactilely identify the matching shape from a group, without visual clues.

14. *Kinesthesia:* Administration of this test can be used to assess the individual's capacity to perceive the position and movement of body parts. The child is asked to duplicate movement patterns with vision occluded. Kinesthesia allows the individual to perform familiar motor activities, such as walking, with a sense of security, and also helps guide the child as he or she tries out new movements and skilled activities, as in sports and crafts. A revised protocol sheet and positioning of the child facing the examiner are noteworthy.

From Ayres AJ[2,3,4]: With adaptation of work from Sandy Adams, University of Florida, 1977.

Continued.

Figure 10-10 cont'd.   Definitions and functional correlates of the sensory integration and praxis tests

15. *Finger Identification:* This is a basic test of tactile sensory awareness. The student must identify which finger of either hand was touched by the examiner, while the subject's vision was occluded. (Note: vision is not occluded while identification is made, only when stimulus is given.) This basic sensory process is protective.

16. *Graphesthesia:* Tests for intersensory integration of tactile discrimination, visual awareness, and fine motor planning. The child must recognize the form of and then duplicate a design drawn on the back of the hand. Vision is occluded when the tester draws designs on the back of the child's hand, but not when the child is duplicating the design. The examiner and child also face each other in the SIPT revision of this test. This complex sensory-motor process allows us to become proficient writers.

17. *Localization of Tactile Stimuli:* This is a test of tactile discriminative ability. The child must point to a spot on his or her arm that was touched by the examiner's pen, with vision occluded. A special pen is provided in the test kit to assure accurate and even presentation of stimuli. This is a basic sensory process that helps individuals with such activities as self-dressing, washing, and hairbrushing.

Figure 10-11 Southern California Sensory Integration tests: clinical observations

Student name: _____

School: _____ Class: _____

Date: _____ Examiner: _____

Date of birth: _____

Chronological age: _____

1. Eye preference for sighting: Offer spy holes at midline. Say, "Look at me through this with one of your eyes."
   a. Student's eye through ring of examiner's thumb and index finger. R_____ L_____
   b. Student's eye through a paper cone to focus on examiner. R_____ L_____
   c. Student's eye through a small hole in large cardboard. R_____ L_____

   Score: 3 = Same as hand preference: R_____ L_____
   2 = Inconsistent
   1 = Opposite
   Comments: _____

2. Eye pursuits: Move pen back and forth, up and down, and diagonally, holding it about 10 to 12 inches from child's eyes at midline. Use child's shoulders, chin, and top of head as landmarks for ends of ranges. Instruct the child to follow the pen with his eyes without moving head. If necessary, examiner, hold child's chin firmly to prevent head movements. To check convergence, begin with pencil at examiner's nose and move it slowly forward to student's nose and then back. Ask child to tell you when he sees "two pens."

   Score: General pursuits:
   3 = Basically smooth, coordinated movements. May show small jerks or hesitations.
   2 = Slight irregularities in most planes, even after child becomes accustomed to testing.
   1 = Unable to follow or loses target; unable to separate eye movements from head movements (normal to 6 years).
   Comments: _____

   Score: Across midline:
   1 = Basically smooth, coordinated movements as above.
   2 = Midline jerk, then refocuses.
   3 = Midline jerk, cannot refocus.
   Comments: _____

   Score: Convergence:
   3 = Basically smooth.
   2 = Movement jerky and unsure.
   1 = Eyes break apart or do not converge.
   0 = Unable to fixate.
   Check eyes together and then independently by first covering one eye, then the other. Observe and note right/left differences.
   L_____ R_____ Both_____
   Comments: _____

3. Forearm rotation: Test for adiadochokinesis, 10 seconds. Sit facing child, both with arms resting in laps. Demonstrate rapid supination and pronation, then ask child to imitate and say: "Do it fast." Count the number of times the palms slap thighs in 10 seconds. Observe for incoordination, and compare right and left scores.
   R_____ times L_____ times
   Score: Bilateral coordination:
   3 = Normal
   2 = One arm slower than other throughout: R L
   1 = Both arms deficient
   Comments: _____

4. Thumb-finger touching: Thumb touches each finger in sequence from index to little and then back in sequence to index finger, repeating several times. Observe speed, coordination, and right-left differences.
   Score: 3 = Performs easily L_____ R_____ Both_____
   2 = Slight irregularities L_____ R_____ Both_____
   1 = Awkward or unable L_____ R_____ Both_____
   Comments: _____

5. Muscle tone: Examiner places student's shoulder, elbow, and hand flexor muscles on stretch. Note degree of hyperextension. Palpate muscles for tone.
   Score: 3 = Normal R/L differences: _____
   2 = Slightly hypotonic
   1 = Definitely hypertonic
   0 = Hypertonic
   Comments: _____

Continued.

6. Cocontraction: Examiner applies force against student's position. Sit facing child. Do not let him stabilize against back of chair. Ask child to "freeze like a statue" and not let you push or pull him. (This should be fully developed by 7 to 8 years of age.)
   Score: 3 = Can withstand moderate resistance.
         2 = Can withstand light resistance.
         1 = Unable to hold against resistance.
         Arm: Student holds examiner's thumbs, with elbows flexed.   3   2   1
         Shoulder: Examiner holds student's hands, elbows straight: 3   2   1
         Neck: Examiner gives force against different planes: 3   2   1
             (Do not expect as much strength as in arms.)
   Comments: _____

7. Flexor postural pattern: Student assumes "curled up" position, arms crossed across chest, ankles crossed, knees and hips flexed, neck flexed forward. Do not allow child to clasp hands behind knees. Examiner applies resistive force at head and knees. Decrease force for children under 6 years.
   Score: 3 = Holds 20 seconds or more with moderate effort.
         2 = Holds 10 to 19 seconds with great exertion.
         1 = Holds less than 10 seconds against resistance.
         0 = Unable to hold against resistance.
   Comments: _____

8. Prone extension postural pattern: Student assumes pivot prone position with arms overhead, slightly abducted, and elbows slightly flexed. Legs should be straight together, fully extended. Have child lift head, arms, and legs off the floor ("Superman" position).

Score: Duration	Quality
3 = Holds 20+ seconds with moderate effort.	3 = Lifts four extremities simultaneously.
2 = Holds 10 to 19 seconds with great exertion.	2 = Lifts arms, then legs, or reverse.
1 = Holds less than 10 seconds.	1 = Lifts one part at a time.
0 = Unable to hold.	0 = Unable to assume position.

   Comments: _____

9. Schilder's Arm Extension Test (AET)
   Part I: Student stands with feet together, arms stretched forward, fingers abducted, and eyes closed. Student counts aloud to 20.
   Check: _____ Able to maintain posture with ease.
           _____ Able to maintain posture but with effort.
           _____ Postural change in arms during count (describe).
                   _____
           _____ Difficulty with assuming posture (describe).
                   _____
           _____ Unable to assume posture.
           _____ Spooning of hands, hyperextension of elbows.
   Comments: _____

   Part II: Student assumes same position, without counting. Examiner turns student's head from side to side.
   Check: _____ Minimal or no rotation of shoulder following head.
           _____ Rotation of shoulder.
           _____ Rotation of shoulder and hips.
           _____ Equilibrium is disturbed.
           _____ Extreme exaggeration of asymmetrical tonic neck reflex attitude.
           _____ Resistance to head movement.
           _____ Facial or verbal manifestations of discomfort.
   Comments: _____

Score: Arm position change:	Equilibrium:
3 = Normal	3 = Normal
2 = Slight Change	2 = Slight loss
1 = Marked change	1 = Marked loss
Head resistance:	Emotional response:
3 = Normal	3 = Stable
2 = Slight resistance	2 = Slight discomfort
1 = Marked resistance	1 = Marked discomfort
Arm raised: R _____ L _____	Elbow hyperextension: R _____ L _____

   Comments _____

Figure 10-11 cont'd.   Southern California Sensory Integration tests: clinical observations

---

10. Choreoathetoid movements: Observe movements of hands during pivot prone and Schilder's AET.
    - 3 = No movements
    - 2 = Slight jerking
    - 1 = Marked response
    - Comments: _____

11. Asymmetrical tonic neck reflex (ATNR): Student asssumes quadruped position, then places right hand on right hip and lifts left leg. Examiner turns student's chin to right shoulder. Reverse position for left side.

    Score: Right ATNR: Left ATNR
    - 4 = Assumes and holds for 10 seconds   4
    - 3 = Slight wobbling but holds 10 seconds   3
    - 2 = Difficulty assuming, holds less than 10 seconds.   2
    - 1 = Needs assistance to assume, cannot maintain   1
    - 0 = Unable to assume posture with assistance   0
    - Comments: _____

12. Space visualization contralateral use score (SVCU):
    FORMULA: SVCU = $30 - I/C$, drop fraction
    Score: 3 = Score of 28 is normal.
    - 2 = Score of 29 indicates use of one side only; questionable deficit on opposite side.
    - 1 = Score of 27 or less suggests lack of adequate dominance for skilled motor tasks.
    - Comments: _____

13. Postrotatory nystagmus test: Spin child 10 times in each direction, 2 seconds per revolution. Have child look up at ceiling at end of each spin. Estimate amount of excursion and duration. Repeat in other direction.
    Score: R _____ mm _____ _____ seconds
    L _____ mm _____ _____ seconds
    - Comments: _____

Adapted from Ayres AJ: Sensory integration and learning disorders, Los Angeles, 1972, Western Psychological Services; and Ayres AJ: Interpreting the Southern California Sensory Integration Tests, Los Angeles, 1976, Western Psychological Services; and Adams S, 1976.

Figure 10-12   Norton's basic motor evaluation

ASSESSMENT CHART: MINIMAL CEREBRAL DYSFUNCTION
Movement and posture with inborn reactions

Name _____ Bd. _____ Patient's clinic _____

0—Cannot assume test posture even after demonstration.
1—Can assume an approximate test posture after demonstration.
2—Can assume test posture in an awkward manner on command.
3—Can assume and sustain test posture in a near normal manner on command (note abnormal details).
4—Normal.

Examiner:

D.A.	Test movements and postures	

Supine
6-7 mo.
	1. Rolls completely over:
	  a. to right.
	  b. to left.
		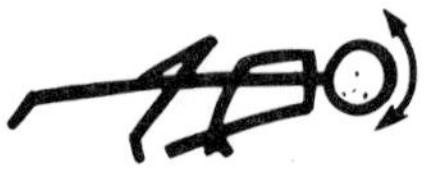

4-10 mo.	2. Pulls hips and knees to chest fully flexed, arms crossed, palms on shoulders, fingers extended.	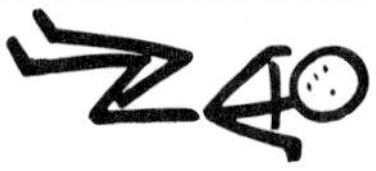

4 mo.	3. With hips, knees fully flexed:
	  a. Extend right leg.
	  b. Extend left leg.
		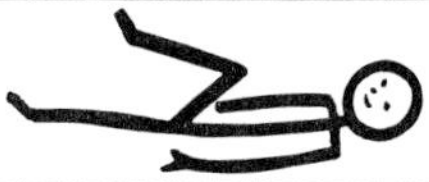

5-7 mo.	4. Head in midline, arms at side, raise head:
	  a. Influence on arms.
	  b. Influence on legs.
		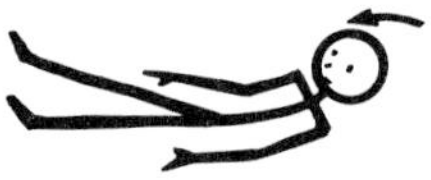

36-60 mo. (3-5 yr.)	5. Pulls up to sit, support on forearms, then by extending elbows.	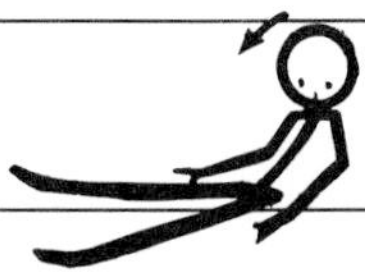

Prone
 	
4-6 mo.
+24 mo.
	6. Extends arms beside head, legs abducted.
	  a. Raises head in midline.
	  b. Supinates forearms (palms toward ceiling).	

+24 mo.	7. Brings arms down beside body, extends arms, palms down.	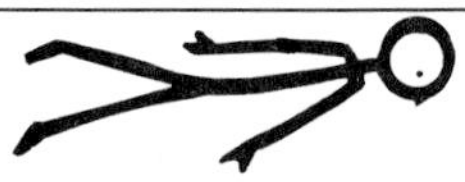
3-6 mo. +36 mo.	8. a. Flex right knee, hips extend. b. Flex left knee, hips extend.	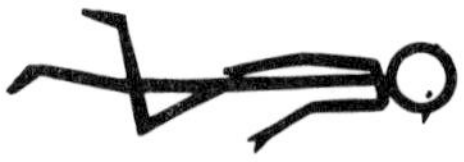
3 mo.	9. a. Support trunk on forearms, upper trunk extended, face vertical. b. Flex knees.	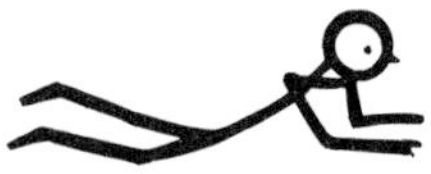

5 mo.
 	
8 mo.
 	
6 mo.
	10. a. Supports trunk on hands with elbows and hips extended, face vertical.
	   b. Flexes neck.
	   c. Extends neck.
	   d. Balance.
		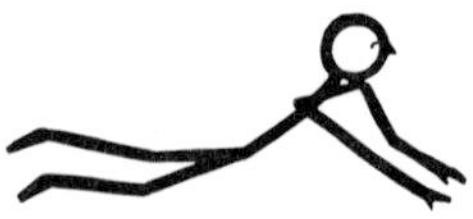

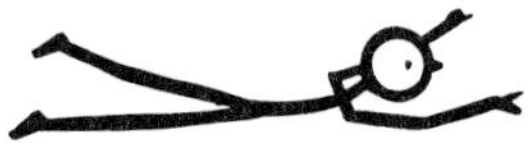

From The American Occupational Therapy Association, Inc, Copyright 1972, vol 26, No 4, p 193, *Minimal Cerebral Dysfunction,* Y Norton.

Figure 10-12 cont'd.   Norton's basic motor evaluation

+ − = Present or absent inborn reactions.
I.R. = Inborn reactions.
* = Equilibrium reactions = learned reactions.
M.&P. = Movements and Posture.
( ) = Retarding influences.
S.T.N.R. = Symmetrical Tonic Neck Reflex.
D.A. = Age that normal responses, movement behavior develop in these positions due to presence or absence of certain basic reflexes and reactions.

Test   **Retest**

Inborn reactions	+	−	Date	Remarks: M.&P.	+	−	Date	Remarks: M.&P.
(Neck righting) Head on body	+	−			+	−		
(Body on body) Body on head			R				R	
Labyrinthine			L				L	
(Tonic neck) Associated reactions (Tonic labyrinthine)								
(Crossed extension) (Tonic labyrinthine)			R				R	
(Tonic Neck)			L				L	
(Tonic) labyrinthine Associated reactions + S.T.N.R.			a				a	
			b				b	
(Tonic) labyrinthine Head on body								
Head on body (Tonic) labyrinthine Landau on floor			a				a	
(Tonic neck)			b				b	
(Neck righting) (Tonic neck) (Tonic labyrinthine)								
(Amphibian)			R				R	
			L				L	
Labyrinthine Optical righting			a				a	
Body on head			b				b	
Labyrinthine Optical			a				a	
(S.T.N.R.)			b				b	
Equilibrium			c				c	
			d				d	

Continued.

Figure 10-12 cont'd.   Norton's basic motor evaluation

Examiner:

D. A.	Test movements and postures	

8 mo.
+9-11 mo.
	11. Moves from prone to sit.
	  a. All fours pushing back.
	  b. Transitional between quadrupedal and adult method:
	    (1) side sit right.
	    (2) side sit left.	

Sitting erect
 	
8 mo.
10 mo.
 	
10 mo.
	12. Sits with soles of feet together, hips flexed and externally rotated to at least 45°.
	  a. Round sit.
	  b. Push laterally: (1) right.
	                    (2) left.
	  c. Balance-extended, flex legs.	

8 mo.
10 mo.
10 mo.
	13. Extends knees, abducts legs: push forward, backward.
	  a. Hips 60°-70°.
	  b. Hips 90°-100°.
	  c. Hips 110°-120°.	

+15 mo.	14. Hangs legs over edge of platform.
	  a. Extends right knee.
	  b. Extends left knee.	

Kneeling and crawling
7 mo.
 	
8 mo.
	15. Gets into four point kneel and rocks (back straight).
	  a. Weight on knees.
	  b. Weight on hands.
	    (1) Neck extended.
	    (2) Neck flexed.
	  c. Crawl.	

9 mo.
36 mo.
	16. Moves to kneel stand, head in mid-position, arms at side. Hips fully extended.
	  a. Push: (1) Forward.
	           (2) Backward.	

10 mo.	17. Moves to half kneel:
	  a. Weight on right knee.
	  b. Weight on left knee.	

Squat 21 mo.	18. Squats heels down, toes not clawed, knees pointing in same direction as toes, hips fully flexed, head in line with trunk. Arms forward.	
Standing and components of walking +15 mo.	19. Stands up. Correct alignment. Feet separated 6″.	

36 mo.	20. Bear weight on one leg.
	  a. Shift weight over right leg: _____ secs.
	  b. Shift weight over left leg: _____ secs.	

+24 mo.
 	
36 mo.
	21. Walks—Adult method.
	  a. Forward.
	  b. Backward.
	  c. Stairs: alternates feet.
	    (1) Up.
	    (2) Down.	

Continued.

Figure 10-12 cont'd. Norton's basic motor evaluation

Test				Retest			
Inborn reactions			Date	Remarks: M.&P.	I.R.	Date	Remarks: M.&P.
Labyrinthine Optical Head on body Body on head (Amphibian) Equilibrium			a			a	
			R			R	
			L			L	
Labyrinthine Optical Protective extension of arms Equilibrium			a			a	
			R			R	
			L			L	
			c			c	
Labyrinthine Optical Protective extension of arms Equilibrium			a			a	
			b			b	
			c			c	
Labyrinthine (Adductor reflex)			R			R	
			L			L	
Labyrinthine Optical (S.T.N.R.) (Asymmetrical T.N.R.) Equilibrium			Rock			Rock	
			Knees			Knees	
			(1) (2)			(1) (2)	
			Crawl			Crawl	
Labyrinthine Optical Protective extension of arms Equilibrium			F			F	
			B			B	
Labyrinthine Optical Equilibrium			R			R	
			L			L	
Labyrinthine Equilibrium							
Labyrinthine Optical Equilibrium							
Labyrinthine Optical Equilibrium			R			R	
			L			L	
Positive Negative Support Equilibrium			a			a	
			b			b	
			c (1) (2)			c (1) (2)	

Continued.

Figure 10-12 cont'd. Norton's basic motor evaluation

HEAD IN MIDLINE FOR POSITIONS

Tests: supine

Test 1

Purpose: To test the level of and ability to roll completely over in both directions.

Instructions: "Roll to your tummy and keep rolling to your back again. Now do it on the other side . . . Lie on your back."

Note: Stiffness. Lack of trunk-pelvis separation (body on body righting). Hyperextended neck in backward roll. Rolls at angle. Normal: Head, hip, top knee slightly flexed in turning over to side.

Test 2 (From position of Test 1)

Purpose: To test for freedom from hypertonicity and lack of associated movement in the supine position.

Instructions: "Pull your knees close up to your chest. Bend your elbows and cross your arms. Put your hands on your shoulders. Raise up your elbows . . . Rest your arms."

Note: Fingers claw. Downward pull of scapular depressors preventing elbows from remaining away from the body. (Children with this difficulty seem to have trouble with writing.) Feet neither inverted nor dorsiflexed.

Test 3 (From position of Test 2)

Purpose: To test for lower extremity differentiation or identify hypertonicity preventing that differentiation.

Instructions: "Put your arms beside your body. Straighten that leg (right). Bend that same knee (right) and straighten the other leg (left) . . . Relax!"

Note: Internal rotation of either leg. Adduction of either thigh. Feet inverted, plantar flexed. Extension of opposite leg when one extends. Back arched. Body asymmetry.

Test 4 (From position of Test 3)

Purpose: To test ability to raise head from the supporting surface and not affect the extremities.

Instructions: "Raise just your head. Put it back down . . . Now relax."

Note: Inability of head to differentiate from the rest of body. Symmetrical tonic neck reflex causing arms to flex and tone to increase in the legs. Feet inverted.

Test 5 (From position of Test 4)

Purpose: To test the ability and method of getting from supine to sit.

Instructions: "Sit up, please . . . Now lie down."

Note: Adult method, 5-year level: symmetry of movement, head forward, bilateral elbow flexion to extension, hips flexing; versus pathology of hypertonicity in back and lower extremities preventing hip flexion as back raises off support. Transitional method: +10-month level: from prone to side sit. Infant method, 8-month level: from quadripedal position to sit. (See illustration: Test 2)

Tests: prone

Test 6

Purpose: To test freedom from hypertonicity in prone.

Instructions: "Get onto your tummy. Straighten your arms beside your head. Raise it. Turn the palms of your hands toward the ceiling. Straighten your fingers . . . Put your head down."

Note: Shoulders and hips: tightness in upper or lower extremities. Inversion of feet. Inability to supinate (after +24 months). Inability to straighten fingers (asymmetry). Hypertonic upper extremity and trunk flexors, adductors, of upper extremity and trunk shoulder girdle depressors and pronators affect ability to do cursive writing. Heavy head: tonic labyrinthine abnormality. Lower extremity tightness can affect the degree of upper extremity freedom of movement.

Test 7 (From position of Test 6)

Purpose: To further test freedom of shoulders and arms from flexor hypertonus in prone.

Instructions: "Bring your arms down straight beside your body. Put the palms of your hands on the mat . . . Now relax."

Note: Freedom of head movement. Influence of head position on tone of extremities (asymmetrical tonic neck reflex), affecting ability in fine skill and possibly figure-ground. Balance, during movement and upright positions. Feet adducted, inverted.

Test 8 (From position of Test 7)

Purpose: To test selective control of hips and knees.

Instructions: "Bend your right knee. Put it down and bend your left knee . . . Now relax."

Note: 90-degree knee flexion with completely extended hips sometime after 36 months. Record hip raising, toppling of leg in inward or outward direction, foot inversion. Tightness at hips and knees affecting balance during movement and in upright positions. Amphibian reactions of forward flexion may be a retarding influence for hip extension, but a precursor for crawl.

Test 9 (From position of Test 8)

Purpose: To test postural control in spinal extension; and with knee flexion.

Instruction: "Pull up onto your elbows. Bend both knees . . . Now straighten your knees."

Note: Inability to place arms at a 90-degree flexion, with slight abduction, forearms straight, hands opened: hypertonicity of adductors, flexors of arms, forearms, and fingers. Toppling to either side. Hip flexion when knees flex. The control in this position is basic to crawl and the beginning use of hands with balance.

Test 10 (From position of Test 9)

Purpose: To test the ability to support weight on extended arms, regardless of the position of the head.

Instructions: "Straighten your elbows. Put your weight on your opened hands. Now bend your neck. Raise your head, (push laterally for balance) . . . Now get onto your tummy."

Note: Inability to carry weight on extended elbows, finger extending with neck flexion, or to bend elbows with neck extension. Leg thrust with neck flexion, (due to symmetrical tonic neck reflex). Hip internal rotation and foot inversion. Lack of equilibrium reactions.

Test 11 (From position of Test 10)

Purpose: To test the ability and method of getting from prone to sit.

Instructions: "Sit up, please . . . Now bring your legs in front."

Note: Symmetry in getting up if the infant method in the quadrupedal position is used. The preferred side that the child turns toward if the transitional method is chosen, or whether the child pushes up to his knees, sits, swings his legs over and forward. (See illustration Test 5).

Figure 10-12 cont'd.   Norton's basic motor evaluation

Tests: sitting erect

Test 12 (From position of Test 11)

Purpose: To test the ability to round sit and the development of lateral protective extension, balance reactions.

Instructions: "Sit up tall. Put the soles of your feet together. Relax your arms (push the child gently and laterally at each shoulder to observe balance and protective extension of the supporting arm with abduction of the opposite arm, and balance reactions as the therapist alternately flexes and extends the legs) . . . Now put your legs out straight."

Note: Inability to balance. The presence or absence of protective extension of arms and the side of the absence. Straight (normal) back versus the need for head forward flexion compensation to prevent backward tipping. Lack of adequate hip flexion and external rotation of the legs.

Test 13 (From position of Test 12)

Purpose: To test balance reactions, protective extension of the arms in long sit.

Instructions: "Separate your legs. Sit up tall and let your arms go limp (push child forward then backward) . . . Now sit at the edge of the platform."

Note: Inability to balance or lack of protective extension of the limbs (elbows extended) when pushed forward, backward. Inadequate amount of hip flexion in forward, straight position. Internal rotation of thighs, foot inversion.

Test 14 (From position of Test 13)

Purpose: To test the ability to extend one leg without associated reactions in the other.

Instructions: "Sit up tall. Raise that (right) leg and straighten your knee. Relax, raise and straighten the other (left) knee. Rest . . . Now get onto your hands and knees."

Note: Any adduction or internal rotation of the other leg when either [first] leg extends. Foot inversions.

Tests: kneeling and crawling

Test 15 (From position of Test 14)

Purpose: To test weight bearing, balance and control in four-point position on open hands, regardless of the position of the head.

Instructions: "Rock backwards. Rock forwards (3 ×). Raise your head. Lower your head. Crawl. . . Now raise up onto your knees."

Note: Lordosis, flexion of elbows when the neck flexes with thrust of lower extremities (symmetrical tonic neck reflex); extension of the elbows only if the neck extends (symmetrical tonic neck reflex); extension of one arm only when the head turns toward that arm (asymmetrical tonic neck reflex); raising of knees off the supporting surface in moving onto extended elbows (symmetrical tonic neck reflex); inversion of feet and asymmetry in crawling.

Test 16 (From position on Test 15)

Purpose: To test for anterior-posterior control of pelvis, trunk and thighs during movement.

Instructions: "Straighten your trunk and hips (push forward, backwards) . . . Remain in that position."

Note: Inability to regain balance without difficulty from forward, backward push. Lack of, or inadequate protective extension of arms. Feet inverted, hips flexed, back lordosed.

Test 17 (From position of Test 16)

Purpose: To test the control of hip rotation, and the effect on the lower extremities; balance.

Instructions: "Raise the left leg, bend the knee, and put your foot down flat. Change legs . . . Squat."

Note: Inadequate flexion of hip, knee, angle of forward leg (more than 90 degrees). Thigh adducted. Balance unstable. Toes constantly clawed. Heel off ground. Lower leg of supporting leg occasionally raised off support, that foot inverted and the hip of the suppporting leg inadequately extended.

Tests: squat

Test 18 (From position of Test 17)

Purpose: To test control of hypertonicity throughout the body.

Instructions: "Squat. Separate your knees. Put your heels down on the floor. Bring your arms forward. Shift weight sideways . . . Now stand up."

Note: Inability to put heels down on the floor. Constant clawing of toes. Tendency to topple backwards, or sideways in movement. Pain behind the knees or in the buttocks or calf of the leg.

Tests: standing, components of walking

Test 19 (From position of Test 18)

Purpose: To test for normal distribution of tone in standing.

Instructions: "Stand up tall. Separate your feet so far (about 6″) . . . Remain in that position."

Note: Inability to extend hips adequately. Excessive lordosis, geno recurvatum. Unequal weight distribution: shoulders of unequal height, spine curved laterally, feet inverted. Balance tenuous.

Test 20 (From position of Test 19)

Purpose: To test the time ability (in seconds) to support the body over one leg.

Instructions: "Shift your weight onto the (right) leg and hold it as long as you can. Do it on the other leg . . . Now stand on both legs."

Note: Time (recorded) in seconds that steady balance can be maintained on either leg. Flexed leg has inadequate hip extension; thigh is internally rotated and adducted; foot inverted. Difficulty in weight shift.

Test 21 (From position of Test 20)

Purpose: To test heel strike and dorsiflexion in forward movement; adult approach: hip extension in backward walk; freedom of upper extremity in stair climb.

Instructions: "Walk forward to that . . . and stop. Walk backwards to me and stop . . . Climb those stairs."

Note: Internal rotation of the thigh, hip-knee flexion, foot inversion; a lack of reciprocal arm movement with rigid spine. Forward walk: alignment of hips, knees, ankles. Dorsiflexion of forward foot on heel strike. Rear leg outwardly rotated at hip; roll off from head of first metatarsal. Slight rotation of trunk. Arms swing freely and alternate with leg movements (right arm with left leg in normal postural control). Backward walk: alignment of hip, knee, ankle or forward leg. Back leg extended, outwardly rotated at hip. Hip extended, knee flexes so that back foot touches first metatarsal, leg somewhat laterally for support. Feet *not* inverted in normal postural control. Climb stairs (without bannister): alternate flexed hip, knee, ankle dorsiflexion. Weight firmly on lower stair. Pulls up onto forward extending leg. Back leg flexed at knee, hip extended, and thigh abducted. Standing leg: leg, foot aligned, arms free in normal postural control. *Not* internally rotated thigh, adducted forward leg, nor inverted feet. (For children of at least 4 years of age.)

11

Instruments to evaluate childhood performance skills

PAT NUSE PRATT
ANNE STEVENS ALLEN
IDA LOU COLEY
LINDA C. STEPHENS
KAREN E. SCHANZENBACHER
RICARDO C. CARRASCO

COMPREHENSIVE DEVELOPMENTAL SCALES
Scope of developmental evaluation

One of the basic components of any occupational therapy assessment for children is a developmental evaluation (Chapter 7). The most common practices are to use standardized tests or criterion-referenced, therapist-made tests that contain items drawn from a variety of standardized tests and from resources in the literature.

Developmental testing is usually thought to measure such early adaptive skills as controlling the head, building block towers, and recognizing pictures. In fact, developmental testing may be more broadly conceptualized as the evaluation of child and adolescent performance in any age-appropriate activity. Therefore a test could, and should, include such items as ordering a hamburger, making one's own bed, getting from class to class, and handing homework in on time. With this concept in mind, the occupational therapist may consider evaluations of schoolwork, prevocational preparation, self-care, and community living activities as logical extensions of the developmental assessment. For purposes of organization, this chapter will separate different types of evaluation. But the continuity between categories of performance evaluation cannot be overemphasized.

Brazelton neonatal behavioral assessment scale (BNBAS)

The Brazelton Neonatal Behavioral Assessment Scale is included here because it most closely approximates a developmental evaluation of the neonate.[8] This test is one of the most commonly used measures of the newborn's socially interactive responses. The scale is designed to look at both the neurological and interactive functions of an infant during the first month of life.

To measure neurological function, the test includes 20 items that evaluate reflexes and other relevant responses:

Plantar grasp	Automatic walking	Tonic deviation of head	Rooting
Hand grasp	Placing	Tonic deviation of eyes	Sucking
Ankle clonus	Incurvation	Nystagmus	Passive movement of arms
Babinski reflex	Crawling	Tonic neck reflex	Passive movement of legs
Standing	Glabella	Moro reflex	

This portion of the scale is as successful for identification of neurological problems in the newborn as a pediatric neurological examination.[41]

The scale also includes 27 items that were designed to measure the neonate's capacity for interaction with the environment and caregivers:

Response decrements to light, rattle, bell, and pinprick.
Orientation: Inanimate visual, inanimate auditory, animate visual, animate auditory, animate visual and auditory.

Alertness	Irritability
General tonus	Activity
Motor maturity	Tremulousness

Pull-to-sit	Startle
Cuddliness	Lability of skin color
Defensive movements	Lability of states
Consolability	Self-quieting activity
Peak of excitement	Hand-mouth facility
Rapidity of build-up	Smiling

These items have been especially useful for demonstrating neonatal behavioral capabilities to parents.[43] When parents understand what their babies are capable of doing through demonstration of the item skills, parental interaction skills may improve.[45] Parental expectations may also increase, a phenomenon that over the long-term can foster the baby's development.[36]

Clinically, the interactions portion of the scale has been used to monitor behaviors between mother and child if either demonstrated early inappropriate skills. Another use that has been explored is the capability of the scale to identify long-range infant temperament and interactive problems. While some preliminary studies have demonstrated potential value in this application, the results are not conclusive.[44]

In summary, Brazelton Neonatal Behavioral Assessment Scale has proved to be an effective predictor of neurological problems, a teaching tool for parents, and an indicator of interactional skills present in the neonate. The scale has also been used extensively in research.

Bayley scales of infant development (BSID)

The Bayley Scales of Infant Development were developed as part of a large-scale longitudinal study of human development carried out by Bayley and associates at the University of California at Berkeley.[39] The scales[5] use typical developmental items to assess mental, motor, and behavior levels of infants and toddlers aged 2 to 30 months. This test battery is an excellent, comprehensive, and well-standardized instrument that requires some advance preparation by the therapist before clinical administration. As with most standardized tests, it tends to be most reliable for the middle of the age range represented. The test uses both performance and parental reports to obtain data and may take several hours to complete. (Any of the three different sections may be used by itself but with a substantial loss of information.) Therefore it is more appropriate to administer the scales to young children through several sessions. A complete test kit of materials and manual are commercially available. Review of the items found for this age range on the Denver Developmental Screening Test form (Chapter 9, Figure 9-10) should give a picture of the types of skills measured by the Bayley tests.

Gesell developmental scales

The Gesell Developmental Scales were developed by Arnold Gesell and his associates at the Yale University Institute for Child Study, beginning in the 1930s. The test items and procedures have been modified and updated through the years.[27] It is helpful to review some of Gesell's concepts (Chapter 3) in preparation for administration of the scales. Several forms are available according to the age level of children from early infancy through 10 years of age.

The test measures performance according to Gesell's behavior patterns: motor, adaptive, language, and personal-social. It also provides developmental levels by months for each of the areas tested. The test has been widely used for diagnostic purposes and is often given by pediatricians as a follow-up to developmental delays identified by the Denver Developmental Screening Test. The kit for this test is commercially available.

Interrater reliability and predictive validity for the Gesell scales are generally excellent. Normative samples for the early schedules (ages birth to 36 months) were large, but there is less information available about parts of the schedules that are used with older children. The user should remember that the tests should be used primarily to determine satisfactory or delayed development of neuromotor and cognitive skills.[27]

Vineland adaptive behavior scales

For many years, the Vineland Social Maturity Scale[14] was the only durable standardized instrument that attempted to measure development from infancy through adolescence. The test was developed by Edgar Doll and colleagues at the Vineland Training Center in New Jersey during the 1920s. However, over the years many of the test items lost their timeliness as a result of cultural changes, and the subjectivity of scoring was questioned.

In response to these problems, Sparrow, Balla, and Cicchetti[38] collaborated to revise the Vineland Social Maturity Scale. The revised edition, called the Vineland Adaptive Behavior Scales, was published in 1987 in three versions: the interview edition—survey form, the interview edition—expanded form, and the classroom edition. The three versions may be used independently or together to measure adaptive behaviors in the four domains of communication, daily living skills, socialization, and motor skills. Each domain also has subdomains. An adaptive behavior composite is the yield of performance in the four domains together. A maladaptive behavior domain is included in the survey and expanded forms as well.

The survey form is most similar to the original Vineland; it is administered to parents or caretakers of individuals aged birth to 18 years, 11 months and low-functioning adults. Information is obtained by interview and provides a general assessment of strengths and weaknesses. The expanded form is also administered to parents and caretakers of the same populations, but provides a more comprehensive and precise assessment and a systematic basis for planning intervention. The classroom edition was developed for children aged 3 years to 12 years, 11 months. It is a questionnaire form that is completed by classroom teachers.

The normative population for the two interview forms comprised a national sample of 3,000 persons who represented the 1980 U.S. census statistics according to variables of sex, race, ethnic group, community size, region of the country, and parents' education levels. In addition, 3,000 students were used to provide the normative data for the classroom edition.[38]

AAMR adaptive behavior scales (ABS)

The AAMR Adaptive Behavior Scales[1,2] also provide comprehensive measures of behavior from infancy through adulthood, although the tests are of more recent origin. These scales are descriptive and provide numerical ratings that may be used to chart progress. Age equivalents for behaviors are not provided. The AAMR Adaptive Behavior Scales are available in two versions. The original test, the AAMR Adaptive Behavior Scales[1] was developed for use in institutional settings and day programs for mentally retarded individuals, and therefore, has a wide age range of behaviors. The public school version, the AAMR Adaptive Behavior Scales—Public School Version,[2] was developed later and measures a narrower age range of behaviors. Both scales are used to record adaptive and maladaptive behaviors.

Both tests have two parts. The first part measures adaptive behavior in the areas of independent functioning, physical development, economic activity, language development, domestic activity, vocational activity, self-direction, responsibility, and socialization. Items are broad and generally do not give the discrete, detailed information about components of activity performance usually preferred by occupational therapists. The second part of the tests identifies an exhaustive array of maladaptive behaviors against which the individual's actual behaviors are compared according to duration, severity, and frequency.

The record review, data-based observation, and informant review are used to obtain information. In general, reports of behaviors must be corroborated by more than one informant for documentation purposes. The AAMR Adaptive Behavior Scales contain many items and can consume a considerable amount of time to complete at the initial assessment. Space is provided in both versions of the protocol booklet for updated assessments (usually conducted annually). In most mental retardation programs the primary recorder for the test is a psychologist or behavior specialist who obtains data from parents and other members of the team who work with the child. Consideration regarding application of findings is generally determined by the entire interdisciplinary team rather than by one individual. Because of the format of the items, behavioral objectives for program plans are easily generated.

Because of length and complexity of requirements regarding documentation of behaviors, these tests are not efficient instruments for use by the occupational therapist who works alone. Typically the therapist will use these tests only when working at a facility that has adopted them as its primary assessment instrument.

Early intervention developmental profile (EIDP)

Under the direction of Schafer and Moersch, an interdisciplinary team at the University of Michigan university affiliated facility spent a number of years developing a comprehensive assessment and practice system for newborn to 3-year-old children. The developmental items for evaluation and early intervention broadly reflect the concerns of occupational, physical, and speech therapists, and psychologists. The Early Intervention Developmental Profile is that part of *Developmental Programming for Infants and Young Children*[35] used to assess skill development over the course of time. The profile is designed to be administered by an interdisciplinary team.

The profile is divided into six sections: perceptual-fine motor, cognition, language, social-emotional, self-care, and gross motor development. The occupational therapist administers the perceptual-fine motor and self-care items. In addition, the therapist may assist with evaluation on the gross motor and cognitive sections. A speech therapist might be best to administer the language items, a physical therapist administers the gross motor section, and a psychologist usually has primary responsibility for the cognitive assessment.

Administration of test items is thoroughly explained in the evaluation manual. References for each item are well documented. Test items are administered to the child until he fails two consecutive items in each major portion of the profile. Basal and ceiling levels of performance determine the range of the child's transitional development at the time of the test. The total time required for test administration may vary from half an hour to several hours. No cumulative score is obtained. Age levels for each performance area are charted on a composite table to yield a profile. Each protocol booklet can be used for several subsequent evaluations, with the composite profile recorded with a different color or line notation each time to document progress.

The Early Intervention Developmental Profile was designed specifically to guide program planning. It is not to be used for diagnostic purposes. Nicely tied into the behavioral items on the profile is a series of intervention activities that can be used to help children achieve skilled performance in subsequent developmental tasks.

Interrater and test-retest reliability studies of the profile used small samples, but with generally excellent results. Significant correlations were found between children's scores on the Early Intervention Developmental Profile, the Bayley Scales of Infant Development, and the Vineland Social Maturity Scale, indicating strong content validity. The sample was small and the test was performed with a clinical population, so findings should be viewed accordingly. The Early Intervention Developmental Profile is best used as a clinical instrument for interdisciplinary team planning. The varied expertise of the team lends itself to more knowledgeable interpretation and application of test findings.[35] This critique of the EIDP is supported by a later analysis of the test, reported by Lydic and Wallace.[30]

Vulpe assessment battery

The Vulpe Assessment Battery was developed by Vulpe[42] under a grant from the Canadian National Institute of Mental Retardation. This test battery is a long and detailed assessment of children's competencies and developmental skills. The battery is used to assess performance in the following areas: basic senses and functions, gross motor behaviors, fine motor behaviors, language behaviors, cognitive processes and specific concepts, organizational behaviors, and activities of daily living. A final component of the battery is assessment of the child's environments. Skills are cross-referenced from one area to another.

Because of its length, administration of the Vulpe Assessment Battery on initial assessment can be time-consuming. However, reevaluation proceeds from the cut-off point fairly quickly, and therefore many therapists believe this justifies the time spent earlier. It may be helpful to administer the test in partnership with another therapist to alternate observation, item presentation, and recording duties. It becomes apparent that as our knowledge of child development and function increases, so does the complexity and length of developmental evaluations. Most comprehensive developmental scales are now best administered cooperatively with one or more professionals to support documentation, to provide expertise in the broad range of areas assessed, and to share the physical and time demands of test administration.

Like many other developmental assessments, the Vulpe Assessment Battery is not considered a true standardized test. Items have been carefully selected and are based on validation through the literature and clinical experience. Interrater reliability for the test is strong, probably because administrative procedures are explained in considerable detail. This latter characteristic of the battery makes it a useful tool for the development of program activities.[42] A comprehensive revision of the Vulpe Assessment is in process; publication is anticipated within 2 years.

Brigance diagnostic inventories

The Brigance Diagnostic Inventories use two elaborate test batteries to assess the functional and academic skill development of children aged newborn through 11 years. The Brigance Diagnostic Inventory of Early Development (IED)[10] is designed for children to 7 years of age and measures psychomotor skills, self-help skills, communication, general knowledge and comprehension, reading skills, printing skills, and math skills. The Brigance Diagnostic Inventory of Basic Skills[9] is administered to elementary school children to evaluate skill development in academic areas. The latter would be less useful to occupational therapists but may be encountered in practice in school systems.

The Brigance Diagnostic IED has been adopted in many education-oriented early intervention programs. Test items are written in behavioral terms and are designed to tie in to programming. Brigance stated that all test items are "norm referenced" for expected age level through extensive review of the literature. Different items are administered through parental report, observation of spontaneous behavior, and specific performance. The packaging of the Brigance test is impressive, and its detail leaves little room for erroneous administration. Experimental editions of the tests were field tested at numerous facilities across the United States, with subsequent refinement of items. Because of its clear detail, including illustrations of appropriate patterns and self-contained instructions in the scoring records, the test is easy, although time-consuming, to administer.[10]

Battelle developmental inventory

The Battelle Developmental Inventory (BDI) is a standardized assessment instrument that was designed for children from birth to 8 years. It consists of 341 significant developmental skills in five domains: personal-social, adaptive, motor, communication, and cognitive. The test battery also includes a screening test that can be administered in 30 minutes or less. The screening and inventory can be administered through presentation of structured items, interview with parents or caregivers, or observation of the child in a natural setting. Some modifications are provided for handicapped children.[4]

The BDI was developed by the Columbus Laboratories of Battelle Memorial Institute to evaluate the effectiveness of the Handicapped Children's Early Education Program under the United States Bureau of Education for the Handicapped. Thousands of items from other developmental tests were collected and analyzed. The final pilot test was administered to a sample of over 500 children. This sample was selected to represent typical demographic characteristics of the total U.S. population. After further refinement, the test was published in 1984. A number of reliability and validity tests have been conducted. Guidubaldi and Perry[20] found a consistent pattern of relationships between the different domains of the BDI and other tests that propose to measure similar developmental functions. It was also found that the BDI was more accurate in predicting first grade achievement than other established test instruments. For this reason, the test is highly regarded and is required for assessment of children who received services funded through the Handicapped Children's Early Education Program.

Hawaii early learning profile

The Hawaii Early Learning Profile (HELP) is a criterion-referenced assessment that measures 685 developmental skills that occur between birth and 3 years of age. Six major areas of function are measured: cognitive, language, gross motor, fine motor, self-help, and social-emotional. The protocol sheets are designed with horizontal bars to illustrate the age range for acquisition of each skill. Primitive or pathologic skills that normally disappear or should not be learned during a child's development are clearly indicated. Examples of these type of items are "rakes tiny objects" and "may refuse foods."[18]

This comprehensive assessment system was designed to monitor the child's ongoing development. The HELP was developed by an interdisciplinary team in the mid-1970s as part of a demonstration project with handicapped infants at the University of Hawaii; it was funded by the U.S. Bureau of Education of the Handicapped.[19] The HELP represents a compilation and synthesis of information from various growth and development scales, standardized tests, research, and project data. An activity guide[19] not only gives directions for testing each skill, but also provides program strategies to develop the skill, with special attention to the older delayed child. Recently an additional checklist was developed for children aged 3 to 6 years. Additional coordinated curricula and home program resources that enhance the usefulness of test findings are available from the publisher.

The test is easily administered with commonly used toys and materials. The horizontal graph format that shows results of testing is easy for parents and non-professionals to understand; it facilitates discussion of a child's delays, especially when gaps or splinter skills occur. However, for reporting purposes, the test sometimes makes it difficult to specify exact levels of function or to document changes because skill acquisition ranges may span several months. For example, "imitates vertical stroke" may occur between 18 to 24 months of age.[18] Therefore, the HELP is most appropriate when used in conjunction with comprehensive clinical and home programming and less useful when only diagnostic assessment is required.

Peabody developmental scales

The Peabody Developmental Motor Scales (PDMS), developed by Folio and Fewell,[17] is a standardized developmental test that measures gross and fine motor skills of children aged birth to 83 months. PDMS items are both norm- and criterion-referenced. The scales are useful for therapeutic and educational programming.

Test results identify levels of achieved, absent, and emerging skills, and pinpoint delayed or aberrant skills in comparison to a normative sample.

The gross motor section of the scale contains 170 items divided into 17 age levels, with 10 items at each level. The fine motor portion includes 112 items divided into 16 age levels, with 6 to 8 items for each age. Age-appropriate items from the combined scale can be administered to a child in 45 to 60 minutes. Raw scores are converted to percentiles, standard and scaled scores, and age equivalents. Although the test was designed for individual administration, the manual includes special instructions for group administration in a station-testing format. In addition, the manual provides special techniques for test administration with handicapped children.

The test kit includes most materials for the fine motor items. Other required materials are commonly available in pediatric settings. No special qualifications are required for test administrators. However, the authors suggest that the tester should be familiar with administration and scoring procedures of the PDMS and other developmental scales and should practice administering the test to at least three children before clinical use.

The normative sample, taken in 1981 to 1982, included 617 children from 20 states who ranged from birth to 83 months of age. Racial distribution was 85.1% white, 7.3% black, and 7.6% Hispanic. Two measures of reliability were used. Test/retest reliability was measured with 38 children from the normative sample who were retested within 1 week. When the same examiner administered and scored the test, correlations of 0.95 and 0.80 were obtained for the gross and fine motor portions, respectively. Inter-rater reliability correlations of 0.97 and 0.94, respectively, were obtained when one person administered and scored the test and a second person observed and scored the test simultaneously.[34]

The test kit also includes a tab-indexed card file of 170 gross and 112 fine motor activities that are referenced to the PDMS test items. The cards provide an instructional curriculum and planning guide for intervention.

Other developmental evaluations

For every test that has been discussed here, there are a dozen tests available commercially, and many times that number of therapist-made tests. Most tests draw on items and use formats in combinations that are based on or similar to tests described here. It is probably best for therapists to become skilled administrators of two or more standardized commercial tests to become familiar with typical and useful test items and response variance. However, with experience, the therapist may wish to develop a personalized series of test items that have proved most useful with a given clinical population and age range. One such format was developed by Carol Leaman to assess preschool and primary elementary school children. Because Leaman had been unable to locate a satisfactory commercial test that included items for this entire age range, she was forced to use two separate standardized assessments. Very often, when testing an older preschool child or a younger primary grade child, she found that items from both tests were needed to accurately assess the developmental level of the individual. Therefore she developed a therapist-made test that spanned the entire age range of her student population, incorporating test items from standardized tests for both age groups. The resultant developmental checklist is shown in Figure 11-1.

EVALUATION OF SPECIFIC PERFORMANCE SKILL CATEGORIES

This section presents measurements of selected tasks of performance in one or more of the occupational activity groups: play, self-maintenance, school-work, and prevocational activities.

Play assessments

Assessment of play and leisure behaviors and skills is a critical component of occupational therapy for children, yet it remains an area with few valid and reliable resources. In an analysis of the literature from 1933 to 1984, Kielhofner and Burris[28] identified and typed nineteen measures for related behaviors. In general, reliability and validity of the identified measures were incomplete. The investigators reported that published instruments could be typed within five categories: developmental assessments of play and leisure, attitude scales related to the meaning and significance of leisure, assessments of play attitudes, measures of play environments, and ethnographic and ecological procedures that yield descriptive data about play and leisure components and hierarchies.

Kielhofner and Burris speculated that the difficulties in developing valid and reliable measures of play are caused by the variable effect of environment on play, the limited boundaries, and subjective and contextual natures of play. The investigators concluded that the assessment of play is in its infancy. They recommended that occupational therapists focus their research efforts on descriptive study of play and employ acceptable scientific test development and evaluation procedures for measures used in such research.

PRESCHOOL PLAY SCALE

The Preschool Play Scale[7] was introduced in Chapter 10 with reference to its usefulness for assessment of psychosocial functions of children in a play situation. The scale is presented here with more detailed discussion, because it serves as a model of an occupational

therapy assessment of this critical area of childhood performance. Furthermore, the scale has been subjected to an increasingly rigorous series of test development and evaluation procedures. In addition to the valuable information it provides about the child's play status, the Preschool Play Scale can be used to identify preferred play experiences for program planning. The scale is shown in Table 11-2 at the end of the chapter and a test analysis is presented in Figure 11-2.

PLAY SKILLS INVENTORY

The Play Skills Inventory is a test battery developed by Hurff[24] at Children's Hospital in Los Angeles. It provides a description of development and play characteristics in four general areas, including sensation, motor function, perception, and intellect. The test has been reported through several sources.[24,25] Materials for the test are not commercially available but may be readily assembled by using instructions from the primary reference.[24] A test analysis is shown in Figure 11-3.

OTHER PLAY ASSESSMENTS

In 1981 Florey[16] published a review of literature related to occupational therapy evaluation of play behaviors and components. She included a table of clinical instruments that had been developed by students of Reilly's occupational behavior theory. Some of these instruments, such as the Preschool Play Scale and Hurff's Play Skills Inventory, have been detailed in these chapters. However, the other instruments discussed by Florey are noteworthy and are included in an adaptation of her table in Table 11-1.

Assessments of self-maintenance skills

Many of the developmental tests described earlier in this chapter provide a good range of self-help and other self-maintenance activities to be assessed by the therapist. However, occupational therapists frequently desire more detailed information about this area of performance than can be obtained from the multicategory tests. In response to this demand, a number of self-care instruments have been developed, although not always subjected to formal test development procedures and publication. Most activities of daily living tests are criterion-referenced and use a graded rating of the individual's ability to perform each task according to the amount of independence demonstrated. For example, a test might use a quasi-ordinal scale and give differential, but arbitrarily defined, points for ability to perform a task (1) without demonstration, (2) after demonstration, (3) with verbal cuing, or (4) with physical assistance. This method is demonstrated by the two self-care assessments shown in Figures 11-4 and 11-6 and discussed here. (Figure 11-6 appears at the end of this chapter).

Figure 11-1 Developmental checklist

Age	Activity	Initial evaluation			Re-evaluation		
		+	+/−	−	+	+/−	−
2.0	Builds tower of 6 to 7 blocks						
2.0	Imitates building a 3-block train						
2.0	Strings 1 to 4 (1 inch) beads						
2.0	Cuts gashes in edge of paper						
2.0	Imitates circular strokes						
2.2	Imitates vertical line within 30 degrees						
2.5	Answers "What do you hear with?"						
2.6	Builds tower of 8 to 9 blocks						
2.6	Adds chimney to train						
2.6	Holds pencil in fingers						
2.6	Makes 2 or more strokes for cross						
2.6	Screws, unscrews top						
2.6	Formboard—3 forms; adapts in 4 trials						
2.6	Gives full name						
2.6	Names 1 to 2 colors						
2.10	Points to teeth and chin on request						
3.0	Builds tower of 9 to 10 blocks						
3.0	Imitates building a 3-block bridge						
3.0	Imitates drawing a horizontal line						
3.0	Imitates drawing a cross crudely						
3.0	Copies a circle						
3.0	Cuts paper in half						
3.0	Puts 10 pellets into bottle in 30 seconds						
3.0	Formboard—3 blocks; no error or correction						
3.0	Names 3 colors						
3.0	Puts together 2 piece puzzle of person						
3.0	Determines size constancy in 3 dimensions						
3.0	Unbuttons medium shirt buttons						
3.6	Copies a 3-block bridge						
3.6	Puts together 3-piece puzzle of person						
3.6	Puts together a 7-piece puzzle						
3.6	Comprehends 3 prepositions (in, on, under)						
3.6	Finds pictures of animals that are alike						
3.8	Points to tongue, neck, arm, knee, thumb						
4.0	Imitates building a 5-cube gate						
4.0	Attempts to cut a straight line						
4.0	Copies a cross						
4.0	Puts 10 pellets into bottle in 25 seconds						
4.0	Puts together a 4-piece puzzle of person						

Reproduced with permission of Carol Leaman, Atlanta, Ga, 1982.

ACTIVITIES OF DAILY LIVING ASSESSMENT: TIME-ORIENTED RECORD

The format for the Activities of Daily Living Assessment: Time-Oriented Record was developed by Coley[11] and associates at the Children's Hospital of Stanford University Medical Center and was reported in 1978. It is a comprehensive assessment of self-maintenance activities organized according to a developmental sequence, and it contains items related to home and hospital living. The test items can be administered and passed during a formal evaluation session or as achievement is observed by the therapist during treatment. Scoring of the test is explained on the forms in Appendix. Again, a quasi-ordinal scale is used. The test record provides the opportunity to differentiate between the child's use of right and left body sides.

Figure 11-1 cont'd. Developmental checklist

Age	Activity	Initial evaluation			Re-evaluation		
		+	+/−	−	+	+/−	−
4.0	Adds 3 parts to incomplete man						
4.0	Determines size constancy in 2 dimensions						
4.0	Knows front and back of clothes						
4.0	Buttons large buttons						
4.2	Imitates square						
4.3	Puts together a 7 piece puzzle in 150 seconds						
4.6	Copies a 5-cube gate						
4.6	Copies a square						
4.6	Prints a few capital letters						
4.6	Counts 4 objects and answers "how many"						
4.6	Knows day and night						
4.6	Knows pictorial likes and differences						
4.6	Knows 4 prepositions						
4.8	Follows 3 commands in proper sequence						
4.8	Puts together a 5-piece puzzle of man						
5.0	Copies a 2-step block						
5.0	Cuts out simple shape with ⅛ inch outline						
5.0	Copies a triangle						
5.0	Prints first name						
5.0	Prints a few numbers						
5.0	Compares textures						
5.0	Buttons medium buttons on shirt						
5.0	Draws house with a door, windows, roof, chimney						
5.4	Judges weights						
5.4	Gives age						
5.6	Prints numbers 1 to 5						
5.6	Knows pictorial likes and differences (9 out of 12)						
5.6	Knows which is bigger, "cat or mouse?"						
5.8	Can form a rectangle of 2 triangular cards						
6.0	Builds 3-step block on demand						
6.0	Copies a diamond						
6.0	Prints most capital letters						
6.0	Prints first and last names						
6.0	Gives name and address						
6.0	Cuts out a simple design						
6.0	Ties shoelaces						
6.0	Buttons small buttons						
6.0	Knows right from left						
6.0	Differentiates morning and afternoon						
6.0	Understands numbers up to 10						

COLERAIN SCHOOL ACTIVITIES OF DAILY LIVING TEST

The Colerain School Activities of Daily Living Test is another useful therapist-made tool and is shown in Figure 11-6 at the end of this chapter. This form is used to assess performance of specific activities that are common expectations of elementary school children. Because the therapists' concern was with performance rather than diagnosis, no developmental levels were as-signed to the test items. It is assumed that the student who can pass every item would be independent in self-care within a school environment. Note the differences in the scoring criteria on this form in comparison to the previous test.

EATING FUNCTION ASSESSMENTS

A number of therapist-made eating assessments have been reported in the literature and at professional con-

Figure 11-2   Preschool Play Scale

Test measures: The scale is used to evaluate observed, spontaneous play behavior of a child and compare this behavior to age-level and age-appropriate behaviors. Expectations of play have been derived primarily through Erikson's theory of child development. Play is assessed through the following dimensions:

1. *Space management:* How the child manages his body and the surrounding space through use of postural mechanisms.
2. *Materials management:* How the child handles objects and materials and the purposes for the use of materials through sensation, process, and result.
3. *Imitation:* How the child understands the world and the child's ability to express feelings through observation and imitation of others.
4. *Participation:* The degree and manner by which the child participates with others in the environment, including cooperation, independence, and dependence.

The first two categories may be used to assess motor, cognitive, and sensory integrative development as well as play performance. The third and fourth categories are particularly useful to assess the psychosocial development of the child.

Population: Knox reported on experimental clinical use of the original scale with a small sample of mentally retarded children.[29] In 1982, Bledsoe and Shepherd[7] revised and retitled the scale, and conducted a small reliability and validity study with a nonrandom sample of 90 normal children. Inter-rater and test-retest reliability results were acceptable, and the test showed variable correlation with other measures of play functions. More recently, Harrison and Kielhofner[22] conducted an experimental study of the scale with a sample of 60 handicapped children. (Severely and profoundly retarded children were not included in the sample.) They found wide ranges of variance in inter-rater and test-retest reliability, as well as concurrent validity, with this population.

Test format:

Content: This is a descriptive, performance-based test that requires access to an adequate play area, test form (see Table 11-2) and pencil for scoring.

Administration: Administration of the test is fairly simple but requires that the examiner observe and record data about the child's play for a specified time period. Bledsoe and Shepherd's procedure[7] included three 30-minute observation sessions, whereas Harrison and Kielhofner's protocol[22] used two 15-minute sessions. Videotape recording, if relatively unobtrusive, is highly recommended. The examiner should be familiar with Erikson's related content and the test item descriptors before observations.

Scoring: The test analysis format provided in the primary reference[29] described behavior but provided no numerical shorthand for grading. A "+" is marked before those statements that best describe observed behavior, and a "−" is marked when the behavior is absent. "NA" and "NE" are used when the opportunity for a behavior does not arise or when a behavior is not evident. Items of special interest are underlined, such as when a child engages in one type of behavior excessively.

Bledsoe and Shepherd's procedure[7] added the use of numerical scores. Raw scores for each section are given an age equivalent at the level of the highest "+" received for each category. A "play age" is derived from the sum of the four category age equivalent scores divided by 4:

$$\frac{(SM+MM+I+P)}{4}$$

Interpretation: Interpretations are determined by comparisons with age level play expectations and are based on the therapist's sound clinical judgment. The test is best used in conjunction with other instruments.

Advantages: The Preschool Play Scale is a descriptive tool that may yield useful information that often cannot be obtained or analyzed through standardized tests. It provides a carefully constructed framework for analysis of situational play behavior.

Disadvantages: The conflicting results of the two reliability and validity studies mentioned here suggest that it may be more difficult to use the test reliably for assessment of handicapped childrens' play behavior. In the Harrison and Kielhofner study,[22] the findings indicated an increasing lag in play age as children approached 6 years (averaging about 3 years delay). This trend could indicate that as handicapped children mature, they are increasingly disadvantaged in chronological age level play activities. Or it could indicate that the PPS is weak in breadth of play description for older children. The latter suggestion is supported somewhat by Harrison and Kielhofner's finding that younger handicapped children (0 to 2 years) showed less or no deficit in play age, when the range of play activities is more limited by a normal child's capacities, experiences, and environments.

A second disadvantage is the absence of a consistent specified time period for observations. Harrison and Kielhofner[22] speculated that their results may have been confounded by their attempt to reduce observation time and therefore make test data collection a more affordable routine. It seems clear that the use of the scale requires competent theoretical and administrative preparation of the examiner and a minimum of two observation periods.

Purchasing information: See references and Table 11-2.

Figure 11-3 Play Skills Inventory

Test measures: The Play Skills Inventory was designed to monitor status of skill development in middle childhood. Specifically, items are designed to elicit data about four areas. Hurff's definitions of these areas include the following:

1. *Sensation:* The ability to identify and detect stimulus change.
2. *Motor:* Includes physical strength, endurance, speed, flexibility, and motor accuracy.
3. *Perception:* The ability to attend selectively to a group of stimuli and to recognize patterns.
4. *Intellect:* The ability to pull past learnings from memory, to select the best solution for a task, to adapt actions to meet the task, and then to reflect on the outcome of the task.

Hurff proposed a model of skill development that used sensation and motor skills as the foundation for the development of, first, perceptual skills and, finally, intellectual skills.

Population: Hurff stated that the test may be administered to children in the range from 8 to 12 years of age. The children who made up her normative sample were all 10 years old.

Test format: This is a criterion-referenced, performance-based test that uses a variety of commercial and therapist-designed games and equipment. Indoor and outdoor activities are included in the 20 items specified. These include, among others, physical fitness test, walking on a balance beam, identification of objects hidden in a picture, size estimates, and building block construction. The entire test battery can be administered in 1 to 2 hours, depending on the child's capabilities.

Administration and scoring information is detailed in the primary reference.[24] A point system and time limit are specified for each test and are used to classify performance as acceptable or unacceptable. Normative data from the sample of 21 subjects were used to determine classifications. A profile is included to record raw scores and interpretation. Interpretation of deficit areas is global, dependent on clusters of unacceptable scores in one or more of the four areas.

Advantages: Because familiar play activities are used, this test is appealing to the age group and tends to elicit optimal performance. Selection of test items by age level appears well grounded. Although it will require some effort to obtain or construct the materials needed for the test, Hurff's descriptions of items are clear.

Disadvantages: The Play Skills Inventory has not been subjected to standard test development procedures. Although considerable literature review was used to determine test items, only 21 subjects were used to determine the final form of the test and provide normative data. Hurff stated that there was no intent to standardize the test. In view of its clinical usefulness, this is unfortunate.

Interpretation is limited and depends more on the therapist's knowledge of Hurff's model, occupational behavior, and child development theory. Therefore, support from stronger standardized tests would be needed to supplement data and impressions obtained from administration of the Play Skills Inventory.

Purchasing information: From Hurff JM: A play skills inventory. In Reilly M, editor: Play as exploratory learning: studies of curiosity behavior, Beverly Hills, Calif, 1974, Sage Publications, Inc.

References: Hurff JM: Am J Occup Ther 34:651, 1980.

---

ferences. In recent years these assessments have become increasingly complex as the knowledge of oral-motor structure and function has expanded and the technology to develop eating and other prespeech mechanisms has expanded. A 1985 literature review of oral-motor assessments by Sparling and Rogers[37] suggested that therapists had become immersed in the technological aspects of eating, and had lost sight of the psychological and sociocultural aspects of the process. They suggested that other factors to consider include the readiness of the child and other persons(s) involved in the process. Readiness factors include: the child's sensory awareness and responsiveness, task orientation and attention, opportunities created to increase the child's skill development, temporal aspects of eating and meals, and interpersonal relationships and behaviors. The Eating Function Assessment form

(Figure 11-4) is a composite of information sought by the occupational therapist who deals with children who have problems in eating. This instrument, developed by Coley, is not all-inclusive. However, it should provide a foundation to begin assessment of such children and may be elaborated on as the examiner's expertise grows.

The eating function assessment form is designed as a checklist, but notations can be added as necessary. For guidance in administration of this assessment, see Chapters 14, 17, 20, and 21.

School readiness tests

School readiness is often assessed through performance on developmental, cognitive, and sensorimotor evaluations. However, therapists will frequently want

Table 11-1   Pilot instruments-guides for play assessment

Name of instrument	Content area	Clinical yield

Guide to play observation
   Age range: not specified
   Author: Florey[15]
	Rules and skills	Interpretation of current play in dimensions of generation of rules, achievement of objective, skilled acts with objects and people, and flexibility of skill

Guide to status of imitation
   Age range: not specified
   Author: deRenne-Stephan[13]
	Imitation	Interpretation of current status of imitative processes in dimensions of child, role models, family organization, and physical environment

Specification for a play milieu
   Age range: not specified
   Author: Takata[40]
	Play	Examination of balance of human, nonhuman, qualitative, and quantitative elements in play milieu

A play agenda
   Age range: birth to 12 years
   Author: Michelman[31]
	Art-games	Specifications for environment, experiences, and activities that promote risk taking and decision making

From The American Occupational Therapy Association, Inc, Copyright 1981, vol 35, No 8, p 520, Studies of Play: Implications for Growth, Development, and for Clinical Practice, L Florey.

additional data on hand use in activities. For this purpose the therapist is referred to the hand function measurements discussed in Chapter 10. In addition, an evaluation of upper extremity function developed by therapists at Colerain Elementary School provides a useful model. This test (Figure 11-7 at the end of this chapter) assists with assessment of preferred hand use, school-related hand activities, prehension patterns, and functional range of motion patterns. Administration and scoring are self-explanatory on the form. Data collected can be used for descriptive purposes in assessment and treatment planning. There is overlap between this therapist-made test and the hand function and other motor tests discussed in Chapter 10. However, the emphasis here is on observed task performance rather than on underlying functions. Components of school readiness discussed in Chapter 16 are also recommended reading.

THE MILLER ASSESSMENT FOR PRESCHOOLERS (MAP)

The Miller Assessment for Preschoolers[32] is a fairly new standardized instrument that shows promise. It was designed by an occupational therapist to determine school readiness and potential learning problems of children aged 2 years, 9 months to 5 years, 8 months. The test may be administered in a short form that measures performance on 27 core items to assess sensory, motor, and cognitive abilities; it examines behavior during the examination in terms of sensory reactivity, social interaction, and attention.[3,32]

A longer version of the test includes a "foundations" section that assesses supplemental characteristics observed during the performance of core items; it also includes a developmental history. The foundations section assesses sensory integration, neurodevelopmental and spatial sequential organization. Miller and Lemerand[33] conducted a study to assess the usefulness of this section because previous tests of such neuromaturational variables had shown questionable useful-

ness. Their results showed little overlap in measurement between the individual areas, but a generally acceptable correlation between the foundations section and total test score. The investigators concluded that the information collected is useful, but they are continuing a longitudinal study for further clarification.

The design and packaging of the MAP are excellent in terms of appeal to children and facilitation of test administration. The test kit, self-contained with all materials, is portable and readily set up in a small area—an advantage to the itinerant therapist. The short form can be administered in 30 minutes. Special continuing education programs are available for therapists who wish to administer this test; these programs are especially recommended for those who will be using the expanded version with the foundations section.[32]

Prevocational tests

A variety of simple to comprehensive tests are available through the literature and commercial resources to assess vocational readiness and skills of adults and older adolescents. Jacobs has compiled detailed information about vocational rehabilitation and occupational therapy assessment for this older population.[26]

It is more difficult to find assessments of developing work attitudes, interests, behaviors, and skills that are suitable for administration with children and adolescents less than 16 years old. (Sixteen years of age is a useful line of demarcation because it signifies the eligibility of an individual for adult vocational rehabilitation services.) The tests included here are clinically useful in work with elementary, middle, and high school students; these tests address the vocational readiness questions asked by occupational therapists.

BLACK'S ADOLESCENT ROLE ASSESSMENT

Black's Adolescent Role Assessment, a semistructured interview, was designed to explore the individual adolescent's progress in the development of oc-

Figure 11-4 A reference form for eating function assessment

Identification of child _____
History: _____
_____

Body position: _____
Abnormal signs: _____
Primitive signs: _____
Normal signs: _____

Oral structures:
Lips: symmetry, retraction, pursing
Teeth: number, caries, abnormal formation, color, position, hygiene
Gingiva: tenderness, inflammation, bleeding, edema, hypertrophy
Tongue: size, position in mouth, deviation, tremors, length of frenulum, scars
Hard, soft palates: clefts, abnormally high arch, abnormal areas of hypertrophy
Uvula: mobility and length
Functional ability:
Suck: movement of tongue, lip prehension
Food: liquid, puree
Utensil: bottle, spoon
Swallow: coordination with respiration, position of lips, amount of drooling
Food: liquid, thickened liquid, puree, lumpy, solid
Drinking: stabilization on rim of cup, movement of jaw, stabilization of jaw, sealing lips
Food: liquid, thickened liquid, Utensil: cup, glass
Biting, chewing: stabilization of jaw, munching pattern
Chewing pattern: up-down, lateral, rotary
Tongue movement: lateral, midline
Food: crunchy, solid
Utensil: fingers, spoon, fork
Straw drinking: position of lips
Hand use:
Palmar grasp, pincer grasp, opposition finger/thumb, hand to mouth reach, hand to mouth control
Developmental level in eating:
Type of food
Skill in using utensils
Cognitive factors: sensory awareness and responsiveness, attention to eating and social process, readiness of child and feeder
Process factors: interaction between child, adults, and peers during meal.
Record:
Time required for feeding
Amount of food intake
Amount of fluid intake
Adaptive equipment: _____
Recommendations for intervention: _____
_____
Expected outcome of intervention: _____
_____

Reprinted with permission of Ida Lou Coley, 1983, Palo Alto, Calif.

cupational role skills. The test was reported in 1976, including format and report forms.[6] A test analysis is shown in Figure 11-5. Unpublished field testing with normal adolescents suggests that the interview can be completed in 1 hour and that comprehensive descriptive information can be obtained if rapport is established early in the interview.

TESTS OF VOCATIONAL INTEREST

Two useful, commercially available tests that are easily administered by occupational therapists in clinical and educational settings are the California Life Goals Evaluation Schedules[21] and the Self-Directed Search.[23] Both tests use a self-assessment format in which the adolescent answers questions related to past and current interests, preferences, and dislikes. The subject can score his own test, and by using obtained scores can identify potentially appropriate vocational choices for further exploration. The therapist's assistance may be needed in the administration of the test with students who are unable to fill out the forms. With either procedure it is helpful to follow up on the testing with task analysis of the prospective job choices. Results can be reviewed with the student to determine the need for further study or training.

WORK PERFORMANCE SKILLS

Other prevocational tests that are of interest to occupational therapists include job samples and timed tests of manual dexterity. There are a number of elaborate commercial work sample evaluation systems that include work samples of varied nature and broad application. These are rarely administered by occupational therapists. Instead, therapists may use the information collected by vocational evaluation programs to assist in planning remedial programs.

However, therapists may wish to construct work samples that will assess client skills in relation to employment prospects in a limited way. For example, if a high school student who is wheelchair bound expresses an interest in teaching, the therapist may wish to assess the student's ability to write on a blackboard, explain a math problem, and move around a school building freely. In this example the work samples are related to the physical demands of a specific job interest, rather than to comprehensive exploration of the student's skills in relation to the broad range of employment possibilities. The example demonstrates a method that is more typical of occupational therapy practice.

Assessment of work skills by occupational therapists usually involves activity analysis of the requirements of a specific job and sampling of the client's abilities to meet those job requirements. Often information from occupational therapy evaluation and treatment is synthesized to relate to job preparedness. Using the example just given, the therapist may note that the student has had difficulty keeping up with academic demands

---

Figure 11-5 Adolescent Role Assessment

Test measures: The Adolescent Role Assessment uses information obtained from self-reports to determine adequacy of development in a variety of occupational roles. Information is gathered that relates to childhood play experiences; adolescent socialization in the family, at school, and with peers; and development of occupational choice and adult work motivation. The assessment is designed to serve as a tool for clinical treatment planning, although its content may also be used for diagnostic purposes by a knowledgeable clinician.

Population: It must be presumed that this evaluation may be used for the entire age range of adolescents. Black reported clinical application with individuals aged 13 to 17.

Test format: The Adolescent Role Assessment is administered as a semistructured interview. Six sets of open-ended questions are provided to open discussion in each of the areas mentioned above. Questions tend to produce information related to actions and feelings. The interviews can generally be completed within 1 hour. Scoring criteria are provided to interpret content elicited through the interview. According to criteria, information about performance in each area is rated with:

+ = Appropriate behavior
0 = Marginal or borderline behavior
− = Inappropriate behavior

A majority of "+" and "0" scores indicates no obvious role dysfunction. However, a majority of "0" and "−" scores indicates a trend of inadequate development that requires intervention.

Advantages: This interview system can yield considerable data about the breadth of developmental performance in the adolescent. Although it was tested clinically by the developer with youths who had emotional and behavioral disorders, its scope lends itself to application with a broader population. The interview questions are carefully formatted in the vernacular to assist in establishing rapport with the teenage client.

Disadvantages: Black cautions that the validity of content obtained is dependent on the truthfulness and cooperation of the individual who is interviewed. In the experimental stage the test was administered as part of an evaluation battery. Black believed that, when combined with data from other evaluation tools, the Adolescent Role Assessment could be used to define clear patterns of behavior. However, it is not clear what the relative value of data from this instrument was in relation to information collected through other tools. The test was initially given to a small group of adolescents, and a case study that relates data from one such application was described by Black. However, there was no follow-up on the results of treatment planned through this evaluative process, nor was any attempt made to establish validity or reliability.

Purchasing information: From Black MM: Am J Occup Ther 30:134, 1976.

---

of his own high school program because of slow writing. If the student has been using a typewriter and tape recorder to aid in his completion of high school work, the therapist must consider how this equipment may be used to meet the demands of college preparation for a teaching career, as well as classroom duties. If it appears that a teaching career is beyond the student's capability, the therapist might work with vocational specialists to develop alternatives for the student.

JACOB'S PREVOCATIONAL SKILLS ASSESSMENT

A unique assessment of vocational development and readiness was developed by Karen Jacobs[26] and the occupational therapy staff at the Little People's School in Massachusetts. This school serves learning disabled children, adolescents, and young adults, with an emphasis on preparation for productive membership in the adult community (see further discussion of this program in Chapter 16.) In response to the assessment needs of younger students, a standard testing procedure, the Jacobs Prevocational Skills Assessment (JPSA), was constructed. The test is suitable for administration to older children and adolescents through age 15 who have uneven levels of function in academic, communication, and manipulative skills. The test includes 15 tasks that represent a range of work skills:

Quality control	Money concepts
Filing	Functional banking
Carpentry assembly	Time concepts
Classification	Work attitudes
Office work	Body scheme
Telephone directory	Leather assembly
Factory work	Food preparation
Environmental mobility	

The work samples are well developed and measure critical skills. Materials needed to replicate, administer, and score the test battery are generally available in occupational therapy environments. Performance of the tasks is timed, with maximum times allowable per task determined by data from a sample of normal adolescents.

Although no validity and reliability studies have been reported at the time of this writing, Jacobs and

Text continued p. 215.

Figure 11-6 Activities of daily living

Name ______________________ Birthdate ______________________
Communication ______________________ Ambulation ______________________

Key: 0 = Totally dependent, cannot perform
1 = Dependent, but can help
2 = Assisted or supervised with fine and gross activities
3 = Assisted or supervised with fine activities
4 = Normal independence for chronological age

I. Feeding activities *Date*

Eat finger food
Pick up and feed self sandwich
Eat with fork
Eat with spoon
Spoon liquids, such as soup
Drink through straw
Drink from cup
Spread butter with knife
Cut soft food
Cut meat
Can eat with standard service
Can eat in normal time

Comments (note special equipment, avoided or modified foods):

II. Dressing activities *Date*

Remove socks
Remove shoes
Remove braces
Remove underpants
Remove bra
Remove trousers
Remove skirt
Remove slip-over garment
Remove cardigan garment
Remove hat
Remove gloves
Remove rubbers, boots
Put on socks
Put on shoes
Put on braces
Put on underpants
Put on bra
Put on trousers
Put on skirt
Put on slip-over garment
Put on cardigan garment
Put on hat
Put on gloves
Put on rubbers, boots

Comments (note special equipment, unusual position):

III. Fastenings *Date*

Large buttons—open
Large buttons—close
Small buttons—open
Small buttons—close
Velcro (TM)—open
Velcro (TM)—close
Snaps—open
Snaps—close
Safety pins—open
Safety pins—close
Zippers—open
Zippers—close
Buckles—open
Buckles—close
Shoelaces—open
Shoelaces—close
Bows—open
Bows—close

Comments (note special equipment, etc.):

IV. Hygienic activities

Operate water faucet
Wring wash cloth
Wash hands
Get into tub
Bathe self in tub
Get out of tub
Apply toothpaste to brush
Brush teeth
Shampoo hair
Comb hair
Clean, trim nails
Use handkerchief
Adjust clothing for toileting
Get on toilet
Use toilet paper
Get off toilet
Flush toilet
Use urinal
Empty urinary appliance
Apply deodorant
Feminine hygiene

Comments (note special equipment, mobility):

Occupational therapist: ______________________

Reprinted with permission of the Columbus Public Schools and Colerain Elementary School, Columbus, Ohio.

Table 11-2   Preschool Play Scale

Child Number _____
Session Number _____
Observer's Initials _____

	0-1 year	1-2 years	2-3 years
Space management	Gross motor activity: reaches; plays with hands and feet; touches hands to feet; crawls; sits with balance; pulls to stand; moves to continue pleasant sensation	Gross motor activity: stands unsupported; sits down; bends and recovers balance; walks and runs—wide stance; climbs low objects; broad movements involving large muscle groups; rides kiddie car	Gross motor activity: beginning integration of entire body in activities—concentrates on complex movements (i.e., throwing, jumping, climbing); pedals tricycle
	Territory: crib; playpen; house	Territory: home, immediate surrounds	Territory: outside; short excursions
	Exploration: of self and objects within reach	Exploration: of all unfamiliar things; oblivious to hazards	Exploration: increased exploration of all unfamiliar objects; very curious
Material management	Manipulation: predominant—handles, mouths toys; brings two objects together; picks up; hits; bangs; shakes	Manipulation: predominant—throws; inserts; pushes; pulls; carries; pounds	Manipulation: remains predominant—feels; pats; dumps; squeezes; fills
	Construction: not evident	Construction: little attempt to make product: relates two objects appropriately (i.e., lid on pot); stacks; takes apart; puts together	Construction: manipulation predominates; scribbles; strings beads; puzzles 4 to 5 pieces
	Interest: people; gazes at faces; follows movements; attends to voices and sounds	Interest: movement of self—explores various kinesthetic and proprioceptive sensations; moving objects (i.e., balls, trucks, pull toys)	Interest: explores new movement patterns (i.e., jumping); toys with moving parts (i.e., dump trucks, jointed dolls); makes messes
	Purpose: sensation or function—uses materials to see, touch, hear, smell, mouth (i.e., rattles, teething rings, colored objects)	Purpose: experiments in movement—practices basic movement patterns (i.e., rock, walk, run); process important	Purpose: process important—less interest in finished product (i.e., scribbles, squeezes play dough); repetition of gross motor skills
Imitation	Attention: follows moving objects with eyes	Attention: rapid shifts	Attention: intense interest; quiet play up to 15 minutes; plays with single object or theme 5 to 10 minutes
	Imitation: of observed facial expressions and physical movement (i.e., smiling, pat-a-cake); emotions (hugs toys)	Imitation: of simple actions; present events and adults—self-related mimicry (i.e., feeds self with spoon)	Imitation: of adult routines with toy-related mimicry (i.e., child feeding doll); toys as agents (i.e., doll feeds self)
	Imagination: not evident	Imagination: imaginary objects (i.e., pretend food on spoon)	Imagination: personifies dolls, stuffed animals; starts having imaginary friends (i.e., animals, persons)
	Dramatization: not evident	Dramatization: not evident	Dramatization: portrays single character
	Music: attends to sounds	Music: sways; listens	Music: responds to music with whole body (i.e., marching, twirling)
	Books: pats; strokes; picks at pictures	Books: handles; points to pictures; begins to name pictures	Books: likes familiar stories; fills in words and phrases
Participation	Type: solitary play (no effort to interact with other children or choose similar activities)	Type: combination of solitary, onlooker play (watches others—speaking but not entering their play)	Type: parallel play (plays beside others, play remains independent, but child situates self among others, enjoys their presence)
	Cooperation: demands personal attention; simple give and take interaction with immediate family or caretaker (i.e., tickling, peek-a-boo); 7 to 10 months—initiates games himself	Cooperation: more complex games with a variety of adults (i.e., hide and seek, chasing); offers toys but is somewhat possessive; persistent	Cooperation: possessive (much snatch and grab, hoarding, no sharing, resists toys being taken away); independent (does not ask for help, initiates own play)
	Language: attends to sounds and voices; babbles; uses razzing sounds	Language: jabbers during play—talks to self, often in sing-song rhythm; uses gestures and words to communicate wants; labels objects	Language: talkative—very little jabber; begins to use words to communicate ideas, information

Revised from Knox, Susan: A Play Scale. In Reilly M, editor: Play as Exploratory Learning, Beverly Hills, 1974, Sage Publications, Inc, Jayne Shepherd, Nancy Bledsoe, 1981.

GROSS MOTOR ACTIVITY: Play involving large muscle groups.
TERRITORY: Physical area used during play.
EXPLORATION: Interest in new environmental experiences.
MANIPULATION: Fine motor play skills.

CONSTRUCTION: Play with materials to make products.
INTEREST: Attention to or involvement in a specific type of activity.
PURPOSE: Goal of an activity.
ATTENTION: Length of time a child independently occupies himself in play.

	The following to be filled in after observations are recorded: Mean ages for dimensions:	Space Management _____ Imitation _____ Material Management _____ Participation ___ Play Age (mean of all dimensions) _____

3-4 years	4-5 years	5-6 years
Gross motor activity: more coordinated body movements, smoother walking, jumping, climbing, running (accelerates, decelerates)	Gross motor activity: increased activity level; can concentrate on goal instead of movement; ease of gross motor ability allows stunts, tests of strength, exaggerated movements; clambers	Gross motor activity: more sedate; good muscle control and balance; hops on one foot; skips; somersaults; skates; lifts self off ground
Territory: home; immediate neighborhood	Territory: neighborhood	Territory: likes to be up off ground
Exploration: interest in new experiences, places, animals, nature	Exploration: anticipates trips, likes change of pace	Exploration: plans and enjoys excursions and trips
Manipulation: small muscle activity—hammers, sorts, inserts small objects (i.e., peg boards); cuts	Manipulation: increasing fine motor control allows quick movements, force, pulling	Manipulation: uses tools to make things (i.e., cuts more precisely); copies; traces; combines various materials
Construction: makes simple products (i.e., blocks, crayons, clay); combines play materials; takes apart; arranges in spatial dimension—design is evident	Construction: predominates—makes products, specific designs evident, builds complex structures; puzzles 10 pieces	Construction: predominates—makes recognizable products; likes small construction, attends to detail (i.e., eyes, nose, fingers apparent in drawings); uses products in play
Interest: anything new; fine motor manipulation of play materials	Interest: takes pride in work (i.e., shows and talks about products, compares with friends, likes pictures displayed); complex ideas	Interest: in reality—manipulation of real life situations (i.e., miniature things); making something useful—props for play; permanence of products; toys that "really work"
Purpose: beginning to show interest in result or finished product	Purpose: product very important—use to express self; exaggerates	Purpose: replicate reality
Attention: longer span—around 30 minutes: plays with single object or theme 5 to 10 minutes	Attention: amuses self up to one hour: plays with single object or theme 10 to 15 minutes	Attention: concentration for long period of time; plays with single object or theme 10 to 15 minutes
Imitation: more complex imitation of real world—part of dramatization	Imitation: more complex imitation of real world as part of dramatization	Imitation: more complex imitation of real world as part of dramatization
Imagination: assumes familiar roles—domestic themes, past experiences	Imagination: prominent—able to use familiar knowledge to construct a novel situation (i.e., expanding on the theme of a story or TV show)	Imagination: prominent—continues to construct new themes but emphasis on reality—reconstruction of real world
Dramatization: imitates simple action and reaction episodes—mirrors experience, emphasis on domestic and animals; portrays multiple characters with feelings (mostly anger and crying); little interest in costumes	Dramatization: role playing for or with others; portrays more complex emotions; sequences stories—themes from domestic to magic; enjoys dress-ups	Dramatization: sequences stories—emphasis on copying what occurs in real world; costumes important; props; puppets
Music: sings simple songs—not necessarily on pitch; plays instruments	Music: sings whole songs on pitch; musical games (i.e., Farmer in the Dell); good rhythm	Music: meaning of songs important; enjoys catchy tunes, songs that tell stories; dances reflect interpretation of music
Books: new or information books: pictures important; relates own experiences to story	Books: listens better—doesn't need physical contact with book; looks at books independently—repeats familiar stories	Books: looks at books independently or with peer; describes picture to tell story; must be credible
Type: associative play (similar activities with groups of 2 to 3, no organization to reach a common goal, more interest in peers than activity)	Type: cooperative (groups of 2 to 3 organized to achieve a goal, i.e., assigns roles for pretend play)	Type: cooperative (groups of 2 to 5, organization of more complex games and dramatic play)
Cooperation: limited—some turn taking: asks for things rather than grabbing; little attempt to control others	Cooperation: takes turns; attempts to control the activities of others (often self-centered, bossy)	Cooperation: social give and take evident (i.e., compromises to facilitate group play); rivalry seen in competitive games
Language: uses words to communicate with peers, interest in new words (repeats them, asks their meaning)	Language: very talkative—plays with words; fabricates—capable of long narratives; questions persistently; communicates with peers to organize activities	Language: very prominent in a socio-dramatic play (uses words as part of play as well as to organize play); interest in present; relevant how, what for questions

IMITATION: Mirroring aspects of cultural environment.
IMAGINATION: Recombining aspects of cultural environment and introducing novelty into a situation.
DRAMATIZATION: Prtetending, assuming roles and sequencing stories.
MUSIC: Response to and use of music.
BOOKS: Response to and use of books.
TYPE: Level of social interaction with others in play.
COOPERATION: Ability to get along with others in play situations.
LANGUAGE: Means of communication with others in play.

Figure 11-7 Evaluation of upper extremity function

Name _____ Date _____

Diagnosis _____

Code: 0 = Unable to perform

    1 = Difficult, accomplished, but only *with* assistance

    2 = Some difficulty, accomplished *without* assistance

    3 = Accomplished with ease

Preferred hand

	Right		Left	
	0	1	2	3
1. Pencil/crayon				
a. Holding and marking randomly _____				
b. Dot to dot _____				
c. Color simple shape _____				
2. Blocks				
a. Tower _____ Number _____				
b. Bridge ____ _____				
c. Train _____				
3. Pegboard				
a. Small (plastic) _____ Time _____				
b. Golf tees _____ Time _____				
c. One-inch diameter _____ Time _____				
4. Safety pin _____				

Comments:

Hand activities

	Right		Left	
	0	1	2	3
1. Scissor cutting				
a. Holding and cutting randomly _____				
b. Straight lines _____				
c. Curved lines _____				
d. Star _____				
2. Pencil sharpening _____				
3. Opening book and turning pages _____				
4. Bead stringing				
1. Large _____ Number _____				
2. Small _____ Number _____				
5. Screwing and unscrewing jar lid _____				
6. Coin from coin purse _____				
7. Telephone _____				

Comments:

Figure 11-7 cont'd.   Evaluation of upper extremity function

Grasp, release, pinch

	Left				Right			
	0	1	2	3	0	1	2	3
1. Spherical grasp (2-inch diameter ball) _____								
Cylindrical grasp (1-inch diameter peg) _____								
2. Hook grasp (Purse or bookbag handle) _____								
3. Active release _____								
Tip pinch (picking up ⅛-inch bead _____								

Lateral pinch (piece of paper) _____ pounds left
_____ pounds right
Palmar pinch (pencil)   _____ pounds left
_____ pounds right

Comments:

Functional UE range of motion

	Left				Right			
	0	1	2	3	0	1	2	3
Reach or touch								
Above head _____								
Top of head _____								
Back of head and neck _____								
Face _____								
Mouth _____								
Shoulders _____								
Waist (putting on belt) _____								
Back (fastening clothes) _____								
Knees _____								
Feet _____								
Floor _____								

Comments:

_____
Occupational therapist

Reprinted with permission of the Columbus Public Schools and Colerain Elementary School, Columbus, Ohio.

staff hypothesize that this test battery measures a student's prevocational readiness in these skill areas:

Fine motor coordination
Eye-hand coordination
Motor planning
Figure-ground
    discrimination
Sorting
Classification
Sequencing
Decision making
Problem solving

Organizational skills
Use of tools
Ability to follow visual
    directions
Ability to follow verbal
    directions
Auditory memory
Visual memory
Conceptual skills
Task focus

A detailed discussion of the critical foundations, construction, administration, and use of test materials, as well as test forms, are contained in the primary reference by Jacobs. The JPSA has been used successfully in its replicated form in public school programs for learning disabled adolescents, and in modified forms with children and adolescents with physical and developmental disabilities (see Chapter 16).

CROMWELL'S PRIMARY PREVOCATIONAL EVALUATION

In 1960 Cromwell[12] published a manual that described the prevocational evaluation program used by occupational therapists at the United Cerebral Palsy Center in Los Angeles County. This assessment system was developed through a 4-year research project and includes three parts: the activities of daily living inventory, manual dexterity test battery, and the prevocational job sample test battery. Norms for performance of both handicapped (persons with cerebral palsy) and nonhandicapped individuals are included for all parts of the assessment system. Cromwell stated that the system was used clinically with individuals aged 14 years and older.

One of the useful features of Cromwell's manual is its survey of a variety of manual dexterity tests. The entire group of tests, which includes both commercial and therapist-designed tests, or the short version can be administered according to the needs and abilities of the individual client. Complete information is included about the construction of manual dexterity and job sample tests so that the therapist can safely apply norms. In addition to the evaluation's usefulness, Cromwell's job sample descriptions provide a model for the development of other task samples. This includes a description of the job sample, materials to be included in the sample kit, instructions for the examiner, instructions for the client, and rating-scoring information with norms. The Manual for Primary Prevocational Evaluation is no longer in print. Because therapists have found parts of it so useful, the author is most generous in allowing individuals to photocopy it and has granted blanket permission for copying in part or in entirety.

SUMMARY

This chapter has reviewed a number of clinically useful instruments that allow an occupational therapist to assess age-related task performance. The tests presented include standardized and criterion-referenced developmental evaluations and assessments of self-maintenance, play, school readiness, and prevocational skills performance. Selections were based on use in the general range of occupational therapy treatment centers rather than on use in highly specialized locales. Although a number of commercial instruments are available for developmental assessment, occupational therapy concerns with activity performance usually require more detailed information about self-maintenance, school readiness, and prevocational skills. The majority of measurement tools used in practice for assessment of these areas are therapist made. Chapter samples of such clinical tools are considered representative and can be adapted to meet the needs of individual therapists and their clients. Credit to the designer of the original format should be retained on any adaptations.

The therapist is reminded that the focus of occupational therapy is on performance of observable everyday activities in the areas discussed. Therefore it is anticipated that the final assessment of a child before his discharge would include one of the tools presented in this chapter to determine progress and achievement of occupational therapy objectives.

STUDY QUESTIONS
Using the resources discussed in this chapter, select four appropriate instruments to use for your assessment of each of the following children:

1. A 2-year-old girl with Down syndrome;
2. A 4-year-old boy with mild cerebral palsy involvement;
3. An 8-year-old girl who has sustained a closed head injury; and
4. A 16-year-old boy with a history of learning disability and drug and alcohol abuse.

Explain why each of the tests you have selected is appropriate. What information do you expect to obtain from administration of each test?

REFERENCES

1. American Association on Mental Retardation: AAMD adaptive behavior scales, Monterey, Calif, 1981, CTB/McGraw-Hill Inc.
2. American Association on Mental Retardation: AAMD adaptive behavior scales—public school version, Monterey, Calif, 1981, CTB/McGraw-Hill Inc.
3. Banus BJ: The Miller assessment for preschoolers (MAP): an introduction and review, Am J Occup Ther 37:333, May 1983.
4. Battelle developmental inventory: examiner's manual, Allen, Tex, 1984, DLM Teaching Resources.
5. Bayley N: Bayley scales of infant development, New York, 1969, The Psychological Corporation.
6. Black MM: Adolescent role assessment, Am J Occup Ther 30:134, February, 1976.
7. Bledsoe NP, and Shepherd JT: A study of reliability and validity of a preschool play scale, Am J Occup Ther 36:783, 1982.
8. Brazelton TB: Neonatal behavioral assessment scales, Philadelphia, 1973, JB Lippincott Co.
9. Brigance AH: Brigance diagnostic inventory of basic skills, Woburn, Mass, 1977, Curriculum Associates, Inc.
10. Brigance AH: Brigance diagnostic inventory of early development, Woburn, Mass, 1978, Curriculum Associates, Inc.
11. Coley IL: Pediatric assessment of self-care activities, St Louis, 1978, The CV Mosby Co.
12. Cromwell FS: Occupational therapist's manual for basic skills assessment or primary prevocational evaluation, Altadena, Calif 1960, Fair Oaks Printing Co. (Available through the author: 1179 Yocum Street, Pasadena, Calif 91103.)
13. deRenne-Stephan C: Imitation: a mechanism of play behavior, Am J Occup Ther 34:95, 1980.
14. Doll EA: Vineland social maturity scale: condensed manual of directions, Circle Pines, Minn, 1965, American Guidance Service, Inc.
15. Florey LL: An approach to play and play development, Am J Occup Ther 25:275, 1971.
16. Florey LL: Studies of play: implications for growth, development, and for clinical practice, Am J Occup Ther 35:519, August, 1981.
17. Folio MR, and Fewell RR: Peabody developmental motor scales and activity cards, Allen, Tex, 1983, DLM Teaching Resources.
18. Furano S, and others: Hawaii early learning profile (HELP) activity guide, Palo Alto, Calif, 1984, VORT Corp.
19. Furano S, and others: HELP chart: Hawaii early learning profile, Palo Alto, Calif, 1987, VORT Corp.
20. Guidubaldi J, and Perry JD: Concurrent and predictive validity of the Batelle developmental inventory at the first grade level, Educ and Psych Measurement 44:977, 1984.
21. Hahn ME: The California life goals evaluation schedules, Los Angeles, 1969, Western Psychological Services.
22. Harrison H, and Kielhofner G: Examining the reliability and validity of the Preschool Play Scale with handicapped children, Am J Occup Ther 40:167, 1986.
23. Holland JL: The self-directed search, Palo Alto, Calif, 1979, Consulting Psychologists Press, Inc.
24. Hurff JM: A play skills inventory. In Reilly M, editor: Play as exploratory learning: studies of curiosity behavior, Beverly Hills, 1974, Sage Publications, Inc.
25. Hurff JM: A play skills inventory: a competency monitoring tool for the 10 year old, Am J Occup Ther 34:651, October 1980.

26. Jacobs K: Occupational therapy: work-related programs and assessments, Boston, 1985, Little, Brown & Co.

27. Kielhofner G, and Burris R: Collecting data on play: a critique of available methods, Occup Ther J Res 4:151, 1984.

28. Knoblock H, and Passaminick: Gessel's manual of developmental diagnosis, revised, New York, 1980, Harper & Row, Publishers, Inc.

29. Knox S: A play scale. In Reilly M, editor: Play as exploratory learning: studies in curiousity behavior, Beverly Hills, 1974, Sage Publications, Inc.

30. Lydic J, and Wallace J: Developmental programming for infants and young children: an analysis, Physical and Occup Ther in Peds 5:59, Winter 1985-86.

31. Michelman S: Play and the deficit child. In Reilly M, editor: Play as exploratory learning: studies of curiousity behavior, Beverly Hills, 1974, Sage Publications, Inc.

32. Miller LJ: Miller assessment for preschoolers: manual, Littleton, Colo, 1982, The Foundation for Knowledge in Development.

33. Miller LJ, and Lemarand PA: Neuro-maturational variables within the Miller assessment for preschoolers, Occup Ther J Res 6:123, 1986.

34. Palisano R, and Lydic J: The Peabody developmental motor scales: an analysis, Physical and Occup Ther in Peds 4:1, 1984.

35. Rogers SJ, and D'Eugenio DB: Assessment and application. In Schafer DS, and Moersch MS, editors: Developmental programming for infants and young children, vol 1, Ann Arbor, 1977, The University of Michigan Press.

36. Snyder C, Eyres FJ, and Barnard E: New findings about mothers' antenatal expectations and their relationship to infant development, Am J Matern Child Nurs 4:354, 1979.

37. Sparling J, and Rogers J: Feeding assessment: development of a biopsychosocial instrument, Occup Ther J Res 6:123, 1986.

38. Sparrow S, Balla D, and Cicchetti D: The Vineland adaptive behavior scales, Circle Pines, Minn, 1987, American Guidance Service.

39. Sprinthall RC, and Sprinthall NA: Educational psychology: a developmental approach, ed 3, Reading, Mass, 1981, Addison-Wesley Publishing Co, Inc.

40. Takata N: The play milieu: a preliminary appraisal, Am J Occup Ther 25:281, 1971.

41. Tronik E, and Brazelton TB: Clinical uses of the Brazelton behavioral assessments. In Firedlander B, Sterit G, and Kirk B, editors: Exceptional infants, volume III: Assessment and intervention, New York, 1975, Brunner/Mazel Inc.

42. Vulpe S: Vulpe assessment battery: developmental assessment/performance analysis/individualized programming for the atypical child, Downsview, Ontario, Canada, 1979, National Institute on Mental Retardation.

43. Walker LO: The Brazelton neonatal behavioral assessment scales. In Humanick SB, editor: Analysis of current assessment strategies in the health care of young children and child-bearing families. Norwalk, Conn, 1982, Appleton/Century Crofts.

44. Waters E, Vaughan BE, and Egeland BR: Individual differences in infant-mother attachment relationship at age one: antecedents in neonatal behavior in an urban, economically disadvantaged sample, Child Dev 51:208, 1980.

45. Widmeyer SM, and Field TM: Effects of Brazelton demonstrations on early interactions of preterm infants and their teenage mothers, Infant Behavior and Development 3:79, 1980.

12

Program planning

PAT NUSE PRATT
ANNE STEVENS ALLEN

INTEGRATION OF EVALUATION FINDINGS

Through the course of formal and informal evaluation, occupational therapists compile extensive information about their young clients. The final, professional component of assessment is to organize, synthesize, and use these data to guide intervention. The American Occupational Therapy Association[2] defines assessment as

. . . the process of determining the need for, nature of, and estimated time of treatment, determining the needed coordination with other persons involved, and documenting these activities.

Organization of data

From the beginning it is helpful to have some concrete tools to assist with the organization of data. Two resources are useful for these purposes. The Uniform Occupational Therapy Evaluation Checklist was adopted by the American Occupational Therapy Association's Representative Assembly in 1981.[2] It was developed with the use of the *Uniform Terminology for Reporting Occupational Therapy Services* and serves as a guide for baseline data collection (Figure 12-2 at the end of this chapter). It is designed to be all inclusive, but each occupational therapy assessment in which this format is used is not expected to reflect all details. Instead, all evaluations should address the major categories. The checklist has proved especially useful in medical settings. Definitions of terminology are available.[2]

The Worksheet for Organizing Data Collection (Figure 12-3 at the end of this chapter) was developed to organize results of assorted evaluative procedures by use of the defined parameters of occupational therapy practice identified by the American Occupational Therapy Association.[2] The terminology used in the worksheet is more in keeping with the model of practice described in Chapter 7, and it is perhaps more suited to educational settings. Information may be transferred from assorted measurements and evaluation resources with "+" and "−" notations regarding perceived strengths and weaknesses in the different areas. This worksheet can be adapted and tailored to the needs of the individual clinician, but the basic components of comprehensive occupational therapy should remain to serve as ticklers for overlooked areas. The worksheet is intended for internal use only; it does not constitute a formal evaluation report.

Interpretation of findings: the professional assessment

Using a sequential thought process that closely approximates that used for general problem analysis (Chapter 7), the therapist mentally compares, contrasts, and ranks the information that has been accumulated about the child. Then, using a written format suitable to the service and agency, evaluation data are reported together with the therapist's interpretation, impressions, conclusions, predictions, and recommendations. The content of this formal assessment may be organized in various ways, but includes the components shown in Figure 12-1.

Part one, the identifying information, is similar to data found in other professional reports. Occupational therapists tend to emphasize more information about developmental history and services previously received by the child. The second section is more elaborate, with its documentation of test results and their interpretation. Through this section the therapist identifies the motor, sensory integrative, cognitive, social and emotional capabilities and limitations of the child. The

> **Figure 12-1** Components of occupational therapy assessment reports
>
> 1. Identification and background information
>   Includes referral source and reason, history, and precautions.
> 2. Assessment
>   Includes tests and measurements administered and results, interpretation of functional and performance status, record of consultation with other service providers, the problem list, and recommendations for occupational therapy services and referral.
> 3. Program plan
>   Includes goals and objectives, general and specific program recommendations, frequency, type, and duration of treatment, expected results, and other options for meeting service needs.

Adapted from American Occupational Therapy Association: Guidelines for occupational therapy documentation, Am J Occup Ther 40:830, 1986.

assessment includes description and discussion of the child's roles, expectations, and life space, including human and environmental resources, alternatives, and inhibiting factors.

Clear assessment of the child's abilities and limitations in performance of related play, self-maintenance, school, and prevocational development or readiness is presented. This component is the most critical part of the occupational therapy record, as the aggregate of other service providers may provide data that overlaps regarding life space and functional status. The occupational therapist, however, is unique in her ability to provide a comprehensive assessment of the child's participation in the broad spectrum of daily living activities and the relation of these different activities to each other and to future development.

The preceding information is mentally gathered to develop a clear, concise *problem list*. This list includes both functional and performance problems of the child, and unless facility policy dictates otherwise, it should not be limited to only those problems that relate to occupational therapy intervention. Rather, the problem list should be used to present the therapist's professional impression of the service needs of the child or adolescent, and to form the basis of collaborative relationships that will mutually foster the resolution of those needs. Therefore, a problem list, presented either as a discrete numerical listing, or a narrative summary of critical findings, might include a variety such as:

1. Unable to feed self without assistance
2. Requires standby physical assistance for all dressing activities

3. Poor visual acuity for reading and other academic requirements
4. Parents unable to transport child to eye clinic appointments

Based on this list and the therapist's awareness of service resources, recommendations are made for occupational therapy and other intervention.

The final component of the written assessment, which is discussed in detail throughout the rest of this chapter, is the *program plan*.[1] This component of the assessment constitutes the therapist's initial recommendations regarding how the child's occupational therapy needs should be met. It is important to emphasize the "initial" concept here, because program plans, however precisely prepared, are subject to modifications by the persons, time, places, things, and actions involved in the service delivery process.

Sample assessment reports

Formal reports of occupational therapy assessment are usually filed in narrative form or on multi-part, multi-paged preprinted forms. At a minimum, the original is retained in agency files and copies are distributed to the parents and the occupational therapist. Often teachers, physicians, and other service providers will request copies as well. Again, agency policies will dictate the number of copies required, as well as due dates. Two sample reports that demonstrate the use of the two formats to present information about the same child are shown in Figures 12-4 and 12-5 at the end of this chapter. The preprinted form was originally adapted from an occupational/physical therapy screening tool designed by Taylor and Christopher,[4] but it has since been considerably revised. This format has been used in school system practice, so it would need further modification for a medically-oriented setting.

THE PROGRAM PLAN
Goals and objectives

Based on the problem list, the therapist prepares goals and objectives for occupational therapy intervention. *Goals* are long-term for the anticipated period of rehabilitation and tend to be written in general terms. In reference to the short problem list presented earlier, examples of goals might be:

1. The child will feed herself using adaptive equipment and standby assistance for food preparation
2. The child will dress herself using adaptive equipment and techniques without assistance
3. In collaboration with the teacher, the therapist will improve the child's access to reading and other written materials
4. The therapist will refer the child's family to social services for assistance with eye clinic transportation

As discussed in Chapter 7, *objectives* are the measurable accomplishments that indicate that a child is making progress on achievement of the desired goals within a specified short period of service delivery. These may be set on a daily, weekly, monthly, quarterly, or annual basis. For example, in an acute care hospital, objectives may relate to what can be done within a 3 day stay, prior to transfer to an outpatient facility. In contrast, in a school system, objectives are often written for the entire school year. Within this time frame, the therapist will consider that some objectives will be achieved earlier and more readily than others, or that meeting one objective will prepare the child to accomplish a task or skill established in another objective.

These readiness and sequential factors tend to distinguish between the short- and long-term program. As discussed previously, the early short-term objectives and program will generally involve improvement in the component functions of behavior that are the foundations of skilled performance. In contrast, longer-term goals, objectives, and program will relate to the child's skilled performance of activities and roles in the play, self-maintenance, school, and vocational development arenas. This does not imply that, for example, a school system therapist would spend the fall and winter working with a child on finger strengthening games only, and then in spring begin handwriting techniques. Instead, it means that the therapist might do a variety of program activities throughout the year, including writing, but that she would expect the child's pinch strength to increase before handwriting skills improve.

Other factors that will affect priority of goals and objectives include issues that are critical to the child, the family, the agency, or other service providers. Very often there is something specific that the child would like to do, or do better, and such an objective needs to be given high priority. Even if sequential factors rule out improvement in the early stages of a program, the child's motivation for achievement is a modulating influence and should be fostered. Graded levels of independence in the desired activity can be set, and cooperation with other "therapist-directed" program components is more likely.

Similarly, parents or other significant persons in the child's life may have needs related to daily management that must be addressed early. For example, a mother who is having difficulty providing any nutrition to her child will require immediate intervention for feeding management, even though a longer-term objective may be to facilitate head control preparatory to improved oral motor function.

Objectives are written in terms of behaviors that will be demonstrated by the child or therapist. It is usually preferable to write objectives about the child's behaviors because this approach more clearly illustrates the content of the program plan. Sometimes, however, objectives related to therapist behaviors are unavoidable. An example of this is when further evaluation or work with parents is indicated. In general, however, as Llorens and Schuster[7] have suggested, behavioral objectives should be measurable and specify what tasks the child is able to perform to demonstrate goal achievement.

The use of broad goals in combination with specific measurable objectives in task performance is now generally required by regulatory bodies involved with occupational therapy services. Goals will be short and clear; for example, they might be written as "Johnny will develop age-appropriate feeding skills." This is adequate, but it would be clearer to say "Johnny will self-feed at the 2-year-old age level."

In contrast, measurable objectives are more elaborate. Each contains three components. First, a *behavioral statement* specifies what the child will do that can be observed. If working on a behavior characteristic that cannot be observed, such as a "healthy self-concept," the therapist must specify an observable behavior that indicates the desired phenomenon. For example, the objective might read, "Sally will smile at herself in the mirror."

In addition, each objective includes at least one *condition statement*. This describes under what conditions the child will accomplish an activity. The third component is a *performance criterion* that denotes how acceptable performance is measured. For example, "Johnny will feed himself (behavioral statement) using a spoon (condition statement) without spilling (performance criterion)."

The example above may be clear to the therapist, who is aware of other variables involved in self-feeding, but it may not be descriptive enough for other personnel to implement a program, or for parents or supervisors who are reviewing a program plan. So it is more common for a typical objective to obtain more than one condition statement and often more than one performance criterion. As a result, the objective becomes: "Johnny will feed himself (behavioral statement) solid foods (condition statement) using a fork or spoon (another condition statement) at lunch in the cafeteria (still another condition) without spilling (a performance criterion) in 20 minutes (a second performance criterion) with no more than two verbal cues (a third performance criterion)." This gives a more precise description of what is expected of the child, as well as how and where he will do it.

An increasing trend, which assists with precision of documentation and measurement of achievement, is the use of a continuum of performance criteria related to the degree of independence that is expected. In other words, the therapist specifies what assistance an individual requires to accomplish a task or demonstrate a function. These criteria, which tend to follow a pattern originated by Vulpe,[12] may be summarized as:

1. The child can generalize the skill or perform the task in any environment
2. The child can perform the skill without assistance, supervision, or use of adapted equipment or techniques in familiar environments
3. The child can perform the skill without assistance or supervision, but requires adaptive equipment or techniques
4. The child requires supervision for safety to perform the skill
5. The child requires standby assistance to perform the skill
6. The child requires some type of direction or cuing (verbal, visual, or physical) to perform the skill
7. The child requires physical assistance to perform the skill
8. The child is unable to perform the skill, but attends to the activity or the caretaker

It is apparent that further gradations exist within this continuum, which are typically expressed in percentages of assistance or numbers of cues required.[11]

SELECTION OF PROGRAM ACTIVITIES AND OTHER MODALITIES
Theoretical considerations

The instrumentation of a program plan is still another of the analytical and correlational processes carried on in the mind of the professional. The ability to mentally engage in this process is derived through the maturation of human cognitive capacities, development of critical thinking skills through preparation in a broad and lengthy course of study in the liberal arts and sciences,[13] and professional preparation in the organization and interpretation of the facts, values, and beliefs of a particular discipline. In occupational therapy, program planning may be conceived as the ongoing outcome of a mental process that compares, contrasts, correlates, and predicts the interaction between the findings of the assessment process, activity analysis, activity adaptation, and what is known and observed about the effects of people, places, time, things, and actions on the therapy process. This latter component of the therapist's knowledge is collectively referred to here as *theoretical considerations*. Because of its modulating effect on program planning, this facet will be explored in more detail.

Occupational therapists have a strong tradition of considering factors that impinge on, facilitate, and inhibit the treatment process. Hopkins and Tiffany[6] have provided the profession with a comprehensive discussion of these critical factors, which include:

1. The *patient* or client, including variables of stress, motivation, the nonhuman world, and cultural implications
2. The *therapist,* including variables of knowledge,

skills, attitudes, and awareness of and ability to use therapeutic relationships
3. The *activity,* including variables of its properties, meanings, and types
4. The *context,* including variables of time, place, people, prevailing ideas, values, beliefs, and technology

Rather than provide a rephrasing of Hopkins and Tiffany's well-organized and thoughtful discussion, it seems more appropriate to move forward with a review of recent literature that develops these factors in relation to program planning for children.

During review of the literature for this second edition, the improvement in quality, volume, and variety of research reported by occupational therapists during the 1980s became apparent. Of particular interest was an increasing amount of critical analysis of program planning variables, especially in relation to occupational therapy for children. Attention to concepts and developments in learning theory is a common theme in these studies.

MOTOR LEARNING

Gliner[6] proposed that occupational therapists examine research related to motor learning. He defined this term as how a skill is learned, controlled, and retained. The three variables of the motor learning process include the actor (child), the task, and the environment, within an ecological framework.

Gliner wrote that of particular concern to occupational therapists are the motor learning aspects of the task environment. The environment includes affordances and structural media. The *affordances* are those aspects of the environment that support performance of the activity, such as cultural expectations, motivating factors, and equipment adaptations. *Structural media* include those characteristics of the human and nonhuman environment that are specific to the learning task or event and provide information to the child about what is learned. This includes stimuli for production of motor responses and feedback related to the efficacy of the produced motor responses.

Because the situational motor response of a human is multiphasic and multidimensional, motor learning theorists advance the term *coordinated structures.* These are variable combinations of motor actions, such as postural changes, speech, glandular secretions, and movement patterns that work together to produce an action in a specific situation. Gliner hypothesized that the occupational therapist's use of purposeful activity facilitates the acquisition and use of coordinated structures. Through engagement in developmentally appropriate and meaningful activity that involves graded steps, repetitions, and motivational factors, the child acquires practice in the use of multiple motor actions together in variable combinations. This contrasts with a "splinter" approach to skill development that merely involves repetition without motivation, meaning, and transferability.[5]

Cognitive and motivational components of programs

In a series of single subject research projects, Campbell, McInerney, and Cooper[3] manipulated variables of motivation, neuromotor treatment procedures, and training context. Their study examined use of standard program approaches with children and adolescents with severe motor handicaps, but their findings and discussion have implications for occupational therapy in general.

The authors speculated that the typical neuromotor treatment approaches used with severely handicapped children have not sufficiently (or systematically) addressed the cognitive and motivational factors involved in facilitating movement patterns and skill development. For example, in the study of an adolescent with cerebral palsy who had minimal hand and arm function, Campbell, McInerney, and Cooper[3] looked at the influence of variable rewards (motivating factors) on frequency of the same motor response. Given the opportunity to use an external switch to operate a fan, receive vibratory stimuli, and operate tape recorders to play mixed or rock music, the adolescent showed the highest rate of switch operation to listen to rock music.

A typical technique in the application of a neuromotor approach is the use of physically guided movement, initiated and controlled by the therapist. The researchers hypothesized that the use of this technique is often guided by the erroneous assumption, in spite of assessment evidence to the contrary, that the child has the normal sensory integrative and motor capacities needed to learn from the physical guidance. Further, they questioned whether the motivation for such a move rested within the therapist or the child. Accordingly, they conducted a study with a preschool child with cerebral palsy and multiple handicaps. The researchers found that the child's frequency of independent use of a reaching movement markedly increased in a social interaction situation, but the frequency was relatively unchanged in a one-to-one therapy situation.

In the final phase of the studies Campbell, McInerney, and Cooper conducted, they examined the context of program activities. The researchers were aware that occupational therapists need to develop transferable concepts rather than splinter skills; therefore, they evaluated program approaches to develop early hand skills with an adolescent with multiple handicaps. An occupational therapy objective for this student was to improve ability to reach for and open objects. Given the proportionally small amount of the student's time spent individually with the occupational therapist, little improvement in these specific skills was noted. As an alternative approach, the investigators looked for a way to develop the desired skills throughout the student's day in a variety of meaningful environments and situations. Together with other staff, they identified objects that could be opened in different times and places, and trained all staff members in the physical guidance techniques used to facilitate the necessary hand and arm patterns. Results of the alternative program approach were a slow but consistent improvement in the student's interest and ability to initiate hand use. The researchers postulated that this improvement resulted from increased opportunities for repetition, practice, and application, and was reinforced by situational motivating factors.[3]

This last component of the Campbell, McInerney, and Cooper studies is interesting because it raises the issue of transfer of "occupational therapy" skills to other service providers. This is an issue that has haunted both members and leadership of the profession for many years. On reflection, the problem is not unique to occupational therapy. The answer appears to lie in an individual resolution of whether the value of the occupational therapist's skills is in the techniques she uses at any given time, or in her ability to develop technology that meet the needs of clients at a given time. In the research studies reported here, the focus was on how best to meet the needs and improve the skills of the children and adolescents.

Zone of potential development

Lyons[8,9] has published some interesting reports related to occupational therapy applications of Vygotsky's theories of cognitive development. Vygotsky's concept of the zone of "proximal" development, also referred to as the zone of potential development, signifies the child's readiness to develop higher cognitive skills under the guidance of a more capable individual. The zone of potential development contrasts with the child's actual independent level of function. Vygotsky believed that the most effective teaching and learning takes place under conditions that take advantage of childrens' problem-solving potential.

In an early review of Vygotsky's theory, Lyons[9] proposed that occupational therapists determine the child's zone of potential development during assessment, and use these findings in program planning, consultation, and treatment. She suggested that it is inappropriate to modify the initial administration procedure of a standardized test, such as a developmental scale, because this invalidates determination of the child's actual level of independent performance. Lyons recommended subsequent readministration of several of the slightly higher-level items the child had previously failed, with attention to the process that was needed to assist the child to successfully perform the items. Lyons speculated that in fact therapists already make these modifications on an intuitive basis, either through altering directions on a standardized test or through construction of many "therapist-made" tests.

However, when such modifications are made on the initial test administration, important information is lost (i.e., the true lower end of the zone of potential development); a lack of awareness of Vygotsky's theory is demonstrated. Lyons noted that the Purdue Perceptual Motor Survey, the Vulpe Assessment Battery, and the Miller Assessment for Preschoolers (see Chapters 10 and 11) exemplify tests that on first administration can yield information about the zone of potential development. Adherence to standard procedures in each of these tests, or a second administration of failed items from other tests, can yield valuable clues to the therapist. Guidance for prognosis of the degree of improvement that may be anticipated would come from comparing the child's independent level of function with her assisted level of function. In addition, records of the child's response to different methods of assistance would suggest which instructional or facilitative approaches could be most effective in treatment. (See also Chapter 20 for Carrasco's discussion of including the child's response to facilitation techniques as part of the assessment process in cerebral palsy.) Finally, Lyons suggested that information about such approaches, as related to cognitive function and academic skill development, could be responsibly shared with teachers or others in situations where availability of occupational therapy services for children is limited.

To follow up her literature review and program suggestions, Lyons[8] reported on a series of research studies that examined types of guidance to facilitate higher levels of independent performance. The skill she studied was the child's ability to pretend to use a familiar object to carry out a familiar action. Previous researchers had found that 4-year-old normal children tend to use their fingers as the pretend object, whereas 5-year-old children position their hands as if they were holding the object. Lyons looked at the comparative effects of using verbal directions only, prior practice with the real objects, prior demonstration of the desired pattern by an adult, and use of pantomine to establish a context for the requested pretend pattern. Her findings, obtained through a series of experiments designed to rule out other variables, clearly established that the children who observed the adult demonstration showed a significantly higher frequency of the mature (5 or more years) pattern. The use of a pantomined context was the next most effective method; this supports the importance of context concepts suggested by Gliner[5] and Campbell et al.[3] It may be hypothesized that, at least for the age group and types of cognition and hand use studied by Lyons, adult demonstration and guidance, within a framework of meaningful, purposeful activity, has a powerful effect on achievement of a child's potential.

Activity analysis

As discussed in Chapter 7, activity analysis and activity adaptation are the core mental processes used by the occupational therapist throughout assessment and programming. These processes are not new to the student of pediatric occupational therapy, and the components of analysis are generally similar to those applied to adults. However, critical components to activity analysis that must be considered when working with children are the developmental antecedents of the functions, skills, and behaviors necessary to engage in each activity. The importance of cognitive and emotional readiness have been stressed, but the variables of the other component functions and the developmental sequence of habits, skills, and behaviors are equally important. Such awareness allows a therapist to develop a program that will be enjoyable and beneficial rather than frustrating and time-consuming. Each of the subsequent chapters about occupational therapy treatment, both generic and specialized, contains examples of activity analysis. The outline for pediatric activity analysis presented in Chapter 7 (Figure 7-3) is useful for review.

Activity adaptation

The third primary task of program planning is to determine the need for and types of activity adaptations to be used to promote the child's highest level of performance. The major types of adaptation techniques presented earlier in this book include alterations of the position of the body or the work (play) surface, the activity process, levels of independent performance, the tools, materials, and equipment used, and the therapeutic relationship.

For purposes of generalization, adaptations to the position of the body or work surface are used when improved physical access is needed. This might occur with limitations in the size of the child, or in strength or joint mobility. Changes in the activity process are most often used when a child is not developmentally ready to accomplish a desired activity independently. Therefore adaptations are made to simplify the activity or to enhance the results of the child's independent effort. Variations in expected levels of performance tend to be used when readiness or levels of function prohibit a child from completing all components of an activity independently. For example, the therapist might have the mother assist a child through portions of a self-care task but require that the child do certain steps of the process herself. Often it is appropriate to return to more practice with an accomplishable, developmentally-antecedent activity or behavior to strengthen the child's ability to learn higher level tasks. Tools, materials, and equipment, including the therapy environment, are adapted to facilitate more independent performance, or to prevent a loss of function or skill. Such adaptations, including the use of commercial adaptive equipment, are made when it appears that some physical characteristics of the child or the activity are interfering with independence. Finally, the therapist becomes a skilled, but caring, "manipulator" of his or her relationship with the child. The therapist, through knowledge of development and the individual child, learns when to push, when to help, and when to let a child slacken his efforts, in an effort to maintain the best levels of motivation and performance.

Numerous examples of activity adaptations are provided in subsequent chapters. Adaptation techniques are discussed at length in Chapter 17. Creativity is the key, and is a special characteristic among occupational therapists.

OPTIONS FOR SERVICE DELIVERY

A number of decisions need to be made to operationalize a comprehensive program. First, the therapist needs to determine what aspects of the program require his specialized knowledge, and thus should be carried out in direct treatment. There are further considerations as well. What activities need to be practiced and reinforced on a routine basis, and therefore lend themselves to implementation by others, with monitoring by the therapist? What objectives can be met with a short period of intense intervention, and therefore can be handled through consultation, "crisis intervention," or adaptive equipment prescription? Where is the best place to teach a child a new skill, and is another place more appropriate for follow-up practice of the new skill? What program activities should be carried out on a conjoint therapy basis with the physical or speech therapist, or another service provider? What is a realistic amount of home programming for an individual family at a given time? Should training for the home program be carried out at the clinic or is a home visit preferable? Should a particular program be carried out by the school-based therapist or the diagnostic agency therapist? Is the necessary equipment available, or will other materials need to be substituted for a period of time? How many times does a child need to practice a task in each therapy session? When should parents observe treatment and when should they be asked to leave their child alone with the therapist? How many times should a treatment modality be tried with a child before its use is abandoned? These and other situational questions need to be addressed and decisions made and documented.

Regardless of how well constructed a program plan is, it is only useful if it meets the needs of the individuals involved in the therapy process. Any therapist can provide personal examples of perfect plans that were never executed. Plans evaporate when a parent's car breaks down, when the teacher forgets to send a child to therapy, when a sudden and severe illness causes regression, or simply in the face of a child's dislike of the "perfect" activity. Any number of seemingly trivial or overwhelmingly tragic circumstances can prevent implementation of occupational therapy services as planned. For example, an occupational therapist, physical therapist, and special education teacher waited for 2 years to obtain an electronic feeder for a girl with severe cerebral palsy. Two weeks before the feeder arrived and the school year ended, the girl sustained a stress fracture of the hip and was placed on bed rest in a body spica cast. The therapists made a home visit to instruct the parents and home aide in correct positioning and to review range of motion techniques. However, the healing hip fracture and cast were extremely painful to the girl, and she cried whenever her family or the aide tried to use the demonstrated program. Reluctant and fearful to press the girl, the family discontinued their efforts, but were embarrassed to recontact the therapists. When the girl returned to school in the fall, her contractures, loss of strength, and diminished postural stability prevented use of the bright new piece of equipment, and further resulted in loss of other functions and skills that had been developed over 3 years.

The two main factors that caused the situation presented above were the lack of therapy services available in the summer and the parents' feelings. These are not atypical factors; as mentioned in Chapter 7, availability, accessibility, and acceptability are key terms in determining what services are actually delivered. Therefore it becomes critical that the therapist look carefully at options for meeting a child's needs, and develop a workable plan in collaboration with others. In the example above, the therapists assumed, from prior positive experiences with these particular parents, that the program recommendations for the summer would be carried out. The parents assumed that the therapists would be upset to learn that the recommendations had been discontinued. In both cases, the untested assumptions of adults had the most serious consequence for the child toward whom all were directing their concern. Had either side set aside its assumptions, and simply contacted the other, the result might have been very different.

It is important to plan alternatives in advance. As Procter states in Chapter 17, emergency plans are important, and may be applied to the service delivery process as well. Open lines of communication are important, particularly with parents and others who are involved in carrying out the daily routines of the child's habilitation program. When, due to vacations, work hours, and other scheduling variations, the primary therapist is unavailable, other resources for assistance need to be available.

COMPONENTS OF THE WRITTEN PLAN

As stated by Pedretti,[10] the importance of a written program plan cannot be overemphasized. Regulatory procedures that govern most agencies for children's services require written plans. However, even in the absence of an agency policy, such documents are needed to refresh the therapist's memory, to train other staff or caregivers, to be used by a substitute therapist, and to document progress and efficacy. A pool of carefully developed program plans also provides an excellent tool for clinical research (see Chapter 31.)

The program plan format shown in Figure 12-6 has been found clinically useful in a number of educational, health care, and private practice settings. The left hand column records activities that are used to meet behavioral objectives. The second column is used to record physical setup of the activity, work surface, and child or adolescent. The adaptations column may be used to specify techniques, equipment, number of repetitions, assistance needed, and similar information. The "comments" section is used as needed, to note a child's response to the activity or communicate other pertinent information, such as safety concerns, to an assistant or other care provider.

Figure 12-2   Uniform occupational therapy evaluation checklist

---

Procedure
I. *Demographic information*
  A. Personal information
    1. Name
    2. Address
    3. Telephone
    4. Date of birth
    5. Age
    6. Sex
  B. Referral-related information
    1. Date of referral
    2. Reason for referral
    3. Referral source
    4. Date client first seen by OT
    5. Diagnosis
    6. Presenting problems/symptoms
    7. Date of onset
    8. Medications
    9. Precautions/complications
    10. Date of evaluation
    11. Evaluator
  C. Personal history
    1. Developmental history
    2. Educational history
    3. Vocational history
    4. Socioeconomic history
    5. Medical history
II. *Skills and performance areas*
  (See the AOTA *Uniform Terminology System for Reporting Occupational Therapy Services,* January, 1979, for definition of categories.)
  A. Independent living/daily living skills and performance
    1. Physical daily living skills
      a. Grooming and hygiene
      b. Feeding/eating
      c. Dressing
      d. Functional mobility
      e. Functional communication
      f. Object manipulation
    2. Psychological/emotional daily living skills
      a. Self-concept/self-identity
      b. Situational coping
      c. Community involvement

  3. Work
    a. Homemaking
    b. Child care/parenting
    c. Employment preparation
  4. Play/leisure
  B. Sensorimotor skills and performance components
    1. Neuromuscular
      a. Reflex integration
      b. Range of motion
      c. Gross and fine coordination
      d. Strength and endurance
    2. Sensory integration
      a. Sensory awareness
      b. Visual-spatial awareness
      c. Body integration
  C. Cognitive skill and performance components
    1. Orientation
    2. Conceptualization/comprehension
      a. Concentration
      b. Attention span
      c. Memory
    3. Cognitive integration
      a. Generalization
      b. Problem solving
  D. Psychosocial skills and performance components
    1. Self-management
      a. Self-expression
      b. Self-control
    2. Dyadic interaction
    3. Group interaction
  E. Therapeutic adaptation
    1. Orthotics
    2. Prosthetics
    3. Assistive/adaptive equipment
  F. Prevention
    1. Energy conservation
    2. Joint protection/body mechanics
    3. Positioning
    4. Coordination of daily living skills

This outline was taken and adapted from the AOTA Uniform Terminology System for Reporting Occupational Therapy Services, prepared by AOTA Commission on Uniform Reporting System Task Force, Rockville, AOTA, January 7, 1979.

From The American Occupational Therapy Association, Inc, Nov 1981, Occupational Therapy Newspaper.

Figure 12-3 Worksheet for organizing data collection

Performance element	Assessment process	Results (+ = Strength; − = Weakness)
Component functions		
Motor function		
Range of motion		
Gross muscle strength		
Muscle tone		
Endurance		
Functional patterns		
Postural stability		
Mobility		
Gross motor skills		
Prehension-manipulation		
Fine motor skills		
Expressive communication		
Sensory integrative function		
Body scheme		
Postural-bilateral integration		
Visual-spatial relationships		
Sensory-motor integration		
Reflex integration		
Visual and auditory functions		
Somatosensory awareness		
Somatosensory perception		
Cognitive function		
Comprehension		
Written communication		
Verbal communication		
Concentration		
Problem-solving		
Time management		
Conceptualization		
Ability to follow directions		
Integration of learning		
Social function		
Dyadic interaction		
Group interaction		
Cooperation and competition		
Task performance with others		
Emotional functions		
Ability to sublimate drives		
Sources of need gratification		
Tolerance for frustration/anxiety		
Impulse control		
Object relations		
Performance skills		
Age-specific developmental tasks		
Role performance		
Self-care		
Home living		
School living		
Community living		
Play		
Schoolwork		
Prevocational development		
Life space data collection		
Life roles		
Significant others		
Environmental requirements		
Cultural requirements		
Role requirements		
Resources		
Barriers to performance		
Alternatives		
Concurrent goals and programs		

Figure 12-4 Case example: narrative report

Date of report: (month, year)

Occupational therapy evaluation
(Any County Schools)

Student: K.X.   Date of birth: XX/XX/80
Parents: Mr. and Mrs. X
School: Any City Elementary School
Class: Kindergarten, Mrs. Teacher

K. is a 6 year, 9-month-old girl who attends the half-day regular kindergarten program at Any City Elementary School. She was referred for occupational therapy evaluation by the psychologist and school personnel because of her delay in fine motor and social skills in classroom activities.

K. has been seen for evaluation one to two times weekly for ½-hour sessions since March 22, 198X. Because of immature social-emotional behavior, she has been difficult to test. Typically, when asked by her teacher or this therapist to leave the classroom with the therapist, K. sits on the floor or continues with her previous activity, avoiding the request. On several occasions she has agreed to come with the therapist when promised a reward. On other occasions it has been necessary to carry her to the classroom used by the therapist. By report of Mrs. Teacher and other school personnel, this behavior pattern is occurring with increasing frequency when K. is directly asked to do something.

In the testing situation K. tends to cooperate fairly well but within a range of manipulative behavior. She refuses most activities initially, but eventually will try most things when a reward is promised. In general, she seems to like the test activities and often becomes engrossed in the activity once she accepts it. It should be noted that it would have been helpful to administer several additional performance tests to K., but her behavior patterns precluded this.

Tests administered: Any County Schools (A.C.S.) Occupational Therapy (O.T.) Developmental Skills Evaluation; Motor Free Test of Visual Perception; Ayres' Clinical Observations; Observation in classroom activities.

General performance skills: K. has been observed in class during pre-academic sessions with Mrs. Teacher in singing and dress up play groups and when working at prewriting and visual perception activities. In singing and in the small group with Mrs. Teacher, she attended but did not participate. In an activity that looked for words that sounded the same, she pointed to the correct answer in her book but resisted answering the teacher. She finally gave the wrong answer even though her finger was still on the correct answer. When working on prewriting and visual perception worksheets, she focused on the task and did not interact with other children at the same learning station. When asked to share learning materials with other children after she had finished with a task, she refused.

K. seemed to enjoy the dress up sessions and interacted more with other children during that time. She spoke with the other children in three-word sentences and tended to alternate between parallel and cooperative play. She tried to put on as many clothes as possible to make herself a fat man, after another child had done the same.

Because this is a half-day program, K. does not eat at school. Parents report that K. is independent in self-feeding with a spoon but requires considerable assistance with cutting, even soft foods. She can put on most clothing with supervision but needs physical assistance with fasteners and shoes. She washes her hands and toilets independently at school. She is unreliable in school hallways without supervision. At home she is generally supervised by other siblings or parents.

Based on expectations of child development and the observations noted above, her behavior was similar to that seen in a 4- to 5-year-old child during the first few weeks of a new preschool or kindergarten program. It is not typical of a child at the end of kindergarten.

Fine motor skills: K. is able to draw horizontal and vertical lines, a cross, circle, and square. She attempts a triangle and diamond, but the results look like her squares. She was able to draw a house with doors, windows, and roof but did not draw a recognizable human figure. She can cut a piece of paper in two, and she attempted to stay on a ¼-inch line with only one deviation. During the cutting activity, she shifted hands several times. Her left hand appears to be more accurate, and she tended to use this hand more in other activities as well. Cutting and prewriting skills appear to be just below the 5-year-old level.

K. is able to button and unbutton large and small buttons. However, her performance is quite slow. She can remove lacing easily but has considerable difficulty inserting the lacing into holes. She could not tie a bow or her shoelaces—skills that are normally expected of a 6-year-old child. Lateral prehension patterns are adequate for manipulation of objects greater than ½-inch but fine tip prehension is not well developed.

Continued.

Figure 12-4 cont'd. Case example: narrative report

Clinical observations: Throughout the testing K. showed a negative reaction to, and actively avoided being touched by, the therapist. It was necessary to eliminate several checks on gross motor function and muscular development that required direct physical manipulation.

Hand and arm functions: Muscle tone is slightly hypotonic, with some loss of cocontraction of arm, shoulder, and neck musculature, Again, she was defensive during this checkout, so results should be viewed accordingly. She was unable to rotate forearms smoothly and rapidly.

Reflex integration: K. was unable to hold the flexor postural and prone extension patterns for the minimum of 10 seconds. During administration of the arm extension test, she showed a slight loss of balance when her eyes were closed. In all patterns tested, she positioned each body part separately; she could not initiate movements with both arms and legs at the same time.

Ocular pursuits: It was noted that K.'s preferred eye is her right, which contrasts with her left preferred hand. She was unable to cooperate with testing of oculomotor function-visual pursuits.

Gross motor functions: Gross motor function and coordination are typical of patterns seen in ambulatory children with Down syndrome. K. has a broad-based, flat-footed gait with minimal reciprocal movement of the arms. Running is slow and lurching.

Sensory motor functions:

Visual perception: On the Motor Free Test of Visual Perception, K. passed 23 of 36 items. She performed best on items that involved simple matching, form constancy, visual memory, and difference discrimination. She had difficulty on items that tested visual figure-ground discrimination and form-in-space visualization. It should be noted that K. often required more than the usual time limit to pass items. She tended to use a lot of finger tracing and verbalization to determine the correct answers.

Visual-motor function: K. easily replicates familiar designs but has difficulty reproducing drawings and constructions of unfamiliar forms. She pushes away such activities, saying that they are "too easy."

Tactile-kinesthetic processing: Formal testing of somatosensory awareness and discrimination was not possible. However, avoidance of touch has been noted on several occasions, and Mrs. Teacher reports similar observations.

Summary and recommendations: K. presently demonstrates the adaptive skill levels associated with a 4- to 5-year-old child. Her language development appears delayed. She requires one-to-one teaching-training situations with considerable repetition to learn new skills. Her social-emotional behavior is inconsistent and immature with peers and manipulative with adults. Although she is likable in a one-to-one situation, her immaturity and manipulative behavior tend to be disruptive in small group and classroom situations.

It would be to K.'s benefit to be placed in a very structured class with a low teacher-student ratio. Although Mrs. Teacher has worked very well with K. this year, it is doubtful that K. could receive the one-to-one attention that she needs in a regular first-grade classroom. Again, it would be to K's benefit to have her primary educational placement with a specialized Educationally Mentally Handicapped (EMH) teacher. Program needs include training in fine and gross motor skills, social skills, and language development. To supplement her special education program, K. could be seen by the occupational therapist one to two times weekly to develop fine motor skills and sensory integration.

198X Occupational therapy goals and objectives

Goals: 1. Improve skills in school-readiness activities
2. Improve sensory processing

Objectives:

1. K. will cut out a simple geometric form along a ⅛-inch line using her dominant hand with no more than three deviations of more than ⅛-inch 80% of the time.
2. K. will draw a six-part human figure using her dominant hand 80% of the time.
3. K. will fasten three ½-inch button closures on a training board within 2 minutes 80% of the time.
4. K. will rotate both forearms simultaneously at least six times in 10 seconds 80% of the time.
5. K. will hold the prone extension pattern for a minimum of 10 seconds 80% of the time.
6. K. will permit the therapist to touch her arms three times in a row with vision occluded 80% of the time.
7. K. will identify the location of tactile stimuli given on her arms within 5 cm accuracy 80% of the time.

Pat Nuse Clark, M.O.T., OTR/L
Occupational Therapist
Any County Schools

Figure 12-5   Case example: printed report form

Occupational therapy evaluation
Any County Schools

Student: K.X.   Date of birth: XX/XX/XX   Chronological age: 6.9 years
Parents: Mr. and Mrs. X
School: Any City Elementary School
Class: Kindergarten, Mrs. Teacher
Meds-precautions: None stated
Referred by: Dr. Psychologist
Reason for referral: Delay in fine motor skills and social skills in classroom activities.
Pertinent history: K. was diagnosed as having Down syndrome at birth. She has been seen in early intervention
    programs since infancy. Her parents are anxious for her to attend a local school.
Tests administered: A.C.S. O.T. Development Skills Evaluation; Motor Free Test of Visual Perception; Ayres' Clinical
    Observations; observation in classroom activities.
Evaluation summary-current levels and recommendations: As stated in narrative report.
Recommended therapy: One to two times a week, 30-minute sessions
Direct: initially   Monitor-skill support: check at midyear
Consult: Therapy not indicated:
Annual goals: As stated in narrative report.
Objectives: As stated in narrative report.

Pat Nuse Clark, M.O.T., OTR/L
Any County Schools

School-related performance skills:
0 = Normal
1 = Slightly impaired-delayed; independent with adaptations
2 = Moderately impaired-delayed; partial dependence
3 = Severely impaired-delayed; complete dependence

1. Self-feeding: uses spoon, needs maximal assistance with cutting	0 <u>1</u> 2 3
2. Dressing: difficulty with fasteners because of fine motor delay	0 <u>1</u> 2 3
3. Grooming and hygiene: needs reminder to leave bathroom	0 <u>1</u> 2 3
4. Toileting:	<u>0</u> 1 2 3
5. Transfers:	<u>0</u> 1 2 3
6. Movement around school: needs supervision.	0 <u>1</u> 2 3
7. Functional communication: uses words, phrases, three-part sentences	0 <u>1</u> 2 3
8. Age-level schoolwork: needs one-to-one training for new concepts	0 1 <u>2</u> 3
9. Age-level play and recreation: tendency toward parallel and imitative play	0 <u>1</u> 2 3

Fine motor skills:
0 = Normal
1 = Slightly impaired or delayed
2 = Limited performance
3 = Unable to perform

Preferred hand: (L) R (dominance not established)

1. Development of prehension-reach: **X**; grasp: **X**; release: **X**; ulnar grasp: ; radial grasp: **X**; tripod: **X**; lateral pinch: **X**; tip pinch: +/−	0 <u>1</u> 2 3
2. Accuracy of preferred hand use:	0 <u>1</u> 2 3
3. Use of nondominant hand: tendency to switch hands in middle of activity—midline?	0 <u>1</u> 2 3
4. Use of hands in bilateral activities:	0 <u>1</u> 2 3
5. Copying geometric figures: horizontal, vertical lines; cross; square; identifies triangle	0 <u>1</u> 2 3
6. Prints-writes: name: **X** letters: numbers: words: sentences: Check if problems noted in letter formation: **X**; spacing: **X**; directionality: **X**	0 1 <u>2</u> 3
7. Cutting skills: ¼-inch: **X** ⅛-inch: ¹⁄₁₆-inch:	0 1 <u>2</u> 3
straight lines: **X**; angles:; curves:	0 <u>1</u> 2 3

Continued.

Figure 12-5 cont'd.   Case example: printed report form

Clinical observations:
0 = Normal
1 = Slightly impaired; needs improvement
2 = Moderately impaired; interferes with skills
3 = severely impaired; prevents performance

1. Hand and arm functions: slightly hypotonic, some loss of cocontraction, unable to rotate forearms
   smoothly   0 1 2 3
2. Reflex integration: Unable to hold flexor and extension postures for 10 seconds; could not
   move body parts simultaneously   0 1 2 3
3. Ocular pursuits: unable to test; right eye preferred   0 1 2 3

Gross motor functions:
4. Oral-motor: lip closure: **X** slightly hypotonic; swallow: **X**; chew: **X**   0 1 2 3
5. Muscle tone: 0 1 2 3
6. Muscle strength: 0 1 2 3
7. Postural stability: 0 1 2 3
8. Balance-equilibrium: 0 1 2 3
9. Developmental skills (check highest pattern used below): Head control: ; rolling: ; creeping: ;
   sitting: ; kneeling: ; half-kneeling: ; standing: ; climbing: ; running: **X**; other: 0 1 2 3
10. Respiratory control: 0 1 2 3
11. Hopping and skipping: 0 1 2 3

Sensory motor functions: vision: adequate; hearing: adequate
1. Visual perception: Scored 23/36 on MFTVF, required additional time, finger tracing   0 1 2 3
2. Visual-motor function: see comments concerning fine motor   0 1 2 3
3. Tactile-kinesthetic processing: unable to test; however, noted defensive responses throughout
   evaluation; teacher agrees   0 1 2 3
4. Bilateral body integration: 0 1 2 3
5. Motor planning: requires considerable repetition to learn new skills   0 1 2 3
6. Vestibular functioning: unable to test; reportedly likes swinging and other vestibular stimulation activities 0 1 2 3

Prevocational skills:
1. Attention span: will stay on task once engaged   0 1 2 3
2. Ability to follow directions: 0 1 2 3
3. Ability to work with others: manipulative with adults, interacts minimally with peers—parallel
   play preferred   0 1 2 3

NOTE: Problems in performance appear to result primarily from: motor impairment (#4); cognitive
impairment (#2); sensory-integrative impairment (#3); behavioral impairment (#1)

Adaptations and equipment needs:
Current status: one-to-one assistance from teacher or aide
    Environmental: recommend at least partial EMH placement
    Splinting: not indicated
    Wheelchair-mobility equipment: not indicated
    Small adaptive equipment: not indicated

Figure 12-6

NAME: _____   DATE: _____

OCCUPATIONAL THERAPY WEEKLY PROGRAM

ACTIVITIES	SET UP	ADAPTATIONS	COMMENTS
(1) (Objective)			
(2)			
(3)			
(4)			

SUMMARY

The program planning process, documented through written assessment reports and program plans, is one of the critical ingredients of professional level occupational therapy. Interpreting assessment results, developing a prioritized problem list of the child's needs, and developing goals and objectives to describe and document the intervention program are important means of communication between the therapist, parents, and other service providers. In addition, the program planning process operationalizes the application of the therapist's knowledge, skills, attitudes, and resources to meet the specific needs of an individual child. As part of this process, the therapist will consider the relationships between the child, his environments, the activity, and therapy practices, including treatment approaches and adaptations. Ongoing analysis and adaptation of the activity process, with special regard to learning factors and situational contexts that are meaningful to the child or adolescent, is a unique contribution of the occupational therapist to the child's comprehensive program.

STUDY QUESTIONS

All of these questions relate to the case example (K.X.) presented in Figures 12-4 and 12-5, narrative and printed report forms.

1. As you review the reports, identify and categorize critical factors (as specified by Hopkins and Tiffany) that the therapist needs to consider for program planning, according to: the patient, the therapist, the activity, and the context. How do the issues discussed by Gliner, Campbell, McInerney, and Cooper, and Lyons relate to this case?
2. K's program was developed for a public school, so problems, goals and objectives were limited to those that could be implemented under the restraints of PL 94-142. As you review this case, identify and prepare two additional problems and related goals that might be implemented in another type of setting.
3. Develop three measurable objectives for each goal above.
4. What information is missing from the report that would help you plan a better program for K.X.?
5. Using the format provided in Figure 12-6, develop a program plan to meet one of the objectives you have prepared and two of the existing objectives from Figure 12-4.

REFERENCES

1. American Occupational Therapy Association: Guidelines for occupational therapy documentation, Am J Occup Ther 40:830, 1986.
2. American Occupational Therapy Association: Uniform terminology for reporting occupational therapy services and uniform occupational therapy evaluation checklist, Occup Ther Newspaper 35:9, 1981.
3. Campbell PH, McInerney WF, and Cooper MA: Therapeutic programming for students with severe handicaps, Am J Occup Ther 38:594, 1984.
4. Gilfoyle EA, editor: Training: occupational therapy educational management in schools: a competency based educational program, module 3, vol II. Rockville, Md, 1980, American Occupational Therapy Association, Inc.
5. Gliner JA: Purposeful activity in motor learning theory: an event approach to motor skill acquisition, Am J Occup Ther 39:28, 1985.
6. Hopkins HL, and Tiffany EG: Occupational therapy: a problem-solving process. In Hopkins HL, and Smith HD: Willard and Spackman's occupational therapy, 6, Philadelphia, 1983, JB Lippincott Co.
7. Llorens LA, and Schuster JA: Occupational therapy sequential client care recording system: a comparative study, Am J Occup Ther 31:367, 1977.
8. Lyons BG: Defining a child's zone of proximal development: evaluation process for treatment planning, Am J Occup Ther 38:446, 1984.
9. Lyons BG: Zone of potential development for 4-year-olds attempting to simulate use of absent objects, Occup Ther J Res 6:33, 1986.
10. Pedretti LW: Occupational therapy practice skills for physical dysfunction, 2, St Louis, 1985, The CV Mosby Co.
11. Uniform data system for medical rehabilitation. Buffalo, NY, 1987, Data Management Service, Department of Rehabilitation Medicine, Buffalo General Hospital (100 High Street, Buffalo, NY, 14203).
12. Vulpe S: Vulpe assessment battery: Developmental assessment performance analysis and individualized programming for the atypical child, Downsview, Ontario, Canada, 1979, National Institute on Mental Retardation.
13. Yerxa EJ, and Sharrott G: Liberal arts: the foundation for occupational therapy education, Am J Occup Ther 40:153, 1986.

PART V

GENERIC OCCUPATIONAL THERAPY: MAJOR AREAS OF CHILDHOOD PERFORMANCE

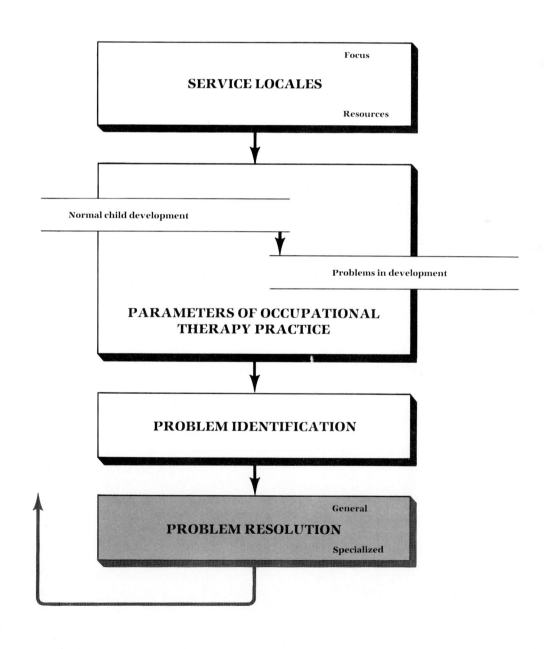

13

Development of hand functions

CHARLOTTE E. EXNER

Hand function is critical to interaction with the environment. Hands allow us to act on our world through contact with our own and others' bodies and through contact with objects. Hands are the "tools" most often used to accomplish work, to play, and to perform self-maintenance tasks. The child who has a disability affecting the hand has less opportunity to take in sensory information from the environment and to experience the effect of his or her actions on the world.

COMPONENTS OF HAND FUNCTION

Effective use of the hands to engage in daily occupational activities is dependent upon a complex interaction of visual perception and fine motor functions. This interaction, referred to as *visual-perceptual-fine motor function,* has four major components: fine motor skills, visual skills, visual perceptual skills, and visual-motor skills. It is recognized that other parts of the body have fine motor skills, but this discussion will refer to the hand only. In addition, it is assumed that the development of visual-perceptual-fine motor function is dependent upon adequate somatosensory and postural functions, and these will not be discussed in detail.

Fine motor skills are those patterns that normally rely on both tactile-proprioceptive and visual information for accuracy. However, fine motor skills may be accomplished without visual feedback if somatosensory functions provide adequate information. The patterns include basic reach, grasp, carry, release, and the more complex skills of in-hand manipulation and bilateral hand use. Brief definitions of these patterns follow.

Reach Movement and stabilization of the arm and hand for the purpose of contacting an object with the hand.
Grasp Attainment of an object with the hand.
Carry The movement of the arm in space for the purpose of transporting a hand-held object from one place to another.

Release The intentional letting go of a hand-held object at a specific time and place.
In-hand manipulation The adjustment of an object within the hand after grasp.
Bilateral hand use The effective use of two hands together to accomplish an activity.

In this discussion, *hand-arm* refers to the interactive movement and stabilization of different parts of the hand and arm to accomplish a fine motor task.

Visual skills are the use of extraocular muscles to direct eye movements. These include the ability to visually fix on a stationary object and the smooth, accurate tracking of a moving target.

Visual perceptual skills are the recognition, discrimination, and processing of sensory information through the eyes and related central nervous system structures. Visual perceptual skills include the identification of shapes, objects, colors, and other qualities; the orientation of objects or shapes in space; and the relationship of objects or shapes to each other.

DEVELOPMENTAL CONCEPTS
Factors that influence the development of hand function

As children mature, they begin to effectively coordinate visual with fine motor skills, and later combine eye-hand coordination with visual perceptual skills.[3] These skills, in conjunction with cognitive and social development, allow the child to engage in increasingly complex activities. Although motor issues are usually given the most attention, many other dimensions of development significantly impact effective hand use. These include the child's culture, social factors, cognitive factors, visual perceptual development, sensory integration, somatosensory function, and visual regard.

CULTURE

In some African cultures the accomplishment of gross motor skills is emphasized over the development of fine manipulative skills.[46] In other cultures, expectations are greater for development of skilled handling of tools, writing, and other fine motor skills. For example, Saeki, Clark, and Azen[41] reported that Japanese children aged 5 to 10 years performed better on the Motor Accuracy Test than did their Japanese-American counterparts. Both of these groups of children were more skilled on the test than Caucasian children.

SOCIAL FACTORS

Lewis[32] found that children who live in poverty may have less access to material goods, such as construction toy sets. These toys involve material handling and require the child to follow directions. The child is asked to associate a visual image of a desired object with the gradual construction of that object. Poor children may also have less opportunity to play with school readiness materials, such as pencils, paints, scissors, paste, and rulers. This again places them at a disadvantage in comparison to peers who have had greater exposure to school materials.

Another social factor that may influence proficiency of hand skills is the child's sex. Gender role stereotyping remains evident in the choice of toys that are given to children. For example, Etaugh et al[16] and Fein et al[22] noted that boys tend to be given and choose constructive and manipulative toys more often than girls. Girls are given and tend to choose dolls and other small materials such as toy housework equipment, paint, crayons, and books. Girls playing with such items may develop similar fine motor tasks, but they do not learn to translate two-dimensional graphic information into three-dimensional constructions. This difference may place girls at a disadvantage in developing complex perceptual-fine motor skills. This disadvantage may be compounded for handicapped children, as their opportunities for independent toy and play selection decrease.

COGNITIVE FUNCTION

In clinical situations, children with short attention spans demonstrate less visual monitoring of hands, tend to perform with speed rather than accuracy, and show less desire for manipulative tasks that require persistence. For this reason, their hand skills are often immature. Children with severe cognitive deficits rarely develop refined in-hand manipulation and bilateral hand use because their conceptual ability does not extend itself to constructive and symbolic play situations.

VISUAL PERCEPTION

Problems in visual perception may or may not be associated with cognitive delays. Regardless, visual perceptual dysfunction affects the child's ability to use tools and relate materials to one another.[4] Thus bilateral manipulative skills are affected to a greater degree than the basic prehension patterns. The child with vi-

sual perceptual deficits may show problems with cutting, coloring and writing, construction, doing puzzles, using fasteners, and brushing teeth.

SENSORY INTEGRATION

The types of sensory integration problems (Chapter 23) that are most likely to influence hand use are tactile defensiveness, poor bilateral integration, and dyspraxia. The defensive child is likely to avoid contact with certain materials, thus limiting exposure to varied objects. Bilateral integration dysfunction limits development of in-hand manipulation and bilateral hand use. Motor planning deficits are often seen in children with fine motor problems. These problems may be associated with poor body scheme (particularly poor awareness of the fingers as individual units) and poor tactile discrimination.[4]

SOMATOSENSORY AWARENESS

Sensory deficits are common in children with cerebral palsy[48] and those with sensory integration disorders.[4] Children with spastic cerebral palsy frequently have deficits in stereognosis, graphesthesia, two-point discrimination, and localization of touch.[30,38] Curry and Exner[12] found that about 70% of a group of preschool children with cerebral palsy showed significantly different tactile preferences from normal children of the same age.

In a study of school-aged children with and without cerebral palsy, Jones[30] found that children with athetoid involvement had significant problems with proprioception. The children with spastic involvement scored just slightly lower on this function than did uninvolved children. Hulme et at[29] found that "clumsy" school-aged children performed significantly more poorly on tests of kinesthesia than did normal children. In the latter study, Hulme et al also found a moderately high correlation between kinesthesia scores and motor skill time scores.

VISUAL REGARD

Fraiberg et al[24] noted that without early intervention, a visual problem can delay the infant's knowledge of his or her own hands as well as awareness of objects that can be reached for and grasped. As a result, reach and grasp skills of visually impaired infants develop later than in sighted children. However, the Fraiberg study noted that once skills are facilitated, they are effectively used by the visually impaired child as long as they are not negatively affected by cognitive or somatosensory problems.

Motor and physical factors in hand development

INTEGRITY OF THE HAND

The integrity of the hand is an important consideration in hand function. Children with congenital hand anomalies may be missing one or more digits, thus significantly affecting the variety of possible prehension patterns. Refined finger movements and in-hand manipulation skills may also be limited or absent. Severe congenital anomalies can affect bilateral hand use. Involvement of the thumb has a more significant effect on hand function development than impairment of any other digit.

RANGE OF JOINT MOTION

Range of joint motion has a significant effect on positioning the arm for hand use and reaching and carrying skills. Effective hand function is also dependent upon adequate mobilization of distal muscle groups that control palmar arches. Limitations in range (Chapters 6 and 24) may occur as a result of abnormal joint structure, muscle weakness, and joint inflammation. Any of the problems that decrease range of motion are likely to affect the child's endurance in fine motor tasks, particularly if the task requires sustained use of the hand in one position or against resistance.

TONE

Tone of muscle groups will affect the stability of parts of the upper extremities during activities as well as the types of movements possible. Tone abnormalities, caused by nervous system impairment, will affect range of joint motion and, in general, will decrease speed of movement. Increased tone tends to result in loss of range; decreased tone results in exaggerated joint range, thereby decreasing stability. Children with fluctuating tone typically have full range, but can maintain joint stability only at the extreme end of a joint position (full flexion or full extension). In addition, movements are less controlled and often appear to be too fast for the task.

Developmental foundations of hand function

This chapter will review and elaborate on information presented in Part II of this text. As discussed in Chapter 3, *gradients of growth* are pertinent to a discussion of hand function development. The proximal-distal progression here refers to the development of some degree of trunk and scapulo-humeral control before the emergence of refined hand function. Additionally, there is a proximal-distal progression in the development of prehension patterns, as palmar holding occurs before finger control of objects. Mass to specific action suggests that less differentiated movement patterns will precede discrete, highly specialized skills. For example, gross, inaccurate reaching will be used first, and gradually be refined and replaced by accurately timed, smooth, direct reaching with effective hand placement. Finally, there is a progression of ulnar to medial to radial control of objects in development of grasp patterns.

Refined movements are also dependent upon the ability to effectively combine *patterns of stability and mobility.*[7] The child must develop the ability to stabilize the trunk effectively and maintain it in an upright position without relying on frequent use of one or both arms to maintain balance. Also, the child sequentially develops patterns of stability and mobility in the scapulo-humeral, elbow, and wrist joints. This permits arm use that is independent from, but effectively used with, trunk movement. Eventually, independent movement and stabilization of the hand and fingers develop.

For normal functioning, joints must be able to stabilize at any point within the normal range of movement and to move within small, medium, or large segments of range. At times during upper extremity fine motor activities, the proximal joints are more stable. Grasping is an example. However, as in carrying, there are times when distal joints are more stable. Occasionally, as in adult handwriting, the elbow, forearm, and wrist joints are stable, while the shoulder and finger joints are mobile.

Another important sequence is the development of straight movement patterns prior to the emergence of controlled rotation patterns. For example, the baby first develops controlled stability and mobility in basic flexion and extension of the shoulder, elbow, and wrist. This is followed by control of internal and external rotation of the shoulder and pronation and supination of the forearm.

In normal development, the infant progresses from gross asymmetrical patterns to generalized symmetries, to mature, voluntarily controlled asymmetrical patterns. This sequence is dependent upon the child's maturing ability to dissociate movements from one another for specialized purposes. The baby uses upper extremities initially in patterns that are not coordinated. Movement of one arm often elicits reflexive, non-purposive reactions in the other arm. Gradually, the baby develops the ability to move the two arms together in the same pattern. As skilled use of symmetrical hand/arm patterns is refined, the baby begins to use the two arms discriminatively for different parts of an activity. For example, an object is stabilized with one hand while the other hand is used to manipulate it. Overflow and associated movements gradually decrease to allow separate but coordinated action of the two hands together.

DEVELOPMENT OF HAND FUNCTION

As in all areas of occupational therapy, academic study of hand skill development and treatment must be supplemented with clinical awareness. Directed observation in practice settings is highly recommended. In addition, it is helpful to try out each of the normal and abnormal movements and patterns described in the text, both as isolated actions and also within the context of activity performance.

Reach

The random arm movements of the newborn are asymmetrical. Soon, however, the baby shows increasing visual regard of the hands and objects close to him. This visual awareness is followed by swiping or batting of objects, with the arm in an abducted position. Objects are rarely grasped, and then only by accident, because the baby is not yet able to sustain an open hand while stabilizing the arm away from the body.

Gradually, a midline orientation of the hands develops. Initially, the hands are held close to the body, but, as visual regard increases, the child holds her hands further away to view them. This pattern precedes the onset of symmetrical bilateral reaching, usually first in supine and then in sitting. Reach is initiated with humeral abduction, partial shoulder internal rotation and elbow extension, forearm pronation, and full finger extension.

As the baby shows increasing dissociation of the two body sides during movement, unilateral reaching begins. Abduction and internal rotation of the shoulder are less prominent, and the hand is usually more open than necessary for the size of the object. As scapular control and trunk stability mature, the baby begins to use shoulder flexion, slight external rotation, full elbow extension, forearm supination, and slight wrist extension during reaching. It should be noted that supination of the forearm is not seen until some external rotation is used to stabilize the humerus. Mature reach is usually seen in conjunction with sustained trunk extension and a slight rotation of the trunk toward the object of interest. Over the next few years, the child will refine this unilateral reaching pattern, increasing accuracy of arm placement and grading of finger extension as appropriate to a specific object (Figure 13-1).

Hand reflexes: foundations of grasp patterns

Twitchell[47] described a series of hand reflexes occurring in the young infant that provide a tactile-proprioceptive foundation for development of purposeful grasp. These reflexes influence the normal baby's hand use and may predominate over the development of more refined hand use in children with central nervous system damage. Although strong influence usually diminishes within the first year, Twitchell found that elements of the hand reflexes may be seen through the preschool years.

The earliest occurring hand reflex is the *traction response.*[47] This is a pattern of strong flexion throughout the upper extremity when the shoulder is passively abducted. This response is present in newborns, and gradually diminishes in strength over the next 5 months.

The *grasp reflex*[47] may be a full reaction or a less complete response, called fractionation of the grasp reflex. When the baby is about 4 weeks old, tactile stimulation to the radial portion of the palm and web space of the thumb elicits a response of thumb and index finger adduction. Over the following weeks, broader con-

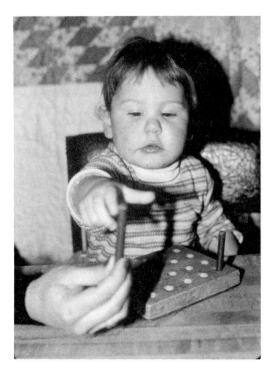

Figure 13-1 This normal child demonstrates reach with trunk rotation, full elbow extension, slight forearm rotation, and wrist stability, yet some degree of excess finger extension before grasp.

Photograph by Ed Exner.

tact with the palm and proximal surface of the fingers is needed to elicit the reflex, but the response is also one of more complete finger flexion and adduction.

By 3 to 4 months, stimulation of the grasp reflex must include proprioceptive and tactile qualities. Contact must originate in the radial part of the palm and move toward the distal part of the baby's hand. The baby responds with rapid, mass finger flexion. If resistance is given to the baby's finger movement, flexion is sustained. This reflex usually disappears by approximately 4 to 5 months of age and more isolated hand use is established.

As the full grasp reflex diminishes, the fractionated pattern occurs. Ammon and Etzel[1] identified the stimulus for this reaction as proprioceptive input to one finger on its palmar surface. Presence of the fractionated reflex is evidenced by flexion of an isolated finger.

The *avoiding reaction*[47] appears in the neonatal period and persists throughout infancy. However, it is not fully integrated until the child is 6 to 7 years old. This reaction occurs in response to stimuli applied to the back of the hand and fingers, the ulnar border of the hand, or the palmar surface of the fingertips. The reflex reaction acts to move the hand away from the stimulation, by pronating or supinating differentially in response to ulnar or radial hand contact.

The *instinctive grasp reaction*[47] helps the baby develop an appropriate orientation of the hand to the object being grasped. The stimulus may be either stationary or moving light touch along either the radial or ulnar side of the hand. At 4 to 5 months, radial contact elicits a slight supination of the forearm, but by 7 to 8 months the hand will grope to find an object presented at either side. By 8 to 10 months, the baby will follow a moving stimulus with her hand.

GRASP

Napier[37] proposed two basic terms to describe hand movements: prehensile and non-prehensile. *Non-prehensile movements* involve pushing or lifting the object with the fingers or entire hand. In contrast, *prehensile movements* involve grasp of an object, and may be further divided according to purpose of the grasp: precision or power. *Precision grasps* are characterized by opposition of the thumb to finger tips to hold an object. *Power grasps* involve the entire hand and are used to resist forces on the object being held. The thumb may be held flexed or adducted to other fingers according to control requirements.

The grasp pattern that is used is usually determined by the intended activity and characteristics of the objects. Small objects are generally held in a precision grasp, primarily due to the large amount of sensory feedback that is available through the fingertips. Medium objects may be held with either pattern, and large objects are held with a power grasp. Napier noted a frequent interplay between precision and power handling of different objects according to the activity process.

A slightly different method of classification, described by Weiss and Flatt,[49] also uses thumb position as a determinant. Grasps with no thumb opposition include hook and power grasps and lateral pinch. The patterns that use thumb opposition include tip and palmar pinches. The palmar pinch category is further divided into standard, spherical, cylindrical, and disc grasps.

The *hook grasp* is used when strength of grasp must be maintained to carry objects. The transverse metacarpal arch is essentially flat, fingers are adducted with flexion at the interphalangeal (IP) joints, and flexion or extension at the metacarpophalangeal (MCP) joints[49] (Figure 13-2).

In contrast, the *power grasp* is often used to control tools or other objects. Maximum power is obtained with horizontal placement of the object in the palm and full thumb and finger flexion.[49] Precision handling with this grasp, for hairbrushing as an example, is facilitated by oblique placement in the hand, more finger extension on the radial side of the hand, and thumb extension and adduction. Thus the object is stabilized with the ulnar side of the hand and controlled for position

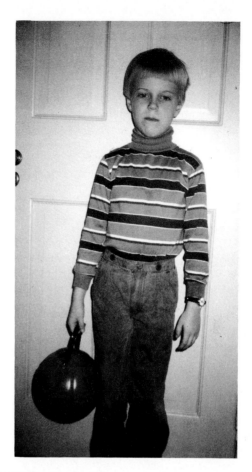

Figure 13-2   Hook grasp.

and use by the radial side of the hand[49] (Figure 13-3).

Lateral pinch is used to exert power on or with a small object. This pattern is characterized by partial thumb adduction, MCP extension, and IP flexion.[49] The index finger is held in a slightly flexed position. The pad of the thumb is placed against the radial side of the index finger at or near the distal interphalangeal (DIP) joint (Figure 13-4).

Tip pinch is characterized by opposition of the thumb and index finger tips, so that a circle is formed[49] (Figure 13-5). All joints of the fingers and thumb are partially flexed. This pinch pattern is used to obtain very small objects.

Patterns of *palmar pinch* include standard, spherical, cylindrical, and disc. In all patterns, the thumb pad is opposed to the pad of at least one finger. The thumb is more adducted and the IP joints of both thumb and fingers are more extended than in tip pinch.

There are two types of *standard* palmar pinch. When the thumb is opposed to the index finger pad only, this pattern may be referred to as pad to pad,[44] standard palmar pinch,[49] two-point pinch,[44] or pincer grasp.[25] Opposition of the thumb simultaneously to index and middle finger pads, providing increased stabil-

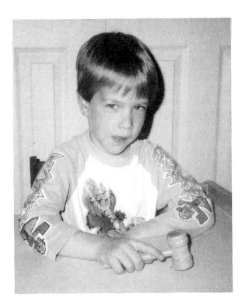

Figure 13-3   Power grasp.

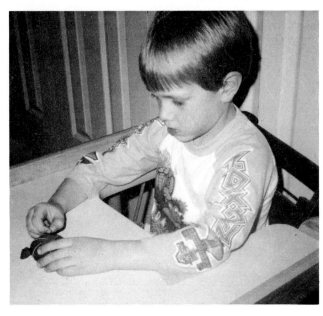

Figure 13-5   Tip pinch. Normal radial grasps, such as tip pinch, are accompanied by slight forearm supination.

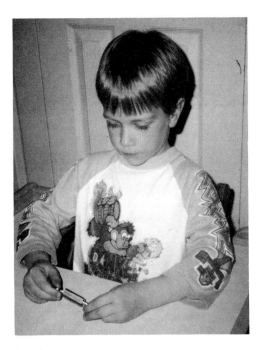

Figure 13-4   Lateral pinch.

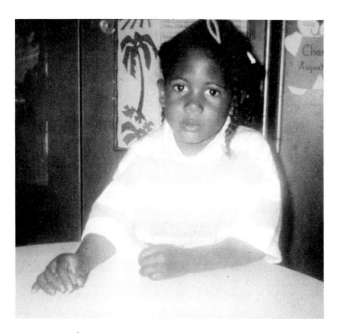

Figure 13-6, A   Pincer grasp.

Courtesy Council Day Care Center, Towson State University, Towson, Md.

ity of prehension, has been called three-point pinch,[44] three jaw chuck,[15] and radial digital grasp[25] (Figure 13-6, *A* and *B*).

Differences in hand posture characterize the other palmar grasps. *Spherical grasp* is marked by significant wrist extension, finger abduction, and even flexion at the MCP and IP joints. Stability of the longitudinal arch is necessary to use this pattern to grasp large objects.

Extension of the transverse arch allows the hypothenar eminence to lift and cup the hand to increase stabilization and control of the object[49] (Figure 13-7).

In the *cylindrical grasp,* the transverse arch is more flattened to allow the fingers to hold against the object.

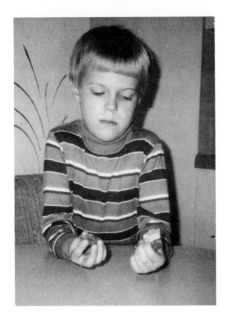

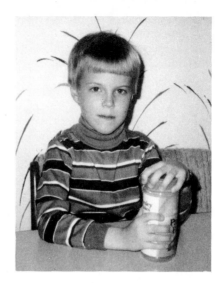

Figure 13-8 The child uses a cylindrical grasp with his right hand and a disc grasp with his left.

Figure 13-6, B This child is using a 3-jaw chuck grasp with his left hand and a variation of this grasp pattern with the right.

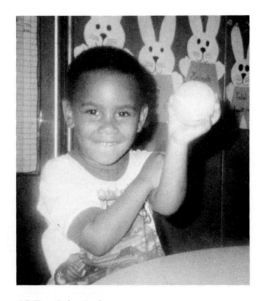

Figure 13-7 Spherical grasp.

Courtesy Council Day Care Center, Towson State University, Towson, Md.

The fingers are only slightly abducted, and IP and MCP joint flexion is graded according to the size of the object. When additional force is required, more of the palmar surface of the hand contacts the object[49] (Figure 13-8).

Disc grasp[49] is characterized by finger abduction that is graded according to the size of the object held,

hyperextension of the MCP joints, and flexion of the IP joints (Figure 13-8). The wrist is more flexed when objects are larger, and only the pads of the fingers contact the object. The amount of thumb extension also increases with object size. The transverse metacarpal arch is flattened in this prehension pattern.

SEQUENTIAL DEVELOPMENT OF GRASP PATTERNS

Initially, the infant is dominated by hand reflexes, alternately opening and closing the hand in response to various sensory stimuli. Gradually, the traction response and grasp reflex decrease, and a voluntary ulnar grasp begins to emerge. Within the next 3 to 4 months, the baby progresses through holding objects with a palmar grasp (see Figures 4-1 and 9-4 in Chapters 4 and 9) and then with a radial palmar pattern. Another progression in the development of grasp is a proximal to distal one, with objects held first in the palm, then on finger surfaces, and finally at the finger pads.[28] These progressions reflect the baby's decreasing flexor tone in the hand and an increased ability to supinate the forearm. During weight-bearing on the upper extremities, the baby gradually moves from a fisted hand posture to one of more finger extension. This pattern appears to contribute to the baby's use of a more open hand during initiation of grasp. Similarly, the baby's growing interest in objects, and desire to attain them, also affect skill in hand use.

At 8 to 9 months, the baby begins to use three-point prehension, a refinement of the radial palmar pattern. Immature two-point prehension begins to emerge soon after, with the fingers held in more extension during reach phase than necessary for the size of the object. The wrist is held in a neutral position, and when the object is grasped, all fingers pull into some degree of flexion. Thus the pattern appears to be a "raking" action, without differential inhibition of movements of fingers on the ulnar side of the hand. Gradually, the baby refines this pattern and achieves more inhibition of the third, fourth, and fifth fingers. The baby's improved sensory awareness and discrimination of the qualities of a desired object, together with increasing wrist and MCP joint stability, result in use of more selective movements. Eventually only the index finger and thumb are extended during grasp initiation (Figure 13-1).

In-hand manipulation

"Manipulation" refers to the general movement of objects or the movement of objects to accomplish a task. The process of adjusting objects within the hand after grasp is called "in-hand manipulation."[19] A related term, "precision handling," means that there is ". . . a change in position of the handled object, either in space or about its own axes"[33] (p. 854). Elliott and Connolly[14] use the term "intrinsic movements of the hand" and define this as use of the fingers to manipulate a hand-held object. It is important to be aware of these different terms for effective communication with families and other professionals.

In-hand manipulation skills have a major impact on efficient and effective accomplishment of fine motor tasks. The child who cannot use a variety of in-hand skills may complete a task, but will appear slow and awkward. Deficiency is likely to have far-reaching effects in self-maintenance, play, school, and vocational readiness skills. The occupational therapist frequently assesses the product of in-hand manipulation, such as the number of beads strung in 30 seconds, the child's ability to button or tie a bow, or the quality and speed of his handwriting. However, the process of manipulation must also be assessed, because treatment to improve the product is often appropriately implemented through strategies to improve the process.

Exner[19] identified three basic categories of in-hand manipulation skills: translation, shift, and rotation. *Translation*[33] is a linear movement of the object from the palm to the fingers or fingers to the palm. Finger-to-palm translation[19] is the more basic pattern, and uses movement from finger extension to flexion. In contrast, palm-to-finger translation requires isolated thumb control and a movement from finger flexion to controlled finger extension. Either type of movement can occur while the person is holding only one object (translation without stabilization) or while he is holding several objects (translation with stabilization).

Shift[19] is a linear movement of the object between or among the fingers. Shift movements may occur in vertical or horizontal directions. For example, an object may be shifted from a proximal to a distal position on the fingers or from the pad of the ring finger to that

of the index finger. Horizontal shift movements are very slight, as in shifting pages to turn only one at a time. Sometimes objects are moved in a linear direction with no change in fingers contacted, as in shifting a pen into position for writing. When shift patterns are used the object usually ends in a position against the pad of one or more fingers. The thumb may be in an opposed position, or slightly adducted with extension of the MCP and IP joints. Shift, like translation, may occur with or without stabilization of other objects in the hand.

Rotation[33] is movement of an object around one or more of its axes. Elliott and Connolly[14] refer to different movements that are similar to rotation, including the "radial roll," "rock," "index roll," "twiddle," "rotary step," and the "interdigital step." Objects may be turned horizontally or end-over-end. These movements occur at the pads of the fingers and require skilled isolation of thumb and finger actions. Thumb opposition is used more in rotation than in translation and shift patterns.[19] At times the thumb is held stable as the fingers rotate an object against its pad. Other times the object is stabilized by the fingers and rotated by the thumb. Picking up and orienting a pen into a mature grasp pattern for writing requires rotation and shift. Other objects may or may not be stabilized in the hand during use of rotation.

DEVELOPMENTAL ASPECTS

Ongoing research by this author[18-20] is directed toward determining a sequence and assessment instrument for in-hand manipulation skill development. Preliminary findings indicate that there are important motor skill prerequisites of in-hand manipulation. These skills include: thumb stability in opposition and abduction, presence of isolated finger use, ability to curve and adjust the distal transverse arch of the palm, and ability to grasp on the finger surfaces. Wrist stability in neutral to extended positions, and the ability to at least partially supinate the forearm also appear important. These findings are supported by related work previously reported by Long et al,[33] Skerik et al,[43] and Napier.[37] Obviously, in-hand manipulation skill progression is influenced by development of tactile discrimination, sensory integration, perception, and cognition.

Carry

Carrying involves a smooth combination of body movements while stabilizing an object in the hand. Small ranges of movements are used and adjusted in accordance with task demands. Cocontraction often occurs in the more distal joints of the wrist and hand. The forearm must have stability in all positions. Similarly, the child must be able to use shoulder rotation patterns effectively with anterior, posterior, and lateral movements of the humerus.

Voluntary release

Voluntary release also depends on control of arm movements. To place an object for release, the arm needs to move into position accurately and then stabilize, as the fingers and thumb extend. Ayres[2] stated that the development of smooth, accurate release of small objects normally takes several years. Initially, release is governed by hand reactions and reflexes, and often objects must be forcibly removed from the baby's hand in the presence of a strong grasp reflex.

As the baby's nondiscriminative responses to tactile and proprioceptive stimuli decrease, and visual control and cognitive development increase, more volitional control of release occurs. This is seen as the baby begins to drop objects, but without intent or accurate placement. As mouthing of objects increases, and the baby becomes more proficient in bringing both hands to midline and playing with them there, the transfer of objects from one hand to another emerges. Initially the object is stabilized in the mouth during transfers, or is pulled out of one hand by the other. Soon the baby begins to freely transfer the object from one hand to another. The object is stabilized by the receiving hand and the releasing hand is fully opened.

Toward the end of the first year of life, the baby begins to release objects without stabilizing with the other hand. The arm is fully extended during release.[11] Shoulder control appears to develop in conjunction with voluntary release as the baby freely drops objects in a circumference. The next step is development of elbow stability in various positions, and the baby begins to release with the elbow in more flexion. The arm or hand is now often stabilized on the surface during release. At about 1 year the objects are released with shoulder, elbow, and wrist stability, but MCP joints re-main unstable during this pattern so the child must still extend the fingers completely (Figure 13-9, *A, B,* and *C*). The release pattern will be refined over the next few years until the child can release small objects with graded extension of the fingers, indicating control over the intrinsic muscle groups of the hand.

Bilateral hand use

As discussed earlier, the normal baby progresses from asymmetry to symmetry to differentiated asymmetrical movements in bilateral hand use. Asymmetrical movements occur up to about 3 months. Symmetrical patterns predominate between 3 and 10 months, when bilateral reach, grasp, and mouthing of the hands and objects occur. These movements are controlled primarily at the shoulder, with the hands engaged at midline. More complex bilateral symmetrical skills, such as catching or bouncing a large ball, will develop later in childhood.

The ability to use differentiated movements begins at about 8 to 10 months. Initially, arm movements are reciprocal or alternating. However, by 12 to 18

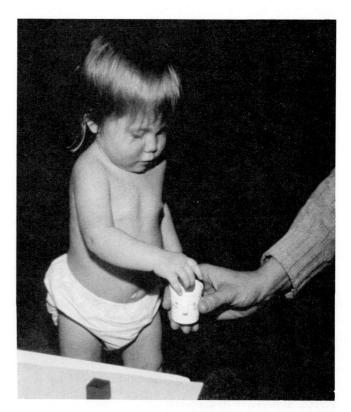

Figure 13-9, B The shoulder, elbow, and wrist are stable and less finger extension occurs with release. The child can release objects into a small container.

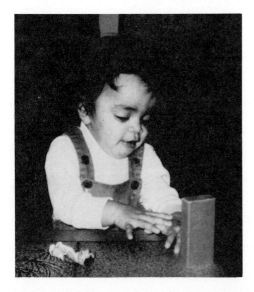

Figure 13-9, A Full finger extension and some wrist movement occur with voluntary release.

Courtesy Kennedy Institute, Baltimore, Md.

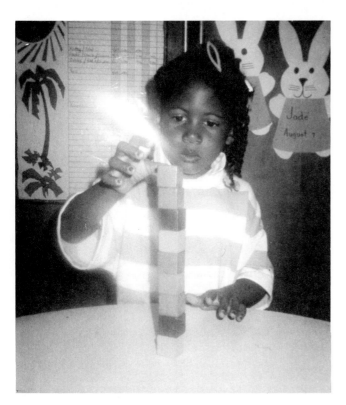

Figure 13-9, C Shoulder, elbow, forearm, wrist, and finger stability combine with perceptual development to promote accurate placement of objects off a surface.

Courtesy Council Day Care Center, Towson State University, Towson, Md.

months, materials are stabilized with and without grasp.[11] For these skills to emerge, the baby must be able to dissociate the two sides of the body and begin to use the two hands simultaneously for different functions. Effective stabilization of materials, of course, also depends on adequate shoulder, elbow, and wrist stability (Figures 13-4, 13-5, 13-6 *B*, and 13-8). Patterns used are similar to those used at the same age level for voluntary release.

Between 18 and 24 months, the child begins to develop skills that are precursors to simultaneous manipulation. Bilateral skill refinement is heavily dependent upon continuing development of reach, grasp, release, and in-hand manipulation skills. Visual-perceptual, cognitive, and motor skill development become more integrated, leading to the child's effective use of motor planning for task performance. Simultaneous manipulation is demonstrated at 2 to 3 years.[11] The mature stage of bilateral hand use, which is the ability to use opposing hand and arm movements for highly differentiated activities such as cutting with scissors, begins to emerge at about 2½ years. Patterns from each stage of

bilateral hand use are applied and refined through different activities throughout the child's development.

TYPICAL PROBLEMS IN THE DEVELOPMENT OF HAND FUNCTION

This section will discuss problems in a generic manner, without reference to a specific disease, disabling condition, or aspect of hand function. Most problems in upper extremity control and hand function result from a combination of contributing factors. Disorders in muscle tone, continued presence of primitive reflexes and reactions, or abnormal coordination of muscle function are the most commonly identified inhibitors of hand skill development and cross diagnostic categories. However, problems may also occur as a result of cognitive, somatosensory, and sensory integrative dysfunction, as well as musculoskeletal weakness and limitations in joint mobility and function. Similarly, each type of problem discussed affects the development of each type of hand function. Significant impairment of the most basic hand functions (reach, grasp, carry, and release) in early childhood will necessarily preclude emergence of more advanced hand skills (in-hand manipulation and bilateral hand use) without intervention.

One of the more common problems is *inadequate isolation of movements*. Children who demonstrate this problem tend to use total patterns of flexion or extension throughout the upper extremities; they are unable to combine wrist extension with finger flexion, or elbow flexion with finger extension. Similarly, the child is unable to perform differentiated motions with each arm and hand. Inadequate isolation of movements is handicapping even in early infancy, as the most basic movements of reach and grasp are affected.

Another common problem is *poorly graded movements*. Usually the extent of a movement is too great for the task, impairing coordination and accuracy of performance. This problem occurs when joint stability in the hand or proximal to the hand is not effective. For example, the child may not be able to hold the elbow in a mid-range of flexion and the wrist in neutral position during a grasp activity. Thus, when initiating the grasp, the child will overflex the fingers in an attempt to obtain the object before the arm posture is lost. Children with poorly graded movements lack the ability to effectively use the middle ranges of movement, and instead use too much flexion, extension, or any other movement. To compensate, some children learn to hold one or more joints in a locked position during attempts at hand use (Figure 13-10). Typical patterns used include internal rotation of the shoulder, elbow extension, forearm pronation, wrist flexion or extension, and hyperextension of the MCP joints. Problems with grading of movement are typically associated with abnormal tone, muscle weakness, or sensory integrative dysfunction. In the latter situation, the child has

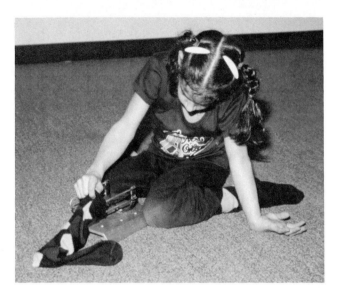

Figure 13-10   This child, who has involuntary movement, demonstrates the attempt to find stability by locking the elbows in extension and by elevating her right shoulder during hand use. She also has difficulty isolating upper extremity movements and using both hands together at midline.

Courtesy Kennedy Institute, Baltimore, Md.

difficulty perceiving and evaluating sensory feedback and so cannot accurately plan the extent of movements needed for a task. Disorders that cause poorly graded movements in infancy will particularly affect the development of effective reach and release, as well as in-hand manipulation and bilateral hand use.

Poor timing of movements may also be a problem. Inadequate timing of muscle contractions leads to the use of movements that are too fast or too slow for the intended purpose. Movements that are too fast also tend to be poorly graded. Disorders of tone or muscle weakness are often the underlying factors in movement that is too slow. Instability at joints tends to cause disordered sequences of hand/arm movements. For example, wrist extension may not be initiated until after grasp, rather than in combination with reach for the object.

A fourth problem that affects hand function is a *disorder in bilateral integration of movements*. This will affect both the normal symmetrical and asymmetrical movements needed to develop and use hand functions. Some children are unable to effectively bring both hands to midline or to maintain use of both hands at midline long enough to accomplish a task. Other children can work symmetrically at midline, but are unable to dissociate movements of the two upper extremities. Therefore, they have difficulty with activities that require refined forms of bilateral hand use.

Many children have difficulty with hand use due to *disorders of trunk movement and control.* Central nervous system dysfunction or generalized muscle weakness way impair development or effective use of equilibrium reactions. Therefore, the child often needs to use one or both arms for support to maintain many sitting or standing positions. This significantly limits bilateral hand use and may also limit the development of fine motor skills in the hand that the child most often uses for support.

Children with trunk instability or abnormal posture also tend to have difficulty with smooth and accurate placement of the hand/arm that is being used for a fine motor task. When the trunk is postured in flexion, functional range of motion in the arm is limited (Figure 13-11). On the other hand, hyperextension of the trunk tends to be accompanied by hyperextension of the humerus. The latter pattern typically causes one of three patterns of shoulder and elbow position: external rotation with elbow flexion, neutral rotation with elbow flexion, or internal rotation with elbow extension. Dominance by any of these arm positions will affect the development of hand skills. Similarly, lateral trunk flexion causes the child to lean to one side, and thus affects the child's ability to use the arm on the flexed side.

Any of the problems described above can contribute to the child's use of *compensatory patterns of movement.* In an effort to increase function, the child seeks another pattern to substitute for movements impaired by the primary problem. For example, the child with weakness or instability may learn to use lateral trunk flexion to increase the height of the arm during reach. Or, a child with increased tone may compensate for limited finger extension by using a tenodesis action. Although these patterns may be effective initially, and in some cases may provide all of the independent function that is available to a child, development of higher level skills may in fact be hindered by continued use of compensatory movements.

TREATMENT STRATEGIES

To reiterate, the occupational therapist needs to consider a variety and combination of motor, cognitive, sensory integrative, and social-emotional issues in the assessment and treatment of children with hand function problems. Assessment has been discussed in Chapters 9 through 12, and should include measures of hand skill development, quality of performance, and process. Treatment to improve hand/arm functions is usually carried out in the following sequence:

Preparation
1. Positioning for postural control and stability
2. Inhibition or facilitation of tone
3. Improvement of joint mobility
4. Activities to improve postural control, particularly with regard to trunk stability and rotation and head control

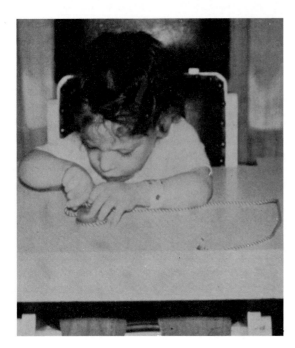

Figure 13-11   Poor trunk stability affects the upper extremity range of motion this child can use. Note her forearm pronation and wrist flexion on the right. She is unable to effectively use a 3-jaw chuck grasp or a pincer on the materials.

Courtesy Kennedy Institute, Baltimore, Md.

5. Intervention to improve proximal control (particularly scapulo-humeral), including weight-bearing
   Hand function development
6. Activities that emphasize isolated arm or hand movements, such as external rotation, supination, and wrist extension
7. Reach, grasp, and release activities
8. Isolated finger movement activities
9. In-hand manipulation activities
10. Bilateral hand use activities
    Carry over
11. Integration of hand skills into functional activities

Not all children need all of the steps of this sequence. In addition, intervention for all areas is rarely done in one treatment session.

Preparation for hand skill development

Many children require preparation of the total body in each treatment session before intervention for a specific hand function is addressed. A primary element of preparation for hand activities is attention to muscle tone and musculoskeletal stability through use of positioning and handling techniques. Head, trunk, and scapular stability and mobility are critical. Weight-bearing activities are also typical components of the preparation program. These are used to improve stability in the scapulo-humeral area or to improve the child's ability to use small, graded ranges of proximal movement.

The child with increased tone throughout the body may need overall inhibition prior to hand treatment activities. Children with high tone in primarily one upper extremity will require specific attention to the involved body side. Finnie[23] suggested several helpful techniques, including the use of very slow rotary movements at the shoulder and forearm. These movements may be performed within a very small range of motion between internal and external rotation of the shoulder and forearm pronation and supination. Movement of the humerus into an abducted position and the elbow into extension at the same time rotary movements are applied is also useful. Sustained holding of a joint in neutral position can also diminish flexor tone.

Upper extremity weight-bearing is particularly useful in treatment because it encourages the child to maintain elbow cocontraction and some degree of wrist extension while engaging in slight weight-shifting. Proprioceptive stimuli are also provided during weight-bearing. The primary focus should be on helping the child increase overall stability, rather than concentrating on achieving full elbow, wrist, or finger extension. Weight-bearing activities can be carried out with the child in prone on forearms, prone on extended arms, side-sitting, or long-sitting, depending on the child's skill level.

Effectively controlling the child who has significant wrist flexion in an upper extremity weight-bearing position is often difficult. The most appropriate positions to use include prone on forearms and sidelying. The therapist can help the child position wrists in neutral, but may not expect extension beyond neutral.

Mildly involved children can often work toward maintaining full finger extension during weight-bearing. However, this may not be feasible for children with moderate or severe involvement. Finger flexion may be permitted during weight-bearing as long as the thumb is not in an abnormal position. If the child's thumb is tightly adducted and flexed, the therapist should use handling techniques prior to weight-bearing. The therapist can use his own hand to provide firm pressure on the first metacarpal and relax the child's hand through slow, small rotary and flexion/extension movements.

Barnes[5] used upper extremity weight-bearing in a multiple baseline study with three children who had cerebral palsy and increased tone. The children ranged from 3 to 5 years. Part of the treatment included unilateral weight-bearing on the child's fully extended arm and hand, with placement on the floor to the front, side, and back of the body during sitting. Each treatment session was 10 minutes long and included the weight-bearing activity and another technique for joint approximation. The quality of the child's reach, grasp, and release was tested while the children sat in their wheelchairs, with objects placed on the wheelchair tray. Data collection for ten trials was carried out immediately following each treatment session. All three children improved in the skills measured. The most significant changes were seen in elbow extension during reach, and wrist extension to or beyond a neutral position during grasp and release.

As shoulder and elbow stability improve, the child should be encouraged to use this stability during reach, grasp, and release. Elbow cocontraction in about 90 degrees of flexion is necessary for effective arm use on a table surface. Cocontraction of the wrist, in at least neutral position, is crucial for hand use. Lauretana, Partan, and Twitchell[31] suggested having the child and therapist push against each other's palms, with wrists extended. Boehme[8] recommended encouraging the child to squeeze the therapist's index and middle fingers while holding the wrist in neutral or slightly extended position. In addition to reinforcing wrist stability, this pattern also facilitates development of intrinsic hand actions. When the wrist is placed in an extended position during squeezing, flexion posturing throughout the entire upper extremity is inhibited. If finger flexor tone increases while using this technique, the therapist can apply firm pressure to the child's hand and use slow, small range rotation of the radial and ulnar parts of the hand in opposition to each other.[8] If a child cannot achieve independent wrist stability during functional activities, a cock-up splint can be used. For guidelines, refer to the discussion of splinting at the end of this chapter.

Children who are weak or clumsy often need only appropriate body positioning to ensure trunk stability prior to emphasis on hand function activities. Traditional muscle strengthening activities against resistance, particularly for wrist extension and cocontraction, are also recommended for problems with strength. Treatment for children with distal weakness may also include the use of dynamic or static splints to support the wrist or encourage finger movements.

Although children with abnormal tone often require intervention for both head/trunk control and hand/arm skill, it is not always effective to combine treatment for both functions. Simultaneous intervention for postural control and hand function can result in poor quality and skill in both areas. This is particularly true early in a child's treatment. Most children need more external trunk support (positioning support and adaptations) during fine motor and eating activities than at other times of the day. Gradually such support may be decreased as postural control and fine motor skill improve.

In addition to intervention to improve motor function, specific attention should be given to the child's sensory functioning. Tactile and proprioceptive contact to the arms and hands may be provided to enhance sensory awareness and discrimination. Stimuli may be provided by lotion, toys, the child's own clothing, or, preferably, active movements of the child's hands, with or without assistance. Normal children, as well as those with developmental dyspraxia, have greater tactile sensitivity when performing an activity that involves active touching rather than being touched.[26] Visual awareness of the hands in conjunction with tactile and proprioceptive input should also be encouraged.

Strategies for reach

When the child initiates little movement, or is unable to open the hand during arm movement, the primary focus of intervention will be on controlled initiation of arm movements. This will include varying arm movements and placing the arm for contact with objects. This type of reaching goal is a priority for children with extremely limited strength and movements or those whose degenerative disease process results in skill regression. It can promote contact with others and be used to activate switches for toys and electronic adapted equipment.

To facilitate arm movements and contact with objects, the therapist must identify the best position to promote postural stability and visual regard. The most commonly used position is sitting, with attention given to head and trunk control, visual regard, and visual tracking.

Children with severe motor involvement need toys and materials that are easy to activate and have no "failure" elements. Such toys include play foam, beans, rice, musical toys that are activated by light touch, and soap bubbles. Best results are usually obtained through proximal handling at the shoulders and upper arms, as the therapist assists the child with movements of either or both arms. Initial emphasis is on general arm movement, then upon hand/arm placement, and finally on finger extension during arm movement as a precursor for reach with grasp.

When children are able to contact objects with some control, the therapist should introduce structured activities to assist the child with using elements of a more normal, mature reaching pattern. Gradually these elements are combined for a smooth direct reach. Sometimes object placement must be varied. For example, initial presentation of objects at a level below the child's shoulder may facilitate the use of shoulder flexion and neutral rotation, rather than abduction and internal rotation. Gradually objects are raised higher as the child develops more control. Lateral reaching may be used to promote shoulder abduction and neutral to external rotation during reach. The child should also be encouraged to reach behind her body, combining humeral hyperextension with controlled internal rotation and various elbow positions. Many children have difficulty with this posterior reaching pattern, which is required in dressing and other daily living skills.

Some children are able to use neutral to slight external shoulder rotation in combination with humeral flexion if provided with a minimal amount of handling at the humerus or elbow (Figure 13-12). However, if such handling techniques are required in order for a child to use a mature reaching pattern, ipsilateral reaching activities are recommended. The child is probably not yet ready to practice reaching across the midline for an object that is positioned far from the body.

To encourage reaching that incorporates neutral to slight external rotation of the shoulder and forearm supination, objects can be oriented vertically. Horizontal orientation and use of large objects tend to encourage forearm pronation. Difficulties with initiating or sustaining forearm supination are often compensated for with abnormal posturing at the trunk, shoulder, elbow, or wrist.

Supination is easiest to use when the elbow is fully flexed and most difficult to use with full elbow extension. Therefore, activities that position the elbow in more than 90 degress of flexion can be used to facilitate supination. If the child can initiate supination, but has poor control of this pattern, he can benefit from activities with the elbow held in 90 degrees, with the forearm stabilized on a surface and an object presented vertically (Figure 13-13). Gradually materials are moved to encourage more elbow extension while maintaining the supinated position. Children with more severe involvement may only be able to achieve about 30 degrees of supination—the minimum amount needed to effectively handle materials on a table. Other children with less motor impairment should be encouraged to obtain at least 90 degrees of supination to accomplish functional activities such as drinking, eating with utensils, or turning a doorknob. It is also helpful to facilitate supination in the non-preferred arm, so that objects can be more effectively stabilized for manipulation by that hand.

Children with muscle weakness will be better able to reach objects when they are provided with a table or tray surface that is at or slightly above elbow height. Mobile arm suspension systems can be used for support and to assist with movements of the child with muscle grades of fair-minus or lower.

Children with attentional or visual impairment should be presented with objects that have high color contrasts or bright solid colors. In the presence of severe visual impairment, initial objects should combine both auditory stimuli and varied textures. If the child has not developed the ability to search for objects, materials should be presented within a confined space or tied to strings so that they can be easily retrieved after dropping.[24]

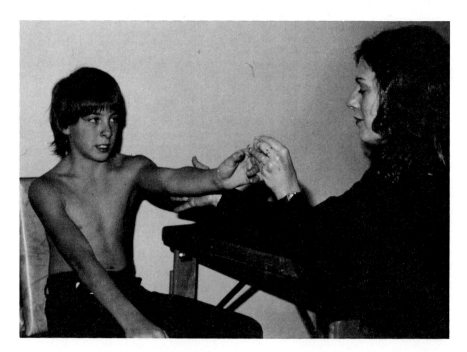

Figure 13-12   Facilitation is provided to prompt use of slight humeral external rotation and forearm supination. The object is held vertically to assist this reaching pattern.

Courtesy Kennedy Institute, Baltimore, Md.

Strategies for grasp

The child who has difficulty opening the hand for grasp may have significantly increased tone, muscle weakness, or joint limitations, or may be avoiding contact with the object. Preparation through handling, positioning, strengthening, splinting, and development of reach with extended fingers is paramount for children with problems in these areas. If sensory avoidance is present, treatment should follow principles appropriate to the child with tactile defensiveness (see Chapter 23). In addition, weight-bearing with the hand closed and graded tactile input are useful. Usually firm objects with smooth surfaces and contours will be tolerated best initially. Maintenance of grasp may also be influenced by sensory impairment, particularly when tactile discrimination is poorly developed. Regardless of the cause of manifestation of a somatosensory deficit, most children seem to benefit from graded sensory input and increasing attention to sensory discrimination. Active exploration of the size, shape, and texture of materials is preferred to passive stimulation imposed by the therapist.

Development of grasp begins with emphasis on grasp alone, rather than combining reach with grasp. Initially, the therapist will ensure that the child's arm is well stabilized when objects are presented. Stability at the wrist in at least neutral extension is critical. The therapist can hold the object first with her fingers, and present the object directly to the child's fingers (Figure 13-14). Positioning the object to promote optimal grasp allows the child to experience success and obtain normal sensory feedback. Later the therapist can place the object in the palm of his own hand, and present it to the child's fingers. This position requires the child to use more wrist, finger, and thumb stability than the earlier activity did.

Once the child can retrieve objects successfully from the therapist's hand, table placement near the child's hand is instituted. As the child progresses, objects may be moved increasingly further from the child's body. Eventually the stability of the table surface for arm support and object presentation are removed. This requires that the child stabilize the arm in space while controlling finger movements. Again, a sequence of object presentation begins close to the child's body and proceeds further away as the child improves in reach and grasp. Continued treatment for grasp will be focused on the development of more refined and other functional prehension patterns that will be used for independent performance of play, school, and self-care activities.

Materials for grasp should be selected with consideration of the child's interests, sensory needs, and motor skills, Properties to consider include size, shape, weight, and texture of objects. Children with severe disabilities need to develop an effective palmar grasp, and if possible, a three-point palmar or lateral pinch. Children with moderate involvement can be expected

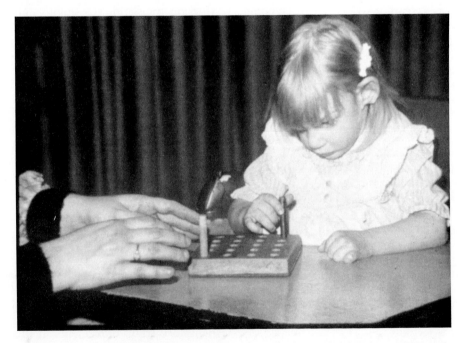

Figure 13-13   Arm support on the surface, elbow flexion, and vertical orientation of materials encourage this child's use of forearm supination. Note this child's lack of spontaneous stabilization of the pegboard with her right hand.

Courtesy Kennedy Institute, Baltimore, Md.

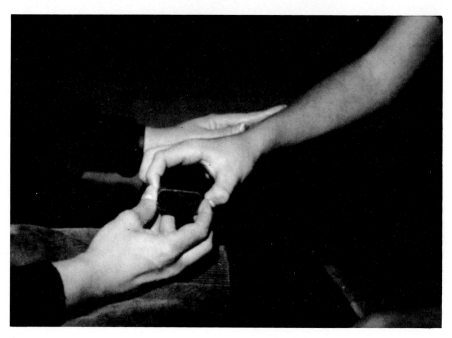

Figure 13-14   The child is assisted with using grasp with thumb opposition and finger pad contact by stabilization of his forearm and presentation of the object directly to his fingers.

Courtesy Kennedy Institute, Baltimore, Md.

to develop the ability to grasp objects using the surface or pads of all fingers (Figure 13-14). The three-point pinch pattern and its variations are more functional in daily living skills than tip or two-point pinch, and should have priority for intervention.

Children with less severe motor disabilities need assistance to use tools and objects of a variety of shapes and sizes. Emphasis may also be placed on inhibiting the ulnar fingers and using only the radial fingers in grasp; this ability is a precursor for power grasp and in-hand manipulation.

When grasp of certain materials cannot be used effectively for a task, adaptations are made. The clumsy child often has more success with sturdy objects that are crush- and break-proof. The child with involuntary movements works better with heavier materials or objects that can be pushed rather than lifted.[23] The child with high tone has more control with medium-sized and medium-weight objects. Children with muscle weakness perform best with lightweight objects. Refer also to Chapter 17.

Strategies for in-hand manipulation

Early treatment for children who are beginning to show readiness for in-hand manipulation can address isolated finger movements and refinement of thumb opposition and isolation. Attention to enhancement of tactile and proprioceptive awareness and discrimination is also helpful.

Treatment activities generally progress from finger to palm translation, to simple shift, to palm to finger translation. Objects that are placed in the radial part of the hand are usually easier to move than those placed in the middle. Ulnar placement is the most challenging. Medium-sized objects are most appropriate in early treatment; other sizes can be worked with later.

After the child shows some skill in translation and shift activities, rotation can be introduced. More difficult skills, addressed later in treatment, include activities that combine translation or shift with rotation. The most difficult activities combine all three patterns in conjunction with stabilization of materials in the hand. See Figure 13-15 for a list of specific preparation and treatment activities for each of the types of in-hand manipulation.

Strategies for carry

Because the child must maintain grasp of an object during the carry phase, wrist extension with sustained finger flexion needs to be emphasized. The therapist should be especially attentive to the child's use of compensatory trunk movements. If these are present, the child may need intervention to improve trunk control in midline and trunk rotation in conjunction with arm movements. The use of adapted positioning equipment to support the trunk in a symmetrical, erect posture is helpful for many children. Stabilization of the shoulder to prevent scapular elevation may also be necessary.

Facilitation of arm movements in a manner similar to that described for reaching will encourage carry patterns of shoulder rotation, stabilized elbow extension, and forearm supination. Most children with increased tone or stability problems have more difficulty carrying small or thin objects. Use of objects that are larger in diameter, such as those adapted with built up handles, can promote wrist extension and management of carrying.

Strategies for voluntary release

Treatment for problems with voluntary release is commonly combined with programs to facilitate reach or grasp. Development of more effective orientation of the arm is similar to methods used for reaching. Promotion of the child's ability to use more distal placement of objects on the fingers during grasp can also allow the child to release the object with more control.

When the child shows dominance of finger flexion, (fisting), initial treatment for release will focus on ability to move the arm while maintaining some finger extension. If the child shows persistent use of tenodesis during release, treatment activities should be structured to improve ability to place objects at midline with the elbow flexed and wrist in neutral. The child's next goal might be to release increasingly smaller objects into containers with openings of decreasing diameters. Subsequent treatment, reflecting the child's improved scapulo-humeral stability and ability to sustain slight forearm supination during release, would address the child's quality and skill in stacking objects.

Children generally have the greatest initial success releasing objects that are medium-sized and firm into containers with large openings. Gradually, as the child progresses in stability and control, smaller objects and openings can be used. When the child can release small objects into openings about twice the size of the object, then softer objects can be presented.

Many children can improve their ability to use wrist extension during release if their elbows are more extended (Figure 13-16). This level of control is similar to that of a baby who releases objects with the arm held in a total extension pattern. Over time, target containers for release of objects can be brought closer to the body, requiring gradually increasing elbow flexion with wrist extension. Sometimes this pattern can be facilitated if containers are set at an angle. Once the child can release medium-sized objects into a container at midline, while maintaining wrist extension to at least neutral, the size of the container opening can be decreased.

The child may need special practice with release activities that require maintenance of the forearm in midposition. Tipping containers that hold other substances, such as a glass of milk, often occurs when a child has difficulty with this pattern.

Figure 13-15   In-hand manipulation treatment activities

PREPARATION ACTIVITIES
General tactile awareness activities
1. using crazy foam
2. using shaving cream
3. putting on hand lotion
4. finger painting

Activities involving primarily proprioception
1. weight-bearing—wheelbarrow, activities on small ball
2. pushing heavy objects (boxes, chairs, benches, small ball if resisted)
3. pulling (tug-of-war)
4. catching/ throwing "heavy" ball
5. pressing different parts of hand into clay
6. pushing fingers into clay or therapy putty
7. pushing shapes out of perforated cardboard
8. tearing packages/boxes open
9. tearing edges off computer paper
10. rolling clay into ball on a surface
11. clapping games

Activities primarily involving tactile discrimination
1. doing finger games/songs
2. playing localization of tactile stimulation games
3. playing finger identification games
4. discriminating objects, with the object stabilized
5. discriminating shapes, with the shape stabilized
6. writing on body and identifying shape, letter, object drawn
7. discriminating textures

SPECIFIC IN-HAND MANIPULATION ACTIVITIES
Translation—fingers to palm without stabilization
1. getting a coin out of a change purse
2. hiding penny in hand (magic trick)
3. crumpling paper
4. taking lid off jar and holding it in palm while getting object out with other hand

Translation—fingers to palm with stabilization
1. getting two or more coins out of change purse, one at a time
2. taking two or more chips off magnetic wand, one at a time
3. picking up pegs/paper clips one at a time, to hold two or more in hand at one time
4. picking up several utensils one at a time, to hold two or more
5. picking up three blocks, one at a time

Translation—palm to fingers without stabilization
1. moving penny from palm to fingers (magic trick)
2. moving chip to fingers to put on magnetic wand
3. moving object to put into container
4. moving lid to put on jar   *Continued.*

Figure 13-15 cont'd. In-hand manipulation treatment activities

---

Translation—palm to fingers with stabilization

1. holding several chips to put on wand one at a time
2. handling money to put into bank, soda machine, gum machine
3. putting one utensil down when holding several in hand
4. holding several game pieces (chips, pegs, markers) during game

Shift without stabilization

1. turning pages in book
2. picking up sheets of paper, tissue paper, or dollar bills
3. separating playing cards
4. flattening a small ball of clay between pads of fingers
5. stringing beads (shifting string and bead as string goes through bead)
6. shifting crayon, pencil, pen for coloring/writing
7. shifting paper in the non-preferred hand while cutting
8. playing with tinkertoys (the long, thin pieces)
9. buttoning
10. lining up snaps for dressing
11. moving cookie while eating
12. adjusting spoon, fork, knife for appropriate use
13. rubbing paint, dirt, tape off pad of finger

Shift with stabilization

1. holding pen and pushing top off with same hand
2. holding chips while flipping one out of fingers
3. holding fabric in hand while attempting to button or snap
4. holding key ring with keys in hand, shifting one for placement in lock

Rotation without stabilization

1. removing/putting on small jar lid
2. putting on/removing bolts from nuts
3. rotation of crayon/pencil—tip oriented ulnarly
4. rotation of crayon/pencil—tip oriented radially
5. removing crayon from box and preparing for writing
6. rotating pen or marker to put top on after writing
7. rotating "weeble" people to put in chairs, bus, boat
8. rotating puzzle piece for placement in board
9. feeling objects or shapes to identify them
10. handling tinkertoy parts in construction of object
11. playing with legos (TM)
12. constructing twisted shapes with pipe cleaners
13. rotating twisties

Rotation with stabilization

1. handling parts of small shape container while rotating shape to put into container
2. holding key ring with keys, rotating correct one for placement in lock

Strategies for bilateral hand use

Difficulties with bilateral hand use tend to result from a combination of problems, of which motor factors may be only one component. Some children with significant cognitive delays cannot attend to two objects simultaneously, so alternating hand use or stabilization combined with manipulation are not possible. Deficits in bilateral integration of the two body sides may be present (see Chapter 23). Impaired sensation may contribute to a lack of attention to one body side. Finally, lack of bilateral motor experience, as in children with hemiplegia or brachial plexus injuries, can cause children to approach all tasks in a one-handed manner.

The focus of treatment goals varies, depending on the severity of the child's disability. Children with muscle weakness can often manage simultaneous manipulation activities well, since these require little hand strength and movement of the arms against gravity. They often need assistance or adaptations to develop the ability to stabilize materials with one hand because this demands more strength in the stabilizing arm.

Children with low tone or involuntary movements can usually achieve the normal sequence of bilateral hand skill development. Therapy should initially focus on improving symmetry and stability and proceed through the developmental progression of bilateral hand use as feasible for the individual child. If influence of involuntary movements is severe, more advanced types of bilateral activities may not be possible without adaptations.

Treatment of the child with significantly increased tone or marked asymmetry will focus primarily on promoting ability to stabilize materials with the more involved upper extremity while manipulating with the more proficient hand/arm. Activities that require stabilization with grasp (rather than stabilization without grasp) are often easier for these children. However, stabilization without grasp may be accomplished without finger extension as long as the child can use his hand in a fisted position with the wrist in neutral to slight extension. Symmetrical bilateral hand use should also receive some attention, particularly if the child's involvement is mild to moderate.

Special handling techniques can promote the child's ability to stabilize while manipulating or to use gross bilateral skills. The therapist can sit behind and stabilize both shoulders to help the child bring and keep both hands at midline. Trunk rotation should also be encouraged so that the child can cross midline more effectively. Treatment for difficulties with simultaneous manipulation is usually addressed through selection and structure of activities rather than use of handling techniques.

Toys and materials selected for program activities must *require* bilateral hand use, particularly in the early phases of treatment. If objects are presented on a slippery surface, the child will have more incentive to stabilize them than if a non-skid surface is used. Ob-

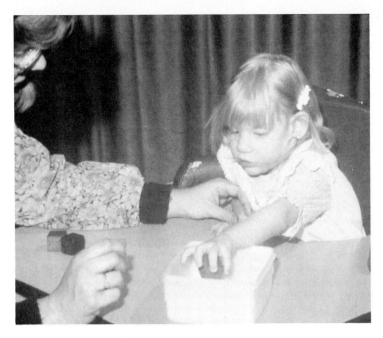

Figure 13-16   Positioning materials to elicit elbow extension during release encourages this child's use of wrist extension.

Courtesy Kennedy Institute, Baltimore, Md.

jects that are too small to be stabilized with the palm and those with an obvious handle are useful when stabilization with grasp is the treatment focus.

Usually materials are placed at midline. However, children with asymmetrical involvement may perform better with objects placed slightly toward the more involved upper extremity. Midline crossing is initiated by positioning objects only a few inches to the left or right of midline. Later objects can be moved further away, and off the surface, to encourage use of trunk rotation. Medium and large objects are generally more appropriate to use in the early phases of treatment.

When a child cannot successfully stabilize materials and does not show potential for this skill in the near future, adaptations should be considered. Non-skid surfaces, and other techniques as described in Chapter 17 (Figure 17-1) can assist in stabilization with table activities. Various commercial adaptations are available to aid accomplishment of other types of bilateral daily living activities with one hand.

SPLINTING FOR CHILDREN

Splinting is often a component of occupational therapy intervention for children with hand function problems. Children who have one or more of the following problems may benefit most:

1. Deformities
2. At risk for developing deformities
3. Increased tone
4. Limited movement of the hand

5. Limitations in functional skills secondary to problems with hand functions

Any one or a combination of these problems may necessitate splinting for a child with severe motor disability as a result of central nervous system damage. Children with moderate motor impairment are less likely to require splinting to prevent or correct a deformity, but are apt to use splints to reduce tone or improve mobility and functional skills. The child with minimal involvement secondary to central nervous system damage may have more difficulty with thumb use than wrist or finger control. Therefore, this child may need a thumb splint to decrease tone or provide stability so that function is enhanced. Children who do not have central nervous system damage may require splint application for any of the above problems except increased tone.

Precautions and indications for splint use

Precautions for splint use are always in order, particularly for young or nonverbal children who have poor sensation or are tactilely defensive. These factors make them vulnerable to skin irritations and pressure problems. Children may be unable to report sensory or motor problems during or following splint application. Therefore, the therapist must carefully instruct the child's parents regarding the wearing schedule, possible problems, and postural changes to note.

Static splints generally require shorter wearing times

than splints that allow hand movement. Initially, children may only tolerate 10 minute application periods. Usually these periods can be gradually increased to alternating 2 hour sessions. If the child has increased tone, maximum wearing time for a static splint is usually 6 to 8 hours per day. However, if splints allow some hand movement and are used to aid accomplishment of functional activities, additional hours may be tolerated. At least a portion of the day or night should be spent without splints.

Not all children with increased tone need night resting splints. In many cases their hands are more relaxed during sleep, and arms and hands can be positioned in neutral by parents. These children are generally not at risk for development of contractures. The child who shows abnormal hand posturing during the day, but not at night, may, however, require daytime splint application to increase function.

Boehme[9] noted that some children have learned to use abnormal patterns of wrist flexion and ulnar deviation or thumb adduction to accomplish their daily activities. If this pattern is inhibited by a splint, the child will tend to compensate by using another abnormal position of the hand or arm. Therefore, before a splint is applied, the therapist must determine whether functional skill patterns that the child has been using will be lost. Treatment to help children develop better quality patterns of hand use should be increased, not decreased, when splints are introduced.

The use of splinting has rarely been questioned regarding applications with children who have muscle weakness, traumatic injury of the hand/arm, or joint inflammation. However, splinting has been more controversial in relation to its applicability to individuals with abnormal tone. Most of the related literature addresses problems of adults with abnormal tone; only three studies[17,34,36] report the use of splints with children. This topic will be explored further in conjunction with splint descriptions.

Types of splints used with children

Splints may be categorized into those that allow hand movement and those that do not. *Static* splints include resting pan splints, other volar and dorsal full hand and wrist splints, spasticity reduction splints, and thumb positioning splints. A second category of splints are considered *dynamic,* in that they assist the child with a particular wrist, finger, or thumb movement. A third type of *special purpose* splint, which is applied to enhance a specific function, may provide stimulation to the hand/arm or assist with stabilization of one or more joints during hand/arm activities.

Doubilet and Polkow[13] and Snook[45] reported case studies suggesting that *spasticity reduction splints* help decrease tone in adults. McPherson[36] used an empirical design to study the effectiveness of Snook's spasticity reduction splint for five severely-profoundly

handicapped adolescents. Splint wearing time was gradually increased from 15 minutes the first day to 2 hours daily by the fourth week. The outcome measure was passive muscle tone at the wrist, which was documented on a daily basis through use of a scale that measured pounds of force when the individual assumed wrist flexion. During the 4 weeks of splint application, the subjects' wrist tone decreased significantly. When they did not wear the splints for a week, their tone increased again. In contrast, Mathiowitz et al[35] found that four adult subjects showed no reduction in tone during or immediately following use of finger spreaders and hard cone splints.

A concern with many spasticity reduction splints is that they control the thumb over the first and second phalanges, but not over the metacarpal. Phelps and Weeks[39] noted that control of the first metacarpal is essential when a thumb-index finger web space contracture is present. Distal force on the thumb can result in ". . . stretch or even rupture of the ulnar collateral ligament of the MP joint of the thumb. . . "[39] (p. 545) as well as subluxation of the MP joint. Because children with spasticity usually demonstrate marked thumb adduction, distal control of the thumb moves the MP and IP joints into hyperextension, but does not abduct or extend the first metacarpal. Thus, if a splint does not control the carpo-metacarpal (CMC) joint of the thumb, joint damage can occur, further impairing thumb and hand use.

Resting pan splints may provide more support to and control of the thumb than some of the spasticity reduction devices. However, splints should be planned and monitored carefully for reactions at the wrist and fingers. The child with moderately increased tone may tolerate a resting splint that holds the wrist in neutral and fingers in slight flexion. However, if flexor spasticity is severe, the child will often pull out of such splints. In this instance, serial splinting that gradually raises the wrist from partial flexion to a more extended or neutral position is indicated. Initially, wrist position should be stabilized in just slightly more extension than the child normally achieves, but still less than neutral.[9] Splints are then adjusted or reconstructed to bring the child progressively toward a more neutral position at the wrist, thumb, and fingers. In general, extension is increased at only the wrist or fingers at one time, to prevent the occurrence of flexion or extension deformities in the fingers.

Other *volar splints,* such as the wrist cock-up, may be used with children who respond to control of wrist flexion but who do not need or cannot tolerate positioning of fingers or thumb simultaneously. The cock-up splint also allows the child to use the hand to perform functional activities. Volar cock-up splints may also require serial refitting to promote progression in controlled finger extension.[42] Ulnar deviation should be controlled by the wrist cock-up as well.

Controversy regarding the use of dorsal vs volar

static splints is long-standing and has yet to be resolved. In general, it appears that *dorsal splints* (Figure 13-17) are most effective with children who have muscle weakness and those with mild to moderately increased tone. Because of their small amount of contact with the volar surface of the hand and forearm, dorsal splints interfere less with sensory input. However, use of dorsal static splints to control abnormal finger position in children with central nervous system deficit is sometimes difficult.

Thumb splints are indicated when a child has difficulty with thumb control but can adequately coordinate movements in other parts of the wrist and hand. Exner and Bonder[17] reported a study of short opponens thumb splint use with twelve children who had cerebral palsy with spastic hemiplegia. The Orthoplast splints controlled the thumb over the first metacarpal and extended onto the distal phalanx (Figure 13-18). Splints were used 8 hours daily for 6 weeks. When tested with the splints off, two children showed improvement in bilateral hand use and three children showed improved grasp. Some children in the study found that wearing the splints on the non-preferred hand interfered with stabilization of materials that could not be grasped.

Reyman[40] reported on construction of a Neoprene Neoplush "sof-splint" for the thumb. Two straight pieces of the material, which is about ¼"-thick and has a slight stretch, were used for Reyman's design. However, this design appears best suited for control of only mildly increased tone. Use of a regular opponens splint pattern, as described above, is more suitable when higher tone is present (Figure 13-19). Hill[27] described other splinting techniques for thumb adduction problems.

Several therapists have explored the effectiveness of other orthotic devices to provide specific types of sensory stimulation, and thereby inhibit or facilitate tone. The hard cone, dowel, and orthokinetic cuff are common examples. Farber and Huss[21] stated that the purpose of the cone was to activate golgi tendon organs through pressure on the finger flexor tendons. Hard cones should be fabricated to the shape of the hand,

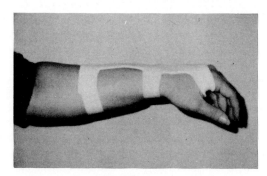

Figure 13-17 Dorsal splint to support the wrist in extension.

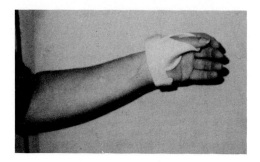

Figure 13-18 Short opponens thumb splint.

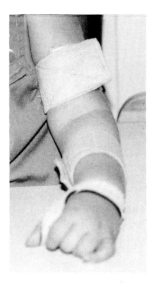

Figure 13-19 A neoplush thumb splint is worn with orthokinetic cuffs on the forearm and arm. Both orthokinetic cuffs are designed to promote extension and inhibit flexion.

with a narrower diameter on the radial side and larger area on the ulnar side.

MacKinnon, Sanderson, and Buchanan[34] introduced the *MacKinnon splint,* a device that uses a dowel stabilized in the child's hand against the metacarpal heads. A piece of rubberized tubing is attached to each end of the dowel and connects to a small band that fastens around the child's wrist. Contact of the dowel with the metacarpal heads is believed to stretch and facilitate the intrinsic muscles of the hand, and inhibit the long finger flexors. MacKinnon et al reported that children with spastic cerebral palsy improved in hand awareness and bilateral hand use and showed a decrease in fisting.

Exner and Bonder[17] modified the MacKinnon splint in the study described in discussion of opponens splints. The forearm piece was enlarged to provide better stabilization (Figure 13-20). No method to improve stabilization of the dowel against the metacarpal heads

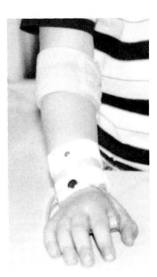

Figure 13-20 MacKinnon splint and forearm orthokinetic cuff.

could be found, so palm placement was substituted. The orthotic was fitted with the child's hand in its most typical wrist position, so that firm dowel contact with the palm could be maintained. (Wrist positioning is not a function of this splint.) Children wore the modified MacKinnon splints 8 hours daily for 6 weeks. Seven of the twelve children showed improvement secondary to use of this splint. Three children improved in both grasp and bilateral hand skills, two improved in grasp only, and two improved in bilateral hand skills alone. The children with improved skills all had moderate to severe upper extremity motor involvement. All children tolerated the splint well, and found that weight-bearing could be accomplished comfortably during application periods.

Several precautions regarding use of the MacKinnon splint should be noted. The splint is usually constructed by attaching aquarium tubing to the dowel with small nails. This method should be used with caution if the child is likely to put objects in his mouth. An alternative is to roll thermoplastic material around the tubing in place of using a dowel. This alternative is not as readily adjustable, however.

Hill[27] noted that some children may experience instability of the upper extremity in conjunction with decreased tone secondary to MacKinnon splint use. Therefore, careful monitoring, particularly in number of weeks for use, is recommended.

Orthokinetic devices are applied to facilitate tone in one muscle group and inhibit tone in the opposing muscles. These cuffs are made of elastic and non-elastic segments. Blashy and Fuchs[6] postulated that the elastic portion activates afferent fibers of skin exteroceptors and possibly the proprioceptors, and thus affects the motor neurons that innervate the muscles underlying the stimulated skin area. It is not clear whether the effectiveness of the device is due to its inhibitory or facilitory functions or a combination of both. However, Blashy and Fuchs[6] noted that orthokinetic cuffs were more effective when tone imbalance between the muscle groups was very pronounced.

The Exner and Bonder[17] study of splint use with twelve cerebral palsied children also tested application of orthokinetic cuffs. Evaluation of effects was tested over a 6 week period, with 8 hours of daily use. Cuffs were placed on the forearm, with the elastic (facilitory) portion over the muscle bellies of the finger and wrist extensors (Figures 13-19 and 13-20). Four children demonstrated improved performance in bilateral hand use, one showed improved grasp skills, and one child improved in both functions. The study indicated that the device helped encourage wrist or finger extension when the child was able to use some active contraction of the muscles being facilitated.

Orthokinetic cuffs are made from three layers of elastic bandage material, with non-stretch fabric sewn into the areas that are to be inhibitory. The cuff should be carefully fitted before final sewing so that it is snug and the elastic portion does not extend onto the muscles to be inhibited. For facilitation of elbow extension, the active (elastic) area of the cuff is placed over the triceps and the inactive area over the biceps. Orthokinetic cuffs can easily be used with other hand splints. They can also be worn during treatment activities.

New splinting techniques have been developed for children with increased tone or contractures. Positioning children who have had head injuries, to prevent loss of range, is particularly important during extensive comatose, semi-comatose, and recovery periods. Inflatable air (pneumatic) splints[27] are used to decrease tone, maintain and increase joint range, and stimulate somatosensory function. Serial casting,[50] dynasplints, and continuous passive range devices are also used to reduce contractures, particularly at the wrist and elbow. Research on these techniques is still in the early stages, and therefore literature is limited.

INTEGRATING DEVELOPMENT OF HAND FUNCTION INTO PLAY, SCHOOLWORK, SELF-MAINTENANCE, AND VOCATIONAL READINESS ACTIVITIES

Goals for hand/arm function should be linked to the child's ability to engage in daily activities. This link is assured if assessment focuses on identifying the child's specific abilities and problems in task performance. The therapist will identify and analyze components of function, including the presence, absence, and effects of hand/arm function deficits. This process has been detailed in Chapters 9 through 12. A sample analysis of an activity that is affected by impairment in hand function is shown in Figure 13-21.

Figure 13-21   Sample analysis of a fine motor
problem

***PROBLEM: UNABLE TO EFFECTIVELY ENGAGE IN
CONSTRUCTIVE MANIPULATIVE PLAY***
Components, subcomponents, and causes

1. Has poorly isolated finger use
   a. Wrist not stable in neutral/extension, uses wrist
      flexion—Possible causes:
      1. Decreased tone in the wrist extensors or
      2. Increased tone in the wrist flexors
   b. MP joints not stable—Possible causes:
      1. Poor cocontraction in the finger
         extensors/flexors associated with low tone
      2. Increased pull of extensor digitorum
   c. Unable to identify finger being touched—
      Resulting from decreased tactile discrimination
   d. Lacks midrange movements of finger
      joints—Possible causes:
      1. Decreased proprioception
      2. Poor cocontraction in MP and IP flexors and
         extensors
      3. Increased tone in the intrinsics and long
         finger flexors
2. Breaks materials often
   a. Drops objects—Possible causes:
      1. Poor tactile and/or poor proprioceptive
         awareness
      2. Poor manipulation of objects resulting from . . .
   b. Crushes materials during handling—Possible
      causes:
      1. Poor proprioceptive awareness of size,
         weight, etc.
      2. Increased finger flexor tone
      3. Associated reactions
      4. Grasp reflex
   c. Breaks materials when attempting to put two
      together—Possible causes:
      1. Poor spatial relations
      2. Grasp unstable as a result of poor wrist
         extension caused by increased flexor tone
      3. Overflow in one upper extremity
      4. Unilateral disregard

One issue to note during functional analysis is that
some children with poor attentional skills may show
fine motor problems secondary to mild motor or somatosensory deficits. However, other children, who superficially appear to have difficulty with hand/arm function, are actually showing impairment secondary to attentional deficit. They lack attention to detail or, in
their attempts to "get through" with the activity, work
too quickly to achieve accuracy.

Most children do not readily generalize skills from
isolated activities presented in therapy to their everyday life activities without assistance. Therefore, activi-

ties for children with hand/arm function problems
should be presented to the child in a meaningful
context.[10] For example, reaching program activities
can be carried out during dressing and hygiene training, or while playing with a toy that has many different
parts. Grasp activities can be incorporated into independent eating and vocational readiness tasks. In-hand
manipulation can be facilitated by having the child
demonstrate materials from his pencil or crayon box,
or through building with construction toys. Voluntary
release can be structured into a game that uses move-
able pieces. Bilateral hand use can be developed
through meal preparation activities, play, and schoolwork. Many other combinations are possible to help
the child develop mature function of hand/arm skills in
conjunction with increasing competence in daily life
activities. Subsequent chapters in this section on generic treatment will provide additional resources for
this aspect of hand function development.

SUMMARY

This chapter has presented a description of the components of hand and arm function that are instrumental
in the performance of play, self-maintenance, schoolwork, and vocational readiness activities. Factors that
influence the development of hand function, as well as
generic types of problems in hand/arm use, were discussed. The normal sequences of development for basic skills of reach, grasp, release, and carry, as well as
advanced functions of in-hand manipulation and bilateral hand use, were presented. Treatment strategies for
development of hand skills were described, as well as
the appropriate uses of splinting with children. Assessment and treatment of hand/arm function problems
should be seen within the context of the child's daily
life tasks.

STUDY QUESTIONS

1. What would be the major considerations for intervention
   with an adolescent who has spastic hemiplegia, demonstrates elbow flexion, forearm pronation, and fisting in the
   non-preferred hand, and who is having difficulty completing manual dexterity tasks in his vocational readiness program?
2. A 5-year-old with marked involuntary movements in the
   upper extremities and poor postural stability would like to
   feed herself. What aspects of arm and hand function would
   you assess to determine if she can do this with or without
   adaptive equipment? What treatment strategies could be
   used to promote the most effective grasp of the spoon and
   cup, and achievement of the plate to mouth pattern? What
   type(s) of splinting could be considered?
3. An 8-year-old has "sloppy" handwriting. How may problems with bilateral hand use and in-hand manipulation
   skills be interacting with short attention span and somatosensory problems to contribute to his handwriting difficulties?
4. What aspects of reach, grasp, release, and bilateral hand
   use should be addressed with a 15-month-old Down syn-

drome baby who shows low tone, and hand function and cognitive skills at 8 to 10 month levels?

5. A 10-year-old girl sustained a head injury 2 months ago. Prior to the accident she was left hand dominant. She is now alert, but has some memory deficits and motor planning problems. She has a left elbow contracture, and shows moderately increased tone in wrist flexion, thumb adduction, and finger flexion. What types of splinting or casting could be considered? How could you determine if the splinting or casting devices are effective treatment?

REFERENCES

1. Ammon JE, and Etzel ME: Sensorimotor organization in reach and prehension, Phys Ther 57:7, 1977.
2. Ayres AJ: Ontogenetic principles in the development of arm and hand function, Am J Occup Ther 8:95, 1954.
3. Ayres AJ: The visual-motor function, Am J Occup Ther 12:130, 1958.
4. Ayres AJ: Sensory integration and the child, Los Angeles, 1979, Western Psychological Services, Inc.
5. Barnes KJ: Improving prehension skills of children with cerebral palsy: a clinical study, Occup Ther J Res 6:227, 1986.
6. Blashy MRM, and Fuchs RL: Orthokinetics: a new receptor facilitation method, Am J Occup Ther 13:226, 1959.
7. Bobath B: Adult hemiplegia; evaluation and treatment, ed 2, London, 1978, Heinemann Educational Books Inc.
8. Boehme R: Improving upper body control, Tucson, Ariz, 1988, Therapy Skill Builders.
9. Boehme RH: NDT advanced course for treatment of the upper extremities, Denver, Colo, 1985.
10. Campbell PH, McInerney WF, and Cooper MA: Therapeutic programming for students with severe handicaps, Am J Occup Ther 37:594, 1984.
11. Connor FP, Williamson GG, and Siepp JM: Movement. In Program Guide for Infants and Toddlers, New York, 1978, Teachers College Press.
12. Curry J, and Exner CE: Comparison of tactile preferences of normal preschool children and preschool children with cerebral palsy, Am J Occup Ther 42:371, 1988.
13. Doubilet L, and Polkow LS: Theory and design of a finger abduction splint for the spastic hand, Am J Occup Ther 31:320, 1977.
14. Elliott JM, and Connolly KJ: A classification of manipulative hand movements, Devel Med Child Neurol 26:283, 1984.
15. Erhardt RP: Erhardt Developmental Prehension Assessment, Laurel, Md, 1982, RAMSCO Publishing Co.
16. Etaugh C, Collins G, and Gerson A: Reinforcement of sex-typed behaviors of 2-year-old children in a nursery school setting, Devel Psych 11:255, 1975.
17. Exner CE, and Bonder BR: Comparative effects of three hand splints on bilateral hand use, grasp, and arm-hand posture in hemiplegic children, Occup Ther J Res 3:75, 1963.
18. Exner CE: Assessment and treatment of in-hand manipulation skills, Sensory Integration Special Interest Section meeting, Amer Occup Ther Assn Annual Conf, Indianapolis, 1987.
19. Exner CE: Manipulation development in normal preschool children, Amer Occup Ther Assn Annual Conf, Minneapolis, 1986.
20. Exner CE: Patterns of in-hand manipulation in preschool children, Amer Occup Ther Assn Annual Conf, Indianapolis, 1987.
21. Farber SD, and Huss J: Sensory motor evaluation and treatment procedures for allied health personnel, Indianapolis, 1973, Indiana Univ–Purdue Univ at Indianapolis.
22. Fein G, et al: Sex stereotypes and preferences in toy choices in 20-month-old boys and girls, Devel Psych 11:527, 1975.
23. Finnie NR: Handling the young cerebral palsied child at home, ed 2, New York, 1975, EP Dutton.
24. Fraiberg SA, Smith M, and Adelson E: An educational program for blind infants, J of Sp Ed 3:121, 1969.
25. Gesell A, and Amatruda CS: Developmental diagnosis, New York, 1947, Harper & Row, Publishers, Inc.
26. Haron M, and Henderson A: Active and passive touch in developmentally dyspraxic and normal boys, Occup Ther J Res 5:101, 1985.
27. Hill SG: Current trends in upper-extremity splinting. In Boehme R, editor: Improving upper body control, Tucson, Ariz, 1988, Therapy Skill Builders.
28. Hohlstein RR: The development of prehension in normal infants, Am J Occup Ther 36:170, 1982.
29. Hulme C, et al: Visual, kinaesthetic and cross modal judgments of length by normal and clumsy children, Devel Med Child Neurol 24:461, 1982.
30. Jones B: The perception of passive joint movements by cerebral palsied children, Devel Med Child Neurol 18:25, 1976.
31. Lauretana MM, Partan DL, and Twitchell TE: Rehabilitation of the upper extremity in infantile spastic hemiparesis, Am J Occup Ther 13:264, 1959.
32. Lewis O: The culture of poverty, Sci Am 215:19, 1966.
33. Long C, et al: Intrinsic-extrinsic muscle control of the hand in power grip and precision handling, J Bone Joint Surg 52-A:853, 1970.
34. MacKinnon J, Sanderson E, and Buchanan J: The MacKinnon splint--a functional hand splint, Canad J Occup Ther 42:157, 1975.
35. Mathiowitz V, Bolding PJ, and Trombly CA: Immediate effects of positioning devices on the normal and spastic hand measured by electromyography, Am J Occup Ther 37:247, 1983.
36. McPherson JJ: Objective evaluation of a splint designed to reduce hypertonicity, Am J Occup Ther 35:184, 1981.
37. Napier JR: The prehensile movements of the human hand, J Bone Joint Surg 38-B:902, 1956.
38. O'Malley PJ, and Griffith JR: Perceptuo-motor dysfunction in the child with hemiplegia, Devel Med Child Neurol 19:172, 1977.
39. Phelps RE, and Weeks PM: Management of thumb-in-palm web space contracture, Am J Occup Ther 30:543, 1976.
40. Reyman J: The sof-splint, Devel Dis Special Interest Section Newsletter, Amer Occup Ther Assn 8:1, 1985.
41. Saeki K, Clark FS, and Azen SP: Performance of Japanese and Japanese-American children on the Motor Accuracy-Revised and Design Copying Tests of the Southern California Sensory Integration Tests, Am J Occup Ther 39:103, 1985.
42. Samilson RL, and Perry J: The orthopedic assessment in cerebral palsy. In Samilson RL, editor: Clinics in developmental medicine, Orthopedic aspects of cerebral palsy: p 35, 1975.
43. Skerik SK, Weiss MW, and Flatt AE: Functional evaluation of congenital hand anomalies, Am J Occup Ther 25:98, 1971.
44. Smith RO, and Benge MW: Pinch and grasp strength: standardization of terminology and protocol, Am J Occup Ther 39:531, 1985.
45. Snook JH: Spasticity reduction splint, Am J Occup Ther 33:648, 1979.
46. Super CM: Environmental effects on motor development: the case of "African infant precocity," Devel Med Child Neurol 18:561, 1976.
47. Twitchell TE: The automatic grasping responses of infants, Neuropsychologics 3:247, 1965.
48. Twitchell TE: Sensation and the motor deficit in cerebral palsy, Clin Orthop 46:55, 1966.

49. Weiss MW, and Flatt AE: Functional evaluation of the congenitally anomalous hand—part II, Am J Occup Ther 25:139, 1971.

50. Yasukawa A, and Hill J: Casting to improve upper extremity function. In Boehme R, editor: Improving upper body control, Tucson, Ariz, 1988, Therapy Skill Builders.

ADDITIONAL READINGS

1. Bairstow PJ, and Laslo JI: Kinaesthetic sensitivity to passive movements and its relationship to motor development and motor control, Devel Med Child Neurol 23:606, 1981.

2. Derevensky JL: Relative contributions of active and passive touch to a child's knowledge of physical objects, Percept Mot Skills 48:1331, 1982.

3. Gilfoyle EM, Grady AP, and Moore JC: The development of purposeful activities and skill. In Children adapt, Thorofare, NJ, 1981, Slack, Inc.

4. Henderson A, and Duncombe L: Development of kinesthetic judgments of angle and distance, Occup Ther J Res 2:131, 1982.

5. Hogg J: Learning, using and generalizing manipulative skills in a preschool classroom by non-handicapped and Down's syndrome children, Ed Psych 1:319, 1981.

6. Loria C: Relationship of proximal and distal function in motor development, Phys Ther 60:167, 1980.

7. Moss SC, and Hogg J: Development of hand function in mentally handicapped and nonhandicapped preschool children. In Mittler PJ, editor: Frontiers of knowledge in mental retardation, Baltimore, 1981, University Park Press.

8. Rosenbloom L, and Horton ME: The maturation of prehension in young children. Devel Med Child Neurol 13:3, 1971.

9. Ruff HS: Infants' manipulative exploration of objects: effects of age and object characteristics, Dev Psychobiol 20:9, 1984.

10. Sand PL, et al: Hand function in children with myelomeningocele, Am J Occup Ther 28:87, 1974.

14

Self-maintenance activities

IDA LOU COLEY
SUSAN A. PROCTER

An early joy of parenthood is to observe the emerging independence of one's child, from the first gestures of holding a rattle to the fine hand manipulations seen in buttoning a shirt. Children are endowed with an innate drive toward mastery of their bodies and their environment.

For most parents their child's evolving competence is an assumed natural order of events, the result of maturation and the influence of surroundings. Occasional regression and unpredictable behaviors presented by children are to be expected as a part of their uniqueness. Overall, independence is an expectation within the family and society at large. When a baby is born with a physical or intellectual disability or acquires one after birth, the disruption in the lives of all family members can be intense.

FAMILY CONSIDERATIONS

Restructuring and adaptation necessarily may stretch over a period of months or years. Today, parents are increasingly expressive about the impact of restructuring lives and about their real needs for knowing the extent of their child's potential. They also express a need to understand the disability, to know specifically what they can do to help their child, and to know where they can receive assistance. They yearn to hear about their child's strengths as they come to grips with the handicap and cope with problems of medical expenses, energy output, time management, and underlying sadness.

Occupational therapists and other professionals are in a strategic position to help parents learn, to help create a partnership in problem solving, to demonstrate techniques that will facilitate care, to provide reading material, and to listen. Timing is an important factor in the adaptation process. Not all families respond to helping gestures offered by professionals. Their responses can be confusing to others and to themselves and may be tempered by a sense of inadequacy, guilt, embarrassment, or anger. They may need counseling and intervention by social service or, to a lesser degree, require reassurance and permission to ask questions again and again: as one parent expressed, "Until I can hear what is being said." Most individuals need time to master information, particularly when under stress.

There are a number of actions a therapist can take to assist a family in gaining a sense of direction:

1. Sharing knowledge of the child's self-maintenance function: what he can do and why he can do some things and not others. Copies of reports written in clear, understandable language help to reinforce verbal information.
2. Clarifying expectations and what responsibilities parents can realistically set for their child in self-care since this is often a source of parental indecision and inconsistency.
3. Outlining realistic programs that family members can carry out according to their capabilities, home environment, and life-style.
4. Presenting equipment options in such a way that parents' consumer rights are recognized and they are supported in making important decisions.

It is only when a therapist can view professional responsibilities as extending beyond the child—in a sense addressing the needs of the family as a whole—that it is possible to maximize the effects of efforts put forth in the child's treatment program. Above all, the desired goal should be to assist the child and family with the business of getting on with living full lives.

BASIC FACTORS
The activity setup

Thoughtful preparation is a first step toward a successful therapeutic session. The therapist must think through and organize the many details involved in assessment and treatment. A good way to begin is to consider immediate goals and then select activities that provide the child with specific experiences. One would want to question, In what order should the therapist introduce tasks? What supplies and equipment are needed? Is the equipment in good working order?

The degree to which the treatment environment influences the child's performance can range from minimal to striking significance. For some children a therapist will want to minimize stimuli and eliminate both visual and auditory distractions. Other children require environmental stimulation from color, music, and objects. The therapist is an influential part of the environment and must consider how to give reinforcement for the child's positive responses.

It is essential to be perceptive to parents and other persons who may be present and to address their needs and concerns, listen, give reassurance, involve them in making observations, and engage them in problem solving. A part of thoughtful preparation is to organize the information they need and have it in written form.

The functional position

An important concept to recognize is that there is no "one" position for function. An individual requires a variety of positions for various activities. Changing positions at intervals provides relief to skin areas and bony prominences and affords important changes in muscle length.

A therapist considers positions that will maximize independent task performance. The child with motor involvement may need to be positioned to break up mass patterns of flexion, extension, and asymmetry. Key points for stability that enable the child to use voluntary movement must be identified. When muscle weakness occurs, the therapist determines where support is needed or, for the child with muscle tightness, whether a preferred and comfortable position is contraindicated.

Looking carefully at the entire body of the child, one asks the following:

Where are the hips, shoulders, and head in relation to the trunk? Will more hip flexion in sitting break up extension patterns (Figure 14-1)?

What things increase trunk stability? Inserting lateral supports? A surface for supporting the feet? Widening the sitting base by abducting the legs?

If more head stability is needed, should the child be placed prone with a roll under his shoulders? Is the roll really under the shoulders or the chest? Are the elbows under the child's shoulders? Check the head position again (Figure 14-2, *A*).

Does positioning in sidelying break up the strong flexion that is dominant in prone and the extension patterns seen in supine? Will a support pillow to the back prevent the child from rolling to the supine position? Will an anterior support pillow prevent rolling to the prone position? Is a roll between the legs needed to prevent adduction of the hips? Will

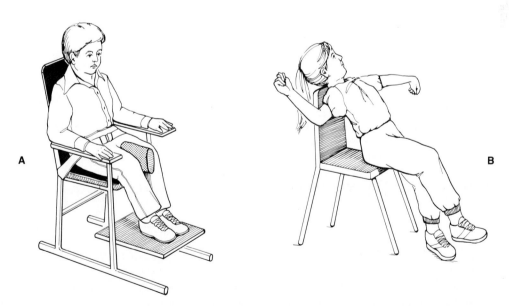

Figure 14-1 Sitting postures. **A,** Correct sitting posture. Weight equally distributed on the sitting base; feet and elbows supported. **B,** Incorrect sitting resulting from a massive extension pattern and an asymmetrical tonic reflex posture.

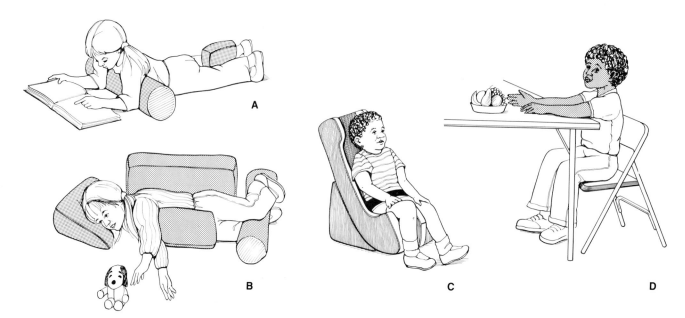

Figure 4-2 Adapted positioning for improved function. **A,** In prone position. **B,** In side-lying position. **C,** Grading sitting balance in a partial recliner. **D,** Increasing postural stability by elevation of working surface.

a small wedge pillow position the head so that the child can see more efficiently with her eyes as her arm reaches out to contact a toy (Figure 14-2, *B*)?

Will reclining the head and trunk prevent the head from falling forward (Figure 14-2, *C*)? Does the position facilitate eye contact between the child and persons in the environment?

The child with weak musculature should be viewed from the standpoint of the forces of gravity and what can be done to provide external support that will allow the use of the available muscle power. Postural security will allow the child to use energy more fully in arm and hand activity.

For the child whose problems are related to muscle tightness, one would need to consider giving required support to prevent persistent abnormal postural alignment, but a therapist should also question whether a continuous position will foster further contracture. Legs may need to be supported in maximal extension, rather than in a position of flexion.

The working surface

Having positioned the child, attention is next directed to the working surface that serves to give support at the elbows and provides an area for the objects the child will touch, manipulate, and use for self-maintenance. Here one looks more closely at the eye, arm, and hand at work and determines the surface height and angle that allow these body parts to work together more efficiently (Figure 14-2, *D*).

EATING
A bond with nurture

An infant's first experiences with eating usually occur in an atmosphere of tenderness. Nutritional nurture becomes a means for bonding between infant and mother and for building a sense of trust: the first stage of psychosocial development. During feeding, eye contact, touching, and talking reinforce the quality of social communication. It is a process of life that should be a part of awareness as attention is given to the more mechanical aspects of eating function.

Throughout this chapter, looking at the entire body and the whole child is emphasized. An experienced therapist put it another way, "When you evaluate an eating problem, be sure you don't just look at the mouth!" Like a camera lens, the trained eye of the clinician moves to view the child, focusing on details of posture, affect, movement, environmental stimuli, then it shifts to a close-up view of specific behaviors such as the subtle retraction of the upper lip as the child looks up at his feeder.

Eating is a complex function resulting in essential nutrition of the body. It requires a high degree of coordination of orofacial musculature and the vital functions of breathing and swallowing. Alternately and within boundaries, food and air share a common space. During eating the child opens his mouth, adjusts his lips, and gathers up the food, masticates it, moves it about in his mouth, forms a bolus, closes his mouth, and moves the bolus to the back of his throat for swallowing. Having an understanding of how eating occurs will clarify the kind of intervention that is needed when there is dysfunction.

Oral motor development

HOW GROWTH AND STRUCTURAL CHANGE AFFECT FUNCTION

The principle that development proceeds from proximal points to distal points applies to eating sequences. Initially consider the neck region as being proximal and the jaw as being distal. While the neonate is acquiring head control and stabilization in the shoulder region, nature provides reflexive mechanisms to assist him with acquiring food and protective mechanisms for his reclining posture.

SUCKING AND SWALLOWING

As the infant's lips grasp and close around the nipple and hold it close to the junction of the hard and soft palates, mucosal folds on the gums assist in sealing off the oral cavity. When the infant's lips develop more muscular control around 3 or 4 months of age, the folds disappear. The infant rhythmically suckles, and his cupped tongue moves in and out to bring the milk to the back of his throat. The tongue and jaw move together simultaneously and are lowered while the mouth is closed, thus creating a negative pressure. In addition, retrusion of the mandible facilitates the efficiency of the stroking action of the tongue.

When the tongue moves back during sucking and comes in contact with the tensed soft palate, the contact causes the milk to be directed into the lateral food channels.[29] The position of the epiglottis also directs the flow laterally. At this time the epiglottis and soft palate are in close approximation, and the larynx is high in close proximity. In this structural relationship the epiglottis provides a breakwater effect, and this protects the air passages. In addition, the tonsils and lymphoid tissue serve to keep the airway open and prevent food from reaching the posterior pharyngeal wall as the infant feeds in a reclining position.[29]

Because the oral cavity is small, the infant's tongue fills it, leaving little space for air to move in and out. But the infant now can breathe through his nose and can suckle, swallow, and breathe at the same time. The centers for these functions are located near one another in the brain stem. They coordinate their functions to allow liquid and air to cross the alimentary and respiratory passages in the pharynx. Respirations of the infant tend to be rapid and are accomplished by an abdominal breathing pattern. The chest at this time is barrel shaped, and there is minimal movement of the rib cage during breathing.

Cheeks are equipped with fatty tissue called *sucking pads,* which give the infant's face a rounded contour. It is thought that the sucking pads lend stability to the buccinator muscle of the cheek and contribute to the rigidity needed to maintain pressure for sucking.[28] The sucking pads also help to steady an unstable temporomandibular joint.

One of the most puzzling areas of dysfunction occurs within the swallowing mechanism. Therapists can observe the movements within the mouth, can check for the gag reflex, can palpate movement of the larynx, but according to some experts, conclusions must be considered an educated guess. What therapists observe is primarily the voluntary oral phase of swallowing. Cineradiography or videofluoroscopy is required for one to know what is happening in the pharyngeal phase.

In the older infant, child, and adult, the process of swallowing begins as a voluntary act and ends with a series of involuntary, automatic events. The time involved in the complicated process, from the oral phase through the pharyngeal phase, is a brief 2 seconds. Morris[23] states

The majority of neurologically impaired children and adults who aspirate do not have an absent swallowing reflex. The reflex may be delayed, but the problem most likely lies with the coordination of the tongue, the lips, the cheeks, and the larynx. They may be unable to take food into the mouth, to maneuver it sufficiently to the back, and to trigger an efficient swallow reflex with appropriate timing of pharyngeal and laryngeal movements (p. 29).

In the *voluntary oral stage* (Figure 14-3, *A*) the tongue moves upward, pushes, strips along the soft palate, and propels the bolus to the back of the tongue. When the bolus reaches the area of the anterior and posterior pillars of fauces at the base of the tongue, the swallow reflex is triggered. Phrenic and intercostal nerves inhibit diaphragm and intercostal muscles, and respiration is inhibited.

In the *involuntary oral stage,* or automatic pharyngeal stage (Figure 14-3, *B*), the back of the tongue elevates and presses against the posterior wall. Meanwhile, the soft palate moves backward and upward, closing off the nasopharynx to prevent food from entering the nose. Simultaneously, the bolus stimulates nerve endings in the mucosal lining of the pharynx, and pharyngeal constrictors squeeze the bolus downward. Bronchial passages are protected by the epiglottis and the valving of the true vocal folds and the false vocal folds. The food passes downward into the esophagus as the cricopharyngeal muscle, or bottom pharyngeal constrictor, relaxes.

In the final *involuntary esophageal stage* the bolus stimulates nerve endings in the walls of the esophagus. Peristaltic movements then squeeze the bolus toward the cardiac sphincter. Relaxation of the cardiac sphincter allows the bolus to pass into the stomach.

FUNCTIONAL CHANGES

As head control and postural stability increase in the neck and shoulder region, structural changes within

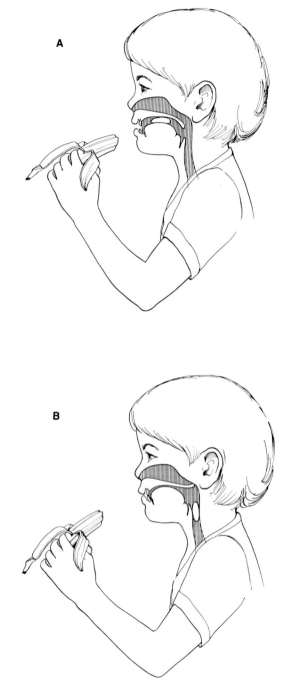

Figure 14-3 Swallowing. **A,** Voluntary oral stage. **B,** Involuntary oral stage.

the oral cavity contribute to functional changes. The mandible enlarges and grows downward, enlarging the space within the mouth. Teeth erupt and will further enlarge the oral space vertically (see Dental development, p. 265). This allows the tongue to move more freely in an up and down sucking pattern. The tongue

grows at the tip differentially, a good example of form following function.[29] It elongates and protrudes naturally to receive and carry semisolids between the gum pads.

With the more mature sucking pattern that now develops, a change in sucking, breathing, and swallowing functions is seen. They no longer occur simultaneously but alternately, and this is related to structural changes. Now the larynx is lower, exposing the airway to a greater degree. This necessitates a more mobile role for the epiglottis, which must move back and down to protect the airway. It is aided in its shielding function by the vocal folds. The soft palate rises to close the nasopharyngeal sphincter, and this interrupts nasal breathing. Now the infant accumulates fluid in his mouth and pauses in sucking and breathing while swallowing.

At 6 months, when the infant begins to spend more time sitting, gravity pushes downward on his body, elongating the thoracic cavity. The ribs, which have been at a right angle with the spine, begin to rotate so that the size of the thorax increases with inhalation. Now breathing is slower but deeper, and this allows babbling and longer, more controlled vocal sounds.

SEMISOLIDS AND THE SPOON

Initially when semisolids are introduced by spoon, there is a choking response as the child learns to handle a new texture and establish coordination between his tongue and pharynx. The food is drawn from the spoon by a suckling in and out movement. By 6 months the child is sucking more often, and the upper lip becomes active, closing down on the spoon. In time the lip will become mobile enough and isolated in movement to remove the food. Spoon-feeding becomes easier as the child learns to draw in his lower lip as the spoon is removed. Later the child's head comes forward to receive the spoon being presented by the feeder.

DRINKING FROM A CUP

The child starts to take liquid from a cup at about 6 months of age. In the first attempts, suckling movements may be evident along with up and down movements of both tongue and jaw. Choking responses are common as the child again learns to coordinate swallowing and breathing. The tip of the tongue may rest under the rim of the cup, and it now begins to elevate with swallowing. At first liquid leaks from the corners of the infant's mouth until he learns to purse his lips. The center of his top lip rises slightly to take in liquid. To maintain liquid in the mouth, the tongue forms a groove, while the cheeks press inward. Now the sucking pads are disappearing, and the cheeks become more mobile and autonomous in movement. To provide more external jaw stability, the child may bite down on the rim of the cup. Drinking will become a smoother function when the muscles around the jaw that control opening and closing can cocontract and the child can control opening.

BITING, CHEWING, AND SOLID FOOD

An infant begins to munch when crackers or cookies are introduced. Munching is the earliest form of chewing, and movements are up and down with mastication aided by a flattening and spreading of the tongue.[23] Because the infant cannot yet stabilize his jaw in a closed position, the feeder must break off the cracker as the infant maintains a bite position. When the infant eats, there is a suckling pattern, often in combination with sucking to move the food to the back of the tongue. A simple protrusion of the tongue may be present as well.

The infant also uses munching when ground food of lumpy texture is introduced. There may be choking again with accommodation to the new stimuli. The added stimulation of lumpy food contributes to the loss of hypersensitivity to touch within the mouth as the child experiences the additional sensory stimulation.

Next there is more movement of the tongue as it rolls the food to the sides. When the bolus is in the center of the tongue, the child may revert to a suckling pattern. The child begins to experiment with mouth play and uses the tongue to wipe food from the upper lip. When the tongue shifts to move food from the sides of the mouth to the middle, the jaw follows in a lateral and diagonal direction. By 12 months, the child may be able to transfer food from the center of the mouth to the sides through coordinated movement, rather than experimental rolling.

Lips too become more mobile and autonomous in movement. The corners begin to draw inward to control the movement of food and to prevent the loss of food or saliva while chewing. By 1 year, drooling is under better control. The upper incisors become useful for cleaning the lower lip of food, as well as providing the child with added sensory equipment to explore food. There are new possibilities for the child to enjoy mealtime as his skill with movement grows. By 2 years, the child chews with his mouth closed as he shifts food from one side of his mouth to the other. Jaw movement for breaking up solids is better controlled and by 3 years, the child shows the mature rotary pattern of chewing that is seen in adults.

HOW REFLEXES AFFECT FUNCTION

The relationship between reflexes and function has been described by Bobath,[4] Illingworth,[19] Peiper,[28] and others. At birth the newborn feeds by a sucking reflex. In 2 or 3 weeks he suckles and is directed to the nipple by a rooting reflex. With tactile stimulation to the perioral skin, including the cheeks and lips, the infant turns toward the stimulus in a food-searching manner. When there is stimulus to the lips, they respond with closing and pouting movements in preparation for sucking. These reflexes can be elicited when the infant is hungry, but they are diminished when he is satiated. The rooting reflex fades by 6 months, and by this time the child is sitting and taking swallows from a cup. He no longer needs the assistance of a reflex in searching out sustenance.

Similarly, the newborn shows a phasic biting reflex. When the newborn's lower gum is stimulated, his jaws open and close with rhythmic up and down movements. This response continues to be present until 3 to 5 months of age and is a component of the early munching pattern. It is gradually replaced by the more controlled volitional bite.

Moro's reflex is present at birth and is demonstrated by a strong abductor-extensor reaction of various parts of the body with loss of support that results in shaking of the head. The reflex fades and is integrated by 6 months when the infant begins to sit erect in a high chair and uses propping reactions of his arms. The startle reaction remains but with diminution. Otherwise, the infant would be unable to maintain sitting stability in the presence of stimuli.

Thus nature provides mechanisms for essential life-sustaining functions. With maturation of the central nervous system, primitive movement is inhibited and brought under control by higher centers. In addition, reactions appear that will be present for a lifetime. The labyrinthine righting reflex, optical righting reflex, propping, and equilibrium reactions assist voluntary, controlled movement that is needed for self-maintenance function.

Dental development

The primary, or deciduous teeth, erupt in a fairly predictable fashion, beginning with upper and lower central incisors. Most infants have a total of two upper and two lower incisor teeth by 7 months of age and thus acquire biting surfaces. Within another 4 months the biting surfaces will widen with the appearance of the lateral incisors. Sometime between 12 and 15 months the anterior (first) molars erupt, coinciding with the occurrence of refined lateral movements for chewing. Posterior (second) molars erupt between 24 to 30 months.

Normally the shedding of primary teeth coincides with the eruption of corresponding secondary teeth, and this begins at the end of early childhood (between 6 and 7 years) with the appearance of the first permanent molars and the loss of the lower incisors. Permanent teeth are usually in place in early adulthood, from ages 17 to 22 (Figure 14-4).

Common problems of eating

Children with impaired neurological functions may show a combination of feeding difficulties that are not

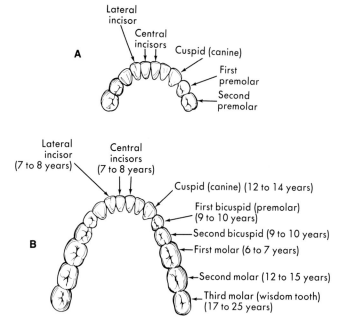

Figure 14-4   Dental development. **A**, Deciduous teeth. **B**, Permanent teeth.

easily identifiable. Motor patterns may be a mixture of abnormal, primitive, and normal signs.

The child's body tone is indicative of the types of problems that may be seen. Newborns with neuromotor impairment are frequently hypotonic. They may show head lag and floppy extremities. Some rigidity may be seen, particularly at times of distress or with feeding. The infant may suck weakly or the sucking action may be arrhythmic and inefficient, resulting in excessive jaw movement and loss of liquid from his mouth. When the infant is in the supine position, gravity may contribute to his tongue retraction, and he may fix his tongue against his palate, making it difficult to accept a nipple. Lack of muscle tone may result in a flattened tongue without the capability of forming a central groove through which liquids can move easily.

As the infant grows and begins to deal with gravity, he must find ways to compensate for his low body tone, and so he tends to lock in postures in his attempts to become functional. As he exerts more and more effort, muscle tone increases, and in time hypertonia may be seen.

Strong extensor tone of the neck, shoulders, and even hips can affect oral mechanisms and result in lip retraction and compensatory pursing, a jaw thrust, and tongue thrust. This is seen in children with spasticity who have difficulty developing isolated and independent oral movement patterns. Massive extension makes it difficult to close the mouth, chew, or use the tongue to move food in the mouth. A strong jaw thrust will inhibit the development of graded jaw movements for

biting and chewing (Figure 14-5, *A*). Lip retraction will prevent use of the upper lip to draw food from the spoon (Figure 14-5, *B*). A tongue thrust will interfere with swallowing (Figure 14-5, *C*).

Children who have fluctuating tone have problems with stability in oral movement. Inefficient movement may result in poor timing, which delays the swallowing reflex, and results in coughing and choking responses. For example, the child may be unable to use his cheeks well in holding the bolus of food on his tongue.

When children have poor hand skills, have difficulty with grasp and cannot direct the hand, and have asymmetry such as is shown with the asymmetrical tonic neck reflex, they are also deprived of opportunities to explore properties with their mouths. It is characteristic of a child at about 5 months of age or earlier to grasp objects voluntarily and bring them to his mouth where he has abundant sensory receptors. This mouthing exploration is one means of reducing the hypersensitivity of the oral cavity. Without oral stimulation, hypersensitivity can contribute to a number of problems, including gagging, greater head extension, lip retraction, tongue thrusting, and jaw thrusting. Additionally, there may be sensitivity of the gums and teeth that trigger a bite reflex. Hypersensitivity may be so great that the child is unable to tolerate stimuli about the face, and he may find textured foods unpleasant.

Abnormal postural tone directly affects respiratory patterns.[18] When there is strong extensor spasticity with the head extended, the shoulders pulled back, even the abdominal muscles contracted, the rib cage becomes flared and flattened over a period of time and reduces the amount of air the child can inhale. The child's breathing is shallow, and his vital capacity is reduced. This, in turn, makes it diffcult for him to sustain vocal production and to vary the sounds produced. Strong flexor spasticity also affects respiration. In this case, the head is lowered and the arms are forward and frequently are held tightly against the rib cage. This position also inhibits deep respiration and results in shallow breathing. When children have extremely low tone, they may develop asynchronous breathing. As they inhale, the sternum is indented and pulled inward. In addition to influencing sustained vocal production, respiratory patterns influence quality, pitch, and loudness of the voice.

Finally, children with neurological impairment may be limited in their means to communicate and unable to indicate by word or gesture that they do not like a food, or that they would like more, or that they are satiated. If tone is low, they may not use facial expression and characteristically may show a sad, droopy face with little emotional affect. Communication is an integral part of the eating environment and should be addressed as part of the program design (Chapter 22).

The following examples are presented to illustrate the questioning process as one seeks to identify the

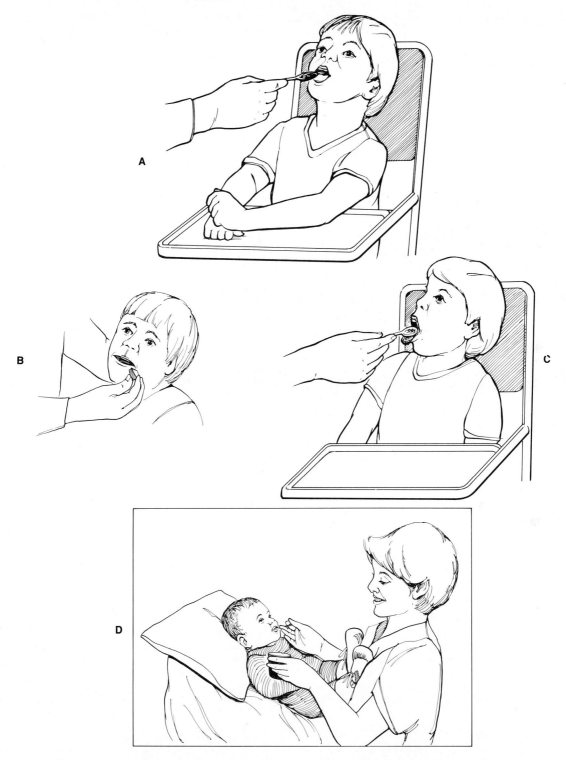

Figure 14-5 Feeding patterns. **A,** Jaw thrust: an abnormal downward movement of the lower jaw to an open position, making it difficult for the child to close his mouth and take in food. **B,** Lip retraction: an abnormal tightening of the lips horizontally, making it difficult for the lips to assist with sucking movements or to remove food from the spoon. **C,** Tongue thrust: an abnormal, forceful protrusion of the tongue from the mouth, causing utensils and food to be ejected. **D,** Symmetrical positioning for feeding with visual contact.

source of the eating problem. Questions and solutions may evolve together.

- Is the infant's difficulty in sucking related to poor tone? Can the nipple be removed from his mouth easily?
- Why can't the bottle be placed in the infant's mouth? Is his tongue retracted? Is it pressing against the hard palate? Does the infant sometimes tend to project his tongue? Is this a compensatory action to prevent obstruction of the airway? What happens if the infant is placed on his stomach?
- Why is the child not able to move food in his mouth? Is his tongue flat and bunched? Can tongue control be improved by changing sensory stimuli during feeding or by presenting textured foods? Is the problem motor oriented, or sensory oriented, or both? Which exerts the greatest influence?
- If the child has an adverse reaction when a spoon is introduced to his mouth—such as lip retraction, tongue thrust, or jaw thrust—will allowing the spoon to remain there longer give the system more time to adjust?
- Does the child bite down on the cup for stabilization or because of a bite reflex?
- Is drooling related to poor tone, positioning, or increased motor output?

Answers may not be immediately available and may require investigation of the effects of changes in stimuli. The selection of remediation techniques will be based on the child's responses, rather than on a single approach. To help therapists organize their questioning process, a summary of observations for eating function is shown in Figure 14-6.

Eating interventions

There are many remediation techniques described in the literature, and some are quite precise. Three approaches have been developed by Farber,[11] Morris,[23] and Mueller.[25] Farber uses neuromuscular facilitation for individuals with oral motor deficits. She suggests stretching the arches of the soft palate and uvula for the hypoactive gag response, using the walking back technique for the hyperactive gag response, vibrating the frenulum and stretching the tongue for tongue thrust, and using vibration and stretch techniques for sucking and swallowing. Morris uses a naturalistic approach and, among other things, looks to the total environment and normal development for therapy guidelines. Mueller advocates positioning and specific handling techniques, including jaw control and normalizing oral tactile sensitivity. All three authorities, plus

---

Figure 14-6   Summary of clinical observations for eating function

Position for eating:
In what position is the child usually fed? How well does the child maintain head and trunk control? Symmetry? Does the effort of eating affect postural tone? How often is adjustment in posture needed?

Response to sensory stimulation and environment:
How does the child respond to firm and light touches on legs, trunk, hands, arms, forehead, cheeks, lips? Does the child tolerate touch to gums, teeth, tongue, palate? To new tastes and textures? To temperatures? To sudden abrupt noises? Use smell to investigate food?

Sucking, swallowing, breast/bottle, spoon, cup:
What type of bottle nipple is used? How well does the infant grasp the nipple? What tongue pattern is used in sucking? Is sucking rhythmical? Is there excessive movement of the jaw with sucking? Does it take over 20 minutes to complete a bottle? Has the infant ever been tube fed?

What tongue pattern is used in sucking semisolids from a spoon? Does the child gag or choke? How well does the child coordinate sucking and swallowing? What is his head position when swallowing? Does the top lip come down on the spoon? Does the child use upper incisors to clean his lower lip?

Do the jaw and tongue move together in drinking?
Does the child choke? Bite down on the rim of the cup? Elevate his tongue tip in swallowing? Can the child purse his lips at the corners? What abnormal patterns interfere with sucking, swallowing, and drinking?

Biting, chewing solids:
Can the child stabilize with jaw closed while a cracker is broken off? Does the child use a munching pattern? Shift food from sides to center? Use his tongue to roll food to the sides of his mouth? Does the child cough and choke? Close his mouth when chewing? Show a rotary chewing pattern? What abnormal patterns interfere with chewing?

Drooling:
Is drooling under control? Is the chin wet or dry? Can the child keep his mouth closed? Does drooling increase with motor activity? With position change?

Respiratory patterns:
Does the child breathe through his nose or mouth? What is the postural tone of trunk, shoulders, and arms? What is the shape of the rib cage? Is the child's voice loud, soft, weak?

Communication:
Does the child communicate verbally? Or nonverbally through eyes, facial expressions, or hand gestures?

others, offer valuable insights, and the reader is encouraged to become acquainted with varying points of view.

Clinicians in the field today are inclined to choose those techniques that they personally have found to be successful and with which they are most comfortable. The techniques included here are among the most commonly used approaches in eating intervention. Among the factors to be considered in a program are positioning; the eating utensils; the types of food in the diet; the normalization of orofacial hypersensitivity; and stabilization and control of the jaw, lips, and tongue for cup drinking, spoon feeding, and chewing.

POSITIONING

This chapter has thus far established the high priority of positioning in promoting more normal function and has emphasized looking at the total body in space. By way of review, specifically one looks for those positions that interrupt the motor pattern of asymmetry and massive hyperextension and hyperflexion. The key points of support are the neck and spine, shoulders, and pelvic area.

A variety of positions for eating are available and useful. It is important that those who feed the child share a common knowledge, understand the child's movement patterns, and recognize those postures that facilitate the child's function and those that interfere with it.

Sitting is the social posture for mealtime communication. Common guidelines include the following:

Keep the head and body aligned in midposition; the head forward in slight flexion; the shoulders slightly forward to bring the hands to midline; the hips flexed to 90 degrees or beyond with the legs slightly abducted and weight evenly distributed.

Avoid extension of the head that interferes with swallowing and elicits abnormal extension patterns in the mouth; asymmetry of the head that can affect the position of the jaw, the arms, the legs, and inhibit the child's visual fields; protraction of the shoulders that can contribute to flexion patterns and involuntary jaw clenching; retraction of the shoulders and extension of the hips that may trigger abnormal extension patterns in the mouth.

Good positioning should be based on what works for the individual child, what normalizes his tone, and what contributes to midline and proximal stabilization. This will permit the child to use the controlled movement available to him for distal refined movements of the jaw, tongue, lips, and the arms and hands.

Infants feed in their parents' arms, feeling the close body and face-to-face contact. When possible, positioning that allows maximal contact with the parent or caretaker is to be encouraged. The parent's comfort in sitting is also a consideration, since feeding may be slow and time-consuming. A quiet uninterrupted time, as free from pressures as a household permits, helps to make the feedings as pleasurable as possible for parent and child.

Through simple adaptation the parent can use a large pillow or wedge to position the infant before her on her lap. The angle of the infant's body can then be adjusted by propping her feet on a stool. The infant's posture can be checked while he feeds, keeping his head slightly flexed in midline, his arms forward and at midline, and his legs slightly apart (Figure 14-5, *D*).

When the infant gains greater head and trunk control and is ready for a more upright posture, feeding can be carried out by sitting across his parent's lap. She can adjust the angle of the infant's hips and give stabilization and support where it is needed by bringing her arm around the infant's back.

When a child is ready to sit in a chair, the caretaker should provide postural security by inserting rolls in the seat if necessary. The child's spine should rest comfortably against the back of the chair, with the seat giving support along the thighs to a point just proximal to the knees, permitting full knee flexion to 90 degrees.

If strapping is necessary to maintain positioning, this should be applied across the pelvis. Added flexion of the hips to inhibit an extension pattern can be obtained by a rolled towel or a reversed wedged pillow under the child's thighs. The elbows should be supported; a tray suits this purpose well. The height of the tray may need to be raised if the child has trunk instability. If the child's legs tend to adduct, a small pillow between his legs will help to maintain abduction. Weight should be distributed evenly on both hips, and symmetry maintained. Feet should be supported, if necessary, by placing a box under the feet.

Prone lying is also an option to consider for the child with severe sucking and swallowing problems. This can be arranged in various ways, including use of a prone board or placement of a wedge pillow on the floor. Sidelying may be useful for a child who has a strong extension pattern in the supine position and a flexion pattern in the prone position.

The ultimate goal is to achieve as much independent movement for function as possible, and this requires practice and freedom to move. Static posture in most cases is not the end point.

FOOD PROPERTIES

Before discussing the selection of food for remediation techniques in eating, food terms according to texture and consistency need to be clarified. The following terms are commonly used:

Thin liquid Water, juice, or milk.
Thickened liquid Liquids thickened with cereal, pureed fruit, or other substances that make them less fluid.
Semisolids that are very smooth Solids that have been blended, strained, or pureed to obtain a smooth, thick consistency.

Semisolids that are lumpy Solids that have been passed through a food grinder or have been blenderized for a smooth and slightly lumpy texture; foods that have not been ground but are lumpy, including scrambled eggs, cottage cheese, and mashed cooked vegetables.

Solids Textures that are firm and tough, such as roast beef; crisp; or soft, such as cheese and skinless weiners that require minimal chewing.

Foods have specific properties that have significance for children with oral motor problems. Thin liquids are harder to manage than thickened ones. Because of their low specific gravity, thin liquids do not excite pressor receptors in the tongue and soft palate and tend to leak into the trachea, causing choking. Some therapists feel that acidic liquids, such as orange juice, increase saliva production; drooling is a common problem for children who lack tone or for some other reason have difficulty keeping their mouths closed. Dairy products, particularly milk rich in casein, produce mucus, which decreases sensation. This complicates the child's management of secretions still further. Above all, these children have difficulty handling mixtures of liquids and solids, as found in minestrone soup. The task of swallowing liquid while continuing to chew solids overburdens the poorly coordinated oral mechanisms.

Children may be able to demonstrate more normal oral patterns and show less coughing and choking when liquids are thickened. This can be done by adding yogurt or baby cereal. Thin purees can also be thickened, and nutritional substances such as bran and wheat germ can be added, depending on the child's tolerance. The thickened liquids slow down the swallowing process and give the child more time to organize the sensory information.

A cracker is usually one of the first solids an infant bites, and because it is soft, it mixes easily with saliva and can be easily swallowed.[2] Soft chicken or turkey pieces are also easily chewed and tend to stick together. Placing soft solids such as cubes of cheese in the sides of the child's mouth increases demands for chewing at a beginning level and also serves to inhibit the immature suckling and sucking patterns that occur when the food is resting on the center of the tongue. Morris[23] believes one should choose foods that put the system slightly under stress and challenge it through sensory input. Smaller, harder particles that do not mix with saliva, such as raisins, require greater manipulation by the tongue and increased chewing ability.

EATING UTENSILS

When determining the utensil that best serves the child's eating function, it is best to have an assortment of various shapes and sizes. This permits one to evaluate a number of them and determine which is more effective for the individual child. Parents appreciate seeing and knowing about products and learning about the availability, merits, and drawbacks of equipment on the market.

When an infant sucks weakly, mothers may attempt to help by enlarging the holes in the nipple. This is never recommended as a procedure, because it tends to elicit undesirable compensatory patterns. The preemie nipple, a soft one that compresses easily, is often selected in the hospital nursery. For an inefficient suck, the NUK nipple offers the advantage of keeping the infant's jaw further open than do regular nipples. This helps the lip maintain contact with the nipple. But the NUK nipple requires greater strength and coordination and may not be appropriate for the infant with a weak suck.[22] Some specialists feel that air swallowing may be prevented to some extent by use of a "banana" or "boat-shaped" feeding bottle that allows a slower, more even flow of milk. The nipple of choice is determined by the infant's response.

In general, spoons with a shallow bowl permit the child to have more success in pulling food from the spoon with the upper lip. The Mothercare line of spoons are functionally satisfactory and attractive. The sturdy plastic material is not vulnerable to shattering. Brittle plastic spoons should never be used with children who have oral motor problems, particularly when they have patterns of jaw clenching or exhibit the tonic bite reflex. For those children who are sensitive to warm and cold sensations, the sturdy plastic spoon offers the advantage of not conducting temperature as readily as a metal spoon. Some therapists and parents prefer the protective feature of the latex-coated spoon, while others feel that the added depth of the latex coating causes children to open their mouths wider. Additionally, they believe that the flexible plastic coating often stimulates a stronger bite reflex.[2]

When introducing cup drinking, many therapists choose to use a small, easily compressible plastic cup that can be held to form a spout. The cutout cup is usually satisfactory in preventing head extension as the cup is tipped for emptying, thus it allows the child to maintain slight flexion of the head. Therapists often choose cups that are translucent so that they, or the parents, can see the liquid levels in the cup, as well as the oral function of the child. Some children need the external stabilization provided by biting down on the rim of the cup. A thick-rimmed cup prevents this adaptation, but such a cup works very well for children not having problems with jaw stabilization.

NORMALIZING OROFACIAL HYPERSENSITIVITY

A guiding principle in reducing sensitivity to stimuli about the face, lips, and mouth cavity is to proceed slowly, kindly, and gently. It is a program that cannot be rushed, for the child's system must be given time to accommodate. The child is likely to be less defensive and apprehensive if tactile stimuli are presented through play, by use of firm, sustained pressure. Stuffed animals of various textures or furry puppets can reduce stress when they are used to converse with the child while taking imaginary journeys along the child's body, proceeding from the extremities toward the child's face, when tolerance for touch increases. Firm rubbing and stroking can be given with a washcloth during bathtime.

In approaching the face and mouth area, a good way to begin is by encouraging the child to explore his mouth with his own hands, providing he does not have a strong tonic bite or jaw clenching. The child may respond to soft squeeze toys that can even be used as utensils when it comes time to introduce food. Another natural activity includes wiping the mouth, but the method for this is to apply a slow, firm pressure in a blotting manner. Using a soft, damp, lukewarm cloth makes the stimulation more tolerable. Toothbrushing is a vigorous way of normalizing sensitivity.

Digital stimulation is a technique that can be used when touch about the face—the forehead, cheeks, and lips—is tolerated. It is introduced at the beginning of feeding to aid the child in accepting the sensory stimulation of food and utensils within his mouth. As an intrusion, the stimulation can be upsetting to the child and must be done slowly in a gradual manner. Again, by using play the therapist or parent can reduce the stress associated with this sensitivity. A suggested way to proceed is to invent a mouth game and during the game rub the child's outer gums on either side (not the front areas). Inner gums are then rubbed in a similar manner, and, if possible, stimulation may be given to the buccal and palatal regions as well. As discussed earlier, increasing food textures is another useful technique for reducing sensitivity.

Some children are sensitive to the point that the sight of an approaching spoon can result in a tongue thrust, jaw thrust, lip retraction, and extension of the head. Generally, tongue thrust should always be inhibited before presenting food in a spoon. This is commonly done by "walking the spoon back on the tongue," using an unfilled spoon. Starting at the anterior half of the tongue, the feeder gives downward pressure with the spoon and holds for a few seconds. This is repeated two or three times while continually moving back toward the middle of the tongue each time. An additional consideration for the child who is hypersensitive to spoon-feeding is to explore the use of a cup. When a child is spoon-fed, the spoon is repetitively inserted for brief periods, bombarding the system. On the other hand, in taking food from a cup, the contact is sustained over a longer period of time.

When a hyperactive gag response is present, stroking the tongue firmly, front to back by using an unfilled spoon is a step toward desensitizing the child's response. It is also helpful to press down on the center of the tongue with the spoon when food is presented to

the mouth and to close the mouth to inhibit the gag response.

A number of interesting techniques have been proposed by therapists working with infants who show sucking problems. When an infant shows an arrhythmic suck, instilling a tempo of one suck per second is attempted by stroking the infant's tongue downward and forward at this tempo. Rocking the infant at a rock per second has also been suggested. When the infant's problem is a weak suck, measures include cuddling in flexion, since sucking is a flexion pattern. A pacifier can be used to facilitate the initiation of the suck, then at intervals semi-solid food by spoon can be introduced for suckling.

JAW CONTROL

Jaw control is a technique in which the therapist or other feeder gives external stabilization to the child's jaw and controls its opening and closing; it is frequently used when there are abnormal extension patterns and poor coordination of oral structures. Initially, a child may only be able to tolerate the control for a short period. It is advisable that the technique be introduced in a therapy session by a therapist, preferably during snacktime. In time the child should be able to accept the control during mealtimes as well. The person providing the jaw control must be aware of the degree of the child's function so that the amount of assistance can be diminished as the child learns to function better.

Essentially, jaw control is given in two ways: sitting beside the child or sitting in front of the child. When sitting beside the child (Figure 14-7, *A*), put one arm around the back of the child's head. Place your index finger on the front of the child's chin; it assists with controlling the lip and jaw. Place your middle finger under the child's chin; it helps in controlling the jaw and closing the mouth. Use your thumb on the side of the child's cheek to stabilize his jaw. Try to position yourself so that you have eye contact with the child.

When sitting in front of the child (Figure 14-7, *B*), place your thumb on the front of the child's chin. Place your middle finger under the child's chin; it helps to control the movement of the jaw. Place your index finger along the side of the child's cheek to stabilize his jaw.

A therapist should always keep in mind that this technique will not work satisfactorily if abnormal oral motor patterns are being triggered by tonic reflex activity in other parts of the body. Careful monitoring of total body position should be maintained while jaw control is given. The technique is used during spoon-eating, drinking, chewing, and swallowing. In addition to observing the steps outlined in the jaw control procedure, the following guidelines also facilitate better function.

With *spoon-feeding,* use a spoon with a shallow

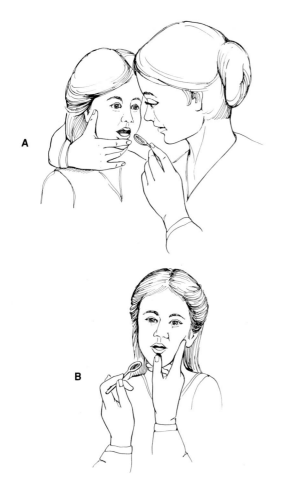

Figure 14-7 Jaw control. **A,** From the side. **B,** From the front.

bowl. Present the spoon at midline. Introduce the spoon slowly, and encourage the child to use his upper lip to clean the spoon.

With *drinking from a cup,* position the child so that his head is slightly forward. Use a cut-out cup if there is head extension. Place enough liquid in the cup so that the child does not need to tip his head back. Close the child's mouth for swallowing.

Closing the lips helps to control drooling, to prevent loss of food from the mouth, to promote better chewing patterns, and to coordinate swallowing. Other techniques for closure include brushing the lips with your fingers, pinching the cheeks lightly, stretching the corners of the mouth, and having the child imitate the sound, "mmmmmm."

A technique sometimes used to teach *swallowing* is to fill a plastic straw halfway with a liquid the child likes. By placing a finger over one end of the straw, the feeder can keep the liquid in the straw. The other end of the straw is then placed in the child's mouth, and the liquid is released on the back of the tongue. To help the child close his mouth and swallow, the feeder gently strokes with a finger the child's throat. Upright posture and slight flexion of the head aid in swallowing. Some therapists have found that sour liquids facilitate swallowing as well.

A child normally acquires tonicity and lip control at about 2 years of age, but to be skillful at *straw drinking,* it may take an additional year or so. A play activity such as blowing bubbles or paper windmills helps the child to learn how to position his lips. Popsicles are useful to facilitate puckering of the lips and drawing in the liquid.

Other ways of managing feeding

In the acute medical setting one encounters a number of conditions that necessitate an alternative way of feeding. Although it is the nurse who is most closely involved in maintaining nutrition, an occupational therapist should be aware of the implications of the measures. Some of the methods of feeding are the following.

MEDICINE DROPPER

The medicine dropper is used with small premature infants who have a good swallowing reflex but who cannot suck with sufficient strength to draw the milk through the nipple or cannot swallow rhythmically as they suck. The tip of the medicine dropper is protected by a piece of rubber tubing. The infant is given a few drops of liquid at a time and allowed to swallow before the bulb is again compressed.

BOTTLE FEEDING

Bottle feeding is used with more mature premature infants or those with an unusually strong suckling swallow reflex.

NONORAL FEEDING

The infant who is unable to suck or swallow, or who becomes fatigued with the effort of nursing, or who is apt to become cyanotic after feeding on the bottle or medicine dropper is fed by *gavage,* a method generally performed by the nursing staff. A catheter is inserted through the child's nostril down into his stomach. The nurse holds a syringe above the infant and slowly pours nutrient into the syringe barrel. After feeding, the tube is cleansed with sterile water. The catheter is changed at least every 4 days. Problems presented by gavage feeding are a reduced gag reflex and irritation to the infant's nose and throat.

The tube poses a real problem to the caregiver who attempts to introduce oral feeding. Since the mouth became the place where the child was poked and investigated by strange objects, it would be understandable that he would reject food or intrusion from oral stimulation. Moreover, when the swallowing reflex is triggered, the back of the tongue elevates and bumps into the tube—a negative reinforcer for oral feeding.

A *gastrostomy* makes it possible to avoid the potential hazards of prolonged nasogastric intubation. It is useful to prevent esophageal reflux and acts as a safety and outlet valve when vomiting occurs.

An incision is made into the abdominal cavity, and a tube is inserted directly into the stomach, halfway down the greater curvature. The tube is sutured firmly to the skin. A syringe is attached to the tube and is elevated for feeding.

Morris[23] points to a number of advantages this system presents. First, the child's clothing covers the area and eliminates the visual evidence of nonoral feeding, reducing the adverse reactions of others in the environment. Most importantly, it leaves the mouth free for oral stimulation while food enters the stomach. The feeder can reinforce the concept that the mouth is an enjoyable place through touching, mouthing, and sound play. Such measures help to prevent the hypersensitivity resulting from understimulation of a body part.

Morris further suggests a gradual progression from tube feeding to oral feeding as the child becomes nutritionally stable. She suggests allowing 20 to 30 minutes for oral feeding with the rest of the meal given by gastrostomy. She stresses the importance of holding, stroking, and engaging the child in other types of communication while the stomach is being filled. She also points to the advantage this system offers in conserving the child's energy, which was formerly required to maintain a borderline existence through oral feeding.

Problems presented by a gastrostomy include infection and skin breakdown.

Hyperalimentation is a medical procedure that introduces highly nutritional solutions directly into the bloodstream. It provides protein and calorie intake sufficient to sustain life and to promote growth in the absence of adequate gastrointestinal tract function. It is used for children with congenital bowel anomalies, extensive burns, intractable diarrhea, and cancer.

To be effective the fluid must contain protein, calories (dextrose), water, vitamins, minerals, and electrolytes. Since the high concentration of the solution makes it irritating to the blood vessel walls, a Silastic catheter through which the fluid is given must be placed into a vein large enough where blood flow is rapid to prevent sclerosis and thrombosis and to dilute the solution before it enters the peripheral circulation.

A surgical procedure is required and consists of inserting a catheter through the jugular vein and threading it down through the superior vena cava. The brachial artery also may be used. The catheter is secured by sutures.

An intravenous pump must be used at all times, since fluid will not drip by gravity. It is a continuously closed system. One of the complications that can occur is yeast and bacterial infection, since the hyperalimentation fluid is an excellent environment for the growth of organisms.

Self-feeding problems resulting from deficits in postural control

Before children are allowed to feed themselves alone, they should be able to swallow liquids and then solids without choking. They will also need a degree of sitting balance and some ability to control head movements.

There comes a time when a child is psychologically ready for self-feeding and desires to try. The dilemma for the therapist is that, although the child may have sufficient control to bring a spoon to his mouth or drink from a cup, his movement may trigger associated reactions leading to abnormal oral mechanisms. It is not unusual to see increased tension in the mouth as a result of the physical effort required in self-feeding.

Mueller[25] believes that when children have already been feeding themselves or are at an age when they feel a strong urge to do so, they should be allowed to pursue self-help efforts. Her approach is to assist them with a minimum of body control through key points, such as the shoulder or wrist, and with jaw control and lip closure for swallowing. She might assist the child with the first few bites by placing her hand over the child's hand as he holds the spoon, then gradually withdraw her help. Using this approach, a therapist gives support at the wrist and elbow, then just at the elbow, and finally the therapist withdraws support, allowing the child to eat unassisted.

Morris[22] gives examples of how associated reactions occurring with self-feeding can be minimized through repositioning and support at key points. Along with the action of a child's bringing a spoon to his mouth, there is overflow into the opposite arm that causes internal rotation and abduction of the shoulder and flexion of the elbow—the result of associated reactions in the arm. This has the effect of reducing the child's oral ability during feeding. When a therapist gives assistance through stabilizing and straightening and outwardly rotating that arm, there is relief of total body tension, and this allows more normal mouth patterns.

Another illustration is when the child attempts to drink from a glass. He brings his head forward and his trunk follows—the result of poor postural control. To compensate, the child stabilizes his elbows on the table and hyperextends his head, instinctively adapting to the effect of gravity as well. The therapist stops or inhibits this tendency to pull into a flexed pattern by providing a type of positional stability through elevating the elbows and thus supporting the shoulders in abduction. Less effort is then exerted by the child in holding the cup, and drinking improves.

Morris[23] also emphasizes that the success of techniques and adaptive equipment depends on the environment of the home and school. One must separate what will work in therapy, from what is possible at home, from what affects the child in a busy, stimulating atmosphere of a classroom or cafeteria. The therapist can convey his or her concerns and work with parents and school personnel in reaching the best possible solutions.

ADAPTIVE EQUIPMENT

To facilitate ease of feeding, one may first consider stabilizing the plate and cup. If the child is unable to grasp, a variety of handles can be evaluated. Some are built up or contoured to fit the hand or have straps to secure the spoon in the hand. To scoop food onto the spoon, the child may need a dish with a raised edge. These "scoop dishes" are available in many commercial designs. They make self-feeding easier by preventing the food from sliding off the plate. To bring the spoon to the mouth, further help may be needed in the form of a curved, extended handle. A cup with a handle on either side may be required initially so that the hands may be used bilaterally for greater stabilization. Mechanical or electric feeders may be appropriate for children who lack the arm and hand control to grasp, fill and bring the spoon to the mouth. The ability to take food from a stationary spoon is a prerequisite for use. Further suggestions for equipment are included in Figure 14-8.

Self-feeding problems resulting from limitations in mobility and strength

Feeding difficulties may arise as the result of contracture, weakness, structural deformity, or lack of body parts. Such problems require a very different approach to feeding than those resulting from incoordination and poor postural tone. Here self-feeding is not so much a matter of remediation as it is of adaptation. To better understand why a child may have difficulties, let us look at the requirements for feeding from the standpoint of range and strength.

PROBLEMS IN RANGE AND ADAPTATION

Beginning with the neck, slight flexion is needed to look down at the table surface and monitor the hand as it manipulates utensils or finger foods. One has only to observe a child with severe involvement of the cervical spine in juvenile arthritis to appreciate how the lack of neck flexion can inhibit the visual field.

We are inclined to take for granted our ability to open and close our mouths and chew food, but this function is dependent on the range of the temporomandibular joint. With joint involvement, feeding can be painful and movement restricted.

The alignment of the vertebral column with its multiple joints can affect the position of the head relative to the body. For example, in severe scoliosis a child may need to support his trunk with at least one arm to maintain balance. This can slow and interfere with his ability to feed.

The elbow joint is the primary junction for bringing the hand to and from the mouth. A 60-degree arc of motion, between 60 degrees of flexion and 120 degrees of extension, is considered functional range. Contractures greater than this arc in either direction can compromise reaching the eating surface and reaching the mouth.

Lack of mobility and fixed contracture in the forearm, wrist, and fingers limit one's ability to grasp a utensil and to hold it at the required angle for food scooping and presentation to the mouth. An example of a feeding problem was presented by an adolescent whose wrist was subluxed and fused in flexion and ulnar deviation. She also had little supination available. This caused the spoon to approach her opposite cheek area rather than her lips. Limitations in supination can also result in spilling as the spoon is elevated.

PROBLEMS IN STRENGTH AND ADAPTATION

A child with weakness will often compensate and seek to stabilize body parts through external support, as in propping elbows on the table to keep the trunk from leaning forward. Then the neck is extended to bring it in line and out of the pull of gravity. Thus the child may tend to exaggerate postures to enlist or eliminate gravity. A child with a high spinal cord injury will sometimes use all available motion in his neck to reach toward a spoon of food with his mouth. By instinct, a child with weakness may first flex the elbow before raising the arm, thereby shortening the lever arm and changing mechanical forces. By raising feeding height, children lacking strength in the shoulder and elbows are able to bring the hand to the mouth by eliminating gravity. A higher surface on which arms are propped also serves to support an unsteady trunk.

Adaptive aids and techniques are among the most useful measures in helping children with these problems achieve greater independence. They offer the therapist the oportunity to work closely with parents and child, to enlist their help in evaluating equipment, and to choose the items that they determine to be the most useful in solving self-maintenance problems in the home setting.

EQUIPMENT CRITERIA

The choice of an adaptive aid is a cooperative decision to be made by the child, parents, and therapists as they evaluate its effectiveness together. Adolescents who are striving to identify with their peer group tend to reject aids that call attention to their disabilities. Younger children are easily frustrated if the aid's use exceeds their coordination abilities, their attention spans, or gadget tolerances. Some criteria to consider in selecting aids include the following:

1. The aid must be developmentally appropriate. It should not exceed the child's ability to manipu-

Figure 14-8 Supporting function through adaptive aids

Function	Adaptive aid
Arm movement	*Suspension sling:* A device to support the upper extremity. Cuffs fit under the elbow and wrist and are spring-suspended from overhead bars. Assisted motions are shoulder horizontal abduction and adduction, shoulder external and internal rotation, shoulder abduction, and elbow flexion and extension.
	Mobile arm support (MAS): A frictionless arm support using the concept of the inclined plane. A trough supports the forearm and connects to a series of movable bars with adjustable stops. The unit fastens to a wheelchair with brackets. The MAS provides movement in space and helps weak shoulder and elbow muscles to position the hand.
	Gooseneck spoon: A spoon is mounted to a gooseneck holder that is clamped to the table edge. The gooseneck provides resistance through the motions of scooping and bringing food on the spoon to the mouth. This can help inhibit extraneous movement and athetosis.
Wrist support	*Cock-up splint:* A simple splint that extends from the distal palmar crease, supports the wrist, and ends two thirds up the distance of the forearm. It stabilizes and positions the wrist to provide mechanical advantage needed by fingers in prehension and grasp.
Grasp	*Universal cuff (utensil holder):* A cuff that fits around the palm, has a pocket for the insertion of handles of utensils, and can be used when grasp is not possible.
	Built-up handle: An enlarged handle that facilitates grasp.
	Modified handle for cup or glass: A projection on the utensil that will accommodate the child's grasping pattern. NOTE: Maintain low center of gravity when weakness is present.
Reach	*Curved handle:* A handle adjusted to angle so that the child can reach his body parts.
	Extended handle: An elongated handle that provides reach. It becomes less stable with length and weight.
	Sandwich holder: A plastic holder with rubber band that grips the sandwich; inserted in universal cuff.
Supination	*Swivel spoon:* Spoon with swivel mechanism that levels the bowl when wrist or finger motion is gone.
Stabilization of equipment or food	*Nonslip mat:* A nonslip plastic material that holds plates and glasses steady.
	Plate guard: A rim that clips onto a plate, provides a "wall" against which food is scooped by the fork or spoon.
	Scoop dish: A plate molded low in front and high in back to facilitate scooping food.
One-handed feeding	*Rocker knife:* A knife with curved blade; cuts with rocking motion provided by one hand. Other aids that can be used are the plate guard and nonslip mat.
Self-feeding	*Electric or battery feeder:* An expensive device that enables self-feeding without using the arms; requires a single motion to control switches; must be set up by caregiver.

late it. Results from its use should be consistent, predictable, and fairly easily obtainable.

2. The aid should have a pleasing color, texture, and odor, with as close to normal appearance as possible and simple, flowing design lines.

3. The aid must be sturdy.

4. The aid should show good mechanical advantage and be well balanced with a low center of gravity.

5. The aid should be easily cleaned and stored.

6. The aid must be economical, replaceable, and easily obtainable.

Behavioral problems in eating and self-feeding

Children with developmental delays or motor difficulties are potential candidates for behavioral problems having to do with food, just as are children with primary emotional behavioral disorders. Parents, anxious about their child's nutritional intake, can easily fall into a pattern of urging, nagging, or bribing their child to eat. When parents are confused about appropriate expectations for their child, they may show even greater inconsistency in approaches and responses and feel even more stress in dealing with their child's behavior. Because no one can make a child eat, the child often assumes control of the feeding environment. Howard[17] stated, "Food becomes the vehicle through which the child expresses his feelings and attempts to gain control over an environment in which he may have little or no control" (p. 580). Moreover, if the child has an early history of being gavage or force fed, he may not have learned to establish a trusting relationship with the individual feeding him. Food may have been a symbol of frustration or conflict rather than love, and it initiates a host of feeding and behavioral problems.

FEEDING BEHAVIORS CAUSING CONCERN

A variety of behaviors can appear. Among the most common are refusal of the child to eat specific foods; bizarre feeding patterns; gagging; vomiting or rumination; unwillingness to finger feed or self-feed; limited attention span at mealtime; and disruptive behavior. Physical conditions that may result from feeding behaviors include slowed growth; in some cases, an excessive weight gain; anemia; lack of appetite or increased appetite; and constipation. These conditions are of concern to parents and professionals alike.

APPROACHES TO CHANGING BEHAVIOR

Professionals use a number of approaches to change eating patterns. One approach is the *mealtime assessment,* where mealtime behaviors of parent and child are observed. O'Neil[26] outlined the method by which interactions are analyzed in terms of the antecedent events, the behavior, and the consequences revolving around eating. Factors that contribute to behaviors include the parents' expression of attitudes, values, interests, beliefs, and their caretaking behaviors. On the child's side, behavior is influenced by intrinsic factors: the child's individual growth patterns, his learning potential, and his ability to incorporate increasingly complex experiences into his current state of thinking and functioning.

A basic concept in behavioral assessment is that behaviors are increased, maintained, or decreased by the consequences that immediately follow them. Through the observational assessment, parent-child mealtime interaction is analyzed according to most frequent eating and noneating behaviors. The team members help parents identify those child behaviors that they wish to change, as well as the appropriate eating behaviors that they wish to foster in their children. From the analysis, team members determine appropriate consequences that affect behavior; this can vary from child to child. Reinforcement and consistency are keystones for success in changing patterns.

Another approach is *teaching feeding behaviors.* This method is appropriate for the child who needs to have the feeding process broken down into sequential steps according to his developmental level. Reinforcement is given when the first step is learned, and other steps are added in succession as skill grows. This technique is sometimes referred to as *shaping. Fading* is a procedure in which one first gives maximal assistance and then withdraws help as the child's skill develops.

THE VALUE OF THE TEAM APPROACH

When behavior interferes with eating function, perhaps one of the most important things to remember is to seek help and collaboration with other professionals: the nutritionist, the social worker, the nurse, and significant others. Feeding is very complex, particularly when viewed within the framework of social interaction. Professionals need to be clear about their roles as they analyze behavior, design programs, and implement steps for change.

Other factors for a therapist to consider
COLLABORATION WITH THE SPEECH PATHOLOGIST

Speech pathologists specialize in identifying specific language deficits and help the occupational therapist in a number of ways. They are able to clarify the interrelationship between breathing patterns and phonation and can detect the fine, discrete coordination required of muscles for articulation. They are highly skillful in diagnosing language difficulties as a result of injury to speech centers and are able to obtain information about children's learning styles.

The *close tie between acquisition of feeding skills and later development of speech* is widely accepted among therapists. Indeed the tie is considered so close that in some settings it is the speech pathologist who evaluates eating problems and carries out the treatment program and consults with the occupational therapist on eye-hand motor function. Two of the leading authorities on eating problems, Morris and Mueller, are specialists in prespeech. Morris[23] believes the relationship between feeding and speech skills remains relatively unexplored and calls for more study. She describes how the function of feeding can be used to facilitate the movement required for speech. First, the child adds movement components before these are built into speech itself. The movements are facilitated at the automatic level, rather than the cognitive level. The therapist provides feedback and sensory awareness and facilitates a more volitional repetition of movement. Both food and the automatic feeding movements can be used to promote easier voicing and wider variety of articulatory movement.

Morris[23] provides examples of how this can be done. As the child approximates his lips to remove food from the spoon, the therapist may focus on the word *more*. The child is then able to immediately experience the proprioceptive feedback from the motor pattern to produce the word *more.*

If the child demonstrates good tongue tip elevation during the swallowing of pureed foods from the spoon, a spoonful of food can be used to reinforce correct tongue tip placement for words beginning with *t, d,* or *n.* Thus feeding movement facilitates speech movement.

Morris[23] emphasizes the *need for communication systems between feeder and child.* For the child who is developmentally above 18 months but unable to speak, Morris suggests such practical measures as a mealtime placemat containing pictures or symbols for concepts such as "more," "no more," "something else," "yummy," and "yuk." An older, nonverbal child with many persons who feed him benefits from a feeding procedure book with photographs that make the feeding process clear to others in terms of the child's comfort and function.

A speech pathologist and occupational therapist have much knowledge to share in mutually promoting functions of eating and speech.

COLLABORATION WITH THE NUTRITIONIST

Nutrients from food provide the raw material that allows the body to function and grow. Thousands of chemical compounds are broken down by the body to provide energy. Nutritionists are able to estimate the amount of nutrients needed for the individual child based on his size and motor dysfunction. Nutritionists understand the nutrient requirements at various stages of growth and identify the critical times for the introduction of foods with a variety of flavors and textures. They provide essential information for a feeding program that encompasses not only the function of the oral motor mechanisms but also the quality and amount of food required for health.

There are many insights to be gained from reviewing *nutritional research.* Some investigators believe the degree to which the mouth area is involved directly affects nutrition and that mouth involvement and general growth closely parallel one another.[28] A high calorie density diet has been recommended for those having poor oral skills. On the other hand, Hammond and others[16] found that the degree of mental retardation impeding self-help skills was a more significant factor in influencing dietary intake than the motor deficits imposed in neurological disorders. While studies may be debatable, they point to the overall effects of nutritional intake.

Two factors that affect children's eating performance are *medication* and *constipation.* Nutritionists can clarify the effects of medication on food intake. Medications can interfere with feeding in a global way: they can alter taste sensation, diminish appetite, promote insatiable appetite, and cause drowsiness. Anticonvulsant drugs prescribed to control seizures increase a child's need for vitamin D, alter folic acid metabolism, and interfere with riboflavin status.

One of the most frequently encountered problems in a disabled child is constipation. Fiber and fluid are important ingredients in ameliorating this common condition. Coarse fibrous foods such as raw fruits and vegetables are helpful, but when a child cannot chew, other preventive measures include the use of well-soaked bran, whole grain cereals, and foods with natural laxative effects.

In summary, there are many questions to present to the nutritionist who can help therapists make the eating program a nutritional model for parents to follow.

COLLABORATION WITH PARENTS

Successful feeding in early infancy is generally regarded as one of the measures of a parent's child-rearing competencies. It is no wonder that a parent can feel threatened by the professional who questions how the child is fed and observes quietly as the parent struggles to place a spoon of food within the child's mouth. A sensitive therapist will recognize the potential for feelings of inadequacy on the part of the parents and will strive to *reinforce those good parenting behaviors observed.* The therapist will exercise caution in intruding on the parenting role, but at the same time present a model for parents to follow. The goal is to improve the child's eating function and also to help parents acquire skill in management and to increase their feelings of competency.

There are *communication measures* to consider that can contribute to the parents' ease and receptiveness. First of all, determine what they perceive as the problem, what they want to change. Explore how this child's development differs from that of siblings. As one begins to investigate positioning, consult with the mother and father regarding the position for feeding that is comfortable for them. During the feeding, observe how well they perceive cues from their child and help them to be aware of communication gestures. Finally, provide the *environmental support* that enables the child and parents to relax, whether this be a quiet, dimly lighted room or one with privacy and freedom from distraction.

Data collection is an important part of the interview. Information is gathered on how long it takes to feed the child, the person or persons responsible for feeding, past successful or unsuccessful methods, utensils used, and whether there are behavioral problems and how they are handled. Investigation includes the kind of responses the child makes to new foods, their texture, smell, and temperature; how the child handles different kinds of food (liquids, semisolids, and solids); what preferences and dislikes exist; and how often the child feeds during the day.

It is unwise to spend the entire time presenting questions to the parents. For that reason, some therapists prefer the use of a questionnaire that parents can complete at their convenience. This allows time to carefully consider their child's eating patterns. Excellent examples of questionnaires are presented in works by Finnie[12] and Morris.[23]

During the evaluation session the therapist can also observe the *feeding environment;* the general atmosphere of parent-child interaction, the techniques used, the parental attitudes toward feeding, and the kinds of positive and negative reinforcing behaviors displayed. Above all, the therapist seeks to involve parents in the problem-solving process (Chapter 8).

TOILETING
Prerequisites for toilet training

In the literature there is a great deal of information and advice for parents on when and how to embark on a toilet training program with their child. Emphasis is rightly placed on the readiness of the parties involved. Certainly, parental attitudes are a strong factor in the ease with which progress is made.

Independent toileting is an important self-maintenance milestone with wide variation among individual children. It carries considerable sociological significance. Self-sufficiency can be a determinant when a school is considering whether to accept a child into a regular classroom program. Like other self-care skills, toileting is a complex task requiring a series of learning subskills. But before embarking on learning, a child must be physically, physiologically, and psychologically ready. Toileting consists of training sphincter reflexes and the volitional holding of urine and feces.

Physiological factors

At birth a newborn voids reflexively and involuntarily. Changes in position, handling by others, and other stimuli can trigger micturition. Voluntary control and restraint of the reflex, which is the method employed when control is established, is not available to the youngster until the spinal tract is myelinated to a level for bowel and bladder control at the lumbar and sacral areas. This is after the child is standing and walking alone. Bowel control precedes control over the bladder, and studies indicate girls are trained an average of 2.46 months earlier than boys.[10] Daytime bowel and bladder training is usually attained by 30 months, but bladder nighttime control may not be accomplished before 5 and 6 years of age.

The child's awareness

Another indication of readiness for toilet training is the child's awareness of discomfort after emptying bowel and bladder, as well as the ability to identify elimination as the cause of discomfort. There must be an awareness that characteristic sensations precede excretion. As early as 10 months the infant may begin to pay attention to the act of voiding. This can be detected by general facial expression and quieting behavior. By 14 months the need to eliminate may be indicated by gesture or action.

Other requirements for toilet training

The methods by which training is introduced vary, but most authorities agree on these fundamentals. First, there should be one or two significant people who are willing to devote time and effort to establishing patterns of toileting, and there must be a communication system between them and the child. Behaviorally, reinforcement is given for success, and harsh punishment for failure is avoided.

A gentle approach to toilet training

Brazelton[5] presents gradual steps for toilet training. He suggests that after 18 months of age, a child can be placed on a potty chair with all his clothing on, avoiding the cold surface of the seat. Introduction can begin pleasantly by talking or reading aloud as the child sits there. Within a week or so one can try having the child sit on the chair without diapers. This is followed by dropping the dirty diaper into the potty chair to build an association between the chair and elimination. Finally, efforts are made to catch the stool or urine while the child sits on the chair, and this is done several times a day. As the child's interest grows, independence can be made easier and more pleasurable if he is dressed in comfortable clothes, including training pants, that allow him to manage clothing adjustment alone.

Brazleton[5] also speaks of the fears that toddlers may experience with toileting and the anxiety they may have associated with giving up the bowel movement as a part of themselves. He points to the value of repetitive play to help children overcome such feelings. Brazelton notes that boys hold back their bowel movements much more frequently than do girls, even as they achieve urine training. He urges patience and reassurance from the parents to help the children relax and to master the task at their own pace.

Because of interest and motivation toward bowel and bladder control, toddlers demonstrate curiosity toward their own and other's genital organs. They observe and feel their own urinary stream and may touch and feel the feces, and touch and manipulate their own genitals. Parents can help a toddler satisfy tactile and perceptual curiosity by providing a simple explanation or by presenting play activities with clay and water and containment and release themes.

Tasks to be mastered

To be truly independent in toileting, the child will need to manage fastenings, get the pants up and down, and in the case of a girl wearing a dress, hold the dress away from the buttocks—subskills usually achieved at about 4 years. Children will need to climb on the toilet and seat themselves. This occurs at about 3 years. By 5 they are successful in cleansing after toileting, and they can wash and dry their hands efficiently without supervision. Progress is accomplished in sequence, according to each child's unique pace of development.

Considerations when posture is unstable

The child with postural control deficits must first acquire sitting balance or do so through the support of equipment. One can readily see that the child with increased tone would have difficulty. This is shown early when the mother attempts to diaper the infant. She may first need to place a pillow under the infant's hips, then flex them and spread the legs apart to break up the strong extensor and adduction patterns in his legs. With unstable sitting posture, the child will have difficulty relaxing and maintaining a position for pressing down and emptying the bowels. It has been said that unless the toilet seat is low enough so that the feet rest firmly on the floor and some flexion of the thighs is possible, the accessory muscles that normally aid in defecation have little opportunity to fulfill their function. Every effort should be made to help the child feel posturally secure. The feet should always be supported, and if the child needs to rely on his hands for balance, toilet bars should be considered.

Finnie[12] offers suggestions for adapting potty chairs and toilet seats for children with poor postural control. For example, she suggests placing the toilet in a corrugated cardboard or wooden box when the child's balance improves. Across the top of the box, attach a bar for the child to hold onto for added security. Commodes that feature such modifications as adjustable legs; safety bars; angled legs for stability; and padded, upholstered, and adjustable backrests and headrests are available on the market. Commodes are also available with seat reducer rings, seat belts, and adjustable footrests.

How range and strength affect function

Children with weakness and limited range of motion face a number of difficulties with toileting. They may not be able to manage fastenings because of hand involvement, or they may have problems in sitting down or getting up from the toilet seat because of hip and knee contracture or quadriceps weakness. In such cases a raised toilet seat is a consideration. Most distressful of all their problems is when they are unable to supinate the hand, flex the wrist, or internally rotate and extend the arm to cleanse after a bowel movement. An anterior approach may be tried. It is important to caution girls against contamination from feces, which can cause vaginitis. If at all possible, girls should wipe the anus from the rear. Solutions to cleansing problems are difficult and often discouraging.

Again, adaptive devices are among the most helpful measures available. A combined bidet and toilet offers a means for total independence. Several models are available that attach to any standard toilet bowl. A self-contained mechanism spray-washes the perineal area with thermostatically controlled warm water, and dries it with a flow of warm air. Controls can be operated with the hand or foot (Figure 14-9). The unit is expensive but is worth considering, particularly for the sensitive adolescent. Other simple, inexpensive aids include various tong devices. Toilet paper holding devices can be clamped to the toilet seat to assist in perineal wiping without the use of hands, for bilateral upper extremity amputees.

Loss of normal excretory function

Children with spinal cord injury or other conditions that produce a full or partial paralysis present a challenge for skin care when there is lack of sensation, and they require special management for bowel and bladder activities. Loss of control over these bodily functions can be infantilizing, producing embarrassment and decreased feelings of esteem. School-age children are characteristically modest about their bodies, and

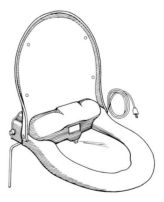

Figure 14-9 An electrically powered toilet bidet makes it possible to clean the perineal area independently without hands or paper.

adolescents are struggling with identity issues and need to be like their peers.

BLADDER CONTROL

There are two types of bladder problems. When there is a lesion in the lumbar region or below, the bladder is flaccid. The reflex arc is not intact, and the bladder has lost all tone. The following terms are used for this condition: the lower motor neuron bladder and the atonic, or areflexic, bladder. When an injury occurs higher, above the level of bladder innervation, the reflex arc remains intact. Thus when the bladder is full, or its contents reach a critical level, it empties by reflex. In this situation the bladder is said to be a reflex bladder, an automatic bladder, or an upper motor neuron bladder. Training programs are undertaken to develop automatic responses in a spastic bladder. Children with a flaccid bladder cannot be trained because the bladder has no tone to empty. To determine if a child is a candidate for training, a number of tests may be carried out to measure the ability of the bladder to expel urine and to hold a particular amount of urine, depending on the size and age of the child.

There are a number of ways to manage urine collection. In boys one of the most common systems is by *condom drainage.* Boys are able to learn to apply and use this system independently, given sitting balance, hand dexterity, and alertness in following the procedure. With this external device system the condom is placed over the penis and is attached to a tube running down the leg to a collection bag that must be emptied at intervals. A common problem is skin breakdown where the condom is attached.

Managing the bladder can be more difficult for girls because of their anatomy. It is sometimes accomplished by an *indwelling catheter.* Boys may use this system as well. A Foley catheter consists of a small rubber tube and a balloon attachment. After the tube is inserted through the urethra to the bladder, the balloon is filled with sterile water, and this serves to keep the catheter in place. The tube drains the urine from the bladder to a collection bag. In some cases the catheter is clamped and unclamped at regular intervals to "train" the bladder to empty by reflex when the contents reach a critical amount. Bladder irrigation is a regular procedure when a catheter is used and is carried out periodically. This is done by injecting a benzalkonium (Zephiran) solution into the catheter to stir up sediment and prevent stopping up the catheter.

The catheter itself increases the likelihood of urinary infection and bladder stones, since it introduces a foreign body into the bladder. For this reason a high fluid intake is considered an important precautionary measure.

Credé's method is sometimes used to expel urine. With this method the hand is placed on the lower abdomen, on or above the bladder, and a gentle pressure downward is given. Balanced bladder function is attained if the amount of urine left in the bladder is 20% of bladder capacity or less. The Credé's method must be carefully executed to prevent reflux. When reflux occurs, urine goes up the ureters and then returns to the bladder, forming a pool for infection.

When urinary tract infection becomes chronic, a *suprapubic catheter* may become the system of choice. Here a catheter is placed directly into the bladder through the abdominal wall. Urine then drains through the catheter tube directly into a urinal bag.

Because of problems from infection and renal stones, an alternative method, *intermittent catheterization,* is increasingly used for management. The catheter is inserted into the bladder every 4 hours, then every 6 hours, to empty its contents and to promote an automatic bladder. It also offers the individual the advantage of being able to carry the catheter inconspicuously in a small bag. Self-catheterization has been successfully taught to children by nurses. A precaution to observe is to restrict fluid intake to prevent bladder distention. When there is partial control of bladder function, girls may wear disposable diapers or incontinence pants that are available in various styles and sizes.

When there are serious difficulties with the muscles or nerves controlling the bladder, congenital malformations of the urinary tract, obstructions, chronic infections, and scarring, physicians may recommend a surgical procedure, the *ileal conduit.* This is a detailed procedure, and children and parents need preparation and explanation. During the surgery a small section of the ileum (a few inches long) is resected, and the remaining ends of the small intestine are rejoined, leaving the digestive system intact. This separated section is then used to form a stoma in the abdominal wall. Ureters are severed near the bladder and are reattached so that the urine drains through the stoma into a collection pouch. The pouch must be emptied at intervals and periodically cleaned and replaced.

The procedure can have a deep psychological effect on children, especially the adolescent, since it represents a change in body image. Parents too express hostility and depression and question whether a daughter may bear children or whether it will impair a boy's masculinity. The surgery itself has no effect on sexual organs or childbearing.

BOWEL CONTROL

A basic principle for success in bowel reeducation is to have a regular, consistent evacuation of the bowel. The time for this is a matter of choice, but there should be a schedule that remains constant. In some cases, suppositories and a warm drink are given before evacuation. This stimulates contractions and relaxation of muscle fibers within the walls of the intestine that move the contents onward. Other techniques include digital stimulation, massage around the anal sphincter, or manual pressure by Credé's method on the abdomen.

Removal of the stool by hand may become necessary. Factors that contribute to ease in elimination include an adequate fluid intake and a regular diet. Stool softeners are sometimes used to maintain a stool of normal form and consistency.

Closely associated with bowel and bladder care is *care of the skin* in the perineal area. Skin should be cleansed thoroughly to protect the tissue against contact with waste matter and to eliminate odor. All children with decreased sensation are susceptible to decubiti, which are pressure sores that occur fairly rapidly when blood vessels are compressed, as around a bony prominence such as the ischial tuberosity. This can result in ischemia, or lack of tissue nourishment. Skin self-care for these children includes daily inspection of the skin by mirror and avoiding sitting in one position for long periods of time. There are also a variety of special cushions on the market designed to prevent tissue trauma.

A number of *surgical procedures* are carried out to construct alternative means for stool collection. One of these is a colostomy. An incision is made in the colon and a fistula, or tubelike passage, is made between the bowel and the abdominal wall. Special bags cover the opening and are emptied as needed. An ileostomy is a similar procedure in which the surgical opening occurs in the lower part of the small intestine.

SOCIAL ENVIRONMENT

To be socially acceptable, a child lacking bowel and bladder control needs to be helped with measures to eliminate odors. Odors can be produced by the collection devices, the collected urine, or stool. Appliances should be changed and cleaned regularly. They can be washed in a commercial cleanser or in a vinegar and water solution. Maintaining a good fluid intake will prevent a strong concentrated urine. If urine is alkaline, it is more likely to have a strong odor. Therefore keeping the urine acidic by drinking cranberry juice will not only cut down on odor, but it also prevents bacteria growth as well.

Of all self-care tasks, toileting may require the most sensitive approach on the part of those who work with the child on a self-maintenance program. Children may deny that they are unable to toilet themselves independently, or they may purposely restrict their fluid intake at school in an effort to avoid the need for elimination. Toileting can be a distressing, unverbalized problem that should be explored with great care after the child feels comfortable with the therapist.

Menstruation

Therapists should also be aware of a young girl's status regarding menstruation, which normally begins between 10 and 17 years of age. In particular, mentally retarded individuals may be viewed by others as never growing up, and their bodies, therefore, are viewed as remaining undeveloped too. Thus adults around mentally retarded adolescents neglect to prepare them for changes in their bodies and the onset of menarche. Consequently, its arrival can be traumatic and frightening. This undeniable indicator of puberty can be distressing to some parents, and their troubled feelings can be conveyed in a confusing way to their child. Families may require support and counselling in ways of giving their child reassuring, understandable explanations.

For the girl with a physical disability, it is also important that first experiences with menstruation be positive ones. Duffy[9] is an informative resource on the subject. She points to the possibility that the menses experience offers the young disabled female an affirmation of equality with her peers. Her body, though different in some ways, is operating normally in an area of particular significance, confirming her identity as a sexual being.

Duffy describes personal experiences of "differently abled" women, their feelings, problems, and solutions. For example, one subject who was cited found that using disposable diapers in the toddler size worked best during her menstrual period, because they were flat rectangles and the sticky tapes on the sides could be used to fasten them to the insides of underpants. Stick-on menstrual pads are also a useful product. Others report on the brands of tampons they find easiest to insert, as well as the best positions for insertion.

Another useful reference is the work of Friedman[13] who provides collective information on techniques and adaptive aids for bilateral high-level upper limb amputees. In general, there is still too little material available in the literature. This indirectly validates the expression of some young disabled persons that in this area of self-care there continues to be a lack of supportive assistance from medical and rehabilitation personnel.

DRESSING

An infant makes a first gesture to cooperate with dressing at about 1 year of age by holding out an arm or a leg while being dressed. By 18 months the child is beginning to remove his socks. At 3 years he is independent with pull-down garments but has some difficulty with turning the heel of a sock and does not know the front of garments from the back. Usually by 4 years of age he can turn clothing right side out and needs little assistance. By 5 years, he dresses with care except for some fastenings and tying bows. Normally it takes 4 years of practice—a combination of experimentation, repetition, and assistance—to master dressing.

It is easily understood that children must have the eye-hand coordination for manipulating fastenings, but in addition they must also have knowledge of their physical selves and how body parts are related.[6] They must know where their bodies are in space. As they attend to dressing tasks, they look at body movements. Kinesthetically they feel the position of their body parts and may even verbalize motor actions aloud. They consciously direct some body movements, whereas other movements are automatic and compensatory, enabling them to maintain equilibrium in the various positions they assume. They are aware of the two sides of their bodies and, because of neurological integration, are able to use their limbs cooperatively and reciprocally.

Children also look at the clothing they will wear and in doing so distinguish boundaries of the clothing article. They visually scan for details, and as the attention and focus of their eyes shift selectively, they separate foreground and background. Discriminatively, they recognize the form and totality of an article of clothing and categorize it as a sweater, shirt, sock, or other item. This is an extension of the sensory process that involves concept formation. Having identified a clothing article, they maintain a visual form constancy of it, even if it is turned upside down. Through experience they accumulate space ideas.

The motor components of dressing—balance, range, strength, and control of movement—can be observed and, consequently, are more readily comprehended. What is less clearly understood are the internal mechanisms at work: the way the child receives and processes sensory information leading to a response in attending to the task at hand.

Common problems
PERCEPTUAL DYSFUNCTION

From the description of the dressing process one can begin to predict some of the problems that may occur with dressing. Among those children having perceptual deficits, difficulties may exist in distinguishing right and left sides of the body, in putting a shoe on the correct foot, or in turning the heel of a sock. A child may be unable to tell the front of his clothing from the back, or identify which leg goes with which pant leg or which sleeve goes with which arm. If one observes closely, there may be evidence that the child avoids crossing the midline by performing dressing tasks on the right side of the body with the right hand and those on the left with the left hand. At the other end of the spectrum, a child will most likely have great difficulty with fastenings and in tying shoelaces, tasks that require the two hands to work together.

INTELLECTUAL LIMITATIONS

Children with mental retardation tend to be chaotic in their organization of perceptual stimuli and, in addition to problems with left-right discrimination, may be unable to make connections with words such as "above," "behind," or "in front of" insofar as their own bodies are concerned.[7] Normally children become aware of these important dualisms between 2 and 3

years of age and are able to attach verbal labels to them between 4 and 5 years. Spatial relations are first mastered in the immediate areas of mouth, vision, and touch, and then they gradually extend out and away from the individual.

The child who has intellectual limitations cannot remember instructions and has a short attention span. Behaviorally there may be a low tolerance for frustration because the child cannot perform and dress himself as quickly as his siblings can. Language skills may be inefficient, which restricts the child's verbal capacity to express his frustration. This may increase when the child is faced with tasks that require fine manipulations. Coordination too may be impaired, as shown in attempts to button, snap, zip, or buckle.

To acquire independence, the child may require a special approach. After making a baseline assessment the therapist carefully analyzes each dressing task into its fine component parts so that the child can progress slowly in steps, in a chaining process, with reinforcement. Excellent examples of task analysis and teaching approaches are given by Copeland and others.[7] Their work is a valuable resource for those working with children who require great patience and consistency over a considerable period of time.

PHYSICAL LIMITATIONS

Children with various conditions may find dressing difficult because of the *coordination* and the range and strength required for pulling clothes on and off and connecting fasteners. Youngsters with arthritis who have painful fingers frequently require assistance during a flare-up of their disease. They may be unable to move their arms freely and to reach to areas of their body. Children with the use of only one hand will find it hard to zip trousers, tie shoelaces, and button shirts or blouses. Dressing is tedious and tiring. In most cases they learn adaptive techniques, often through their own experimentation. Children with abnormal muscle tone and retained postural reflexes often have difficulty balancing themselves or positioning their bodies while donning and removing clothing. Limited dexterity may also interfere with dressing. Tasks can be made easier by using simple measures such as proper positioning, dressing the involved extremity first, or by using adaptive aids such as button hooks, rings on zippers, one-handed shoe fasteners, or Velcro closures (Figure 14-10).

Dressing infants and dysfunctional children

Although the common approach to dressing an infant is to do so while he is lying supine, the supine position frequently increases extensor tone in those infants with neurological impairment. For that reason, some therapists advocate placing the infant prone

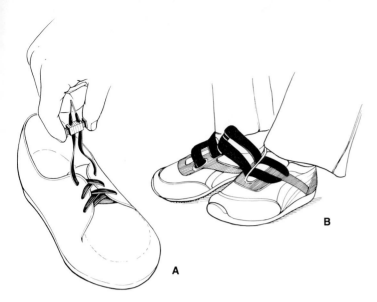

Figure 14-10 These shoelace fasteners can be managed with one hand. **A,** Spring tension blocks. **B,** Velcro.

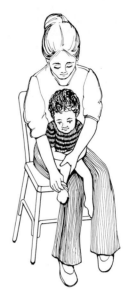

Figure 14-11 When dressing the child who is hypertonic, carefully flex the hip and knee before putting on socks and shoes.

across one's knees with the infant's hips flexed and abducted, thus breaking up the extensor-adduction tone. As soon as the infant gains head and trunk control, there are advantages to the sitting position, with the infant's back resting against and supported by the caregiver's trunk. In this arrangement the infant has an opportunity to observe his body. Knowledge of the physical self is to be encouraged whenever possible. As early as 14 months some infants begin to point to a named body part.

During dressing, the caregiver carefully bends the infants hips and knees before putting on his shoes and socks (Figure 14-11), and brings the infant's shoulders forward before putting his arm through a sleeve. Attention is continually directed to positioning and to keeping the body in symmetrical alignment. When a child achieves sitting balance, a good way to proceed with dressing is to place the child on the floor and later on a low stool, continuing to provide support where needed from the back. Orientation to the body and its various parts should remain a focus in the social interaction. The caregiver can help the child understand how his body relates to his clothes and to the various positions—the arm goes through a sleeve and the head goes through the neck of a garment. There are many perceptual concepts to be explored and learned as a part of the dressing procedure.

When the child is older and heavier, there may be no alternative but to dress him while he is lying supine. Placing a hard pillow under the child's head, thus raising his shoulders a little, will make it easier to bring his arms forward and to bend his hips and knees. If it is

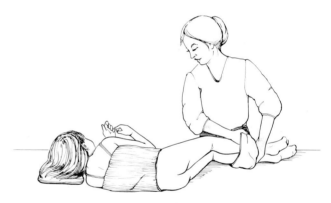

Figure 14-12 Sidelying may decrease tone and make dressing easier.

possible to maintain the child in a sidelying position, this posture may make it easier to bring his shoulders and head forward, to bring his arm forward, and to straighten his elbow (Figure 14-12).

Self-dressing techniques
A DEVELOPMENTAL APPROACH

Gesell[14] described with amusing accuracy the child learning backward rather than forward. Characteristically, one undresses before he dresses. This is an important guideline in setting expectations. Self-dressing can be introduced in a natural way, at bedtime, by allowing the child to complete the final step in pulling off a garment. Similarly, when the child becomes more goal directed and motivated to be independent, he is ready to try the more difficult tasks of learning to put on clothing. Again, the caregiver can begin by putting the garment on the child and then allowing the child to complete the action. Gradually the child learns to do a little more, eventually accomplishing mastery.

POSITIONING AND SUPPORT

The child who has hand skills but poor balance may be able to take advantage of the function he possesses when he is in a sidelying position with the effect of gravity lessened. For the child who can sit but is unstable, a corner of two adjoining walls or a corner seat on the floor may provide enough postural support for independent dressing. Finnie[12] suggests using chairs as supporting devices while the child either kneels on the floor or stands holding on, particularly when balancing on one leg, as when pulling on pants.

Associated reactions may occur as the child starts to use both hands. Thus one hand may be needed for holding on, while the other hand performs the task. Many dressing tasks require bilateral use of the hands. It is learned too that balance is more fragile as one reaches out with the arms, and this occurs frequently when donning overhead garments and reaching to the periphery of the body.

SPECIAL TECHNIQUES AND ADAPTIVE EQUIPMENT

When planning a dressing program, a therapist can assist the child and parents by refining procedures. Additionally, a part of good therapy is to increase the options for function by opening up a variety of ways to solve problems from which child and parents may choose. Perhaps the parents will elect to change the selection of clothing, finding this a better solution. Such a flexible approach has been suggested by Orelove and Gibbons.[27]

The following outline offers choices in problem solving, either through clothing selection and changes or by use of a technique or adaptive equipment that is feasible for the child.

Pull-up garments. Clothing aids that facilitate independence include loops sewn inside the waistbands of pants and skirts to assist with pulling; elasticized waistbands, provided the bands do not restrict pulling movements; and pressure tape as a substitute for conventional fastenings. If zippers are used, consider enlarging the grasping surface by adding a metal ring or fabric loop. A dressing stick may be used when limited range of motion of the lower extremities or trunk hinders donning pants or other articles of clothing that are pulled onto and up the legs.

As previously noted, Finnie[12] advises that the task of donning garments will be difficult for the child who is unstable in standing or when required to balance on one foot. Sitting or lying on the floor is to be encouraged so that once the feet are through the pant legs or

skirt band, the child can roll to either side while pulling up the waistband. If trunk balance allows, the child may kneel to pull up the garment once the waistband is above the knees. Having a chair close by is useful for support.

Pullover garments. The most important feature for ease in donning pullover shirts and sweaters is an easy opening for the head. It should be a neckline that expands, such as one made of rib-knit fabric. Again, consider flexible, elasticized waistbands and large sleeve openings. Stretchy knit fabrics allow children to experiment with movements as they gradually become more efficient in dressing.

For perceptual orientation it is helpful to have the child lay the garment on lap, floor, or table, front side down. Then, reaching out and opening the bottom of the garment, one arm can be pushed into the corresponding, or ipsilateral, sleeve, followed by the arm on the other side. After the arms are in the sleeves, the bottom of the garment can then be grasped with one hand and pulled over the head.

If the fabric has sufficient give and the child has adequate trunk balance, an alternate technique is simply to pull the garment over the head and then hold a sleeve open with one hand while pushing the other arm through. Repeat for the other side. An important point for making dressing easier is *always put clothing on the affected limb first.*

Front-opening garments. Selecting sleeves as loose as possible also applies to front-opening shirts, jackets, and sweater. Fullness in the back of the garment through pleats, gathers, or gussets will allow more freedom in movement.

One of the most common techniques used by children with coordination or weakness problems is flipping the garment over the head. This is done by laying the garment on the lap, floor, or table, front side up, with the neck of the garment closest to the body. The child then puts an arm in each sleeve, working each down until the hand is visible. The next step is to duck the head forward while extending the arms over the head. Shrugging the shoulders and pulling down with the arms will help the garment fall down into place.

Buttons. If a child is learning to dress, avoid buttons in the early stage of training by selecting pullover styles or by sewing buttons on the right side of the garment and using pressure tape for fastening. When buttoning is introduced, provide flat buttons large enough to grasp and ones that are not sewn tightly. Buttons with shanks may be easier to grasp. The location of buttons will affect the child's success in fastening. They should be easy to see, posssibly of a contrasting color, and easy to reach. Have the child begin buttoning with the bottom button so that it is possible to see the hands working. Having once secured the bottom button, it becomes easier to line up the other ones. Clothing adaptations are often helpful. Velcro may be sewn onto the garment behind the button and on top of the button hole as an adapted closure. Buttons on sleeve cuffs may be sewn on with elastic thread to allow the buttoned cuff to stretch open enough for the hand to slide through.

Zippers. A useful reminder is to test a zipper at the time a garment is purchased to be sure it glides easily. In general, nylon coil zippers are pliable and less likely to snag than metal ones.

When the child attempts to zip, give instructions on how to make the zipper taut by holding the garment below the zipper with one hand while pulling up the zipper tab with the other. To pull up a side zipper with one hand, hold the bottom of the zipper by leaning against a steady table or a wall. Zipper openings may also be adapted with Velcro to minimize the fine dexterity demands of the task. Zipper rings and zipper pull handle devices can facilitate grasp of the tab while working the zipper.

Socks. Children are frequently frustrated when attempting to don socks because the socks may be too tight and unyielding or the tops may be edged with tight elastic. Soft, stretchy fabric and a larger size alleviate strain in pulling. Tube socks eliminate problems with heel placement. Sewing loops on both sides of the socks may make them easier to pull into place. A stocking aid may be used by the older child for applying socks or hosiery when trunk and leg flexion are limited. This device often proves to be frustrating to children and also requires considerable ankle mobility. A technique that makes sock donning more successful for the child is folding or rolling down the upper part of the sock over the foot portion so that the toes can be placed directly into the foot of the sock.

Shoes. Styles that provide a broad, long opening will help children who have limited ankle motion. Tabs at the heel help the child to pull. Pressure-sensitive tape closures eliminate lacing and tying.

As previously suggested, shoes can be put on more easily if the leg is flexed and toes are pointing down. As the foot slides forward, encourage the child to push down at the heel. Keep the laces very loose when donning the shoe during the training period. Long-handled shoehorns are helpful, as are the tabs on the heels of some sport shoes.

Special considerations in clothing
FOR EASE IN TOILETING

For children who wear diapers, a full-length crotch opening with a zipper or Velcro closure will make changes easier. Girls may enjoy wearing wraparound skirts, and these are easy to put on and adjust for toileting. When children wear leg bags, they can reach and drain them with greater ease when their pants have zippers or Velcro along the seams.

FOR USE OF CRUTCHES

Children who use full-length crutches may tend to pull and tear their sleeves. Features to consider are double-stitched underarm seams or sleeves with gussets, knit inserts, or action pleats.

FOR CHILDREN SITTING

Most clothing is made for individuals in a standing position. For those who spend long hours in a wheelchair, the sitting position can cause pulling and strain on some areas of the garment and a surplus of fabric in others. Alterations can be made to provide more comfort in sitting, and directions to do so are presented by Kennedy[20] and Kernaleguen.[21] In general, moderate fullness in both skirts and trousers is recommended for children in wheelchairs.

FOR CHILDREN WEARING BRACES

The child who wears a brace may need to have clothing reinforced to protect against rubbing. Ideas include sewing fabric patches inside the garment where friction will occur and reinforcing all seams that will receive stress.

Adapted clothing

Increased attention to the needs of the disabled individual has been shown over the last decade, with some adaptive clothing becoming available through catalogue supply companies. Because of marketing volume, there is a limited range of choice and a higher cost per item factor, but a beginning has been made to provide attractive, functional clothing.

Even more promising is the literature with practical suggestions for those with sewing skills. Kernaleguen[21] presents sewing instructions for a variety of garments and aids. She is a strong advocate of providing attractive, fashionable clothing for the disabled, and she stresses that clothing should meet functional requirements, yet conform in appearance to peer group standards and fashion trends. Modifications should be inconspicuous, and, in general, the appearance of the clothing should not single out the wearer in any way. When possible, clothing should conceal the handicap or at least not attract attention to it. The clothing should contribute to the wearer's sense of well-being. Functionally the design of the clothing should enable the wearer to take care of personal needs as much as possible, help maintain proper body temperature, and provide freedom of movement.

GROOMING AND HYGIENE

Good grooming habits are important for all children but take on added significance for the disabled. At an early age the child with a disability needs to be encouraged and helped to achieve cleanliness.

Bathing

Bathing should be a pleasurable activity, but for the parent of a child who lacks balance it can be a tedious task that requires constant attention and alertness. The work involved multiplies as the child grows and becomes larger and heavier.

Finnie[12] outlines a number of measures to make bathing easier. As has been stressed repeatedly, positioning and handling are prime considerations. The child with a strong startle reaction should receive special mention, since triggering the reaction can result in sudden loss of balance. Keeping the child's head and arms forward before lifting and maintaining them there while lowering the child into the tub are advisable. Finnie suggests handling the child slowly and gently, and when the child is old enough, telling him what is going to happen next, including turning the water faucets on and off and draining water from the tub. It is a good idea to drain the tub and wrap the child in a towel before lifting him from the tub.

Making the child feel safe and secure can also be aided by special equipment that gives the support needed. There are bath hammocks that fully hold the body and enable the parent to wash the child thoroughly (Figure 14-13, *A*). A simple, inexpensive way for giving security is to use a plastic laundry basket lined with foam at its bottom (Figure 14-13, *B*). Commercially, a light, inconspicuous bath support (Figure 14-13, *C*) offers good design features. The front half of the padded support ring swings open for easy entry and then locks securely, holding the child at the chest to give trunk stability. Various kinds of bath seats and shower benches are available for the older child to aid bathtub seating and transfers (Figure 14-13, *D*).

For the seriously involved youngster lying supine in the tub in shallow water, a horseshoe-shaped inflatable bath collar (Figure 14-13, *E*) serves to support the neck and keep the child's head above water level. A bath stretcher is constructed like a cot and fits inside the bathtub to provide full body support. It can be set up at the tub rim level or mid tub level to minimize the caregiver's bending while transferring and bathing the child. It is usually used with a hand-held shower head.

Some parents and children find a hand-held shower head useful in removing soap suds. A long-handled bath brush or sponge helps in reaching body parts. Children with limited grasp may be able to wash themselves with a bathmitt. If a child is unable to extend his fingers for washing, the parent may try to facilitate relaxation by stroking downward on the top of the child's hand with a washcloth and then trying to flex the wrist. As a last measure the parent could straighten each finger, beginning with the little finger.[8]

Nonslip bath mats are essential for safety, both beside the tub and in the tub. Grab bars and their placement require careful thought and planning in each individual case.

The parents' safety also should be addressed. They should be cautioned to protect their backs and be taught good body mechanics. To lessen strain, it is best for the adult to sit on a stool beside the tub or kneel on a cushion. Lifting is done with knees bent and the back straight, using the legs for power.

Oral hygiene

Toothbrushing can be especially difficult for the child with sensitivity. For that and other reasons, when assistance is given, the teeth should be brushed slowly and gently. This will help to prevent fear of the toothbrush. A small, soft brush is easier to move around in the mouth, especially if the child has a tongue thrust or gag reflex. When gums are tender, a soft sponge tip called a toothette can be substituted for a brush. This is a disposable product.

If a child has problems with a weak grasp, the handle can be enlarged with sponge rubber, or, if necessary, a Velcro strap can be added. When the difficulty is a matter of wrist coordination and arm movement, an electric toothbrush can be evaluated for use. This proves to be a good solution in some cases, but the unit may be too heavy for every child to manage. Some electric brushes have dual controls, moving from side to side and up and down, which allows for good cleaning of teeth and gums. To help with managing toothpaste, a long handle attached to the bottom of the tube helps in squeezing paste onto the brush.

Hair care

A simple style and good haircut are among the easiest ways to facilitate hair care, but children will want to identify with their peers and observe current fads. It is sometimes less tiring and gives greater stability when the child supports both arms on a table while combing or brushing his hair. A large comb or a brush with a thick handle may be easier for the child to use. A mirror at the proper height should be placed so that progress with personal grooming can be checked. When the child is unable to reach his head, extended handles can be tried. A hose attached to the faucet helps when washing hair over a basin or tub. If flexibility of the neck is a problem, a plastic shampoo tray can be fitted around the neck to direct water and suds away from the face.

Fingernail care

Caring for fingernails is often a trial for any child but is especially difficult when there are coordination problems or when the child has use of only one hand. Two styles of nailbrushes are useful. One is suction based and is used by rubbing the nails across the brush. The other has a curved handle that fits over one hand and then can be used to brush the nails of the other. A child may be able to file his fingernails if an emery board is taped to the edge of a table.

Confidence in one's appearance is essential to an in-

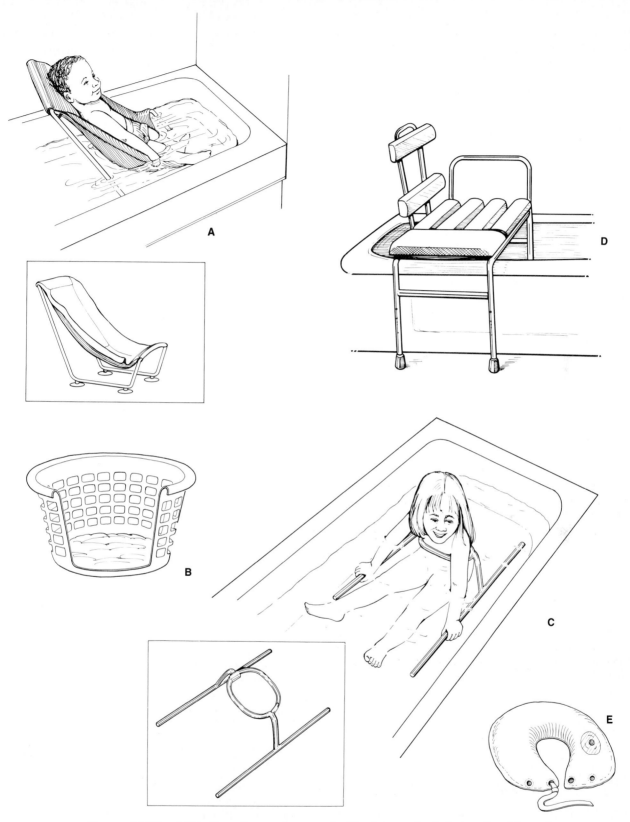

Figure 14-13 Adapted seating equipment. **A,** The hammock chair is adjustable and equipped with oversized suction feet. It fully supports the child who has no sitting balance and poor head control. **B,** The front of a plastic laundry basket is cut out to allow room for the child's legs. The basket gives security during first baths in a large tub. **C,** The trunk support is lightweight and compact and fits all bathtubs. **D,** The shower bench aids seating and transfers. **E,** The inflatable bath collar can be used when the child is either supine or prone.

dividual's sense of worth. Good grooming and attractive clothing are strong allies in inviting positive responses from others. When children present an acceptable image to their cultural group, they in turn potentially receive stable, consistent, clear messages that help to shape a healthy self-concept.

Adolescent skills

Adolescence begins at the onset of puberty and continues until adulthood. It is a period of remarkable growth toward physical and sexual maturity as well as emotional and social maturity. The physiological changes that occur at puberty are due in part to the increased output of hormones by the pituitary gland. Boys and girls develop pubic and axillary hair. Facial hair develops on boys along with body hair on the chest and legs. Body hair develops also on the legs of girls. In boys and girls alike, the skin becomes coarser with larger pores. The sebaceous glands become more active, producing oily secretions. The composition of sweat is altered and becomes stronger in odor. New self-maintenance tasks emerge with these physical changes.

Shaving is often simplified with the use of an electric razor. Although it is heavier, it can be safer to use and requires less precision. It also eliminates shaving soap and the need to handle blades. Electric razors can be adapted with holders for those with weak or impaired grasp. Light-weight disposable safety razors eliminate blade changing and can be easily adapted with built-up handles to facilitate grasp or with long handle to accommodate limited reach or range of motion.

Regular bathing and more frequent face washing are important to manage increased body secretions and skin conditions accompanying adolescence. Use of deodorant, perfumes, and facial ointments for excessive oils or acne becomes important. Girls become interested in using makeup. The therapist often becomes involved in adapting self-care product containers to permit independent use. To accommodate weak grasp, jar lids may be left loose. Transferring ointments to pump containers can reduce the hand dexterity needed to use the product. Lipstick or mascara tubes can be built up with foam rubber or tape for ease of handling.

MOBILITY

SUSAN A. PROCTER

The mobility of a child has a tremendous impact on his life experiences and overall development. The ability to move from one point in space to another enables the child to get to know his world and the people and objects in it. Mobility enhances physical development, perception, social interaction, autonomy, and knowledge of the environment. When a child's mobility is impaired, other areas of development can become delayed secondary to limited access to people, objects, and events. For instance, the child who is unable to roll or crawl over to his toys will forgo opportunities to manipulate and explore them unless they are brought to him. The child who takes 20 minutes to propel a wheelchair to class and is fatigued on arrival misses parts of class and has expended energy that might otherwise go toward learning. The child who cannot effectively move toward his playmates, siblings, and parents is prevented from enjoying self-directed social experiences.

The therapist plays an important role by helping children develop independent and device-assisted mobility appropriate to developmental age level and physical, functional, and social needs. The therapist evaluates the performance capabilities of the children; their home, school, and community environments; and the desires of the parents. This information enables the therapist to select the system of mobility practical for the individual children, the families, and those people who interact with them on a daily basis.

Normal developmental sequence of mobility

Knowledge of the normal developmental sequence of mobility forms the basis for therapeutic intervention. In the course of normal development, children acquire postural and movement patterns that are the basis for functional mobility. Mobility develops first in a horizontal relationship to the floor. In an orderly sequential pattern children assume new postures and movement patterns leading to upright positions and vertical relationships in their movement in space.

Rolling is the first form of mobility that allows the child to change position in the horizontal plane. The ability to pivot on the abdomen to change position develops and is soon followed by the forward prone progression of crawling. As postural stability, righting, and equilibrium reactions mature, the child develops the ability to move onto all fours to creep. The rotational movement pattern from quadruped to sitting allows the child to attain the first independent vertical posture. When sitting can be maintained independently, the hands are free for object manipulation and tool use. From sitting, the child returns to his hands and knees to move through space. From all fours, progress is made to tall kneeling by holding onto furniture or the wall for stability. Moving further upward, the child develops the ability to pull to the standing position by using his arms and hands to attain and hold the vertical position. Mobility in the upright plane progresses from sideways cruising to walking by holding onto objects in the environment. The child then develops the ability to free his hands from external support and achieves independent standing and walking.

Mobility impairment resulting from disease or disability may limit the child's capabilities at any stage during the developmental progression of movement from rolling to walking. The degree of impairment is primarily determined by biological factors such as nervous system functioning, strength, coordination, physical structure, and cognitive functioning. Factors that can either facilitate or limit the ability or desire to move include the availability of experiences, activities, time, space, and assistive devices to augment mobility. Thus a combination of biological and environmental factors influence the functional level of mobility the child will attain.

Children need to develop effective methods of mobility in various physical settings to derive maximal benefit from childhood experiences. They learn by moving around and getting into situations where they can manipulate and explore, thereby experiencing the consequences of their actions. Participating as a member of a group, taking responsibility in school and at home, enjoying play with peers, and becoming independent are natural sequences to exploration.[1] Many children with disabilities learn adaptive ways to move by rolling or crawling. However, when the child's own abilities are insufficient to meet functional and environmental needs, assistive devices are used to help the child in a particular developmental stage to parallel or simulate the normal mobility milestones.[3,24,31]

Mobility for the nonambulatory child

Depending on the extent and severity of the disability, children who are nonambulatory move on the floor by using various patterns of rolling, crawling, creeping, or scooting in the seated position. Assistive devices, such as strollers and wheelchairs, expand the mobility capability of the child to traverse longer distances at home, at school, and in the community where floor-oriented mobility is not functional. Describing adaptive mobility and device-assisted mobility within the developmental sequence helps to point out the functional significance to the child.

ROLLING

The child who can roll is able to change position from prone to supine and to move on the floor. Rolling as a mobility mode is useful for making positional changes in bed regardless of age or disability. As a primary method of mobility, it is most suitable for short distance movement in indoor settings. The youngster who is eager to be amused and stimulated but who has severe limitations in moving toward and manipulating what he wants can have a more enriched environment when toys are placed on the floor with him and play activities are brought to him.

PRONE PROGRESS, CRAWLING

The child who crawls can go farther than one who rolls. Crawling is most functional on environmental surfaces where friction and abrasion forces are minimal, since the child has contact with the floor at his abdomen, arms, and legs. For example, the vinyl kitchen floor or the carpeted family room floor is more suitable for crawling than the asphalt driveway or playground. Mobility devices for children who are at the functional stage of crawling include scooterboards and crawligators that support the trunk close to the floor while allowing arm and leg use (Figure 14-14, *A*). Such devices can be homemade or purchased from therapy equipment catalogues for children. These devices are best used on hard surfaces that allow the small caster wheels to roll without excessive resistance. Some larger, ball casters are safer and roll with greater ease on carpets. The child's hands should be kept well in front of the wheels so that the device cannot roll over them. Supervised use of the device is important when the child cannot get on and off independently.[30]

CREEPING ON HANDS AND KNEES

Once off the abdomen, the child can venture further. Although rolling and crawling allow short distance mobility, for instance, within a room, the child who creeps independently may have wider access to the house and yard. Assistive devices for creeping are

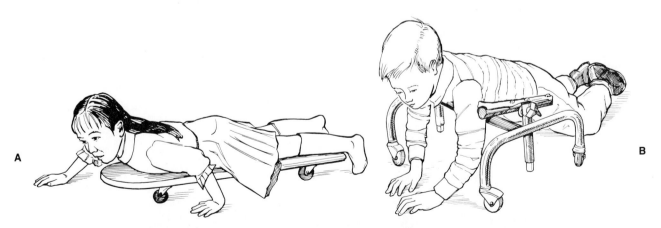

Figure 14-14 Mobility devices. **A,** For crawling children. **B,** For creeping children.

available. These support the trunk far enough off the ground to allow use of the arms in an extended position for weight bearing and use of the legs for weight bearing on the knees (Figure 14-14, *B*). They are best used in a training mode versus a functional mode. The child who creeps is often capable of attaining a sitting position by rotating onto the buttocks or by sitting back on the lower legs. These functional positions could be restricted by a creeping assistive device.

MOBILITY IN SITTING

Scooting on the buttocks while sitting on the floor is a mobility pattern used by some children who have adequate sitting balance, upper extremity strength, and control to move the body. The child may take weight on extended arms, unweighting the buttocks, sliding either forward or backward along the floor. Many children with physical disabilities such as meningomyelocele or traumatic paraplegia mobilize themselves using this pattern. Children who have some volitional leg function will assist their movement with their hips and feet. The upright position is more conducive to functional activities. Caster carts and wheelmobiles are available to facilitate floor-based mobility in the seated position. With these devices the child is seated in a long sitting position just off the floor. They are propelled by pushing wheels that are attached to the base in line with the child's shoulders (Figure 14-15).

Children whose mobility capabilities are floorbound will use these patterns and mobility devices for floor-oriented play in most settings where other children are frequently playing on the floor. Normal developmental progression and activity interests take the nondisabled child from floor-based activities to higher areas involving sitting on furniture, participating in table-level activities, standing during play, walking. The disabled child also has these needs and desires to be higher in space to pursue age-appropriate activities at a height and speed similar to those of peers. Children who are

unable to achieve this through standing and walking will need mobility aids that provide support and mobility in the seated position. The growing child becomes larger and heavier and more difficult to lift off the floor. This too influences the transition from floor-oriented mobility devices to devices that place the child at a higher level (Figure 14-16).

WHEELCHAIR MOBILITY

Identification of the appropriate wheelchair is based on evaluation of a broad spectrum of factors, including the ability of the child, concurrent developmental tasks, environmental settings, and desires of significant others who interact with the child. The occupational therapist, the child, the parents, the physical therapist, the teacher, and other team members have valuable information to offer regarding the child's abilities and needs that will contribute to the selection of the device that will provide maximal function. The medical equipment dealer is an excellent source of information regarding new or improved items and features that may help solve unique problems relevant to the child's needs. Rehabilitation engineers may be called upon to develop or modify equipment for special needs.

A wide variety of wheelchairs from different manufacturers are available for children. They may generally be categorized as the following:

1. Transport chairs, such as strollers and travel chairs, designed to be pushed by others
2. Manual wheelchairs propelled by the child or pushed by others
3. Power wheelchairs for those children who have insufficient strength, coordination, or endurance to propel a wheelchair manually, but who have the control and judgment to use power mobility safely.

Young children (under age 3) are often transported in *strollers* designed for the normal population of infants and toddlers. Strollers are frequently used for

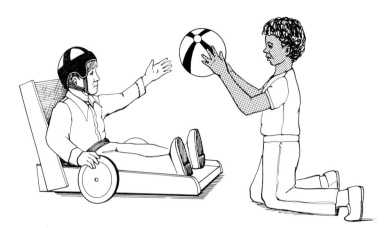

Figure 14-15 A caster cart provides seating and mobility for floor-oriented play.

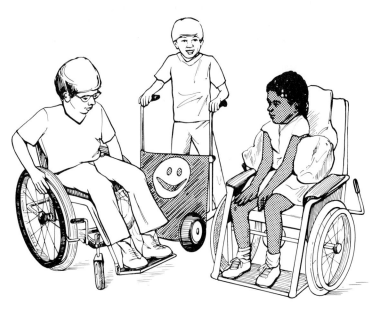

Figure 14-16 Higher level mobility devices.

transportation outdoors or in the community where carrying the child is impractical for the parents and the child's own method of mobility is inadequate for the distance or terrain. The umbrella stroller is popular because of the convenience, portability, and "normal" appearance. However, children with postural control problems are generally not supported adequately by the sling seats used in these strollers. The semireclined seat angle places the child in a passive position rather than upright, and this may hinder spontaneous postural responses, the feeling of comfort and security, and the ability to view the surroundings. Large strollers for children who have outgrown regular strollers are available from medical equipment vendors and are easily portable. The occupational therapist often helps the family adapt the stroller with solid seats and backs that provide improved postural support and seat angle for the child.

Travel chairs are highly specialized stroller systems with rear wheel retractor units that provide several adjustments of seat angle. For car travel the rear wheels fully retract to allow placement of the chair on a car seat while the child is still sitting in the device. These chairs are designed for the severely involved child who has positioning needs. The chairs come with a wide variety of accessory options to provide postural support and control, including solid seat and back units; knee abduction units; lateral supports for the trunk, hips, and thighs; head rests; trunk harnesses; and lap trays. Travel chairs provide postural stabilization and alignment during hand use activities, feeding, and transportation. Their capability of doubling as both car seat and wheelchair offers versatility. These systems are pushed and operated by others, making them appropriate only

for children who are not capable of wheeling themselves. The chair should be tried in the family's car before purchase because some chairs do not fit on the seats of some vehicles. In most cars they will only fit on the front passenger seat.

Children who have sufficient upper extremity strength and control for self-propulsion are candidates for *manual wheelchairs*. Children around the age of 3 reach the size necessary to fit into Tiny Tot models offered by the major wheelchair manufacturing companies. Recently smaller chairs have become available for younger children who are ready to propel themselves. Most wheelchair companies have a series of models to meet the average size and functional needs of the growing individual from preschool to adolescent to adult. Modifications to meet individual requirements can be made by selecting different styles of armrests, footrests, wheel hand-rim options, and positioning accessories. The wheelchair size may be custom modified by upholstery, frame construction, or the addition of seat inserts. Selection of the appropriate size chair is based on body measurements and consideration of functional needs. The following measurements, taken while the child is in the seated position, determine the relationship between the size of the child and the chair (Figure 14-17).

1. Hip width: The measurement at the widest point across the hips or thighs plus 2 inches determines the width of the chair seat.
2. Leg length: The measurement from behind the knee to behind the buttocks determines the seat depth. For children there should be a clearance of 1 inch from behind the knee to the front edge of the seat.

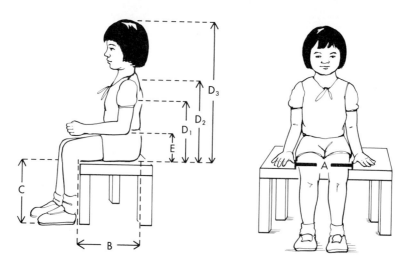

Figure 14-17   Measurements for the wheelchair. *A,* Hip width; *B,* leg length; *C,* foreleg length; D_1, seat base to axilla; D_2, seat base to top of shoulders; D_3, seat base to top of head; *E,* arm height.

3. Foreleg length: The measurement from the heel to under the thigh determines the height of the footrest system for foot support and weight bearing under the thighs.
4. Back height: Depending on the upper torso support needs of the child, the following measurements determine the seat's back height.
   a. Seat base to axilla: For children who require standard support.
   b. Seat base to top of shoulders: For children with additional trunk support needs.
   c. Seat base to top of head: For children who require head support.
5. Arm height: The measurement from the seat base to the elbow with the arm flexed determines the height of the armrests.
6. Seat height: The distance from the floor to the top of the seat base determines the seat height.

Functional activities that will be performed in the wheelchair have implications for the style of wheelchair and selection of components. For example, an ultralight model is necessary to increase the wheeling efficiency of the child or to help the parent who frequently lifts the chair in and out of the car. Removable armrests are needed for sliding transfers. Desk-type arms are an important feature for children who need to get close to tables for schoolwork, feeding, and play activities. Adjustable height arm rests are helpful for children using wheelchair lap trays as they allow adjustment of the work surface height for optimum performance. The height of the seat base from the floor is critical for those doing standing transfers, and it affects access to tables and desks. Swing away and removable footrests facilitate standing transfers and getting close to counters. Home accessibility can be enhanced by removing the footrests in tight spots such as bathrooms and hallways.

Wheelchair accessories can enhance function. A book bag can be used to carry school materials and personal items so that arms and hands are free for wheeling. Lap trays provide a play or work surface on the wheelchair.

Power wheelchairs should be considered for the child who is physically unable to propel a manual chair. Those who need to limit energy expenditure and joint stress, or whose wheeling capabilities prevent them from going fast enough or far enough to meet their needs for functional activities and exploration, are also candidates for power wheelchairs.[32] The child's physical control, endurance, cognitive abilities, visual and perceptual skills, and judgment are essential considerations for safe use of power mobility. Assessment of the home, school, and community environments where the chair will be used, how it will be transported, and who will be responsible for its maintenance help to determine the feasibility of power mobility and will influence the type of system selected for a given individual.[3]

Most power wheelchairs are configured like manual chairs with the addition of electronic component systems, control unit, batteries. They can be purchased as a complete power system from a variety of manufacturers. Separate power add-on systems designed to convert standard manual wheelchairs to electric wheelchairs are also available. Most models are equipped with a joystick for right- or left-hand use. Special controllers, electronic systems, or adaptations can be made for those who have insufficient upper extremity coordination or strength to manipulate the standard joystick. Joystick adaptation includes special knobs to promote grasp, templates to guide directional control, and special mounting and modifications to allow operation by the chin, head, or foot.

Other control systems drive the power wheelchairs through puff-sip codes which designate directional mobility of the chair. An array of single switches can be used to drive a wheelchair. Each switch corresponds to a direction, and when each is activated, the chair moves in either the foreward direction, right turn, reverse, or left turn. Switch arrays can be operated by hand, arm, head, or feet. Those with reliable control of a single movement can operate a power wheelchair through activation of a single switch on a directional scanning interface system. Voice and sonar control systems are being developed but are not ready for commercial application.

Frequently additional equipment, such as a van with a lift and tie-down system or ramps for the home, must be acquired to maximize the child's wheelchair use and independence. Such environmental modifications need careful consideration during the assessment process so that the family may plan to acquire additional systems that support the independent mobility of their child. Portable electric wheelchairs that can be dismantled and folded for transportation may be selected when a van and lift are not available. Those using power wheelchairs often have a manual wheelchair for use when the power system is being serviced or when the situation will not accommodate the electric wheelchair. There are also power units that can be placed on and removed from a manual wheelchair, allowing one wheelchair frame to be used for both manual and power mobility.

Mobility for the ambulatory child
WALKING BY HOLDING ON

The child who has adequate postural control and stability to stand and take steps while holding on to some support will use this method of mobility in the home or classroom where walls and furniture are available for the external stability needed to stay upright. The child's mobility is limited by the environment unless ambulation aids are provided. Orthotic devices, such as a shoe insert to stabilize the foot; an ankle foot orthosis (AFO); knee ankle foot orthosis (KAFO); or additional appliances that provide control at the hips, pelvis, and trunk, may be used to stabilize and align the lower extremities for ambulation according to the needs of the child. Walkers, crutches, and canes may be used to aid balance during ambulation. Children who can functionally use such ambulation aids are able to venture into open areas to determine their own route through space in contrast to being limited to the route determined by fixtures in the environment.

WALKING INDEPENDENTLY

The achievement of independent ambulation enables the child to move about with his hands free from body support functions. The disabled child often uses an abnormal gait pattern. Orthotic devices may be needed to align or support the lower extremity joints to improve the pattern. Those with congenital limb deficiency or amputation use prosthetic devices to achieve independent ambulation. The functional use of independent or device-assisted ambulation depends on the effort and energy it consumes, the time it takes to get from one place to another, and the distance that can be covered. Short-distance ambulatory children may walk within the home, school, and neighborhood, but use a wheelchair for long-distance community mobility.

• • •

Parents and professionals strive for a delicate balance with any adaptive aid, whether for mobility or for tasks such as eating or dressing. In general, aids should help children use their own skills as much as possible. Aids should not become substitutes for the children's efforts to learn to do things on their own.

Parents and professionals together need to observe children in their environments to clarify the goals to be accomplished with the particular aid. Once the goals have been established, efforts can be directed toward finding equipment that can be adapted to meet the goals. Regardless of what equipment is purchased, an ongoing review of the individual child's use of the equipment is essential to assess its value and to review whether modifications or changes need to be made.

SUMMARY

This chapter discussed the ways in which occupational therapists can help a child become more independent. The processes of eating, toileting, dressing, and grooming were described, both from the aspect of evaluation and from that of training. Normal development of mobility and methods for building a child's ability to get around independently were also discussed. The child's treatment program must include the needs of the family as a whole. Adaptive equipment must be acceptable to the child's self-image and to the family's finances and life-style.

STUDY QUESTIONS
1. List and briefly describe five strategies that can be used by an occupational therapist for improving feeding function.
2. List four physical problems that could interfere with dressing. Identify an adaptive technique or assistive device to enhance dressing function for each condition.
3. Place in order the following developmental skills required for toileting:
   a. Management of clothing
   b. Perineal cleansing
   c. Awareness of voiding
   d. Ability to sit on the toilet

   What occupational therapy interventions could be used at each stage?

4. Identify a reason for using each of the following mobility aids:
   a. Scooterboard
   b. Caster cart
   c. Manual wheelchair
   d. Power wheelchair
5. What positions may be used to facilitate the child's independent performance of the following activities: (name at least two positions for each)
   a. Drinking from a cup
   b. Perineal cleansing
   c. Putting on trousers
   d. Blowing dry one's hair

   Try doing these activities yourself in the adapted positions. Are the results qualitatively different?

REFERENCES

1. Bergen AC: Positioning the client with central nervous system deficits, New York, 1982, Valhalla Rehabilitation Publishers, Ltd.
2. Bigge J: Teaching individuals with physical and multiple disabilities, ed 2, Columbus, Ohio, 1982, Charles E Merrill Publishing Co.
3. Bleck EE, and Nagel DA: Physical handicapped children; a medical atlas for teachers, New York, 1982, Grune & Stratton, Inc.
4. Bobath K: The motor deficit in patients with cerebral palsy, London, 1966, William Heinemann, Ltd.
5. Brazelton TB: Toddlers and parents, New York, 1974, Dell Publishing Co, Inc.
6. Coley L: Pediatric assessment of self-care activities, St Louis, 1978, The CV Mosby Co.
7. Copeland M, and others: Occupational therapy for mentally retarded children, Baltimore, 1976, University Park Press.
8. Doyle P, and others: Helping the severely handicapped child, New York, 1979, Thomas Y Crowell Co, Inc.
9. Duffy Y: All things possible, Ann Arbor, Mich, 1981, AJ Garvin & Associates.
10. Erickson ML: Assessment and management of developmental changes in children, St Louis, 1976, The CV Mosby Co.
11. Farber S: Sensorimotor evaluation and treatment procedures for allied health personnel, Indianapolis, 1974, The Indiana University Foundation.
12. Finnie N: Handling the young cerebral palsied child at home, ed 2, New York, 1975, Dutton-Sunrise, Inc.
13. Friedman L: Toileting self-care methods for bilateral high level upper limb amputees, Prosthet Orthot Int 4:29, 1980.
14. Gesell A: The first five years of life—a guide to the study of the pre-school child, New York, 1940, Harper & Row, Publishers, Inc.
15. Hale G: The source book for the disabled, New York, 1979, Paddington Press, Ltd.
16. Hammond MI, Lewis MN, and Johnson EW: A nutritional study of cerebral palsied children, J Am Diet Assoc 49:196, 1966.
17. Howard B: Nutritional support of the developmentally disabled child. In Suskind R, editor: Textbook of pediatric nutrition, New York, 1981, Raven Press.
18. Howison M, Perella J, and Gordon D: Cerebral palsy. In Hopkins H, and Smith H, editors: Willard and Spackman's occupational therapy, ed 5, Philadelphia, 1978, JB Lippincott Co.
19. Illingworth RS: The development of the infant and young child—normal and abnormal, ed 3, Baltimore, 1966, Williams & Wilkins.
20. Kennedy E: Dressing with pride, vol 1, Groton, Conn, 1981, PRIDE Foundation, Inc.
21. Kernaleguen A: Clothing designs for the handicapped, Edmonton, 1978, The University of Alberta Press.
22. Measuring the patient, Los Angeles, 1979, Everest & Jennings.
23. Morris SE: The normal acquisition of oral feeding skills: implications for assessment and treatment, New York, 1982, Therapeutic Media, Inc.
24. Motlock WM: Mobility for spinal cord impaired spina bifida patients, Paper presented at Conference on Mobility Aids, Toronto, 1974.
25. Mueller H: Facilitating feeding and prespeech. In Pearson P, and Williams, CA, editors: Physical therapy services in the developmental disabilities, Springfield, Ill, 1972, Charles C Thomas, Publisher.
26. O'Neil S: Behavior management of feeding. In Pipes P: Nutrition in infancy and childhood, St Louis, 1977, The CV Mosby Co.
27. Orelove F, and Gibbons S: A guide to independent dressing, Except Parent 1981.
28. Peiper A: Cerebral function in infancy and childhood, New York, 1963, Consultants Bureau Enterprises, Inc.
29. Pipes P: Nutrition in infancy and childhood, St Louis, 1977, The CV Mosby Co
30. Robinault IP: Functional aids for the multiply handicapped, New York, 1973, Harper & Row, Publishers, Inc.
31. Swinyard C: The child with spina bifida, Chicago, 1980, Spina Bifida Association of America.
32. Treffler E, and Cook H: Powered mobility for children, Knoxville, 1979, University of Tennessee Center for the Health Sciences, Rehabilitation Engineering Center.

15

Play and recreational activities

PAT NUSE PRATT

This chapter addresses play as a generic modality and one outcome of occupational therapy intervention. A conservative estimate, based on clinical observations, is that at least half of occupational therapy services for children are delivered through the medium of play. Play is the preeminent occupational behavior of childhood and, as such, constitutes a major concern of occupational therapy. Services may be expected to promote the development of play behavior, as well as use play as the primary modality to facilitate change in the motor, sensory integrative, cognitive, emotional, and social functions of children. In observations of pediatric practice, play can readily be identified as the tie that binds occupational therapy assessment and treatment together.

SCOPE OF PLAY IN OCCUPATIONAL THERAPY

A thorough review of literature on play is impossible within the constraints of this chapter, but the references and suggested readings should prove helpful. For organizational purposes, however, a discussion of the scope of play in occupational therapy is warranted.

The theoretical foundation that is generally adopted for discussion of play is Reilly's explanation of play as an appreciative learning system[26] (Chapter 3). However, practice in occupational therapy demands more than a theoretical explanation of play. What is needed is a way to classify the myriad of toys and activities that can assist the therapist with selection of appropriate play experiences according to the interests, capacities, needs, and ages of children seen in treatment. For this purpose, the works of Florey,[6] Michelman,[18,19] and Takata[30] provide a useful background.

Florey: a classification of play

Florey[6] defined play as the action on human and nonhuman objects that is engaged in for its own sake.

Her concept that play is intrinsically motivated and rewarding was gleaned from, and continues to be supported by, a comprehensive review of play theories.[3,29] Florey[6] further described play as a learning process. This concept has been differentiated somewhat by other theorists. Piaget, as cited by Flavell,[4] defined play as those actions of the child that are dominated by assimilation, that is, when the child is able to direct actions with established mental schemes. In contrast, Piaget believed that playful actions that were dominated by accommodation are more properly described as imitation. Hutt[11] proposed a taxonomy of play that nicely integrates Piagetian theory with the more global view of Florey. Hutt stipulated that there are two major categories of play. *Epistemic play* behaviors are concerned with the acquisition of new information and knowledge. *Ludic play* includes those behaviors that are dominated by use of past experiences. This differentiation can be useful to the occupational therapist for selection and adaptation of activities.

Florey[6] developed a classification system that organizes the developmental sequence of play behaviors according to variations in actions with human and nonhuman objects. Actions with human objects include play with parents, peers, significant others, and the child's own body. Nonhuman objects are divided into three groups according to the inherent properties of the object for change as a result of the child's actions. Type I objects include creative and unstructured media that can be directly changed by the playful actions of the child. Objects that can be changed when combined with other objects are classified as Type II. Objects that maintain their original form in relatively stable condition regardless of play actions, such as bicycles and dolls, are referred to as Type III. Florey indicated through her classification that differential and preferential engagement in play with human and nonhuman objects will vary over the course of time. For example, during the preschool years, play with human objects is often directed toward the self and family. As the child matures, more action is directed toward peers and away from the self and parents. Similarly, involvement with an increasingly broad range of nonhuman objects occurs as the child ages.

Takata: a taxonomy of play

In work that enriches concepts of play presented earlier by Florey,[5,6] Takata[30] sought to identify critical patterns and representations of play and relate these to age and milieu. This was accomplished through the construction of a two-directional taxonomy that can be used to examine the content of play and to help prescribe areas for intervention. The taxonomy's elements will be reviewed here, and its content described through discussion in the practice section of this chapter.

Takata proposed that play evolves through a sequence of age-related *epochs,* and Takata characterized these in an integration of concepts developed by Piaget, Erikson, and Florey. Each epoch has representative elements, which Takata identified as materials, actions, people, and setting. The epochs are the following:
1. Sensorimotor epoch: During the period from birth to 24 months, the play of the child is characterized by exploration and manipulation of the self, parents, siblings, significant others, and common objects in the environment. The child engages in play for its sensory experience and comes to know the basic actions and sensory properties of people and things.
2. Symbolic and simple constructive epoch: Through the emergence and refinement of language, the child develops symbols for the actions and properties that he discovered during the sensory motor period. The ability to communicate through symbols, coupled with increasing gross and fine motor capacity, allows the child to construct relationships between objects. Relationships are established through the child's sensorimotor experiences but are extended through the developing imagination of the child.
3. Dramatic, complex constructive, and pregame epoch: The 4- to 7-year-old child learns to act out concepts and experiences through play and begins to put concepts together to form elementary rules of actions. Dramatic play replaces imaginative fantasy, since the child now knows better what is likely to happen. The putting together of objects through construction becomes increasingly important as the child's ability to represent reality increases. Peer interaction becomes pivotal as the child begins to test the validity of constructs and skills. This period is transitional from exploratory to competency play as defined by Reilly.[25]
4. Game epoch: The elementary school child is driven by the urge to control the actions of objects and events. Occupation in game playing predominates, because such activities offer the child increasingly complex variations of rules and thus increase the child's sense of control and mastery. Rules prescribe ways of doing things and show the child a way to increase competence. Competence is measured through competitive play with peers.
5. Recreation epoch: The play behavior of the adolescent assumes a more mature form through involvement in recreational activities. The balance of occupation has shifted in the direction of work, and recreation allows the refinement of skills and interactions that will relate to or support the youth's performance in adult roles. The games and social activities of recreation demonstrate increasingly sophisticated rules, role functions, and patterns of cooperation with the team or group.

This play taxonomy was originally designed to be used in conjunction with Takata's play history (Chapter 9). The data on play and environment can be contrasted against the requisites defined by the taxonomy to identify the play status of the child. Areas of acceptable development and risk are highlighted.

Michelman: creative growth

The elements of symbolic and constructive play discussed by Takata and Florey were explored further in Michelman's study[18] of the development of children's creative interests. Michelman[18] wrote

Art is a language of symbols and non-verbal communication. The child who freely explores with creative art media absorbs information through his senses which he assimilates and recasts into new symbolic forms (p. 88).

Drawing on the work of Lowenfield, Michelman identified six stages of creative growth and symbol formation that show differentiated development of human, color, and design schemata with stage-specific representation, motivation, media, and methods. Creative activities promote the self-expression of the child and are less rule-bound than other types of play behaviors. In a later work Michelman[19] proposed more specifically that creative interests are the route to intellectual growth.

A MODEL OF PLAY IN OCCUPATIONAL THERAPY

By using the studies of Florey, Takata, and Michelman in combination with Reilly's theoretical explanation of play and the other theoretical approaches discussed elsewhere in this text, a model of play in occupational therapy can be constructed. As an example, a developmental model of play activities is presented in

Figures 15-1 to 15-5. This model provides an overview of play that is organized according to major types of play, and it analyzes some of the generic modalities of occupational therapy that are related to play. By using these tables, the therapist can determine what types of play experiences are most appropriate to the child's age and functional status.

Each major category of play activities is characteristic of an age group. However, it must be emphasized that engagement in play varies with the mood and mo-

---

Figure 15-1 Exploratory play

1. *Description:* Play-recreational experiences through which the child develops a body scheme, sensory integrative and motor skills, and concepts of sensory characteristics and actions of human and nonhuman objects.
2. *Properties of activities:*
   a. Tools, materials, and equipment
      Child's own body
      Significant others
      Environmental textures
      "Infant" toys with distinct sensory characteristics and actions
      Everyday household objects
   b. Human and object relationships:
      Strongest relationships occur through play between child and parents.
      Egocentric relationships occur with nonhuman objects as an extension of the child.
   c. Characteristic age level is newborn through 2 years.
3. *Representative toys and activities:*
   a. Newborn to two years:

Auditory toys: Rattles, play piano, and so on	Mobiles	Scarves, brightly colored
Balls: All sizes and textures	Pop-up toys	Scooters, scooter boards
Bells	Pots and pans	See N' Say
Blocks	Pull-and-push toys	Sensory play with parents
Busy boxes	Rolling, crawling, cruising activities	Spice bottles, empty
Containers and nesting toys	Sand and water toys and activities	Squeeze toys
Hammers and pegs		Teething toys
Inflatables		Textured surfaces

   b. Two to four years:

Amusement park rides	Magnets	Sand and water toys
Balance-rocker boards	Play tunnel	Seesaw
Blowing bubbles	Rocking horse	Slides
Finger paints	Rolling in the grass	Swings
Inflatables	Running	Tricycle riding

   c. Four to seven:

Amusement park rides	Obstacle courses	Simple woodwork
Balance beam	Playground equipment	Swimming
Bicycles and tricycle riding	Rocker boards	Swinging equipment
Dot-to-dot line drawings	Sand and water play	Tracing, templates
Inflatables	Scooter boards	Trampolines
Magnets	Simon Says	Visual perception worksheets
Mazes		

   d. Seven to twelve years:

Amusement park rides	Mazes	Simon Says
Dot-to-dot line drawings	"New" games	Stilts
Hopscotch	Parachute games	Swimming and water play
Hula hoops	Playground equipment	Throwing games
Jump rope	Obstacle courses	Visual perception worksheets
Kite-flying	Rough and tumble play	

   e. Adolescence:

Amusement park rides	Gymnastics	Swimming and water play
Calisthenics	Jogging, running	Wrestling
Dancing		

Figure 15-2   Symbolic play

1. *Description:* Play and recreational experiences through which the child formulates, tests, classifies, and refines ideas, feelings, and combined actions. Associated with the development of language.
2. *Properties of activities:*
   a. Tools, materials, and equipment:
      Gross motor play equipment
      Simple construction toys
      Simple art materials
      Toys for fantasy-imaginative play
   b. Human and object relationships:
      Play with peers begins with parallel imitation and develops into cooperative interaction.
      Parents validate products of play.
      Objects are given importance according to the child's ability to symbolize, control, change, and master.
   c. Characteristic age level is 2 to 4 years.
3. *Representative toys and activities:*
   a. Newborn to two years:

Dolls and stuffed animals	Mirrors	Scribbling with crayons
Imitative hand-body games	1- to 3-piece form	Shape boxes
Language play with parents	puzzles	

   b. Two to four years:

Abacus	Dolls and stuffed animals	Put-together toys
Beads	Dollhouses	Puzzles
Blocks	Dramatic songs	Records
Cars, trucks, trains	"Dress up" materials	Sewing cards
Chalk and blackboard activities	Hand puppets	Simple storybooks
Clay, modeling dough	Household play items	Space stations
Colorforms	Miniature figures	Stacking toys
Construction kits	Musical instruments	Toy telephone
Crayons, paints, paper	Nesting toys	Tricycle riding

   c. Four to seven years:

Action figures	"Dress up" materials	Play house or store
Arts and crafts materials	Lemonade stands	Puppets
Building sets	Musical instruments	Records
Dolls and stuffed animals	Papier-mâché	Storybooks
Dramatic play		

   d. Seven to twelve years:

Action figures	Computer games	Mime
Arts and crafts materials	Mad libs	Reading materials
Charades		

   e. Adolescence:

Arts and crafts materials	Decorative arts	Mime
Charades	Diaries	Plays and skits
Computer programming	"Feelings" games	Role-playing

tivation of the child. The competitive 8-year-old, for example, may well be found reading to stuffed animals as a respite from vigorous peer group play. The organization of the charts, therefore, is also designed to show a developmental progression of toys and activities in each category of play. There is recognizable overlap between many of the representative activities of each category, because analysis will indicate that each toy or play experience can serve several functions for the child. The examples of play activities are representative rather than all-inclusive. They should be interpreted and supplemented by knowledge gained from visiting toy stores and toy departments, observing children in play situations, and reviewing activity books for children in bookstores.

Use of the model for program planning

When considering assessment results, the therapist can determine which activities would help to meet intervention goals. For example, if a 4-year-old child has problems with fine motor function, the therapist would select symbolic and creative activities appropriate to the 4- to 7-year old age range (Figure 15-6). If an 8-

Figure 15-3 Creative play and interests

1. *Description:* Play and recreational experiences through which the child refines sensory, motor, cognitive, and social skills; explores combinations of actions on multiple objects; and develops interests and competencies that will promote performance of school-related and work-related activities.
2. *Properties of activities:*
   a. Tools, materials, and equipment:
      Arts and crafts
      Complex construction toys
      Dramatic play materials
      Household activities such as cooking, simple woodwork, pet care, and gardening
   b. Human and object relationships:
      Play begins in cooperative peer groups, with gradual emergence of competitive atmosphere; peer validation of play products becomes increasingly important.
      Parents assist and validate in the absence of peers.
      Nonhuman objects are valued according to outcome of play.
   c. Characteristic age level is 4 to 7 years.
3. *Representative toys and activities:*
   a. Newborn to two years:
      Blocks
      Crayon scribbling
      Pop beads
   b. Two to four years:
      Bead stringing
      Finger painting
      Mobile making
   c. Four to seven years:

Baking cookies	Gardening	Simple weaving—placemats, pot holders
Bicycle riding	Painting	Simple woodworking
Craft kits	Paperdolls	Stencils
Cutting and pasting		

   d. Seven to twelve years:

Cooking	Drawing	Painting
Crafts	Model kits	Science experiments
Decorative arts	Needle arts	Woodworking

   e. Adolescence:
      Crafts: jewelry making, woodworking, metalworking
      Creative writing
      Fine and decorative arts

year-old child is developmentally delayed, the therapist might work toward engagement of the child in competitive games and activities at a slightly lower age level (Figure 15-7 on p. 302). The teenager who has become withdrawn might be directed toward some of the symbolic and creative activities appropriate to adolescence. This model is designed to appeal to the developmental interest level of the child or adolescent, as discussed by Frantzen,[7] and at the same time provide a wide range of therapeutically useful modalities.

PROGRAM DEVELOPMENT
Adaptation of play activities

Adaptation of play activities to promote the child's involvement, enjoyment, and success is another ele-

ment of play in occupational therapy. Adaptations may be made to the position of the body and work surface; to the activity process itself; to the expectations for performance; and to the tools, materials, and equipment used in the activity process. In addition, the therapist can use different interpersonal relationships to promote activity performance. Specific adaptive equipment and physical techniques are also used to enable the individual to participate in a larger range of activities. Ideas for activity adaptation may be found throughout this text in relation to specific problems. Procter presents a wealth of ideas for adaptations of play activities (Chapter 17) and Cummings' use of computers for play experiences (Chapter 22) will also prove valuable. Therefore, only selected activities will be discussed at this time. Suggestions

---

Figure 15-4   Games

---

1. Description: Play and recreational experiences that have distinct rules and involve skill development and social interaction in a competitive atmosphere. Actions and results of actions are compared against those of peers.

2. Properties of activities:
    a. Tools, materials, and equipment:
       Sports equipment that requires refined control of gross and fine motor actions
       Table games
       Perceptual-motor games
       Cognitive-language games
    b. Human and object relationships:
       Peer relationship is most important.
       Attachment to nonhuman objects that are important in games in which the child can successfully compete.
    c. Characteristic age level is 7 to 12 years.

3. Representative toys and activities:
    a. Newborn to two years:
       Sensory-motor games with rules, for example, peekaboo
    b. Two to four years:

Checkers	Matching card games
Dominoes	Simple classification board games
Lotto	

    c. Four to seven years:

Same as above	Organized outdoor games at age level
Bicycle or tricycle races	Scooter board races

    d. Seven to twelve years:

Arcade games	Collections	Ping-Pong
Board games	Computer games	Roller-skating and ice-skating
Card games	Field days: races, tug-of-war	School plays, performances
Checkers	Hangman	Team sports
Clubs	Jacks, marbles	Trading cards
	Jump rope	

    e. Adolescence:
       Individual or team competition
       School political activities
       Team sports

---

will be presented through case examples and program reports from the literature.

MOTOR FUNCTION

Very often motor impairment may prevent the child's full participation in play. Through knowledgeable selection of activities, in cooperation with the child's interests and capacities, the occupational therapist can design a treatment program that will improve motor function and at the same time promote continuity in the child's development of play and related skills. The techniques that are used most with children who have motor problems include adaptation of position (of the body and work surface) and adaptation of the tools, materials, and equipment that are used for an activity.

CASE STUDY

Donna is an 8-year-old girl with moderate spastic hemiplegia who was referred to occupational therapy for improvement of gross and fine motor skills. Assessment indicated that her typical play behaviors were at the level of symbolic activities, although she was interested in participating in more creative play and games. She was able to use her uninvolved left hand in all fine prehension patterns, but precise manipulative ability was generally poor. She had difficulty drawing geometric figures, her printing was crude, and she needed assistance to hold paper when cutting. Results of her independent attempts in these activities were generally poor. Although her involved right hand was used fairly well as a gross assist and was relaxed at rest, she tended to become tight during concentrated efforts. In such instances, she became frustrated because she would lose control over her right hand as an assist.

Donna's sensory integrative function appeared slightly depressed, with fair localization of tactile and proprioceptive stimuli. Equilibrium responses were adequate against mild resistance, but she needed support to maintain positions against moderate resistance. So-

Figure 15-5   Recreation

1. *Description:* Play-leisure experiences that allow the youth to explore complex interests and roles to develop a sense of self-identity and achievement.
2. *Properties of activities:*
   a. Tools, materials, and equipment:
      Arts and crafts
      Collections
      Organized interest group activities
      Social activities
      Sports
   b. Human and object relationships:
      Peer group is still important for sharing of interests.
      Validation of outcome by self is increasingly important.
      Objects may have sentimental value but are viewed realistically.
   c. Characteristic age level is adolescence.

3. *Representative toys and activities:*
   a. Newborn to two years:
      Activities from other categories that represent individual interests and preferences
   b. Two to four years:
      Same as above
   c. Four to seven years:
      Same as above
   d. Seven to twelve years:
      Same as above
   e. Adolescence:

Collections	Musical instruments
Crafts	Performing arts
Dancing	Singing and choir
Decorative arts	Spectator sports
Fine arts	Social sports
Hiking and camping	Team sports
Individual sports	

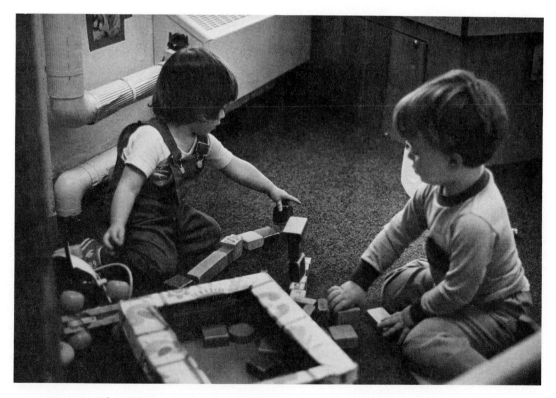

Figure 15-6   Preschool children develop fine motor, language, and role skills through play with toys that represent common objects.

From Weiser MG: Group care and education of infants and toddlers, St Louis, 1982, The CV Mosby Co.

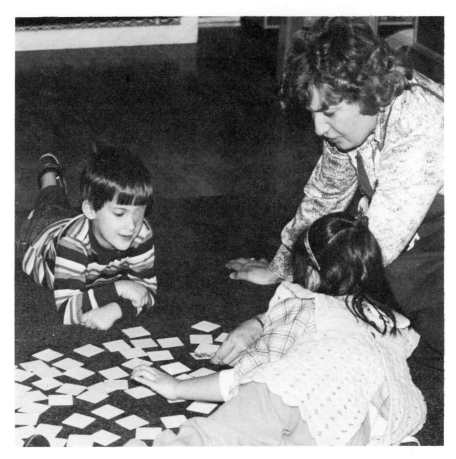

Figure 15-7   School-age children can strengthen visual processing skills through competitive game play.

From Hendrick J: The whole child: early education for the eighties, ed 3, St Louis, 1984, The CV Mosby Co.

cial skills were well developed. Although her articulation was not always clear, her speech and language development were generally age-appropriate. She related well to others in her class and seemed to have a loving relationship with her divorced mother and siblings.

General goals of occupational therapy were to strengthen gross and fine motor skills to improve performance in schoolwork and age-appropriate play activities. Because of her age, she received her occupational therapy services two times weekly as a member of a group that included three age-mates who had similar problems. As a general rule, the group worked on creative activities once a week, with an emphasis on development of fine motor skills. The other weekly session was reserved for gross motor play through competitive activities.

One favorite activity was the puppet show, which was chosen to strengthen fine motor skills and symbolic representation. The therapist prepared two side outlines of simple animal shapes for felt hand puppets. The two sides were fastened together with a few paper clips over a slightly smaller cardboard template and set up in a table clamp. Donna sewed her puppet together by using a large needle and yarn in her left hand and by using the right hand to stabilize the edge near her stitches. Although she was unable to handle the felt with scissors, she traced and cut out paper patterns for the puppet's facial features. When the puppets were completed, the children worked together to develop a skit to present to the rest of their class.

Because each of the children had weak balance and underdeveloped gross motor control of their uninvolved arms, the therapist designed a beanbag toss game that would allow them to compete with each other and strengthen their gross motor skills. Together with the therapist, the children developed a set of rules that would govern the actions and scoring of the game. A rocker board was used for sitting, knee-standing, and standing. Each child was responsible for positioning the rocker board behind the starting line before each throw. Target distances ranged from 5 to 10 feet and were increased as individual improvement was noted.

Initially, the target was a large square area on the floor that was bordered by masking tape. As the children became more proficient, the target was changed to a hula hoop, and later to a wastebasket. Donna began by using an underhand toss, and she progressed to an overhand throw. An overriding concern of the group was that each child should compete fairly with the others. Consequently, the children modified the rules according to the performance capacity of each group member. For example, because Donna was the best thrower in the group, her starting line was placed 1 foot behind the others. Each child's positions on the rocker board varied according to his postural stability.

Teenagers with handicapping conditions are often restricted from participation in recreational activities due to safety considerations, lack of motor control, and environmental access difficulties. Therapists who work with these youth are challenged to locate, analyze, and adapt recreational opportunities to simultaneously promote development and improve motor function. Peganoff[23] reported on the use of an aquatics program for a 14-year-old girl with cerebral palsy. The program developed for the girl required special arrangements for pool use, adaptation of methods for entry and exit from the pool, and physically assisted use of the hemiparetic arm and leg. The therapeutic aquatics program lasted for 8 weeks, with sessions held twice weekly.

The immediate effects of the program, in its function as a therapeutic modality, were improvements in gross and fine motor control, self-image, and spontaneous increase in self-care skills. A long-term effect was the girl's continued participation in swimming for recreation.

SENSORY INTEGRATIVE FUNCTION

Chapter 23 will present a thorough discussion of the activities that are used in sensory integrative therapy. As mentioned previously, much of this therapy is provided through the medium of play. Mack, Lindquist, and Parham[17] published a detailed study of the interactive relationship between play and sensory integrative treatment. They emphasized that sensory-motor play experiences normally mature through a hierarchical sequence of exploratory, symbolic, and creative activities. However, when the sensory integrative functions are inadequate, the child's ability to engage in more complex and mature forms of play is impaired.

Two critical areas for adaptation of play with such a child include the relationship between the child and the therapist, and the structure of tools, materials, and equipment in the play environment. Lindquist, Mack, and Parham[15] recommended that the therapist serve as a role model (Figure 15-8). When children lack the organization to direct their actions in new situations or with new play materials, they tend to withdraw from the activity. For example, the therapist can demonstrate how to get onto and ride a scooter board to a child whose interest in the play equipment results in

awkward frustration. The therapist also serves as an extension of the child's body, helping the child to monitor movements. Once on the scooter board, or a piece of suspended equipment, the child may lack the capacity to make postural adjustments as his body shifts with the movement of the equipment. The resulting postural insecurity changes the activity from a playful to a fearful experience. Verbal and physical cuing can be helpful in this instance. As the child's organization improves, the therapist may ask the child to explain what body parts must be moved to make postural adjustments.

Knickerbocker[14] also suggested that the therapist should serve as a role model, but in a more nondirective manner. Knickerbocker asked children to show what they could do when a piece of sensory motor play equipment was initially introduced to them. If a child demonstrated reluctance to approach the new play object, Knickerbocker advocated quiet play with the object by the therapist.

Structure of the play environment is always an important element of occupational therapy, because materials and equipment must always be organized to elicit maximal responses from children. However, the child with sensory integrative impairment has special needs for environmental structure because of diminished ability to handle competing stimuli. The treatment area or room can be attractive but sparse. Although a monotone barrenness can be depressing to a child, it is useful to set up the area with a minimum of colors. Cool but clear colors are usually manageable. Equipment should be neatly stored in closed cabinets whenever possible. It is helpful to have an open but raised shelf to hold the materials for a daily treatment session. Decorations on the walls should be neatly arranged, and too many decorations and distractible ones should be avoided. Treatment duration for each session should be determined by the child's ability to handle changing stimuli. Often two or three activities within a half hour are all that can be accomplished successfully by the child. Finally, sessions should be scheduled so that interruptions are held to a minimum.

In recent years, a number of studies have been reported that correlate sensory integrative programming with the developmental aspects of play. Anderson[1] reviewed findings in infant development and made concrete recommendations regarding what types of stimuli are best processed by the premature infant. Visual forms should be red or black on white backgrounds, and are best presented in low lighting. Mirrors, significant faces, and mobiles are also appropriate. Tactile and proprioceptive stimuli are critical, with an emphasis on physically guided movements that allow the infant to explore his own body. Light touch stimuli are contraindicated. Anderson recommended swaddling the baby at the end of the session, with hands positioned near the mouth to promote oral motor exploration.

Anderson also noted the importance of vestibular in-

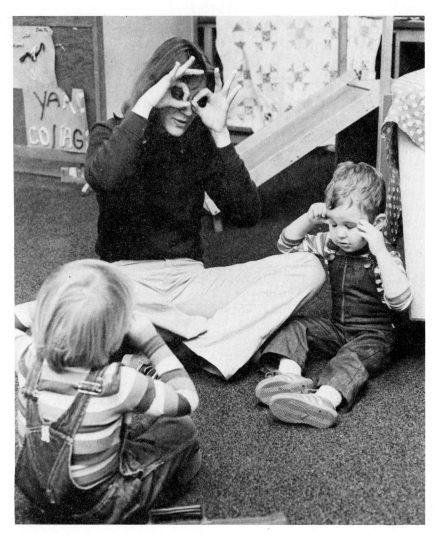

Figure 15-8   The therapist as role model.

From Weizer MG: Group care and education of infants and toddlers, St Louis, 1982, The CV Mosby Co.

put, suggesting that the child be swaddled and rocked in various body planes and positions. It is helpful for the therapist to sit on a gym ball while gently rocking the swaddled child, to promote a sense of postural unity. Auditory stimuli should be presented with great care, and only when the infant is calm. Soft sounds and a high-pitched voice appear to be the best tolerated forms.

Moyer[20] recommended varieties of more mature activities to promote sensory integration of adolescents. Students can have pillow fights, a traditional teen activity, while standing on rocker boards or balance beams. Competitive exercise groups, soccer, and bicycling can also be adapted to provide controlled sensory input and promote postural adjustments and praxis.

As alluded to previously, it is important for occupational therapists to provide play activities that can be accomplished with a sense of success. This key ingredient can make the difference between a child who is intrinsically motivated to try out new play experiences[5,15] and a child who endures a program of meaningless, although potentially therapeutic, activities. Again, before developing a program, to achieve the preferred outcome, it is necessary to carefully assess performance skills and interests and to measure sensory-integrative functioning. The representative exploratory activities shown in Figure 15-1 on p. 297 provide a broad variety of suggestions for treatment. Each can be adapted to provide challenging and positive age-appropriate, play-learning experiences for the child or adolescent.

COGNITIVE FUNCTION

If the principles espoused by Piaget, Reilly, and Florey are accepted, then it is axiomatic that play experiences are critical to cognitive development and learning. The entire complement of play categories, activities, and toys presented in Figures 15-1 through 15-5 provides a range of self-directed experiences that will sharpen and expand the child's mind.

The mental development of children may be permanently impaired by neurological and metabolic problems. In such instances, special education services, including occupational therapy, will be needed to promote the child's achievement of optimal mental growth. However, therapists need to be aware that any problem that temporarily or permanently restricts the child's ability to engage in learning experiences can result in delay or depression of cognitive development. For this reason, therapists need to concentrate on the cognitive process and outcomes of treatment experiences for all children. Occupational therapists should select and grade treatment activities within the operative capabilities of the child.

Accordingly, the teaching skills of the therapist, in concert with knowledgeable activity analysis, will be of special importance to programs for children with cognitive impairment. The therapist's role-modeling as a player can assist the child's development of action schemes. Through imitation, the child can try out behaviors that have been demonstrated by the therapist.

One useful teaching technique is called *chaining*.[28] Through an activity analysis, the therapist identifies the sequence of steps required in an activity. Then the activity is taught to the child through his mastery of each successive step in the sequence. Although this basic method, called *forward chaining*, is often successful, its opposite, *reverse chaining*, tends to be more productive when cognitive impairment is present. In reverse chaining the therapist and the child work through the activity sequence together, with the child assisting as possible. But the child is expected to perform the last step independently. When the last step is mastered, then the next-to-last step becomes the new target step for independent performance. From clinical practice, it appears that reverse chaining is more engaging to the child, because it allows the child more exposure to the complete process so that learning takes place through repetition. In addition, the child's experiences of success are tied into the outcome of the process. This appears to maintain higher levels of interest in the activity.

Sharp[27] developed a very useful series of Piagetian tasks that can be adapted for use in occupational therapy. Most of the activities are designed to support the development of classification, seriation, and conservation, and are typical of the symbolic play-learning experiences of the preschool and elementary school-aged child. Materials are prepared by the therapist from items readily available. For example, the children can play with glasses of water to develop volume conservation concepts or arrange shapes to form faces and objects. The activities are graded in a developmental sequence so that learning that is accrued from some of the earlier games will enable the child to master later activities more readily. Sharp[27] is an excellent resource for any occupational therapy program.

Rubin and others[26] reported a program for the remediation of cognitive-perceptual-motor dysfunction in primary grade children that emphasized skill development through exploratory, symbolic, and creative play and educational experiences. The activity program followed a developmental progression that allowed the children to proceed from mastered activities to more challenging ones. The investigators' approach to intervention also included the removal of the child from stress-evoking and stress-producing experiences in school on a part-time basis to obtain optimal results. The investigators found that children who participated in this program for one semester were able to return to home and to school with excellent adjustment and preparation for educational experiences.

Analysis of any toy or activity will suggest cognitive components. Color-matching games, for example, require the development of sensorimotor schema of color likes and differences. However, the child must also have a beginning ability to remember sequences of actions and to differentiate between a personal marker and markers of others and, for example, that a particular motion will cause an arrow to spin. These classification and causation operations may be expected and promoted in 4- to 5-year-old children. Children 3 years of age would have more difficulty playing such a game and would be likely to lose interest.

In Chapter 16, Stephens provides a clinical example of a jump rope activity that was unsuccessful because it was beyond the cognitive integration of the children for whom it was designed. She found it advisable to drop the activity entirely and concentrate on antecedent developmental skills. This type of situation will occur in practice daily; for every activity that is successful, there is likely to be another that is less so. Therapists need to remember that, although children's maturation follows a progressive course, there is a spiraling, cyclical nature to development that results in uneven functional states. This appears to be particularly true of cognitive development, because fluctuations of mood, restfulness, and other physical factors can influence the sharpness of the child's operative capabilities.

Construction toys offer a wide range of variations according to the cognitive development of the child. Young children engaged in exploratory play may examine the sensory and action characteristics of simple colored cubes and blocks. At this stage, blocks may be knocked, manipulated, dropped, banged together to produce noises, and placed side by side. Demonstration of the latter pattern on a repeated, purposive basis may be an indication of the child's transition to symbolic play. At this point, blocks take on additional characteristics through their relationships to each other and to the child's mental images. Through symbolic constructions, blocks become parts of a whole and are put together in increasingly complex patterns to represent real or imagined objects. As the child's fine manipulative skills increase, and schemata for interactions multiply, simple blocks are replaced by construction toys that have different shapes and properties. The variety of construction sets that are commercially available seems infinite, from shapes with simple projections that allow pieces to connect at random, to elaborate kits containing wheels, motors, connectors, and specialized parts. Even adolescents and adults may play for hours with the advanced technical kits.

EMOTIONAL FUNCTION

Clinical observations show children who are experiencing emotional difficulty to be characterized by diminished and regressed play behaviors. Children who are withdrawn usually withdraw from play as well. Children who demonstrate acting-out behaviors may use play objects in the course of such episodes, but the actions with such objects are not likely to be described as play. When children with emotional problems do play, their play tends to be perseverative, and the play objects are more appropriate to younger children. These observations indicate that engagement in play serves as a barometer of the emotional status of children.

Adaptation of play activities for the child with emotional problems is often accomplished through structure of the play environment and therapeutic relationship. Axline[2] reported on the use of a Rogerian form of play therapy with young children. She chose toys that, in general, lent themselves to symbolic play, such as action figures, dolls and dollhouses, and water play items. Toys that did not elicit feelings and expression were not used in the program. As children explored, played with toys, and talked about their play, Axline used nondirective techniques to focus, clarify, and enhance the child's expressive capacity.

Goldstein[8] discussed the use of sensory integrative group treatment in a child psychiatry practice. The children were referred to therapy for treatment of secondary emotional symptoms, with poor self-esteem noted as the most common problem. Goldstein felt that a group program would decrease the children's feelings of isolation and incompetence by providing the opportunity to participate in a true peer play situation. Under the therapist's guidance, opportunities of healthy interaction, dealing with feelings, and developing a sense of competence among like children were structured.

Goldstein[8] provided some specific guidelines for therapists who seek to enhance emotional function through play experiences.

1. Make groups as homogeneous as possible, with no more than four children.
2. Set clear limits and expectations.
3. Plan several activities to reach each goal and allow the children to choose from the options.
4. Avoid quiet, one-to-one competitive situations.

Vandenberg and Kielhofner[32] reported on the occupational therapy treatment of a 13-year-old boy with a diagnosis of adolescent adjustment reaction who demonstrated a tendency to withdraw from new situations. The boy resisted initial efforts to participate in a ceramics activity. Subsequently, the occupational therapist began to play with the clay, thus providing a role model for the boy. When the therapist dropped the clay, the situation was handled in a playful manner, subtly indicating to the boy that mistakes in new situations were permissible. Through this experience and subsequent treatment sessions with clay and other craft activities, the boy developed the capacity to approach and explore new situations with a sense of control and satisfaction. In this case, the therapist's structure of the interpersonal relationship was subtle. The choice of clay, a medium that lends itself to many different uses and forms, was complemented by the structuring of a playful atmosphere.

Llorens and Rubin[16] reported on a graded program of play activities that was used by occupational therapy for treatment of children with emotional disturbances. The core of the program was the children's involvement in activity groups. The "basic skills group" for children aged 6 to 12 emphasized free exploratory play with sensory-motor toys. When a child chose to play with an unfamiliar toy, the therapist instructed the child in one way to play with it. This technique was used, first, to provide the child with a successful play experience with the new toy and, second, through the success experience, to stimulate the child's motivation to explore the toy further and develop additional skills.

The "skill development group" was more structured, with specific training in performance of symbolic and creative activities. The children worked on projects in a large group. Although specific expectations for project completion were established, children were permitted to perform at their own individual rates. Interactive experiences with the other children in the group were fostered by the therapist.

The "advanced group" used craft activities and was highly structured. The therapist adopted the role of a teacher. Children were expected to work cooperatively and maintain a level of performance with the rest of the group. Activities ranged from structured kits to materials that demanded original designs. Increasingly complex techniques were taught through units, and children were graded on their productions.

Through this program, which used a variety of play

activities that are similar to those shown in Figures 15-1 through 15-5, the children progressed from free play to highly structured play. Expectations for performance were initially self-directed, with gradual increases in external controls. Play progressed from being parallel, to cooperative, to competitive. This program demonstrates well how occupational therapy can provide a microcosm of developmental play experiences for children.

SOCIAL FUNCTION

Many of children's social skills are developed through play experiences. The occupational therapist needs to be alert to this and to structure play situations to provide opportunities for social development.

Parten[22] was one of the early investigators of play. She identified six levels of social interaction in play that are generally regarded as definitive. As reported by Neumann,[21] the six levels are:

1. Unoccupied: Playing with own body, random activity.
2. Onlooker: Watching others, but not entering into the situation.
3. Solitary: Plays with toys differently from children within speaking distance; interest centered on own play; independent activity.
4. Parallel: Plays independently, but beside and not with others (Figure 15-9).
5. Associative: Group play with overt recognition by group members of common activity, interest, and personal association.
6. Cooperative: Most highly organized group activity; division of labor; group is organized to achieve some goal; control by one or more children (p. 97).

Through unoccupied play and the child's awareness of parental reactions to sensory exploration, the child begins to develop a sense of what actions are socially appealing. As the child watches the play and actions of others, she stores mental images for future consideration and imitation. Onlooker play is not limited to the very young child. It is apt to occur in novel situations, as when the child observes another playing with a new toy. In therapy the actions of the therapist with an unfamiliar toy may be repeated in the child's first experience with the object.

The child's play with a new object will often be solitary as the child obtains firsthand knowledge of characteristics and actions of the toy. The child may then imitate behaviors that were previously observed. Social behaviors in relation to sharing and cooperation are developed through parallel play experiences. Here also modeling and imitation are important, because the child will tend to do what he sees others do. The therapist can help by establishing simple rules for behavior and following up by clarifying to the individual child what behaviors are appropriate or not. Children will often want to play with a toy that another child is using. The therapist can develop skills of sharing and cooperation by structuring time limits and suggesting ways that two children can play together with the desired toy.

Associative and cooperative play experiences are

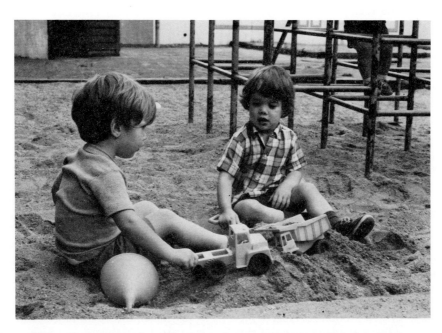

Figure 15-9   Exploratory play with sand and toy trucks in a parallel play situation.

From Weiser MG: Group care and education of infants and toddlers, St Louis, 1982, The CV Mosby Co.

easily promoted in the occupational therapy program. Craft projects and games are well suited to the development of interactive planning, decision making, and role-taking. In addition, children must take turns with tools and materials and develop and follow other cooperative rules. In the clinical example presented earlier, a group of children made felt hand puppets. Although adequate tools could have been made available, the therapist structured the situation to promote social skill development by providing a limited number of scissors, needles, and bottles of glue. The children had to pace their own work to share. The subsequent puppet show was written by the children, each taking turns to contribute lines for one's puppet character and offering ideas for each others' characters. Through this process the individual child's involvement was directed from his own puppet to the success of the group project.

The importance of play programs

In 1972 Gray[10] discussed the effects of hospitalization on work-play behavior. She proposed that, to a greater or lesser degree, the medical focus on the individual's disability and related intervention overrides concern for the life that has been disrupted. Through the course of intervention practices, the individual may experience loss of self-care, social, work, time, play, and decision-making skills. She speculated that these losses may be more of an impediment to the individual's recovery than the initial medical condition.

Although Gray's focus was on the hospitalized individual, her concepts may be readily applied to any individual who experiences a disabling condition. The well-meant reactions of significant others in a child's life tend to "do for" the child (Chapter 16). In addition, the child is often isolated from the mainstream of childhood play and interactions. Therefore it becomes increasingly important for occupational therapists to provide the types of play experiences that promote skill development in the areas cited by Gray.

Gralewicz[9] conducted a study that compared the play of small samples of nonhandicapped children and multihandicapped children who were 3 to 5 years old. Observations of play were recorded in the children's homes by their parents. Gralewicz found that the nonhandicapped children spent significantly more time playing, had more play companions, and engaged in a wider variety of play activities than the handicapped children. In addition, although data were not statistically significant, the multihandicapped children spent more time engaged in no observable activity at all.

A later study by Kielhofner and others[13] examined the differences in play of three nonhospitalized preschool children and three hospitalized children of similar ages who had spent more than 60% of their lives in hospitals. The children were videotaped at play in a hospital playroom and in a standardized play environment in which selected play objects were specifically set up before all videotape sessions. The investigators found significant differences in the level of play development and the playfulness of the children. The nonhospitalized children were more advanced. The investigators noted that the hospitalized children used toys more simply, rather than trying out a variety of actions, and that they usually did not engage in symbolic and interconnected play activities.

Johnson and Deitz[12] noted that mothers of preschool children spent an average of 11.7 hours daily caring for the physical needs of children with disabling conditions, in contrast to 4.1 hours per day for these activities with non-handicapped children. These findings indicate that mothers of handicapped children have a markedly decreased amount of time to spend nurturing and playing with their children.

These studies indicate that the children who are seen by occupational therapists in both educational and medical settings are likely to demonstrate deficiencies in both quality and quantity of play experiences. Therefore it is important that the therapist provide opportunities for children to engage in play for its own sake, exclusive of objectives for improvement of specific functional correlates. This may be done through the organization of hospital play programs, in-school and after-school play groups, and free play periods as part of occupational therapy treatment sessions. The role of the therapist as a player is critical. In the study described previously, Kielhofner and others[13] found that the attitude and engagement of adults in the play situation had specific effects on the playfulness of the children.

In addition, therapists can share their knowledge and appreciation of play and its developmental correlates with parents (Chapter 8). Again, the focus and range of play materials and experiences presented in Figures 15-1 through 15-5 may be useful for such purposes. Toys and materials can be demonstrated and made available for loan. Formal and informal parent education sessions, with opportunities for demonstration and practice, can be a productive addition to the occupational therapy service. Any program that results in the improvement of the play skills of the child may be considered a significant achievement.

Tessler[31] developed a structured approach in recommending home exploratory play activities for infants. Structure is based on the interaction between stimulus needs and maturation of the child's motor control, and is divided into four stages:

1. The newborn is gaining oculomotor control; therefore, visually interesting objects and stimulating toys are recommended for this age.
2. As children gain more hand and upper trunk control and begin to develop hand-arm use, toys should combine visual or auditory stimuli with properties that promote hand action (mobiles, mirrors, squeeze toys).

3. As trunk and finger control improves, Tessler encourages parents to provide children with elementary cause and effect toys, such as busy boxes, jack in the boxes, and musical toys.

4. As the infant develops increased mobility and is ready for standing and walking with support, Tessler recommends objects and games that encourage planning and postural adjustments, such as simple take apart and put together toys.

Rast[24] cautioned therapists to remember that the "goal-oriented, externally controlled aspects of the therapy situation (can) conflict with the essence of play itself" (p. 30). Successful use of play situations and activities for promoting development and functional gains is therefore dependent on the therapist's knowledgeable use of theory and modalities. This must be combined with a trained sense of when to emphasize "therapeutic" aims and when to step back and allow the intrinsic nature of play to direct its own course.

SUMMARY

This chapter presented play as a generic modality in occupational therapy practice with children. Although play activities have long been used because of their therapeutic characteristics, occupational behavior theory has generated a renewed attention to the merits of play for its own sake. Based on the theoretical framework of play that was proposed by Reilly (Chapter 3), other occupational therapists like Florey, Takata, and Michelman have examined the development and content of play behaviors. Their ideas have been incorporated in this chapter in the development of a model of play development and activities for occupational therapy.

With this developmental model as a guide, occupational therapy programs may be planned and carried out that use play as both an adaptive modality and outcome of therapeutic intervention. Adaptation of play activities according to the functional needs of children was discussed in relation to the enhancement of motor, sensory-integrative, cognitive, emotional, and social skills. In addition, therapists were challenged to ensure the adequacy of play experiences for healthy development. Play is the preeminent occupational behavior of childhood and, as such, is a primary focus and modality for occupational therapists who work with this age group.

STUDY QUESTIONS

1. Using Florey's typology for classification of objects, determine whether the activities for the 2- to 4-year-old child listed in Figure 15-2 are Type I, II, or III. Is there a predominance of any type of play object for that age group? Why?

2. Using the tables shown in Figures 15-1 through 15-5, choose three activities that might be used to initiate treatment for each of the following children:
   a. Suzanne, 8 months old, with Down syndrome

   b. Fred, 8 years old, diagnosed with autism
   c. Mickey, 18 years old, with spastic hemiparesis secondary to cerebral palsy

3. For each child mentioned above, select a fourth activity that is age-appropriate, but would be difficult for the child because of his disability. How could you adapt the activity so that it could be engaged in more readily?

4. You have been asked to develop materials for a toy lending library to serve parents of handicapped children in a small rural school system. The system serves children from 3 to 18 years of age. You have $300. How would you spend the money, and why?

REFERENCES

1. Anderson J: Sensory intervention with the pre-term infant in the neonatal intensive care unit, Am J Occup Ther 40:19, 1986.
2. Axline, VM: Play therapy, New York, 1969, Ballantine Books, Inc.
3. Bruner JS, Jolly A, and Sylva K: Play: its role in development and evolution, New York, 1976, Basic Books, Inc, Publishers.
4. Flavell JH: Cognitive development, Englewood Cliffs, NJ, 1977, Prentice-Hall, Inc.
5. Florey L: Intrinsic motivation: the dynamics of occupational therapy theory, Am J Occup Ther 23:319, 1969.
6. Florey L: An approach to play and play development, Am J Occup Ther 25:275, 1971.
7. Frantzen J: Toys . . . the tools of children, Chicago, 1957, National Easter Seal Society for Crippled Children and Adults.
8. Goldstein PK: Sensory integration groups—an effective treatment modality in child psychiatry, AOTA, SISIS Newsletter, VI (1), 1983.
9. Gralewicz A: Play deprivation in multihandicapped children, Am J Occup Ther 27:70, 1973.
10. Gray M: Effects of hospitalization on work-play behavior, Am J Occup Ther 26:180, 1972.
11. Hutt C: Exploration and play (#2). In Sutton-Smith B, editor: Play and learning, New York, 1979, Gardner Press, Inc.
12. Johnson CB, and Deitz JC: Time use of mothers with preschool children in a pilot study, Am J Occup Ther 39:578, 1985.
13. Kielhofner G, and others: Comparison of play behavior in non-hospitalized and hospitalized children, Am J Occup Ther 37:305, 1983.
14. Knickerbocker BM: A holistic approach to the treatment of learning disorders, Thorofare, NJ, 1980, Charles B Slack, Inc.
15. Lindquist JE, Mack W, and Parham LD: A synthesis of occupational behavior and sensory integration concepts in theory and practice. Part 2: clinical applications, Am J Occup Ther 36:433, 1982.
16. Llorens LA, and Rubin EZ: Developing ego functions in disturbed children: occupational therapy in milieu, Detroit, 1967, Wayne State University Press.
17. Mack W, Lindquist JE, and Parham LD: A synthesis of occupational behavior and sensory integration concepts in theory and practice. Part 1: theoretical foundations, Am J Occup Ther 36:365, 1982.
18. Michelman SM: Research in symbol formation and creative growth. In West WL, editor: Occupational therapy functions in interdisciplinary programs for children, Rockville, MD, 1969, Maternal and Child Health Service, United States Department of Health, Education, and Welfare.
19. Michelman SM: Play and the deficit child. In Reilly M, editor: Play as exploratory learning: studies in curiosity behavior, Beverly Hills, Calif, 1974, Sage Publications, Inc.

20. Moyer B: Suggestions for adolescents, AOTA, SISIS Newsletter II (1) 1979.
21. Neumann EA: The elements of play, New York, 1971, MSS Information Corp.
22. Parten MB: Social play among school children, J Abnorm Psychol 28:136, 1933.
23. Peganoff SA: The use of aquatics with cerebral palsied adolescents, Am J Occup Ther 38:469, 1984.
24. Rast M: Play and therapy, play or therapy? In AOTA, DDSIS, Play: a skill for life. 1 Rockville, Md, 1986, AOTA, Inc.
25. Reilly M, editor: Play as exploratory learning: studies in curiosity behavior, Beverly Hills, Calif, 1974, Sage Publications, Inc.
26. Rubin EZ, and others: Cognitive-perceptual-motor dysfunction: from research to practice, Detroit, 1972, Wayne State University Press.
27. Sharp E: Thinking is child's play, New York, 1969, Avon Books.
28. Sieg KW: Applying the behavioral model to the occupational therapy model, Am J Occup Ther 28:421, 1974.
29. Sutton-Smith B, editor: Play and learning, New York, 1979, Gardner Press, Inc.
30. Takata N: Play as prescription. In Reilly M, editor: Play as exploratory learning: studies in curiosity behavior, Beverly Hills, Calif, 1974, Sage Publications, Inc.
31. Tessler E: A developmental approach to home activities for infants, AOTA, DDSIS, Newsletter I (2) 1978.
32. Vandenberg B, and Kielhofner G: Play in evolution, culture, and individual adaptation: implications for therapy, Am J Occup Ther 36:20, 1982.

SUGGESTED READINGS

Play theory

Chance P: Learning through play, New York, 1979, Gardner Press, Inc.
Ellis MJ, and Scholtz GJL: Activity and play of children, Englewood Cliffs, NJ, 1978, Prentice-Hall, Inc.
Kielhofner G: A model of human occupation. Part 2: ontogenesis from the perspective of temporal adaptation, Am J Occup Ther 34:657, 1980.
Kielhofner G, Burke JP, and Igi CH: A model of human occupaton. Part 4: assessment and intervention, Am J Occup Ther 34:777, 1980.
Levy J: Play behavior, New York, 1978, John Wiley & Sons, Inc.
Parent LH: Effects of a low-stimulus environment on behavior, Am J Occup Ther 32:19, 1978.
Robinson AL: Play: the arena for acquisition of rules for competent behavior, Am J Occup Ther 31:248, 1977.
Takata N: The play milieu: a preliminary appraisal, Am J Occup Ther 25:281, 1971.
Takata N: Introduction to a series: occupational behavior research for pediatric practice, Am J Occup Ther 34:11, 1980.
Wehman P, and Abramson M: Three theoretical approaches to play: applications for exceptional children, Am J Occup Ther 30:551, 1976.

Play programs

Azarnoff P, and Flegal S: A pediatric play program: developing a therapeutic play program for children in medical settings, Springfield, Ill, 1975, Charles C Thomas, Publisher.
Frost JL, and Klein BL: Children's play and playgrounds, Boston, 1979; Allyn & Bacon, Inc.
Moersch MS: Training the deaf-blind child, Am J Occup Ther 31:425, 1977.
Morris AG: Nationally speaking: parent education in well-baby care: a new role for the occupational therapist, Am J Occup Ther 32:75, 1978.
Wehman P, and Marchant J: Improving free play skills of severely retarded children, Am J Occup Ther 32:100, 1978.

Play as a modality

AOTA Dev Dis Spec Int Sec: Play: a skill for life. Rockville, Md, 1986, AOTA, Inc.
Burnell DP: Egocentric speech: an adaptive function applied to developmental disabilities in occupational therapy, Am J Occup Ther 33:169, 1979.
Day S: Mother-infant activities as providers of sensory stimulation, Am J Occup Ther 36:579, 1982.
DeGangi G, Hurley L, and Linscheid TR: Toward a methodology of the short-term effects of neurodevelopmental treatment, Am J Occup Ther 37:479, 1983.
Fahl MA: Emotionally disturbed children: effects of cooperative and competitive activity on peer interaction, Am J Occup Ther 24:31, 1970.
Farmer R: A musical activities program with young psychotic girls, Am J Occup Ther 17:116, 1963.
Hindmarsh W: Play diagnosis and play therapy, Am J Occup Ther 33:770, 1979.
Kohler ES: The effect of activity/environment on emotionally disturbed children, Am J Occup Ther 34:446, 1980.
Llorens LA: Fingerpainting with an obsessive-compulsive organically-damaged child, Am J Occup Ther 17:120, 1963.
McKibbin EH: An interdisciplinary program for retarded children and their families, Am J Occup Ther 26:125, 1972.
Montgomery P, and Richter E: Sensorimotor integration for developmentally disabled children: a handbook, Los Angeles, 1977, Western Psychological Services.
Orem RC: Montessori and the special child, New York, 1969, Capricorn Books.
Price A: Juvenile rheumatoid arthritis and occupational therapy, Am J Occup Ther 19:249, 1965.
Rugel RP, and others: The use of operant conditioning with a physically disabled child, Am J Occup Ther 25:247, 1971.
Tyler NB, and Kahn N: A home treatment form for the cerebral-palsied child, Am J Occup Ther 30:437, 1976.
Tyler NB, Kogan KL, and Turner P: Interpersonal components of therapy with young cerebral palsied, Am J Occup Ther 28:395, 1974.

16

School work tasks and vocational readiness

LINDA C. STEPHENS
PAT NUSE PRATT

DEVELOPING SCHOOL READINESS SKILLS

LINDA C. STEPHENS

Readiness factors

The occupational therapist who works with young children often must help them to cope adequately with schoolwork tasks. To do this, the child needs to develop academic readiness skills. These are the skills that educators deem important as foundations for learning academic skills such as reading and writing. Readiness has been described as the achieving of subskills along with the developmental maturity to integrate these subskills into a desired new skill.[21] The following is a discussion of motor, emotional, social, auditory-language, visual perception, and cognitive skills.

MOTOR SKILLS

Adequate physical developmental and physical health are considered important aspects of school readiness.[25] In the United States children generally enter an academic setting at age 6 and are assumed to have achieved physical readiness because of their chronological age. According to the Gesell Institute,[2] the average 6-year-old can stand on each foot alternately, make a 32-inch broad jump, catch a beanbag with hands only, tie shoelaces, and copy a divided rectangle. The 6-year-old likes to draw, color, paint, cut and paste, and can print most numerals from 1 to 11. In a study of prekindergarten screening,[10] the information processing of body awareness and motor control was considered to be an important predictor of readiness

for first grade. This study also identified children with high activity levels to be less likely to be ready for first grade.

Table 16-1 presents a developmental sequence of sensory integrative skills. The items in the third column can be considered functional readiness skills that are necessary for adequate performance of the activities listed in column four. Of particular importance as academic readiness functions are eye-hand coordination and ocular motor control.

EMOTIONAL SKILLS

Important emotional readiness skills include emotional stability and self-reliance.[25] Some normal 6-year-olds may not have developed this emotional maturity. The 6-year-old has been described as tumultuous and violently emotional, "typically brash and aggressive, ready for new adventure, falsely sure of himself" (p. 39).[18] To be ready for academic learning, the child should have achieved some degree of mastery of environment and developed feelings of adequacy (Table 16-1). Aggressive behavior has been identified as a factor likely to interfere with school readiness.[10] The abilities to self-direct and actively participate in schoolwork tasks are also important in the learning process.[21]

SOCIAL SKILLS

A child needs to develop the ability to function as a member of a group and to relate appropriately to authority figures to function in a formal learning environment. This social maturity has been identified as a preentrance variable necessary for school success.[25] Attentive behavior is another predictor of readiness for first grade.[10]

Table 16-1 Sensory integration development

The inherent function of the nervous system and information from the senses of	Are used to develop	These sensorimotor abilities are utilized to learn more concrete concepts and to develop	Use of these abilities develops an automatic level of function in
Touch	Body scheme	Eye-hand coordination	Reading
Movement	Reflex maturation	Ocular motor control	Writing
Gravity	Center of gravity awareness	Postural adjustments	Spelling
Vision	Motor planning ability	Auditory-language skills	Number work
Hearing	Postural balance	Visual-spatial perception	Problem solving
Smell	Awareness of two sides of the body	Emotional stability	Sequencing
Pain	Balance between the protective and	Mastery of environment	Ability to conceptualize
Temperature	discriminative sensory systems	Feelings of adequacy	Independent work
		Behavioral control	Spontaneous play
			Creativity
			Ability to form meaningful personal relationships

From The American Occupational Therapy Association, Inc, Copyright 1980, Totems, vol 3, p. 37, Gilfoyle EM, and Hays MA.

AUDITORY/LANGUAGE SKILLS

Another important area of development is auditory-language function. Information processing of language and verbal reasoning ability have been identified as prerequisites for first grade. Verbal reasoning is defined as the ability to understand and express language.[10]

VISUAL PERCEPTION SKILLS

Some maturity of visual perception is a necessary factor in school readiness. There is evidence that the child who enters school with delayed perceptual development never catches up with his peers in academic achievement, although perceptual processing ability is believed to be fully developed by age 9.[26] Information processing in the visual perceptual-motor domain has been identified as one of the major factors that can predict readiness for the first grade. Adequate perceptual discrimination and visual-spatial perception are considered necessary for the development of reading and writing skills.[25]

COGNITIVE SKILLS

Cognitive function is also considered to be a school readiness factor. A child needs to have acquired a body of knowledge through experience and to be able to attach meaning to that experience. Information processing in the areas of auditory-language skills, perceptual-motor skills, and body awareness must have meaning for the child to benefit from formal educational experiences.

Learning is considered to be a natural function of human beings; it takes place throughout life in and out of the classroom. Children approach new tasks eagerly and enthusiastically, enjoying the challenge of novelty. Jensen[21] stated that "children do not have to be cajoled, persuaded, coerced, manipulated, or tricked into learning. Given the appropriate conditions, including readiness, children simply learn" (p. 7). The child whose development is delayed, or whose ability to learn is impeded by a physical or cognitive handicap, is also eager to learn. The challenge for the occupational therapist is to provide the appropriate conditions and activities to enable the child to learn at his own level. In this way the child can be helped to develop the necessary readiness skills for academic work.

Functional components of schoolwork tasks: subskill development

ACADEMIC LEARNING

Academic learning is a complex process that generally depends on the development of the readiness skills discussed earlier. In addition, the performance of specific academic tasks depends on the development of specific functional capacities and developmentally antecedent skills, or subskills. For example, a child who is attempting to print letters must have developed the abilities to maintain a sitting position at the desk or table and to grip a pencil or crayon. The child must also have sufficient eye-hand coordination and motor planning ability to direct the movement of the pencil; sufficient motor control to keep pencil marks in the appropriate space; and adequate visual perception, including perceptual constancy, spatial perception, and directionality. In addition, the child must have achieved a level of cognitive maturity that allows him to put together the subskills and abstract concepts needed to print letters. This is called integrated learning.[21]

It is possible that a child might have all the necessary subskills for a task, yet be unable to integrate them for successful performance. For example, a therapist recently attempted to teach two girls how to jump rope. Both girls were 11; one was mildly retarded and the other was learning disabled. Both girls were eager to learn to jump rope. The task was analyzed and broken down into subskills: standing, standing balance on one foot, jumping, jumping over a rope, jumping over a moving rope, and turning the rope with the arms. Each subskill was practiced and mastered. However, neither girl was able to achieve the necessary integration required to put the subskills together and jump rope independently.

When working with children to develop subskills, the therapist often reaches points at which the children's functioning seems to be limited by developmental level or integrative ability. It is of little benefit, and indeed might cause harm, to have the child continue to repeat the subskills in an attempt to learn the higher level skill. In the example given earlier, after several unsuccessful sessions, the jumping rope activity was deleted from the occupational therapy program unless requested by the girls. Meanwhile, other activities were substituted to help the girls develop integrated motor functioning. Perhaps later these girls will be ready to try again, or having mastered the subskills, they may try it on their own when they are developmentally ready.

EMOTIONAL FACTORS

It is important to consider emotional factors when planning occupational therapy programs to prepare a child to cope with schoolwork tasks. *Motivation* is a critical factor. Given the appropriate tasks, most children are eager and motivated to learn without extrinsic rewards. Some children, however, are considered unmotivated when presented with tasks that are beyond their capacities. When instruction persists beyond the child's level of learning, there seems to be a lack of motivation, and psychological turnoff may result.

This turnoff inhibits behaviors that promote learning, even learning for which the child is ready.[21] A teacher complained that a child in his multihandicapped class was unmotivated. The child did not finish her work, appeared uninterested, and persisted in printing her letters backward. The teacher insisted on completion of assignments and set up a reward system for good performance, using gummed stars and stickers. When the occupational therapist evaluated the child, the child was found to have a severe visual perception deficit. The occupational therapy program was planned, using simple perceptual activities and progressing to more complex ones in a small group setting. The child not only worked hard and enjoyed the activities, but also asked for more as homework. Was this an unmotivated child, or had she merely withdrawn from the usual presentation of tasks beyond her readiness level? Jensen[21] stated that "the most effective reinforcement for learning . . . is the child's own perception of his increasing mastery of the skill he is trying to acquire" (p. 7).

Another important emotional component is *self-di-*

rection. Ayres,[3] in discussing the art of therapy, stated that "the most therapeutic situation is that in which the child's inner urge for action and growth drives him towards a response that furthers maturation and integration" (p. 256). The skillful and effective therapist takes cues from the child and his approach to various activities. The self-directed child works with the activity presented by the therapist, needing little encouragement to perform. This child often repeats the activity a number of times, adding variations to it that require even greater organization and integration.

The therapist can frequently learn a great deal about the child by observing free play. Often the child chooses activities that are therapeutically appropriate and that provide both a challenge for growth and learning and also the opportunity for mastery. Certain other activities may be avoided, however, either because the child is not developmentally ready, or because earlier experiences with those activities have resulted in turnoff. The most effective therapy is a program that provides some guidance and structure, yet gives the child freedom to exercise self-direction.

Closely related is the concept of *active involvement.* For change to take place, positive emotional involvement with the activity is needed. The child who is coerced or performs an activity under threat of punishment may meet the requirements of the adult but never become actively involved in the therapy session. When a child works only because of extrinsic factors (that is, a reward, therapist's praise, or mother's insistence), it is extremely difficult for the therapist to determine if the activities are appropriate or to plan a progressively challenging program.

The child who lacks emotional involvement therefore poses a challenge to the occupational therapist. Frequently such children are older and have experienced failure repeatedly. They find it more comfortable to refuse an activity and experience the therapist's disapproval than to risk further failure and reinforce their feelings of inadequacy.

It is essential to work closely with parents when trying to develop active involvement of the child. If the therapist can find out what is important to a child or, for example, what aspect of the disability is particularly bothersome, then this can be used as a starting point for therapy. Sometimes a structured reward program that uses rewards that are meaningful to the child is necessary to encourage the child's cooperation at the beginning of therapy. As the child experiences successes in developmentally appropriate activity performance, the extrinsic reward program can be diminished gradually.

SPLINTER SKILLS

Often, through repetitive training or imitation, children learn to perform certain skilled actions without adequate development of subskills. Such splinter skills are characterized by an inability to generalize and the tendency to lose a skill if it is not practiced. A common example may be found among preschoolers who learn to recite numbers by rote but who are unable to count objects and forget the labels or sequence during a summer vacation.

Although reliance on splinter skill training should be avoided, this method may be useful on occasion in therapy. Most children are highly motivated to learn skills that they see their peers performing and will persist in their own attempts to imitate the behaviors. One intelligent boy with severe athetosis learned to ride a bicycle after many bumps and bruises, although he continued to walk with great difficulty and had no other functional hand to use. Other children seen in practice who have extremely poor eye-hand coordination manage to become very adept at electronic video games.

Training to develop splinter skills as part of the occupational therapy program can help make a child more independent, or it can boost self-esteem. Learning to tie shoelaces is a good example. Some children can learn this skill by repetition, even though they do not have an adequate foundation of subskills and could not tie a bow anywhere else. Learning the splinter skill gives the child a sense of accomplishment and avoids the embarrassment of having untied shoes or having to ask the teacher for help. Of course, it is important to continue a comprehensive treatment program that will develop underlying functional capacities and developmentally antecedent skills so that the child will continue to progress in an integrated manner.

ATTENTION SPAN

Attention span is generally defined as the length of time a person attends to a task. Often the evaluation of a child's performance capacities will include a subjective appraisal of his attention span. The therapist (or teacher) observes the child's ability to attend to a task and compares this with the duration and nature of attention seen among other children of the same chronological age on the same task. Thus a child is often said to have a short attention span if he quickly becomes bored or distracted from a task. Efforts can then be concentrated on increasing the attention span. Making a subjective judgment that a child has a short attention span may be superficial and inaccurate. The therapist must question whether the presenting problem impairs the child's ability to attend or whether the activities are inappropriate. Most children become bored with and quickly distracted from activities for which there are no adequate subskills. The following case studies will illustrate this point.

CASE STUDY 1

Allen is a 7-year-old boy in a psychoeducational center for children with emotional and behavioral problems. He was referred to occupational therapy for evaluation and was described as hyperactive and distractible with a short attention span. He was difficult to test, because he concentrated very little on assessment activities presented, and he constantly turned around to grab something else. Several times he darted out of the room and ran down the hall. However, during administration of a standard developmental evaluation, the therapist presented him with a small bottle with a screw top and pellets inside. Allen sat quietly at the table, unscrewing the top, dumping pellets out, and putting them back inside the bottle. He would have continued longer if time had permitted. (Putting pellets in a bottle and dumping them out demonstrates a developmental level of approximately 15 months; screwing a 1-inch top is a developmental level seen at approximately 3½ years.) Does this child have a short attention span, or is his development delayed below age expectancy?

CASE STUDY 2

Kent is an 8-year-old boy who spends half a day in a language disorders class, and the rest of his school day is spent in a class for behavioral disorders. He was referred for an occupational therapy evaluation and was also described as hyperactive and distractible with a short attention span. Kent attempted the assessment activities presented by the therapist but constantly looked around the room, stopping his activity to point and ask, "What's that?" When attempting gross motor activities, he frequently halted and ran to an object in the room. He fingered things excessively and went quickly from one object to another. Kent had many splinter skills (that is, he could print his name but could not copy a cross) and showed uneven developmental levels.

It is interesting to compare these two children. Allen's attention span deficit appeared to be, in part, a result of being expected to perform activities for which he was not developmentally ready. The occupational therapy program for this child should emphasize developmentally appropriate activities and treatment of other deficits found in the assessment process. In contrast, Kent's evaluation revealed that he probably had a sensory integrative deficit that prevented him from screening out irrelevant stimuli to concentrate on a task. The occupational therapy program for Kent would use a sensory integrative approach to deal with functional deficits. For each of these boys the poor attention span was only one symptom of the child's dysfunction. Therefore treatment was geared toward remediation of the dysfunction, rather than merely working to increase the attention span. Remediation of the dysfunction would have the effect of increasing the attention span.

Developing readiness skills: program goals

The occupational therapist can help young children develop school readiness skills in a number of ways by using selected activities. Many young children with handicaps become accustomed to being the center of a family's attention and to having things done for them. They do not have the social maturity, independent work skills, willingness to share, or ability to take turns that is needed to function in both formal and informal groups.

Table 16-2 Eye-hand coordination activities

Activity	Adaptations	Purposes
PUNCH THE BALL Hold stick with both hands and punch small ball suspended by string (Figure 16-1).	Use cutoff broomstick or long cardboard tube. Try to hit spot marked on wall. Hit while prone or supine. Two children hit ball to each other.	Bilateral coordination Eye tracking Motor planning
BLEACH BOTTLE TOSS Make scoop from bleach bottle. Attach wiffle ball with string (Figure 16-2).	Toss in air and catch in scoop. Use unattached ball. Toss ball to another child to catch. Catch ball in scoop while sitting on T-stool or while walking across room.	Motor planning Eye tracking
BEAD STRINGING	Use varying sizes of beads. Pick out all one shape or color. Copy sequence of beads on another string or on pattern card.	Bilateral coordination Fingertip pinch Grasp and release Figure-ground perception Form perception Sequencing
RUBBER BAND BOARD Make board with rows of nails sticking up 1 to 2 inches. Use colored rubber bands.	Stretch rubber band from one nail to another. Make rows of horizontal, vertical or diagonal bands. Copy pattern card. Superimpose rubber bands over shape made by another rubber band. Try to find hidden shape.	Bilateral coordination Fingertip pinch Form constancy Spatial relationships Figure-ground perception

By using group activity programs, the occupational therapist can help the young handicapped child develop these subskills that are needed in school settings.

The therapist, in guiding the child to complete a project that might be either a block tower or a clay figure, helps the child develop other skills that are important for schoolwork. Manipulating materials to make a tangible object helps a child gain mastery over the environment and develop feelings of adequacy. The development of self-reliance not only aids in performance of activities of daily living, but also promotes the child's feelings of capability.

By using carefully planned activities, the therapist helps the child attach meaning to experiences. Physically handicapped children do not have the spontaneous opportunities to explore their environments that normally developing children have. Sensory stimuli and physical activity are needed to promote body awareness and motor control that are prerequisites for academic work.

The therapist can also provide the child with opportunities for problem solving. Often the dependent status of a child with handicaps precludes experiences in making choices, repetition of trial and error, and taking responsibility for one's decisions. The child needs to experiment with different ways of doing activities and to develop the capacity to predict the results of various actions.

RECOMMENDED PROGRAM ACTIVITIES

The pediatric occupational therapist has an infinite variety of activities to use for planning and directing programs to develop school readiness skills. Many traditional childhood games can be used or adapted to meet defined needs. The therapist can also get many ideas by observing normal preschool children at play and determining what developmental needs are met by the activities seen. Why do young children love to play in large boxes? Why does the toddler enjoy playing with Mom's pots and pans, and what variations does he introduce into the play? Activity analysis, guided by an understanding of child development, can help the therapist relate the use of these everyday activities to the needs of special children.

The following listed material describes a sample of games and activities that can be used with children in treatment programs. The emphasis here is on developing school readiness skills that every child needs, regardless of the presenting problem or disability. Activities for specialized treatment are not included here but may be found in Part VI. In recent years the number of commercially available products for therapists to use in

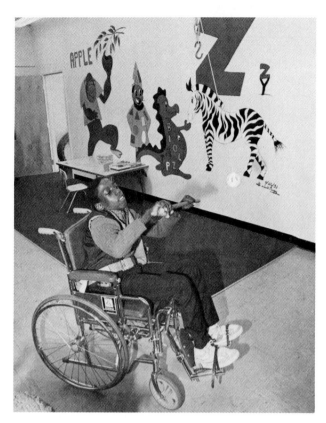

Figure 16-1   This eye-hand coordination activity is positioned to encourage trunk and arm extension.

Courtesy Atlanta Public Schools, Atlanta, Ga.

pediatric programs has increased dramatically. Some of the companies offering these products, as well as some useful commercial program packages, are listed in educational catalogs. However, the therapy program can be adequately equipped at little expense. Basic materials and equipment might include the following:

Balls of several sizes	Rope (a 50-foot clothes-
Beanbags	line is good)
Cardboard cartons of	Large wooden, plastic,
various sizes	or cardboard blocks
Carpet samples	Velcro dart board
Beads to string (large	Crayons and large
and small)	marking pens,
Pegboards and pegs	assorted
(large and small)	Children's scissors,
One-inch cubes in	assorted
colors	Paper, assorted
Formboards with various	
shapes	

With the above materials and thoughtful activity analysis, the variety of program ideas is limited only to the therapist's imagination. Tables 16-2 and 16-3 and Figure 16-3 show some sample activities and suggested adaptations that can be used for various purposes in occupational therapy programs.

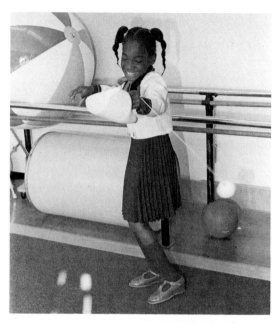

Figure 16-2   This girl demonstrates use of the bleach bottle scoop.

Courtesy Atlanta Public Schools, Atlanta, Ga.

SCHOOLWORK PROBLEMS

The occupational therapist is frequently asked to evaluate and remedy certain functional problems that interfere with a child's ability to perform schoolwork activities. The most common reasons for referral are (1) uncertain hand dominance, (2) poor visual perception, (3) problems with handwriting, and (4) inadequate ability to use scissors.

Hand dominance

Although a preference for one hand may be evident early in life, hand dominance is often not evident until a child reaches school-age, and it is not stabilized until age 7.[3] Hand preference and dominance, are indications of a well-established maturation and differentiation of the two cerebral hemispheres. In general, there is a hereditary predisposition toward hand preference. Of all children with two left-handed parents, 42% will be left-handed. Of children having one left-handed parent, 17% will be left-handed. When both parents are right-handed, only 2% of the children will be left-handed.[5]

The significance of cross dominance (right-handed and left-eyed, or vice versa) has probably been over-emphasized as a contributing factor to learning problems. It is estimated that as many as 50% of normal children exhibit cross dominance.[5]

However, in an academic setting, the child must learn to write. If the child does not show a clear hand preference, then it becomes necessary to make a decision regarding hand use so that the child can keep up with the rest of the class. The occupational therapist may be asked to provide data on which a decision can be based and also to provide program activities to aid the child in establishing hand dominance.

One of the first things that the therapist must consider is that lack of established dominance may be a symptom of a more pervasive dysfunction. Children who lack a cerebral dominance may also display inadequate postural mechanisms, hesitancy to cross the midline of the body, a tendency to use each hand on its own side of space, and other indications of an underlying neurodevelopmental problem. Ayres[3] recommended investigating the underlying causes, ameliorating them, and allowing the brain to establish its own dominance.

ASSESSMENT

As a practical matter, however, it is sometimes necessary to make a decision regarding handedness for classroom activities while therapy is progressing. The therapist who has been trained to administer the Sensory Integration and Praxis Test battery can obtain useful information through this instrument. The comparison of differences between right-hand and left-hand scores on the Motor Accuracy Tests and left-right differences on the somatosensory tests can be especially helpful when detecting dominance trends.[3]

Knickerbocker[22] offers several methods of assessing hand dominance in children. Timed hammering and coloring samples offer data regarding efficiency of hand use through observation of hand and shoulder control, facial stress, overflow, attempts to change hands, and finished sample products.

PROGRAM ACTIVITIES

Lack of hand dominance in school-aged children rarely occurs as an isolated phenomenon. Therapy for this problem must occur in conjunction with remediation of the underlying dysfunction. However, activities for exploring dominance, such as those suggested by Knickerbocker[22] (hammering, pounding clay, punching bags, and so on), are also helpful in establishing dominance.

Visual perception

Adequate development of visual perception is crucial, not only for academic learning, but also for coping with and adapting to the environment. Ayres[3] suggested that visual perception is one of four interactive sensory integrative and motor functions that are essential to survival:

1. Perception of gravity and motion through space
2. Extraocular muscle control
3. Locomotion and postural responses
4. Visual perception of space

This section will present a developmental sequence of visual perception and a description of types of visual perceptual dysfunctions to guide the therapist in planning intervention for children with these problems. It is beyond the scope of this chapter to present various theories of dysfunction, nor will the countless research studies related to visual perception be reviewed. Methods of assessing visual perception are found in Chapters 10 and 23, and intervention for visual perception problems associated with sensory integrative dysfunction is discussed in Chapter 23.

SEQUENCE OF VISUAL PERCEPTION DEVELOPMENT

At birth the infant has rudimentary visual fixation ability and brief reflexive tracking ability.[4] Even very young infants have some shape perception and are particularly aware of the human face. Infants as young as 1 week have a differential response to patterns. Complex designs, such as the bull's eye, stripes, and checkerboard squares, receive more attention from the infant than simple circles and triangles.[7]

The infant of 2 months or younger has the ability to organize visual information in a meaningful manner. There is some evidence to indicate that visual form perception results from an interaction of innate ability, maturation, and learning, with a critical period for the development of a given visual behavior.[7] At the critical period, or age, the child is physically and mentally ready to develop the perceptual function with little or no training.

In the developmental process of organizing space the child first acquires a concept of vertical dimensions, followed by horizontal dimensions. Oblique and diagonal dimensions are more complex, and perception of these spatial coordinates matures later. The 3- to 4-year-old child can distinguish vertical lines from horizontal ones but is unable to discriminate vertical, horizontal, and oblique lines until about age 6.[5] The ability to discriminate between asymmetrical numbers and letters, such as *b* and *d* and *p* and *q*, does not mature until around age 7.[5,18]

The ability to recognize shapes and forms matures much earlier than the visual motor ability to draw those shapes, or the cognitive-language function of labeling the same. Around 15 months the child begins to make random marks and scribbles on writing surfaces. Most 3-year-olds are able to draw a circle.

The Gesell Institute[18] found that children could draw certain geometric forms at the following ages:

Circle: 3 years
Square: 4 to 5½ years
Cross: 4 years
Triangle: 5 years
Divided rectangle: 6 to 7 years
Diamond: 7 years

Preschoolers and primary grade children continue the developmental process of organizing and defining concepts of form and space by drawing pictures to represent the world around them. Circles with sticks (oblique lines) radiating from them are "suns," squares are

Table 16-3 Gross motor activities

Activity	Adaptations	Purposes
PASS THE BEANBAG	Imitate manner that beanbag is passed (for example, under one leg, behind back). Sit on floor or on T-stools. Use only right or left hand. Play "hot potato." Person holding beanbag when music stops is loser.	Grasp and release Cross midline of body Motor planning Sitting balance Body scheme Right-left discrimination
ANIMAL WALKS (FIGURE 16-3)	Use for relay races or "Mother may I." Include in obstacle course. Walk along rope or line on floor. Do it blindfolded.	Motor planninng Bilateral integration Body scheme
CROSS THE RIVER Child must step on "stepping stones" to "cross the river" (walk across room) without "getting feet wet" (missing stepping stone and putting foot on floor) (Figure 16-4).	Use carpet squares, cardboard pieces, tape marks, and so on, for stepping stones. Jump or hop on squares. Color code for right and left. Vary placement of squares. Step on rope laid across floor. Walk across by stepping in shoe boxes.	Motor planning Cross midline of body Balance Bilateral integration Right-left discrimination
OBSTACLE COURSE Arrange course to go over, under, around, through, between, and so on (Figure 16-5).	Examples: under chair or table; step in boxes; roll on carpet or mat; step between rows of blocks; jump over boxes; crawl around desk; and so on.	Motor planning Body scheme Bilateral integration Tactile input Sequencing
HOPSCOTCH	Use jumps instead of hops. Reduce size or number of squares. Use beanbag as marker.	Motor planning Equilibrium Sequencing Bilateral integration
HIT THE TARGET Throw beanbag or ball in box or trash can, or use Velcro dartboard (Figure 16-6).	Throw from different positions: all fours, prone, and so on. Sit on T-stools. Throw with both hands simultaneously. Cross midline when throwing. Throw while swinging. Throw with right or left on command.	Motor planning Eye-hand coordination Crossing midline Sitting balance Right-left discrimination

houses with triangle roofs, and two vertical lines with circles are trees.

VISUAL PERCEPTION PROBLEMS

Perception may be defined as the ability to recognize, differentiate, and ascribe meaning to information received from the senses. Visual perception can be categorized into several areas: figure-ground perception, size and shape constancy, position in space perception, and spatial relationships.

Figure-ground perception is the ability to differentiate a stimulus from its background or the ability to attend to one stimulus without being distracted by irrelevant visual stimuli around it. Children with figure-ground problems may have difficulty attending to a word on a printed page because they cannot block out other words around it. Inattentive, distractible children may feel compelled to respond to visual stimuli around them (such as a colorful bulletin board or movement in the room) rather than attend to the task at hand.

Size and shape constancy are important aspects of perception that allow a person to develop stability and consistency in the visual world. *Size constancy* enables a person to make assumptions regarding the size of an object, even though visual stimuli may vary under different circumstances. A visual image of a car in the distance is much smaller than the image of the same car at close range, yet the person knows that the actual sizes

Figure 16-3 Animal walks

Frog jump	Squat on floor, placing hands on floor in front of you. Move both hands forward, then bring feet up to hands in jumping motion (remain in squatting position).
Bear walk	With hands and feet on floor, move right arm and leg forward simultaneously, then move left arm and leg. If this is too difficult, try it on hands and knees (homolateral creeping).
Inchworm	Squat on floor with hands in front. Keeping feet stable, walk hands forward as far as you can so that you are stretched out. Then keep hands stable and walk feet up to hands back to squatting position.
Elephant walk	Bend over with arms dangling toward floor. Clasp hands together to form trunk. Maintain position while walking, swinging trunk from side to side.
Kangaroo jump	Squat on floor, hands at sides. Raise up and jump forward, sinking back into squatting position as you land.
Crab walk	Lean back and put hands on floor (supine with buttocks off floor). Walk backwards, using hands and feet alternately.
Duck walk	Squat on floor with hands at sides. Remain in position while walking (waddling) forward.

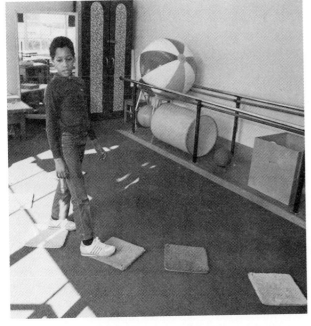

Figure 16-4 Stepping on rug squares can be a challenging motor planning activity.

Courtesy Atlanta Public Schools, Atlanta, Ga.

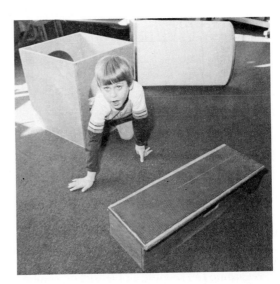

Figure 16-5 This obstacle course requires the child to go through the box and jump down from the step.

Courtesy Atlanta Public Schools, Atlanta, Ga.

of the cars are similar. In fact, as adults we learn to gauge speed and the distance between cars by the varying size of the distorted visual image of the cars. *Shape constancy* enables the person to recognize objects even when there are differences in orientation or detail. Children with perceptual constancy problems may have difficulty recognizing geometric shapes presented in different sizes or orientations in space. This interferes with the child's ability to organize and classify perceptual experi-

ences for meaningful cognitive operations (Piaget, Chapter 3). This may result in a problem recognizing letters or words in different styles of print or in making the transition from printed letters to cursive ones.

Position in space perception is the ability to perceive the relationship of an object to the self.[8] This perceptual ability is important in understanding directional language concepts such as *in, out, up, down, in front of, behind, left,* and *right.* Children with problems of position in space perception may have difficulty differentiating among objects that differ because of their direction in space. They will also have diffi-

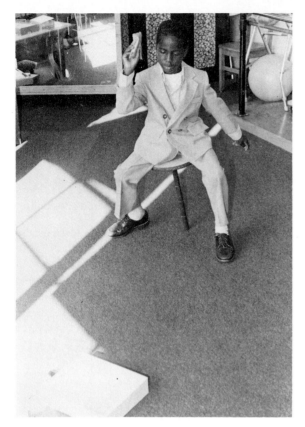

Figure 16-6 The addition of a T-stool adds an element of balance to a beanbag game.

Courtesy Atlanta Public Schools, Atlanta, Ga.

culty planning their actions in relation to the objects around them. These children may continue to show letter reversals past the age of 8, or they may be confused regarding the sequence of letters or numbers in a word or math problem. For example, they may read *was* instead of *saw.* Such children may also have difficulty with the left-to-right, top-to-bottom orientation needed for reading and writing.

The perception of positions of two or more objects in relation to each other and to oneself is called *spatial relationships.* Dysfunction in this area impairs the individual's ability to make judgments when moving through space, because the individual cannot tell if there is sufficient space to walk between two objects. The child might have difficulty catching a ball, because he cannot prepare his body in relation to the ball's movement through space. Adequate spatial relationships are necessary for writing and spacing words and letters on the paper.

OCCUPATIONAL THERAPY INTERVENTION

Visual perception problems are frequently encountered among the handicapped children with whom the occupational therapist works. Such children can benefit

most from the activities discussed in this section. However, it is recommended that the treatment for learning disabled children who have visual perceptual difficulties follow the sensory integrative model presented in Chapter 23. Ayres[3] wrote that "irregularity in development of form and space perception is seldom seen independently of other sensory integrative problems" (p. 191) in the learning disabled population. Other children such as those with cerebral palsy, spina bifida, mental retardation, and behavioral disorders should be able to improve their capacity in schoolwork performance through the use of a simple visual perception training program.

Many gross motor activities and games that are used to improve movement and body scheme will also aid in developing basic visual perception abilities. Examples are the following:

Simon Says: Imitating body postures to develop position in space perception and spatial relationships.

Hokeypokey: Concepts of right and left directionality.

Obstacle course: Position in space concepts of *in, on, through, around,* and so on.

Many activities for eye-hand coordination help develop visual perception (Table 16-2). Additional activities for visual perception are shown in Table 16-4.

Handwriting

Occupational therapists concerned with developing independent living skills and functional hand use are often involved in program planning for children with significant handwriting problems. A discussion of the developmental stages in writing and some approaches to remediation are presented here.

Cratty[5] described a series of stages of written expression through which children progress:

1. Holding a writing instrument; making marks on paper and other surfaces
2. Crude scribbling and random marks
3. Reaction to stimuli on paper; the child may "balance out" a figure on one side of the paper with lines or scribbles on the other side
4. Drawing of simple geometric figures such as crude spirals and crosses
5. Drawing of more exact geometric figures; combining two or more figures
6. Drawing of objects familiar to the child, such as people, houses, trees
7. Printing and cursive writing
8. Drawing of three-dimensional figures and pictures.

OCCUPATIONAL THERAPY INTERVENTION

Children who are referred to occupational therapy for handwriting problems generally are those who have experienced difficulty after having had regular classroom instruction or children whose physical handicaps make it difficult for them to benefit from the usual

Table 16-4 Activities for visual perception

Materials	Figure-ground discrimination	Shape constancy	Position in space	Spatial relationships
Beads to string— assorted sizes, shapes, and colors	Pick out all one color (or shape) from box of assorted beads	String beads of one shape that vary in size or color	String beads in specified sequence (red, blue, yellow or square, circle, oval)	Copy pattern card showing different shapes and sizes
Blocks (1-inch color cubes)	Arrange blocks of one color in a pattern with several colors surrounding it; identify pattern		Copy set of four, six, or nine blocks with colors in correct positions	Copy pattern cards showing three-dimensional block designs
Puzzles	Puzzles with figures having competing background	Formboard puzzles; outline of one shape or picture	Puzzles of graded difficulty requiring rotation to fit in hole	Interlocking puzzles
Pegboards of different sizes	Pick out one color or size from box of assorted pegs	Make different shapes for child to copy on pegboard (square, rectangle, etc.)	Copy pegboard patterns emphasizing left and right, top and bottom	Copy abstract pegboard patterns from pattern cards

instructional techniques. It is the educator's responsibility to teach handwriting skills. The occupational therapist's role is to determine underlying postural, motor, sensory integrative, or perceptual deficits that might interfere with the development of legible handwriting.

Evaluation of the child with handwriting difficulties should begin with observation of the child's attempts to write. Several areas should be assessed.

Postural control and stability are important prerequisites for writing. The child's position at the desk should be observed to determine if the trunk is stable and erect without the need for external support, such as leaning on the desk top. Does the child achieve the stability necessary to dissociate the movement of the arm from the trunk? Does the child maintain the head in an erect position at midline or is it tilted or supported by desk top or the child's arm? Are the feet firmly on the floor, swinging freely in the air, or under the seated child? How does the muscle tone affect postural stability?

Quality of movement is assessed while the child is forming letters on the paper. Is the movement fluid, or stiff and choppy? Does the child attempt to "draw"

each letter or is there evidence of automatic motion? Does the child experience motor planning problems such as confusion of direction of stroke, stops and starts, incorrect formation of the letter?

Sensory integrative problems frequently interfere with the development of handwriting skills. Poor bilateral coordination could result in lack of stabilization of the paper with the nondominant hand and reluctance to cross the midline of the body. Poor kinesthetic awareness causes some children to grip the pencil too tightly or to put so much pressure on the pencil that the point breaks. Price[31] reported that many of the children referred to her with handwriting problems had sensory integrative deficits including tactile defensive behaviors, poor postural control, and gross motor dyspraxia.

Physical handicaps may require specific adaptations to enable the child to learn handwriting skills. These include special pencil holders and devices to stabilize paper. It is also imperative to position the child appropriately to achieve necessary stabilization for writing (Figure 16-7).

Appropriate remediation of handwriting problems depends on underlying causes as identified in the occupational therapist's evaluation. Maddox[23] gives suggestions for postural preparation for writing that include influencing muscle tone, improving proximal joint stability, disassociating hand from forearm, and improving distal fingertip control. Several authors have developed specific programs for improving handwriting skills. The methods described by Olsen,[29] Knickerbocker,[22] and Frostig and Horne[9] are summarized here.

Olsen[29] described a method of teaching both printing and cursive writing that emphasizes letter formation. Olsen specified readiness skills needed before learning writing. She presented a logical method of teaching writing based on the kinds of strokes used in each letter. The use of specially prepared paper that has large spaces, directional orientation cues, and simple lines is recommended. This method has proved to be especially useful with older children who have already learned how to write but who are unable to write legibly because of poor eye-hand coordination and improper formation of letters.

Knickerbocker[22] described a program for developing writing skills that stressed the development of sensorimotor skills as prerequisites for learning to write. The progression from gross motor coordination and sensory functioning to fine movements of the dominant hand is described in the program plans which include a section on manuscript printing and cursive writing. This section spans "the development of pencil skills from the early scribbling stage and beginning finger prehension of preschoolers to the refinements of script writing" (p. 223).[22] In Knickerbocker's approach, large writing motions are initially used with scribble board activities, bimanual circles, templates, and large figure eight patterns. Such motion patterns help develop the basic motions for formation of letters in writing. Directional orientation of letters and numbers is emphasized with specific training in letter formation and sequential patterns of movement.

Frostig and Horne[9] described an approach for teaching writing in which premanuscript exercises and precursive writing activities are presented to help the child practice the basic components of letters and numbers. For example, "cat's tails" become the stroke for the printed *j* and *g*, while "giant's upper teeth" are the basic motions for the cursive *i* and *u*. The use of grids is recommended to aid the child in producing letters correctly without reversals. Frostig and Horne mentioned the need for adequate form perception and form constancy before developing the ability to form letters correctly.

Cutting with scissors

Children in kindergarten and primary grades are frequently involved in coloring, cutting, and pasting activities. These are necessary readiness skills that also promote visual-motor coordination and perception. The occupational therapist often includes cutting activities as part of programs to improve eye-hand coordination or fine motor function (Figure 16-8).

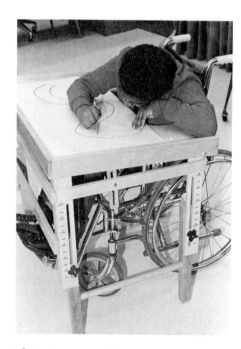

Figure 16-7 Proper positioning is essential for this prewriting activity.

Courtesy Atlanta Public Schools, Atlanta, Ga.

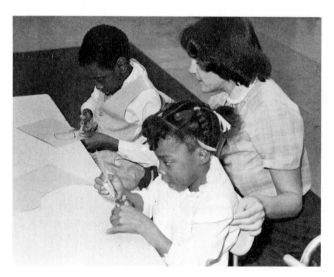

Figure 16-8 Cutting activities are often used as part of programs to improve eye-hand coordination or fine motor function.

Courtesy Atlanta Public Schools, Atlanta, Ga.

DEVELOPMENTAL SEQUENCE

When the motor and perceptual functions of a child have developed normally in the first 2 years, cutting skills will generally progress in the following manner[4]:

2 years: Holds scissors with fingers in correct holes.

2½ years: Holds paper with nondominant hand; makes snips or single cuts.

3 years: Makes continuous straight cut close to or on the line to cut paper in two.

4 years: Cuts along lines to cut out triangle.

5 years: Cuts curved lines; cuts out circle.

6 years: Cuts cardboard and cloth.

7 years: Cuts out complex designs and pictures.

OCCUPATIONAL THERAPY INTERVENTION

Careful assessment of the child's scissor-cutting skills is necessary before occupational therapy can be planned. Is the child correctly positioned and supported sufficiently for optimal hand use? Is the child developmentally ready for the activity? Does the child have sufficient supination to hold the scissors correctly? Is there sufficient isolation and differentiation of movement of the fingers to open and close the scissors?

The therapist can then make decisions regarding appropriate activities and adaptations for the child. Although some left-handed children can use regular right-handed scissors, left-handed scissors are preferable. Right-handed scissors cause pressure and pain in the metacarpophalangeal thumb joint area of left-handers, and under the best of conditions this can reduce motivation for cutting activities.

A number of types of special training scissors are available from educational supply companies. One type has a large, single loop to control the blades rather than smaller finger loops, and it is useful for children with immature fine motor control. Cutting is achieved by using gross grasp and a squeezing motion on the loop. Other training scissors have extra loops for the therapist to control the scissor movement. For some children it may be necessary to use some type of holding device to facilitate one-handed cutting.

Using scissors is not only important as a developmental and school readiness skill, but also as a life skill necessary for independent living. Graded cutting activities can be included as part of a prevocational program. For example, a retarded, blind teenager progressed from snipping rolls of therapy putty, to cutting small pieces off a strip of paper, to cutting yarn for a weaving project. The overall goal was to develop adequate prevocational skills for employment in a sheltered workshop setting.

PROGRAM EXAMPLE

An effective program to develop cutting skills that is interesting to children has been developed by Carol Leaman, Fulton County School System, Ga. Initial testing of cutting skills is done to identify:

1. *The width of line that the child can stay within while cutting.* This may be ½ inch, ¼ inch, ⅛ inch or ¹⁄₁₆ inch. Normal performance is demonstrated when a child can cut along a ¹⁄₁₆ inch line with few deviations.

2. *The form of line that the child is able to control hand movements to cut.* These are sequenced from straight lines, to angles, to corners, to large and small curves. The ability to cut along all of these forms constitutes normal performance.

3. *The number of deviations from the line (into the white space of paper) made by the child during testing on the width and form of line that represents the upper limits of cutting skills.* This precise measurement of cutting skills assists both with the formulation of objectives and the plan of treatment activities. Variations in training scissors and other adaptive techniques are made according to the cause of the child's cutting problems.

A series of geometric shapes that uses the described line forms are preprinted with different line widths. Each child is presented with a booklet of pictures that uses the same basic geometric shapes and coloring to produce animal cartoons. The child selects a cartoon to copy and then colors in the geometric shape with specified line width that is used for that cartoon. Shapes are then cut out and pasted to construction paper; coloring completes the cartoon details (Figure 16-9). This activity aids in the development of writing skills as well when necessary adaptations are made in the selection of drawing and coloring tools. Leftover paper from the geometric forms are taped together and deviations are checked in red pencil to maintain a record of skill development. Original cartoons can also be made with the shapes according to the skills of the child. Children like this activity, because they have a finished product to share with their parents that has been more enjoyable to perform than rote cutting exercises on strips of paper.

VOCATIONAL READINESS

PAT NUSE PRATT

Vocational development processes in early and middle childhood

It is generally agreed that the ability to work constitutes a primary indication of mature adult functioning in our society. Therefore a major goal of the growing child's socialization is to develop work attitudes, goals, and behavior. This is particularly true of the formalized socialization experiences that occur within educational institutions.

However, most vocationally oriented instruction begins at the junior high and high school levels. In most instances, satisfactory performance of related classwork is dependent on the prior development of adequate

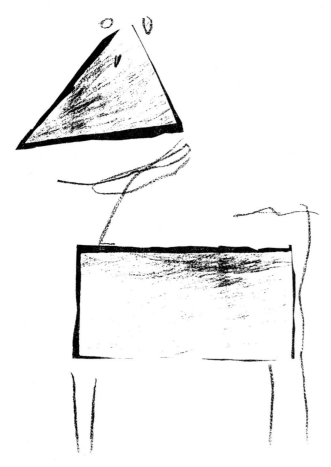

Figure 16-9 Sample of cartoon made by cutting and coloring.

manipulative, cognitive, and interpersonal skills. For adolescents with chronic developmental, physical, or emotional disorders, such instructional programs can be particularly stressful, because the assumed foundation of skills is generally not well developed. The youth with an acute condition may have less difficulty with developmentally antecedent skills but still be limited in participation in vocationally oriented classwork by the constraints of a presenting problem.

Clinical observations

Observation from occupational therapy practice suggests that the difficulty encountered by children with chronic disabilities is caused by a paucity of appropriate play and vocational readiness experiences during the preschool and elementary school years. People around a handicapped child tend to "do for" him or her, thus eliminating opportunities for decision making, problem solving, and development of perceptual, manipulative, and interpersonal skills to develop to full capacity. Parents frequently place a larger burden of household chores on other siblings because of the more extensive care needs of the handicapped child. Too often they tend to overlook the possible assignment of feasible household responsibilities to the handicapped child. In fact, both teachers and parents often relieve the handicapped child of many of his achieved self-care tasks in the interest of time. Although children with emotional or behavioral problems may be expected to assume more self-care and household responsibilities than the child with motor impairment, expectations are still limited by time, tolerance, and temperament. The short-term result of these childrearing methods is that the child never acquires enough practice to become proficient in those tasks for which he has the capacity.

The described problems are coupled with fewer opportunities for free play experiences with other children. The child with behavioral or emotional problems tends to be rejected by his peers because of his poor play skills. The child who has an acute illness or injury may have, through hospitalization or confinement at home, severely diminished play experiences. The child with motor impairment is dependent on others to transport him to playmates. Increased time spent on self-maintenance and transportation activities results in less time available for play. In addition, because the child cannot engage in many of the play activities of neighborhood peers, he may be excluded from other activities for which capability does exist. Often the simple fact that a child does not attend the local school or preschool is enough to preclude development of play relationships with other children in a neighborhood. The end result of these limiting factors is often a disabled adolescent who is poorly prepared to enter the competitive labor market.

The following section will identify some of the specific differences in the vocational development experiences of handicapped and nonhandicapped children in early and middle childhood. Examination of such differences will allow the therapist to design pediatric occupational therapy programs that can help to promote more adequate vocational development. A continuum of prevocational programming and recommended modalities are also proposed.

Development of work behaviors

Regrettably, there is only minimal information available that is specifically related to prevocational and vocational development of handicapped children during the preschool and elementary school years. Occupational therapy is the only discipline that has a history of identifying this early development as important, yet there is little clinical research to support our hypotheses. Pertinent information is available, however, about general vocational development and vocationally oriented programs for handicapped adolescents. There is also a large body of research related to attitudes toward handicapped children that has bearing on the problems described earlier.

VOCATIONAL DEVELOPMENT

There is general agreement among theorists of work behavior that vocational development is already in process during middle childhood. Ginzberg and others[11] identified middle childhood as a fantasy period for occupational choice, in which the child daydreams and role-plays with future possibilities. At about 10 years of age the child enters a tentative stage of occupational choice, and begins to consider vocational opportunities in terms of personal interests, skills, and values. By late adolescence the choice process becomes realistic. The older teenager is able to more accurately determine his capabilities and interests in terms of job options and settle on a specialized course of vocational skill development.

Super[37] proposed that the first stage of vocational exploration occurs in early adolescence, with the recognition of a number of possible vocational choices. Both Super[37] and Ginzberg and others[11] believed that more realistic matching of vocational interests and aptitudes occurs later in the teen years. However, Roe[34] proposed that the antecedents of occupational interests and aptitudes could be found in the activities and relationships of preschool children.

Super,[37] Ginzberg,[11] and Roe[34] all agree that vocational readiness begins in early childhood, and involves specific characteristics.[7] These include:

1. Identification with a worker. This usually occurs as part of the process of gender role identification with the same sex parent during preschool years.
2. Learning to get along with peers. This happens during preschool and elementary school years.
3. Development of basic habits of industry. This aspect begins in elementary school. The child is literally assaulted by the education system, with the need to work, produce, and contribute to the class, team, group, or system. This pressure is reinforced by parents.
4. Learning to adjust to authority. This facet of vocational development begins in infancy as the parents' influence systematizes and schedules the basic bodily functions of the child into routines of eating, playing, toileting, dressing, sleeping. This organization of behavior continues through school system experiences where "discipline" is a primary emphasis.
5. Learning about work and its varieties. Again, this aspect of vocational development begins in infancy—when a parent is "not there" he is usually "at work." When parents cannot respond immediately to the infant's or preschooler's demand for attention, it is usually because the parent is "working." Learning about the varieties of work is strongly influenced by the child's access to the community and proceeds in the preschool and early elementary preoperational years as the child is increasingly aware of people who are workers. For the preoperational child, workers

are identified most readily when their appearance gives a specific concrete indication of what they do, such as uniformed personnel. Although the child can identify the worker by appearance, work tasks are a product of the child's fantasy. During fourth through seventh grades, the child becomes more aware of job-related tasks and tries them out during play. For the adolescent, abstract operations as well as an increased schemata for work tasks and processes allow the youth to look more in-depth at varieties of work without concrete observation.

6. Development of the concept of the self as a worker. This is a continuous process, reinforced by years of hearing statements like "you did good work" and "what are you going to do when you grow up?" Structured extracurricular activities and household and neighborhood chores are critical to the development of the worker self-concept. Society rewards productivity. The growing child and adolescent learns that if he wants something it may not automatically be given—it has to be earned.

Through this course of vocational development, the child acquires and refines work habits and skills.[32] These include: 1) Work attitudes; 2) values related to punctuality, attendance, appearance; 3) attitudes toward authority figures; 4) differentiated views of peers as playmates, coworkers and resources; 5) production rates including speed, quantity, and knowing when to increase and decrease productivity; 6) manual and perceptual motor skills; 7) ability to attend to and concentrate on tasks; 8) basic independent living skills; 9) endurance or work tolerance. These nine areas are particularly important to occupational therapists as they constitute vocational readiness. Occupational therapists are often asked to provide information about a student's performance in these areas to teachers, guidance and vocational rehabilitation counselors.

One of the most comprehensive and recent texts on work behavior is by Neff,[27] who was interested in vocational rehabilitation of psychiatric clients. Neff believed that work is a learned behavior, and that immediately on entry into school, children are socialized into being productive. They develop a need to achieve that is reinforced by families.

Hershenson[16] proposed that work adjustment involves three domains that develop in the following sequence:

1. Work personality, including self-concept and personal motivation for work
2. Work competencies, including habits, physical, cognitive, and interpersonal emotional and social skills
3. Work goals that are specific and appropriate

There are some differences in Hershenson's model when applied to handicapped individuals, which will be discussed later in this chapter.

In a cross-sectional study of children's knowledge, attitudes, and experiences of work, Goldstein and Oldham[13] surveyed 905 children in first, third, fifth, and seventh grades. They found that children were very aware of work behaviors, even in first grade, although their knowledge became increasingly specific and realistic by seventh grade. Of particular interest was their finding that most of the children already had direct, personal work experiences. Even first graders typically had at least two household chores for which they were held responsible. Many had been paid for chores that assisted neighbors, such as feeding pets or helping with gardening.

CONTRIBUTIONS OF PLAY TO WORK

In the field of occupational therapy, play is viewed as the exploratory arena for the development of work skills, competencies, and roles[33] (Chapter 3). Shannon[36] stated that

Play provides for the development of the child's physical and intellectual capabilities and is therefore a major force in shaping self-concept. Play teaches discipline, responsibility, and citizenship. Cooperation, competition, loyalty, and respect for others are learned in the play milieu. Play encourages risk-taking, trial and error, and commitment, essential to the development of problem-solving or decision-making skills. Play also provides for identification with the worker role through the simulated experiences of role-playing and day dreaming (p. 290).

Play fosters the development of initiative and creativity, as well as the acquisiton of tool use, language, and other cultural skills. Because of the nature of play, the child has the opportunity to try out, practice, repeat, select, and consolidate skills, patterns, and routines. One of the most critical elements is the developmental progression of interaction with peers from onlooker to role-differentiated play and recreation. Through childhood play the rules of space, actions, and things are determined. Through the performance of the self-maintenance and schoolwork tasks of childhood, the work personality, vocational readiness, and survival skills are developed. These integrate in the child's understanding of himself and his environment.

During adolescence, role differentiation and role taking are critical tasks. These are developed through the youth's leisure experiences, games and recreation, and through work-related experiences of household chores, formal education, and occupational choice activities.

In essence, play and childhood chores promote the development of a foundation of readiness skills commonly regarded as being prevocational. This includes such elements as motor, sensory-integrative, and cognitive skills for task performance, problem solving, ability to follow directions and work with others, and decision-making.

PREVOCATIONAL PROGRAMS FOR HANDICAPPED ADOLESCENTS

Although there is an abundance of literature related to vocational rehabilitation of handicapped adults, only recently has attention turned to programs for youth. Hershenson[16] stated that a handicapping condition affects work competencies and that this in turn reflects back on components of the work personality. Because an individual does not have adequate competencies for the work environment, self-concept and motivation to work are affected. The self-concept does not include identification with the worker role, and motivation to work is hindered by expectation of failure. Although Hershenson's remarks were related to the adult with an acquired disability, his concepts seem applicable to children with chronic disabilities.

Similarly, Neff[27] defined work as a learned complex of behaviors and stated that

An early disability may have the effect of denying the person those experiences, interactions, and environmental pressures which gradually transform most of us from nonworking children to working adults. . . . They have either never learned to play the role of a worker or have been desocialized for so long a period that the work role has become alien (p. 264).

Most reports of work-oriented programs for handicapped youth are available to high school students only. In a comprehensive review of services for adolescents, Goldberg[12] declared the need for enriched prevocational experiences. He reported on a number of new programs in the metropolitan New York City area that included field trips to businesses and industries, part-time work experiences, and counseling. Perhaps the best developed of these programs was under the direction of Haraguchi[15] at the New York University Institute of Rehabilitation Medicine. Although the program was designed to serve adolescents only, similar types of experiences seem feasible for younger age groups. Haraguchi[15] noted that

The family has no immediate experience with living life as a disabled person. . . . They are often more likely to try to protect a more vulnerable disabled teen from additional physical harm and the stresses of life than to urge the teenager to creatively make maximum use of his or her assets (p. 76).

This statement supports speculations made earlier regarding parental limitations of the handicapped child's activity competencies. This should not be misconstrued as a negative attitude toward parents; the behaviors noted are typically demonstrated by concerned and caring parents.

ATTITUDES

No reports have been found that investigated early prevocational development among preschool and elementary school-aged handicapped children. However, another body of relevant literature is concerned with attitudes of others toward disabled children as play-mates and classmates. Westervelt and Turnbull[38] reported on a review of such attitudinal studies and concluded that as the physical or behavioral manifestations of a child's disability increase, so does the child's social isolation.

Popp and Fu[30] asked normal preschool children to indicate whether handicapped and nonhandicapped children could participate in a variety of play and self-care activities. The children were shown a series of line drawings accompanied by audiotaped verbal descriptions. The subjects were then asked to point to one of two pictures of children (nonhandicapped and wheelchair-confined or walking with a crutch) to indicate which child was capable of performing the activity. Popp and Fu found that, to a significant degree, even preschool children judged the handicapped child as being less capable. Even more pertinent was the fact that when the subjects had the opportunity to choose a representational child as playmate for the various activities, they most frequently chose the least disabled child.

It may be concluded that a child with a chronic or severe disability who manifests many observable signs of the disabling condition is likely to suffer from a deprivation of play and other socialization experiences that normally promote vocational development. Occupational therapy appears to be the only human service discipline that has historically demonstrated a concern with programming related to this phenomenon before the adolescent years of the handicapped youth. Particularly for children who experience chronic disabilities, it seems clear that vocational readiness programs should be instituted at the time that they normally would or should occur in childhood. The same readiness skills for schoolwork that were discussed earlier permit the maturation of vocational readiness. It may be hypothesized that prevocational programming for handicapped children that begins at the high school level is too late to achieve even minimally adequate results.

Activities to promote prevocational skill development in early and middle childhood

Shannon[36] developed an inventory of occupational choice skills that rates an individual's experience with various play and household chore activities that are believed to promote self-discovery, decision-making skills, and work role experimentation. Activities included playing with erector sets, painting, dramatic play, caring for pets, and many others. Although the ratings that Shannon presented are inadequately normed, it is believed that the chosen activities do constitute an appropriate variety of prevocational development experiences for the elementary school-aged child. These activities can form the basis of a prevocational program for children when combined with some

Figure 16-10   Composite list of play-leisure and household activities that promote vocational development

1. Construction sets: erector sets, Tinkertoys, Lego sets
2. Toy cars and trucks
3. Doll play
4. Household odds and ends
5. Toy tools
6. Handcrafts
7. Collections
8. Dress up
9. Cops and robbers
10. Doctor-nurse-patient
11. Space fantasy games
12. Other dramatic play
13. Races
14. Contests
15. Model building
16. Photography
17. Playing cards
18. Sketching
19. Drawing and coloring books
20. Painting
21. Scrabble
22. Dramatics
23. Musical instruments
24. Creative writing
25. Inventions
26. Experiments
27. Video games and computer play
28. Soccer
29. Basketball
30. Baseball and softball
31. Aerobic exercises and dancing
32. Care for pets
33. Care for younger siblings
34. Help with housework
35. Clean own room
36. Make own bed
37. Wash and dry dishes; help load dishwasher
38. Remove trash
39. Help with yardwork
40. Set dinner table
41. Prepare simple foods
42. Run errands for parents
43. Do chores for neighbors and teachers

Adapted from Goldstein B, and Oldham J: Children and work: a study of socialization, New Brunswick, NJ, 1979, Transaction Books; and Shannon P: Occupational choice: decision-making play. In Reilly M, editor: Play as exploratory learning: studies in curiosity behavior, Beverly Hills, Calif, 1974, Sage Publications, Inc.

of the activities identified by Goldstein and Oldham[13] as routine chores of children. Figure 16-10 provides a composite list of activities from these two sources, with the addition of computer play. Certainly, not every child will perform all of these activities because of variable interests and capabilities. However, activity adaptation by the occupational therapist should enable each child to participate in a number of these choices.

HOUSEHOLD ACTIVITIES THAT PROMOTE VOCATIONAL DEVELOPMENT

One of the critical elements will be persuading parents and teachers to use the adapted activities in the daily routine of a child. For example, a child in a wheelchair might easily carry daily attendance sheets from the teacher to the principal's office. A child at home can sort through fresh fruits as easily from bed as at the kitchen table, if parents are alerted to the relationship of such activities to future vocational skill development. Similarly, the parents of a developmentally disabled child may need periodic encouragement to continue their efforts to involve the child in self-care activities, with the reminder that skill development comes through prolonged repetition.

CRAFTS AND VOCATIONAL DEVELOPMENT

Handicrafts offer an excellent medium for occupational therapy programming to develop work skills of school age children. Crafts offer the therapist the opportunity to structure vocational readiness skill development within a playful experience for children. Crafts can be adapted to teach a variety of work routines including assembly line production. Crafts give a reward. Crafts are marketable—children can take and fill orders for their projects. Many of the activities that are typically classified as arts and crafts were once the cottage industries of American society and still provide employment to people in many countries including our own. Children like to do crafts. Their motivation to do and make things is particularly evident with crafts such as leather kits, simple jewelry making, popsicle stick projects, embroidery, ceramics, and the ubiquitous plastic-lacing activities. Figure 16-11 details the task analysis objectives for a prevocational program that was designed for a group of 8- to 10-year-old children in a class for severe learning disability. For the 2 years before initiation of this program, the children participated in individual and small group occupational therapy programs that emphasized sensory integrative and academic skill development. The occupational therapists felt that these children could not wait until high school to begin programs that would relate to career development, so they chose to shift the focus of therapy services.

The goal of the next yearlong program was to begin to develop prevocational skills, and the medium chosen was stringing alphabet bead bracelets. This activity

---

Figure 16-11   Prevocational program objectives for elementary school children with learning disabilities

Annual goal: The student will complete several prevocational skill development activities that will use elementary marketing, taking written orders, measuring, sequencing, money skills, counting, adding, construction, and fine motor dexterity. Activities will be completed with decreasing supervision and assistance and increasing accuracy.*

Media: Prevocational work task kits and projects, including alphabet bead bracelets and necklaces and rainbow link belts. Graded puzzles will also be used as enabling activities for practice of skills.

Objectives: The student will:
1. Correctly count and record the number of all parts in a designated set of 1 to 20 parts, with 90% accuracy
2. Correctly identify and record the type and number of missing parts in a designated set of 1 to 15 parts, with 80% accuracy
3. Follow a three- to five-part verbal instruction sequence through completion of a designated task, using written cuing, with 80% accuracy
4. Complete two product samples with 100% accuracy, and 90% independence of assistance from the therapist
5. Approach at least five customers, following a prescribed verbal sequence with 90% accuracy
6. Measure size of product for individual customer orders, using a string and measuring instrument, with 100% accuracy and minimal assistance from the therapist
7. Plan out and place parts of product in correct sequence to prepare for construction of order, with 100% accuracy and minimal assistance
8. Complete five orders, with 100% accuracy and minimal assistance
9. Count the number of components used in the product, and by using price of 1 cent per component, determine cost of product and write out a "bill for service," with 100% accuracy and minimal assistance
10. Return to customer for payment by following a prescribed verbal sequence, with 90% accuracy and minimal assistance from the therapist.

Courtesy Carol Leaman, OTR, Fulton County Schools, Atlanta, Ga.
*Percentages for accuracy and independence are varied according to the ability of each child in the group.

was selected because of its appropriateness to the sensory-integrative and academic status of the children, and because it lent itself to practice of a wide range of vocationally useful skills. A review of the objectives (Figure 16-11) indicates that to complete the alphabet bead bracelet project the children were involved with elementary marketing as they approached school staff to show samples and take written orders. Their measuring skills helped determine the proper length for the finished bracelet, and their money concepts and money-changing skills were developed as well. The development of sorting, counting, sequencing, and math skills was also intrinsic to the activity. Finally, the actual production of the bracelets strengthened prehension and manipulative abilities of the hand and challenged visual and tactile perception. As the program progressed, the success of its objectives was increasingly apparent through improved interest levels, self-confidence, and organization of work.

Another group of elementary school children was seen by the occupational therapist in a self-contained class for orthopedically handicapped students. The children ranged in age from 6 to 10. An excellent collaborative relationship with the special education teacher resulted in the development of a daily work skill period. The occupational therapist was responsible for selecting the activities, preparing program plans, making evaluations, and adapting the group activity for each child. In addition, the therapist supervised the group two times weekly. On the other days, the teacher and aide supervised the group and recorded children's progress mastery of each step. The therapist's written plans included name and description of the activity, date started and completed, purpose of the activity, including functional and vocational development goals. Special adaptations and process steps were clearly delineated. Through the year, the children manufactured and sold (or gave as gifts) mosaic tile trivets, place mats, hand woven wall hangings, and Christmas ornaments. The quality of the crafts was remarkably good.

COMPUTER SKILLS

Another important component of vocational skill development for today's children is computer use. In the majority of schools observed in clinical practice, most elementary school children have hands on experience with computers that begins at the kindergarten level. Regretfully, similar opportunities are often lacking for disabled children, particularly those with multiple handicaps. The long-term result of this is an even greater handicap for the individual as an adult who has no computer skills. Considering how much computers are a part of modern work life in all areas of industry, this is a critical handicap.

Accordingly, the occupational therapist with skills in facilitating computer access for the handicapped (Chapters 17 and 22) can play an important role. At a minimum, students can learn to input data through a computer keyboard. Simple activities such as putting one's name and the alphabet on display, using Logo and playing computer games serve as valuable experiences in the introduction to computers. Inexpensive interface cards are available to convert the computer for external switch control. Also, there are a variety of switches that can be adapted for computer use with play, language, cognitive, and motor skill applications.

Vocationally oriented occupational therapy with older children and adolescents

PREREQUISITES FOR VOCATIONAL TRAINING

In an unpublished paper Sarkes,[35] a vocational educator, prescribed a list of readiness skills expected of entering students before the initiation of specific job skill training. This list included awareness of and adherence to safety rules, work motivation, understanding of the importance and purpose of work, ability to follow rules, positive self-image, and specific perceptual and motor skills needed for job performance. Table 16-5 contrasts these criteria with areas of a standard occupational therapy assessment through which vocational readiness data can be obtained. Specialized prevocational evaluation instruments are discussed in Chapter 11, along with a number of tests that can be used to elicit relevant information. However, most useful information can be obtained within the format of an ordinary occupational therapy assessment, if the therapist looks at the data in terms of these criteria.

THE LITTLE PEOPLE'S LEARNING PREP SCHOOL

A unique and well-developed program for vocational readiness of children and adolescents has been established at the Little People's Learning Prep Schools. These programs have been reported in detail by Jacobs.[19,20] In addition to the student's academic program, "the majority of learning experiences provided have a direct relationship to career or prevocational development" (p. 230).[19] Students in the elementary and middle school ages participate in occupational therapy groups including commercial cookie production, school store and library operations, year book publication, small craft businesses, and cashiering. Funds for the programs are raised by the students in an annual arts and crafts fair and other school fund raising activities. As the students progress to the high school levels, their course work includes specific job training in cashier work, child care, clerical work, building maintenance, automotive and bicycle maintenance, and similar levels of employment. Additional workshops are offered in carpentry, food service, graphic arts, horticulture, and photography. Work study and apprentice training programs are also utilized. Occupational therapists are involved at the high school level and at the

Table 16-5 Comparison of prerequisites for vocational training with data collected through a standard occupational therapy evaluation

Factor	Occupational therapy evaluation items
Awareness of and adherence to safety rules	Judgment
	Ability to follow directions
	Problem-solving ability
	Knowledge of safety rules
Work motivation	Psychological functions
	Performance motivation
	Social and cognitive functions
Understanding the importance and purpose of work	Same as above, plus—
	General pattern of activity involvement
	Independence in self-care, home, and community living skills
	Ability to describe purpose of work
Ability to follow rules	Cognitive functions
	Same as first section above
Positive self-image	Psychological functions
Perceptional motor skills needed in vocational arena	Sensory-integrative functions
	Motor functions
	Activity analysis

Adapted from Sarkes, A: Unpublished paper presented to the Cobb County School System, Marietta, GA, 1979.

management and marketing levels. In addition, the school provides job placement services for its graduates.

Detailed study of the Little People's Learning Prep School Program is merited because it serves as a model of what can be done with long-term planning and allocation of resources. It is a noteworthy example of how a creative occupational therapist can apply knowledge of human occupation and the needs of a special population and marshall community support to meet these needs.

OCCUPATIONAL THERAPY PROGRAM OBJECTIVES

It should be reiterated that occupational therapy services should be directed to developing readiness for vocational exploration and training. There are a number of well-trained disciplines that can provide specific training for job performance. Occupational therapy is not one of these. Instead, the focus of the occupational therapist is on total task performance within the developmental requirements of the individual's daily routine. For the adolescent this includes preparation for the worker role. In the middle (junior high) and high school levels, most curricula provide opportunities to explore different vocational opportunities and develop specific work skills. Related services may include guidance counseling, industrial arts, vocational education, career days, cooperative work experiences, home economics, and office or library aide programs. School systems typically require several related courses and offer other options as electives.

In a discussion of occupational therapy and vocational education, Creighton[6] noted that the therapist is best qualified to provide the following services: task analysis of specific job training activities for student placement purposes, pretraining assessment of student skills, and modification of equipment and facilities. These services may be used in the computer labs, home economics and typing rooms, as well as in sheltered workshops and day training centers. An American Occupational Therapy Association position paper[1] on the role of occupational therapists in vocational rehabilitation stressed that services should be used to ensure the potential worker's smooth transition from the evaluation phase to the work environment. Again, this rests on the therapist's use of the processes of activity analysis and activity adaptation.

CONTINUUM OF OCCUPATIONAL THERAPY SERVICES

The suggestions from Sarkes[35] and Creighton[6] may be used to support the development of a continuum of occupational therapy services in prevocational and vocational skill development. At the beginning of the continuum, which is directed toward promoting independence in self-maintenance skills, the occupational therapist is heavily involved in the planning and training aspects of the program. However, as the adolescent participates more in specific work-related training and performance, the therapist's role becomes more consultative.

1. Increasing independence in self-maintenance skills. As part of gaining independence in the world of work, the adolescent is first expected to assume increasing responsibility for self-reliance in personal care, home management, school responsibilities, community living, and communicating for himself. Occupational therapists can provide practice experiences in related activities for the child or adolescent with a disability in cooperation with other service providers in an educational or rehabilitative setting. The therapist can ensure that the youth can make telephone calls, order food from a fast-food restaurant, establish a morning routine for personal care and household chores, and get from one place to another by using appropriate transportation resources.

Nochajski and Gordon,[28] reported on the use of an adapted form of Trivial Pursuit to teach community living skills to adults with developmental disabilities. A similar program could readily be used with adolescents. Questions related to six categories of survival skills were used for the game. The categories were: functional signs, domestics and measurements, health and safety, time and money, social skills, and public services and occupations.

2. Developing work skills through leisure activity groups. Assuming that not all adolescents will have had the benefit of a vocationally oriented rehabilitative program during elementary school years, the therapist may often need to intervene at the middle and high school levels. The focus of treatment is to develop those same skills identified by Sarkes[35] and discussed earlier. Again, the use of craft activities and graded individual and group chores can be adapted and used.

At a training center a group of young adults with severe cognitive impairment were referred to the occupational therapist. Their age range was 18 to 23 years, and all were independent in ambulation or wheelchair locomotion. Several had lived at home exclusively and participated through the years in training center programs directed toward developing partial independence in feeding, developmental, and perceptual-motor activities. Others had participated in similar programs at a state residential facility for the retarded before discharge in a deinstitutionalization phase. The training center had a well-established sheltered workshop program doing industrial subcontracts on a piecework basis. However, the referred group members were unable to adapt to this program because of their poorly developed work skills.

The therapist felt that a daily program was needed that would allow the clients to learn to produce tangible objects. A group program was chosen that had gradually increasing requirements for adherence to rules and independent task performance. The training center aides were instructed in the use of various structured, repetitive crafts, such as mosaic tile designs and leather link belts. Initial sessions were held for 30 minutes daily, including time for clean up of work space. As general abilities improved, the sessions were lengthened to one hour daily, and clients were expected to help prepare materials as well as clean up cooperatively. The program continued well over a year for a number of clients before they were able to transfer to the subcontract program. Rather than using a variety of activities, this program concentrated on developing increased skill in performance of a small number of tasks. This focus seemed more appropriate to the repetitive nature of piecework jobs that would be done in the sheltered workshop. The therapist monitored the program on a twice monthly basis and spent additional on-site time with staff training and client evaluation.

Goldstein and Collins[14] developed an interesting program for hospitalized adolescents with acute and chronic diseases, including leukemia and chronic renal failure. The initial program goals were related to improving social and emotional functions, but a variety of work skills were developed through the process. Five teenagers worked together to develop video tapes about hospital routines that were later shown to other children on admission. The "production crew" learned about film-making equipment, preproduction tasks, including the development of a story board, and differentiated roles and tasks in film production.

3. Improve function in specific work activities. As the adolescent reaches the point of specific vocational education-preparation, the therapist's role becomes generally consultative. The selection and the direction of training activities are likely to be done by a rehabilitation specialist, industrial arts teacher, or other personnel specialized in job skill training. The occupational therapist is called on when problems arise in the performance of training activities that appear generally appropriate to the client. The occupational therapist's use of activity analysis according to functional components of task performance may assist in the selection and grading of work assignments to improve quality and productivity.

Often the occupational therapist is asked to assist with adapting the job so that it can be at least partially performed by the client without assistance. This may involve adapting the position of the body, work surface, or task materials; grading the tools, materials, or equipment that are used to do a job; altering the training methods or work process to meet the capabilities of the client; or establishing graded sublevels of expected task performance (Chapter 7). Very often the therapist merely needs to help design a "jig," that is, a small piece of equipment that will assist the work trainee in doing a specified task.

For example, a young man placed in the sheltered workshop program discussed earlier was hemiplegic. The primary subcontract of the workshop was packaging parts for silk flower kits in small plastic bags. Trainees who had use of both hands would hold the bags open with one hand while sorting and stuffing with the other. Because the hemiplegic hand of this trainee was immobile, he had tried to work one-handed without much success. Because he was highly motivated to produce, and had attained a high production rate on previous subcontracts, the trainee became highly frustrated and began a pattern of absences. The case was referred to the occupational therapist who designed a simple Orthoplast jig to hold the plastic bags upright and open. Within one day the young man learned how to use the jig efficiently enough to match piecework rates of other trainees.

Occasionally a client in job training or preparation requires specific remedial programming to improve his function before he can satisfactorily meet the demands of one or more tasks. In such instances it may require backing away from the specific vocational preparation program to concentrate on improving component functions. The occupational therapy treatment program will be time-limited: activities should be age-appropriate and clearly related to subsequent performance of the desired work.

CASE STUDY 3

A 19-year-old college student had grown up in a small town where her family was well-known. She participated throughout her school years in church-related activities. She reported that she had always had difficulty with academic work, but, with family and teacher assistance, she graduated from high school. She chose a career in religious education and attended a small junior college for her first 2 years because her fiancé was going there. Because of various external social pressures, she decided to earn her associate degree in arts and sciences before transferring to another school for her junior and senior years in religious education. She was referred to the occupational therapist by another therapist at the end of her freshman year.

Confronted by the demands for technical reading and writing, as well as time-limited tests in the sciences and math, the student experienced overwhelming failure in her freshman courses. After reviewing the student's self-reported history and observing her postural patterns, the occupational therapist decided to thoroughly assess her work interests, sensory-integrative function, and study skills. The therapist referred the student to speech therapy evaluation of cognitive language development and auditory perceptual functions. Evaluation results indicated that the student had impaired postural and bilateral integration, including poorly developed dominance, visual figure-ground discrimination deficits, and very poor auditory and visual memory. Her chosen occupation as a religious teacher was well in line with her interests and capabilities, and it appeared that the required coursework for her junior and senior years would be manageable. However, results of the vocational interest tests indicated that her associate degree curriculum courses were far removed from areas that interested her.

The combined occupational and speech therapy programs included a modified Montgomery-Richter[24] home program to improve postural and bilateral integration. Every 2 weeks the therapist would demonstrate a set of exercises to the student and send materials home with her with check-off instruction charts to document the exercises that she practiced 15 minutes daily. The activities began at the apedal level in prone and supine positions and progressed to the standing position in which balance activities on one foot were to be done. To provide a higher level of difficulty, selected activities from the first 8-week sequence were then to be done on a large inflatable. The student reported that she often did the activities with her roommate, and both girls tended to think of it as a physical fitness program rather than an occupational therapy program.

In addition to the home exercise program, treatment activities also included giving the student drills to improve her auditory and visual memory and giving her assistance with developing her study skills. The student was advised to meet with professors of courses to review reading and writing requirements before selecting courses for registration. By underlining sentences as she read, the student eliminated some of the difficulties she had with figure-ground discrimination and visual memory. A number of other compensatory methods were suggested and adopted, and the student's grades gradually improved. She was discharged at the end of her sophomore year after 6 months of therapy with the option to return if she had difficulty meeting academic requirements of the religious education curriculum.

PLANNING AHEAD FOR VOCATIONAL DEVELOPMENT

Developing work-related skills is a long-term process, even for normally functioning children. Parents have to make conscious decisions about when to require independence of their children, when to assign them a new responsibility, and when to intervene in their interactive play situation. The occupational therapist who intervenes in this process with children who have handicaps must create and simulate developmental experiences. This requires working and planning ahead with other service providers, agencies, work-related resources, and parents.

Most often services will be provided in coordination with educational facilities and staff. In an average high school, space and curriculum schedules are determined 1 or more years in advance. Practically speaking, this means that, although an occupational therapist may decide that a group of physically handicapped high school students need to learn to make sandwiches, the home economics room and teacher may not be available for such a program until the following year, if that soon. Industrial arts classes cannot be readily moved from an inaccessible basement, even if they are nominally open to students with any disability. A whole year may be necessary to survey vocational resources in a school and community before the therapist can begin to develop a program framework to present to administrators. Transportation, teacher, and room resources and schedules; alternatives to on-site programs; and capital improvement costs need to be considered. Useful alternatives include area vocational-technical schools, state vocational rehabilitation programs, and state independent living programs. These agencies are already developed to assist with the handicapped teenager, but each has individual constraints in service delivery. The therapist and colleagues are faced with sorting through resources and needs, and they must use careful planning to design a program continuum that will foster the development of work readiness.

SUMMARY

This chapter has presented an overview of school and prevocational skills that are considered basic outcomes of occupational therapy programs for all children. The therapist has a responsibility to ensure that children will be prepared to undertake the requirements of appropriate academic and vocational training opportunities. To ensure children's preparedness for schoolwork, the occupational therapy program will emphasize the development of visual perception skills, cutting skills, and writing skills, as well as the establishment of hand dominance. Occupational therapists are aware that these skills also support the development of vocational abilities, and they design programs that provide graded experiences to promote work skills and knowledge of occupational choices. This is accomplished through activity selection in general occupational therapy programs for preschool and school-aged children, as well as in specific, vocationally oriented programs for adolescents. Occupational therapy services in vocational programs include increasing independence in self-maintenance activities, developing work skills through leisure activity programs, and improving function in specific work activities. Collaboration with teachers and vocational specialists is basic to service delivery.

STUDY QUESTIONS

1. Identify the six school readiness factors. Contrast these with factors that influence vocational readiness. What physical, environmental, and sociocultural aspects of development will promote school and vocational readiness? What types of situations/conditions will impede readiness?
2. As a therapist responsible for treating an 8-year-old child with spina bifida, what concerns would you have related to her ability to carry out academic tasks? What types of program activities might you select for direct treatment sessions? What adaptations would you recommend for the teacher to use?
3. You have been asked to make recommendations for a system wide special education program that seeks to improve its students' vocational readiness. The school system, based in a residential county near a large industrial city, serves special education students from 3 to 21 years of age. Make five recommendations for each level of education including: preschool, elementary, middle, and high schools.

REFERENCES

1. American Occupational Therapy Asociation, Inc: Official position paper: the role of occupational therapy in the vocational rehabilitation process, Am J Occup Ther 34:881, 1980.
2. Ames LB, and others: The Gesell Institute's child from one to six, New York, 1979, Harper & Row, Publishers, Inc.
3. Ayres AJ: Sensory integration and learning disorders, Los Angeles, 1975, Westrn Psychological Services.
4. Brigance A: Brigance Diagnostic Inventory of Early Development, North Billerica, Mass, 1978, Curriculum Associates, Inc.
5. Cratty BJ: Perceptual and motor development in infants and children, New York, 1970, Macmillan, Inc.
6. Creighton C: The school therapist and vocational education, Am J Occup Ther 33:373, 1979.
7. Creighton C: Career development theory. In Kirkland M, and Robertson SC: Planning and implementing vocational readiness in occupational therapy, Rockville, Md, 1985, The American Occupational Therapy Association.
8. Fantz RL: The origin of form perception, Sci Am 204:66, 1961.
9. Frostig M, and Horne D: Frostig Program for Development of Visual Perception, Chicago, 1963, Follett Publishing Co.
10. Gallerani MO, and Reinherz, H: Prekindergarten screening: how well does it predict readiness for first grade? Psychol Sch 19:175, 1982.
11. Ginzberg E, and others: Occupational choice: an approach to a general theory, New York, 1956, Columbia University Press.
12. Goldberg RT: Toward an understanding of the rehabilitation of the disabled adolescent, Rehabil Lit 42:66, 1981.
13. Goldstein B, and Oldham J: Children and work: a study of socialization, New Brunswick, NJ, 1979, Transaction Books.
14. Goldstein N, and Collins T: Making videotapes: an activity for hospitalized adolescents. Am J Occup Ther, 36(8):530, 1982.
15. Haraguchi RS: Developing programs meeting the special needs of disabled adolescents, Rehabil Lit 42:75, 1981
16. Hershenson DB: Work adjustments, disability, and the three R's of vocational rehabilitation: a conceptual model, Rehabil Couns Bull 26:91, 1981.
17. Ilg FL, and Ames LB: The Gesell Institute's child behavior, New York 1981, Harper & Row, Publishers.
18. Ilg FL, and Ames LB: School readiness, New York, 1965, Harper & Row, Publishers, Inc.
19. Jacobs K: Occupational therapy: work-related programs and assessments. Boston, 1985, Little, Brown & Co.
20. Jacobs K: The Little People's Learning Prep School. In Kirkland M, and Robertson SC: Planning and implementing vocational readiness in occupational therapy, Rockville, Md. 1985, The American Occupational Therapy Association.
21. Jensen AR: Understanding readiness: an occasional paper, Urbana, Ill, 1969, ERIC Clearinghouse on Early Childhood Education.
22. Knickerbocker B: A holistic approach to the treatment of learning disorders, Thorofare, NJ, 1980, Slack, Inc.
23. Maddox V: Postural preparation for writing, Dev Disabil Spec Interest Section Newsletter 9:3, Sept 1986.
24. Montgomery P, and Richter E: Sensorimotor integration for developmentally disabled children: a handbook, Los Angeles, 1978, Western Psychological Services.
25. Moore RS, and others: School can wait, Provo, Utah, 1979, Brigham Young University Press.
26. Morency A, and Wepman J: Early perceptual ability and later school achievement, Elemen Sch J 73:823, 1973.
27. Neff WS: Work and human behavior, ed 2, Chicago, 1977, Aldine Publishing Co.
28. Nochajski SB, and Gordon CY: The use of Trivial Pursuit in teaching community living skills to adults with developmental disabilities, Am J Occup Ther 41(1):10, 1987.
29. Olsen JZ: Handwriting without tears, Brookfield, Ill, 1980, Fred Sammons, Inc.
30. Popp RA, and Fu V: Preschool children's understanding of children with orthopedic disabilities and their expectations, J Psychol 107:77, 1981.
31. Price A: Applying sensory integration to handwriting problems, Dev Dis Spec Int Section Newsletter 9:4, Sept 1986.
32. Reed KL: Values orientation in occupational therapy and vocational readiness. In Kirkland M, and Robertson SC: Planning and

implementing vocational readiness in occupational therapy, Rockville, Md, 1985, The American Occupational Therapy Association.

33. Reilly M: Play as exploratory learning: studies in curiosity behavior, Beverly Hills, Calif, 1974, Sage Publications, Inc.

34. Roe A: The psychology of occupations, New York, 1951, John Wiley & Sons, Inc.

35. Sarkes A: Unpublished paper presented to the Cobb County School Systems, Marietta, Ga, 1979.

36. Shannon P: Occupational choice: decision-making play. In Reilly M, editor: Play as exploratory learning: studies in curiosity behavior, Beverly Hills, Calif, 1974, Sage Publications, Inc.

37. Super DE: The psychology of careers: an introduction to vocational development, New York, 1957, Harper & Row, Publishers.

38. Westervelt VD, and Turnbull AP: Children's attitudes towards physically handicapped peers and intervention approaches for attitude change, Phys Ther 60:896, 1980.

17

Adaptations for independent living

SUSAN A. PROCTER

Children develop increasing levels of independence and self-reliance as they grow. This natural process is an interplay between biological, social, and environmental parameters; the individual's physical, cognitive, and social abilities interact with the structure, events, and persons in the environment. The foundations of independent living skills begin in infancy and are refined, with nurturing, time, and opportunity, through various stages of development and mastery to functional independence. Attainment of independent living skills is generally believed to be critical to the development of a positive self-image.

Occupational therapists help children develop independent living skills through direct instruction, facilitation, and motivation of the individual. Through observation and evaluation of the child's performance, limitations that prevent independent function are identified and alternative ways of accomplishing tasks are developed.

ADAPTATION FOR RESTORATION OF FUNCTION

Adaptations allow the child to learn to perform a task or skill more independently. When total independence is not possible, parts of the task can be delegated to devices or other persons to achieve more autonomy in a given area of performance. This chapter discusses ways of enabling children to participate in a broad spectrum of daily living skills through preparation of the individual, adaptation of the activity process, and structuring of the environment.

Adaptation of position
THE BODY

Good body positioning enhances function. The ability to move into position for a particular task is the starting point of an activity. Children with disorders of posture and movement often lack sufficient control to assume or maintain stable postures during activity performance and benefit from positioning adaptations. Ward[28] notes that appropriate positioning maximizes symmetrical alignment of the skeleton, prepares children for movement, provides support that can free the hands for manipulation, allows participation in activities at a variety of developmental levels, and maximizes access to the environment.

External support can be provided through the use of standard or special furniture, seating systems for wheelchairs, and use of physical handling techniques. These mechanisms support the child's posture and improve functional potential. Positioning systems can maintain symmetry of body parts and facilitate bilateral movement patterns. Skeletal alignment with the appropriate orientation in space helps muscles work in a more balanced manner. Primitive or pathological postural reflexes and unequal pull of muscles on joints can be mediated. Maximizing the child's ability to balance and shift weight with less effort can facilitate a variety of functional movement patterns. More normalized sensory feedback can be elicited and will aid in learning new patterns of movement.

There are a variety of body positions for daily living tasks. Lying, sitting, and standing are the major positions used, with numerous options in each. It is important to provide various postural alternatives so that children can experience themselves in different spatial relationships and thus develop a perceptual set for spatial orientation.[28] When possible, use the most "normal" position for a given activity, employing adaptations as needed to stabilize the body for function. Alternative body positions may be necessary adaptations to compensate for physical limitations in strength, joint movement, control, or endurance.

THE WORK SURFACE

The work surface can be conceptualized as any surface in the immediate environment that supports the child, materials, tools, and assistive devices in an activity. For example, the floor supports the child and toys during play activities. Adding a positioning wedge to facilitate body positioning changes the orientation of the child to the floor and the toys. Boundaries of the work space can be set by a play pen. Various textures and colors can be added to the work surface/play area to increase stimulation.

There are many other ways to adapt the work surface to enhance or modify an activity and the child's performance. Characteristics that are amenable to adaptation include height, angle of incline, size, distance from the body, distance from other work areas, and general accessibility of a work surface. Changes in these characteristics can enhance the child's function in varied ways, such as improving arm support, increasing the visual orientation of a task, adapting seat height for transfers, or improving table height for wheelchair access.

Adaptation of the activity process

Task analysis helps identify the component processes and subskills of an activity. The therapist examines each component or subskill in relation to the child's level of development and performance capabilities to identify the need for adaptations. The goal is to develop adaptations that promote independent participation to the fullest extent for the child.

ACTIVITY LEVEL

The level or complexity of an activity needs to be considered from the standpoint of the developmental, physical, cognitive, and social skills required for successful completion. It is not uncommon for discrepancies to exist among these parameters. For example, a child may comprehend and be socially ready for a task but lack the physical dexterity to perform it. In this case, the cognitive level of the activity would be age-appropriate but adaptations would be needed to compensate for the motor requirements.

GRADING

Grading is the adaptation of a task or portions of a task to fit the child's capabilities. Component skills of the activity can be rated and varied according to their degree of ease or difficulty for the child. Those skills that the child is capable of performing should be practiced independently. He may be assisted with difficult portions of the task. There are many ways to grade an activity according to qualities—gross to fine, light to heavy, and simple to complex. Quantitative grading may include gradually decreasing the amount of time used to complete an activity, or gradually increasing the number of steps for which the child is held responsible while decreasing the amount of assistance given by another person.

EXPECTATIONS FOR INDEPENDENT PERFORMANCE

It is important that performance expectations be realistic. Goals should correspond to age and ability levels of the child, and be compatible with the child's environment, ethnic, and social background. Expectations of the teacher, parent, and therapist may vary because of each person's different frames of reference. Thus, collaboration with family and other professionals is important so that expectations can be discussed, brought into perspective, and established on a consistent basis.

Although independent performance is highly valued, complete self-reliance in a task may not be achievable or even desirable if the task requires too much time and energy, or if it exacerbates abnormal behaviors or movement patterns. Dependency in some tasks is appropriate at times and may permit completion of other, more readily achieved independent living skills.

CASE STUDY

Dan is a high school student with excellent grades. He is wheelchair-independent for classroom changes within the standard 5 minute time limits. However, Dan's physical therapist became concerned that his crutch-walking skills were not being maintained in the school environment. The occupational therapist recommended against changes due to possible effects on peer interaction and schoolwork. However, the parents and team decided to have Dan practice his crutch-walking between classes for one quarter session. During the trial quarter, it was noted that travel between classes took 15 to 20 minutes, requiring that Dan leave each class 5 minutes early and arrive 5 to 10 minues late. Dan required more assistance from his special education teacher to keep up with his schoolwork, and was angry about his loss of social interaction during classroom changes. At the end of the quarter, Dan's grades were barely passing and he was frequently absent from school.

This case example clearly demonstrates how exercise of an unrealistic level of independence in one task (mobility by crutch-walking) can decrease performance in other areas.

Adaptations to tools, materials, and equipment

Our living environment is filled with useful tools, materials, and equipment. We cook and eat with utensils, sit in chairs, read books, magazines, and the newspaper, and write with pen and paper. An important role of the occupational therapist is to make adaptations to the tools and hardware of our everyday environment to enable or enhance a child's function. Typical adaptations are discussed in detail in the continuing sections of this chapter.

Special adaptation techniques
ASSISTIVE DEVICES

A myriad of special devices is available through equipment vendors, catalogs, and specialty and department stores. These aids range from simple to complex, inexpensive to costly, and have varying quality. The therapist must maintain and update knowledge of available devices and be able to search out equipment for unique or specific problems. The occupational therapist may fabricate devices directly or collaborate with skilled craftsmen, orthotists, or rehabilitation engineers who make custom equipment. To be worthwhile, an assistive device should:

1. Enhance function without being cumbersome
2. Be acceptable to the child and family
3. Be practical for the environment(s) in which it is used
4. Be durable
5. Have a system of maintenance or replacement with continued use
6. Meet the cost constraints of the family or purchasing agency

It is imperative that selection of devices be guided by systematic evaluation of the child's abilities and analysis of limitations. Environmental assessment and collaboration with others who interact with the child and the equipment is also important. Trial use of a device is highly recommended to demonstrate its value to the child and primary caretakers.[10]

ENVIRONMENTAL STRUCTURE

Both the physical environment and conditions within it may be adapted to support optimal function in living skills. Architectural elements and equipment in the physical environment may need to be changed, modified, or rearranged to enhance independence. Ramps may be installed to facilitate wheelchair access. The family computer may be moved to a more accessible location so that the wheelchair-dependent child can use it for homework. Environmental conditions such as the amount of visual or auditory stimuli may need to be altered to improve attention to tasks. Since changes to the environment will affect other persons and activities that take place in the same space, the therapist must consider these interrelationships to arrive at workable solutions.

PHYSICAL TECHNIQUES

The child's ability to accomplish tasks using alternate physical techniques should be explored to reduce reliance on other persons or impractical assistive devices. This search involves creative teamwork between the therapist and the child. A prompt from the therapist, "Now, how can you do this? . . ." often taps the child's motivation to find a way. The therapist, observing and analyzing the child's attempts, will guide and adapt the most promising efforts toward success.

Alternative physical techniques or substitute movement patterns need to be practiced in therapy until they become functional. For example, the child with bilateral upper extremity amputation learns to use her feet to write or fold clothes as an adapted physical technique. New movement patterns may be needed to use an assistive device. For instance, the youngster is taught to hook an arm on the wheelchair push handle to increase stability while he leans over to get a mixing bowl from a low shelf. Or, the child mentioned previously would learn to use existing trunk and shoulder movements to operate a prosthetic arm before learning to write with the device.

STRATEGIES FOR FACILITATING INDEPENDENT LIVING SKILLS

Independent living skills are discussed in this chapter as areas of functional performance that depend on the integration of many subskills. Pertinent skills of infancy and early childhood include play and self-maintenance activities. In late childhood and adolescence, schoolwork, household skills, leisure pursuits, and community activities become important areas of independent living. The therapist must take a holistic perspective to see how the component subskills and conditions of the environment are integrated to yield a functional level of achievement for the child. For each area of performance the therapist considers the child's current abilities and identifies skills that will improve with practice. She analyzes how the environment can be arranged to allow the child to perform at an optimal level. Tasks must also be structured so that the child can accomplish them in a reasonable amount of time with reasonable effort. Finally, skills must be integrated effectively into the family, classroom, or other life situations, and adapted to meet the needs and skills of the caregiver and the child.

Intervention within a developmental continuum

The theorists discussed in Chapters 3 and 4 found that skills tend to develop in chronological order and that early skills form the basis for future skills. These findings support the need for early occupational therapy intervention to initiate skill development and a continuum of intervention to promote acquisition of further developmentally appropriate skills.

Therapy objectives for very young children will differ from those established for older children because of the changes in the child's abilities and interest levels. For example, intervention with the play of the infant or preschooler may be directed toward developing adaptations that enhance exploratory and sensorimotor experiences. In contrast, play intervention with the school-aged child might include adaptations for participation in team sports and rule games such as Monopoly. In the performance area of school skills, the occupational therapist might focus on pencil and paper adaptations for the first grade child who is learning to form letters. For the high school student who must produce essays in class, intervention with written communication might instead be directed toward adapted computer use.

Intervention strategies
MATCHING TO FUNCTIONAL CAPACITIES AND SKILL LEVELS

The child's physical abilities and cognitive function influence the potential for independence and type of intervention possible. Interest level and motivation are strong forces that can allow children to attain levels of performance that are either above or below expectations. Highly motivated children generally improve their functional level with adaptations to activities, equipment, and the environment. A follow-up study of patients with cerebral palsy by Cohen and Kohn[9] demonstrated that, in general, intelligence was positively correlated with independent function. However, those subjects who had severe physical disabilities remained more dependent regardless of intelligence.

MATCHING TO CAREGIVER'S SKILLS

Children grow up with the assistance, support, and guidance of caregivers. Parents are typically the primary caregivers who are with the child most consistently. Teachers, aides, attendants, baby-sitters, and day care staff have a shorter term of involvement and usually change throughout the child's life.

The abilities and available time these significant others have to assist and encourage the child to function with adapted activities, materials, and equipment must be considered. Their levels of understanding have a bearing on how instructions should be presented. Some caregivers will require only verbal instruction, while others will require visual aids, written instruction, and training to effectively assist the child. Levels of motivation should also be assessed. If motivation is low, additional encouragement over longer periods of time is needed, or the therapist may need to alter goals and objectives to incorporate those that are of value to the caregiver. The physical abilities of caregivers also influence the kind of assistance they provide. The number of caregivers available in a particular environment, such as the student-teacher ratio or the number of attendants who can assist the child in a group foster home, should be considered. Adaptations are best kept simple in situations where time is at a premium and a variety of persons is involved.

MATCHING TO THE CHILD'S ENVIRONMENT

Evaluation of the child's home, school, and community environments is important because these are the settings where tasks are performed. Any form of intervention, whether assistive device or adapted technique, influences and is influenced by the environment in which it is used. The environmental "fit" of a recommended device or technique should be considered in terms of space, structural requirements, and interaction with other objects and persons. As mentioned previously, modifications or structural adaptations may be needed and related costs of time, expense, and energy need to be weighed to determine feasibility. The most effective means for evaluating an environment is an on-site visit. If this is not possible, the therapist should get a good description from the child and her significant others. It is helpful to obtain pictures and informally drawn floor plans and pertinent measurements.

ADAPTATIONS FOR PLAY EXPERIENCES

For many children, the ability to enjoy and progress through the various stages of play development depends greatly on the adaptations that can be made. The occupational therapist can help the child, family, and school teachers establish ways of participating in independent and cooperative play through adaptations of positioning, materials, and the environment (Figure 17-1).

Enhancing independent manipulation and exploration
POSITIONING FOR PLAY

Children play in an interesting and endless variety of positions. Much of early childhood play takes place on the floor. Wedges for supine and prone lying, sidelying positioners, corner chairs, and other floor sitting devices can help the child with poor postural reactions and control. Finnie[13] illustrated and described how parents or therapists can use their bodies (chest, thighs, abdomen, and lap) to position the cerebral palsied child for play.

Children can also be placed with their backs against the wall or base of the sofa, or sit into the corner of a room or contoured area formed by sofa back cushions. Stable seating can be achieved through properly fitted children's chairs, wheelchairs, bolster seats, or chair and table sets that provide full thigh support, back support, and foot support. Additional positioning components may be needed to further enhance posture and control. Play in standing position can be facilitated by use of standing tables, prone standers, and orthotic standers.

Children who require postural support for play typically have difficulty moving into and out of positions for play. If the activity involves movement, consider mobility systems with positioning components (see Chapter 14, section on mobility).

Toys and their adaptations
STANDARD TOYS

The therapist can help the child and family select standard toys that are appropriate to the child's cognitive level and other performance capacities. The toy should promote the exploratory process so that the

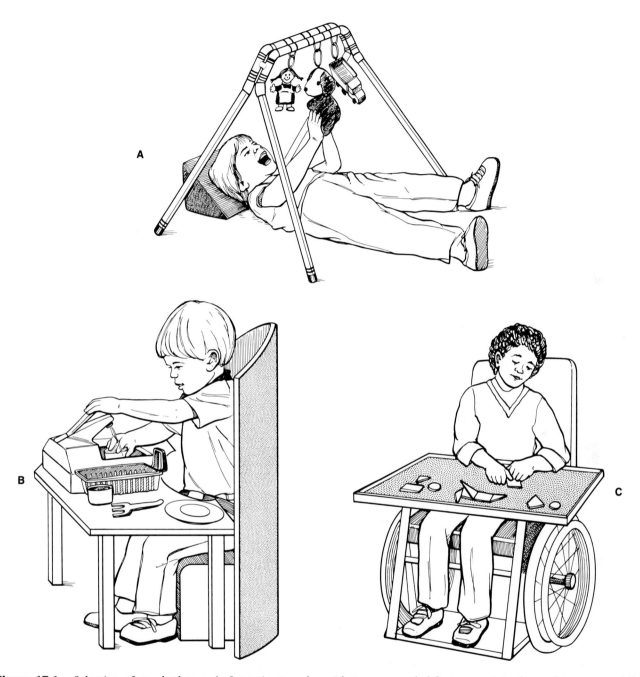

Figure 17-1 Selection of standard toys. **A,** Sensorimotor play with toys suspended from an activity frame, for a young child with limited upper extremity control and poor sitting posture. **B,** Imaginative play with a sink set, featuring sturdy construction, stable base, and large sized play pieces that are easy to grasp. **C,** Constructive play at a magnetic play set that permits the child to manipulate pieces by sliding them on the magnetic surface.

sensorimotor, symbolic, and constructive aspects of play are addressed (see Chapter 15, Figures 15-1 through 15-3). Toy concepts should be simple enough for the child to understand, yet complex enough to provide a challenge and opportunity for achievement. Toy selection guides help the therapist and parent. Sinker[25] of the national Lekotek Play Library program has compiled a particularly useful resource guide of toys that have been field-tested with children who have special needs.

TOY AND PLAY ADAPTATIONS

The occupational therapist is a key professional to make adaptations to toys and locate appropriate adapted toys through special catalogs for the child. The most common needs are stabilization of play materials and facilitation of grasp, manipulation, and access to toys.

Motorically involved children, particularly those with athetoid movements, often displace toys when attempting to manipulate them. Or, when conditions of hemiplegia or quadriplegia are present, one side of the body may be impaired to the point that the child cannot effectively stabilize toys for play. Examples of some effective techniques and equipment for holding objects are described in Figure 17-2.

When grasp or dexterity limitations interfere with play, several adaptations are possible. The addition of handles to toys can permit sustained grasp and orientation of the toy (Figure 17-3, *A*). Extensions made from splinting materials or tongue depressors can help a child operate levers and switches on toys (Figure 17-3, *B*). Straps may be added to attach the toy directly to the hand (Figure 17-3, *C*). Pressure-sensitive hook and loop tapes may help children hold objects in hand mitts (Figure 17-3, *D*). Toys with handles, such as xylophone strikers or hammers, can be built up with small foam balls, cylindrical foam padding from therapy supply catalogs, or with cylindrical foam hair curlers, to facilitate grasp.

Isolation of the index finger is needed for pressing the keys of toy telephones, pianos, and the wide variety of electronic toys with keyboards. A mitt or glove that maintains all fingers in flexion while allowing extension of the index finger is useful when a child's fingers typically fan out in extension or show extraneous movement. Splint material can also be used to support index finger position. Hand-held pointers, including wooden dowels with built up handles, pencils inserted into universal cuffs, or custom fabricated hand splints with pointer extensions, can also be used.

Carlson[8] developed a playboard that incorporates some of the adaptations. It was designed for children whose motor problems affect their ability to play. Toys that associate with each other in play schemes are attached to a lap tray. Examples include toy furniture from various rooms in a house or farm sets. Some pieces are bolted down permanently and other pieces are fixed in routed tracks so that they can be moved

Figure 17-2	Stabilization materials, procedures, and applications
Tape	Generally a temporary solution. Can be applied quickly as need arises, is inexpensive, and readily available in households, schools, and therapy units. Duct tape is very sturdy, with good holding power. Masking and cellophane tapes are less sturdy, but widely used.
Non-slip pressure-sensitive matting	This can be ordered through therapy supply catalogs in rolls or pads and is becoming available to the public in kitchen stores. Minimizes slipping and sliding of objects with large bases that are placed on it. Small pieces can be glued to small objects to aid stabilization. These products rely on friction between materials for stabilization.
Suction cup holders	These holding aids are widely available in both stores and through therapy supply catalogs. Single-faced suction cups are generally permanently applied to a toy or object. Double-faced suction cups can be set up where suction is needed between the object and work surface.
C-clamps	These are readily available and suitable for securing flat objects to lap trays, table edges, and other surfaces.
Tacking putty	This product is sold for sticking posters onto a wall and is quite useful for holding lightweight objects on tables, lap trays, angle boards, walls, etc.
Pressure-sensitive hook and loop tapes	These tapes can be glued to the base of toys and other objects, and to play or work surfaces for stabilization. Soft loop tape can be used on areas that will contact the child's skin or clothing.
Wing nuts and bolts	In some cases it is possible to bolt toys and other objects to a table surface through holes drilled through the object and holding surface. This stabilizes objects more permanently.
Magnets	Magnets that are affixed to a toy can aid stabilization in metallic surfaces such as refrigerator doors, metal tables, and magnetic play boards.
L-brackets	These hardware store items are particularly effective for stabilizing items in an upright plane. Holes are drilled in both the work or play surface and the toy or other object to correspond with the L-bracket holes. Objects are then secured with nuts and bolts.
Soldering clamps	Small clamps are mounted to free-standing bases that are weighted, suction-cupped, or use clamps for stability. These are best used to hold small items for intricate play, hobbies, or work.
Elastic or webbing straps	Straps can be attached to toys to tie them down, or to play or work surfaces to secure flat objects.

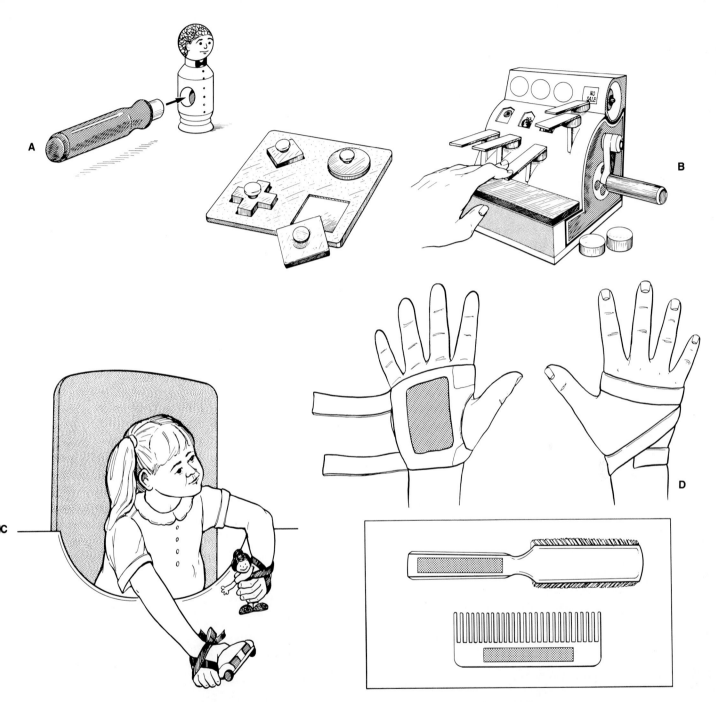

Figure 17-3   Adaptations for play. **A,** Handles and knobs can facilitate grasp. **B,** Lever extensions permit operation of the toy with less force and control. **C,** If grasp is nonfunctional, small toys may be strapped to the hand. **D,** If grasp is nonfunctional, a Velcro mitt may be used.

around without falling off the board. Other movable pieces are strapped to the child's hand. Such a setup can stimulate imaginative and symbolic play.

Older children develop interests in cooperative and competitive rule games such as cards or checkers. "The combination of pleasure, social skills and learning that these games can promote emphasizes the need for adapting them for children with disabilities who have the mental abilities to participate successfully"[20] (p. 39). Card holders and automatic shufflers can be used. Playing cards with extra large markings help the child with impared vision or visual perceptual deficits. If manipulation of the game materials is impossible, the player can signal to a partner to manipulate her game pieces after she has decided on her move.

The technology of electronics has dramatically increased play opportunities for the child who has extremely limited motor control. Battery operated toys, microprocessors, and computers can be adapted for use with special switches and controllers. Many adaptations to meet the needs of this population have become commercially available. Battery operated toys can be modified to use a remote switch through the addition of a battery adapter or interrupter (Figure 17-4). Burkhardt,[6,7] Wright and Nomura,[29] and Vanderheiden[27] present excellent information on how to make or order battery adapters, switches, and toys.

The computer is becoming more accessible to children with physical and developmental limitations through use of special software, hardware, and interfaces. At this writing, most play and early learning programs are written for the Apple computer. The advantages of computer use include its ability to provide highly motivating visual and auditory feedback and consistent reinforcement of cause and effect.

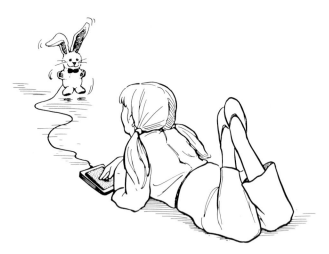

Figure 17-4   Battery operated toys can be fitted with large on/off switches for use by children with limited motor control.

Adaptations for the computer are needed for those who cannot access a standard keyboard. A switch adapter interface allows a single switch to be used with special "single switch" software such as the Motor Training Games by Schwejda. The Adaptive Firmware card by Adaptive Peripherals, Inc. allows standard software to be accessed by a single switch using a scanning method of selection or by an expanded membrane keyboard. Special package programs, such as Exploratory Play and Representational Play by Peal and the UCLA/LAUSD Microcomputer Team Software, which are being field-tested, are designed to stimulate language and concept acquisition through computer play experiences. Computer games against oneself or another player are manipulated through the keyboard, joystick, or game paddle. The computer can be used for art, using the Logo program to command a turtle to draw lines on the screen. Graphic pads and mouse interfaces are used with various software to create and color computer pictures.[3,4]

Adaptations to play areas and surfaces

Accessibility of toys and play experiences often must be structured for the child who has difficulty moving toward toys and playmates. Toys must be moved to the immobile child. Presentation for a range of toys in varying locations near the child is beneficial for stimulation of limited movement capabilities. Toys can be placed so that the child can select one and reach it by rolling, crawling, or using a wheelchair, and simultaneously facilitate initiation and self-direction.

Keeping toys within reach can effectively prolong independent play and reduce the frustration of toys that "get away." One mother discovered that placing a hula hoop around her small son's body and his toys as he played on the floor was a workable solution. Lap trays and tables with rims can also be used, particularly with toys that cannot be stabilized. Angle play surfaces can allow gravity to return a toy to a child after it is knocked away.

Participation in group skill activities

Children 3 to 5 years old begin to participate in and benefit from group and peer interaction. Access to group play is complicated for the disabled child, who may have difficulty getting to other children or their play areas. Even when such children are physically close to their normal agemates, slower movements and responses handicap the speed of their play interactions. Often the disabled child is left behind as able bodied peers run off to the next play situation.

Independent mobility is of prime importance for making group play accessible and for maintaining contact as the activity moves about in the environment. Structuring the group play situation is also helpful.

Group play periods can be scheduled in group therapy and school programs to enhance integration. A peer "helper" can be appointed from the group to assist with disabled child as needed. Refer also to the section on mobility in Chapter 14.

ADAPTATION OF THE HOME ENVIRONMENT TO FOSTER INDEPENDENCE

Home is where an individual has the most control over the arrangement of her environment and living routines. It is a place to relax, play, and work, and serves as a base for excursions into the outside world. Because most living skills are practiced in the home, it is a very important environment for occupational therapy intervention. Architectural adaptations, assistive devices that promote independent function, and arrangement and organization of the living areas will be considered. In some households, it may be possible to make major changes to meet specific needs, but most families must make adaptations on a limited budget. In the case of a rented house or apartment, changes must comply with restrictions set by a landlord.

Environmental adaptations
INDEPENDENT ENTRANCE AND EXIT

The entrance to a home is often an architectural barrier for children who cannot go up or down stairs, turn door knobs, use keys to unlock doors, or open heavy doors. These problems become barriers to independence as children reach school age and in other respects have the judgment and mobility to move around the house and neighborhood. Wheelchair users are particularly handicapped by the architectural structures encountered at most home entrances.

STAIRS

Ambulatory children with difficulty managing stairs can be assisted by a hand railing to provide balance and leverage. Half steps may be built in to reduce the distance the leg must be moved while ascending or descending stairs.

Ramps are most commonly used for adapting short sets of steps for wheelchair users. Standards cited by Hale[14] and Russell[21] are commonly accepted. The recommended standard for ramp gradient is 12 feet of length per 1 foot of rise to allow the wheelchair to be propelled or pushed safely. Low curbs at the base edges of the ramp and handrails are also important for safety. The width standard is 3 feet, with a landing at the top that is large enough to securely park a wheelchair while opening the door. For inward opening doors a 3 foot square landing is sufficient; a 5 foot length is recommended for entrances with outward opening doors. Surfaces should be slip-resistant when wet.

The design of a ramp will depend on its necessary length and available space. A zigzag style may be necessary for long ramps with limited yard space. A side or rear entrance can be ramped if front entrances are not amenable. Ramps are often made by family members or friends experienced in construction, or may be installed by a contractor. Portable ramps made of metal channels, aluminum mesh, or heavy duty plastic are available from equipment vendors, and may be the best solution for the rented dwelling or the family that moves frequently.

Large flights of steps cannot be ramped, so alternatives are needed. Some large cities have houses that resemble flats with 15 to 20 stairs leading up to a house that is built on top of the garage. Small in-home elevators or stair lift platforms that move up and down a staircase on tracks may be installed. Both are expensive options, but may be desirable for the family whose child becomes bigger and heavier with age and cannot be easily carried.

DOORS

To permit free wheelchair, walker, or crutch-walking clearance, the recommended minimum door frame opening is 31 inches; however, 33 inches is preferable.[21] Clearance through a door should be measured between the two nearest points, usually the inner side of the door jamb and the medial edge of the door when opened. If door width needs to be increased, the family can install step-back hinges that allow a door to swing free from the frame to lie flat against the wall. Sufficient wall space must be available for this modification. Structural changes, such as widening the doorway opening, should be considered for critical rooms such as the bathroom. When managing doors is difficult from a wheelchair, it may be feasible to rehang the door so that it opens in the opposite direction. Interior doors can be removed and replaced with a curtain, pocket door, or folding door. Electric door openers are available, but are expensive to install.

Doorknob adaptations may be needed for those children with weak or poor grasp. Lever door handles are the best alternative when feasible because they can be operated with either gross arm or foot movements. Standard round doorknobs may be converted with lever extensions that snap or bolt onto the existing hardware (Figure 17-5, *A*). Portable doorknob turners, available from adaptive equipment vendors, can increase the independence of the older, more responsible child (Figure 17-5, *B*).

Key use can be impossible in the presence of impaired hand function. The addition of a thermoplastic or metal extension to the grasp and turn surface of the key can increase leverage (Figure 17-5, *C*). Electric door openers and locks that operate through activation of a single switch or remote control, such as garage door openers, are also useful.

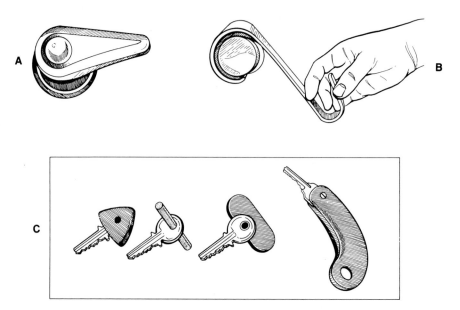

Figure 17-5   Devices for opening doors. **A,** A rubber knob extension that snaps on to the doorknobs. **B,** A portable door knob turner. **C,** Key adaptations that increase leverage for turning.

The bathroom

The bathroom is usually the most inaccessible room in the house, yet it is one of the most essential. The floor space inside is rarely sufficient to permit turning a wheelchair for tub or toilet transfers. Adaptation possibilities include remodeling, selecting assistive devices, or devising alternative strategies to enhance independence. Adaptation to provide privacy is particularly important for the older child and adolescent. Caretaker needs must also be addressed, as the child becomes heavier and more difficult to assist.

ASSISTIVE DEVICES

Most assistive devices for the toilet aid transfers and seating. Small children often need reducer rings to decrease the size of the toilet seat opening and thus improve sitting support. A step in front of the toilet helps small children get onto it. Safety rails that attach to the toilet or wall may assist balance so that the child can safely be left in privacy. Free-standing commodes may be used by the child who has outgrown small training potties. Units that roll into place over the toilet may be useful when wheelchair access to the bathroom is impossible.

Bathtub transfers can be assisted by the use of tub chair or bench. One bathing device can be filled with warm water from the faucet, becoming a rigid seat to aid transfers. The bather then opens a valve with a pull-string, and as the water drains into the tub the bather descends into the water. To exit, the unit is refilled with tub water and raises the bather to the level of the tub edge. Although this unit is expensive, it is efficient

and eliminates a number of safety hazards. For the heavier child or caretaker with back problems, a hydraulic patient lifter may be necessary.

ROOM MODIFICATIONS

The child in a wheelchair can attain more independence through structural modifications of the bathroom and fixtures. Floor space enlarged to permit wheelchair mobility is desirable. The sink can be mounted lower, with a cabinet or open space underneath it for wheelchair access. Pipes and drains should be insulated to protect the child's legs, particularly if sensory impairment is present. Single lever faucets that require only light pressure to control temperature and flow of water are easier to operate for children with hand impairment.

Toilet height and space to set the wheelchair should be specific to the child, but must include consideration of future growth and use by others. Bathtubs should be equipped with sturdy grab bars. Stall showers may be designed or converted to permit access to a mobile shower chair. The curb of a shower stall can be removed and replaced with an incline slope to contain the water. It is also possible in some bathrooms to ramp the shower stall curb and build up the floor of the shower to curb height. Glass shower enclosures should be replaced with shower curtains.

ALTERNATIVE STRATEGIES

In some situations, bathroom accessibility is impossible, or modifications are either not affordable or not permitted. Bedside commodes may be used for toileting in the child's bedroom. These may be a preferred option for any child with paraplegia or meningomyelocele who needs longer time for bowel movements. This option leaves bathrooms free for other family members. Urinals can save trips to the bathroom and can be used in the seated position by both boys and girls.

Bathing alternatives are more complicated. Some children take full baths once or twice weekly with sponge baths in between. Another alternative is to use an inflatable bed top bathtub that is filled with water from the nearest source and suction drained afterward.

The bedroom

The child's bedroom is the setting for sleep, play, homework, and clothing storage, as well as her own personal space. Independence can be enhanced by carefully selecting the most appropriate bedroom for the child with special needs. A child with limited strength and ability, or one who uses a wheelchair, may prefer a downstairs bedroom. This enables more direct access and avoids the need for daily trips on the staircase. Rooms with the widest doorways or the most maneuvering space around doorways are also important. Furniture should be arranged with mobility and transfers in mind. Pieces of furniture can be moved closer together to assist the child who needs external stability for walking.

THE BED

A firm mattress provides good body support and facilitates transfers and bed mobility. The height of the bed from the floor also affects ease of transfers. If increased height is needed, blocks can be secured to the legs. To reduce height, legs can be sawed off. A hospital bed with electric controls may provide the best solution for the child with limited mobility. Height is adjustable and head and foot sections can be raised and lowered to facilitate bed mobility and positioning.

Assistive devices can be attached to standard or hospital beds. An overhead trapeze can aid in sitting up, weight shifts, exercises, and transfers. Similarly, straps, rope ladders, or bed rails secured to the bed frame can improve mobility in bed.

BEDROOM STORAGE

Toys, clothes, and personal belongings should be accessible considering the child's range of reach and mobility. A lowered closet pole may make it easier to obtain clothing independently. A wall mounted shoe rack or elevated shelf can be used for shoes or other items normally kept on the floor. The most important clothes can be kept in drawers that are between knee and shoulder level. Russell[21] recommends adapting drawers with glides for easier opening, or bolting dressers to walls for stability when drawers are pulled.

BEDROOM WORK STATION

Desk activities of homework, art, tinkering, and other hobbies often take place in the child's room. Good seating is essential. As discussed in Chapter 14, good seating implies adequate back support with seat depth and height that permit foot support and independent transfers. The work table or desk should be stable with dimensions that relate to the height of the chair and the child in it. Ideally, the child's elbows should be level with the table top when seated. However, a higher surface may increase stability for some children. Height may be modified with wooden blocks and leg extenders or saws.

Other living areas

Children will need many of the same adaptations throughout other parts of the house that are typically used by disabled adults. Special considerations are needed, particularly in regard to the child's size, anticipated physical growth, and developmental needs. Some of the adaptations that are more specific to the needs of children and adolescents are listed below.

Useful adaptations for other home living areas

Kitchen	Countertop access via bar stool, standing frame, or prone stander
	Location of frequently used utensils and food in low cupboards to improve access
	Food preparation or clean-up while seated at the table if countertop is inaccessible
	Avoid stacking heavy bowls and pans
	Use time and energy saving devices such as microwave ovens with large touch controls, food processors, electric mixers, and blenders
	Use other adapted kitchen aids and utensils
Dining room	Use adapted chairs for posture control and proper seat height
	Use a wheelchair laptray as an eating surface
Variable areas	Use push-button telephones, wall-mounted at lower heights for access and stability
	Use special telephone functions such as automatic dialing, speaker phone, or receiver amplification available through the special services division of the local telephone company
	Use environmental control switches, remote units, or systems for lights and appliances
	Avoid use of thick pile carpet or throw rugs to optimize mobility

Emergency alert and call systems

Children with impaired mobility, dexterity, or communication skills, and those with life support systems need more frequent monitoring both day and night. Intercom systems assist parents with this responsibility and give the child a way to initiate calls for help or social interaction. Call switches or buzzers that attach to the bed or wheelchair can also provide an independent means of seeking assistance from individuals in other rooms. A variety of portable intercoms is available at electronic supply stores and children's stores.

Many parents fear leaving their older disabled children at home alone. The fear of fire from which the child cannot escape, the child falling or getting caught in one spot, or having a medical emergency or an urgent personal need (like going to the bathroom) are common concerns. Typical consequences are that either the parents' activities are curtailed or the child is taken everywhere. Children with immature judgment cannot be left unsupervised on life support systems. However, the parents' inability to leave the child is often due to the fact that effective emergency alert or escape mechanisms have not been established. This is of particular concern with teenagers who really want and need the opportunity to be alone at home to develop more independence.

Access to the telephone and the ability to get out of the house are key skills. An accessible telephone station, combined with knowledge of how to contact emergency services or a designated helper, are of prime importance. Some parents call in at regular intervals to check on their children. If the child's speech is unintelligible over the telephone, prerecorded emergency messages in clear speech can be set up on a tape recorder. As an alternative, an augmentative communication system can be used. Emergency alert systems, worn as pendants or stabilized on wheelchairs, can be purchased with a service that places emergency calls when the system is activated. Outside alarms that can be heard in the neighborhood can be used to summon assistance. Arrangements and alternatives must be carfully planned and made in advance. An attendant or visiting nurse can come to the house at prescribed intervals to assist with specific functions such as toileting. The ability to get out of the house is most directly influenced by the child's ability to get to the door, open it, and get out. Please refer to this chapter's section on independent entrance and exit for specific information.

ADAPTATIONS FOR INDEPENDENCE AT SCHOOL

With the advent of PL 94-142, integration of disabled students into the least restrictive environment has "mainstreamed" many children into classes with teachers who are untrained in management of handicapping conditions. In addition, special education classes have been relocated to "regular" schools that often have architectural barriers. The therapist can give valuable input regarding adaptation of the school and classroom environments and materials. Typical areas for intervention include mobility, positioning, written communication, handling classroom materials and tools, adaptation of activities to promote participation, and management of toileting, feeding, and other self-maintenance activities. Coordination with school staff is essential because the recommendations of the occupational therapist will often be carried out on a daily basis by teachers and aides. Their understanding of the objectives and benefits of the recommendations is crucial. Input from the teacher will help clarify what is and is not possible to implement in the classroom and school setting.

Architectural barriers

The therapist begins by evaluating the locations where the child's school activities take place. The school teacher and principal should be involved because they will ultimately be the ones to advocate and obtain funds for any necessary adaptations.

Entrance to the school involves getting past the curb at street side, the main door through which the student will enter, any doors that connect hallways or lead to bathrooms and classrooms, and stairways. Fire and safety regulations for both normal and handicapped students must be considered. Additional curb cuts may have to be installed for wheelchair users. If doors are too heavy for the child to manage, arrangements must be made for doors to be left open or for able bodied students to open them, since it is rarely possible to modify school doors (particularly fire doors). Thresholds and stairs are common, especially in older schools, and should be ramped according to the standards described previously. Thorough consultation with the principal and custodial staff is essential.

Distances between classrooms and other rooms such as the cafeteria and bathrooms should be evaluated to determine travel time requirements and potential for fatigue. Additional time may be needed for class changes. Appropriate mobility devices such as power wheelchairs permit the student to get about at a functional speed that is commensurate with peers. For an individual student, careful planning of room assignments that are in proximity and avoid stair use is a strategy that also requires the action of school administrators.

Bathrooms may require modifications such as enlarged stalls and grab bar installation. Mirrors and towel dispensers may require remounting at a lower level. Classroom furniture may need to be rearranged to accommodate a wheelchair or other special equipment.

Classroom furniture and workstation adaptations

The existing furniture may need to be adapted or special equipment purchased to support the student's best function. The goals of intervention are to ensure that the student has:

1. Adequate postural support
2. Good orientation of the body to the work surface and school materials
3. Good body and visual orientation to the teacher
4. Ability to get to and leave workstations as independently as possible
5. Physical integration with other classmates

Adaptations of existing equipment

CLASSROOM SEATING

Chair height may need to be modified so that the feet are supported to enhance postural stability and facilitate transfers. If seat height must be raised, a foot rest should be provided. Chair legs can be sawed off or built up with blocks or leg extenders.

The occupational therapist often fabricates positioning units for standard classroom chairs to enhance posture, fine motor performance, and the ability to attend (Figure 17-6). One or more of the following adaptations may be necessary. Seat back height and seat depth can be modified as needed. Seat belt may be added to stabilize the pelvis or chest. If more stability is needed, a wedge cushion or anti-thrust seat made from high density foam or ethafoam can be added to the seat base to prevent hip extension. Small foam lumbar pads are useful for children with spontaneous trunk righting. These adaptations encourage a more neutral pelvic position and erect spine. Lateral trunk supports are often needed for children with impaired trunk righting, equilibrium, and alignment. Lateral hip and thigh pads are helpful in centralizing the pelvis and maintaining a neutral thigh position. Abductor units are useful for limiting hip adduction or asymmetrical hip position but should never be used to hold the child back in the seat. Contour seat backs behind the scapula can help mediate spinal hyperextension and shoulder retraction.

TABLES AND DESKS

The height may be adjusted for wheelchair access or to correct work surface height. If a desk storage compartment interferes with leg clearance, another desk or small table without underneath storage should be located. If equipment such as a typewriter or computer is used on top of the desk, additional surface space is often needed and table height requires adjustment so that the level of the keyboard is appropriate to the child. When several students share a computer or typewriter, the best solution is to use a height adjustable table. If this is not feasible, the correct orientation of the student to the keyboard can be attained through chair adaptations.

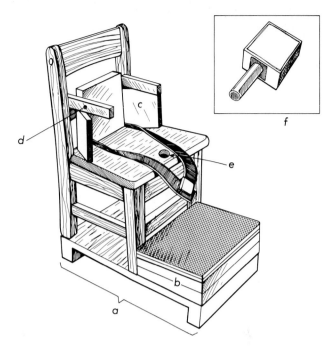

Figure 17-6 Adaptation of a wooden classroom chair. *a*, Seat height is increased by adding a platform to accommodate table height. *b*, A foot rest supports the feet. *c*, A wing-back insert and seat belt help stabilize the pelvis. *d*, Lateral supports for increased trunk stability. *e*, A hole (*e*) drilled in the seat accepts an abduction post (*f*).

Commercially available equipment

Adjustable classroom chairs with positioning components are available, as are tables with cut outs that provide increased arm support and orientation of the trunk. Tables with adjustable angle tops, such as drafting tables, permit further adaptability of the work surface (Figure 17-7). Children who have their own wheelchairs will benefit from seat inserts if they have difficulty maintaining appropriate posture for classwork.

Increasing independence in classroom skills

WRITING DEVICES

Grasp can be facilitated by building up handles with foam or rubber materials (Figure 17-8A), or by using large marking pens or primary pencils. The tripod (three-point pinch) position is encouraged by a number of writing aids available from therapy equipment suppliers or can be made by the therapist from thermoplastic materials (Figure 17-8B). The child who cannot use a tripod position can use devices that accommodate to wrist and finger positions (Figure 17-8C). Some

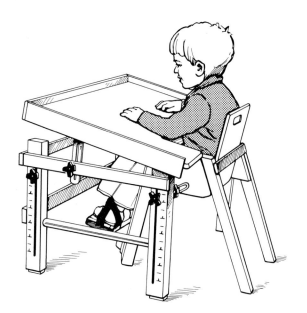

Figure 17-7 A commercially available chair with positioning components and a desk with an adjustable height and adjustable inclined work surface.

children must use other parts of their bodies to write. Headwands and mouthsticks can be used to hold writing tools, often in conjunction with angled writing surfaces (Figure 17-8, *D*).

When stabilization of the paper is difficult, some of the methods presented in Figure 17-2 may be used. As alternatives, the therapist may recommend clip boards with pressure-sensitive matting on the bottom, use of a writing tablet rather than single sheets of paper, or a one-handed writing board available from therapy suppliers.

Typewriters and computers

Children who are cognitively able to manipulate letters and numbers but who have dysfunctional handwriting are candidates for use of electric typewriters and computers. Early use of these devices is advocated for children with severe motor impairment. For example, as students in the primary grades are learning to form letters on training paper, the student with severe writing impairment learns to use the typewriter or computer to type letters and spaces. Older children whose handwriting continues to be large and poorly formed, or who are too slow to keep up with the rest of the class, will also benefit from using this equipment.

Error correction features are essential on electric typewriters to avoid the need for correction fluid or tape. Major brands of typewriters can be fitted with keyguards that usually can be ordered directly from the manufacturer. Large knobs that retrofit to the platen turn knob can aid inserting and positioning paper. Fan fold computer paper can also be used, so that

the carriage is always filled (see section on computer access for keyboard adaptations). Portable electronic typewriters with small memory capabilities for correcting and editing are widely available. These tend to be quieter than electric typewriters, have a self-contained battery source, and are light and small enough to fit on a laptray or school desk. These features make them ideal for mainstreamed students who change classes and need a typewriter in each class.

While the computer has superceded many of the typewriter's capabilities, the latter continues to be very valuable in school. Typewriters are particularly useful for completing workbook and worksheet assignments. Pages can be cut out of workbooks. The typewriter is less efficient for math because of borrowing and carrying functions that require movement to the left of the page.

The computer gives the student many capabilities through selection of hardware and software. The basic computer hardware system includes the computer with keyboard, one or two disk drives, a monitor, and a printer. Word processing software permits the student to compose and edit on the monitor, and print out a final copy. Computers can be adapted for access by students who are physically unable to use the standard keyboard.

Computer access

Often the therapist is challenged to assist the child who cannot use a keyboard, turn on the system, or load the disk drive due to incoordination, weakness, or visual impairment. Figure 17-9 presents a summary of some typical keyboard adaptations.

KEYBOARD ACCESS TOOLS

When the student has difficulty isolating the index finger to press keys, a number of adaptations are possible. Children with gross palmar grasp may use a hand-held pointer such as a dowel or the eraser end of an unsharpened pencil, providing that their best control is with the forearm in a neutral position. If the child's forearm is more pronated, then the pointer should be angled (Figure 17-10, *A*). If the student cannot grasp the pointer, it can be strapped to the hand. Keyboard mittens, made out of stockinette tubing or sock material, can isolate one finger for typing and prevent accidental involvement of other fingers (Figure 17-10, *B*). Commercially available devices include universal cuffs, palmar clips with pockets, and slip-on typing aids.

Headwands that extend from the forehead or chin line may be used by the student with fair to good head control (Figure 17-10, *C*). Mouth sticks can be used by children with good oral-motor control and fair to good head control. Key latches and special placement of the computer are necessary when using these devices. Keyguards may also help.

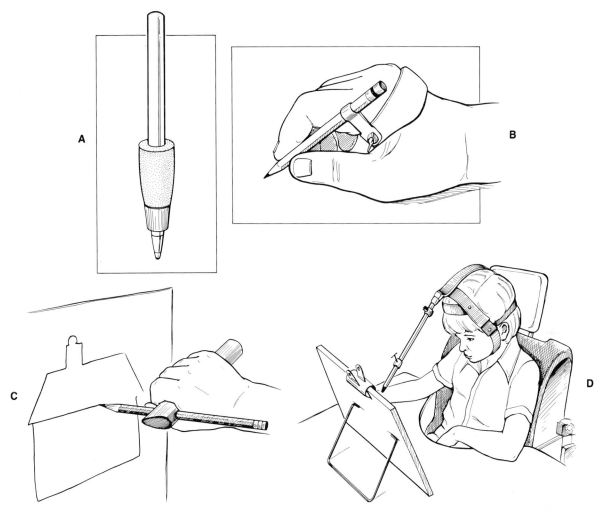

Figure 17-8 Adaptations to writing tools. **A,** A foam cylinder can be used to build up grasp surface. **B,** This adaptation encourages the tripod grasp of a pencil. **C,** This adaptation accommodates grasp and wrist position. **D,** A headwand with felt-tip pen attached is used for marking in a workbook that has been clipped to a slantboard.

ALTERNATIVE ACCESS METHODS

When direct access to a keyboard is not possible for severely physically involved students, alternative access methods are sought. These usually require adaptation of computer hardware and software.

Direct selection is the fastest way to access the computer. Expanded keyboards or small keypads are alternate direct input devices that may be used in combination with a keyboard emulation interface. These adaptations plug into the computer so that all functions can be performed using the alternate input device (Figure 17-11 on p. 352). Expanded keyboards are useful for children who have large or excessive range of movement, but limited accuracy. In contrast, small keypads are best used by students with good accuracy and limited movement range.

Most microcomputer-based augmentative communication systems can be used as interfaces to computers. The two systems must be compatible, and a keyboard emulating interface is required to make the communication system function as the keyboard of the computer. Any selection strategy used for the communication device, such as direct selection with an optical pointer or single switch scanning, will then work to access computer functions.

New technologies, as discussed by Brandenburg and Vanderheiden[4,5] have increased the options for direct selection. The Headmaster is an alternate input device that uses head motion and a sip and puff switch to select letters and functions. Voice entry systems recognize spoken letters or words and display these on the computer provided that consistent speech quality is available. An eye gaze system has recently been developed that translates eye movements for computer access.

If direct select options cannot be used, use of a single or dual input switch can access computer functions through a scanning method of selection. This is a slower technique that requires a relatively high level of cognitive function and attention. The Adaptive Firmware Card again serves as the interface between computer and switch functions. This interface utilizes the

---

Figure 17-9   Computer and typewriter keyboard adaptations

Key latch	For children who are able to use only one finger, a headwand, or mouthstick. This device locks the "shift" and "control" keys to allow simultaneous activation of another key.	Arm support systems	Wrist rests or arm supports can be secured in front of the keyboard when motor weakness or extraneous movements are present. Supports may be continuous with the front of the keyboard or raised. These systems are effective in increasing speed, accuracy, and endurance. Overhead slings and mobile arm supports may also be used.
Key guard	Used to improve accuracy when the student has difficulty hitting one key at a time. Acts as a guide for finger placement and resting surface for the hand. Typical errors that indicate the need for a keyguard: frequently hitting the keys next to desired letters or unintentionally activating other keys with other fingers or parts of the hand due to uncontrolled motion. Most commercial keyguards have a latching feature for the "control" and "shift" keys.	Disabling the repeat function	Sustained pressure on keys usually results in continuous repetition of the letter. Students with slow reactions or poorly moderated downward pressure activate repeat functions, often with frustrating results. Software and hardware can be altered to prevent this. Contact special services divisions of computer manufacturers for assistance.
Special placement of the keyboard	One-handed typists and children who have difficulty crossing the midline often benefit from offset placement of the keyboard toward the dominant hand. Placing the keyboard on an inclined surface may facilitate key selection.		

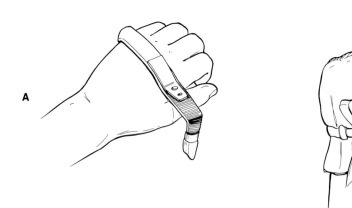

Figure 17-10   Keyboard access tools. **A,** Angled pointer accommodates for forearm and palmar grasp. **B,** Mitten isolates one finger. **C,** Headwand is used to access the keyboard that is adapted with a keyguard.

bottom two lines of the video display as an alphabet array. The cursor scans the letters in chunks at a rate that is established according to the student's switch control speed. When the cursor highlights the desired group of letters, the child activates the switch. The cursor then scans the group of letters, one at a time, and the student activates the switch again when the desired individual letter is highlighted.

There are several other alternate input devices, such as the Tetrascan, Zygo 100, and other microprocessor communication systems that allow access to the computer through scanning. Although interfacing is more complex, these devices have more flexibility regarding the style of scanning and the way the alphabet can be configured to enhance speed. A typical adaptation substitutes arrangement by frequency of letter use for alphabetical order.

COMPUTER SYSTEM OPERATION

Power on/off switches on computers, printers, and monitors are often difficult or inaccessible to children with limited reach and coordination. An external power strip can be used so that the entire system can be turned on or off with the switch on the strip. Some computers have retrofit front switch kits available. Handling of diskettes can be facilitated with the addition of a platform set in front of the disk drive to help guide the diskette into place. The use of two disk drives or a hard disk drive can reduce the need for disk handling.

Management of classroom materials

Holding, manipulating, or carrying books and papers can be very difficult and result in destruction of the

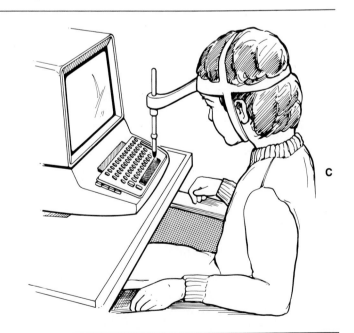

c

materials. Students with severe motor or visual limitations will need to have materials set up for them to reduce handling requirements. Bookstands can be used to hold written materials at the proper angle and to hold books open. Page turning can be assisted with the eraser tip of a pencil, a rubber finger tip cover, or a headwand or mouthstick with rubber tip to increase friction. Electric or battery operated page turners can greatly enhance the independence of severely physically involved students. These devices hold the book open and use a single switch or switch array to turn pages. Back packs can be used to carry books to free both arms for use in mobility functions. Papers or worksheets can be held on stenographers' stands or easels.

Note-taking

Alternatives to note-taking include photocopying the notes of a classmate or tape recording lectures. Rather than taping an entire lecture, students can record only pertinent segments by using the switch control on the microphone. Portable electronic typewriters or small augmentative communication devices are also useful for note-taking.

Self-maintenance activities at school

Equipment adaptations and special techniques for self-maintenance activities such as eating, toileting, and managing clothes, should also be addressed by the occupational therapist. Refer to Chapter 14 for review.

Adapted physical education

The therapist often consults with the adaptive physical education specialist regarding the capabilities of students and activity and equipment adaptations to enhance participation. The adaptive physical education specialist is well versed in adapting sports equipment and games, such as bowling frames and batting tees. However, the therapist is more likely to be called upon to address special individual problems, such as adapting a Ping-Pong paddle to facilitate grasp.

INDEPENDENCE IN THE COMMUNITY
Transportation

Mobility and function in the community are critical to the child's development and to the family's ability to be active outside the home. Community participation ranges from the early stages when the child accompanies her parents on errands to the time when the child goes out on her own. Transportation of the special child must be addressed from both functional and safety standpoints. Furthermore, when new equipment is selected for a child, the methods used for home, school, and community mobility should be

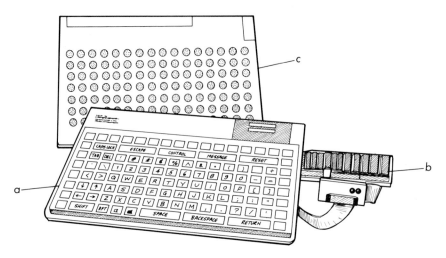

Figure 17-11 Alternate input device; *a*, An expanded membrane keyboard, *b*, the Adaptive Firmware Card, and *c*, a keyguard.

considered to ensure that the device can be transported as necessary with the child.

THE FAMILY VEHICLE

Over 40 states have safety laws requiring children to use restraint systems while traveling in cars. Commercial car seats are useful for many disabled children who are small enough to fit into them. Other children who have skeletal deformities, poor head or trunk control, spica casts, or abduction braces will often need modifications of commercial seats to increase access, support, comfort, and protection. Simple modifications that do not alter the structure of the car seat can be made by the therapist. These might include adding foam or towel rolls to improve lateral control, or adding closed cell foam positioning inserts to the inside shell.

The Automotive Safety for Children Program (James Whitcomb Riley Hospital for Children, Indianapolis) has developed a car seat modification for children in hip abduction casts. This adaptation involves cutting away the lower side of the plastic shell, placing a firm pad under and behind the pelvis, and adjusting the harness.[3,12] Shaw[24] recommends that therapists work closely with manufacturers or qualified engineers for structural modifications, as such changes always affect the safety features of restraints.

Children who have outgrown standard commercial car seats, yet have not developed adequate sitting balance, may use the Britax or Carrie car seats designed specifically for larger disabled children. Transport/travel type wheelchairs such as STC or Orthokinetics that are designed to be used also as car seats are an option for some children. Restraint harnesses, such as the Whitworth Vest or the E-Z-On Vest by Rupert, attach to the regular car or school bus seat and help restrain children with postural or behavior problems.[15,24]

Older, heavier children who cannot manage car transfers may benefit from free-standing portable or special car lifters.

Vans enable children to ride seated in their wheelchairs. Vans are especially helpful for children in power wheelchairs that do not dismantle or fold. It is essential that the van be equipped with a wheelchair restraint system that secures the frame to the floor. Additionally, a child's seat belt that attaches to the wheelchair frame is necessary. Restraints should be applied over skeletal regions such as the pelvis and shoulders, rather than over the soft abdominal area. Facing the front or rear of a vehicle is safer than sideway placement. Rear head restraint is necessary to prevent backward head excursion.[22] Ramps or power van lifts are needed to transfer the child into the vehicle.

SCHOOL TRANSPORTATION

Rules and equipment for transporting disabled children and their equipment vary among school bus companies. The occupational therapist facilitates school transportation in the equipment selection process by making sure that wheelchairs, laptrays, communication systems, and other devices meet the requirements of the individual school system. Wheelchairs should have sufficient positioning controls to maintain the child's posture throughout the bus ride and should have a bag to contain belongings safely. The therapist's role often involves working with school transportation officials regarding safety issues and helping to solve special problems for individual children.

PUBLIC TRANSPORTATION

Few communities have accessible rapid transit programs for the disabled. Many, however, have "Dial a

Ride" type programs that provide door to door bus or van service. This is typically arranged in advance by telephone. Children who are able to board buses or rapid rail systems must learn important skills such as handling money and tickets, using transit schedules, and identifying correct buses, trains, and stops.

INDEPENDENT DRIVING

The therapist usually consults with adapted driving program specialists unless she has had specialized training in driving adaptations and instruction. Strength, range of motion, sensation, coordination, reach, reaction time, balance, and perceptual abilities must be considered in functional terms related to driving. Automobile adaptations for the teenage driver who is handicapped range from simple add-on components to those that convert a car or van permanently. Add-on adaptations that will not affect others' use of the car are preferred when feasible. Steering knobs facilitate grasp and turning the wheel. Built up brakes and accelerator pedals or left-footed accelerators are useful. Right or left hand controls, or relocation of the horn and dimmer switches are examples of other adaptations for the family auto. The therapist also deals with techniques to transfer the teen driver and equipment such as wheelchairs into and out of the car.

Community activities and skills

Shopping, eating in restaurants, banking, and attending sports and recreational events involve many similar skills. These include mobility, communication with strangers, handling money and packages, and functional reading and writing. Adaptations may be needed to assist children with these requirements of community living. Falvey[11] advocates teaching the use of strategies and adaptations on site in community environments. Using assistive devices in public will depend on their degree of portability, ease of use, and attitudes of the child and family. Therefore, careful selection and training, as well as counseling, are important aspects of occupational therapy intervention.

COMMUNITY MOBILITY

Factors to consider include other people and crowds, street crossings, use of personal or public transportation and elevators, and architectural barriers. Occupational therapy may involve selecting the most appropriate mobility device or techniques and training the child in a variety of community settings. For example, the child in a power wheelchair should learn to use the high speed setting to cover long distances where there are few maneuvering obstacles, but to use the slow speed when driving around persons and obstacles. If curb cuts are not available at corners, the wheelchair user must learn to look for driveway cuts to get onto and off the street. If the child cannot reach elevator controls a reacher may help.

COMMUNICATION WITH STRANGERS

This skill is needed to place orders in restaurants, ask for directions, or conduct a banking or shopping transaction. Augmentative communication systems help children whose speech is nonfunctional. Communication systems for public use must be portable, readily accessed by the child, and understandable to others in a community setting. Systems range from handmade picture boards that are specific to a community task, such as ordering fast food, to comprehensive synthesized speech output systems. Refer to Chapter 22 for a comprehensive discussion of augmentative communication.

ADAPTATIONS FOR LEISURE AND RECREATIONAL ACTIVITIES

Participation in leisure and recreational interests benefits the individual both physically and emotionally through enjoyment, exercise, competition, and meeting other people. The therapist helps the child develop skills, recommends equipment and adaptations, and refers the child and family to appropriate resources to enhance participation. Many individual activities, such as hobbies, can be adapted to suit the child's needs using the methods described throughout this and other chapters, and will not be discussed further here.

Group activities

Schools, churches, and community recreation departments have many organized youth activity groups that offer excellent opportunities for disabled children. Although most programs are integrated with able bodied children, some groups are designed specifically for the youth with special needs. Although the trend is for all children to participate in local troops, the Girl Scouts, Camp Fire Girls, and Boy Scouts will set up special troops in schools and camps. Optimum participation can be facilitated through the use of assistive devices and techniques. The therapist may confer with the child, parent, or group leader regarding adaptations specific to the group's activities.

PLAYGROUND SPORTS

Equipment such as swings, teeter-totters, merry-go-rounds, and bars are common to community and school playgrounds, as are games such as volleyball, basketball, four square, and handball. Some newer playgrounds are adapted with platform swings that accommodate wheelchairs, but most older ones do not. A wheelchair can be placed on a large merry-go-round, and car seats or one-piece adapted seating systems may be hooked onto swing chains with heavy load adapter brackets. Children with slow reaction time can play volleyball over a low net with a balloon. Basketball can be adapted for play with a large ball and low hoop. Batting tees can be used for baseball. The use of adapted tricycles and bicycles on playgrounds can provide faster mobility in a normal manner that promotes group and independent play.

ORGANIZED AND SPECTATOR SPORTS

Sports equipment, performance techniques, and game rules may need to be modified to permit full participation by a special child.[26] Many sports are learned at home or school. Community agencies such as recreation departments have integrated special programs for the disabled. Recreational events such as the Special Olympics and the National Wheelchair Basketball Championships take place at regional and national levels as well. Athletic and recreational departments are the primary resources for these programs, but the occupational therapist may assist with individual adaptations.

Many of the recent wheelchair design improvements can be traced to wheelchair sports. Cambered wheels, lighter and stronger aluminum and titanium frame materials, precision wheel bearings, adjustable rear axles, and quick release wheels were introduced to improve athletic performance. Good equipment is essential for participation in all wheelchair athletics, including basketball, track and field, and tennis. National organizations for wheelchair sports can provide information regarding training and competition. (A list of these associations and their addresses precedes the Summary at the end of this chapter.) In addition, *Sports and Spokes* and *Accent on Living* magazines have regular articles about participation in different sports.

Most stadiums and arenas have special seating areas for persons in wheelchairs or those who cannot climb stairs. The number of special seats is usually limited, and access is often via different routes, so advance arrangements are necessary.

WATER SPORTS

Many children with disabilities achieve greater freedom and flexibility of movement in water than on land. Swimming is the skill common to all water sports and recreation. Flotation devices to keep the head above water and other equipment, such as hand paddles and flippers, assist safety and movement. Pool lifts that transfer the swimmer from a wheelchair and ramps that lead to the water promote access. The American National Red Cross has adapted aquatics programs that provide lessons and information about accessible pools.

Boating requires mastery of swimming and use of a flotation device. Flat bottom boats are more stable and may even accommodate a wheelchair. Safety harnesses are available for sailing. Children who require cushions for skin protection can often use air-filled pillows in boats. Custom seats can be fabricated for kayaks to sta-

bilize the pelvis of the adolescent with excellent upper body control but impaired hip and low trunk function. Special skis are available for water skiing in the seated position.

Individual outdoor sports
SKIING

A sled ski resembling a kayak can be used by children with paraplegia or diplegia, provided that upper body control is good. These devices have two runners molded onto the bottom surface and are balanced by the skier by means of short forearm ski poles that have little skis on the end. Beginners are tethered to a ski instructor or parent and guided down the slope until they are sufficiently skilled to ski independently. Lower extremity amputee skiers use two forearm braced outrigger skis to give them a three-point balance (Figure 17-12). Upper extremity amputees can ski with one or no poles. Blind skiers may be accompanied by a sighted companion who provides directions by verbal command or a tether. Adapted recreational skiing and lessons are now available in more areas with ski programs for the disabled such as Alpine Meadows in California and Winter Park in Colorado. Toboggans can be used just about anywhere in the snow, provided that safety considerations are addressed. For resources on winter sports, refer to the list of sporting associations in Figure 17-13.

FISHING

Adaptations are often needed to stabilize fishing rods. Devices such as EZ Cast attach to the wheelchair

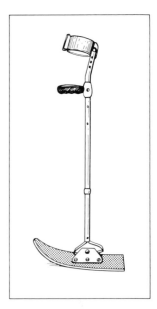

Figure 17-12 An outrigger ski with forearm support is used by the lower extremity amputee for stability and balance while skiing.

arm and assist casting and reeling with limited use of one arm. Lightweight trunk belts and harnesses can also be used to mount rods.

HORSEBACK RIDING

Horseback riding has become one of the most popular and enjoyable adapted sports for children with mental or physical handicaps. Many communities have stables that offer riding lessons to the disabled. Mounting platforms that place the child at saddle level are often equipped with ramps for wheelchairs. Adapted saddles with hand holds, back rests, and harness systems to stabilize the rider are typically found in adapted programs. Fleece covered or padded seats are available for children with sensory impairment who are at risk of pressure sores. A rein-bar that attaches to the saddle permits control with one hand. Protective helmets and safety stirrups are usually worn.

Figure 17-13 Information about adapted sports and recreation can be obtained from these associations:

SPORTS ASSOCIATIONS

GENERAL

National Handicapped Sports and Recreation Association
Capital Hill Station
P.O. Box 18664
Denver, Colorado 80218

Special Olympics, Inc.
Joseph P. Kennedy Jr. Foundation
1701 K Street NW, Suite 215
Washington, D.C. 20006

National Wheelchair Athletic Association
40-24 62nd Street
Woodside, New York 11377

Adapted Sports Association
6832 Marlette
Marlette, Michigan 48453

ACTIVITY-RELATED

National Foundation for Wheelchair Tennis
3055 Birch Street
Newport Beach, California 92660

American Water Ski Association
P.O. Box 191
Winter Haven, Florida 33880

Handicapped Boaters Association
P.O. Box 1134 Ansonia Station
New York, New York 11023

North American Riding for the Handicapped Association
Box 100
Ashburn, Virginia 22011

Disabled Sportsmen of America
P.O. Box 26
Vinton, Virginia 24170

National Wheelchair Softball Association
P.O. Box 737
Sioux Falls, South Dakota 57101

National Wheelchair Basketball Association
110 Seaton Building
University of Kentucky
Lexington, Kentucky 40506

DISABILITY-RELATED

United States Association for Blind Athletes
55 W. California Avenue
Beach Haven Park, New Jersey 08008

American Athletic Association of the Deaf
3916 Lantern Drive
Silver Spring, Maryland 20902

United State Deaf Skiers Association
159 Davis Avenue
Hackensack, New Jersey 07601

International Committee of the Silent Sports
Gallaudet College
Florida Ave. and 7th St. NE
Washington, D.C. 20002

Amputee Sports Association
11705 Merch Boulevard
Savannah, Georgia 31406

National Association of Sports for Cerebral Palsy
United Cerebral Palsy Association
66 E. 34th Street
New York, New York 10016

OUTDOOR RECREATION

National Park Service
Division of Special Programs and Populations
U.S. Dept. of the Interior
Washington, D.C. 20240

American Camping Association
Bradford Woods
Martinsville, Indiana 46151

The Committee for the Promotion of Camping for the Handicapped
Bradford Woods
5040 State Road 76 North
Martinsville, Indiana 46151

Vacations

Vacations are a part of the family's special times together and enhance the child's social, intellectual, and cultural development. However, traveling with a child who has a lot of equipment or who needs special attention can be complicated. Advance planning and use of resources are required to ensure a successful trip. To obtain information on accessible travel, contact state and local departments of tourism, commerce, economic development, and parks and recreation. Major cities have information available through their convention and visitors bureaus and Easter Seal Societies.

TRANSPORTATION BY BUS, TRAIN, OR PLANE

Large major transportation systems accommodate disabled passengers with boarding priority and special seating. Different companies and transportation modes have varying amenities, so it is necessary to compare policies in advance. In most cases, handicapped persons cannot sit in their wheelchairs on planes and trains, making it difficult to use the restroom. Wet cell batteries for electric wheelchairs cannot be transported on airplanes. Airports are typically newer and more accessible than train or bus stations, but advance checks on accessibility are advised before taking a trip.

LODGING

Automobile associations publish information on the accessibility of hotels and highway service areas. Most hotels and motels have a limited number of guest rooms specially equipped for the handicapped, but their functional attributes vary. It is important to make advance reservations.

SUMMER CAMPS

Camps provide opportunities for the child to spend time away from home and for family respite. A directory of special camps is available from the Easter Seal Society. If the child is mainstreamed into a regular camp program, the counselor and director must be aware of and plan for the child's special needs.

NATIONAL PARKS AND SPECIAL FACILITIES FOR THE HANDICAPPED

A national park guide for the handicapped identifies the parks with paved trails and wheechair accessible campsites. The U.S. Forest Service also has barrier-free camps that can be located by consulting the field office in a local community or the national office in Washington, D.C. A number of private organizations also support adapted camping. The list of sporting associations in Figure 17-13 includes resources for these activities.

SUMMARY

This chapter discussed methods of enhancing independent living skills through adaptations of the activity process, tools, and materials, and through preparation of the individual. The areas of early childhood play, schoolwork, home living skills, community skills, and recreation and leisure were presented. Occupational therapy intervention must be appropriate to the child's developmental level, functional capacity, and life environments, with consideration of parents, other caretakers and the child's motivation. The importance of positioning and orientation of the child to the work surface and task were stressed. Examples of assistive devices, adapted techniques, and environmental modifications to increase the level of independent functioning were presented.

STUDY QUESTIONS

1. Discuss the importance of the relationship between the child and the work or play surface.
2. Discuss methods of increasing the independent play of a 3-year-old child who has gross grasp and release hand patterns but poor sitting balance, through adaptation of position, toys, and the environment.
3. Describe five possible modifications to the home environment for a child who uses a wheelchair full time and requires physical assistance with transfers.
4. Describe three possible adaptations for a school program in each of the following areas:
   a. Written communication
   b. Computer access
   c. Architectural barriers.
5. Give examples of adaptations for the following community or recreation activities: transportation, horseback riding, and swimming.

REFERENCES AND RELATED READINGS

1. Bergen A, and Colangelo C: Positioning the client with central nervous system deficits: the wheelchair and other adapted equipment, Valhalla, NY, 1982, Valhalla Rehabilitation Publications, LTD.
2. Biggie JL: Teaching individuals with physical and multiple disabilities, Columbus, Ohio, 1982, Bell and Howell Co.
3. Brandenburg S, and Vanderheiden G: Communication, control and computer access for disabled and elderly individuals, resource book 1: communication aids, Boston, 1987, College-Hill Press.
4. Brandenburg S, and Vanderheiden G: Communication, control, and computer access for disabled and elderly individuals, resource book 3: software and hardware, Boston, 1987, College-Hill Press.
5. Bull MJ: Safety seat use for children with hip dislocation, Pediatrics 77:873, 1986.
6. Burkhardt LJ: Homemade battery devices for severely handicapped children with suggested activities. College Park, Md, 1980, Linda J. Burkhardt.
7. Burkhardt LJ: More homemade battery devices for severely handicapped children with suggested activities, College Park, Md, 1982, Linda J Burkhardt.
8. Carlson F: Prattle and play, Omaha, Neb, 1982, University of Nebraska Medical Center.
9. Cohen P, and Kohn JG: Follow-up study of patients with cerebral palsy, Western J of Med 130:6, 1979.
10. Enders A: Technology for independent living sourcebook, Washington, DC, 1984, Association for the Advancement of Rehabilitation Technology.
11. Falvey M: Community based curriculum: instructional strategies

for students with severe handicaps, Baltimore, MD, 1986, Paul H Brookes Publishing Co.

12. Feller N, and others: A multidisciplinary approach to developing safe transportation for children with special needs, Orthopedic Nursing 5:25, 1986.
13. Finnie NR: Handling the young cerebral palsied child at home, New York, 1968, EP Dutton.
14. Hale G: The source book for the disabled, New York, 1979, Paddington Press Ltd.
15. Holland S: Car safety for special children, The Exceptional Parent, October, 1983.
16. Jones ML: Home care for the chronically ill or disabled child, New York, 1981, Harper and Row, Publishers, Inc.
17. Lefchez R, and Winslow B: Design for independent living, New York, 1979, Watson-Guptill Publications.
18. Munoz PJ: The significance of fostering play development in handicapped children. In: Play: a skill for life: selected readings related to occupational therapy. Rockville, Md, 1986, Developmental Disabilities Special Interest Section, The American Occupational Therapy Association, Inc.
19. Musselwhite C: Adaptive play for special needs children, San Diego, 1986, College-Hill Press.
20. Rast M: Play and therapy, play or therapy? In: Play: a skill for life: selected readings related to occupational therapy, Rockville, Md, 1986, Developmental Disabilities Special Interest Section, The American Occupational Therapy Association, Inc.
21. Russell P: The wheelchair child, Englewood, NJ, 1985, Prentice Hall.
22. Schneider LW: Protection for the severely disabled—a new challenge in occupant restraint, International Symposium of Occupant Protection, 1981.
23. Seligman A: On the cognitive component of learned helplessness and depression, Psych of Learning and Motivation 13:219, 1979.
24. Shaw G: Vehicular transport safety for the child with disabilities, Am J Occup Ther 41:35, 1987.
25. Sinker M: Toys for growing: a guide to toys that develop skills, Chicago, 1986, Year Book Medical Publishing, Inc.
26. Sports for disabled individuals, Rehab Brief 4: Jan 26, 1981.
27. Vanderheiden GC: Toy modification (personal communication), Madison, Wisconsin, 1986, University of Wisconsin-Madison.
28. Ward D: Positioning the handicapped child for function, St Louis, 1983, Diane E. Ward, OTR.
29. Wright C, and Nomura M: From toys to computers: access for the physically disabled child, San Jose, Calif, 1985, Christine Wright and Mari Nomura.

PART
VI

SPECIALIZED OCCUPATIONAL THERAPY SERVICES

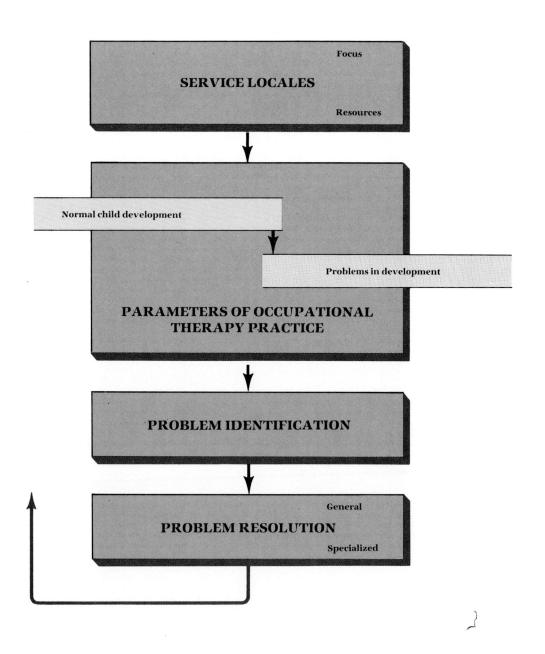

18

High-risk infants

JUDITH PELLETIER SEHNAL
ALISA PALMERI

Advances in medical technology have resulted in higher survival rates for gestationally younger, smaller, and sicker infants.[30,46] Improvements in obstetrics now enable medical and nursing staffs to monitor infants through complicated gestations, to postpone premature births, and to make difficult or high-risk deliveries safer for both mother and infant. Concurrent improvements in pediatrics have increased the ability to prolong and maintain the lives of sick infants. One of the by-products of such medical advances has been the development of special care nurseries that are equipped to provide specialized treatments needed by these high-risk infants.

CONCEPT OF RISK
Identification of infants at risk

A number of biological and sociological factors that appear to indicate high-risk status have been identified in the literature.[64] Concern with early identification of these factors has resulted in the development of several screening devices. These include Parmelee's Obstetric Complications Scale,[42] which is used to predict the effect of maternal factors on the unborn child. The Apgar Scoring System[40,63] (Chapter 9) is used to assess fetal and perinatal factors. A number of developmental and neurobehavioral assessments, such as the Brazelton Neonatal Behavioral Assessment Scale[10] (Chapter 11), the Dubowitz Neurological Assessment of the Preterm and Full-term Newborn Infant,[20] and Als' Assessment of Preterm Infant Behavior (APIB),[2] are used to monitor the progress of the infant beyond the delivery room.

High predictive value of neurological and neurobehavioral assessments of newborns has not been well established.[63] Instead, it appears that long-term outcome depends on a large number of variables. Examples include severity of an initial traumatic insult, plasticity of the central nervous system, potential for re-

covery, and hereditary and environmental (including socioeconomic) factors. Research in this area continues in an effort to provide comprehensive, accurate, and useful assessment of the newborn.

Who is at risk?

The term *at risk* has been discussed at length in Chapter 6. For purposes of this chapter, it shall refer to an infant who has suffered prenatal or perinatal complications that might contribute to later developmental delays or deficits.[22,32] Such infants have a certain probability of showing sensory-motor deficits or cognitive handicaps in childhood.[48]

Traditionally, birth weight and gestational age have been major determinants of the risk status of the newborn.[40] Concern with these factors has given rise to the terms *small for gestational age (SGA), appropriate for gestational age (AGA),* and *large for gestational age (LGA),* as well as *preterm, term,* and *postterm.* In general, the shorter the gestation period, or the lower the birth weight, the greater the infant's risk status.[17]

Without the addition of other complications, shortened gestations per se are not necessarily risk-producing. However, a preterm delivery may be symptomatic of dysfunction in the maternal, fetal, or placental systems. It is these complications that can interfere with a smooth transition from fetal to extrauterine life.[25] The more common medical problems to which premature infants are susceptible vary according to the degree of prematurity (Table 18-1). Other medical problems of high-risk infants that are not necessarily related to prematurity are described in Table 18-2.

Because of the variety of individual differences, as well as the variations in postnatal complications, it is difficult to make generalizations regarding the developmental outcome of preterm infants. Variable defini-

Table 18-1   Common medical problems of premature infants

	Description	Potential associated disorders of developmental significance
RESPIRATORY		
Respiratory distress syndrome (RDS)	A respiratory disorder that affects immature lungs and is characterized by grunting, retractions, nasal flaring, tachypnea, and cyanosis.	May require prolonged mechanical ventilation that results in decreased movement, decreased stimulation or interaction, and decreased parent-infant interaction. There is an increased incidence of neurodevelopmental deficits in infants who have required prolonged ventilation resulting from respiratory complications. Abnormal tone/movement patterns (e.g., increased trunk/neck extension, shoulder retraction, decreased shoulder girdle stability) may be evident. The infant may also develop secondary feeding problems.
Atelectasis	Incomplete expansion of lungs at birth resulting from poor development of lung tissue and weak respiratory muscles.	
Hyaline membrane disease (HMD)	A respiratory disorder in which there is inadequate amount of pulmonary surfactant lining the terminal respiratory units of the mature fetal lung, and subsequently inadequate fetal lung development.	
Bronchopulmonary dysplasia (BPD)	A chronic lung disease characterized by abnormal development of the lung and bronchi that occurs in many survivors of respiratory therapy for HMD.	Increased incidence of hospitalization secondary to lower respiratory infections. Increased incidence of asthma and asthma-like conditions.
Meconium aspiration	Inspiration of meconium, a fetal fecal substance passed during delivery when hypoxia occurs; can result in obstruction of the airway, interference with gas exchange, and respiratory distress.	
Apnea	The transient cessation of breathing.	
CARDIOVASCULAR		
Patent ductus arteriosus (PDA)	Failure of the fetal heart openings to close. The most common cause of congestive heart failure in the newborn.	Inadequate nutrition resulting from fluid restriction. There is a risk of chronic pulmonary abnormalities with prolonged ventilation.
Hemorrhage	Bleeding resulting from deficiency of several clotting factors in the blood combined with the fragility of the capillary walls, especially in small vessels as in the brain, which leads to intraventricular or intracranial hemorrhage.	Neurological insults and subsequent neurodevelopmental deficits.
METABOLIC		
Hyperbilirubinemia	An excess of bilirubin (a red bile pigment) in the blood causing infants to appear jaundiced.	Neurological deficits in severe cases.
Metabolic acidosis	A pathological condition resulting from accumulation of acid or loss of base in the body, characterized by decreased pH.	Jitteriness. Neurological deficits in severe cases.
Hypocalcemia	Reduction of the blood calcium below normal.	Jitteriness, convulsions.
Hypoglycemia	An abnormally diminished content of glucose in the blood.	Hyperirritability, jitteriness, apnea, cyanosis, irregular respiration, convulsions.
NUTRITIONAL AND GASTROINTESTINAL		
Necrotizing enterocolitis (NEC)	An acute superficial necrosis of the mucosa of the small intestine and colon characterized by profound shock and dehydration.	Long-term feeding problems and behavioral complications.

Table 18-1 cont'd.   Common medical problems of premature infants

TEMPERATURE REGULATION

Subnormal body temperature	Results from poor heat production or increased heat loss. Cold exposure can cause an increased metabolic rate and oxygen consumption with subsequent acidosis, apnea, hypoglycemia, and pulmonary hemorrhage.	Possible neurological deficits in severe cases.

IMMUNITY

Pneumonia	Inflammation of the lungs.	Respiratory distress, temperature instability, acidosis, poor feeding, lethargy, seizures. Potential hearing loss secondary to ototoxic antibiotic medication.
Septicemia	Presence in the blood of bacterial toxins.	
Meningitis	Inflammation of meninges of the brain.	
Urinary tract infection (UTI)	Infection of the urinary tract.	

OPHTHALMOLOGICAL

Retrolental fibroplasia (RLF)	Characterized by the presence of opaque tissue behind the lens, leading to retinal detachment and arrest of eye growth; generally attributed to use of high concentrations of oxygen in the care of the premature infant.	Myopia, strabismus, poor central acuity, retinal detachment, blindness. Problems with depth perception.

Adapted from Dorland's illustrated medical dictionary, ed 25, Philadelphia, 1974, WB Saunders Co; and Paxson C: Van Leeuwen's newborn medicine, ed 2, Chicago, 1979, Year Book Medical Publishers, Inc.

tional criteria of prematurity in different studies in the literature[9,13,58,59] have led to the investigation of heterogeneous populations, and therefore comparisons of these studies are difficult to make. However, it is evident that young, sick preterm infants are a vulnerable group who may be at risk for neurodevelopmental deficits.

Although *at risk* and *vulnerable* are often used interchangeably in this and other writings, some authors do make a differentiation.[65] In such instances, vulnerability refers to those intrinsic characteristics of the infant that increase susceptibility to complications, and at risk is related to extrinsic, environmental factors. These distinctions are supported by increasing evidence from follow-up analysis of groups of preterm infants at older ages. The literature suggests that as the child ages, perinatal factors assume considerably less importance, while environmental factors become more significant. There is reason to believe that the detrimental effects of prematurity are exacerbated in nonsupportive environments and ameliorated in supportive, caregiving environments.[17,18,61] Retrospective studies now indicate that the four factors that relate to subsequent deficits include social conditions, as well as anorexia, delivery complications, and prematurity.[61]

Despite a rich body of literature, a well-developed conceptual model of risk remains elusive.[37] A combination of prenatal, perinatal, postnatal, and genetic conditions offers the best definition of cause. Recent data show that the proportion of children who demonstrate serious sequelae as a result of preterm birth is markedly reduced from prior years. While studies indicate continuing problem areas, such as learning disabilities, we cannot clearly identify causal mechanisms, early precursors, or onset periods. What has become more apparent is that the hazards and stresses that were thought to have specific, definitive, and direct influences on development are in fact more complex in their interactions and effects.

Research on early intervention

The significance of early identification of risk status lies in the implication that early intervention may lead to improved function and outcome. Much has been written on the effects of early experiences on behavior, especially with regard to the nature-nurture controversy, the plasticity of the central nervous system, critical periods, and effects of sensory stimulation and deprivation. General conclusions from a review of the literature are that:

1. The vulnerability and responsiveness of the innate elements of the central nervous system are heightened during critical periods.
2. The significance of both stimulation and deprivation varies with the type, length, and time of the experience, as well as other factors.

One view that may be postulated is that the preterm infant who is placed in an Isolette is deprived of the opportunity to complete fetal maturation in the protected environment of the womb and is deprived of its

Table 18-2 Other common medical problems of high-risk infants

	Description	Potential associated disorders of developmental significance
NEUROLOGICAL		
Asphyxia	Anoxia and increased carbon dioxide tension in blood and tissues.	Abnormal tone, poor interactive skills, irritability, feeding problems, decreased spontaneous movement. Cerebral palsy, mental retardation, developmental disabilities, and related problems.
Intraventricular hemorrhage (IVH)	Bleeding into the ventricles of the brain.	
Seizures		
CONGENITAL ANOMALIES		
Trisomies	Presence of an additional chromosome of one type in an otherwise diploid cell, as in Down syndrome.	Abnormal muscle tone; mental retardation.
Limb deficiencies	Absence at birth of a portion of one or more of the extremities.	Temporary movement and functional disorders.
Cleft lip or palate	Longitudinal opening or fissure (occurring in the embryo) in the lip or palate.	Feeding problems, speech difficulties.
Tracheal-esophageal fistula	Abnormal passage or communication between trachea and esophagus.	Feeding problems.
BIRTH WEIGHT		
Small for gestational age (SGA)	Weight for age falls in the 0 to 10th percentile range.	Impaired attachment process. Jittery, irritable.
Large for gestational age (LGA)	Weight for age falls in the 90th to 100th percentile range.	Frequently poor tone.
BIRTH TRAUMA		
Head injuries		Neurological sequelae, depending on nature of injury.
Nerve injuries		
Fractures		Temporarily impaired movement.
OTHER		
Substance abuse (maternal)		Jitteriness. Irritability. Impaired attachment.
Failure to thrive		Feeding or behavioral problems. Abnormal muscle tone, head growth. Developmental delay.

Adapted from Dorland's illustrated medical dictionary, ed 25, Philadelphia, 1974, WB Saunders Co; and Paxson C: Van Leeuwen's newborn medicine, ed 2, Chicago, 1979, Year Book Medical Publishers, Inc.

normal intrauterine sensory experiences as well. Moreover, life in an Isolette deprives the infant of many human interactions and the opportunity to receive organized stimuli. Such deprivations may contribute to later problems. In contrast, it may be hypothesized that the infant in an Isolette is exposed to additional, different experiences, particularly of a visual and auditory nature, that can affect behavioral development in a detrimental way.[70] Although no definitive body of knowledge clearly supports either proposal, it seems clear that deprivation or experience must be considered within the context of the infant's maturational level. This means that the immature infant may be more susceptible to the negative effects of either deprivation or disorganized, inappropriate or excessive stimuli of various types. However, the same infant can

benefit from an organized plan of graded stimulation. This concept can be applied both neurologically and behaviorally, and requires thorough knowledge of the embryological development of the central nervous system, as well as postnatal neurobehavioral development.[38,44,47,60]

It is also apparent that extrauterine experience influences development. Review of the literature seems to indicate positive effects of infant stimulation programs with preterm babies.[23,24,33,62,70] However, because of variations in research design, types of stimulation provided to study groups, and measurement techniques, it is difficult to draw specific conclusions. More research is necessary with clearly defined groups, special attention to individual differences, and measurement of responses at multiple age periods. The most critical issue at this time is the identification of more specific types of intervention that are appropriate for each particular infant.

THE NEONATAL INTENSIVE CARE UNIT

The neonatal intensive care unit is a busy, often crowded place where the atmosphere is frequently high-pressured.[39] Emergency life-and-death decisions are interspersed throughout the daily care routines for infants. A visitor to the unit is immediately struck by the complicated equipment (Figures 18-1 to 18-4). Each infant lies in an open warmer, an Isolette, or a crib. The open warmer allows easy access to the infant during the initial period after admission to the unit when many medical interventions are necessary. It also contains a heat source to keep the infant warm. The Isolette provides a neutral thermal environment for temperature maintenance, and as a contained area it allows the provision of supplementary oxygen when necessary. Mechanical ventilatory assistance (via respirator use) can be provided to infants in open warmers or in Isolettes. Once the infant is able to maintain his own body temperature and to tolerate room air, he will be moved to an open crib. Parents and staff then have easier access to the infant, and the infant can be more easily moved to other locations within the unit or outside the unit, for example, to and from the par-

ents' visiting room. Often attempts are made by parents and staff to personalize each infant's space through placement of toys and pictures.

There is an abundance of additional equipment that is used in caring for these infants and that adds to the complexity of the unit. Ventilators provide respiratory assistance to infants who are unable to sustain adequate respiratory patterns on their own. Cardiac monitors, apnea monitors, and oxygen monitors assist the staff with constant monitoring of vital signs. Since many infants are unable to receive adequate nutrition orally because of illness or immaturity, volumetric infusion pumps may be used to provide nutritional requirements through continuous nasojejunal (tube) feedings or through central alimentation (intravenously).

While some of the additional equipment has a diagnostic purpose (for example, the transilluminator, portable x-ray machine, electroencephalography [EEG] and ultrasound equipment), other equipment (for example, bright lights that provide phototherapy in the treatment of hyperbilirubinemia) is used in the treatment of specific medical problems. The infant himself, being necessarily attached to some of this equipment, most likely has skin electrodes placed on him to monitor his heart rate; may have an intravenous tube; may be on a respirator; or may have an orogastric or nasogastric tube in place for feeding. Obviously the effect

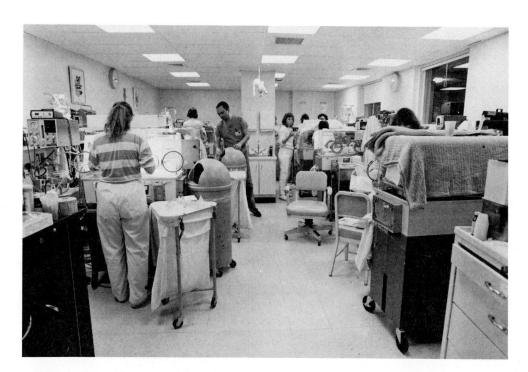

Figure 18-1   The neonatal intensive care unit.

Photo by Gregory Kriss, courtesy Neonatal Intensive Care Unit, University of Connecticut Health Center's John N. Dempsey Hospital, Farmington, Conn.

Cardiac monitor   Respirator   Oxygen monitor (T-com)

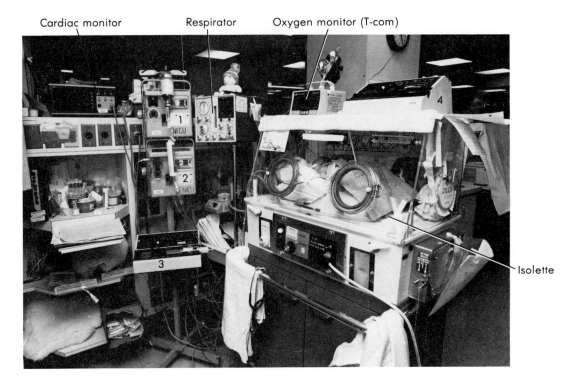

Isolette

1, 2, 3, 4-infusion pumps

Figure 18-2   Isolette and other neonatal equipment as indicated: *a,* Isolette; *b,* cardiac monitor; *c,* oxygen monitor (T-com); *d,* respirator; *e,* infusion pumps.

Photo by Gregory Kriss, courtesy Neonatal Intensive Care Unit, University of Connecticut Health Center's John N. Dempsey Hospital, Farmington, Conn.

may be overwhelming for parents who are already faced with the stress of the unexpected birth or an ill or premature infant.

Although the environment of the nursery is lifesaving, it can also be potentially overstimulating to the infant. The intense medical care required by the sicker infants often necessitates bright lighting around the clock. The various sounds and alarm signals of monitors and ventilators combine with ringing telephones, voices of staff and visitors, and cries of infants to maintain a fairly high noise level. The infants are also subjected to a variety of procedures, such as multiple examinations, radiography, and other tests including blood work, some tube feedings, and surgery, that can be considered invasive.

The general activity level of the nursery is high because of the multitude of services required by the infants. The subsequent number of personnel involved may include physicians, nurses, respiratory therapists, occupational therapists, physical therapists, x-ray and EEG technicians, aides, unit clerks, and volunteers. The number of people in the unit at any given time may be increased intermittently by the presence of parents taking advantage of the 24-hour visiting privileges.

Although the primary focus on the neonatal intensive care unit historically may have been on medical care for survival, growing concern has developed regarding more qualitative issues, many of which relate directly or indirectly to the ultimate question of developmental outcome. What are the long-term effects of the medical problems that caused the infant's hospitalization in an intensive care unit? What effect might such a difficult introduction to life have on growth and development? What is the role of early experiences and, in this case, the early experiences provided by prolonged hospitalization? How does the infant respond to the many and varied sensory stimuli, such as bright lights and loud noises, provided in the special care nursery? And what kinds of interventions or environmental adaptations can we make to provide the infant with an optimal setting for growth and development?

OCCUPATIONAL THERAPY INTERVENTION
Practice settings

With the increasing recognition of the importance of early identification and treatment of developmental

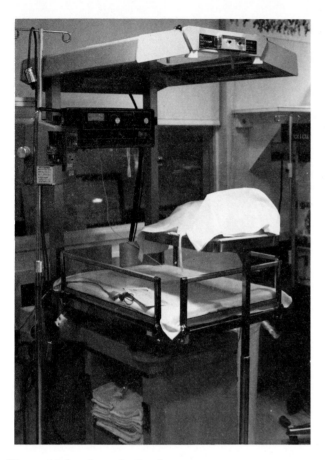

Figure 18-3 Open (radiant) warmer.

Photo courtesy Neonatal Intensive Care Unit, University of Connecticut Health Center's John N. Dempsey Hospital, Farmington, Conn.

risk factors, the services of allied health professionals, especially occupational and physical therapists, have been more consistently employed at facilities providing health care for high-risk infants. Earliest contact with these infants is made in the neonatal intensive care unit. Most neonatal intensive care units are attached to larger medical centers that can provide a variety of specialized services and follow-up care. After the initial intensive care hospitalization, infants requiring long-term hospitalization, but not continued intensive care, may be transferred to another unit within the facility such as a pediatric inpatient floor where occupational therapy services may continue to be provided. Further follow-up care is provided after discharge through the neonatal follow-up clinic. Here the services of an occupational therapist may be employed to provide developmental assessment at regular intervals during the early years of life. Typically, follow-up visits might be scheduled at the ages of 4, 8, 12, 18, and 24 months and annually until school age.

Because of the high level of technology required,

special care nurseries most often function on a regional basis. This means that admissions to a particular nursery may be from a widespread geographical region. Therefore, although a certain percentage of infants come from the immediate local area, a number of others are from outlying areas and have either been transported to the unit shortly after birth or have been delivered at the unit's medical center after maternal transport. Since parental visiting is often more difficult in these cases, the goal with such infants who need continued medical care is to transfer them back to local hospitals as soon as medically advisable. Therefore the length of stay at the neonatal intensive care unit or its related step-down nursery may be relatively short. Follow-up occupational therapy services may be necessary at the outlying hospital.

A certain number of infants seen in the neonatal intensive care unit have specific and identifiable deficits that may require continued intervention after discharge from the hospital. In some cases occupational therapy services can be provided on an outpatient basis at the medical center where often the same neonatal therapist can follow the child. In other cases occupational therapy services are most efficiently provided through local early intervention programs.

Role of the occupational therapist

In whatever setting, the multiple and varied needs of high-risk infants necessitates the involvement of a variety of professionals: physicians (including neonatologists, neurologists, ophthalmologists, and often other medical specialists), audiologists, nurses, occupational therapists, sometimes physical therapists, and social workers. Continuous interaction among these professionals is essential to providing complete and efficient care.

Because the professionals involved must work so closely, there is at times an overlap of specific caregiving roles. A concrete example is feeding. Although feeding is routinely an integral part of the nurse's role in caring for the infant, it often becomes a primary concern to the occupational therapist when the infant is having some difficulty in this area. The occupational therapist, nurse, and parents must collaborate in dealing with the problem. However, the specific responsibilities of the occupational therapist can be identified and categorized into four major areas: assessment, consultation, referral, and intervention. This categorization is applicable to both inpatient work in the neonatal intensive care unit itself and to follow-up care of infants after their discharge from the hospital. The individual importance of each area may vary in different settings.

ASSESSMENT

A primary service provided by the occupational therapist in the neonatal intensive care unit is assess-

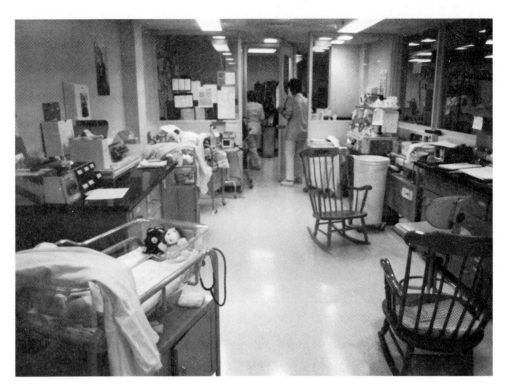

Figure 18-4　Newborn step-down nursery houses "graduates" of the neonatal intensive care unit. Of note are the more open environment, the quieter atmosphere, and open foreground.

Photo courtesy Neonatal Nursery, University of Connecticut Health Center's John N. Dempsey Hospital, Farmington, Conn.

ment (Figure 18-5). When the infant reaches a point of medical stability, initial evaluation from a developmental perspective can begin. A single evaluation visit is almost never satisfactory, and repeat visits invariably provide valuable additional information from which to determine a more accurate overall picture of the infant. For very small or young infants it is often impossible to complete a full developmental assessment in one visit because of the infant's intolerance of prolonged handling and stimulation. In this sense, *prolonged* may be a matter of only a few minutes.

Developmental assessment is also a primary role of the occupational therapist in the follow-up clinic. A transdisciplinary model for assessing young children is appropriate, efficient, and effective with this population. While sensory, perceptual, and motor competency may be of primary interest to the occupational therapist, it is important that the occupational therapist be able to expand the scope of the evaluation to gain a more global understanding of the child in the context of the family. Specific assessment techniques are discussed later in this chapter.

CONSULTATION

As information is gathered through the assessment process, sharing this information with parents and other staff and, at the same time, making suggestions for encouraging or facilitating appropriate responses and inhibiting abnormal responses becomes perhaps the second most important role of the occupational therapist. In this way the occupational therapist fulfills the role of consultant. Interventions that are appropriate for infants often fit best into routine caretaking procedures. Such interventions are more effective when provided on a consistent basis in a relaxed environment. Providing the infant's consistent caretakers—parents and nurses—with the information and skill that will benefit that infant may be the most efficient use of the therapist's time and the most effective means of reaching the infant. Specific areas often addressed are positioning, feeding, sensory stimulation, and motor development.

While in most settings a social worker will be available to help parents work through their feelings of anger, rejection, and mourning, it is not unusual for the occupational therapist to be called on to fill such a role. Working with the parents may involve helping them deal with their feelings of helplessness by providing them with instructions for specific activities that can be therapeutic. Involvement with the infant through such activities may assist them in overcoming feelings of helplessness, hopelessness, and the fear that

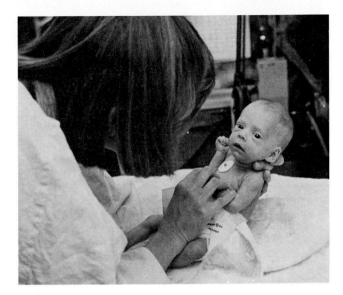

Figure 18-5 Assessment of premature infant.

Photo by Gregory Kriss, courtesy Neonatal Intensive Care Unit, University of Connecticut Health Center's John N. Dempsey Hospital, Farmington, Conn.

can be generated because of the infant's apparent fragility. Such therapeutic activities may include simple acts such as gentle stroking, slow rocking, or holding (cuddling). Experience shows that parents are in general very eager to actively contribute to their infant's care by providing developmentally relevant stimulation, and they are pleased to find that many of their own attempts to reach their infant through touching, holding, and cuddling are in fact appropriate and beneficial. In addition, the occupational therapist is often the most appropriate resource person to answer the many questions posed by parents regarding the current and future development of their infant. This can be done individually or in a group. Parents' groups afford the opportunity for parents to voice their questions and share their concerns among other parents whose infants are at various stages in their neonatal course. In this way the group can be a supportive and helpful resource to its participants. Developmental issues can be addressed by the occupational therapist at parent group meetings.

REFERRAL

Specific neurodevelopmental deficits that are interfering with normal function and development—for example, increased or decreased muscle tone, abnormal reflex activity, lack of alertness, and feeding problems—are identified in some infants during the course of their hospitalization. When these deficits continue at the time of discharge, it is appropriate to refer the infant for treatment after discharge. Questions regarding parental ability to provide nurturing experiences for their infant are also appropriate reasons for referral.

The parents' own desire to have ongoing guidance/information regarding their infant's development may be reason for referral as well. Most often such referrals are made to local early intervention programs and more specifically to the home-based infant program component. Infants being discharged to other hospitals may need referrals for occupational therapy follow-up through those hospitals.

INTERVENTION

There are some instances when direct intervention, other than assessment, is necessary. For example, an occupational therapist can be most effective in working directly with an infant who is medically and developmentally ready for feeding but experiencing difficulty because of poor sucking, swallowing, or some other neuromuscular, behavioral, or structural disorder. Other areas of direct treatment or intervention include organization of sensory stimuli for a specific sensorimotor deficit, positioning, facilitation and inhibition techniques, and range of motion for immobilized infants. In all cases, infants are assessed individually, and treatment programs are prescribed based on specific needs.

It is important to note that direct treatment never occurs in isolation. In any case in which direct treatment is necessary, it is always appropriate and also necessary to consult with staff and parents to assure carryover of the techniques prescribed and to facilitate continuity of care for the infant.

Characteristics of the therapist

Completion of an accredited professional curriculum is a basic requirement for eligibility for employment in a facility treating high-risk infants. Prior pediatric experience should be a prerequisite. Furthermore, given the nature and complexity of this field, it is recommended that therapists contemplating employment in such a setting become further acquainted with the field of fetal and infant development, as well as the psychology of parent-infant relationships.

The neonatal intensive care unit can be a demanding, stressful, and often unpredictable place. Although there is a certain amount of regularity in the routine care of the infant in the nursery, these routines are subject to unexpected change for a variety of reasons. Because of the nature and severity of the medical problems of many of these infants, the infants themselves are often unpredictable. As such, working with high-risk infants requires flexibility on the part of the therapist. It is necessary to coordinate occupational therapy visits with medical procedures, feeding schedules, and parent visits. It is absolutely essential to maintain a working relationship with the many other professionals involved, as well as with parents.

A final suggestion is that therapists working in intensive care nurseries should continue to see normal infants periodically to maintain an appropriate perspective regarding the developmental process.

NEONATAL ASSESSMENT

During the last 20 years our understanding of the newborn has undergone a tremendous change. Instead of being considered helpless, passive, reflex-bound and capable of little more than eating, sleeping, and crying, newborns are now considered to possess a number of well-organized behaviors and to be capable of molding their own environments. What then are some of the inborn capacities that the newborn child brings into the world?

The traditional, standardized neurological examination, such as that of Prechtl and Beintema,[54] was the prevalent tool available for looking at newborns. It considered only the physical and neurological status of the infant. With the increasing recognition of innate behavioral capacities, interactive behaviors and organized responses of the newborn are now recognized to be as significant as the neurological findings. Pioneering work in identifying, organizing, and quantifying these behavioral components has been done by Brazelton, culminating with his Neonatal Behavioral Assessment Scale.[10]

As medical technology improved, the focus shifted to the increasing numbers of low birth weight, preterm infants and the surviving distressed infants who filled the intensive care nurseries. Although the primary concerns regarding these infants will always be survival with minimal medical complications and subsequently adequate growth, more attention is being given to the preterm infant's *adaptive* behaviors[3] and his ability to meet the challenge of the extrauterine environment. The Assessment of Preterm Infant Behavior (APIB)[2] is an assessment tool created for research purposes. It defines and organizes these behavioral findings into a meaningful and useful schema. These, as well as some other measures, will be described more fully later in this chapter.

General considerations

A number of considerations apply to the administration of assessments in general. Any examination, however noninvasive, should be recognized as having a potential impact on the infant. While the goal of the examination is to gather valuable clinical information, for the infant the experience can be either therapeutic or stressful. Therefore procedures may have to be modified and carefully administered, depending on the individual infant's particular medical problems.

In addition to the infant's clinical problems, there are additional elements that need to be considered before each examination and noted to aid in the interpretation of findings:

1. State of the infant at the time of examination by use of Brazelton's definition of six states of sleep and arousal.[10]
2. Timing of the examination in relation to feeding. Specific recommendations may vary with each measure. About two thirds of the way between one feeding and the next, irrespective of the frequency of feeding, is generally considered an advisable time for many infants. However, this may not be true of the very premature infant who may be more likely to become alert one-half hour just before feeding.
3. Medication. Some drugs are frequently used in the intensive care nursery; their effects may vary according to amount and time of administration in relation to examination.
4. Unusual physical or environmental conditions. This includes many elements such as intravenous tubing or other elements the examiner feels may have a limiting effect on the examination.

There is general agreement in the literature that a single examination may, at best, offer a glimpse of an infant's clinical state. Repeated examinations, whether partial or complete, offer a much greater opportunity for accurate assessment and are preferred whenever possible, for it is the cumulative data over time that serve diagnostic and monitoring tasks of the occupational therapist.

In summary, a complete assessment should include:

1. Pertinent medical information, including history, physical and neurological data, and a list of present problems
2. Reported observations, as related by staff and parents
3. Observations of the infant at rest and during routine procedures, such as feeding, and diapering
4. Results of the examination
5. Summary of findings with a resulting impression

Specific neonatal assessments

There are a number of infant assessments available that require varying degrees of expertise and training. The specific type of assessment performed by occupational therapists may vary, depending on the needs within each nursery. Some of the more well-known tools with which the therapist should become familiar are described here.

The Brazelton Neonatal Behavioral Assessment Scale[10] was designed for the purpose of measuring the interactive capacity of the full-term infant. It differs from many other measures in that it strives to bring out the best of the rich repertoire of interactive behaviors of the newborn. Thus the examiner is encouraged to make every effort in that direction, rather than be bound to format. The scale measures the newborn's capacity to habituate to stimuli, regulate changes in state of consciousness (sleep and arousal), and respond to both animate and inanimate objects. It also measures the neuromotor integrity and physiological stability of the newborn. The scoring system is complex with 27 behavioral items to be scored on a 9-point scale and 20 reflex items scored on a 3-point scale. Reliability training is recommended for formal use of this scale.

The Neurological Assessment of the Preterm and Full-term Newborn Infant developed by Dubowitz and Dubowitz[20] is a comprehensive scale designed to measure the functional state of the central nervous system of the preterm and full-term infant. It considers the various stages of neurological maturation of the premature infant, as well as interactive capacity of the newborn. This assessment was found to be more comprehensive than the classical neurological assessments like that of Prechtl and Beintema[54] because of the addition of the interactive behavior component. Directions and scoring are well-illustrated and simplified to make it more accessible for routine examinations by medical staff.

The Assessments of Preterm Infant Behavior (APIB)[2], which was based on Brazelton's work, is a rather complex instrument designed for research purposes. It requires extensive training for its administration and scoring. The underlying concepts, however, contribute very valuable information regarding the preterm infant's early stages of behavioral organization. It also provides a rich and comprehensive description of the vast array of observations in the physiological, motor, attentional-interactive, and regulatory systems, and general state of the infant by interpreting and organizing them meaningfully. The scale is divided into six packages, each one placing specific graded demands on the infant and measuring the effect of these on a number of subsystems.

Other neonatal assessments not described here include the Clinical Assessment of Gestational Age in the Newborn Infant,[19] the Neurological Examination of the Full-term Newborn Infant,[53] and the Graham Rosenblith Behavioral Examination for Newborns.[57]

Although there are no published or formal occupational therapy assessments of the newborn, the following was developed to meet the needs of the occupational therapists at the University of Connecticut Health Center intensive care nursery. The Occupational Therapy Neonatal Assessment (OTNA) represents one system of organizing a number of findings that are considered relevant and appropriate to the role of the occupational therapist in the intensive care nursery. Many of the items are derived from Brazelton's work.[10] A number of other authors[1,48,65,67] have contributed to our understanding of the significance of developmental assessment findings. The assessment form of the Occupational Therapy Neonatal Assessment (not provided here) is divided into four parts, each one outlined and clarified:

1. Part 1 includes any pertinent medical history and information about the infant.
   a. Name, sex, and date of birth
   b. Gestational age (GA) and weight at birth
   c. Conceptional age: Refers to gestational age plus time in weeks since birth.
   d. Prenatal complications: Refers to any fetal or maternal factors, such as maternal history of drug abuse or intrauterine growth retardation of the fetus, which have occurred before the birth process and are likely to be related to the infant's present state.
   e. Birth information: Refers to the type of delivery and any complications at or around the time of birth.
   f. Apgar scores: Refers to the scoring system devised by Apgar.[6]
   g. Medical complications: Refers to any of the common medical problems listed in Table 18-1 and their supporting diagnostic data.
   h. Present medication
   i. Other factors affecting assessment
2. Part 2 consists of the list of observations made during the examination. It is separate from the rest, and it may be used for repeated or periodic examinations.
   a. Habituation: Refers to the "infant's capacity to decrease responses to repeated disturbing stimuli."[10] Lack of this function may be indicative of hyperexcitability of the central nervous system and should be considered worrisome.
   b. State transitions or patterns: State refers to the infant's state of consciousness. There are six states as defined by Brazelton that cover the continuum between sleep and crying. Observations regarding rapidity of buildup and smoothness in transition between one state and another, as well as observations regarding regularity and predictability of sleep-wake cycles, are noted here. It is not uncommon for preterm infants to have irregular sleep patterns. Such information may be particularly helpful to parents.
   c. Alertness: Refers to state four according to Brazelton's scale,[10] a period when the infant is most available to interactive behavior. Periods of alertness may vary from fleeting moments, which is characteristic of the very premature infant, to sustained periods exhibited by the more intact and mature infant.
   d. Orienting behavior: Refers to the infant's capacity to turn toward the examiner (or other person) in response to a combination of sensory stimuli. An orienting response may be useful in facilitating the attachment process for infants with decreased visual and auditory responses.
   e. Consolability: Refers to the infant's capacity to quiet following a period of crying. The degree of intervention necessary to help the infant to quiet is usually noted, and it may be indicative of the infant's ability to regulate state changes.
   f. Sensory responses: Auditory, visual, tactile, vestibular, pain, and olfactory. The infant's responses

in each of the sensory systems are considered separately. For the visual and auditory responses, animate or inanimate stimuli may be presented. Observations regarding the tactile and vestibular senses are arrived at by noting the infant's responses to handling and changes in position during the examination. Observations regarding pain can be reported by nurses. A bottle of common extract such as orange or mint can be used to assess olfactory responses.

g. Muscle tone: Passive and active; trunk and shoulders; lower extremities; and upper extremities. Passive tone refers to the infant's position at rest as described by Dubowitz.[19] Active tone refers to the infant's general tone following handling. There is usually a significant change in tone in response to a number of sensory experiences. Proximal muscles (trunk, neck, and shoulders) are examined separately from the extremities. Consistent signs of asymmetries as well as hypertonia or hypotonia are described.

h. Motor responses: Spontaneous activity, quality of movements, and reflexes. Spontaneous activity refers to the amount or frequency of activity exhibited by the infant in between specific maneuvers. Jittery, flailing, smooth, clonic, and organized movements are terms used in describing the quality of movements. A number of neonatal reflexes as described by Barnes, Crutchfield, and Heriza[7] are tested. These include the asymmetrical tonic neck reflex (ATNR), Moro reflex, gag reflex, rooting reflex, sucking-swallowing, palmar grasp, plantar grasp, Galant reflex (trunk incurvation), positive support, stepping, and placing. Deep tendon reflexes are also evaluated. Absent or significant decrease in motor response is often seen in very distressed infants.

i. Feeding: Refers to the infant's ability to take adequate amounts of nutritive liquid by sucking (at times observations may be initiated before actual use of a nipple). All aspects of feeding are considered, including appropriate oral reflexes, muscle tone, and interactive behavior.

j. Medication: It is important to record medications being administered, particularly those that may have an effect on the assessment.

k. Observations/precautions: Any other factors that may affect the assessment are recorded. Precautions are included.

l. Impressions: The information gathered is summarized and interpreted.

m. Recommendations.

3. Part 3 includes pertinent family and social information.

   a. Family information including names, addresses, and phone numbers.

   b. Family composition including ages and relationships of significant others.

c. Significant information about the family including availability of family members for visits to the nursery.

4. Part 4 provides space for a summarizing descriptive paragraph.

   a. Summary

   b. Disposition

In addition to the general considerations discussed earlier, there are some specific guidelines for using Part 2 of the Occupational Therapy Neonatal Assessment regarding procedure and scoring. Although the items are listed in the sequence in which they are usually presented to the infant, the examiner need not feel bound to the order or the number of items to be presented at any given time. Descriptive scoring is used in this form, although a quantifiable scale could be added.

Indications for use of assessment measures

Although each individual test may have been designed for a specific purpose, the examination of the infant and the findings may be used to implement a number of different objectives.

DIAGNOSTIC CONSIDERATIONS

Diagnostic interpretation of findings is never an easy task, particularly with preterm or distressed infants whose changes in status are very unpredictable and occur more rapidly than in any other newborn population. As indicated before, findings derived from a single examination should be interpreted with more caution than those derived from repeated observations over time. It is not uncommon for the examiner to encounter variations of responses in the same infant, but the cumulative data will help to identify the typical as well as the optimal responses of any given infant. This approach will require scheduling flexibility and may be less efficient, but in the end it will provide more reliable and useful information for discharge planning.

Although most therapists agree that the continuum between what is considered normal and abnormal cannot be easily defined, some guidelines for recognizing this continuum in relation to infants are necessary.

1. Normal: This qualifier should be used to describe all those findings that are consistent with the expected level of function for the conceptional age (the gestational age of the infant at birth with the number of weeks since birth added to it) of the infant. For information regarding age-appropriate behaviors, reference can be made to a variety of authors who have described the normal process of development (Chapter 4).

2. Worrisome or suspect: This term should be used to describe most of the findings that are not considered appropriate for conceptional age. They may range from minimal to significant.

3. Abnormal: This term should be used only with

observations obtained from repeated examinations over a prolonged period of time to describe the pathological extreme of any given response. This term should be used preferably when observations are supported by additional diagnostic data, for example, electroencephalography or computerized tomography (CT scan).

CONSIDERATIONS FOR REFERRAL

The plasticity of the central nervous system and its ability to recover from a number of insults is the basis for most of the therapeutic intervention theories. Recent advances regarding fetal development of the central nervous system suggest periods when certain neurological functions may be more vulnerable[31] and therefore more susceptible to trauma. With the information available to date, it has not been possible to predict the severity or degree of the sequelae. However, some of the findings suggest the possibility of problems in certain functional areas such as with hypotonia, which is likely to affect motor development.

Yet, like many other professionals involved in the discharge planning of the vulnerable or at-risk infant, the occupational therapist is often asked to make decisions regarding intervention, implying a predictive value to the assessment information.

Both abnormal and worrisome findings should be considered valid reasons for recommending therapeutic or other intervention. Thus, depending on the degree and nature of the problems, as well as on parental preference, the therapist may recommend: (1) making a referral for early intervention, (2) instructing parents until a later reassessment, or (3) recommending an early follow-up appointment. The importance of considering the readiness of the parents when making discharge plans cannot be overemphasized. The parents' understanding of the nature and ramifications of the problem, as well as their psychological readiness, will play an important role in making the referral more meaningful and acceptable to the family. The eventual success or failure of intervention may depend on the family's attitude and understanding.

THERAPEUTIC CONSIDERATIONS FOR THE INFANT AND PARENTS

Intrinsic to each examination is its therapeutic potential. This is often not given due consideration by those whose primary objective is to gather accurate and sufficient observation. It is possible, however, to carry out examinations that provide the infant with a positive and organizing experience. Recognizing the many and varied signs of stress that may be very subtle in the preterm infant is the first step in that direction. Allowing for sufficient time between maneuvers to permit the infant to reorganize himself and to return to an "available" state[3] is one technique that will more likely result in a therapeutic experience.

Widmayer and Field[74] describe how enriching an experience it is for parents to observe the assessment of their infant with the use of the Brazelton scale. In fact, it has been described as the single most useful form of intervention with some parents who are considered to be at risk for disturbances in the attachment process. While this is generally true in the case of healthy term infants, there are also many instances when it can be beneficial in the neonatal intensive care unit. It is important that the therapist recognize that such an experience, while informative, may be distressing or delightful, depending on the parents' interpretation of responses and their general perception of their infant. It is advisable to omit certain items when examining preterm or distressed infants in front of their parents because of their obvious distressful effect. This may include response to painful stimuli and a number of reflexes including the gag and Moro reflexes.

Specific maneuvers from various test items can be used to teach parents ways of eliciting certain responses in their infants. For example, alertness can be increased with vestibular stimulation. With infants who are exhibiting some worrisome findings, such as obligatory assymetrical tonic neck reflex, irritability, and inefficient sucking, the examination may provide an opportunity to give the parents suggestions for positioning and other facilitating or inhibiting techniques that may be appropriate to the situation.

Although research considerations will not be discussed here, the opportunities for research in the field of neonatology are vast and should be considered by the occupational therapist engaged in observing infant behavior.

CONSIDERATIONS FOR INTERVENTION WITH HIGH-RISK INFANTS
Precautions

Two major considerations must be taken into account in dealing with the high-risk infant: temperature regulation and stress tolerance. Cold exposure can cause increase in metabolic rate and oxygen consumption with resulting increase in oxygen requirement, acidosis, apnea, hypoglycemia, and possibly pulmonary hemorrhage. To keep the infant warm, it may be necessary to be sure he is adequately covered when out of the Isolette. Or, in some cases, it may be necessary to work with the infant inside the Isolette.

Many high-risk infants can tolerate only limited amounts of handling or stimulation. Therefore the therapist must be sensitive to each infant's level of tolerance and must watch for signs of stress. At the point of occurrence of one or more of these signs, it may be necessary to terminate the assessment or treatment at least temporarily. Unnecessary stress or fatigue should be avoided.

Signs of stress in the high-risk infant:
1. Physiological
   a. Color changes including circumoral cyanosis and mottling of the skin

b. Marked increase or decrease in respiratory rate or rhythm
c. Change in heart rate (bradycardia or tachycardia)
2. Gastrointestinal
   a. Spitting or vomiting
   b. Hiccups
   c. Bowel movement
3. Motor
   a. Unexpected or sudden changes in muscle tone (limpness or stiffening)
   b. Sudden changes in quality of movement (jittery, flailing, disorganized movements)
4. Behavioral
   a. Sudden fussiness
   b. Gaze aversion

Guidelines for intervention

There is much controversy in the literature regarding the effectiveness of "infant stimulation." There is some evidence that supplemental stimulation has positive clinical and developmental effects. There is also evidence that eliminating some noxious stimuli and organizing caretaking activities may have positive effects. However, there is not enough data as to the type, amount, and timing of such experiences that would be of most benefit for each infant.[4] It is apparent that the answers to these questions will vary for each infant and his individual needs. In any case, it would seem desirable to provide treatment to encourage developmentally appropriate responses and to reduce inappropriate responses. This type of approach to intervention with developmentally vulnerable infants has been referred to as "developmental support."[68]

The goals of early developmental support as such are to "1) enhance parent/infant interaction thus providing a secure base for a future parent/child relationship; 2) facilitate the infant's own adjustments to his environment; and 3) facilitate the infant's acquisition of developmental skills" (p. 3).[68] In a more specific sense, we might add to this list the facilitation of normal patterns of movement and muscle tone, as well as the enhancement of appropriate sensory and motor responses. Specific intervention techniques, outlined in the following sections, can be accomplished at different levels by therapists, parents, and nurses. These suggestions are by no means all-inclusive. It should be remembered that each infant must be considered individually, and only those techniques appropriate to each infant's gestational age, medical status, and central nervous system maturity should be used.

LEVEL OF ALERTNESS

Premature infants spend the greatest portion of each day in a sleep state. There are, however, brief periods of alertness that occur periodically. It is during these periods of alertness that the infant is available for interaction with caregivers and ready to receive some type of sensory stimulation, particularly visual stimulation. With maturation, the normal developmental process allows for increasingly frequent and more sustained periods of alertness. For many high-risk infants, this process is delayed, altered, or interrupted. Small for gestational age infants and infants who have suffered specific neurological insults frequently fall into this group of infants who demonstrate less than optimal levels of alertness.

At one end of the continuum may be infants with infrequent or lack of sustained periods of alertness. These infants may also be difficult to arouse. At the other extreme, an infant may be hyperexcitable, hyperresponsive, or hyperirritable. These infants commonly experience significant difficulties in the interactive area. Self-quieting behaviors, such as hand-to-mouth movements and positional changes, may also be diminished. In either case, the result of deficits in the ability to sustain alert periods can include interactive difficulties, feeding problems, and sensorimotor deficits.

Intervention guidelines for arousal and state transition (alertness)
1. To facilitate a quiet-alert state.
   a. Swaddle.
   b. Gently restrain flailing arms across chest.
   c. Work in dimly lit, quiet room.
   d. Gently rock into a more upright position.
2. To facilitate self-quieting and behavioral organization.
   a. Swaddle.
   b. Help infant suck on his hand, fingers, or on a pacifier.
   c. Reduce level of stimulation in the environment (lights, sounds).
3. To bring infant to an alert state.
   a. Unwrap.
   b. Bring to semi-upright position.
   c. Provide sensory stimulation through voice, touch, and movement.

MUSCLE TONE

Muscle tone develops in a caudocephalic (toe to head) direction and is a function of maturity of the neuromuscular system. The more immature infant is characterized by hypotonia or reduced muscle tone (Figure 18-6). Because of this hypotonia, the premature infant assumes a relatively extended posture that, with the added effects of gravity, leads to the development of a predominance of extensor tone. The full-term infant is born in a flexed posture with a predominance of flexor tone (Figure 18-7). The premature infant rarely develops this same degree of flexor tone but can still develop normally.

High-risk infants (term and premature) are often prone to abnormal tone patterns.[28,29] These abnormalities may result from prolonged immobility resulting from medical complications, from specific neuromus-

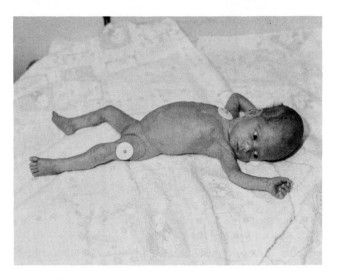

Figure 18-6   Premature infant, resting posture.

Photo by Gregory Kriss, courtesy Neonatal Intensive Care Unit, University of Connecticut Health Center's John N. Dempsey Hospital, Farmington, Conn.

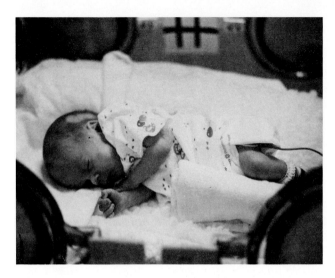

Figure 18-8   Supportive position in sidelying.

Photo by Gregory Kriss, courtesy Neonatal Intensive Care Unit, University of Connecticut Health Center's John N. Dempsey Hospital, Farmington, Conn.

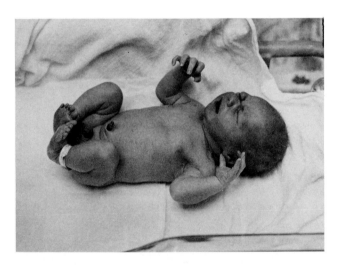

Figure 18-7   Full-term infant, resting posture.

Photo by Gregory Kriss, courtesy Neonatal Intensive Care Unit, University of Connecticut Health Center's John N. Dempsey Hospital, Farmington, Conn.

cular disorders, or from other causes. Persistence of abnormal postures can interfere with later development of normal head control, oculomotor skills, eye-hand coordination, mobility, interpersonal interaction, sitting, and standing. It is therefore essential to interrupt abnormal posture patterns through positioning and other techniques. Many of these techniques are appropriate also for the normally developing premature infant (the growing preemie) to facilitate the development of flexor tone and prevent the development of abnormal patterns that may potentially result from the imbalance of flexor and extensor tone. It should be noted that many of these positioning techniques also have an organizing effect on the behavior of the infant and subsequently allow better potential for self-quieting, developing body awareness, and developing organized movement patterns.

Intervention guidelines for muscle tone

1. To facilitate the development of flexor tone and prevent overstretching of joints resulting from generalized decreased tone.
   a. Position in sidelying. Use rolled blanket behind infant's head and trunk. For additional support, add smaller roll in front of infant's chest and abdomen over which top leg can be placed (Figure 18-8). A blanket over infant and tucked under mattress will keep infant in position.
   b. Place infant in semiflexed position in the supine position. The low tone infant will need considerable support. Place infant on a blanket, each end of which has been rolled. Place rolled diaper under bottom of blanket to support knees. Individual blanket rolls, as illustrated in Figure 18-9 can also be used. It is customary to cover these rolls with a blanket or sheepskin sheet to form a "blanket cradle." Side rolls will support head near midline. Keep shoulders semiprotracted, and prevent external rotation of lower extremities (frog-leg position). Can use stuffed animals instead of rolls.
   c. In infant seat, rolled blankets should also be used at sides to keep head in midline and prevent ex-

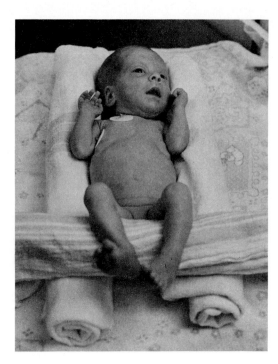

Figure 18-9 Supportive components in supine position.

Photo by Gregory Kriss, courtesy Neonatal Intensive Care Unit, University of Connecticut Health Center's John N. Dempsey Hospital, Farmington, Conn.

cessive abduction and external rotation of upper and lower extremities, as well as retraction of shoulders.

d. Swaddle.

e. Place rolled diaper under chest and hip area to facilitate flexion in the prone position.

FEEDING

Although sucking and swallowing begin very early in fetal life, it is not until 32 to 34 weeks gestational age that a coordinated pattern of sucking and swallowing is strong enough and can be sustained for a long enough period to allow adequate nutritional intake. (This does not imply that preterm infants should be introduced to the nipple at this time.) Medical complications and certain treatment procedures may interfere with this process. Immature infants who require tube feedings or nonnutritive treatment procedures, such as suctioning, may develop hypersensitivity in the oral area, which may develop into later feeding problems (refusal of nipple). Normal sucking patterns may be interrupted by medical equipment used in treatment, for example, the endotracheal tube that is placed in the provision of mechanical ventilatory support. Sucking that does occur may disappear because of lack of use or lack of reward from use. An acutely ill infant may not be able to suck and swallow because of poor tone or rapid fatigue. Other infants may lack the muscle coordina-

tion required for sucking because of neurological or other impairments, or both. The potential causes for impaired oral feeding with an infant who is otherwise medically and gestationally ready are many and varied.[14] Some fairly simple facilitation techniques can be easily incorporated into the infant's routine care to facilitate the normal development of sucking and at the same time perhaps enhance the digestive process in general.

Intervention guidelines for feeding

1. To facilitate sucking-swallowing in premature infants.
    a. Encourage sucking during tube feedings (pacifier).
2. To facilitate use of the nipple for the infant who is developmentally ready for oral feeding.
    a. Position infant semireclined with head in neutral, arms and shoulders forward, and lower extremities semi-flexed (swallowing will be difficult if not impossible if the head or neck is excessively flexed or extended).
    b. Select nipple of appropriate size for the infant's mouth and of the appropriate resiliency to allow moderate flow of liquid into the mouth.
3. To prevent fatigue.
    a. Allow rest periods in between sucking bursts. Do not push too hard. Rest periods are normal.
4. To facilitate sucking when infant appears unresponsive but not fatigued.
    a. Gently move nipple partially in and out of mouth.
    b. Rotate nipple in mouth.
    c. Stroke firmly under chin (back to front) during feeding.
    d. When indicated, provide supportive jaw control by placing your thumb and index finger on either side of the mandible with your middle finger flexed under the infant's chin.
5. To facilitate swallow.
    a. Stroke gums to increase saliva flow and facilitate swallow.
    b. Stroke *gently,* bilaterally on front of throat.
6. To facilitate lip closure.
    a. Intraoral and perioral stimulation before feeding (stroking, tapping, quick stretch to lips).
    b. Supportive jaw control as described above.
7. To reduce tongue thrust.
    a. Supply firm pressure by finger or nipple on tongue.
    b. Avoid stimulation of tip of tongue when approaching mouth with nipple.

SENSORY RESPONSES

One of the first questions asked by many parents is "When will my baby be able to see?" We know that full-term infants are able to visually fixate on and follow objects and that they prefer faces to objects. This behavior is very rewarding to parents and others who are interacting with the infant. This ability is not consistently seen in premature infants, and some high-risk infants actually tend to exhibit more gaze-averting behavior. As a result, parents' interactions with their high-risk infants often are not rewarding and can be frustrating. Their concern can be alleviated somewhat by the knowledge of the course of normal development in this area and perhaps by suggestions of activities to enhance the infant's alertness and visual responsiveness.

The high-risk infant can be hyperresponsive or hyporesponsive to other types of sensory stimulation. Some infants appear to be oversensitive to sound, touch, or movement. Others appear to respond very little, if at all, to these types of input. Olfaction is another sensory function that is often overlooked. Close observation is necessary in this area. In some cases, carefully graded presentation of such stimulation singly or in various combinations, perhaps coupled with environmental adaptations, may enhance appropriate sensory responses. In addition, various types of sensory stimuli can be used in treatment to enhance appropriate functional responses in many cases. For example, tactile stimuli can be used to enhance muscle tone; olfactory stimuli can be used in the treatment of feeding disorders.

Intervention guidelines for sensory responses

1. To decrease hypersensitivity to touch or movement.
   a. Avoid sudden movements.
   b. Approach infant in slow, gentle manner.
   c. Swaddle.
   d. Touch with pressure rather than light touch.
   e. Gradual introduction of graded tactile stimuli.
2. To decrease hypersensitivity to sound.
   a. Avoid loud noises that may startle infant, for example, slamming Isolette porthole doors.
   b. Gradually introduce different sounds—use musical toys.
3. To increase visual responses.
   a. Place toys in Isolette in infant's line of vision.
   b. Encourage parents, staff, and others to move their faces in infant's line of vision when interacting with infant.

Intervention guidelines for other responses

1. To facilitate parent-infant interaction.
   a. Encourage early, active involvement of parents by teaching them developmentally appropriate stimulation techniques, for example, stroking, rocking, oral facilitation.
   b. Encourage positioning during feeding that allows eye-to-eye contact.
   c. Demonstrate to parents the infant's interactional capacities as they develop.
   d. Allow for the parents' expression of negative feelings.
2. To prevent flattening of the head from prolonged positioning on one side.
   a. Support head closer to midline by using props at various points of contact (use rolled blankets, stuffed animals, etc.).

CASE STUDY

Susie was born at a local hospital at 30 weeks' gestational age after a pregnancy that was uncomplicated until the onset of premature labor. The delivery was vaginal with breech presentation. Apgar scores were 1 at 1 minute, and 5 at 5 minutes. Birth weight, length, and head circumference were appropriate for gestational age. Susie was transported to the neonatal intensive care unit because of prematurity and respiratory distress.

Susie required mechanical ventilatory support for 2½ months because of chronic lung disease. She remained on supplementary oxygen after extubation and after discharge from the hospital. She developed cardiac problems shortly after birth and went into respiratory arrest at 10 days of age. Initial diagnosis was patent ductus arteriosus, which was resolved without surgical treatment, but cardiomegaly persisted. Intermittent seizurelike activity was noted early on, and treatment consisted of anticonvulsant medication. Although initial electroencephalograms and CT scans were abnormal (showing evidence of an intraventricular hemorrhage), at the time of discharge both were within normal limits, and head circumference was growing appropriately. Grade II-III retrolental fibroplasia was diagnosed by the ophthalmologist, but it was improving by discharge time. Results of audiology evaluation were age-appropriate. Susie also had hyperbilirubinemia, which was treated with phototherapy.

In summary, Susie's major perinatal problems included prematurity; breech presentation, respiratory distress, hyaline membrane disease with bronchopulmonary dysplasia (chronic lung disease); respiratory arrest; recurrent cardiac arrhythmia; cor pulmonale; patent ductus arteriosus; intraventricular hemorrhage; asphyxia; and retrolental fibroplasia. Among the procedures used in her treatment were endotracheal intubation, oxygen therapy, mechanical assisted ventilation, umbilical catheterization, echocardiogram, electrocardiogram, electroencephalogram, CT scan, phototherapy, lumbar puncture, multiple blood gas tests, and multiple medications.

Susie was referred to occupational therapy 6 weeks after birth (at 36 weeks conceptional age) because of concern about motor development and general level of responsiveness resulting from her complicated medical course and apparent neurological symptoms. Initial assessment was limited, because she was on a respirator at the time. Muscle tone was generally decreased with the exception of increased trunk and neck extensor tone noted during intermittent arching. Findings were discussed with the nursing staff, and various methods of positioning were suggested to decrease trunk arching and to maintain Susie in a more functional position by facilitating a semiflexed posture.

Susie was followed almost daily over the next several weeks so that organized patterns of sensory stimulation, maintenance of appropriate positioning, and continuing evaluation could be provided. The parents were involved early, and the results of the evaluation as well as treatment recommendations were discussed. The parents were eager to participate in Susie's care in anyway they could, and they were responsive to the suggestions made.

Susie had early problems with nutrition secondary to fluid restriction imposed during treatment of cardiac problems. She was maintained on intravenous hyperalimentation until 3 to 4 weeks after birth when nasojejunal feedings were begun. Approximately 2½ months after birth intermittent orogastric feedings were started, and oral feedings began soon after at 3 months. Susie initially had some difficulty accepting the nipple, as well as difficulty handling the fluid once in her mouth. She frequently gagged on the formula. During this time occupational therapy goals were expanded to include improvement of feeding skills. Susie's treatment program included oral facilitation techniques and positioning recommendations (semiupright, semiflexed with extremities toward midline), since she continued to assume a position of neck and trunk hyperextension, which is not a suitable feeding position. Changes were made in the consistency of the formula (by thickening it with rice cereal) to facilitate the swallowing process. She made slow progress but finally began to accept all feedings orally. She continued, however, to be a slow feeder.

In summary, the major focus of occupational therapy with Susie centered on the following areas:

1. *Personal-social-emotional.* As a long-term patient, Susie was generally at high risk for developmental problems in this area. The active participation of her parents was very important in this regard. Additional concerns during her hospitalization included decreased level of alertness, decreased interactive ability, and decreased tolerance for interaction-stimulation. The gradual introduction of playful handling at times other than feeding times and the gentle introduction of various types of stimulation, such as slow rocking, were used by her parents, therapist, and nurses in an effort to improve her function in this area.

2. *Orientation.* Because of early inconsistent auditory and visual responsiveness and the subsequent diagnosis of retrolental fibroplasia, there was a period of serious concern in this area. It was suggested that Susie have toys in her Isolette and that auditory stimuli be combined with visual stimuli in approaching her, for example, using combined face and voice or musical toys. Concern was resolved by discharge time, and Susie was following face and objects 180 degrees and responding appropriately to sounds. Some strabismus did continue but was later corrected by surgery.

3. *Motor development.* Trunk arching; generally decreased tone with increased extensor tone during arching and later increased extensor tone in the lower extremities; decreased head control with poor trunk and neck stability; and some tongue thrusting were some of the specific findings leading to concern in this area. Parents and staff followed through with suggested activities, such as positioning, swaddling, and playing with her in the reclined position and later in the more upright position. These activities aimed to reduce the effects of the motor problems that continued at the time of discharge.

4. *Feeding.* Intermittent tongue thrusting, apparently increased oral sensitivity with refusal of the nipple, and gagging on formula led to concern in this area. Perioral and intraoral stimulation and other oral facilitation techniques were coupled with changes in formula consistency to improve feeding ability. Basic positioning during feeding was also addressed. By discharge time, Susie was feeding slowly but acceptably.

After a long and complicated medical course, Susie was discharged home 6 months after birth at which time she was 3½ months corrected age. Muscle tone continued to be slightly decreased with continued intermittent trunk arching. Head control was poor to fair. Reflex responses were generally within normal limits; however, bilateral sustained ankle clonus continued. Sensory responses (including visual, auditory, tactile, and vestibular) were within normal limits. Although periods of lethargy continued, general level of alertness had improved, and Susie was able to maintain sustained periods of alertness at times. Activity level remained low to moderate. She had begun to coo and make sounds, but no laughing or squealing was noted. She had established consistent hand-to-mouth movement with insertion of her thumb in her mouth. There was no midline hand activity. She had begun to show interest in toys and reached for them with no grasp.

Follow-up plans included participation in a neonatal follow-up clinic with the first visit scheduled 1 month after discharge (earlier than the routine 4-month visit), referral to a home-based early intervention program, and cardiac and ophthalmological follow-ups.

At the time of her last follow-up clinic visit, Susie was chronologically 2½ years old. Following hospital discharge she had five rehospitalizations for respiratory problems and one for corrective eye surgery (for bilateral strabismus). Home visits by team members of the early intervention program to which she was referred were discontinued after about 1 year but were reinstituted about 1 year after that. She made slow but consistent developmental progress, monitored through regularly scheduled visits to the neonatal follow-up clinic.

Susie was then ambulating independently, feeding herself (preferred finger foods but was able to use a fork and spoon), saying a few words (some clearly understood), and was developing appropriate self-care and social skills. A generalized developmental delay of about 4 to 6 months was apparent at this point. Poor fine motor skills, poor eye-hand coordination, continued decreased muscle tone, and speech delay were signs of generalized delay. The poor quality of many of these skills, rather than their existence or nonexistence, contributed to her developmental findings.

Susie's parents were considering preschool nursery placement to provide for her programming needs and to help all three of them (Susie, Mom, and Dad) with the separation-individuation process. After the age of 3 special services will continue through the local school system.

SUMMARY

In considering the role of the occupational therapist with the high-risk infant, the controversy that exists over the effectiveness of early intervention must be recognized, particularly as it relates to the growing involvement of allied health professionals in nurseries and neonatal intensive care units. The neonatal intensive care unit is a busy, at times hectic, stressful place where the greatest precautions must be taken to protect vulnerable infants already at considerable risk because of prematurity and medical problems.

Although attention to the infant's medical status and survival rightfully takes priority, it should not be to the exclusion of other needs more closely related to the quality of life. While there are genetic and maturational bases for individual differences in both rate and pattern of development, there is growing evidence that environmental conditions during the prenatal and perinatal periods and the early years of life have a determining impact on the intellectual, affective, and sensorimotor development of the human infant. This is particularly relevant for the increasing numbers of infants born at risk with central nervous system dysfunction associated with such conditions as malnutrition, drug effects, prematurity infection, respiratory distress, and hyperbilirubinemia. Initially the high-risk infant is exposed to a somewhat distorted somatosensory environment, and often the crucial mother-infant interaction is severely disrupted. Both somatosensory experience and maternal-infant attachment have been identified as playing crucial roles in infant development.

Although further research is needed in this area, the implication is that the environment must make available the right type of stimulation at the right time for the optimal development of the infant. The role of the health care provider, in particular the occupational therapist, is to provide organization in the amount, quality, and kinds of stimulation to maximize developmental potential. For intervention to be consistently effective, it must be individualized to the requirements of each situation.

Occupational therapists have extensive knowledge of developmental processes and the sensory systems influencing those processes. They can contribute to the neonatal intensive care unit primarily by providing (1) individual assessment from a neurodevelopmental perspective, identifying the infant's unique pattern of strengths and vulnerabilities in terms of both rate and adequacy of developmental trends; (2) consultation with other nursery staff to adapt the environment and manipulate the infant's early experiences with the understanding of his needs and response capabilities to provide for optimal development; (3) consultation with parents to give additional information at their level regarding the neurodevelopmental status of their infant, to provide support to facilitate parent-infant attachment, and to use parents as the primary intervenors; (4) information to the team to assist in the early identification of risk status and the potential need for early intervention both on the unit and in the community after discharge (making referrals to community agencies as appropriate); and (5) direct service in cases of "functional deficits" (for example, feeding disorders, specific neurological deficits, and orthopedic deformities), therapeutic programs, and instruction of parents and staff on appropriate therapeutic techniques. With these considerations in mind, the role of

an occupational therapist on the neonatal intensive care unit is a positive step toward the delivery of more comprehensive health care.

STUDY QUESTIONS

1. What is the occupational therapist's role in the neonatal intensive care unit and why is it important?
2. Are infants in the neonatal care unit under- or over-stimulated? Explain.
3. Name five signs of stress to consider in working with high-risk infants. Indicate why consideration of signs of stress is important.

REFERENCES AND SELECTED READINGS

1. Als H, and Brazelton B: A new model of assessing behavioral organization in preterm and full-term infants. J Am Acad Child Psychiatry 20:239, 1981.
2. Als H, and others: Manual for the Assessment of Preterm Infant Behavior (API). In Fitzgerald H, Lester B, and Yogman M, editors: Theory and research in behavioral pediatrics, vol 1, New York, Plenum Publishing Corp. (In press)
3. Als H, and others: Toward a research instrument for the Assessment of Preterm Infants' Behavior (APIB). In Fitzgerald H, Lester B, and Yogman M, editors: Theory and research in behavioral pediatrics, vol 1, New York, 1982, Plenum Publishing Corp.
4. Anderson J: Sensory intervention with the preterm infant in the neonatal intensive care unit, Am J Occup Ther 40:19, 1986.
5. Andre-Thomas AJ, and others: The neurological examination of the infant, Little Club Clinics in Developmental Medicine, No 1, 1960.
6. Apgar V: A proposal for a new method of evaluation of the newborn infant, Curr Res Anesthes Analges 32:260, 1953.
7. Barnes M, Crutchfield C, and Heriza C: The neurophysiologic basis of patient treatment. Vol II: Reflexes in motor development, Morgantown, WV, 1979, Stokesville Publishing Co.
8. Bowlby J: Grief and mourning in infancy and early childhood, Psychoanal Study Child 15:9, 1960.
9. Braine M, and others: Factors associated with impairment of the early development of the prematures, Society for Research in Child Development, Monograph No 31, vol 4, 1966.
10. Brazelton TB: Neonatal Behavioral Assessment Scale, Philadelphia, 1973, JB Lippincott Co.
11. Bronfenbrenner U: When is infant stimulation effective? In Glass, D, editor: Environmental influences, New York, 1968, Rockefeller Press.
12. Bronfenbrenner U: Is early intervention effective? In Ffiedlander B, Sterritt G, and Kirk G, editors: Exceptional infant, vol 3, New York, 1975, Brunner/Mazel, Inc.
13. Caputo D, and Mandell V: Consequences of low birth weight, Dev Psychol 3:373, 1970.
14. Daniels H and others: Mechanisms of feeding efficiency in preterm infants, J Pediatr Gastroenterol Nutr 5:593, 1986.
15. Dorland's illustrated medical dictionary, ed 25, Philadelphia, 1974, WB Saunders Co.
16. Drillien C: The incidence of mental and physical handicaps in school age children of very low birth weight, Pediatrics 27:452, 1961.
17. Drillien C: The growth and development of the prematurely born infant, Baltimore, 1964, Williams & Wilkins.
18. Drillien C: Causes of handicap in the low weight infant. In Jonxis J, Visser H, and Troelstra J, editors: Aspects of prematurity and dysmaturity, Leiden, Holland, 1976, Stenfert Droese.

19. Dubowitz L, Dubowitz V, and Goldberg C: Clinical assessment of gestational age in the newborn infant, J Pediatr 1:10, 1979.
20. Dubowitz L, and Dubowitz V: The neurological assessment of the preterm and full-term newborn infant, Philadelphia, 1981, JB Lippincott Co.
21. Erikson E: Childhood and society, New York, 1963, WW Norton & Co, Inc.
22. Field T: Infants born at risk, New York, 1979, Medical and Scientific Books.
23. Field T: Supplemental stimulation of preterm neonates. Early Hum Dev 4:301, 1980.
24. Field T and others: Tactile/kinesthetic stimulation effects on preterm neonates, Pediatrics 77:654, 1986.
25. Field T, Dempsey J, and Shuman H: Developmental follow-up of pre- and post-term infants. In Friedman S, and Sigman M, editors: Preterm birth and psychological development, New York, 1981, Academic Press, Inc.
26. Francis-Williams J, and Davies P: Very low birth weight and later intelligence, Dev Med Child Neurol 16:709, 1974.
27. Freud A: The concept of developmental lines, Psychoanal Study Child 18:245, 1963.
28. Georgieff M, and Bernbaum J: Abnormal shoulder girdle muscle tone in premature infants during their first 18 months, Pediatrics 77:664, 1986.
29. Georgieff M, and others: Abnormal truncal muscle tone as a useful early marker for developmental delay in low birthweight infants, Pediatrics 77:659, 1986.
30. Gerdes J, and others: Improved survival and short-term outcome of inborn "micropremies," Clin Ped 25:391, 1980.
31. Gilfoyle E, Grady A, and Moore J: Children adapt, Thorofare, NJ, 1981, Charles B Slack, Inc.
32. Harel S and Anastaslow N, editors: The at-risk infant. Baltimore, 1985, Brookes Publishing Co.
33. Harrison L: Effects of early supplemental stimulation programs for premature infants: review of the literature, Mat Child Nurs J 14:69, 1985.
34. Haskins R, Finkelstein N, and Stedman D: Infant stimulation programs and their effects, Pediatr Ann 7:2, 1978.
35. Hommers M, and Kendall A: The prognosis of the very low-birth weight infant, Dev Med Child Neurol 18:745, 1976.
36. Knoblock H, and Pasamanick B: Prospective studies in the epidemiology of reproductive casuality: methods, findings and some implications, Merrill-Palmer Q 12:27, 1966.
37. Kopp C, and Parmalee A: Prenatal and perinatal influences on infant behavior. In Osofsky J, editor: Handbook of infant development, New York, 1979, John Wiley & Sons, Inc.
38. Langworthy O: Development of behavior patterns and myelinization of the nervous system in the human fetus and infant. Contrib Embryol 24:139, 1933.
39. Lawson K, Daum C, and Turkewitz G: Environmental characteristics of a neonatal intensive care unit, Child Dev 48:1633, 1977.
40. Lipsitt L, and Field T: Perinatal influences on the behavior of full-term newborns. In Lipsitt L, and Field T, editors: Infant behavior and development: perinatal risk and newborn behavior, Norwood, NJ, 1982, Oblex Publishing Corp.
41. Lipton R, and Provence S: Infants in institutions, New York, 1962, International Universities Press.
42. Littman B, and Parmelee A: Obstetric Complications Scale (a modification of the Prechtl Obstetrics Optimality Scale) and the Postnatal Complications Scale. Unpublished manuscript, 1964.
43. Lubchenco L, and others: Sequelae of premature birth: evaluation of premature infants of low birth weight at ten years of age, Am J Dis Child 106:101, 1963.
44. Moore J: Concepts from the neurobehavioral sciences in relation to rehabilitation of the mentally and/or physically handicapped, Dubuque, Iowa, 1973, Kendall/Hunt Publishing Co.
45. The nature and nurture of behavior, Readings from Scientific American, San Francisco, 1973, WH Freeman and Co, Publishers.
46. Page K: Predictors of outcome of low birth weight infants, a review of the literature and methodological issues, Phys Ther 66:1252, 1986.
47. Parmelee A: Neurophysiological and behavioral organization of premature infants in the first months of life, Biol Psychiatry 10:501, 1975.
48. Parmelee A: Early intervention for preterm infants. In Brown C, editor: Infants at risk: assessment and intervention for health care professionals and parents, Piscataway, NJ, 1981, Johnson & Johnson.
49. Parmelee A, and Heber A: Who is the risk infant?, Clin Obstet Gynecol 16:376, 1973.
50. Parker S, and Brazelton B: Newborn behavioral assessment: research prediction and clinical uses, Child Today 10:2, 1981.
51. Paxson C: Van Leeuwen's newborn medicine, ed 2, Chicago, 1979, Year Book Medical Publishers, Inc.
52. Phillips M: Prediction of scholastic performance from perinatal and infant development indices, Dissert Abstr Int 33:526, 1972.
53. Prechtl H: The neurological examination of the full-term newborn infant, ed 3, Philadelphia, 1977, JB Lippincott Co.
54. Prechtl H, and Beintema D: The neurological examination of the full-term newborn infant, Little Club Clin Dev Med 12:entire issue, 1964.
55. Rabinovitch M, Bibace R, and Caplan H: Sequelae of prematurity: psychological test findings, Can Med Assoc J 84:822, 1961.
56. Rausch P: A tactile and kinesthetic stimulation program for premature infants. In Brown C editor: The many facets of touch, Skillman, NJ, 1984, Johnson & Johnson.
57. Rosenblith J: The Graham/Rosenblith behavioral examination for newborns: prognostic value and practical issues. In Osofsky J, editor: The handbook of infant development, New York, 1979, John Wiley & Sons, Inc.
58. Ross G: Consistency and change in the development of premature infants weighing less than 1501 grams at birth, Pediatrics 76:885, 1985.
59. Rubin R, Rosenblatt C, and Balow B: Psychological and educational sequelae of prematurity, Pediatrics 52:352, 1973.
60. Saint-Anne Dargassies S: Neurological maturation of the premature infant of 28 to 41 weeks gestational age. In Falkner F, editor: Human development, Philadelphia, 1966, WB Saunders Co.
61. Sameroff A, and Chandler M: Reproductive risks and the continuum of caretaking casuality. In Horowitz F, and others, editors: review of child development research, vol 4, Chicago, 1975, University of Chicago Press.
62. Schaefer M, Hatcher R, and Barglow P: Prematurity and infant stimulation: a review of research, Child Psychiatry Hum Dev 10:199, 1980.
63. Self P, and Horowitz F: The behavioral assessment of the neonate: an overview. In Osofsky J, editor: The handbook of infant development, New York, 1979, John Wiley & Sons, Inc.
64. Sell E: Follow-up of the high risk newborn—a practical approach, Springfield, Ill, 1980, Charles C Thomas, Publisher.
65. Solnit A, and Provence S: Vulnerability and risk in early childhood. In Osofsky J, editor: The handbook of infant development, New York, 1979, John Wiley & Sons, Inc.
66. Taub H, Caputo D, and Goldstein K: Toward a modification of the indices of neonatal prematurity, Percept Mot Skills 40:43, 1975.

67. Thoman E: Affective communications as the prelude and context for language learning. In Schiefelbisch R, and Bricker D, editors: Early language: acquisition and intervention, Baltimore, 1980, University Park Press.

68. Thurber S, and Armstrong L: Nurses' guide—developmental support of low birth weight infants, Houston, 1982, St. Luke's Episcopal Hospital.

69. Tjossen T: Early intervention: issues and approaches, In Tjossen T, editor: Intervention strategies for high risk infants and young children, Baltimore, 1976, University Park Press.

70. Touwen B: The preterm infant in the extrauterine environment: implications for neurology, Early Hum Dev 4:287, 1980.

71. Turkewitz G, and Kenny P: The role of developmental limitations of sensory input on sensory/perceptual organization, Dev Behav Pediatr 6:242, 1985.

72. Usher R: The special problems of the premature infant. In Avery G, editor: Neonatology—pathophysiology and management of the newborn, Philadelphia, 1981, JB Lippincott Co.

73. Usher R, Allen A, and McLean F: Risk of respiratory distress syndrome related to gestational age, route of delivery, and maternal diabetes, Am J Obstet Gynecol 111:826, 1971.

74. Widmayer S, and Field T: Effects of Brazelton demonstration on early interactions of preterm infants and their teenage mothers, Infant Behav Dev 3:1980.

75. Wiener G: Psychologic correlates of premature birth: a review, J Nerv Ment Dis 134:129, 1962.

19

Early intervention and preschool programs

LINDA C. STEPHENS
SUSAN K. TAUBER

WHAT IS EARLY INTERVENTION?

The term "early intervention" connotes different meanings to different professionals. In this chapter "early" refers to a child's development from birth until 5 years of age with the most critical period occurring between birth and 3 years of age. "Intervention" refers to program implementation designed to maintain or enhance the child's development in a specific area of competence, particularly when the child is at risk for developmental delays or disabilities.[24] "Early intervention" is also used here to describe medical and educational services offered to established, environmental, or biological at-risk children from birth to preschool years. Intervention strategies and programs are intended to prevent or ameliorate developmental delays and deformities, maximize each child's potential, and assist the family in adjusting to the challenges of daily living both in the home and in the community.

Established risk children are those with diagnosed disorders known to result in developmental delays and disabilities. Children with Down syndrome, spina bifida, cerebral palsy, and muscular dystrophy are classic examples. *Environmental risk* children are biologically sound but are at risk for delayed development due to limited or inexperienced maternal and family care and limited opportunity for social and physical stimulation. *Biological risk* children have a history of prenatal, perinatal, neonatal, and early developmental occurrences related to suspected biological impairment to the central nervous system that increases the probability of later developmental disabilities. Prematurity, low birth weight, neonatal seizures, anoxia, and apnea are biological risk factors.[13,36] Some children may be considered at risk in more than one category,

further increasing the potential for delays in sensorimotor, cognitive, language, or psychosocial development.

HISTORICAL PERSPECTIVE OF THE OCCUPATIONAL THERAPIST'S ROLE IN EARLY INTERVENTION

Occupational therapists have been working in pediatric intervention programs since the early 1950s. Many of the early programs were in traditional acute care facilities for children with biological impairments resulting from trauma or illness. The emphasis of treatment in occupational therapy was to ameliorate motor dysfunction and to facilitate independent living skills, socialization, perceptual-motor functioning, and communication in inpatient and outpatient settings.[32] Occupational therapists also worked in residential institutions or chronic care facilities where they were involved with custodial care programs for severely and profoundly handicapped children. The number of occupational therapists who work in community settings has increased greatly since the mid-1970s with the trend toward deinstitutionalization.

The move toward community-based intervention provided greater opportunity for family involvement. Some parents became advocates for their children, formed parent groups, and demanded adequate services for them. As a result, many programs have developed in nontraditional settings, such as therapeutic preschools, day care centers, and other nonmedical facilities. In these settings, the occupational therapist's role is often one of facilitating total developmental functioning within the family and teaching skills to parents and other caregivers, rather than focusing on the development of isolated motor skills.

The number of intervention programs increased in the 1960s and '70s as a result of three major factors: (1) medical advances, especially in neonatal care and survival (see Chapter 18), (2) parental involvement and advocacy (see Chapter 8), and (3) federal legislation. The role of the occupational therapist changed, too. Occupational therapists began treating children and infants at younger ages, including children with complex medical conditions.

Another significant change in the 1970s, prompted by federal incentive grants, was the inclusion of some developmentally disabled children of preschool age in traditional school settings. It became imperative for school therapists to become aware of and to understand educational theories, strategies and practices as well as similarities and differences between occupational therapy and special education. This is particularly true within the preschool population in which there is a great amount of overlap due to the synergistic process of sensorimotor, psychosocial, and cognitive development.

REVIEW OF THE LITERATURE

Although many studies concerning the efficacy of early intervention have been in the literature for at least 20 years, the effectiveness of these programs is still being challenged.[27] Problems in methodology are the major issues surrounding the efficacy question. These problems include the following:[4,5]

1. Difficulty in defining a population because of the smaller number and heterogeneous nature of handicapped children
2. Lack of appropriate assessment tools for young children with a wide variety of handicapping conditions
3. Difficulty in assigning control groups due to variability of handicaps and ethical concerns
4. Possibility of misleading conclusions due to changes occurring in variables other than those measured
5. Lack of funding for research in early intervention programs

Little material in the literature specifically addresses occupational therapy intervention with young children in preschool educational settings. This is not surprising since the provision of related services in early childhood special education programs is a recent innovation.

A few studies refer directly to the effectiveness of occupational therapy in early intervention programs for children with developmental disabilities,[1,13,19] and several refer indirectly through the mention of the effectiveness of multidisciplinary intervention.[3,6,23] Ferry[16], on the other hand, questions the effectiveness of sensory integrative and neurodevelopmental approaches, yet cites the possible contribution of occupational therapy and physical therapy with a hypotonic infant. Meisels' rebuttal[27] to Ferry concludes that the "primary intervention target should not be the child, but the child within the context of the family"[27] (p. 8).

There is a great deal of literature related to early intervention services for the medically at risk or handicapped child. The majority of this literature comes from the fields of psychology and education and to a lesser degree the field of medicine. This research can be grouped into three classifications:[30]

1. Early historical studies of institutionalized mentally retarded children and developmentally delayed children from nonstimulating environments who were given intervention to facilitate growth and development
2. Studies on early intervention or enrichment with children from low income or culturally disadvantaged environments[1]
3. Efficacy studies of early intervention programs for handicapped or at risk infants and young children.

The latter includes most of the more recent literature of the 1980s. Casto and Mastropieri,[10] in a meta-analysis of the efficacy of early intervention with handicapped preschoolers, reviewed 74 efficacy studies. They concluded that (1) overall, early intervention programs for handicapped preschoolers are effective; (2) the longer, more intense programs are more effective for handicapped population but are not related to effectiveness for disadvantaged population; (3) structured programs are more effective with disadvantaged population though this is not well supported for handicapped population; (4) limited data support the premise that "earlier is better;" (5) parents are effective as "intervenors" but their involvement is not essential to intervention success; (6) data are still needed to show the longitudinal benefits of early intervention for the handicapped population.

Strain and Smith[34] and Dunst and Snyder[15] refute these findings on the basis that the results of the meta-analysis research are misleading and have methodological, procedural, statistical, and conceptual problems. They point out that Casto and Mastropieri have compared programs that vary widely as to setting, intervention approaches, types of children, and qualifications of service providers. In their rebuttal to Strain and Smith, Casto and Mastropieri[11] acknowledge that early intervention is effective and encourage further research to address the issue of age of onset and parental involvement. Gallagher[18] suggests moving on from postulating the effectiveness of early intervention to documenting the types of intervention that work best in various settings and with different types of children.

According to Crocker and Nelson, the success of early intervention appears relative to the severity of the biological or constitutional deficit.[12] Children with severe deficits may respond less favorably to intervention programs. However, early intervention programs positively affect family acceptance and knowledge of their child, especially in feeding, play, and handling techniques.[12]

In spite of the many problems in conducting acceptable clinical research in early intervention settings, it is critical to do so. In this way, occupational therapists can document their role in early intervention and can provide data to support the value of their contributions.

LEGISLATION

Legislation for early intervention programs grew out of the belief that early intervention is effective in ameliorating or eliminating later handicapping conditions and is cost-effective to taxpayers.[35] This belief, together with strong parent advocacy, led to federal commitment to early intervention through the enactment of legislation that provided funding for experimental model programs. An early legislative initiative was the Handicapped Children's Early Education Assistance Act (HCEEP) PL 90-538 in 1968. This act provided funds for experimental projects for handicapped children from birth to 8 years and their families.

Further support for early intervention came in 1975 with the Education for All Handicapped Children Act (PL 94-142); this act encouraged services for handicapped children from 3 to 5 years of age and mandated the provision of educational services to all school-aged handicapped children. States were required to provide services for preschool handicapped children to the same extent that educational services were available to other preschool children in the state. Federal Act PL 94-142 also established Child Find, a service to identify at risk and handicapped children beginning at birth. The Preschool Incentive Grant (section 619) of PL 94-142 encouraged the expansion of services to young handicapped children by offering incentive dollars.

The Preschool Incentive Act (PL 99-457) was enacted in 1986. It replaced the Preschool Incentive Grant Program of PL 94-142, reauthorized funding for special education and related services to preschoolers 3 to 5 years old with handicaps, and supported the establishment of early intervention programs for infants from birth to 2 years. This legislation emphasizes the need for medical and educational services and identifies occupational therapy as a primary service independent of medical, health, and special education services. Interagency cooperation is stressed, along with a multidisciplinary team approach. Primary early intervention services named in the legislation are occupational therapy, physical therapy, speech therapy, counseling, and family training. Intervention focuses on both the child and the family, which is consistent with the basic philosophy of pediatric occupational therapy.[21]

In addition to the above programs administered through the Department of Education, the Department of Health and Human Resources also administers programs for handicapped preschoolers. DHR provides funds for Head Start and Home Start programs through the Administration for Children, Youth and Families. The Bureau of Maternal and Child Health and National Institute of Health support research for the chronically ill child.

THE EARLY INTERVENTION TEAM

The success of an early intervention program depends largely upon the integration of the child's individual program components into a comprehensive system carried out by a cooperative team of professionals. The overall roles of these professionals are discussed in Chapter 2.

Teamwork is critical because of the interrelated nature of the problems of the developing child and the need for skills and resources from many professionals to meet the needs of both child and family. *The emphasis of intervention should be the child within the family unit, rather than the child alone.* The problems of the child within the family, his relationship with family members and his variety of needs, sometimes require the expertise and thoughtful cooperation of many professionals. This interprofessional collaboration can be called by various names and work in a variety of configurations. The authors have found useful the terms *multidisciplinary, interdisciplinary,* and *transdisciplinary* when referring to these interprofessional endeavors.

Team approaches
MULTIDISCIPLINARY

This approach evolved from the medical model in which multiple professionals evaluated the child and made recommendations.[30] In this type of approach, several professionals may be directly or indirectly involved with the child and family, but do not necessarily consult or interact with each other.[28] Often, services are provided through several locations. Generally one person, such as the parent or physician, acts as case manager.

INTERDISCIPLINARY

The interdisciplinary approach to treatment is a more cooperative and interactive approach consisting of a team composed of professionals from several disciplines involved with the child, usually at the same location. These professionals have continuing direct involvement with the child and collaborate with each other in carrying out the child's program. Even though evaluations are performed independently by each discipline, program planning occurs as a result of group consensus. Implementation is specific to each discipline and may be executed outside the environment in which the child is expected to perform.

Each member of an interdisciplinary team is accountable to the team as a whole. Often one of the team members acts as case manager to implement and manage a tracking system to avoid fragmentation or duplication of services. To ensure the success of this approach, the team members must respect each other's roles and not enter into a "power play" for control. This requires a willingness to share expertise and knowledge and to assume responsibility to be accountable for intervention procedures.

TRANSDICIPLINARY

In the transdisciplinary approach various disciplines interact as a team but one member is usually designated to provide direct intervention with other team members who act as consultants. *Role release* occurs when one professional relinquishes some of his or her functions to another professional. All team members contribute to assessment, program planning, and intervention, but the designated person is empowered by the team to perform functions that are normally outside the bounds of his or her profession. This approach is described by Giangreco as "indirect, integrated, and decentralized;" it limits the number of people carrying out a program but makes use of the expertise of a variety of professionals[20] (p. 9).

For example, a 2-year-old child with spina bifida was evaluated by a transdisciplinary team. The child lived in an isolated rural area and the family had no transportation to a treatment center. The team decided to provide home services with the physical therapist as the direct service provider. The occupational therapist, speech pathologist, and early childhood specialist each taught the physical therapist certain techniques to use for feeding, language stimulation, and cognitive development. As a result, the physical therapist was able to provide a wide variety of intervention strategies on her weekly visits, which freed other team members to work with other children.

Ottenbacher[29] warns of several obstacles to the transdisciplinary approach. These obstacles include differing value systems, issues of professional and legal liability, variable background education of designated service providers, and inconsistent mastery of skills practiced through role release.

Regardless of which approach is used, effective teamwork does not come easily. It requires a flexible administration based on a sound philosophical framework, and honest, hard work on the part of each team member.

PARENTS AS PART OF THE TEAM

The literature includes much evidence to support parent involvement as a predictor of child development.[4,27] It is therefore natural to include parents as integral members of their child's treatment team. The degree of participation generally decreases as the child becomes older and enters school. In the birth to 2-year-old category, parents usually must assume primary responsibility for integrating and coordinating services unless they are part of a comprehensive program model. In early childhood special education programs the focus of parents' participation shifts from total to partial responsibility with emphasis more on the child's daily activities and accomplishments and not only on instructional needs.[30]

It is advantageous for parents to become involved in daily classroom activities ranging from participation in special events to observing how each professional delivers services within the program setting. This allows them to understand more fully the "whys" and "hows" of each discipline so that the skills learned in school can be generalized to home and vice versa.

One of the most valuable roles of the parent team member is to support other parents of at risk or handicapped children. Parents may be involved in community programs for increasing awareness and acceptance of issues related to early childhood intervention and in fundraising efforts. They can act as effective community liaisons. Finally, parents are the persons most familiar with their child and are valuable as members of the assessment and evaluation teams. (For a detailed discussion of parent involvement, see Chapter 8.)

MODELS FOR EARLY INTERVENTION

Occupational therapists provide services to infants and young children in a variety of ways in many different settings (Figure 19-1). The *parent-child* model focuses on direct therapy to the child with concurrent instruction to the parent so that he or she can follow through on treatment techniques. The *pull-out* model involves removing a child or small group of children from a larger group to give them direct therapy. Information is usually relayed to the parent. In either of these models consultation can be given to the parent or to the teacher to enable that person to be more effective with the child. In the *environmental* model the therapist elicits changes in the child by structuring the child's environment (for example, classroom, daycare group) while the family is given information. When changes are facilitated in the child by working with the family and the total environment (such as housing, nutrition, child care) it can be considered an *ecological* model. In each of these examples the occupational therapist functions as a team member in one of the approaches discussed earlier. See Chapter 29 for a discussion of service delivery methods such as direct service and consultation.

Models of intervention

For some infants or young children, the traditional individual treatment approach to intervention is

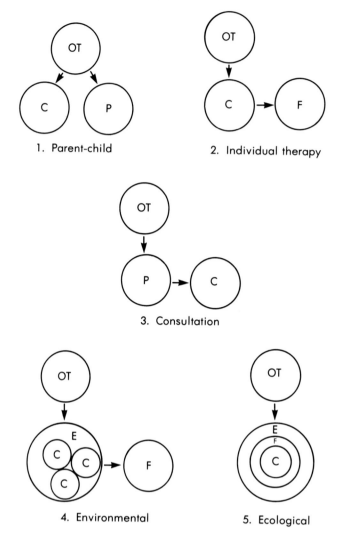

Figure 19-1   Focus of occupational therapy in various models of intervention.
C = child; P = parent; F = family; E = environment.

the most effective. In this approach, the therapist works with the child on a one-to-one basis for a specified length of time (for example, 30 minutes twice a week).

PARENT-CHILD MODEL

In some cases, the focus on intervention may be the child and parent as a unit. In this model the parent is usually instructed in home management techniques, observes the occupational therapist handling the child, and perhaps works with the therapist in problem-solving approaches to ameliorate the child's deficits. With either the parent-child or pull-out model the emphasis is on the identification of specific problems, delays, or handicapping conditions, followed by treatment designed to address those concerns. Monitoring

of the home program and the parent as a therapist are also components of this approach.

PULL-OUT MODEL

When children are located in groups, such as those found in a preschool, daycare center, or residential facility, the *pull-out* model is commonly used to provide treatment. In this model the child is removed from the group and taken to a separate location, such as a therapy room, for treatment. This can be done on either an individual or small group basis. Focus of intervention is on the remediation of identified deficits and on facilitation of appropriate functioning upon return to the group. The parents or other primary caregivers are not usually present, but information is provided to them. This model provides respite care for the families be-

Table 19-1 Models of early intervention

	Parent-Child	**Pull-Out**	**Environmental**	**Ecological**
FOCUS	Child and parent	Child Consultation to parent and teacher	Child within environment (home, classroom). Family involvement	Family, social systems
APPROACH	Remediation of deficits	Remediation of deficits	Total functioning within environment	Change in environment indirectly facilitates change in child
COMPONENTS	Individual treatment Parent/child interaction Parent as therapist	Individual or group treatment Home program for follow-up	Intervention occurs within environment Facilitation of change in strong areas as well as weak	Change in family support systems Improve environmental factors (housing, nutrition, etc.)
LOCATION	Home Clinic/therapy room Mobile unit	Clinic/therapy room Regular or special preschool Residential	Home Regular or special preschool Residential	Home/neighborhood Residential

cause it relieves the caregiver of the constant responsibility of caring for the handicapped child.

ENVIRONMENTAL MODEL

Another way of addressing the needs of young handicapped or developmentally delayed children is by focusing on the provision of an *environment* that facilitates function rather than focusing on specific deficits to be remediated. This can be achieved with small groups of children in a special preschool setting. With this approach the child is encouraged to function to the maximum in all developmental areas (motor, cognition, social, communication, self-help) in an environment that facilitates the mastery of skills and the development of self-esteem. The child's deficits or handicaps are not ignored in this approach, but they are minimized as the child functions within the special environment. Occupational therapy, physical therapy, and speech therapy goals can be coordinated through a single activity rather than having to be addressed separately in individual treatment sessions (Figure 19-2). For example, at lunch speech goals can be addressed by requiring the child to ask for food. At the same time the child is encouraged to improve self-feeding skills (occupational therapy goals) and is placed in adapted seating designed to improve trunk and head control (occupational therapy and physical therapy goals).

There is some support in the literature for the efficacy of an environmental focus for children with some types of deficits. Casto and Mastropieri, in reviewing early intervention studies, conclude that the more highly structured programs are associated with effective outcomes with economically and socially disad-

vantaged children.[10] The use of play along with high levels of structure, consistency, and intensity were more effective than traditional remediation for a group of autistic and severely emotionally handicapped children.[30] Sparling described the use of art and drama with neurologically impaired preschoolers and found greater gains in performance on developmental tests than with the use of intense one-to-one neurodevelopmental or cognitive approaches.[33]

ECOLOGICAL MODEL

Another form of early intervention is to make changes in the child indirectly by addressing total family needs. This method has been termed the *ecological* approach. Family needs such as housing, nutrition, employment, and support systems are addressed in an effort to strengthen family functioning to the benefit of all family members. Umansky describes this approach in dealing with the isolation of families of children with handicaps and the difficulty in normalizing the family's approach to the child.[37] Bailey used a functional model of family intervention and addressed child variables, family needs, and parent-child interaction.[2] By strengthening the total family unit and improving interactions within the family, the child is able to function more effectively.

Dunst provided intervention to entire families, which he termed "Proactive Empowerment through Partnerships."[14] This program included two transdisciplinary teams of professionals (including occupational therapists) that provided services in the home as well as support groups and other family services. In addition, another component of the program included ten special projects. These were such groups as lending li-

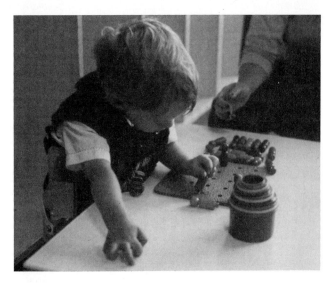

Figure 19-2   This child develops standing tolerance, weight-bearing, fine motor control, and the cognitive skills of matching and sorting in this activity.

brary and toy exchange, workshops for siblings, volunteer programs, respite care, support groups, preschool programs, and parent training. The conclusion was that "early intervention, when conceptualized in social systems terms, has broad-based impacts upon child, parent, and family behavior"[14] (p. 197). (For a comparison of early intervention models, refer to Table 19-1 on the preceding page.)

Location for intervention

Occupational therapists provide services for children from birth to 5 years of age in a number of different settings ranging from institutional settings such as a hospital, residential facility, or rehabilitation center to the child's home (Table 19-1.) As increased numbers of mothers enter the work force, more young children are cared for in daycare centers and preschools. Some children who are at risk or have developmental delays or handicaps may receive therapy services in these settings.

Growing evidence of the efficacy of early intervention has led to the development of greater numbers of special preschools for children at risk. Innovative service approaches have been developed, especially in sparsely populated rural areas. Magrun and Tigges described the use of a converted bus to provide early intervention services in rural New York.[26] This mobile unit was taken to various locations convenient to the families. Therapy was provided using a transdisciplinary approach with shared space.

CASE EXAMPLE

The most effective focus of intervention depends to a large extent on the presenting problems of the child. A 4-year-old boy with severe sensory integrative dysfunction and gravitational insecurity most likely would benefit from individual therapy sessions and probably would work more effectively with the therapist if the mother were not present. However, for an 8-month-old girl with spastic quadriparesis, the most effective focus of treatment might be on the mother's management of the infant. In this case the mother needs to learn handling, positioning, and feeding techniques. In addition she needs emotional support and encouragement from regular contact with the occupational therapist. A 3-year-old boy with Down syndrome might benefit most from a special preschool environment that requires him to develop self-help skills, perform sensorimotor tasks, and relate appropriately to children and adults in a supportive encouraging setting (environmental approach).

An early intervention program that illustrates some of the above models is the Adaptive Learning Center in Atlanta, Georgia. This center provides therapeutic services to children from birth through 6 years using an environmental approach with a combination interdisciplinary and transdisciplinary professional team. In this setting therapists and teachers work with the child interactively and cooperatively within a structured environment (the classroom). Occupational therapy, physical therapy, speech pathology, and special education are synthesized into one harmonious and integrated program that addresses the individual needs of the child and family. Parent involvement is an integral component for successfully generalizing skills from school to home and vice versa.

The therapeutic preschool is divided into classes, each having no more than six children. A child may attend 2, 3, or 5 days a week, according to individual need. Within the 4-hour day each class receives a session of occupational therapy, speech therapy, special education, and physical therapy or recreational therapy. Teacher, assistant, and therapist work closely together within the group to help each child achieve her goals. Weekly team meetings and constant interaction of all team members precludes duplication of functions. Role release occurs when one team member implements techniques learned from another team member. Skills and information from all disciplines are combined to generalize individual therapy goals into practical classroom and home routines. Role release and acceptance occur only as a result of mutual team readiness and consent.

This therapeutic preschool exemplifies the environmental model because the child functions within a total structure designed to enhance performance in all developmental areas. These more functional behaviors are reinforced as they are carried over to the home and other less structured environments. Rather than being removed or set apart to receive therapy, the child finds therapeutic activities to be a part of the normal day. As the day progresses, the teacher is able to integrate various therapy skills into other aspects of the child's program. For example, the occupational therapist might be working on self-help skills but this becomes a joint effort as the teacher also teaches and reinforces those skills in the bathroom, at mealtime, and when preparing to go home. The children also benefit from frequent casual contact with non-handicapped children in a "normal" preschool in the same building.

THE OCCUPATIONAL THERAPIST'S ROLE
Problem identification

The occupational therapist in a preschool setting is involved in an identification process that reflects both medical and educational models. The therapist must address not only the child's abilities and deficits, but specifically the adaptation of the child into the total environment, including both the home and preschool. There are three basic components to the problem identification process: screening, assessment, and reevaluation.

SCREENING

Preschool screenings provide general information with the purpose of identifying children who are not functioning within normal developmental parameters and who may be candidates for early intervention programs.

The occupational therapy screening may consist of both formal and informal evaluations and can be done either individually or as part of a team. Occupational therapy screenings of preschoolers are concerned with social-emotional development, self-help and adaptive behaviors (feeding, toileting, dressing, attending skills), visual-motor and neuromotor development, and parent/child and teacher/child interaction. Screenings for very young children (from birth to 3 years) rely more on medical, family, and environmental factors; developmental skills have greater importance for 3 to 5 year olds.[30] Screenings should be done in a relatively quiet environment, should be efficient, and require only a single contact with child and parent. Some examples of screening tools used by occupational therapists for a preschool population are Denver Developmental Screening Test (DDST), short version of Miller Assessment for Preschoolers (MAP), Battelle Developmental Inventory Screening Test (BDI/S), and the Milani-Camparetti Neuromotor Screening Test. Children should *not* be labeled nor should treatment plans be made as a result of a screening test alone.

ASSESSMENT

The purpose of assessment is to identify levels of functioning and specific deficits to determine appropri-

ate intervention. This should be coordinated with other professionals, particularly the early childhood educator, and with the parent. Professional roles often overlap, but rather than being a duplication, it may contribute to a broader perspective of the child's abilities. For instance, both the occupational therapist and special education teacher could assess social-emotional behaviors but from different perspectives. The occupational therapist may assess quality of interaction between child, teacher, and peers from the standpoint of physical functioning and sensorimotor skills; the teacher may assess level of group interaction within a classroom as well as quality of cognitive skills and behavior.

REEVALUATION

Reevaluation is the process of determining whether a child has made gains in response to the intervention program. The child is retested and results are compared to those of the initial evaluation. In this way it can be determined if goals have been met and if the intervention provided to the child has been effective in facilitating change. The purpose of reevaluation is to measure the child's response to the program and to provide appropriate information for decision-making regarding the extent and type of further intervention. Consideration of reevaluation data from several children is helpful in reviewing the overall intervention program and in making administrative changes (see Chapter 31).

Diagnostic categories
LABELS AND CATEGORIES

Specific areas or disabilites are referred to as "categories." Though labeling young children is discouraged by most professionals, the concept of categories serves a purpose. First, it establishes an advocacy group to help a certain population of children, such as the Down Syndrome Association. Second, it identifies a specific set of characteristics associated with needs and problems of the various exceptionality categories. Third, it encourages research on causes, diagnosis, and treatment of a particular category. Finally, it allows for a convenient mode of communication.

While diagnostic labels may be appropriate for school-age children, many problems are associated with categorizing young children, especially those from birth through 3 years. First of all, it is difficult for the physician to make a differential diagnosis for a child who exhibits characteristics associated with several diagnostic categories. "Developmental delay" is frequently the only medical diagnosis given to the preschool child, particularly the birth through 3 years population. Fortunately, in most states, preschool age children do not need a label or category as a prerequisite for receiving special education and related services.

A second problem with categories is the detrimental effect that labeling often has on the young child and the family. Teachers and families often fall prey to the "self-fullfilling prophecy" in which parents and teachers have certain expectations based on the label. As a result, the child often acts according to the expectations, thus fulfilling the prophecy. For an example, the family of a 2-year-old boy was told that the child was mentally retarded. Consequently the family expected nothing from the child, catered to his every whim, and tolerated unruly behaviors because the perceptions of the family were that retarded persons were totally helpless. With training and higher expectations, the child could learn simple self-help skills and control his behavior.

Another danger associated with categorization is making a premature judgment. Is the problem a result of a specific impairment or caused by immature development? Because of the problems categorization presents, preschool handicapped children are often grouped by using developmental levels within specific domains, such as fine motor or communication.

Most early childhood special education programs are noncategorical and are geared to the child's functional behaviors.[25] However, though preschool children are not grouped according to categories, disabilities common to this population include mental retardation, attention deficit disorders, behavioral and emotional disorders, physical impairments such as cerebral palsy and spina bifida, visual impairments, auditory impairments, and speech and language disorders.

Problem resolution

TREATMENT APPROACHES

There are numerous approaches that the occupational therapist can use to soften the effects of handicapping conditions on a young child or to stimulate the development of the child at risk for delays. After an assessment is completed and areas of strengths and weaknesses identified, the occupational therapist plans goals and objectives of intervention. The therapist then chooses a treatment approach that will enable the child to reach those goals.

Developmental approach. Of primary importance for infants and young children is a *developmental* approach. Occupational therapists must have a thorough knowledge of normal child development including the sequence of developmental stages. Occupational therapists provide treatment activities for the child that are consistent with the child's developmental level, as determined by the assessment, and that encourage the child to reach the next stage of development (see Chapters 3 and 4 for developmental principles, theories, and process). When the child's developmental growth is uneven sometimes it is a challenge for the occupational therapist to stimulate improved function in the weak areas.

For example, a 4-year-old boy's cognitive function was on a 3½ year level, but his social and fine motor functioning was on a 2 year level. The occupational therapy activity planned for him was a "play town" that consisted of a large plastic sheet with streets, houses and trees drawn on it. The child was set up in a parallel play situation in which he played next to, but not interactively with, the other children. He was encouraged to roll his cars on the "road" as it wound around the floor and to stack small blocks to make houses and buildings. He made up stories about the people in his cars and their destinations in the town. In that way he was able to use his higher level cognitive ability while improving his lower level social and motor skills (Figure 19-3).

Specialized approach. Sometimes the diagnosis and identified deficits in a child will indicate the need for a *specialized* approach. Some examples are neurodevelopmental approaches (see Chapter 20), sensory integration (see Chapter 23), and oral-motor facilitation (see Chapter 14). When these approaches are used treatment still must be consistent with the child's developmental levels (Figures 19-4 and 19-5).

Group approach. It is often effective with young children to use a *group* approach. Sometimes a child who is reluctant or uncooperative in an individual setting will join other children who are eagerly participating in an activity. The child benefits from observing other children and can be guided by an adult into variations of the activity to meet individual needs. An ideal group size is four to five children with two adults. In this way each child can benefit from the group yet

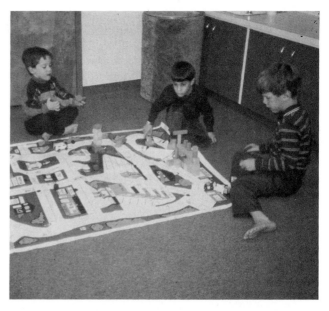

Figure 19-3   These children participate in this activity on several levels of fine motor ability, social interaction, and cognition.

have enough adult attention to stay on task. With more than one adult the group can continue to function even if one child has disruptive behaviors or needs individual assistance.

Different individual goals can be met by using one activity within a group setting. For example, finger painting was planned for a group of 2- and 3-year-old children. One child had tactile defensiveness, and for him the purpose of the activity was to tolerate the tactile input provided by a messy activity. Another child with cerebral palsy needed the activity to facilitate active finger extension and decreased grasp reflex. The fine motor goal for another child was to draw circular, horizontal, and vertical lines, which was accomplished by using the index finger in the paint. Still another delayed child needed sensorimotor exploration and stimulation. For her, a small amount of sand was added to a portion of paint to increase the tactile stimulation (Figure 19-6).

USE OF PLAY

Play is a natural and important part of childhood; it provides intrinsic rewards, provides an opportunity for mastery of the environment, and is pleasurable. Play activities that are consistent with the child's developmental levels and that appeal to the child's natural interests and curiosity can be powerful treatment tools. Play not only provides a means of exploring the environment but gives the opportunity for repetition for skill mastery. The play of young children can be categorized as exploratory play, symbolic play, creative play, games, and recreation (see Chapter 15).

Exploratory play activities can be used to stimulate specific responses from a child. Through the use of a playful approach and carefully selected developmentally appropriate toys, the occupational therapist can encourage an unresponsive developmentally delayed infant to touch, reach, manipulate, and explore tactile qualities of the toy.

An example of *symbolic play* that is popular with many children is "dress up," where the child puts on adult clothing or costumes and pretends to take on various roles. This activity, especially in a group, is more effective in teaching self-help skills than an individual therapy session in which the child practices putting on a shirt or working on a button board (Figure 19-7).

Creative play encompasses art activities such as painting, cutting, pasting, drawing, and coloring, and can meet treatment goals in a variety of ways. Clay and play dough provide additional creative and manipulative experiences. Simple dramatics and creative movement can also be used effectively as part of occupational therapy.

When play is used as treatment, it is usually structured, or directed by the therapist. Unstructured or free play opportunities are also important in two ways: (1) It allows children to practice and integrate skills into their total functioning; (2) it allows therapists to observe what a child chooses to play with and how he plays without adult direction—important clues as to the effectiveness of treatment.

An important component of play is toys; many toys are improvised by the child from sticks and stones,

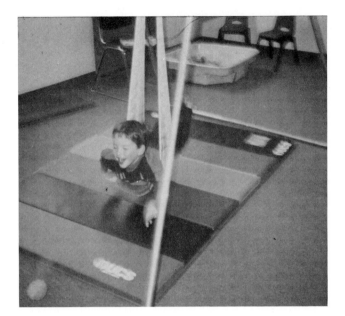

Figure 19-4 Sensory integration is a specialized approach that is effective with some children.

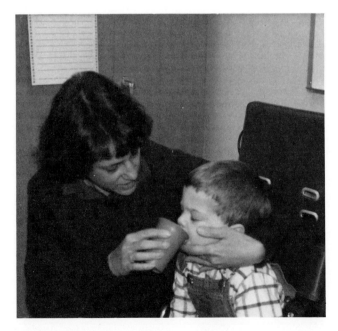

Figure 19-5 Jaw control helps this child improve oral-motor function.

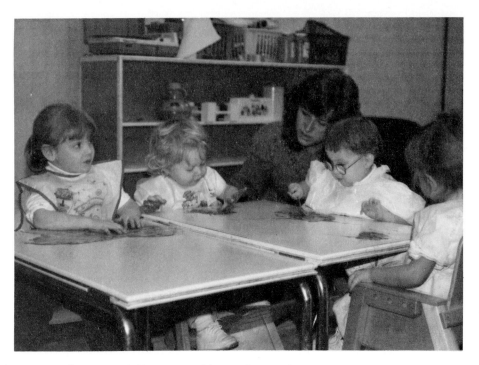

Figure 19-6   These children use pudding as finger paint.

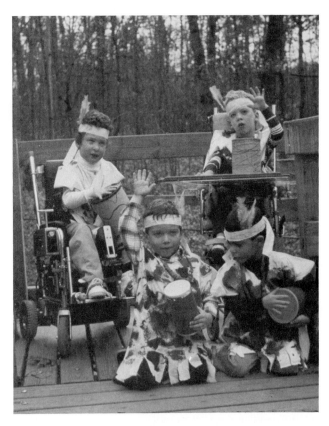

Figure 19-7   An Indian theme provides an opportunity to develop self-dressing skill and fine motor skill through painting the costume and making the accessories.

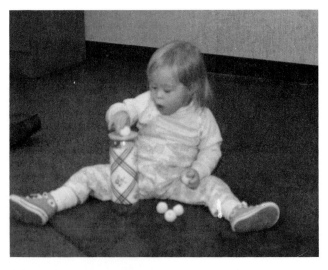

Figure 19-8   This child enjoys a toy made from a tennis ball can and styrofoam balls.

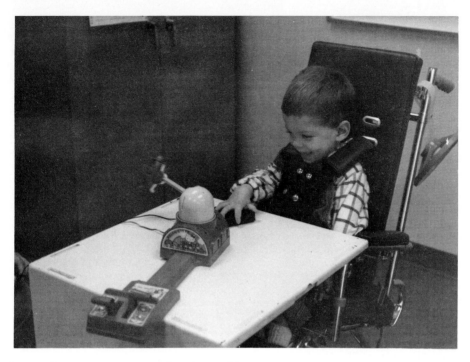

Figure 19-9   A pressure switch activates this toy.

pots and pans, or they can be made by parents from common household materials (Figure 19-8). The reader is referred to several excellent books with instructions for making toys.[9,17,22]

Occupational therapists can adapt toys effectively by using various types of switches for battery operated toys. A pressure switch is effective in helping children gain greater control of arm and hand motion (Figure 19-9). These skills will eventually lead to use of an augmentative communication system and to the use of a computer for academics. The reader is referred to Burkhardt[7,8] for clear instructions on switch adaptations.

The following case history illustrates the process o problem identification and treatment of a child in an early intervention center.

CASE STUDY

At the time of referral to the Adaptive Learning Center, Timmy was an 8-month-old infant. He was diagnosed with left hemiparesis resulting from head trauma at birth. History included a full-term pregnancy with no complications.

Timmy's first visit to the center was for screening to determine if a full evaluation was appropriate. The center's director, an occupational therapist, administered several screening tests which included observation of behaviors, administration of test items, and interview of parents. Timmy was accompanied by both parents, who remained in the testing room during the screening. Results of screening showed passing scores in fine motor (using the right hand only), personal-social, and cognitive areas, but failing scores in gross

motor, adaptive (including self-help), and communication areas. He was referred for a team assessment.

The assessment team included an occupational therapist, a physical therapist, a speech therapist, and a specialist in early childhood education. The entire battery of the Battelle Developmental Inventory was administered. The entire team, plus the parents, remained in the room during the test session. Rather than having each team member administer a portion of the test separately, they worked together to observe the child's responses so that fewer strangers handled the child. For example, the teacher administered the cognitive portions of the test, but the occupational therapist observed how the infant handled toys and materials and asked the teacher to try for specific responses in the fine motor area. In the same manner the speech therapist made note of vocalizations and response to sound and language. The parents supplied information so that the team could take into consideration typical functioning at home as well as the 1-hour sample during assessment.

The assessment team decided that Timmy could benefit from individual occupational, physical, and speech therapy given in 30-minute sessions once a week with parent and child. It was noted in the interpretation that the fine motor score represented function on the unaffected side and that Timmy was not using his affected left upper extremity at all.

Both of Timmy's parents were employed full-time, so mother and father alternated weeks in bringing Timmy for therapy and in attending therapy sessions. A home program was given at the parents' request, but they had limited time in which to work with Timmy at home. Each of the therapists made a consultation visit to Timmy's day care center and made suggestions to day care personnel. Although these persons were willing and eager to help Timmy, they were unable to give him much special attention because of the number of children they cared for. However, they did try to follow through on feeding techniques and began to expect Timmy to move on his own rather than to be carried across a room.

Timmy made considerable progress in 6 months of individual therapy. He had learned to creep, was feeding himself finger foods, and was using the left hand as a gross assist in play activities. Language was emerging with some meaningful approximations of words. However, he sometimes refused to cooperate in therapy sessions and there was inconsistent carry-over between home and day care center. Therapists and parents decided that Timmy would benefit from the infant class in the center's therapeutic preschool.

Timmy spent 4 hours in the preschool setting each day. The remainder of the day was spent in the center's day care program. Timmy's preschool hours were structured with consistent expectations from all staff and with an integrated program of all therapies and special education. Timmy's class of four children received each of the therapies as a group; their teacher was involved in each session. There was overlap and reinforcement of all goals by each professional involved with Timmy.

Timmy spent 2 years in the special preschool program. A comprehensive reevaluation was done each year and an individual therapy/education plan was written. An update and summary of progress was reported at least every 6 months. Each therapist maintained daily data sheets to document progress. The parents were involved in the preschool program, attended parent meetings and training, and occasionally offered volunteer help for special events.

When Timmy was almost 3 years old, reevaluation showed that he was functioning close to age level in all areas. Coordinated movement of the left arm and leg continued to be a problem, although he was able to achieve most age-level tasks. Timmy had displayed some temper tantrums in class and his teacher felt that he was bored with children who were cognitively much slower. It was decided that Timmy no longer needed the restricted environment of a special preschool, although he continued to need occupational and physical therapy. Timmy entered a regular preschool and continued his therapy on a weekly basis at the center.

This case illustrates how different approaches and models of early intervention can meet the changing needs of the developing child. Timmy moved from the parent-infant model to an environmental approach, and finally to individual therapy. It is anticipated that when Timmy enters public school in kindergarten he will need only consultative services. Because Timmy received early intervention he was better able to incorporate movement of the affected left arm and leg into his developing motor skills. In addition, he achieved close to normal functioning in part because the expectations of all around him were that he function as independently as possible appropriate to his age.

SUMMARY

This chapter discussed occupational therapy in early intervention for handicapped and at risk children from birth through 5 years. A historical perspective of occupational therapy's role was presented as well as a review of literature in this area. Legislative influences were discussed. The occupational therapist works in a number of settings with this population and can use a variety of approaches, including parent-child, pull-out, environmental, and ecological. The early intervention team includes a number of professionals who work together as a multidisciplinary, interdisciplinary, or transdisciplinary team. Methods of screening, evaluating, and treating the infant and young child were presented. Understanding the family's adjustment, attitude, and ability to cope with the young handicapped child are crucial in effective intervention.

STUDY QUESTONS

1. Describe and give examples of three different risk factors of children seen in early intervention settings.
2. Why is quality research difficult in the area of early intervention?
3. Describe similarities and differences among the four models of early intervention. When legislation and recent trends are considered, which model do you think will become most prevalent? Why?
4. Give some examples of types of problems of young children that could be treated with a group developmental approach. What are some activities that could be used?

REFERENCES

1. Atkins J, and Kaplan M: Model services for handicapped infants, Third Year Report #8039.
2. Bailey DB, and others: Family-focused intervention: a functional model for planning, implementing and evaluating individualized family services in early intervention. J Div for Early Child 10:156, 1986.
3. Bailey EJ, and Bricker D: The efficacy of early intervention for severely handicapped infants and young children. Topics in Early Child Spec Ed 4:30, 1984.
4. Beckman PJ, and Burke PJ: Early childhood special education: state of the art. Topics in Early Child Spec Ed 4(3):19, 1984.
5. Bricker D: The effectiveness of early intervention with handicapped and medically at risk children. J Child in Con Soc 17:51, 1984.
6. Browder JA: The pediatrician's orientation to infant stimulation programs. Pediatrics 67:42, 1981.
7. Burkhardt LJ: Homemade battery powered toys and educational devices for severely handicapped children. RD 1 Box 124, Millville, Pa, 1982.
8. Burkhardt LJ: More homemade battery devices for severely handicapped children with suggested activities. RD 1 Box 124, Millville, Pa, 1982.
9. Burtt KG, and Kalkstein K: Smart toys for babies from birth to two. New York, 1981, Harper & Row, Publishers, Inc.
10. Casto G, and Mastropieri MA: The efficacy of early intervention programs: a meta-analysis. Except Child 52:417, Feb 1986.
11. Casto G, and Mastropieri MA: Strain and Smith do protest too much: a response. Except Child 53:3, 266, 1987.
12. Crocker AC, and Nelson RP: Mental retardation. In Levine MD, editor: Developmental Behavioral Pediatrics, Philadelphia, 1983, WB Saunders Co.
13. Denoff E: Current status of infant stimulation or enrichment programs for children with developmental disabilities. Pediatrics 67:34, 1981.
14. Dunst CJ: Rethinking early intervention. Anal & Inter in Del Dev 5:165, 1985.

15. Dunst CJ, and Snyder SW: A critique of the Utah State University early intervention meta-analysis research. Except Child 53:269, 1987.

16. Ferry PC: On growing new neurons: are early intervention programs effective? Pediatrics 67:38, 1981.

17. Fisher JJ: Toys to grow with infants and toddlers. New York, 1986, The Putnam Publishing Group, Inc.

18. Gallagher JJ: Policy issues in the new mandate for early education for the handicapped, Keynote Address, National Early Childhood Conference on Children with Special Needs, Denver, Colo, Nov 3, 1987.

19. George NM, and others: A prevention and early intervention mental health program for disadvantaged pre-school children. Am J Occup Ther 36:99, 1982.

20. Giangreco MF: Delivery of therapeutic services in special education programs for learners with severe handicaps. Phys Occup Ther in Ped 6:5, Summer 1986.

21. GLAD Bulletin. Rockville, Md, American Occupational Therapy Association, 1986.

22. Goldberg S: Teaching with toys. Ann Arbor, University of Michigan Press.

23. Hanson MJ: An analysis of the effects of early intervention services for infants & toddlers with moderate and severe handicaps. Topics in Early Child Spec Ed 5:36, 1985.

24. Kysela GM, and others: Early intervention programs with handicapped children. Unpublished paper presented to Annual Convention of American Psychologists Association, Montreal, 1980.

25. Lerner J: Special education for the early childhood years. New Jersey, 1981, Prentice-Hall, Inc.

26. Magrun WM, and Tigges KN: A transdisciplinary mobile intervention program for rural areas. Am J Occup Ther 36:90, 1982.

27. Meisels SJ: The efficacy of early intervention: why are we still asking this question? Topics in Early Child Spec Ed 5:1, Feb 1985.

28. Orelove FP, and Sobsey D: Educating children with multiple disabilities: a transdisciplinary approach. Baltimore, Md, 1987, Paul H Brookes Publishing Co.

29. Ottenbacher K: Transdisciplinary service delivery in school environment: some limitations. Phys Occup Ther in Pediat 3:9, 1983.

30. Peterson NL: Early intervention for handicapped and at-risk children. Denver, 1987, Love Publishing Co.

31. Rogers SJ, and others: An approach for enhancing the symbolic communicative interpersonal functioning of young children with autism or severe emotional handicaps. J Div Early Child 10:135, 1986.

32. Roles and functions of occupational therapy in early childhood intervention. Am J Occup Ther 40:835, 1986.

33. Sparling JW, and others: Play techniques with neurologically impaired preschoolers, Am J Occup Ther 38:603, Sep. 1984.

34. Strain PS, and Smith BJ: A counter-interpretation of early intervention effects: A response to Castro and Mastropieri. Except Child 53:260, 1987.

35. Swan W: Efficacy studies in early childhood special education: an overview. J Div Early Child 4:1, 1981.

36. Tjossem TD: Intervention strategies for high risk infants and young children. Baltimore, Md, 1976, University Park Press.

37. Umansky W: More than a teacher: an approach to meeting children's special needs. Child Ed 58:155, Jan 1982.

20

Children with cerebral palsy

RICARDO C. CARRASCO
WITH CONTRIBUTIONS BY NANCY POWELL*

Historical Review

The scientific study of cerebral palsy has evolved from focal orthopedic surgical procedures to the current interdisciplinary treatment approaches. Interest about the condition began when the physician Cazauvielh first published an article on cerebral paralysis in 1827.[15] However, collaborations on post-poliomyelitis surgical procedures between European orthopedists Delpach and Little set the stage for modern cerebral palsy intervention. In 1861, Little[37] published an article that related abnormal perinatal and paranatal events to developmental deficits. As a result, other physicians became interested in what was to be known as "Little's disease."

During the early twentieth century, Bronson Crothers incorporated physical therapy and psychological treatment to supplement surgical intervention.[39] Wtih other professionals on his team, Crothers ushered in the beginning of interdisciplinary intervention. Using Crothers' multispecialty approach, another orthopedist named William Phelps established a comprehensive rehabilitation center in Maryland.[51] Phelps differed from Crothers' primarily surgical orientation by prescribing exercise, muscle training, and bracing. Phelps is credited with coining the term "cerebral palsy" to distinguish the condition from mental retardation.[29] In 1947, the American Academy for Cerebral Palsy was formed to join the major medical specializations with related allied health services. In New York, the establishment of several programs modeled after Phelps' Maryland clinic led to a state, and eventually a national, United Cerebral Palsy Association, which now has local chapters throughout the United States.[72]

Occupational therapy has played a vital role in the development of interdisciplinary management of children with cerebral palsy. As early as 1929, occupational therapists provided treatment in schools and other settings, using activities to promote bimanual performance, proper positioning, muscle strengthening, play, and academic skills.[48] in 1950, Abbott[1] noted and described the variety of neuromuscular restoration techniques developed by Fay, Kabat, and Phelps that occupational therapists were beginning to use. Concurrent with neuromuscular approaches, occupational therapy was aimed at activity to correct upper extremity movement patterns and to establish "the habits of arm use in play"[25] (p. 65). Specifically, treatment was given in the sitting position by use of:

1. Repetitive motion and conditioning for the spastic child
2. Eye-hand coordination activities for the ataxic child
3. Relaxation followed by motion for the athetoid child

Wheelchair position and self-care training were also stressed.[25,38] Toys were adapted to encourage specific movements, increase hand coordination, and motivate the child to productive self-care and other hand functions.

Since the 1950s, occupational therapy intervention in the developmental, occupational, and self-care functions of children with cerebral palsy has expanded. Developments in occupational therapy theoretical models, treatment approaches, and techniques, as well as innovations in adapted activities and therapeutic equipment technology have had their impact. Bax[6] noted that during the 1970s there were major advances in the early diagnosis and assessment of cerebral palsy. However, as discussed later, the effectiveness of these different intervention methods remains inconclusive.

---

*The editors gratefully acknowledge Dr. Powell's review of the literature, particularly in relation to the developmental effects of cerebral palsy and the major intervention approaches.

To provide optimal occupational therapy services to the child or adolescent with cerebral palsy, the practitioner needs to understand not only the diagnosis and treatment of specific symptoms, but also the role of interdisciplinary management. The therapist is cautioned against stereotypical or generalized application of inflexible diagnostic and treatment procedures. A highly individualized, problem-solving approach must be used to prescribe activity experiences that are tailored to fit each child.

The remaining purposes of this chapter are to:

1. Discuss the scope and effects of cerebral palsy on child and adolescent development
2. Discuss occupational therapy intervention approaches to cerebral palsy
3. Provide examples of intervention through clinical case studies

Scope of the problem

Since its inception, the term "cerebral palsy" has been given various descriptions that have resulted in a definitional quandary. Traditional medically-oriented definitions describe cerebral palsy as "a nonprogressive lesion of the brain occurring before, at, or soon after birth that interferes with the normal development of the immature brain"[29] (p. 664). This approach is misleading to both parents and professionals, because it does not address the functional effects of cerebral palsy. Although the brain lesion is normally nonprogressive, resulting impairments in motor and other functions change over time.

This chapter proposes to define cerebral palsy by combining elements from Bax[6] and Bobath.[10] *Cerebral palsy is a disorder of movement and posture that is caused by a nonprogressive brain lesion that occurs in utero, during, or shortly after birth and is expressed through variable impairments in the coordination of muscle action and sensation.*

Characteristically, the child with cerebral palsy shows impaired ability to maintain normal postures due to a lack of muscle coactivation and the development of abnormal movement compensations. These compensatory patterns develop over the course of time, as disruptions to the child's center of gravity, as well as other sensory stimuli, result in impaired motor and postural responses. For example, the child's poor head control, resulting from poor coactivation of cervical flexors and extensors, causes the center of gravity to move anteriorly; this results in compensatory reactions in the thoracic and lumbar spine as the child attempts to stay upright in space. Likewise, hyperreactive responses to tactile, visual, or auditory stimuli may result in fluctuations of muscle tone that often adversely affect postural control and further diminish participation in meaningful activities.

Sensations that are registered and integrated through normal movement patterns are organizing[3]

and allow for the refinement of movements into more complex performance.[23] Initially, the sensory motor patterns are centrally programmed and expressed through postural reactions. The expression of postural reactions is limited only by the infant's range of motion, which is imposed by prevailing physiologic flexor tone and neonatal anatomic configurations. Responses to the specific stimuli are stereotypical and are mediated automatically through the lower centers of the central nervous system.[22] For example, the asymmetrical tonic neck reflex (ATNR) is elicited more fully in the 2-month-old infant than in an older child, because tone is generally lower and coactivation of the opposing muscle groups is immature. The limbs of the face and skull sides move with obligatory extension and flexion when the head-turning stimulus is introduced.

Through regulation of reflexes and reactions, the child's central nervous system matures and begins to regulate the "degree, strength, balance, and distribution of muscle tone"[22] (p. 26). Without this regulation, the child will experience difficulty in performing automatic movements. Critical to optimal development of postural behavior is the sequential interaction and coordination of the postural reflexes. Eventually, the integration of reflexes into higher level righting, protective, and equilibrium reactions form a solid foundation for skilled and coordinated movements in work, self-care, and play or leisure.

During normal movements, the brain registers sensory feedback from weight-bearing and weight-shifting experiences. The child develops a stable base for performing cognitive and interactive tasks without having to think consciously about maintaining a particular position. This process is reversed when experienced by a child with cerebral palsy. The sensory feedback from compensatory movements feeds into more compensations. Inaccurate feedback leads to further distortions of movements and sensation, contractures, and deformities, together with adverse influences on the psychological and prevocational development of the child.

Classification of cerebral palsy

The locale of the lesion affects the development and quality of movement patterns present in the child with cerebral palsy. Because of its influence on muscle tone, cerebral palsy with *spasticity* indicates a fixed lesion in the motor cortex. Lesions in the basal ganglia typically cause fluctuations in muscle tone that are described as *athetosis* or dystonia. Cerebellar damage tends to produce the unstable movements characteristic of the *ataxic* child.

The variability of the movement and postural disorder may be classified according to which limbs are affected. Involvement of one extremity is commonly referred to as monoplegia, upper and lower extremities on one side as hemiplegia, both lower extremities as paraplegia, and all limbs as quadriplegia. When the child demonstrates quadriplegia with mild upper extremity involvement and more significant impairment in lower extremity function, this is called diplegia.

Several classifications of cerebral palsy have been developed according to quality of tone, disorder distribution, and even locale of brain lesions.[21,43,50] A combination of these classifications is featured in Table 20-1. Characteristics are described according to quality and distribution of muscle tone, range of motion, quality of movement, presence of reflexes and reactions, oral motor problems, associated problems, and personality characteristics. Among these classifications, the incidence of athetosis has decreased in recent years because of advances in prenatal care, such as routine blood incompatibility tests.[58]

EFFECTS ON CHILD DEVELOPMENT
Occupational behavior

Through sensorimotor exploration and experimentation, the child learns about the internal and external environment.[52] These experiences enhance cognitive and psychosocial development. The neonate responds to stimuli through postural behaviors programmed in the immature brain.[22] During the feeding process for example, the infant uses the rooting response to turn her head toward the feeding source. Together the rooting response and reflexive grasp on the caretaker's fingers can lead to eye contact with the caretaker. At the same time, the caretaker's body provides comforting warmth.[4] Because of the movement problems associated with cerebral palsy, this bonding process becomes potentially stressful for both the child and the caretaker. If oral motor function is inadequate, the child becomes frustrated because her hunger is not satisfied, secondary to inefficient sucking and swallowing. The frustrated child fusses and cries, leading to frustration on the part of the caretaker.

Florey discussed Reilly's theory of play behavior in Chapter 3. Cerebral palsy (CP) may restrict exploratory behaviors such as object manipulation and locomotion. Knox[35] pointed out that a disability can inhibit exploration, and delay or limit the discovery of meanings of objects, motions, and people, and the assessment of one's assets and limitations. Competence and adaptation are skewed by faulty feedback from both the environment and the child's actions. Children with cerebral palsy often do not persist in mastering difficult motor tasks. This can affect feelings of self-reliance and self-confidence. Difficulties in exploratory and competency behavior have a cumulative effect on achievement behavior. Gunn[27] noted a relationship between the inability of the handicapped child to play and decreased ability to cope with novel, complex, or dissonant situations.

Takata[63] described aspects of play deprivation of multi-handicapped children. These include:
1. Sedentary and passive experience
2. Limited access to or lack of available materials
3. Emphasis on motor behavior
4. Parental expectations that are too high or too low

Adverse effects of cerebral palsy can also be seen in delays or compensatory movement patterns during manipulative tasks. As a result, the development of prehension and vision for meaningful exploration of toys, objects, and persons is decreased.[19] Impaired development of the concepts, abstractions, and generalizations that normally arise from such concrete explorations can result in diminished understanding of permanence and causal relationships related to objects and persons. Play then becomes distorted and does not enhance the spiral pattern of maturation.[41] The primarily sensorimotor disorder has thus spilled over to cognitive and psychosocial domains, potentially adversely affecting academic and prevocational development.

As the child gets older, the effects of cerebral palsy go beyond movement and sensation. Table 20-2 summarizes the impact on occupational behavior. The child needs equipment and environmental adaptations for independence in self-care, academic performance, and work preparation. The focus switches to environmental controls, barrier-free settings, self-care, school, and recreational equipment, community resource availability, geographic and economic management, and issues of personal hygiene and sexual expression. Nothing can be taken for granted, and in most instances, engagement in normal developmental activities requires extra effort and intervention strategies.

A motor and sensation disorder such as cerebral palsy may interfere with the development of skills and habits related to occupational choice, role, and socialization. Matsutsuyu[40] emphasized the aim of occupational therapy as "one of identifying the nature of adaptations . . . needed to maintain, support, or raise the daily living performance of patients in their current life roles" (p. 292).

Adaptation

Ayres,[4] King,[31] and others[32,33] have explained adaptation as a goal of therapeutic intervention. King[31] noted that individual adaptation involves active participation, responsiveness to environmental demands, outcome orientation, and self-reinforcement. The goals of individual adaptation are described as enhancement of personal survival and actualization of potential. Kleiman and Bulkley[33] have expanded the adaptation concept to a continuum. On one end are basic homeostatic reactions, including survival mechanisms such as reflexes and breathing. Next are the adaptive responses that are active, self-reinforcing, goal-directed, and inte-

Table 20-1 Cerebral palsy classifications

	Severe spasticity	Moderate spasticity	Mild spasticity
QUALITY OF TONE	Severely increased tone; flexor and extensor cocontraction are constant; tone is high at rest, asleep or awake; tone pattern is more proximal than distal.	Moderately increased tone; near normal at rest but increases with excitement, movement attempts, effort, emotion, speech, sudden stretch; agonists and distal muscles more spastic.	Mildly increased or normal tone at rest; increases with effort or attempts to move or attempts at quicker movements.
DISTRIBUTION OF TONE	Quadriplegia, but can also be diplegia or paraplegia.	Same as severe spasticity.	Same as severe spasticity, but more diplegia and hemiplegia.
RANGE OF MOTION	Abnormal patterns can lead to scoliosis, kyphosis, hip/knee/finger deformity; forearm pronation contracture, hip subluxation, heel cord subluxation with equinovarus or equinovalgus; decreased trunk, shoulder and pelvic girdle mobility; limited midrange control where cocontraction is least balanced.	More available movement and more flexor/ extensor imbalance can lead to kyphosis, lordosis, hip subluxations or dislocations, hip and knee flexion contractures; tight hip internal rotators and adductors; heel cord shortening and foot rotation.	Limitations seen more distally; minimal deformities.
QUALITY OF MOVEMENT	Decreased midrange, voluntary and involuntary movements; slow and labored stereotypical movements.	May be able to walk; stereotypical, asymmetrical, more associated reactions, total movement synergies.	Often able to walk; seems driven to move; often a challenge to treat due to many movements; increased ranges with a variety of other movements, some stereotypical.
REFLEXES AND REACTIONS	Obligatory primitive reflexes (Positive support, ATNR, STNR, neck righting); protective, righting and equilibrium reactions are often absent.	Strong primitive reflexes — Moro, startle, TNR, TLR, positive support prominent; decreased neck righting; associated reactions strong; righting may be present, but equilibrium reaction develops to sitting and kneeling.	Primitive reflexes used for functional purposes and not obligatory; righting, protective and equilibrium reactions delayed, but not established; may not get higher level reactions.
ORAL MOTOR	Immobile, rigid chest; shallow respiration and forced expiration; lip retraction with decreased lip closure and tongue thrust; communication through forced expiration.	Not as involved as severe spasticity.	Increased mobility, thus more respiratory function for phonation; shortness of breath limits sentence length; better ability to dissociate mouth parts, but poor lip closure causes drooling.
ASSOCIATED PROBLEMS	Seizures; cortical blindness; deafness; mental retardation; prone to upper respiratory tract infection (URTI); malnutrition.	Seizures; MR; perceptual motor problems; imbalance of eye musculature.	Seizures; less MR; perceptual problems.
PERSONALITY CHARACTERISTICS	Passive, dependent; resistant and adapts poorly to change; anxious and fearful of being moved; generally less frustrated than athetoid.	A lesser picture of severe spasticity.	More frustrated and critical about self due to awareness of better performance; more patient than children of same age.

Table 20-1 Cerebral palsy classifications—cont'd

	Pure athetosis	Athetosis with spasticity	Athetosis with tonic spasms
QUALITY OF TONE	Fluctuation of tone from low to normal; no or little spasticity; no coactivation of flexors and extensors.	Fluctuates from normal to high; some ability to stabilize proximally; moderate proximal spasticity and distal athetosis.	Unpredictable tone changes from low to very high; either all flexion or extension of extremities.
DISTRIBUTION OF TONE	Quadriplegia with occasional hemiplegia.	Same as athetosis.	Quadriplegia, hemiplegia, or monoplegia.
RANGE OF MOTION	Transient subluxation of joints such as shoulders and fingers; may see valgus on feet or knees; rarely any deformities.	Incidence of scoliosis; some flexion deformities at hips, elbows and knees; usually full ROM proximally/hypermobile distally.	More pronounced scoliosis; more dislocation of arm due to flailing spasm; possible kyphoscoliosis, hip dislocation on skull side, flexion contracture on hips/knees, subluxation of hips, fingers, or lower jaw.
QUALITY OF MOVEMENT	Writhing involuntary movements; seen more distal than proximal; no change with intention to move; many fixation attempts due to decreased ability to stabilize.	Decreased ability to grade movements; decreased midline control and selective movement; proximal stability and distal choreoathetosis; varies with case.	Extreme tonic spasm without voluntary control; some involuntary movement, distal more than proximal.
REFLEXES & REACTIONS	Primitive reflexes not usually obligatory or evoked; protective and equilibrium reactions usually present but involuntary movements affect grading.	TNR/TLR strong but intermittent and modified by involuntary movements; equilibrium reactions when present are unreliable and may or may not be used.	Strong ATNR, STNR, TLR; protective & equilibrium reactions absent during spasm, otherwise present, unreliable or absent.
ORAL MOTOR	Fluctuations adversely affect gross and fine motor performance; volume of speech may go up or down with breath; feeding may be decreased due to instability and tongue/jaw/swallow incoordination.	Difficulty with head control, thus decreased oral motor, strained speech; decreased coordination of suck/swallow, resulting in decreased feeding and speech.	Feeding may be difficult because aspiration is unpredictable; severe language and speech impairment due to decreased control.
ASSOCIATED PROBLEMS	Hearing loss; less mental retardation.	Same as athetosis.	Same as athetosis.
PERSONALITY CHARACTERISTICS	Emotional lability; less fearful of movement; more outgoing, but tends to be frustrated.	Same as athetosis.	Same as athetosis.

grated actions, such as grasping. Adaptive skills are next on the continuum, and include combinations and repetition of adaptive responses. Playing baseball is an example of using adaptive skills. Finally, at the other end of the continuum are large, complex behavioral units called adaptive patterns, such as balanced leisure time activity.

Depending on the severity of the motor handicap, the child with cerebral palsy will need variable amounts of intervention to achieve the goals of individ-

Table 20-1   Cerebral palsy classifications—cont'd

	Choreoathetosis	Flaccid	Ataxia
QUALITY OF TONE	Constant fluctuations from low to high with no co-contraction; jerky involuntary movements more proximal than distal.	Fluctuating, markedly low muscle tone; seen at birth or toddler initially as flaccid; later classified as spastic, athetoid or ataxic.	Ranges from near normal to normal; when increased tone is present, usually involves lower extremity flexion.
DISTRIBUTION OF TONE	Quadriplegia.	Quadriplegia.	Quadriplegia.
RANGE OF MOTION	Many involuntary movements with extreme ranges but no control at midrange; deformities rare, but tendency for shoulder and finger subluxation.	Hypermobile joints tend to sublux; flat chest; later range limitations due to limited movement.	Range is usually not a problem; when present, decreased range is in flexion.
QUALITY OF MOVEMENT	Wide movement ranges with no gradation; jerky movements more proximal than distal; no selective movement or fixation of movement; weak hands and fingers.	Ungraded movements; slow movements difficult; many static postures as if hanging on to anatomical structures instead of active control.	Lack point of stability so coactivation is difficult; use primitive rather than abnormal patterns, hence gross, total patterns; incoordination, thus dysmetria disdiadochokinesia, tremors at rest, symmetrical problems.
REFLEXES & REACTIONS	Intermittent TNR; righting and equilibrium reactions present to some extent, but abnormal coordination. Abnormal upper extremity protective extension but often absent.	Usually less reactive due to decreased tone; righting is delayed; delayed protective extension more available than equilibrium reaction.	May develop righting reactions but uncoordinated, exaggerated and poorly used; equilibrium reactions when developed are not coordinated; needs wide base of support because of poor weight shift.
ORAL MOTOR	Facial grimaces; dysarthria; irregular breathing; difficulty in sustaining phonation; poor intra- and extra-oral surfaces.	Quiet soft voice due to decreased respiration; delayed speech; increased drooling; often expressionless face.	Speech is monotone, very slow; uses teeth to stabilize tongue or hold cup to mouth when drinking; decreased articulation.
ASSOCIATED PROBLEMS	Same as athetosis.	Obesity; sensory impairment; URTI.	Nystagmus; mental retardation; sensory problems; uses vision for righting and as reference point for movement.
PERSONALITY CHARACTERISTICS	Same as athetosis.	Visually attentive; cannot move, therefore, are "good" babies; decreased motivation.	Does not like to move.

ual adaptation. Difficulty at each point along the continuum is possible. The reactions linked to basic survival may be impaired, such as breathing and feeding reflexes. Adaptive responses may be hampered by incoordinated movements, becoming too laborious to be functional. Often, very few adaptive skills, such as playing games, can be executed in a normal manner. Without intervention, many children will achieve only limited success and independence in adaptive patterns such as leisure time utilization.

Psychosocial development

Verluys[73] described the effects of chronic illness, some of which pertain to the child or adolescent with cerebral palsy. Problems include reduced self-esteem,

Table 20-2 Effects of cerebral palsy on occupational behavior

Age	Critical Variables	Occupational Behavior Limitations
Infancy and Early Childhood	Sensorimotor exploration, repetition, and imitation	Self-care areas of feeding, toileting and play; academic preparation in sensorimotor, cognitive, and psychosocial areas
Middle and Late Childhood	Fundamental skills, role models, tools and symbols, peer groups	Self-care areas of feeding, toileting, hygiene, communication, geographical orientation and mobility; academic performance; environmental manipulation; relationships
Adolescence	Identity, autonomy, competence, and achievement	Independence in self-care areas of feeding, hygiene, and home management; vocational exploration and identification; participation in interest areas; relationships; independent environmental manipulation and exploration

security, independence, and social contacts. The ability to manipulate and cope with the environment and the behavior of others can be impaired.[37] Therefore, social adjustment is threatened, and the ability to establish effective relationships with peers and adults is impaired.

Abnormal motor behavior can interfere with developing an adequate self-concept, and the perception of the child's needs, feelings, physical performance abilities, and sexuality may be disrupted. Coping with stress and solving life problems may be difficult for the child with cerebral palsy. Because he frequently has difficulty with self-expression, he is likely to be hindered in learning how to deal with social organizational norms. Adjusting behavior to situational demands is often a problem area for children with cerebral palsy if they are limited in opportunities to develop a flexible repertoire of behavioral responses in different environments.

In summary, because of deprivation of play experiences and limitations imposed by sensory and motor deficits, the child with cerebral palsy is likely to have difficulty with developmental tasks. The severity of the motor disorder, the number of associated deficits, family support, and the child's health and educational service providers will all affect the child's play development and subsequent acquisition of self-care and work-related skills. The occupational therapist must be sensitive to the overall process of the child's development throughout the assessment and treatment process.

OCCUPATIONAL THERAPY ASSESSMENT IN CEREBRAL PALSY

Developments in research and technology have made earlier intervention possible for the child with a definite or at-risk diagnosis of cerebral palsy.[36] Current information about early diagnosis and treatment resulted from intensive investigations of early developmental stages. (See also Chapters 18 and 19.) Milani-Comparetti[42] proposed the presence of fetal competencies that correlate with neonatal behaviors. Through fetal examination, Milani-Comparetti identified abilities for active participation during the birth process. Thus the presence of fetal abilities can serve as indicators for potential of fetal stress during the birth process.

In 1980, Bly[8] identified normal and abnormal blocks of development from birth to 12 months of age. She suggested that compensatory movements are normally used by infants and toddlers during their initial attempts at upright positions and transitional movements. The compensations result from lack of control over the initial phases of movement. Eventually the maturation of postural control permits the development of more discrete movement patterns. However, the persistence of compensatory movements, characteristic of cerebral palsy, may lead to an abnormal "block" to motor development. These blocks can result in permanently distorted movement patterns if not remediated. For example, scapular adduction is present during the infant's early practice in independent sitting and standing. However, persistence of adducted scapular patterns may lead to decreased upper trunk mobility and decreased scapulohumeral dissociation. When the latter occurs, the scapula and humerus tend to move as a unit, thereby limiting humeral range in activities such as overhead reach used in combing hair.

Assessment instruments

Such progressive patterns of dysfunction are typical among children with cerebral palsy. Therefore assessment of the child with cerebral palsy takes more than identification of developmental milestones. Developmental scales are desirable, but qualitative components of function must also be identified.[58] Selecting appropriate instruments varies according to the child's chronological and developmental age, diagnosis, referral reasons, the family's priorities, agency operating procedures, and the therapist's expertise, as well as the presence and composition of the interdisciplinary team. Many of the tests and measurements described in Chapters 9 through 11 may be appropriately used for assessment of children with cerebral palsy. Other useful instruments are featured in Table 20-3. Since not every instrument was specifically designed for administration to the child with cerebral palsy, findings should be interpreted accordingly.

Several instruments were specifically designed for children with cerebral palsy or at risk for the disease. The Erhardt Developmental Hand, Feeding, and Vision assessments[18,20] were developed through longitudinal studies that examined reflexive and voluntary aspects of the three functions. The Erhardt assessments and accompanying manuals are helpful for prescribing treatment as well. The Stratton Evaluation of Oral Function in Feeding[62] was proposed to establish a baseline of observable oral behaviors upon which management and change can be measured. The Movement Assessment of Infants (MAI)[36] provides an evaluation protocol to examine muscle tone, primitive reflexes, automatic reactions, and volitional movement patterns of children from birth to 12 months of age. Normative data are available for children to 6 months.[16] The Pre-Speech Assessment Scale developed by Morris,[45] identifies oral motor functions and related areas, and provides a measure of gains or losses during treatment. Use of the Pre-Speech Assessment Scale requires specialized training, preferably certification in Neurodevelopmental Treatment (NDT), because of the complexity of assessment issues. In a later publication, Morris and Klein[44] featured reproducible record keeping forms that are used to chronicle prefeeding and movement patterns demonstrated by children with central nervous system deficit.

Traditional movement pattern evaluations and adaptations[60] investigate the child's ability to oppose the pull of gravity during specific imposed postures. The therapist then makes assumptions about whether such flexion or extension patterns can be applied in the performance of occupational tasks. In other words, these tests assess task performance through observation of static postures in situations that may be meaningless to the child. The tests measure muscular coactivation against gravity, but do not necessarily evaluate transitional components of movement or presence of midrange control. In addition, they do not test the child's cognitive or interactive responses.

Traditional manual muscle testing procedures may not elicit cooperation from dysfunctioning children.

Pact, Sirotkin-Roses, and Beatus[47] suggest that functional muscle strength can be demonstrated during play. However, the therapist needs to be familiar with the performance of non-dysfunctioning children, and should pay attention to range of motion, rhythm of movements, and symmetry of performance during play.

Key issues in assessment

Evaluation of the child or adolescent with cerebral palsy combines the application of scientific skills with consideration of sensory, sequential neurodevelopmental, and anatomical and kineseological issues. *Sensory issues* involve the occupational therapist's awareness that abnormal movement will feed into abnormal sensory feedback. Abnormal sensorimotor patterns from an immature and dysfunctioning central nervous system can result in a downward rather than upward spiral in movement development. Thus the child acquires the distorted postures typically seen in cerebral palsy. A dysfunctional central nervous system can result in behaviors that give an impression of hyposensitivity or hypersensitivity to vestibular, somatosensory, visual, auditory, olfactory, or even gustatory systems.

Sequential neurodevelopmental issues of cerebral palsy assessment involve the application of basic principles such as proximodistal, cephalocaudal, and gross to fine gradients of development. For example, righting and equilibrium reactions tend to develop before situationally responsive movements. The hips, trunk, neck, and shoulders need to be stable before performing the rotational and fine distal prehension patterns necessary for writing.

Anatomical and kineseological issues require the application of basic sciences to look at the performance of joints and muscles in motion. Knowledge of oral motor structure, development, and function, sensory integration, scapulohumeral rhythm, and normal gait patterns is necessary for analyzing the child's movements during performance of occupational tasks. Skills in observation and expedient problem solving are necessary to assess balance of tone, alignment, and coordination of structural key points, reliability of righting and equilibrium reactions, and the ability to impose mobility on stability.

Normal postures and movements are only possible with normal muscle coactivation, which in turn is dependent upon balanced muscle tone. Abnormal or asymmetrical distributions of tone will result in abnormal or asymmetrical postures and movements. When abnormal postural alignment is corrected, muscle tone is also altered and more normal movement patterns are elicited.

Another important element is the alignment and coordination of structural *key points*. This requires the alignment of the head, shoulders and hips in relation to the spine, and secondarily, the elbows and knees in re-

Table 20-3 Additional instruments for assessment of children and adolescents with cerebral palsy†

Name of test	Age range	Specified test population	Sensorimotor
Auditory Discrimination Test	5 to 8 years	Learning/speech problems	
Callier-Asuza Scale	Children to age 7	Blind, multi-handicapped	X
CP Movement Assessment	Birth to 5 yr	CP	X
Crawford Small Parts Dexterity Test	Adol-adult	CNS trauma work disability	X
Dubowitz Neurological Assessment	Preterm and Term Infants	At-risk infants	X
*Erhardt Developmental Vision Assessments	Varies	CP or CNS insult	X
Meeting Street School Screening Test	K to Gr 1	LD	X
Peabody Picture Vocabulary Test (PPVT)	2½-18 yr	CP, autistic, nonverbal	
Peabody Picture Vocabulary Test Revised (PPVT-R)	2.6 to 40-11	CP, autistic, nonverbal	
*Pre-Speech Assessment	Birth to 2 yr	Damage, cleft palate, spina bifida, Down syndrome, LD	X
Response to Sensory Input (Ayres/Ornitz)	Nonspecific	Autism, decreased/increased sensory registration	X
Sequenced Inventory of Communication Development	4 to 48 mos	Developmental delay	
Teacher Questionnaire on Sensorimotor Behavior	4 to school age	LD, DD, emotional problems, CP	X

*Need special training, certification, educational qualifications
†See chapters 9, 10, and 11 for other appropriate tests.
S, self-care; *P*, play; *W*, work.

lation to the shoulders and hips. Together, correct alignment at key points provides a stable base for more distal coordinated movements of the extremities, eyes, and mouth.

The reliability of righting and equilibrium reactions is dependent on the coordination of vestibular, somatosensory, visual, and sometimes auditory systems, and the ability to respond automatically with balance reactions to a weight shift. Difficulty with responses to gravitational stimuli can result in fear or avoidance responses. The imposition of distal mobility on proximal stability requires the coordination of all sensory input to sustain quality performance. Attention to task can be enhanced by an automatic and stable base of postural support.

Obervational analysis of the child's movements, use of sensory modalities, and performance in activity environments is discussed in Chapter 9. (See Figure 9-6 for a checklist.) Observing the child in activities that require transitions to various positions, such as supine to prone or prone to sit, is particularly useful.

In addition, it is also critical to observe a child's *reaction to handling*. This allows the therapist to compare pre- and post-handling reactions, movement pat-

terns, and skill of performance, and improves the quality of treatment handling. If parents are present during the evaluation, explaining the test results in relation to therapeutic goals and procedures becomes an easier task. The therapist should first observe a child's performance of tasks without therapeutic handling (facilitation of normal components of movement and sensation). Then, the therapist may impose some handling techniques and observe the child's reaction to the handling and performance of tasks. Did the child maintain a balanced control of coactivating muscles or did imbalance recur in the flexors and extensors? Did the rotational components on the trunk remain or disappear with the imposed tasks? What were the predominant movement and sensation compensations?

TYPICAL PROBLEMS ASSOCIATED WITH CEREBRAL PALSY

One of the principal goals of the assessment is to identify problems that require occupational therapy intervention. It has been emphasized that the child's improvements in occupational performance are going to

Cognitive	Psycho-social	Occupational performance	Source
X			Western Psychol Svcs (WPS) 12301 Wilshire Blvd, Los Angeles, CA 90025
X	X		Robert Stillman, Ph.D Callier Str. for Communication Disorders, U of Texas–Dallas 1966 Inwood Rd, Dallas, TX 75235
			OT for Phys Dis (Trombly)
		W	Psychological Corp. 304 East 45th St, New York, NY 10017
			Illingworth, Dev. of Infant & Young Child Churchill-Livingstone
			Erhardt, Developmental Hand Dysfunctions, RAMSCO Publishing
X		W	Crippled Children & Adults of Rhode Island, Meeting Str. School, 333 Grotto Ave Providence, RI 02906
X			AGS American Guidance Service, Circle Pines, MN 55014
X			AGS American Guidance Service, Circle Pines, MN 55014
		S	Oral Motor Function and Dysfunction in Children (Wislon) U of NC, Chapel Hill, NC
			AJOT Vol 34, #6 June, 1980
X		S P	WPS
X	X	W P S	Carrasco, RC, Medical College of GA-EF 102 Augusta, GA 30912

be heavily dependent on preparatory intervention with movement and sensory disturbances. To review, these problems relate to muscle tone quality, distribution, and symmetry, movement compensations, and sensory reactivity. These have been discussed generally, but a more detailed understanding of specific patterns is necessary for knowledgeable evaluation and treatment.

Muscle tone

Muscle tone disturbances are expressed in the following manner:
1. Either extensors or flexors predominate
2. Muscle action is too weak, secondary to low tone, to oppose the pull of gravity
3. A combination of extensor or flexor dominance and decreased opposition to gravity
4. Tone fluctuations, resulting in unreliable movements
5. Asymmetrical coactivation (left vs. right body side)
6. Tone distribution variations among extremities

These tone disturbances can eventually lead to loss of joint range, if not contractures, subluxation, and increased compensatory movements. Many children who initially have low tone may later exhibit high tone or spasticity when performing tasks, particularly those that require exteroceptive or proprioceptive stimuli. Muscle tone distribution disturbances, depending on the CNS lesion site, can involve upper and lower extremities, or right-left body side tone variations. This often results in neglect of and compensatory movements by both affected and unaffected limbs, subsequently affecting occupational task performance.

Bly's study of movement development[8] identified compensatory patterns normally seen in young children. The following abnormal patterns of movement and sensory compensations are synthesized from Bly,[8] Ayres and Tickle,[5] and Ward,[74] as well as observations from clinical practice. Movement compensations may be seen in the spine, shoulder girdle, upper extremities, wrist and hand, hips, and lower extremities. As specific problems are reviewed in sequence, it is clear that each pattern can successively cause movement compensations at other anatomical sites.

Movement compensations in the spine

Cervical hyperextension (approximately C1-C4). Lack of flexor or extensor development can adversely affect cervical, shoulder, and thoracic mobility as well as muscle development. If not remediated, exaggeration of the spinal curve, kyphosis, or lordosis can result. With the neck in a hyperextended position, midline gaze is decreased, as is efficient use of other sensory systems. This results in decreased orientation to sights and sounds for environmental, object, and personal exploration. Tabletop activities require increased effort, and hygiene and dressing activities from the neck down are performed with difficulty.

Spinal asymmetry at the cervical level is caused by abnormal cervical extension and lack of antigravity flexor development. The inability to move out of this posture can lead to persistence of an obligatory ATNR. Asymmetry can go down the spine, increasing the possibility of scoliosis, hip dislocation, and asymmetry in the shoulder girdle and upper extremities. Visual field deficits, decreased midline control, impaired body scheme, limited body exploration by the upper extremities, and decreased auditory localization during daily activities can result.

Decreased thoracic spine mobility results from lack of scapular stability or increased thoracic extension. Lateral mobility of the thoracic region will be limited. To compensate for these limitations, scapular hypermobility may develop. If there is too much thoracic extension without lateral flexion, scapular abduction may be used abnormally. During weight-bearing, both the medial and inferior borders of the scapula may tip posteriorly. Functional effects of decreased thoracic spine mobility include limitations in overhead reach for dressing and other activities.

Lumbar spine extension typically accompanies weak cocontraction of the abdominals. Additionally, the anatomical configuration of the thoracolumbar spine is susceptible to hyperextension. As a result, hip flexors do not elongate during the first year, further impairing abdominal flexor development. The "Paradox of the Psoas Muscle" is a kineseological phenomenon that occurs and reinforces the pull of the lumbar spine into extension and worsens the imbalance between abdominals and back extensors. Resulting limitations in lumbar flexion affect gait, dressing, and bathing.

Movement compensations of the shoulder girdle

Scapular compensations include abnormal patterns of adduction and abduction. Compensatory use of *scapular adduction* results from lack of thoracic extension or poor head and neck flexor control. Though normally present in the initial phases of prone weight-bearing, sitting, standing, or walking situations, persistent lack of flexor control can cause the scapulae to be maintained in adduction and downward rotation. This in turn limits forward shoulder flexion. Children sometimes use scapular adduction to increase thoracic extension, but the resulting pattern is abnormal. Scapular

adduction is also sometimes used with clavicular and scapular elevation to compensate for lack of cervical flexor antigravity control. This causes the shoulder girdle to serve as a strut to assist with head control, and decreases effectiveness of forward reach and midline manipulation. There is also decreased toy and body exploration and difficulty with bilateral tasks; spinal asymmetry and scapulohumeral association are reinforced.

The scapulae may also move around the ribcage into upward rotation and *abduction*. During task involvement, this pattern may reinforce thoracic hyperextension. This puts the shoulder in a disadvantaged position and limits range for protective responses and assumption of the sidelying position. As a result, there are increased risks of falling unprotected and limitations in positions for play and leisure activities. Persistence of this pattern may limit the length of the scapular muscles, thus maintaining the position of clavicular and scapular elevation. Decreased scapulohumeral dissociation, breathing, and communication problems may occur.

Decreased scapulohumeral dissociation has been mentioned already and is associated with limitations in rolling and forward reach in prone at about 3 to 4 months. Increased scapular mobility on the rib cage results in "winging" on the inferior border near the axillae while the child is in prone weight-bearing. This causes a disruption of the scapulohumeral rhythm. To compensate for diminished overhead reach, lateral trunk flexion is used. Bilateral hand function is limited as one body side goes up while the other pulls down into more lateral flexion and humeral abduction.

Decreased clavicular mobility is also caused by the combination of decreased neck flexor/extensor cocontraction development and decreased scapulohumeral dissociation. Because of its limited mobility, the clavicle is characteristically elevated and impinges on distal rotation and forward flexion at 90 degrees. This affects placement of the hand and upper extremity in space during daily activities. Posterior dislocation of the clavicle at the sternoclavicular joint can occur during overhead reach. Clavicular assistance during breathing and speech is decreased and vital capacity may be compromised.

Movement compensations of the upper extremity

Humeral extension and abduction results in limitations to scapular mobility and shoulder flexion and depression. There is decreased lateral weight shift in prone, and thoracic mobility may be reduced. This compensatory pattern is usually accompanied by persistent elbow flexion, limiting elbow extension. The latter prevents forearm supination during reach; therefore, primitive grasping and other prehension patterns must be used, with limited accuracy and grading of movements. This compensatory pattern can affect hair combing, dressing, and even spoon to mouth skills.

Humeral internal rotation results from impaired development of shoulder external rotation and is usually paired with shoulder elevation. Increased scapular adduction and humeral hyperextension are also demonstrated. In weight-bearing, elbow flexion is increased with pronation to the radial side. As a result, antigravity reach over the head is difficult. Primitive rotation of the head also occurs during prone weight-bearing.

Elbow flexion results from adduction or poor mobility of the scapula. Humeral abduction and hyperextension, pronation of the forearm, and ulnar deviation of the wrist are often exhibited. This results in decreased reaching, hand placement, and grasp skills, as well as impaired upper limb sequencing.

Forearm pronation, accompanied by internal rotation of the humerus, limits forearm supination. Persistence of this compensation can result in subluxation of the radial head. Attempts to use an extremely pronated forearm result in increased ulnar deviation during reach. Functional effects include difficulty with forearm supination when weight-bearing or reaching into space, limitations in unilateral manipulation and dexterity, and impairment in feeding, other self-care, and palm-to-palm activities.

Movement compensations of the wrist and hand

Wrist flexion may be accompanied by shortening of wrist flexors resulting from decreased weight-bearing, but it can also occur when wrist extensors are overstretched. Depending on tone quality, flexion contractures can develop. Increased ulnar deviation and decreased strength of finger flexors can result. Supination of the forearm is also more difficult because of impaired wrist extension and radial deviation.

Ulnar deviation of the wrist is pronounced when wrist extensors are weak, and reduces forearm supination and wrist circumduction. This compensation can also lead to thumb adduction.

Metacarpophalangeal (MCP/MP) hyperextension often accompanies wrist extension and can result in swan neck deformity, with the possibility of subluxed MP joints. Abduction of fingers is increased, so hand activities are not refined. The child may use extension to compensate for impaired ability to grade finger movements. this compensatory pattern can decrease palmar mobility to accommodate or shape around objects.

Thumb adduction at the carpometacarpal (CMC) and MP joints can accompany decreased wrist flexion, ulnar deviation, and MP hyperextension and, long-term, can result in subluxation of the MP joints into the palm. This deformity can only be corrected surgically. The finger web spaces tighten, so prehension of large objects is decreased, and fine prehension patterns are impaired. There is a tendency toward instability at distal joints that limits fine motor skills and dexterity.

Movement compensation of the hips and lower extremities

Hip flexion results from persistence of lumbar extension and anterior pelvic tilt. Decreased developmental elongation of hip extensors can result in mechanical changes in the hip joint. The gluteus medius cannot abduct the hip when hip flexion is greater than 40 degrees. The mechanical disadvantage also limits internal rotation, extension, and adduction of the hip. The insertion of the gluteus medius may slip laterally. Hip flexion dominance will limit ambulation and self-care skills significantly.

Femoral antiversion may accompany hip flexion, resulting in increased internal rotation of the femur with overstretched external rotators and extensors. Even with the developmental anterior movement of the acetabulum, femoral antiversion with genu valgus on pronated feet can occur. The resulting tendency is to "bunny hop" during ambulatory attempts, especially when the influence of the symmetrical tonic neck reflex is strong. "W-sitting" is also characteristic and places increased stress on the knees.

Genu valgus typically accompanies limitations in hip extension, external rotation, and hamstring tightness. This results in decreased bone molding, bunny hopping, and w-sitting, with deterioration of the medial surface of the knee. Extension contractures with subtalar joint laxity and forefoot valgus and abduction can occur. Walking further complicates this compensation if appropriate intervention is not instituted.

Displacement of the patella is caused by tight hip flexors. Ambulation is limited by the child's decreased ability to extend the knee. The patella slips off the condyles and thus is at a mechanical disadvantage.

Ankle plantar flexion is due to increased unilateral or bilateral lower extremity tone. The subtalar joint tends to fall medially and eventually shortens the Achilles tendon. As the talus slips medially and forward, the calcaneus can slip laterally. Thus active ankle dorsiflexion is impossible and forefoot varus and abduction occurs. This pattern limits ambulation, but corrective shoes or orthotics are helpful.

Excessive subtalar joint inversion accompanies rotation of the distal end of the tibia. The top of the calcaneus slips laterally, and the talus slips laterally and posteriorly, causing ankle inversion, hindfoot varus, and forefoot valgus. This compensatory pattern can also benefit from corrective shoes or orthotics.

Sensory reactivity problems

Vestibular hyperresponsiveness or hyporesponsiveness arises from diminished or inconsistent registration of vestibular stimuli. Achievement of vertical head position becomes a critical problem for some children. (Note that some children with habitual neck hyperextension may not be able to tolerate true vertical head position, so sensory causes must be differentiated from motor.) Reliance on other sensory systems, such as visual, may be used to maintain an upright position against gravity. Slight weight shifts or changes in posture may trigger increased tone. Development of righting, equilibrium, and protective extension reactions may be compromised secondary to diminished registration and integration of vestibular stimuli. Some children may compensate by maintaining constant motion, with decreased midline control and sequencing of movement.

Occupational tasks that require changes in head position or weight shifts, and provide fewer visual cues for postures, such as dressing or bathing, may be avoided or performed inefficiently. This can result in frustration and poor hygiene. There is decreased body feedback on postural alignment, direction, and position during task performance, and increased risk of falling without protection.

Somatosensory hyperresponsiveness or hyporesponsiveness is caused by dominance of the spinothalamic system in processing tactile information. The mediating effects of the dorsal column lemniscal system are diminished. It is possible that tactile hypersensitivity is a learned behavior that results from prior hyposensitivity. Initially, because of diminished sensation, pain may not be registered in time for the child to withdraw from the specific painful stimulus. As a compensatory pattern, the child begins to withdraw from any stimulus. Behavior follows a pattern of avoidance or withdrawal from tactile stimuli, especially on palmar, oral-facial, and ventral trunk areas. There may be inconsistent preferences for textures. Withdrawal from sensation may trigger increased tone. Because of diminished awareness of pain, the child has a delayed response to touch, and tactile localization may be compromised. Intervention may require adaptations for predictability of seating surfaces, approach from the front instead of the back, and use of the child's preferred clothing textures. Constant attention to imposed texture may lead to inefficient energy consumption and fatigue, resulting in decreased energy for participation in tasks that might be integrating. Tactile hyporesponsiveness may require use of extra safety measures for seating systems and in living environments.

Increased sensitivity to pressure or stretch on muscles, tendons, or ligaments, as well as sensitivity to gravitational changes, may also be present. Postural preferences that reduce weight-bearing and weight-shifting from critical areas, as in hemiplegia, may result in shortening of the affected side. Use of avoidance patterns may further reduce registration of body direction, position, alignment, part relationships, and force or direction of movements. Direct handling or adapta-

tions to equalize weight-bearing, and to encourage weight shift for static and dynamic positions, will be necessary during tasks. Caution is necessary when the child is using heavy toys or tools. Reduced ability to preposition body parts for activities, decreased anticipation of postural changes, and decreased cooperation with passive changes in position can further limit the child's performance of daily tasks.

Visual hyperresponsiveness or hyporesponsiveness can result from impaired visual discrimination, space, and form perception. However, it may also stem from decreased control of head position, or from somatosensory or auditory hypersensitivity. Limited alerting and orienting to relevant visual stimuli may further compromise visual perceptual development or cause a passiveness to the visual environment. The child will need intensive visual perception registration and selection management. It may be necessary to adapt the environment to reduce extraneous stimuli or to improve head control before visual remediation activities can commence.

Auditory hyperresponsiveness or hyporesponsiveness is expressed as abnormal sensitivity to sounds, secondary to impaired registration, discrimination, sequencing, memory, or closure. The child appears distracted by background or "white" noise, and may respond with hyperverbalization. Accompanying tactile defensiveness is possible. Increased attention to background noise, up to and including sounds of fluorescent bulbs or the refrigerator, may diminish attention to visual tasks. Functional communication may be decreased, compromising language formation and abstraction. Diminished auditory registration may result in blunt affect during communication. It may be helpful to exercise extra caution during community outings, as well as when the child is using sharp tools and objects.

APPLICATION OF SELECTED APPROACHES TO CEREBRAL PALSY INTERVENTION

Over the years, several major approaches to occupational therapy intervention for children with cerebral palsy have evolved. These approaches may be classified according to the scientific principles from which they were derived. The classifications are: neurological, orthopedic, and pragmatic.

Neurological approaches

Price[54] described major approaches that share a neurological orientation. These include the sensory motor, perceptual motor, and sensory integrative approaches. The *sensory motor approaches* proposed by the Bobaths (Neurodevelopmental Treatment/NDT)[12] and Rood[55] have been widely accepted, and can be distinguished by their emphasis on motor behavior, posture, and the sensory stimuli and feedback mechanisms of movement. Because these approaches, particularly NDT, are used so extensively, additional discussion of their concepts follows this general introduction to neurological approaches. Other sensory motor approaches include proproprioceptive neuromuscular facilitation (PNF), as developed by Knott and Voss,[34] and the Brunstromm methods.[13] Although these latter methods were originally designed for adult intervention, they offer possibilities for pediatric adaptations.

Perceptual motor approaches rely on the use of cognitive skills to remediate deficits in specific areas,[4] and are often used by occupational therapists in school systems to support the educational process (see Chapter 16). Specific activities are used to remediate deficient skill areas such as balance or visual perception. For example, a child with poor balance may practice walking on a balance beam, tandem walking on a line, or walking up and down stairs. Visual figure ground problems may be addressed by having a child color spaces in worksheets that feature a predominating figure against competing background shapes. Caution must be used with perceptual motor approaches. First, there is the possibility of splinter skill development. A typical example of splinter skill development is the ataxic child who can ride a bicycle, but cannot walk straight. Second, repeated use of some activities such as walking on a line may train the child to specific items on standard developmental tests.

Talbot and Junkala[64] investigated whether auditorially augmented feedback (using electronic perceptual motor training equipment) could improve the eye/hand coordination of 59 students with cerebral palsy. The subjects' mean age was 14 years, 3 months. Subjects were pretested using the Southern California Motor Accuracy Test (MAC) and then randomly divided into three groups. The first group participated in training exercises that provided auditorially augmented feedback while tracing line drawings. The second group also traced line drawings, but did not receive auditory feedback. The third group served as controls. Two post-test sessions were implemented at 3 month intervals. The first post-test showed significantly superior performance by the feedback group. However, although the second post-test results showed similar performance patterns, between group differences were no longer significant.

Price[54] stated that Ayres' *sensory integration approach*,[3,4] if used with caution, can be applied to cerebral palsy intervention, because of its emphasis on the organization of sensory information for adaptive responses (see Chapter 23). The strong emphasis on vestibular function, which has a significant role in cerebral palsy, can be an asset for many children with milder involvement. However, the practitioner needs to be aware of limitations regarding use of sensory integra-

tion testing for children with cerebral palsy, as well as watchful for negative influences on muscle tone during treatment.

Neurodevelopmental treatment (NDT)

In 1967, the Bobaths[9] outlined the aims of neurodevelopmental treatment to include development of normal postural tone and reactions, prevention or reduction of abnormal postural tone and reactions, and the prevention of contractures and deformities. NDT *handling*, as the techniques are called, has evolved from the use of static reflex inhibiting patterns that were used to counteract abnormal tonic reflex activities and modify postural tone. Currently, NDT requires *dynamic handling*, which incorporates the use of the child's active graded, transitional movements with the therapist's facilitation of normal movement patterns. Active normal movement patterns are facilitated at specific *key points*, usually the head, neck, shoulders, and hips. Sometimes more distal points, such as the elbows, wrists, and knees, can be used if stability is maintained at the more proximal points. Active movement patterns require weight shifts in different developmental and transitional positions, such as rolling from supine to prone. Through facilitation of active weight shifts, corrected righting and equilibrium reactions are promoted. As these reactions mature, the child can spend less energy on postural stability and more on meaningful tasks.

Dynamic handling incorporates vestibular, proprioceptive, and tactile stimulation to facilitate coactivation of muscle groups. Occupational therapists and others typically apply NDT while the child is engaged in developmentally appropriate activities using toys and selected equipment such as therapy balls or nesting/cruising benches. For selected children with low tone and impaired reciprocal movement, Bobath and Bobath[11] recommend: weight-bearing, pressure, and resistance; placing and holding; and tapping.

Weight-bearing involves weight shift to obtain automatic adjustments of the trunk and limbs. *Placing* is the passive movement of a limb with minimal support into a position that the child holds. *Holding* is the child's maintenance of body limb control after being placed into a specific position. When combined with placing, *tapping* by the therapist, a basic neuromuscular facilitation technique, helps to increase muscle tone and activate antagonists to spastic muscles. A sweeping motion in the direction of the desired movement helps to activate synergists. Caution must be employed in using these techniques to prevent triggering spasticity by stimulating abnormal muscle activity. Diligent observation and expedient problem-solving must be exercised when facilitation techniques are used. A technique such as tapping may facilitate coactivation in one child and be inhibitory to another.

NDT practice also emphasizes interdisciplinary orientation and cooperation. Although much can be gained from academic study of the neurodevelopmental principles of the approach, its application requires skilled motor behavior on the part of the practitioner that can only be gained through clinical training. Theory and certification courses on the application of NDT are given throughout the United States and British Commonwealth countries on a regular basis. During the course, participants review normal and abnormal progressions of movement and other relevant areas of development, practice handling techniques with each other, and learn to implement NDT technology through the modalities of their individual disciplines. Sessions for treatment with dysfunctioning children allow for applicaton of learned techniques. In addition to 8-week certification courses for occupational, physical, and speech therapists, courses for teachers are also scheduled regularly. NDT faculty include occupational, physical, and speech therapists who have completed rigorous postgraduate academic and clinical training before instructor certification.

Advanced specialty courses for such areas as joint mobilization, infant treatment, hand, and oral/motor function are also available for NDT certified as well as other therapists. Qualifications for courses, necessary due to availability of space, include previous and anticipated clinical experience with children with cerebral palsy or other CNS dysfunctions, and attendance of previous NDT courses.

Rood techniques

Rood[55] proposed that evaluation should focus on identification of the child's levels of motor control in the following abilities:

1. The muscles to contract through range of motion with reciprocal inhibition of antagonist muscles
2. The muscles around a joint to contract simultaneously to provide stability
3. The proximal muscles to contract to do heavy work superimposed on distal cocontraction
4. The proximal muscles to stabilize while distal muscles move

Rood treatment is based on the premise that motor patterns arise from the use of fundamental neonatal reflex patterns, and evolve through sensory experiences into the highest control available on the conscious cortical level. There are four major components of treatment. The first is normalization of tone and desired muscular responses through application of specific sensory stimulation. For example, strong gravitational stimuli, such as swinging the child through space, are used to facilitate righting reactions. Second, treatment is designed to facilitate the child's progression through the developmental progression of sensorimotor control. Therefore, rocking in quadruped would be facilitated before creeping. Third, all movements required

of the child during treatment must be purposeful. Passive or isolated movement is contraindicated. Finally, the principle of repetition is applied to strengthen and consolidate normal movement patterns of mobility and stability.

The orthopedic approach

The orthopedic aspects of occupational therapy for the child with cerebral palsy are related to the biomechanical approach used in physical dysfunction as described by Trombly and Scott[68] and Trombly.[67] This approach uses kinematic and kinetic assessment and treatment for orthopedic problems. Emphasis is on improving range of motion, strength, and endurance as necessary components of movement that allow the child to perform functional life tasks (see also Chapter 24). This approach is best applied with cerebral palsied children who have developed fair voluntary motor control.

Often the orthopedic approach is used by occupational therapists when children have concurrent surgical treatment. Therapists must exercise close coordination of treatment with an orthopedic surgeon during the preoperative and postoperative phases of care. Green[26] noted that orthopedic surgery is aimed at changing the "relative agonist-antagonist action and to establish better balance of muscle power" (p. 3). The objectives for performing surgery with children who have cerebral palsy may include:

1. To increase or correct joint function[56]
2. To improve hygiene[7]
3. To improve cosmetic appearance[7,24]
4. To assist in the psychological adjustment of the child and the parents[75]

Although orthopedists may also endorse nonsurgical methods of case, such as the neurological approaches, most believe that surgery has a definite place in cerebral palsy management. Goldner[24] and Zancolli and Zancolli[75] stated that for carefully selected patients, upper extremity surgery can be helpful. However, Goldner[24] cautioned that most children with cerebral palsy are not surgery candidates because they can adapt to their motor deficit and improvements secondary to surgery are limited. Pollack[53] reviewed the results of surgery in cerebral palsy and reported that in one group of patients who had upper extremity procedures, 36.8% had results that were considered failures. Observations from clinical practice indicate that, because of the continuing influence of abnormal tone, which cannot be surgically moved like a muscle, surgical procedures often require repetition after several years to maintain joint mobility. Although occupational therapists may be involved with the orthopedic management of the lower extremities, the degree of this involvement varies among settings. Orthopedic surgeons[28,75] state that children with pure spastic paralysis are the best candidates for surgery. However, children must have some voluntary control over the spastic muscles that are to be operated on to ensure functional results.

The pragmatic approach

Most occupational therapists use a combination of treatment approaches determined on a case-to-case basis. In addition to concepts and technology derived through neurological and orthopedic approaches, pragmatists incorporate ideas from other theories.

The research base using pragmatic and other approaches in occupational therapy intervention for cerebral palsied children is limited and contains some contradictory evidence. Parette and Hourcade[49] reviewed 20 years of intervention research related to gross and fine motor progress of young children with cerebral palsy. The study proposed that, before drawing conclusions regarding the effectiveness of intervention, several internal factors of the research studies required consideration. These factors included weak research designs with poorly defined variables and effects, lack of standard and sensitive instruments to detect significant changes, and limitations in central group designs.

An early study by Tyler and Kogan[69] attempted to assess the effects of occupational therapy, including NDT and other modalities, on children's use of upper extremities in manipulative and self-help skills. The research examined 77 children with various types of cerebral palsy, aged 10 months to 6 years; they were tested at 9 and 15 month intervals. Gain scores were analyzed in relation to age, pre-test scores, measured intelligence, diagnosis, history of previous therapy, and amount of therapy received. Results indicated that intelligence quotient (IQ) was not related to gain scores. Other tentative findings were that children who were less involved, younger, or had received less than 1 year of treatment previously made greater gains. The amount of therapy received during the study period was related to higher gain scores in self-help skills. Generalization of these results is difficult because no control group was used and the specific therapy protocol was not indicated.

Carlsen[14] conducted a pilot study that compared the effectiveness of two occupational therapy approaches—one emphasizing sensory motor facilitation and the other a functional skills program. Twelve young children with cerebral palsy were matched for developmental age and type of motor involvement and randomly assigned to treatment groups. Pre- and post-testing used the Denver Developmental Screening Test (DDST) and the Bayley Scales of Infant Development (BSID). The facilitation treatment consisted of activities to promote sensory organization, postural stability, and controlled movement. The functional treatment consisted of positioning, adaptive hand skills, and self-care skills training. After 6 weeks of treatment in the clinic and daily home programs, post-testing was implemented. The children in the facilitation group made significant improvement on the BSID and the gross motor subsection of the DDST. The facilitation group also had greater gains on the DDST personal-social, fine motor-adaptive, and language subtests, although results were not statistically significant. Study results indicated "that for the age group studied, a program that is primarily based on facilitation of gross sensorimotor integration, but does not exclude training in fine motor activities, may be the most effective"[14] (p. 272). The lack of a control group and blind evaluation were stated limitations of the study.

Norton[46] reported a study that evaluated a combination of sensory integration and NDT approaches. She found that three children diagnosed as profoundly retarded with multiple handicaps achieved higher developmental levels in posture, emotion, perception, and cognition. Treatment consisted of handling, positioning, arousal stimulation, respiratory and pre-feeding facilitation, and vestibular and tactile stimulation, and was administered by the children's mothers for 9 months. Small sample size and lack of a control group are limitations to generalizing these results.

Scherzer, Mike, and Ilson[57] gathered data on 22 infants under 18 months of age who had definite or presumed diagnoses of cerebral palsy. In a double-blind study, an experimental group received physical therapy consisting of positioning, movement to inhibit abnormal reflexes and facilitate normal motor development, and a home program. The control group received only passive range of motion exercises. Medical and physical therapy evaluations of motor status, social maturation, and ease of home management revealed a definite correlation between change and experimental group status. The investigators found a trend of more positive change in children of higher intelligence.

Studies aimed at assessing the vestibular function of children with cerebral palsy show similar inconclusive findings. Torok and Perlstein[66] found that, of 518 children with cerebral palsy, 34% had vestibular abnormalities. Hyposensitivity was most common among those with spastic hemiplegia. These findings may have prompted other investigators to question whether treatment that emphasized vestibular system stimulation would affect the motor behavior of children with cerebral palsy.

A group of 23 preambulatory children with cerebral palsy, aged 2 to 6 years, were evaluated on gross motor and reflex tests by Chee, Kreutzberg, and Clark.[17] Twelve children were assigned to a group that received treatment to stimulate vertical and horizontal semicircular canals for 4 weeks. Two control groups were established. One group received no treatment and the remaining children were handled but received no specific vestibular stimulation. The experimental group showed greater gains on post-tests. In addition, subjective assessment by therapists and mothers indicated that these children showed more improvement in equilibrium, gross motor control, alertness, curiosity, and social-emotional status.

A similar study by Sellick and Over[59] involving 20 children with cerebral palsy, aged 8 to 56 months, did not support the findings of Chee, Kreutzberg, and Clark.[17] In the Sellick and Over[59] study, the treatment group that received controlled vestibular stimulation for 4 weeks showed no significant improvement on the Bayley Scales of Infant Development when compared to a control group. The chidren were post-tested in the week following treatment and 3 months later.

Ayres[2] conducted a study of children with learning disability and choreoathetosis, a motor disorder characterized by mild involuntary motions that interfere with fine motor coordination. She found no significant differences in improvement in eye-hand coordination between a group who received sensory integrative therapy and a control group who received no therapy.

In summary, the research investigating effectiveness of different and combined approaches for treatment of children with cerebral palsy presents contradictory evidence. Although each study has flaws in methodology, as a group they indicate a trend toward improvement through the use of sensory motor approaches.

Current trends and research in cerebral palsy intervention

Much of the current research is directed toward examining more comprehensive aspects of living with cerebral palsy. Although much of the previous work cited has related to preschoolers, the needs of the older child and adolescent are now being addressed. The focus and findings of the following studies help put treatment into perspective within the broader, long-term focus of community living.

Research by Imperio, Cullinan, and Riklan[30] suggested that disabled young adults may be at a higher risk for developing a maladaptive personality. A representative group of subjects with mild physical dysfunction, including cerebral palsy, showed a trend toward greater social-emotional pathology. The investigators recommended the use of counseling and psychotherapy that includes particular attention to the areas of sex role behavior and adaptation.

In a report on public and professional attitudes toward the sexual and emotional needs of the handicapped, Shearer[61] described the lack of sex education for physically handicapped children in schools and at home. She stated that handicapped children are denied knowledge about their own sexuality and the means of expressing sexual and emotional needs. Her findings indicated that society prefers to keep handicapped persons in a child-like state, thereby ignoring sexual needs.

Teplin, Howard, and O'Connor[65] studied self-concept of young children with cerebral palsy. Two measures of self-concept were adapted and administered to 15 mainstreamed children, aged 4 to 8 years, and to a control group of nondysfunctioning children. Findings indicated a tendency for the handicapped children to have lower self-concepts. Teacher ratings of the two groups also indicated perception of a lower self-concept among the handicapped children. The authors concluded that self-concept, and its subsequent effect on self-esteem, is a critical factor to address in the primary grades, particularly for boys.

Tyler, Kogan, and Turner[71] studied interpersonal behaviors between young children with cerebral palsy and their parents during therapy. They found that mothers displayed a controlling and negative affect in therapy sessions that was not evident during play. Children also demonstrated greater negative behavior during therapy. The investigators speculated that children with cerebral palsy were delayed in their interactive abilities. This delay interferes with the establishment of a normal mother/child relationship and may be exacerbated by too much emphasis on therapy for motor behaviors. They concluded that professionals need to assess the mother/child relationship carefully before determining a mother's role in therapy.

A later study by Tyler and Kogan[70] investigated the effect of behavioral instruction given to mothers of children with cerebral palsy. By analyzing behaviors recorded on videotape, they found that 8 weeks of behavioral instruction was sufficient to reduce stressful and conflicted interaction. Most of the change was shown by mothers (rather than children), and the change was maintained as long as 1 year later. There was no gradual decrease in expression of positive feelings. The authors concluded that "physically handicapped children have a more difficult time participating in reciprocal interaction" (p. 155) and that the mothers experience nonrewarding one-way interactions that do not progress to two-way at as rapid a rate as they would with able-bodied children. They speculated that mothers may cope by using various forms of disengaging behavior with their handicapped child.

These studies indicate that occupational therapists must maintain a holistic approach to treatment of children and adolescents with cerebral palsy. Rather than focusing narrowly on posture and tone, therapists must remain in touch with how their treatment relates to a child's present and future life needs. Collaborative relationships with other service providers and family are critical to meeting the child's overall developmental needs.

OCCUPATIONAL THERAPY TREATMENT METHODS

To illustrate the use of occupational therapy intervention methodology, this information is presented in a series of developmentally sequenced case studies. Featured cases include data on sensorimotor, cognitive, psychosocial, and occupational performance areas. Additionally, a general statement regarding response to sensory and motor facilitation is reported for comparison. Each subject represents different classifications of cerebral palsy involvement, as well as various assessment and intervention methodologies. Different settings are represented. Review of Chapters 13 through 17 regarding treatment modalities, adaptations, and illustrations is recommended.

CASE STUDY 1:

Shirley, 4 months old, suspected cerebral palsy.

SETTING:

Occupational therapy department, general hospital.

BRIEF HISTORY:

Shirley was delivered 1 month prematurely by caesarian section. The premature delivery was a result of fetal distress related to meconium aspiration. Shirley remained in the neonatal intensive care unit for 10 days for treatment of respiratory distress. Shirley lived with her biological parents. Both her mother and father were college graduates. The father worked during the day and her mother stayed home to take care of Shirley and two older children.

RESULTS OF INITIAL ASSESSMENT;

Sensorimotor: Joint range of motion was within normal limits for age. Muscle tone was hypertonic in relation to Movement Assessment of Infants (MAI) criteria for passivity, consistency, and extensibility. MAI total performance suggested high risk for a cerebral palsy impression.

Presenting Reflexes: Flexor withdrawal, crossed extension, remnants of Galant, palmar and plantar grasp, Moro and components of the asymmetrical tonic neck reflex with slight extremity extension of the face side.

Righting Reactions: Prone and supine suspension elicited slow but present righting reactions; vertical suspension response was not present laterally. *Equilibrium reactions* in prone and in supine positions consisted of slight lateral flexion and minimal head righting, more pronounced toward the right.

Gross Motor: Peabody Developmental Motor Scales (PDMS) skills were at birth to 1 month level with few emerging skills at 2 months. In prone position, Shirley maintained a primarily flexed posture but could achieve neck extension to 50 degrees with some cervical rotation to the right and slow rotation to the left. Also present was occasional reciprocal kicking of lower extermity. Occasionally, Shirley rolled from prone to supine position. When supine, Shirley maintained head in midline for a few seconds or when shoulders were elevated; otherwise, she held her head to the left or right. Also in supine, Shirley moved her hand toward, but not quite to her mouth.

While sidelying, Shirley occasionally rolled to prone or supine with gravity assistance. In supported sitting, her back was fully rounded and her head was passively flexed into gravity with minimal attempts to lift her head.

Fine Motor: PDMS showed skills at birth to 1 month with few emerging skills at 2 months. Shirley showed decreased spontaneous movements of the upper extremity. Shirley focused on faces, auditory toys, or brightly colored objects held approximately 12 inches from her eyes and tracked horizontally to 90 degrees from midline. This was inconsistent to midline. Grasp of objects was primarily reflexive and grasp was maintained for 10 to 15 seconds before involuntary release.

Oral Motor: Inspection showed a slightly high palate. Oral reflexes were appropriately integrated except for weak rooting, phasic bite, and suckle/swallow. Also present during bottle-feeding was decreased mouth closure, which caused milk spillage.

Sensory Integration/Perceptual: Tactile, vestibular, and proprioceptive responses were reflexive or emerging but slow to occur (see presenting reflexes this section). Auditory and visual acuity were within normal limits but slow to occur.

Cognitive: Reflexive responses to the environment were stated in the sensorimotor section. Toys were visually regarded only when presented in front of the eyes. Shirley responded and oriented to sounds, to mother's face, voice, and movements.

Psychosocial: Shirley showed vague recognition of her mother's voice and face and was comforted by firm or light touch and stroking, rocking, and cuddling. She appeared to maintain eye contact during bottle-feeding while on her mother's lap.

Occupational Performance: Bottle-feeding showed emerging anticipation of bottle and use of available suckle/swallow. Suck was arrhythmical, weak and unsustained. There was much spillage due to decreased mouth closure. There was reduced intake (4 to 6 ounces) and increased number of feeding sessions (12/day). Sleep cycle consisted of several short naps during the day and waking 3 to 4 times at night. Response to toys consisted of minimal orienting responses to sounds such as rattles, to bright colors, to mother's face, and to toys brought in front of her eyes. Movement in play was limited.

General Performance After Facilitation: Facilitation of movement components and sensation showed increased orientation to the environment and improved balance of postural tone and slight inhibition of primitive reflexes.

Strengths: (1) Responsiveness to movement and sensory facilitation and (2) bonding with mother.

Problem:

Occupational performance:	Behavior:	Component function:
Inefficient eating	Increased feeding sessions required	Delayed motor development

Eating is a basic occupational task that poses a problem for both Shirley and her parents. Her inefficiency in eating has resulted in a need for increased numbers of feedings, especially at night. Specifically, impaired eating performance resulted from decreased mouth closure and inefficient suck/swallow secondary to decreased coactivation of the oral musculature as well as that of the whole body. Generally, Shirley's delay in both gross and fine motor development was traced to four factors: an imbalance in postural control related to a hypertonic muscle tone, brainstem and spinal level reflexes that are inappropriate for age, delayed acquisition of cortical level equilibrium responses, and inconsistent responses to sensory stimuli. Cognitive and psychosocial components were also compromised as a result of inconsistent responses to sensation and movement.

Long-term goal:

Shirley will eat 11 or more ounces of food and liquids on a regular daily schedule at the end of 6 months.

Short-term objective sequence:

(1) Shirley will drink 7 to 8 ounces of milk from a bottle per feeding with minimal spillage at the end of 2 months; (2) Shirley will drink 9 to 10 ounces of milk from a bottle without spillage, or alternate pureed food from a cup or spoon with minimal spillage, at the end of 4 months; and (3) Shirley will eat 11 or more ounces of food and liquids with no spillage at 6 months.

Treatment activities:

Preparatory Postural Management: Using age-appropriate toys, and preferably with a parent present, balance of general postural tone was facilitated. In Shirley's case, residual flexor tone and decreased sensory responsivity have impaired both the development of extension and the true antigravity flexion that effectively coactivates muscles in various positions. For example, posture was managed by facilitating coactivation of cervical musculature (necessary for head righting and eventually for equilibrium reactions) by putting Shirley into semi-supine position on the therapist's lap and by facilitating lateral, anteroposterior, and eventually diagonal weight shifts through corresponding shifts of the therapist's lap. Necessary support was provided posteriorly and laterally on scapulae and upper arms. The semi-supine position allowed the elongation of the cervical and upper trunk extensors, preparing them for coactivation with antigravity flexors. Movements in the semi-supine position allowed various weight-bearing experiences that paved the way to various weight shifts necessary for facilitation of proximal stability. Visual gaze was directed by talking to Shirley, by making head movements, or by making facial expressions as necessary. Shirley progressed to sitting on the mat with lateral, anteroposterior and diagonal weight shifts facilitated from the shoulders. Visual gaze was directed by using a hanging toy or one presented by the parent.

Alternate position: The therapist knelt on the mat forming a wedgelike structure with his thighs. Shirley was positioned semi-supine on the therapist's lap with her head lower than her body to facilitate elongation of neck extensors. Using hips as key points, Shirley's hands were held to the side (close to the hips) and games of touching feet close to the head, to the body, or to the side were played while simultaneously verbalizing the procedure in playful language to the child. When necessary, Shirley's shoulders were depressed bilaterally in this position to elongate shoulder elevators and to minimize compensatory shoulder elevation. Therapist made playful sounds and directed Shirley's visual gaze to feet, to toy, or to therapist's face.

Postural management progressed so that feeding and other activity positions used independent sitting at 10 months.

Direct eating management considered feeding position, food quantity, food types, and eating utensils. However, the progression of activities and components of treatment depended on achieving the background postural control and sensory responsiveness required by the more refined oral motor control of eating. For example, progression of the feeding position from the semi-supine or sidelying position during bottle-feeding to independent sitting in a high chair while eating pureed food required independent sitting. Food intake was monitored through the parents and observed during feeding breaks during therapy sessions. Postural management as well as focal oral motor management resulted not only in improved mouth closure but also in the progression from a suckle to a true suck during bottle-feeding. Oral motor management consisted of selecting a longer rubber nipple with smaller holes. The special nipple slowed down the milk flow, and required more work from Shirley. Manual jaw assist during bottle-feeding was performed during therapy and at home to facilitate a suckling pattern initially and later a true suck. At 6 months of age, pureed foods and milk or juice thickened with rice cereal were introduced. Shirley responded to the new texture and consistency by reverting to the previous arhythmical, weak, and unsustained suckle pattern. She showed anticipation of the presented spoon but did not actively use her lips to assist in food removal. Firm pressure on the upper lip facilitated upper lip contraction. The new food texture and consistency elicited increased tone that disturbed Shirley's sitting balance and resulted in withdrawal from the stimulus. The reaction was corrected with coaxing as well as proper facilitaion of normal sitting components.

Home program:

Parents were encouraged to implement the above activities at home as often as possible and to incorporate the procedures into daily activities—changing diapers, bathing, and feeding. During bottle-feeding, for example, Shirley was positioned on lap or infant seat, facing her mother for direct visual gaze. Manual assists on cheeks and lips were used to facilitate lip closure and sequential suckle/swallow pattern.

CASE STUDY 2:

John: Initial evaluation at 18 months and progress evaluation at 28 months, cerebral palsy with diplegia secondary to Seckel's syndrome.

SETTING:

Developmental center.

BRIEF HISTORY:

John was born at term with microcephaly secondary to Seckel's syndrome. He had been seen since birth by an interdisciplinary team at a local hospital. John showed a history of delayed motor development, increased muscle tone, and lack of cooperation during treatment. Both parents had 10 years of education. Father was retired from the military because of age and a disability acquired during his service. Mother was in her middle 40s and worked on a day care staff. The father had been taking John to therapy consistently since birth.

Initial and progress evaluations administered at 18 and 28 months, respectively, are plotted for comparison in chart form on pp. 416 and 417 in this chapter.

General Performance After Facilitation at 18 months: Facilitation could not be assessed at initial evaluation due to lack of cooperation. Facilitation during therapy sessions showed positive responses.

Strengths: (1) Developmentally appropriate gross and fine motor abilities, and (2) Righting and equilibrium reactions are present but slow to occur and incomplete.

Problem:

Occupational performance:	Behavior:	Component function:
Limited Play	Decreased object, position, and personal interaction.	Delayed sensorimotor, cognitive, and psychosocial development.

John had a limited repertoire of play positions, object interactions, and personal interactions. His limited play repertoire appeared to result from sensorimotor dysfunctions. Decreased righting and equilibrium reactions limited John's ability to perform transitional movements and to assume and maintain static play positions. Decreased registration of vestibular, tactile, and proprioceptive input were exhibited by: Weak balance and protective extension reactions; compensatory postural and tactile reactions such as cervical hyperextension/shoulder elevation; inappropriate release of hand-held objects. Compensatory patterns were evident in ambulation. Personal interaction was limited to those individuals John trusted, including his father. John's father was slightly protective because, as John's caretaker, the boy's postural requirements were predictable to him. John's "safe" environment further limited sensorimotor and cognitive development.

Long-term goal:

John will walk backward a distance of 10 feet while pulling a toy, using appropriate movement components without falling 3 out of 5 trials in 6 months.

Short-term objective sequence:

(1) John will walk forward a distance of 5 feet using a narrower base of support and using appropriate movement components without falling 3 out of 5 trials in 2 months: (2) John will push a toy cart or wheelchair to a distance of 5 feet using appropriate movement components without falling 3 of 5 trials in 4 months; and (3) John will bimanually snap off a pop bead without falling backwards and using appropriate movement components 3 out of 5 trials in 6 months.

Treatment activities:

Preparatory Psychosocial Management: Consistent team and parent cooperation was planned to familiarize John with the structure of the center's therapeutic program. John's arrival at the center with his parent was planned shortly before circle time, when other children (and sometimes parents) sat around in a circle and sang action songs or recited nursery rhymes. Slowly children were "weaned" from their parents' presence by imposing progressively shorter periods of parent visits until the parent did not come to circle time at all. This approach proved effective until therapists took John to individual therapy sessions with various and increasing demands. As demands increased, so did crying and uncooperative behavior. The therapist used timeout, withdrawing play materials and attention, until crying stopped or when John indicated he wanted to continue. After 3 months of this behavior management program John was willing to interact with each therapist individually and with other children during the circle group. As increased cooperation was elicited, developmentally appropriate toys were prescribed for John, to encourage him to become more acquainted with the environment and to increase his repertoire of familiar play materials.

Postural Management: As interaction with toys, materials, and therapists increased, a postural treatment regimen started. This included:
1. Facilitation of vestibular and somatosensory responses on a minitrampoline, a rocking horse, a hammock, and a vestibular board. John was allowed to select and activate the equipment. The therapist provided focal tapping or vibratory stimuli of specific muscle groups as needed — for example, abdominals when standing/rocking with a lordotic curve, gluteus medius/minimus when doing lateral weight shifts on the trampoline while dancing to music.
2. Facilitation of normal movement components by including transitional movements during play (for example, creeping up graduated benches to reach for toys on top and placing them in a basket below on the mat).

Direct Play Management:

Circle time included activities like singing and passing the ball to the next person. Action songs included Spider Song, and clothing and body parts identification together with therapists and other children. Object manipulation started with textured playdough in various colors. Playdough activities incorporated sensory and movement components and were performed at the table or during postural management routines. Play progressed from activities that strengthened proximal control (shoulders, hips, trunk) areas but also facilitated distal control using isolated finger movements (pulling small pieces out of dough and putting pieces in a container).

Home Program:

Activities included sitting in a parent's lap in a rocking chair or on the outdoor swing, exploring various food textures, playing with toys checked out from the agency toy library, and consistent use of AFOs.

CASE STUDY 3:

Reneé: 36 months, cerebral palsy with ataxic behaviors

SETTING:

Developmental center toddler program.

BRIEF HISTORY:

Reneé was born at term without complications. Her parents reported that Reneé was a fussy infant, crying when rocked or cuddled. They also reported difficulty with her feeding due to decreased coordination of breathing and swallowing. Gross and fine motor development was reportedly delayed, as stated in previous medical reports. Before coming to the developmental center a year ago, Reneé received services from an infant stimulation program at a U.S. military dependents school in the Pacific region. Reneé's father was a commissioned officer with the U.S. Air Force and her mother worked part-time at the Air Force recreational center. Reports indicated that both parents had been consistently cooperative in attending therapy sessions and in carrying out home programs.

Initial evaluation results:

Sensorimotor: Active and passive joint range of motion were within normal limits except for cervical, lumbar, digital, and knee active hyperextension. Muscle tone fluctuated, increasing with movement, effort and stress, with possibly underlying low tone in the trunk and proximal joint muscles, and less hypotonia in distal lower extremity joints. Primitive

Comparison of initial and progress evaluations for John

INITIAL EVALUATION (at 18 months)

Sensorimotor

ACTIVE AND PASSIVE JOINT RANGE OF MOTION were within normal limits except for increased active foot pronation, decreased hip extension and elbow extension. Mildly *hypotonic extremities* were evident with active hyperextension of the neck and the digits, accompanied by lordosis and lack of trunk rotation during activities; feet were pronated. Slightly increased tone was present in the oral area, evident in lip pursing and tightening during activity.

Residual Reflexes present were weak palmar and plantar grasp. Blink and pupillary reactions were age-appropriate.

Righting Reactions showed delayed reaction time in prone, more so in supine and in vertical suspension.

Protective Extension Responses were present to all directions in sitting but slow in standing.

Equilibrium Reactions in sitting and standing showed delayed reaction time and incomplete in relation to upper and lower extremity responses and trunk rotation components.

PDMS Gross Motor skills were at 15 months. From sitting, John can roll a ball positioned between legs away from the body, creep, but prefers to walk with one hand support up and down stairs. Creeping is done on fisted hands, resulting in decreased palmar contact with floor. High kneeling showed decreased balance. Decreased balance was also evident when turning around, picking up a toy from the floor, or when doing an under/overhand throw.

Gait was wide-based so that hips were slightly abducted, externally rotated and flexed, upper extremities were in high guard position (shoulder extension, abduction and external rotation, elbow flexion, wrist extension and pronation). Hands went into a fisted position when walking or when losing balance.

PDMS Fine Motor skills were at 10 months. In sitting, John reached for 1-inch cubes, candy pellets and pegs, but used a raking movement of digits instead of isolated use of thumb, index and middle fingers. Reaching for rings in a peg was bimanual. Release of pellets and cubes into a container when done was assisted by wrist flexion and accompanying shoulder elevation. Release otherwise was to the side. "Crumpling presented bond paper" and "reach for rings from a peg" were done bimanually with accompanying neck hyperextension and shoulder elevation. John reached for spoon or crayon, doodled with crayon and banged spoon on a table, but did not attempt to imitate stirring spoon in cup. John picked up all presented three pegs from board and poked index finger on board holes.

Oral Motor performance showed integrated primitive oral reflexes with some slight suck/swallow incoordination, resulting in occasional choking. Occasional suckling was evident when eating crackers. Also evident was slight hypersensitivity to some food textures such as hard crackers and crunchy raw vegetables such as carrots.

PROGRESS EVALUATION (at 28 months)

Sensorimotor

ACTIVE AND PASSIVE RANGE OF MOTION were within normal limits. *Active* hip and elbow extension had increasd while foot pronation was managed through AFOs. Improvement was evident in balanced control of muscle tone in extremities and trunk and oral area, with occasional hyperextension of neck, lordosis, and decreased rotation with effort.

Residual Reflexes: Palmar and plantar grasp were integrated.

Righting Reactions in prone, supine and vertical suspension showed improvement in all areas.

Protective Extension Responses showed consistent upper extremity responses in sitting but slow lower extremity staggering responses in standing.

Equilibrium reactions showed faster head righting response but upper extremity and trunk rotational components were still slow.

PDMS Gross Motor skills are at the 17-month level. John can sit to stand from plantigrade (or bear walk position), creep on open hands, walk up and down steps holding on to the rail, kneel stand for 5 seconds without support, throw a ball underhand in standing and walk sideways for 2 feet without losing balance. Attempts at heel to toe walking were unsuccessful.

Standing base in walking was narrower with decreased hip abduction and external rotation. Increased hip extension was also evident. Arms during walking were held slightly lower, showing decreased shoulder extension, abduction, and external rotation. Elbow was approximately 120 degrees extension but wrist was still in extension and pronation. Hands did not consistently go into a fisted position with attempts to regain balance.

PDMS Fine Motor skills were at 15 months. Evident fine motor improvement: increased isolation of finger movements and decreased presence of compensatory neck and shoulder movements during reach for cubes, candy pellets, pegs, and rings. Increased poking on board and other small holes was evident. (Parents were warned about electrical outlets.) Objects such as pellets, cubes, or torn paper were released more consistently into presented containers and with decreased compensatory movements. John showed interest in stirring spoon into a cup but was inconsistent.

Decreased incoordination of suck/swallow was evident, as was decreased suckling of crackers, and increased tolerance of various food textures. John showed playfulness during snack and meals, offering food to caretaker.

Sensory Integration/Perceptual performance showed delayed or slow responses to vestibular stimuli, evidenced by balance loss in high kneel and during gross motor activities. Slight fear was evident upon change of head position. Tactile hypersensitivity was evident in the oral area relative to food textures and in the body relative to clothing textures.

Cognitive performance showed rapid shifts of attention to visual, tactile, and auditory stimuli. Movements were rapid and lacked control and direction. Experimentation with and exploration of toys was limited to pounding on table. Verbal interaction consisted of monosyllables or crying, assisted by pointing.

Psychosocial performance showed marked hesitation to interact with anyone other than parents. John cried throughout the testing session. When crying stopped, John required full attention from at least one staff person. Cooperation was elicited by having John sit on caretaker's lap during evaluation. John accepted some food items from his father but not from his mother.

Occupational performance during *play* showed a limited repertoire of object interaction and play positions. Play during evaluation and as reported was performed on parent's lap. *Self-care* performance and parent report showed inconsistency in toilet training and inability to communicate toileting needs.

Feeding: John showed a slight hypersensitivity to food textures as reported in the Oral Motor Section. Cooperation during dressing was evident in donning and doffing loose-fitting shirts.

Improved balance in sitting and high kneel and gross motor performance, decreased hypersensitivity to touch and improved proprioception. Learning spatial perception was evident in shape and form recognition during games, and release of shapes, forms, and small and relatively large objects into containers. Decreased release to the side.

Decreased inattention was evident with more meaningful and longer manipulation, experimentation and exploration of toys. Slight withdrawal from unfamiliar textures and toys was still evident but John required less prodding to participate. Verbal interaction contained more words but words were muttered.

Decreased clinging behavior was evident. Crying was minimized to times when frustrated and upon arrival for therapy. Caretaker was not present during session. Various types of food were acceptable from both parents.

Play showed increased exploration, experimentation and manipulation of the environment and objects as stated in Sensory Perceptual section. Also evident was improvement in imitative and imaginative play.

Feeding performance showed improved acceptance of various food textures and improved utilization of utensils. DRESSING performance showed ability to don and doff loose-fitting shirts with minimal assistance. Socks could be doffed if heels were exposed.

reflexes were all integrated except for a mild symmetrical tonic neck response. Righting reactions were slightly slow in occurring, more so to the left with panic reactions consisting of holding on tight, increase in muscle tone and crying during labyrinthine righting reactions testing. Equilibrium reactions in prone and supine were accompanied by fear reactions and were incomplete in relation to trunk lateral extension on the weight-bearing side. Sitting equilibrium reactions, although accompanied by fear reactions, were present to the right but slow to occur and incomplete relative to lateral extension of the weight-bearing side. Downward parachute reactions of upper extremity were slow to occur bilaterally. Lateral and backward protective reactions were slow to occur and incomplete in relation to head righting responses. Hand fisting associated reaction was evident during chewing, using eating utensils, and gross motor activities.

Gross Motor: PDMS skills were at the 25 month level. Reneé could roll from supine to prone sequentially, could assume sitting position with some trunk rotation by pivoting over left but not over right upper extremity. In the prone position, Reneé could maintain 45 degree neck extension with weight-bearing on flexed elbows and forearms; however, shoulders were elevated and protracted, and hips slightly flexed. Due to shoulder elevation, weight shift to reach for toy while weight-bearing on one arm was difficult. While independently standing on a wide base of support, Reneé could inconsistently throw small and big Nerf balls but with compensatory movements in the shoulders, slight loss of balance and poor timing when releasing the ball. Due to poor release

timing and incoordination of sequenced movements, ball occasionally ended up short of target or not released at all.

Wide-based gait showed an immature weight shift or no lengthening of the trunk on the weight-bearing side. Arms were held up in a high guard position or with shoulders slightly elevated and extended, elbows flexed to 90 degrees, forearm pronated and hands slightly fisted, therefore allowing no upper extremity reciprocation. Loss of balance occurred while walking and when performing other gross motor tasks, usually when vision was directed other than straight ahead. The imbalance resulted in falling and attempted creeping. Creeping showed residual influence of the symmetrical tonic neck reflex or "bunny-hopping," which consisted of upper extremity extension and lower extremity flexion upon head extension and vice versa.

Fine Motor: PDMS skills were at the 20-month level when attempting age-appropriate tasks. However, general performance was diminished or unsuccessful when balance was lost. Accuracy in tasks such as pegs and shapes into board, cube stacking, stringing, or popping was adversely affected by fast movement attempts and incoordination. Crayon was grasped with forearm in pronation, thumb and index toward paper, three remaining fingers around the crayon. Scribbles were arbitrary and were not distinguishable as specific lines or shapes. Given time and some stabilizing support on the trunk, Reneé was able to perform better in these tasks.

Oral motor performance showed age-appropriate skills in feeding. These skills diminished when postural responses were required. There was slight inconsistency of food lateralization and mouth closure while eating and occasional inco-ordination of swallowing, breathing, and making sounds. Speech was monosyllabic with increased effort needed to make sounds that were throaty. Coordinating breathing with speech was difficult.

Sensory Integration and Perceptual: Responses were slow, inefficient, and fearful to vestibular stimuli such as maintaining balance while standing on unstable surfaces, while walking, while standing, while being passively moved around, or while focusing on an activity. Slight tactile hyper-sensitivity was evident in the oral area; however, firm pressure was tolerated when the mouth was wiped firmly with a handtowel or when touched from the front instead of the back. Localization to sound was present but movement to orient body to the sound was inconsistent. Slight difficulty in understanding verbal directions was evident.

Cognitive: Attention was decreased especially when postural control was challenged and when responses required redirecting visual gaze from one stimulus to another. Trial and error experimentation was evident with some toys such as a busy box. Reneé attempted different ways to make the object come out of the box; however, frustration level was low, resulting in banging the toy when unsuccessful or in discontinuation of toy manipulation. Also evident was searching for hidden objects, exhibited by lifting a piece of cloth to find object hidden by first piece of cloth but not by second. Imitation of actions such as pat-a-cake was slow and limited to times when postural support around the trunk was provided. Imitation of speech sounds was slow and labored. Reneé recognized parents' names, familiar objects, and pictures; however, Reneé had difficulty verbalizing names of familiar people, objects, and pictures.

Psychosocial performance showed no hesitation to interact with examiners but there were occasional switches of attention to look at her parents. There were attempts to manipulate the situation by cooperating most in simple tasks that required minimal postural demands and by switching attention to other objects and to parents. Parents reported that when with other children, solitary type or onlooker play was predominant with emerging enjoyment of being with other children. Verbal interaction was limited both receptively and expressively unless encouraged.

Occupational performance during *eating* showed slight tactile sensitivity to food textures and to passive mouth wiping. However, Reneé preferred performing these eating-related tasks using her hands, left more than right. She was frustrated easily when using a spoon or drinking from a cup and made generous spills. Given postural support around the trunk, Reneé could pull off shoelaces, shoes, and socks. She could take off shirts and pants with minimal assistance in sequencing the activity and maximal assistance when vision was occluded when pulling off shirt. She needed partial to maximal assistance in putting on the above clothing items. *Toileting* report from parents showed that Reneé could sit on the training potty seat on a regular schedule and would indicate need to eliminate. She had occasional accidents and would communicate that her pants were messy. *Play* was exploratory and mostly solitary with emerging skills at wanting to watch and maybe participate in peer play. However, low frustration level when manipulating or experimenting with toys got in the way of peer participation or extended play with toys.

General Performance After Sensorimotor Facilitation: Reneé's movement components and postural reactions showed improvement except when vision was occluded during testing or when removing shirt.

Strengths: (1) Positive response to sensorimotor facilitation; (2) developmentally appropriate gross and fine motor abilities; (3) trial and error experimentation with toys; and (4) cooperative and friendly demeanor.

Problem:

Occupational performance:	Behavior:	Component function:
Delayed self-feeding	Frustration with utensil use	Delayed gross and fine motor development, delayed sensory integration development.

Reneé's major occupational problem was the delayed acquisition of the skills to use utensils during eating. Other self-care or play concerns also showed as much need for integrated component function as utensil use, but would probably be more easily achieved with consistent behavior management, attention to Reneé's constant need for visual cues, and attention from the caretaker. Reneé's limitations in eating utensil use related both to sensory and motor concerns. Due to delayed acquisition of gross and fine motor skills, postural background and discrete manipulation by hands were compromised, especially in tool use. Sensory hyperreactivity, especially around the oral area, prevented experimentation with textures or eating utensils.

Long-term goal:

Reneé will bring food to mouth using a spoon held with palm up using appropriate movement patterns, without spilling 3 out of 5 times within 12 months.

Short-term objective sequence:

(1) Reneé will scoop food toward the body from a scoop bowl using a spoon held with a pronated grasp and appropriate movement patterns without spilling 3 out of 5 times within 3 months; (2) Reneé will bring food to mouth with spoon held palm down or with a pronated grasp and appropriate movement pattern without spilling within 6 months; and (3) Reneé will scoop food toward the body from a scoop bowl using a spoon held in a supinated grasp (palm facing up) using appropriate movement patterns and without spilling within 9 months.

Treatment activities:

Preparatory Postural and Sensory Management: Reneé's fear of movement, of unstable surfaces, of occlusion of vision, and of being touched indicated a strong need for sensory and postural preparation. After being exposed to various toys, equipment, textures, and work surfaces, Reneé selected her most preferred modalities — the mat, the nesting benches, and a basket of toys. The mat was close to the floor, as were most of the benches. The basket contained many surprises. During treatment Reneé usually initiated removing the lid from the basket and pulling out various textured objects such as small quilted cubes, bandana size fabric samples, and paper towel rolls covered with various textures. While Reneé was involved with activities such as stacking blocks or quilted cubes, the therapist facilitated equilibrium responses when the child made transitions to sitting or kneeling. Mature weight shift was encouraged by stabilizing one body side, for example, in sitting or in sidelying, to facilitate lengthening of the weight-bearing side. When possible, usually at the beginning of a session, drumming or banging on the table games were performed to sensitize specific body parts. Activities such as busy box that required forearm pronation and supination as well as finger dissociation were prescribed. During snack time, Reneé's gums were desensitized with the therapist's fingers or pretend toothbrush games. Dress up games were used to introduce various clothing textures and to allow the therapist to provide desensitization to proximal and ventral body areas as well as extraoral areas.

Direct Self-Feeding Management: Preparatory postural and sensory integration management allowed for progressive self-feeding management. General and focal densensitization in ventral and oral areas allowed for introduction of increasingly varied food textures and consistencies. Initially, changes in texture and consistency not only resulted in increased occurrence of tone fluctuations but elicited a gag reflex. When this occurred, the therapist lowered expectations to the previous level. Management was followed at home. Activities for pronation, supination and weight-bearing paved the way to appropriate grasp of eating utensils and increased shoulder stability for distal hand use.

Home Program: Consisted of performing games such as those indicated earlier, and using play materials with various textures from the agency toy library.

SUMMARY

This chapter has presented an introduction to occupational therapy management of children and adolescents with cerebral palsy. An overview of historical developments in medical and occupational therapy intervention was included. A functional definition of cerebral palsy and characteristics of motor, sensory, and associated deficits were presented in narrative and chart form. Effects of cerebral palsy on development and occupational performance were discussed. Key issues in assessment, including sensory, sequential neurological, and anatomical and kineseological considerations, were described, and appropriate instruments reviewed. Causes and performance effects of tonal abnormalities and compensatory postural and sensory patterns were stressed. Approaches to treatment, with emphasis on Bobaths' neurodevelopmental therapy, were reviewed, as well as pertinent research. Three case studies were presented to illustrate occupational therapy management and application of technology for different ages and problems.

STUDY QUESTIONS

1. A 5-year-old boy named Craig with moderate left side hemiparesis has been referred to you. He has never had occupational therapy before and you have never worked with a child with cerebral palsy. Several days before his first appointment, you review this chapter to prepare yourself to work with him. Given his age and diagnosis, what in particular would you review from this chapter? From other portions of the text?

2. Craig has been referred from a Head Start program. Their report indicates that he has been demonstrating disruptive behavior in the classroom. Problems cited include poor attention, constant and uncontrolled movements, excessive verbalization, and a tendency to hurt himself and others during disruptive episodes. What methods and instruments will you choose to assess his current status and program needs?

3. After completing your evaluation sessions, you find that Craig demonstrates the following characteristics:
   a. Delayed and incomplete protective extension of the arms and equilibrium reactions to the left side
   b. Difficulty with transitional movements, especially related to left side body control
   c. Fine motor skills with the right hand are at the 28 month level, and he shows little volitional use of the left hand to perform bilateral activities
   d. Although Craig verbalized extensively, speech production was labored and a tendency to drool was noted
   e. Generalized sensory integrative dysfunction
   f. Poor stabilization of proximal joints, with LUE habitually held in the flexed "high guard" posture, the left foot pronated, and minimal trunk rotation
   g. Marked preference for vestibular and somatosensory stimulation activities
   h. Age-appropriate self-feeding skills, but resistance to self-dressing and toilet training
   i. Solitary play for short periods of time with blocks, hammers, and busy box, with emerging interest in play with other children
   j. Good response to sensory motor facilitation indicated by increased use of left arm and hand and increased activity attention

   Given this information, develop two long-term goals for Craig for his first year of treatment. Plan a sequence of short-term objectives to support the long-term goals.

4. What preparation activities would be useful for your initial treatment session? What types of toys, games, and other activities would be appropriate to achieve each of the short-term objectives?

5. What recommendations would you make to Craig's parents, who live in a rural area and are unable to attend therapy sessions? What program suggestions would you give to Craig's Head Start teacher?

REFERENCES

1. Abbott M: Present day trends in cerebral palsy, Am J Occup Ther 4:53, 1950.
2. Ayres AJ: Effects of sensory integrative therapy on the coordination of children with choreoathetoid movements, American Occupational Therapy Association 31:291, 1977.
3. Ayres AJ: Sensory integration and learning disorders, Los Angeles, 1972, Western Psychological Services.
4. Ayres AJ: Sensory integration and the child, Los Angeles, 1983, Western Psychological Services.

5. Ayres AJ, and Tickle LS: Hyper-responsivity to touch and vestibular stimuli as a predictor of positive response to sensory integration procedures by autistic children, Am Occup Ther 34:6, 1980.

6. Bax M: Management of cerebral palsy, Dev Med Child Neurol 23:703, 1981.

7. Bleck E: Orthopedic management of cerebral palsy, Saunders Monographs in Clinical Orthopedics, vol II, Philadelphia, 1979, WB Saunders Co.

8. Bly L: The components of normal movement during the first year of life. In Slaton DS: Development of movement in infancy, Chapel Hill, 1980, University of North Carolina.

9. Bobath B: The very early treatment of cerebral palsy, Dev Med Child Neurol 9:373, 1967.

10. Bobath K: A neurophysiological basis for the treatment of cerebral palsy, Philadelphia, 1980, JB Lippincott Co.

11. Bobath K, and Bobath B: Cerebral palsy. In Pearson PH, and Williams CE, editors: Physical therapy services in the developmental disabilities, Springfield, Ill, 1972, Charles C Thomas, Publisher.

12. Bobath K, and Bobath B: The treatment of cerebral palsy based on the analysis of the patient's motor behavior, Br J Phys Med 15:107, 1952.

13. Brunstromm S: Movement therapy in hemiplegia, New York, 1970, Harper and Row, Publishers, Inc.

14. Carlsen PN: Comparison of the two occupational therapy approaches for treating the young cerebral palsied child, Am J Occup Ther 29:267, 1975.

15. Cazauvielh J; Recherches sur l'agenesie cerebral et la paralysie congeniale, Arch Gen Med, 1827.

16. CDMRC, University of Washington, Personal communication.

17. Chee F, Kreutzberg J, and Clark D: Semicircular canal stimulation in cerebral palsied children, Phys Ther 58:1071, 1978.

18. Erhardt RP: Developmental Feeding Sequences, Laurel, Md, 1986, RAMSCO Publishing Co.

19. Erhardt RP: Developmental hand dysfunction: theory, assessment, treatment, Laurel, MD, 1982, RAMSCO Publishing Co.

20. Erhardt RP: Developmental vision assessment, Laurel, Md, 1986, RAMSCO Publishing Co.

21. Fay T: Cerebral palsy: medical considerations and clasification, Am J Psych 107:180, 1950.

22. Fiorentino MR: A basis for sensorimotor development — normal and abnormal, Springfield, Ill, 1981, Charles C Thomas, Publisher.

23. Gilfoyle EM, Grady AP, and Moore JC: Children adapt, Thorofare, NJ, 1981, Slack, Inc.

24. Goldner JL: The upper extremity in cerebral palsy. In Samilson RL, editor: Orthopedic aspects of cerebral palsy, Clinics in Developmental Medicine, Nos 52/53, London, 1975, Heineman Educational Books Inc.

25. Grayson E: Occupational therapy for the cerebral palsied baby, Am J Occup Ther 6:64, 1950.

26. Green W: Historical notes — the past generation. In Samilson RL, editor: Orthopedic aspects of cerebral palsy, Clinics in Developmental Medicine Nos 52/53, London, 1975, Heinemann Educational Books Inc.

27. Gunn S: Play as occupation: implications for the handicapped, Am J Occup Ther 29:222, 1975.

28. Hoffer M: Cerebral palsy. In Green D, editor: Operative hand surgery, New York, 1982, Churchill-Livingstone.

29. Howison MV: Occupational therapy with children — cerebral palsy. In Hopkins H, and Smith H, editors: Willard and Spackman's Occupational therapy, Philadelphia, 1983, JB Lippincott Co.

30. Imperio A, Cullinan T, and Riklan M: Characteristics associated with cerebral palsy and dystonia musculorum deformans, Percept Mot Skills 48:1002, 1979.

31. King LJ: Toward a science of adaptive responses, Am J Occup Ther 32:429, 1978.

32. Kiss R: Occupational therapy. In Cruickshank W, editor: Cebral palsy: a development disability, ed 3, Syracuse, NY, 1976, Syracuse University Press.

33. Kleiman B, and Bulkley B: Some implications of a science of adaptive responses, Am J Occup Ther 36:15, 1982.

34. Knott M, and Voss DE: Proprioceptive neuromuscular facilitation, New York, 1968, Harper and Row, Publishers, Inc.

35. Knox S: A play scale. In Reilly M: Play as exploratory learning: studies in curiosity behavior, Beverly Hills, Calif, 1974, Sage Publications, Inc.

36. Larson AH, and others: Movement assessment of infants — a manual, Seattle, 1980, CDMRC University of Washington.

37. Little W: On the influence of abnormal parturition, difficult labours, premature birth, and asphyxia neonatorum on the mental and physical condition of the child especially in relation to deformities, Trans Obst Soc London 3:293, 1861.

38. Livingston D: Achievement recording for the cerebral palsied, Am J Occup Ther 4:66, 1950.

39. Lord E: Children handicappaed by cerebral palsy, New York, 1937, Commonwealth Press Inc.

40. Matsutsuyu J: Occupational behavior—a perspective on work and play, Am J Occup Ther 15:291, 1971.

41. Michelman SS: Play and the deficit child. In Reilly M, editor: Play as exploratory learning — studies of curiosity behavior, Beverly Hills, Calif, 1974, Sage Publications Inc.

42. Milani-Comparetti A: Pattern analysis of normal and abnormal development: the fetus, the newborn, the child. In Slaton DS, editor: Development of movement in infancy, Chapel Hill, 1980, University of North Carolina.

43. Minear W: A classification of cerebral palsy, Pediatrics 18:84, 1956.

44. Morris SE, and Klein MD: Pre-feeding skills: a comprehensive resource for feeding development, Tucson, 1987, Therapy Skill Builders.

45. Morris SE: Assessment of children with oral-motor dysfunction, a neurodevelopmental approach. In Wilson JM, editor: Oral motor function and dysfunction in children. Chapel Hill, 1977, University of North Carolina.

46. Norton Y: Neurodevelopment and sensory integration for the profoundly retarded multiply handicapped child, Am J Occup Ther 19:93, 1975.

47. Pact V, Sirotkin-Roses, and Beatus J: The muscle testing handbook, Boston, 1984, Little, Brown & Co.

48. Paisley S: Occupational therapy treatment for a group of spastic cases: children under twelve years of age, Occup Ther Rehabil 8:83, 1929.

49. Parette HP, and Hourcade JJ: A review of therapeutic intervention research on gross and fine motor progress in young children with cerebral palsy, Am J Occup Ther 38:7, 1984.

50. Phelps W: Etiology and diagnostic classification of cerebral palsy. In Proceedings of the cerebral palsy institute, New York Association for the Aid of Crippled Children, 1950.

51. Phelps W: The treatment of cerebral palsies, J Bone Joint Surg 22:1004, 1940.

52. Piaget J: Les stades du developpment intellectuel de l"enfant et de l'Adolescent. In Maier HW, editor: Three theories of child development: the contributions of Erik H Erikson, Jean Piaget, and Robert R Sears. New York, 1969, Harper and Row, Publishers, Inc.

53. Pollack G: Assessment of the results of surgery in cerebral plasy.

In Samilson RL, editor: Orthopedic aspects of cerebral palsy, Clinics in Developmental Medicine Nos 52/53, London, 1957, Heineman Educational Books Inc.

54. Price A: The issue— neurotherapy and specialization, Am J Occup Ther 34:810, 1980.

55. Rood M: The use of sensory receptors to activate, facilitate, and to inhibit motor responses, autonomic, and somatic in developmental sequence. In Sattely C, editor: Approaches to the treatment of patients with neuromuscular dysfunction, Dubuque, IA, 1962, WC Brown Group.

56. Samilson RL, and Perry J: The orthopedic assessment in cerebral palsy. In Samilson RL, editor: Orthopedic aspects of cerebral palsy, Clinics in Developmental Medicine Nos 52/53, London, 1975, Heinemann Educational Medical Books Inc.

57. Scherzer AL, Mike V, and Ilson, J: Physical therapy as a determinant of change in the cerebral palsied infant, Pediatrics 58:47, 1976.

58. Scherzer AL, and Tscharnuter I: Early diagnosis and therapy in cerebral palsy: a primer of infant developmental problems, New York, 1982, Mercel Dekker Inc.

59. Sellick K, and Over R: Effects of vestibular stimulation on motor development of cerebral-palsied chidren, Dev Med Child Neurol 22:476, 1980.

60. Semans S, and others: A cerebral palsy assessment chart. In the child with central nervous system deficit, Children's Bureau Publications, Washington, DC, 1965, US Government Printing Office.

61. Shearer A: A right to love?, London, 1972, The Spastics Society, The National Association for Mental Health.

62. Stratton M: Behavioral assessment scale of oral function in feeding, Am J Occup Ther 35:11, 1981.

63. Takata N: The play milieu—a preliminary appraisal, Am J Occup Ther 25:281, 1971.

64. Talbot ML, and Junkala, J: The effects of auditorially augmented feedback in the eye-hand coordination of students with cerebral palsy, Am J Occup Ther 35:8, 1981.

65. Teplin S, Howard J, and O'Connor M: Self-concept of young children with cerebral palsy, Dev Med Child Neurol 23:730, 1981.

66. Torok N, and Perlstein M: Vestibular findings in cerebral palsy, Ann Otol Rhinol Laryngol 71:51, 1962.

67. Trombly CA, editor: Occupational therapy for physical dysfunction, ed 2, Baltimore, 1983, Williams & Wilkins.

68. Trombly CA, and Scott AD: Occupational therapy for physical dysfunction, Baltimore, MD, 1977, Williams & Wilkins.

69. Tyler N, and Kogan K: Measuring the effectiveness of occupational therapy in the treatment of cerebral palsy, Am J Occup Ther 19:8, 1965.

70. Tyler N, and Kogan K: Reduction of stress between mothers and their handicapped children, Am J Occup Ther 31:151, 1977.

71. Tyler N, Kogan K, and Turner P: Interpersonal components of therapy with youn cerebral palsied, Am J Occup Ther 28:395, 1974.

72. United Cerebral Palsy: The story of UCP, New York, 1949.

73. Verluys H: Psychosocial adjustment to physical disability. In Trombly C, editor: Occupational therapy for physical dysfunction, ed 2, Baltimore, Md, 1983, Williams & Wilkins.

74. Ward DE: Positioning the handicapped child for function, St Louis, MO, 1983, available from DE Ward, 316 Carmel Drive, St Louis MO 63119.

75. Zancolli EA, and Zancolli ER: Surgical management of the hemiplegic hand in cerebral palsy, Surg Clin North Am 61:395, 1981.

21

Children with mental retardation

M. JEANETTE MARTIN

The retarded individual is a person who, by an error in the developmental process or by severe trauma, is unable to perform adaptive living skills well enough to compete with the majority of independent human beings in society. The American Association on Mental Retardation (AAMR)* defines mental retardation:[8]

Mental retardation refers to significantly subaverage general intellectual functioning existing concurrently with deficits in adaptive behavior and manifested during the developmental period.

The retardation process is an interruption in the person's sensory, motor, or cognitive growth that may occur as early as the first trimester of development. The retarded individual may develop at a slowed rate through the sensorimotor, preoperational, and possibly the concrete stage of development as described by Piaget, but the inability to quickly process cognitive areas of thinking, understanding, and acting based on logical progression will not allow the individual to reach the formal operational stage of development. Mental retardation is a broad diagnostic category and may include the person who is physically and cognitively impaired or one who has as few as one or two deficits in effectively adapting to the social demands of his environment.

The caretakers and the caregivers for the mentally retarded individuals have throughout history attempted to explain these individuals and locate the reasons for their lack of adaptive living skills. The general problem of mental retardation has been explained in a historical vein by various authors.[9,19,21,23] It has been only in the last 150 years that a positive, progressive approach has been taken in caring for the retarded. Before the early 1800s the retarded person was ridiculed, ignored, or sheltered. In the past 50 years the caretaker and the caregiver roles have gradually

*Formerly the American Association on Mental Deficiency (AAMD).

changed to the roles of trainer, teacher, counselor, or houseparent. Retarded individuals are now expected to learn and develop to the limits of their ability, while society is expected to accept them to the extent of these abilities.

Researchers are gradually redefining the set of causative factors for retardation. It is now evident that the retarded may be clustered into two general and somewhat dissimilar groupings: the clinical-organic causes and the cultural-related causes. However, this division is not clear-cut or simple. There is great impact on both groups by the interactive consequences of prenatal and postnatal nutrition and infections, as well as the effects of postnatal, somatic experiences. Researchers have identified at least 200 types of medical problems associated with mental retardation.[5,6,14,20] The causes of these problems have been identified, and extensive research efforts have helped to ameliorate many predisposing conditions. For example, early diagnosis of conditions such as phenylketonuria (PKU) can, by the use of medication and special diets, offset severe and profound mental retardation to a large degree. Prenatal and postnatal surgery has been performed to sidestep the effects of hydrocephalus; and surgery has also helped the retarded person with orthopedic problems and other birth defects.

SETTINGS FOR PRACTICE

Any one of the 6 million retarded persons may be found in community agencies, including:

1. The neonatal nursery with babies at "high risk" who require specific sensory stimulation, special handling techniques, and parent training
2. The early developmental evaluation and screening programs where cytogenetic screening and family counseling are provided
3. The preschool training centers for at-risk or developmentally delayed children

4. The "developmental home" where the retarded person is housed with a foster family who provides special training and care
5. The schools, either in the special education classes, or as mainstreamed students
6. The sheltered workshop or adult training center
7. The residential institution that may be privately or publicly operated
8. The group home where two or more retarded persons live under the supervision of a house-parent
9. The training apartment or cluster apartment complex where one or more retarded persons live and are visited regularly by a counselor or sponsor
10. The skilled nursing facility that cares for the retarded person requiring physical care on a 24-hour, long-term basis.

The occupational therapist or the certified occupational therapy assistant may serve the retarded population in any one or more of these settings, depending on the needs of the retarded person. The occupational therapist with postgraduate education in handling newborns and training parents can provide direct services in the neonatal nursery and in the early developmental evaluation and screening programs. With experience in consultation and training, the therapist can help develop and monitor individualized programs and refer children to preschool training centers and to developmental homes. The school therapist provides support services to mainstreamed retarded persons (Chapter 29). In sheltered workshops, adult training centers, residential institutions known as state schools, developmental centers or retardation centers, and in skilled nursing facilities, certified occupational therapy assistants give much of the daily care and training under the supervision of the occupational therapist. Occasional direct or indirect services from the occupational therapist may be needed in independent living situations such as the group home or cluster apartment complex.

Local chapters of the Association for Retarded Citizens (ARC) and state chapters of the American Association on Mental Retardation provide information and service opportunities for the occupational therapist. The Association for Retarded Citizens was founded as a parent interest group but has grown to include many important legislative and service functions. The local chapters make a powerful contribution to public education regarding the prevention of birth defects and the location of services when assistance is required.[7]

OCCUPATIONAL THERAPY IN MENTAL RETARDATION SERVICES

Mentally retarded persons will always require some measure of mental or physical assistance from the more capable members of society. Occupational therapy offers appropriate evaluation and habilitative treatment or training to facilitate the development and readiness of retarded persons so that they may master and maintain the use of a range of adaptive living skills.[3]

The general goals of an occupational therapy program in mental retardation include but are not limited to:

1. Facilitating development in areas where physical and emotional delays exist
2. Minimizing the disabling effects of a physical handicap
3. Developing attitudes and skills basic to independent functioning

Each retarded person should have the opportunity to develop innate capacities to his full potential. As discussed throughout this text, task occupation is an integral part of normal living. It is an important, natural means through which relationships occur and feelings may be expressed. Purposeful activity is the agent through which human beings learn and develop. Occupational therapy emphasizes coordinated performance of the entire psychomotor system. In physical restoration there is an interdependence between emotions, intellect, and physical functioning. The useful objects constructed while using corrective hand splints; the games played while learning to tolerate longer periods of standing; the completion of a series of sheltered work-shop assembly tasks while learning to control the motor patterns appropriate to good eye-hand coordination; or the simple meals cooked while learning independent living skills are all symbols of occupational therapy. Intangible tools of occupational therapy include planning skills, the sharing of tools and equipment of natural relationships, and satisfaction, which is necessary for a healthy self-image. Activity requires involvement. It develops a sense of self as a contributing participant rather than a recipient.

Activity adaptation

To be involved in an activity the retarded person may need special positioning devices attached to the bed or wheelchair. Articles used in performing activities of daily living may be modified to provide the multi-handicapped retarded person with the assistance necessary to perform self-care and household or vocational tasks. Testing the retarded person's physical capacities to perform vocational tasks should be accompanied by a critical review of the architectural barriers of the work place.

As treatment of the retarded person progresses, the person assumes more of the responsibility for the direction of treatment under the guidance of the therapist, the parent, or the direct caregiver. The therapist gradually provides less direct care of the retarded person and more indirect care by monitoring skills learned or changes made in the treatment program.

Referral

The retarded person may be referred for occupational therapy by any advocate who is aware of problems and the potential for intervention or assistance. The request for help could originate from the parent, physician, school personnel, hospital staff, social worker, court personnel, volunteer agency, or others. The referral may be as simple as a verbal request, or it may be written in great detail.

Service to the retarded person is considered longitudinal in scope, that is, the occupational therapist does not cause an abrupt change or interruption in the person's rhythm of daily life. Instead, intervention is designed to enhance the current life pattern through assessment and treatment that is integral to it. Therefore the occupational therapist will place the retarded person's physical age, developmental level, adaptive living skills, potential, and environmental conditions into perspective when the referral is acknowledged and the person undergoes screening for services.

Screening

The use of a screening tool enables the occupational therapist to determine if the referral is appropriate for services, what those services may be, or whether further assessment is required. The screening tool establishes a general developmental range or capability level in adaptive living skills.[7] Screening tools may be standardized, nonstandardized, or developed in a specific referral location or agency to handle special areas of competency. To obtain basic information, the occupational therapist may use a variety of screening tools, including: (1) Denver Developmental Screening Test (Chapter 9), (2) Milani-Comparetti Neurodevelopmental Screening Examination (Chapter 10), or (3) nonstandardized screening tools. Often it may be more appropriate to develop a screening process that uses the operational definitions common to the specific agency. On the assumption that it is more informative to have a retarded individual demonstrate his abilities in real situations rather than in office interviews, the occupational therapy department of the Georgia Retardation Center developed assessment instruments specific to its population and environment (Figures 21-2 through 21-6). These instruments are a screening tool, tests for ADL (activities of daily living) in food preparation, and an outline for occupational therapy evaluations.

If occupational therapy is indicated, the parent, guardian, or court advocate must give written permission to proceed with services. This is done to protect the rights of the retarded person. In many agencies permission to proceed with evaluation and services is covered in the admission agreement, provided that the occupational therapist is a regular staff member. The occupational therapist should inform the retarded person's primary physician when the screening discloses a physical problem. As manager of the retarded person's physical welfare, the primary physician is responsible for directing and documenting changes in physical care.

Assessment

The retarded person benefits from comprehensive assessment that uses the special evaluation tools of each interdisciplinary team member. A more complete picture of the individual's capabilities and splinter skills will emerge so that an effective program can be developed by the team to capitalize on and expand those abilities. The occupational therapist looks at the results of standardized and nonstandardized tests, checklists, observation of performance, and communication from all persons who directly take care of the retarded person to develop a meaningful evaluation. The evaluation team should use an adaptive behavioral scale at this stage.[7] This type of test can serve as a good place to store raw data over a period of time and can serve as a retest vehicle so that change over several years is clearly seen.

VULPE ASSESSMENT BATTERY

The Vulpe Assessment Battery[22] is a useful tool for therapists who are learning to evaluate retarded persons. Developed for the atypical child, it includes developmental assessments, performance analyses, and examples of individual program plans (see Figure 21-7, a sample page from the Vulpe battery). This battery covers test items for events from birth to 6 years of age in the adaptive living areas of basic senses and functions; gross and fine motor behaviors; language behaviors; cognitive behaviors; organizational behaviors; activities of daily living; and the behaviors of the caregiver in the person's living environment.

TIME SERIES OBSERVATIONS

Time series observations are effective for baseline evaluation, because the retarded person is in familiar surroundings using media and materials common to her daily routine. From three to five separate observations by the same evaluator of performance of activities of daily living such as dressing, toileting, and self-feeding should provide sufficient data regarding level of competency and problems in physical motor performance and emotional growth.

When evaluating a retarded person who is over the chronological age of 6, the occupational therapist may need to select evaluation tools that focus on a specific area of daily living skills. Dressing, feeding, and toileting assessments are better done by observation over a period of a week or more with documentation of each observation. These pieces of information, with data obtained by other evaluators, can present a true picture of the retarded person's strengths and weaknesses in adaptive living skills.

Tests tailored specifically to adult skills should be reviewed carefully for applicability to the retarded population. The Adult Skills Evaluation Survey[10] addresses fine motor skills, perceptual skills, academic skills, and living skills. These areas are germane to the work activity programs used by all retarded persons.

Behavior during evaluation

Until the retarded person has formed an acceptable level of a relationship with the evaluator, he will tend to have difficulty in testing situations. At the first testing session, the retarded person may be very cooperative or may reject any or all test items. This rejection or defensive reaction is often the result of the person's difficulty in dealing with new situations and sensory experiences. With careful and considerate negotiating,[12] the occupational therapist may gradually break down the barriers of the retarded person's "personal space" and fear. The evaluator often needs to place the test item within the context of the environment and the current behavior of the retarded person. In addition, the individual may need to learn the test item over several sessions before the formal testing. The testing process might be accomplished as quickly as one session, but it usually requires three to five sessions to get acceptable levels of performance. For this reason, it is more expedient to begin assessment by using observation and group interaction before using individual testing. Through observation it is possible to define the usual range of a person's general behavior, whether socially cooperative or maladaptive. Does the person demonstrate stereotypic, self-stimulating, or self-abusive movements in a group situation? Does he take food or toys from another person, or does he share with others?

Team or composite evaluations

In some agencies the baseline evaluation is administered jointly by the professional staff by use of one tool that is limited to the scope of the program activities available at that agency. This type of evaluation is often self-limiting because it does not reflect each retarded person's potential or the possible areas for program growth in the agency. Also, it does not allow for indicators of potential future problem areas A great disservice could be done to the retarded person when only one test, such as the AAMR Adaptive Behavior Scale,[7] is used as a comprehensive evaluation. Achievement in skills that do not relate directly to the test items; indications for therapeutic intervention and revision of physical positioning; and ability to profit from sensory experiences are not addressed by a test such as this one.

Because each person is unique, extensive evaluation into problem areas should be done to pinpoint the exact focus of treatment or training. It benefits the re-

tarded person to be evaluated by specialists in all areas of adaptive living. Two or more professional staff members could conduct assessment in a specialized area to investigate associated problems in depth and to develop a task analysis or a treatment or training program designed for the individual. For example, the occupational therapist and the speech and special education teacher could develop an effective treatment or training program in the agency or school setting for the adaptive feeding area (see Figure 21-7).

Program planning

The appropriate format and outline for documentation of information gathered or developed by the occupational therapist is found in the Uniform Terminology for Reporting Occupational Therapy Services[2] and those portions of the Uniform Occupational Therapy Evaluation Checklist[3] that apply. It is recommended that the report format be consistent with headings of specific reporting areas underlined (Figure 21-4). The evaluator need use only the relevant topics in the report. This type of report format is easy for other mental retardation workers to follow, and it makes possible a quick chart audit (Chapter 31).

In addition to these guidelines, the occupational therapist should report specific program recommendations in the format used by the agency so that they are included in the team recommendations for the treatment or training program. For example, all individualized education programs (IEPs) must be written within 1 month after referral of the child to special education, and annually thereafter. The interdisciplinary program plan (IPP) is used in day and institutional programs for the mentally retarded. The IPP is written by the team for the annual review of a retarded person monitored by an agency. It generally requires a broad view of each area of adaptive living, touching on skills such as body control, communication, self-help, social behaviors, effective use of time, basic knowledge or practical skills, and general health care.

It is for these reasons that the occupational therapist's report should clearly define the timeliness of occupational therapy services and whether these services should be direct or indirect. The IPP should state the specific treatment items, if any, that must be delivered by occupational therapy staff members; list those training skills to be taught by any professional staff; and state the due date for any follow-up evaluation.

Treatment or training

The occupational therapist who provides treatment or training services seldom, if ever, works in isolation with the retarded person. Interdependence of the professional staff strengthens the effectiveness and quality of the training program for the retarded person. The addition of parents and paraprofessional workers aids the day-to-day consistency needed to reinforce and maintain an effective action-oriented program.

In general, an educational model is used for the delivery of mental retardation services (Chapter 29). The members of the interdisciplinary program team, including the occupational therapist, share supporting roles. The size of this team varies with the type and location of the facility or agency. With contributions of information from as many sources as possible, the team develops a plan of training or treatment activities on behalf of the retarded person. This specifically designed program is a list of adaptive living skills described by tasks, each with operational definitions written in behavioral terms. Progress or lack of progress is determined after data collected on task performance are reviewed. When the plan calls for a treatment or a service to be performed by a staff member directly for the retarded person, this is listed as a "staff activity" in the written program. In the interdisciplinary setting, progress reports are submitted monthly by the occupational therapist and excerpts are taken and combined with other reports to develop a monthly summary of progress.

When developing a program of treatment or training for the retarded person, the occupational therapist has many good resources available, including the resource packet on mental retardation developed by the American Occupational Therapy Association's Division of Professional Development.[4] The chapters of Part V of this text provide the foundation for program areas and methods that are used with children who are mentally retarded. In addition, related specialty chapters in this section (VI) will provide guidelines for programming for the child whose multiple handicaps include mental retardation. The occupational therapist can also draw from other guidelines and resource packets such as those for physical disabilities, prevocational evaluation and training, adaptive equipment, and mental health to fully cover the many areas of adaptive living that apply to the retarded person's program.

Adaptive equipment

All of the aids and devices required by the retarded person for adaptive living are grouped under the general heading of adaptive equipment. The standards of the Accreditation Council on Services for People with Developmental Disabilities[1] categorize types of adaptive equipment under a variety of headings, including physical development and health assessment, behavior management, and mobility. These standards assure that the facilities and agencies have the services and programs necessary for providing adequate care and training of the retarded individual. Items of adaptive equipment are categorized by purpose and location of use. For example, a padded and modified helmet could be used either as a protective device or as part of an approved behavior training program.

During the habilitation, education, and training process, the aids and devices necessary to enable the individual to learn self-help tasks may be considered adaptive equipment. These items include the clothing adapted for dressing training; electronic, environmental control systems; specialized communication devices; specialized devices used in self-feeding, dressing, and other tasks performed as activities of daily living; and the architectural modifications that allow for increased independence in living tasks. Recent technology has opened the door to the use of switches commanded by the slightest touch or movement of air. When connected to toys or aids to daily living, these switches can enable the retarded person with extensive physical handicaps to have some control over his environment. Once aware of the ability to make something happen, the individual may be able to add other tasks or events to increase his level of functional performance.

When a referral for an adapted device is received, it is necessary for the therapist to have a clear understanding of the retarded person's problems, the living situations in which the adapted device is to be used, the number of caregivers to be instructed in the use of the device, and a working knowledge of the sources of supply of a variety of devices. Also, the occupational therapist is expected to have a working acquaintance with federal guidelines and requirements for accessible design in order to request and describe the exact location for placement of adapted equipment. It is up to the therapist to know what items are needed and to be able to write specifications clearly so that the exact item needed is received. The requisition and delivery processes usually take more than a month, so it may be necessary to assemble a temporary device to begin the training procedure.

Once adaptive equipment is obtained, accountability for these items must be considered. Because these items are vital to the retarded person's habilitation program, each must be listed in permanent records as part of the individual's program. Equipment should be inventoried periodically, and its use should be monitored during programming (Figure 21-2). Unless another person is responsible for repairing adaptive devices, this is to be handled by the therapist. Those items of adapted equipment used by the retarded person should be listed prominently in the written program, and all persons working with that person should be aware that the items exist, why and how they are used, and how to maintain them properly. Appropriate photographs make a useful addition to the record.

Discharge

When retarded individuals meet the criteria for change of placement, the persons responsible for their care develop a plan for that change. The group of responsible persons might include the parent, guardian, program planning team, and the court representative or retarded individual. Any changes in placement should be planned before the change date and in sufficient time to allow for adequate preparation. Discharge to a less or more restrictive environment requires that the occupational therapist write a summary of previous treatment or training, including any recommendations for care that can be handled in the forthcoming placement.

MANAGEMENT OF OCCUPATIONAL THERAPY SERVICES

The variety of duties required of the occupational therapist demands the use of a complex but flexible schedule. Priorities may vary from day to day. For example, the retarded person with self-abusive seizure episodes that involve injurious falls will have an immediate need for head-protective or other body-fitting devices to protect against injury. These unexpected events and others will interrupt any set schedule. Generally, though, it is possible to establish a regular and specific period at least every other week to reevaluate individuals before their annual review meetings. The occupational therapist working in or for any agency will also need to designate time each month to prepare progress summaries. Usually the caseload of retarded clients is so varied that it is imperative to reassess all current tasks and decide whether a change in the schedule is needed to accomplish a change in programming. Such recommendations must be presented to and decided by the team because of the complex nature of each individual's schedule.

Behavioral data collection

A clear understanding of the various types and uses for data collection is essential for objective reporting. This collection of data may refer to:
1. *Frequency:* a count of the number of times a behavior occurs
2. *Rate:* a count of how often a behavior occurs per unit of time
3. *Durations:* a measure of how long each instance of a behavior lasts
4. *Instantaneous time sampling:* a gross estimate of how much of the time a person is engaged in the behavior, rather than a precise measure of it
5. *Interval recording:* a method in which the observation period is divided into intervals of equal length and continuous observation is maintained (Chapters 10 and 12)

Research

Work in the field of mental retardation lends itself to clinical research. Questions arise about why a particular technique was successful for one individual's training program and not another's, why a retarded person with a particular medical diagnosis responds better to one training technique than another, or why one system of monitoring care provider activities is more successful than another. The answers to these and other questions may be found through the scientific inquiry procedures known as research.[13] This method is set in an orderly process that includes:
1. A statement of the question
2. A review of prior research in that area
3. A selection and explanation of the procedure to be used
4. A listing of operational definitions
5. A description of the person or group to be studied
6. A clarification of the method of collecting data
7. The specific procedures for analyzing the data
8. A statement of the hypothesis
9. An objective report of the results of the research methodology
10. The conclusions drawn by the researcher

Perhaps the most practical and useful research methods for the occupational therapist to use to verify treatment or training with the mentally retarded are the single case design and the time series design.[17,18] The single case design and the time series design are valuable to the clinician in mental retardation because these models allow for individual differences, provide an excellent way to integrate practice and research, and allow the therapist to ask and answer most of the scientifically important questions raised in the clinical environment. In the short term these designs help the therapist to make assessment and treatment decisions. In the long term it appears that the continuity of clinical science depends on the generation of data from on-line clinical work rather than the laboratory.

Other types of research designs also have value in mental retardation research. In fact, important work has been done by occupational therapists acting as technical assistants to other members of the interdisciplinary team during drug studies, biofeedback studies, and others. A major benefit of interdisciplinary research is the continuing education and role expansion of all interdisciplinary team members. Examples of these efforts may be found in the literature. The Office of Professional Research Services of the American Occupational Therapy Foundation is committed to assisting the occupational therapist with research efforts and will provide the names and addresses of nearby research consultants.

Staff development or in-service training

The treatment or training aspect of occupational therapy services does not end with the therapist-student dyad. To maintain the newly acquired skills in his repertoire of adaptive behaviors, the individual needs encouragement and prompting from daily care providers to perform this skill. The providers may be parents, other relatives, teachers and aides, direct care staff, houseparents, other professional staff, or any other persons whose participation is relevant to meeting the needs of an individual.

Instruction of other care providers demands the use of group training methods beyond the basic training methods in the occupational therapy undergraduate curriculum. The instructional analysis and the lesson plan are two teaching methods that produce effective results. *The instructional analysis* contains the (1) instructional objective, (2) desired learning outcome, and (3) main points of discussion. In addition, a method of recording the names of participants and a method for follow-up or monitoring the skill learned by the caregiver should be included in the instructional analysis. One or more instructional objectives may be developed as a part of the instructional analysis. When writing the instructional objectives, it should be remembered that a therapist's own knowledge of the subject matter limits what can be taught and learned and that participants will have a variety of prior learning experiences in the topic area. The length of time necessary to provide instruction will vary, and the physical surroundings of the instructional setting will affect the learning experience. Each instructional objective should include a clear reference to the needs of the participants; present a simple, limited topic; adjust for the level of learning or understanding of the participant; and have a purpose or value to the participant. Development of topic areas and use of the same outline and lesson plan will diminish the time needed to prepare for subsequent training sessions. Also, as personnel change, each new care provider receives every part of skill training needed to train the retarded person exactly as his predecessor.

When writing the instructional analysis, include the following:

1. *Topic.* State the general topic area.
2. *Course.* State the specific title.
3. *Time.* State the expected length of instruction.
4. *Objective.* State the skill to be learned.

Then make two columns listing the desired learning outcomes on one side, and list the main points briefly on the other side.

The *lesson plan* is a detailed version of the instructional analysis, and it may contain the following list and procedure:

1. *Topic.* State the general topic area.
2. *Course.* State the specific title.
3. *Time.* State the expected length of instruction.
4. *Objective.* State the skill to be learned.
5. *Materials and equipment.* List all audiovisuals, demonstration items, writing materials, and handout materials.
6. *Presentation.*
   a. Introduce yourself by name and area of expertise.
   b. Establish the interest of the audience by discussing the topic area in general.
   c. Review the specifics and measurable desired learning outcomes with the audience.
   d. Proceed with the narrative portion of the presentation, using audiovisual and other media.
   e. Summarize the points or procedure taught.
7. *Examination.* Present a written test or have each participant demonstrate skill in the topic lesson.
8. *Documentation of training.* Before the audience leaves the classroom area, they should sign a roster for attendance records.
9. *Follow-up.* Develop a procedure for direct supervisors to monitor the application of the new skill in the work setting.

Monitoring programs

When monitoring the treatment or training program, the occupational therapist should write out the program, describing the techniques to be used; consult with the person who will train the retarded individual; demonstrate the techniques; record the training session; and check periodically that the training techniques are used as designed.

CASE STUDY

Occupational therapy evaluation

I. Personal information:
   Todd, age 9.5 years.
II. Referral information: The Butler County Training Center requested evaluation and training in preparation for mainstreaming into the local classroom.
III. Personal history
   A. Developmental history: Todd was a very miserable baby before his thoracotomy. After surgery, he often smiled. He began to roll over at 4 years and to push himself around the floor by using his feet at 5 years. He does not sit independently or feed himself. At the age of 7 toilet training was attempted with no success.
   B. Educational history: Todd was kept at home until age 6 when he began attending the training center. He enjoys watching other children play. Because he is severely handicapped, formal testing has not been possible. His expressive communication is limited to head shaking for yes or no and to the sounds "mama" or "papa" when he is calm.
   C. Medical history: Todd is the second of three children. He was placed in an incubator at birth because of respiratory problems. At 8 weeks a thoracotomy was done on his left lung. During this procedure he suffered three cardiac arrests. He has a history of asthmatic attacks and seizures. The primary physician reports that he seems to see and hear. His head control is good; trunk control is poor; the right upper and lower extremities have less function than the left extremities. The right upper extremity is held in flexion pattern. The left upper extremity has severe flexion and ulnar deviation of the wrist. There is a 2-inch shortening of the right lower extremity, and both feet

are in minimal varus position. Medical diagnosis on referral is profound psychomotor retardation, cause undetermined.

IV. Skills and performance areas

A. *Independent living: daily living skills and performance*

1. *Physical daily living skills:* Todd requires total assistance.

2. *Psychological:* Emotional daily living skills; Todd nods his head yes to recognizing his image in a mirror.

3. *Play:* Todd enjoys all visual and auditory entertainment.

B. *Sensorimotor skills and performance components*

1. *Neuromuscular performance components*

a. *Reflex integration:* The Milani-Comparetti Screening Tool revealed the following personal baseline results:

(1) Primitive reflexes: 5 months of normal development

(2) Righting reactions: 7 months of normal development

(3) Parachute reactions: 4.5 months of normal development.

b. *Range of motion:* Severe spasticity and high diazepam (Valium) dosage precludes accurate measures of passive range of motion. Functional range of motion of upper extremity is not evident because of severe contractures and very poor muscle tone. (*Note: See physical therapy report for arc of passive motion of joints.*) Todd does not have the physical capacity to tolerate prone (face-down) positioning.

2. *Sensory integration*

a. Sensory awareness: Todd responds appropriately to pinprick, rough surfaces, and soft surfaces on extremities.

b. Visual: Spatial awareness was not tested.

3. *Cognitive skill and performance components*

a. Todd responds with head nod or shaking when direct questions are posed. This communication method does not allow for problem solving.

b. His attention span is average for his physical age.

4. *Psychosocial skills and performance components*

a. Self-management: Todd flings out his arms or legs to get attention from passerby.

b. Group interaction: Todd watches other children and staff.

5. *Therapeutic adaptation:* Todd has been using a standard wheelchair in junior size.

Proposed direct or indirect client needs from occupational therapy

(Note: Inform the primary physician of your recommendations.)

I. Positioning for function and therapeutic goals

A. Bed or mat

With the attending physical therapist, select the optimum right and left sidelying positions using wedges, pillows, or a molded orthosis.

B. Wheelchair adaptations

With the attending physical therapist and any other concerned individual, determine the type of mechanical supports needed to place Todd in the best functional, seated position. Consider the use of firm seat and back inserts; removable L-shaped thigh and hip pads; and a lapboard with a raised support pad at the waist cut-out. With the attending speech pathologist, determine the communication devices that can be placed for function on the lapboard (Figure 21-1).

C. Classroom environment

With the classroom teacher, determine physical placement for Todd's wheelchair and other positioning equipment so that he can attend to the teacher. Determine which feeding devices Todd will use, obtain them, and instruct his feeder how to use them with Todd.

D. Home environment

With Todd's direct caregiver, assess his functional use

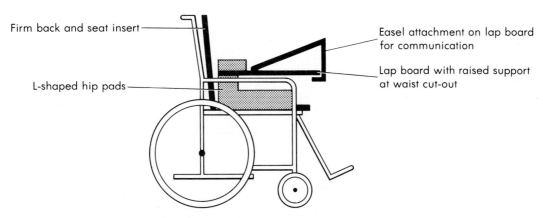

Firm back and seat insert

Easel attachment on lap board for communication

Lap board with raised support at waist cut-out

L-shaped hip pads

Figure 21-1 Todd's adaptations: firm back and seat insert; L-shaped hip pads; lapboard with raised support at waist cut-out; easel attachment on lapboard for communication.

of his living arrangements. Check for architectural barriers or obstacles to his transportation, group activities, and hygiene.

II. Activities of daily living skills
   A. Adapt toileting devices for home and for school.
   B. Adapt bathing devices for home.
   C. Assess oral motor skills and develop training program.
   D. Refer dental hygiene to his dentist.

III. Body control
   A. Develop program of relaxation techniques.
   B. In conjunction with the physical therapist or the therapeutic recreation staff, develop general physical conditioning program to be used at school.

IV. In-service training: Train home and school personnel who work with Todd in each of the techniques he has learned and in the proper use of his special aids and devices. Include copies of his home program in his occupational therapy department client record.

V. Follow-through: If Todd is not under the care of the school occupational therapist, set up a follow-up visit within 1 year.

SUMMARY

The mentally retarded person has significantly subaverage general intellectual function that exists concurrently with deficits in adaptive behavior. Occupational therapy can make an important contribution to the development of the retarded person where physical and emotional delays exist; can aid in minimizing the disabling effects of a physical handicap; and can provide treatment or training to develop attitudes and skills basic to independent function. As an active member of the treatment team, the occupational therapist provides the evaluation, habilitative treatment or training and follow-up of the retarded person so that she will be able to master and maintain adaptive living skills.

STUDY QUESTIONS

1. Describe and discuss deficits in adaptive behavior that affect the lives of mentally retarded persons.
2. How does an occupational therapist contribute to the development of a mentally retarded child in whom physical and emotional delays exist?
3. Discuss evaluation as it applies to the mentally retarded. How does it differ from the evaluation of those children in the normal range of mental development?
4. Plan the occupational therapy intervention for Mary, a 9-year-old minimally involved Down syndrome child who has just entered the first grade.

REFERENCES

1. Accreditation Council on Services for People with Developmental Disabilities: Standards for services for people with developmental disabilities, Boston, Mass, 1987, The Accreditation Council.
2. American Occupational Therapy Association, Inc, AOTA Commission on Practice: Uniform terminology for reporting occupational therapy services, Rockville, Md, 1979.
3. American Occupational Therapy Association, Inc, AOTA Commission on Practice: Uniform occupational therapy evaluation checklist, Rockville, Md, 1981.
4. American Occupational Therapy Association, Inc, Division of Professional Development: Mental retardation, Resource packet, Rockville, Md, 1986.
5. Baroff GS: Mental retardation: Nature, cause, and management, Washington, DC, 1986, Hemisphere Publishing Co.
6. Buda FB: The neurology of developmental disabilities, Springfield, Ill, 1981, Charles C Thomas, Publisher.
7. Fogelman CJ, editor: AAMD Adaptive Behavior Scale, rev ed, Washington, DC, 1975, American Association on Mental Retardation.
8. Grossman HJ, editor: Classification in mental retardation, Washington, DC, 1983, American Association on Mental Retardation.
9. Halpern AS: Mental retardation. In Stolov WC, editor: Handbook of severe disability, Washington, DC, 1981, US Department of Education, Rehabilitation Services Administration.
10. Herrick JT, and Lowe HE: The adult skills evaluation survey for persons with mental retardation, Pasadena, Calif, 1985, New Opportunity Workshops, Inc.
11. Hill BK, and Lakin CK: Classification of residential facilities for individuals with mental retardation, Mental Retardation, 24:107, 1986.
12. Huss AM: Touch with care or a caring touch, Am J Occup Ther 31(1):11, 1977.
13. Jantzen AC: Research: the practical approach for occupational therapy, Laurel, Md, 1981, RAMSCO Publishing Co.
14. Koch R: Bio-medical problems in mental retardation . . . a review. Unpublished paper presented at the National Prevention Showcase and Forum, Atlanta, Sept 15-17, 1982, President's Committee on Mental Retardation.
15. Lederman EF: Occupational therapy in mental retardation, Springfield, Ill, 1984, Charles C Thomas, Publisher.
16. Lyons M, Kielhofner G, and Kavanagh M: Mental retardation. In Kielhofner G, editor: A model of human occupation theory and application, Baltimore, 1985, Williams & Wilkins.
17. Ottenbacher KJ: Evaluating clinical change: strategies for occupational and physical therapists, Baltimore, 1986, Williams & Wilkins.
18. Payton OD: Research: The validation of clinical practice, Philadelphia, 1971, FA Davis Co.
19. Scheerenberger RC: A history of mental retardation, Baltimore, 1982, Brookes Publishing Co.
20. Scheiner AP, and Abroms IF: The practical management of the developmentally disabled child, St Louis, 1980, The CV Mosby Co.
21. Sebelist RM: Mental retardation. In Hopkins HL, and Smith JD, editors: Willard and Spackman's occupational therapy, ed 5, Philadelphia, 1978, JB Lippincott Co.
22. Vulpe SG: Vulpe Assessment Battery, rev ed, Laurel, Md, 1987, RAMSCO Publishing Co.
23. Wright N: Total rehabilitation, Boston, 1981, Little, Brown & Co.

SUGGESTED READINGS

Books

Bergen A: Selected equipment for pediatric rehabilitation, Valhalla, NY, 1975, Blythedale Children's Hospital.

Bernstein FS, Ziarnik JP, and Rudreed EH: Behavioral habilitation through proactive programming, Baltimore, 1982, Brookes Publishing Co.

Copeland M, Ford L, and Salon N: Occupational therapy for mentally retarded children, Baltimore, 1976, University Park Press.

Finnie N: Handling the young cerebral palsied child at home, New York, 1970, EP Dutton & Co, Inc.

Frank J: Resource guide to protective aids, Washington, DC, 1979, George Washington University.

Fraser BA, Hensinger R, and Phelps JA: Physical management of multiple handicaps—a professional's guide, Baltimore, 1987, Brookes Publishing Co.

High EC, editor: Resource guide to habilitative techniques and aids for cerebral palsied persons of all ages, Washington, DC, 1979, George Washington University.

Hoffmann R: How to build special furniture and equipment for handicapped children, Springfield, Ill, 1970, Charles C Thomas, Publisher.

Macey P: Mobilizing multiply handicapped children, Lawrence, Kan, 1974, University of Kansas.

Morris SE: Program guidelines for children with feeding problems, Edison, NJ, 1977, Childcraft Education Corp.

Robinalt I: Functional aids for the multiply handicapped, Hagerstown, Md, 1973, Harper & Row, Publishers, Inc.

US Architectural and Transportation Barriers Compliance Board: A guidebook to: the minimum federal guidelines and requirements for accessible design, Washington, DC, 1981, US Government Printing Office.

Ward DE: Positioning the handicapped child for function, rev ed 2, St Louis, Mo, 1984, Phoenix Press, Inc.

Articles

Berdslee GR: Fieldwork experience in mental retardation, Am J Occup Ther 30:656, 1976.

Bonadonna P: Effects of a vestibular stimulation program on stereotypic rocking behavior, Am J Occup Ther 35:775, 1981.

Bright T, Bittick K, and Fleeman B: Reduction of self-injurious behavior using sensory integrative techniques, Am J Occup Ther 35:167, 1981.

Clark FA, and others: A comparison of operant and sensory integrative methods of developmental parameters in profoundly retarded adults, Am J Occup Ther 32:86, 1978.

DeMars P: Training adult retardates for private enterprise, Am J Occup Ther 29:39, 1975.

Esenther SE: Developmental coaching of the Down syndrome infant, Am J Occup Ther 38:440, 1984.

Gisel EG, Lange LJ, and Niman CW: Chewing cycles in 4- and 5-year-old Down's syndrome children: a comparison of eating efficacy with normals, Am J Occup Ther 38:666, 1984.

Gisel EG, Lange LJ, and Niman CW: Tongue movements in 4- and 5-year-old Down's syndrome children during eating: a comparison with normal children, Am J Occup Ther 38:660, 1984.

Goldman L: Behavioral skills for employment of the intellectually handicapped, Am J Occup Ther 29:539, 1975.

Huff DM, and Harris SC: Using sensorimotor integrative treatment with mentally retarded adults, Am J Occup Ther 41:227, 1987.

Hurff JM, Poulsen MK, Van Hoven J, and Olson S: A library skills program serving adults with mental retardation: an interdisciplinary approach, Am J Occup Ther 39:233, 1985

Hurff J: Gaming technique: an assessment and training tool for individuals with learning deficits, Am J Occup Ther 35:728, 1981.

Kantner R, Kantner B, and Clark D: Vestibular stimulation effect on language development in mentally retarded, Am J Occup Ther 36:36, 1982.

Kielhofner G: The temporal dimension in the lives of retarded adults: a problem of interaction and intervention, Am J Occup Ther 33:161, 1979.

Kielhofner G, and Miyake S: The therapeutic use of games with mentally retarded adults, Am J Occup Ther 33:161, 1979.

Kielhofner G, and Takata N: A study of mentally retarded persons: applied research in occupational therapy, Am J Occup Ther 34:252, 1980.

Lederman E: O.T. with the mentally retarded: Special concerns for a special population, Occup Therapy Forum 2:8, 1987.

Ling-Fong Zee-Chen E, and Hardman M: Postrotary nystagmus response in children with Down's syndrome, Am J Occup Ther 37:260, 1983.

Mann W, and Sobsey R: Feeding program for the institutionalized mentally retarded, Am J Occup Ther 29:397, 1975.

Martin MJ: Shoulder mobility in the older mentally retarded adult. In Vulpe SG, editor: Proceedings of the occupational therapy for maternal and child health conference, volume II, 1987, United States Department of Health and Human Services.

McCracken A: Tactile function of educable mentally retarded children, Am J Occup Ther 29:397, 1975.

McCracken A: Drool control and tongue thrust therapy for the mentally retarded, Am J Occup Ther 32:79, 1978.

Norton Y: Neurodevelopment and sensory integration for the profoundly retarded multiply handicapped child, Am J Occup Ther 29:93, 1975.

Resman M: Effect of sensory stimulation on eye contact in profoundly retarded adult, Am J Occup Ther 35:3, 1981.

Shalik LD, and Shalik H: Cluster homes: a community for profoundly and severely retarded persons, Am J Occup Ther 41:222, 1987.

Shuer J, Clark F, and Azen S: Vestibular function in mildly mentally retarded adults, Am J Occup Ther 34:664, 1980.

Stephan RA: Audiotape instruction of face-washing skills for an adult with mental retardation, Am J Occup Ther 41:3, 1987.

Storey K, Bates P, McGhee N, and Dycus S: Reducing the self-stimulatory behavior of a profoundly retarded female through sensory awareness training, Am J Occup Ther 38:510, 1984.

Weber N: Chaining strategies for teaching sequenced motor tasks to mentally retarded adults, Am J Occup Ther 32:385, 1978.

Webster P: Occupational role development in the young adult with mild mental retardation, Am J Occup Ther 34:13, 1980.

Weeks Z: Effects of the vestibular system on human development. Part 2: effects of vestibular stimulation on mentally retarded, emotionally disturbed and learning-disabled individuals, Am J Occup Ther 33:450, 1979.

Wehman P, and Marchant J: Improving free play skills of severely retarded children, Am J Occup Ther 32:100, 1978.

White J: Stimulus box for the profoundly mentally retarded. Am J Occup Ther 30:167, 1976.

Figure 21-2   Georgia Retardation Center outline for occupational therapy evaluations

---

OCCUPATIONAL THERAPY EVALUATION

Date: _____

Diagnosis: (EXAMPLE: This is an 11--year-old female with the medical diagnosis of profound mental retardation secondary to cranial-cerebral injury sustained in an automobile accident, spastic quadriplegia, major motor seizures, visual handicaps.)

Summary of previous therapy:

General behavior:

Tests used: (could include these or others)

              Range of motion   Developmental

              Gross and fine motor Skilled observation

Gross motor:

Fine motor:

Handedness:

Sensory integration:

Self-help

Adaptive equipment: positioning, feeding, wheelchair

Summary:

Recommendations for placement:

RECOMMENDATIONS FOR TRAINING

1. a. Occupational therapy services are not appropriate for this resident.
   b. Indirect occupational therapy services are appropriate for this resident. (These services will be indicated on the resident activity and staff functions list in his program, since these activities are not appropriate for behavioral objectives.)
   c. Direct occupational therapy services are appropriate for this resident. These services are appropriate for behavioral objectives.
   d. Direct occupational therapy services are appropriate for this resident. These services will be indicated on the resident activities and staff functions list in his program, since these activities are not appropriate for behavioral objectives.
2. Discipline specific goals: None

                   or

   Discipline specific goals: Resident will increase wrist range of motion 15 degrees by December, 19XX through exercise program 3 times a week and wearing of wrist splint 8 hours daily.

   Discipline specific goals: Resident's adaptive equipment will be reviewed annually and repaired as needed.
3. General recommendations for program team:
   Self-help skills: Resident will learn to place button through buttonhole.
4. If occupational therapy services are not currently appropriate: The next occupational therapy evaluation will be done at the request of the primary physician or the program team.

   If indirect or direct occupational therapy services are appropriate: The next occupational therapy evaluation will be done for the annual review of this resident on _____

                                            _____

                                                Signature

Figure 21-3   Georgia Retardation Center resident record of habilitation and adaptive devices

---

Date: _____   **Identification**

FUNCTION:

Orthotic, Prosthetic Devices: Devices used in habilitation/rehabilitation, i.e., splints, braces, polypropylene jackets

Mobility device: Wheelchairs, etc.

Mechanical supports: Achieve proper body position, i.e., adaptations to wheelchair or other devices/ furniture for support, etc.

ADL devices: Activities of daily living, i.e., adapted feeding devices, special communication devices, etc.

Protective devices: Identified medical need or adjunct to behavioral programming, i.e., mitts, protective clothing, protective headgear.

Item #	Device	Date	Reason for Device	When used	Therapist	Initial

Figure 21-4 Georgia Retardation Center Occupational Therapy Service screening tool

Resident: _____

Unit and section: _____

Evaluator: _____

Social Security no.: _____

Birthdate: _____

KEY FOR I AND II:

1 = Cannot do at all
2 = Can do partly with assistance
3 = Can do all, but needs assistance
4 = Can do alone with spoken directions
5 = Can do alone

Hand preference: L R
Color-blind: Yes No

I. GROSS MOTOR SKILLS (CHECK ONE)

1	2	3	4	5	Skills	Comments
					1. Sits down and gets up from floor	
					2. Rolls over (log roll)	
					3. Gets on hands and knees	
					4. Crawls	
					5. Crawls reciprocally	
					6. Walks	
					7. Runs	
					8. Balances on one foot—seconds: ( )L; ( )R	
					9. Hops on left foot	
					10. Hops on right foot	
					11. Skips	
					12. Jumps over stick (both feet)	
					13. Rolls ball	
					14. Catches ball (two hands)	
					15. Catches beanbag (left)	
					16. Catches beanbag (right)	
					17. Throws ball (two hands)	
					18. Throws ball (left)	
					19. Throws ball (right)	
					20. Bounces ball (dribble): ( ) times	
					21. Jumps rope (turns his own): ( ) times	
					22. Other	

Comments: _____

Continued.

II. HAND COORDINATION (CHECK ONE.)

1	2	3	4	5	Skills	Comments
					1. Looks at objects	
					2. Reaches for object	
					3. Grasp (left)	
					4. Grasp (right)	
					5. Lateral pinch (paper) preferred hand; L R	
					6. Palmar pinch (straight fingers) preferred hand: L R	
					7. Three-finger pinch (peg)	
					8. Tip prehension (small bead)	
					9. Holds crayon—how:	
					10. Scribbles with crayon	
					11. Traces with crayon	
					12. Transfers block from one hand to other	
					13. Puts block in box	
					14. Puts peg in hole (½-inch)	
					15. Strings large bead	
					16. Other	

Comments: _____

_____

III. EYE COORDINATION (USE X OR * UNDER EACH.)

Left	Both	Right	Skills	Comments
			1. Focus: ( ) seconds	
			2. Track ⟷	
			3. Track ↕	
			4. Track ↘	
			5. Track ↗	
			6. Track ○	
			7. Track toward nose	
			8. Track from nose	
			9. Two point •—•	
			10. Two point ❘	
			11. Two point ╲	
			12. Two point ╱	
			13. Two point to and from nose	

Comments: _____

_____

Figure 21-4   Georgia Retardation Center Occupational Therapy Service screening tool—cont'd

IV. PERCEPTUAL MOTOR SKILL (CHECK YES OR NO.)

Yes	No	Skills	Comments
		1. Matches ○	
		2. Matches □	
		3. Matches △	
		4. Copies ———	
		5. Copies |	
		6. Copies \	
		7. Copies /	
		8. Copies ○	

Comments: _____

_____

V. IMITATION (DO NOT GIVE SPOKEN INSTRUCTIONS EXCEPT TO TELL A STUDENT TO DO WHAT YOU ARE DOING. CHECK YES OR NO.)

Yes	No	Skills	Comments
		1. Raise two arms out straight, shoulder high	
		2. Clap hands	
		3. Wave good-bye	
		4. Pick up object	
		5. Touch the floor	
		6. Raise one hand over head	

Comments: _____

_____

VI. COOPERATION AND FOLLOWING DIRECTIONS (CHECK ONE.)

	1. Will not hold still, pay attention, or listen to directions
	2. Does not usually follow directions
	3. Tries to follow directions, but needs help
	4. Tries but needs reminders or encouragement
	5. Follows directions usually

Comments: _____

_____

Continued.

Figure 21-4   Georgia Retardation Center Occupational Therapy Service screening tool—cont'd

VII. SELF-FEEDING (USE * IN YES COLUMN FOR INITIAL EVALUATION IF THEY CAN; USE X IN NO COLUMN FOR INITIAL EVALUATION IF THEY CANNOT; USE DATE IN YES COLUMN LATER WHEN THEY MASTER THE SKILL.)
HAND PREFERENCE: L R

Yes	No	(If no, explain problem, present method, and present equipment.)
		1. Lip closure
		2. Sucking (straw)
		3. Swallowing
		4. Chewing
		5. Finger feeding
		6. Grasp (spoon)
		7. Arm control (scoop and spoon to mouth)
		8. Feeds self
		9. Regular food
		10. Regular plate or tray
		11. Regular glass or paper cup
		12. Regular spoon
		13. Regular fork
		14. Cuts food with spoon
		15. Cuts food with fork
		16. Cuts food with knife
		17. Uses napkin
		18. Special diet
		19. Other

Comments: _____

_____

PROBLEMS (USE SAME DIRECTIONS AS SPECIFIED IN SELF-FEEDING.)

Yes	No	
		1. Tongue thrust
		2. Drooling
		3. Poor appetite
		4. Does not want to feed self
		5. Messy eater
		6. Throws food
		7. Other

Figure 21-5 Georgia Retardation Center Occupational Therapy Department ADL
in food preparation skills

Resident names:

Session no.: _____
1. _____
Date: _____
2. _____
Staff: _____
3. _____
4. _____
5. _____
6. _____
7. _____

Resident No.

		1	2	3	4	5	6	7
Preparing to cook	Washes hands							
	Dries hands							
	Puts on apron							
	Sits at table							
Utensil recognition	Recognizes cutting knife							
	Large spoon							
	Frying pan							
	Bowl							
	Saucepan							
Kitchen appliances recognition	Locates oven							
	Sink							
	Refrigerator							
Fine motor	Spreads with knife							
	Stirs batter with spoon							
	Cuts with knife							
Setting table	Puts silver at place							
	Puts plates							
	Puts glasses							
Eating	Waits for others to begin							
	Serves self food							
	Passes food							
	Uses napkin							
	Uses condiments							
Clean up	Cleans off table							
	Washes dishes							
	Dries dishes							
	Puts dishes away							
	Vacuums							

Figure 21-6   Georgia Retardation Center Occupational Therapy Department ADL
in area of food preparation

Name: _____ Birthdate: _____ Unit: _____
Diagnosis: _____
Precautions: _____ Examiner: _____
Hand preference: _____ Eye dominance: _____ Eye level: _____
Wheelchair: _____ Walker: _____ Ambulatory: _____
Other adaptive devices: _____
Food restrictions: _____

Vertical reach:	**Right UE**	**Left UE**		**Right UE**	**Left UE**
Comfortable—up	_____ inches	_____ inches	Maximal	_____ inches	_____ inches
Comfortable—down	_____ inches	_____ inches	Maximal	_____ inches	_____ inches

Horizontal reach:

	Right UE	Left UE		Right UE	Left UE
Comfortable—forward	_____ inches	_____ inches	Maximal	_____ inches	_____ inches
Comfortable—sideways	_____ inches	_____ inches	Maximal	_____ inches	_____ inches

Two-handed control: Gross-grade _____ Fine-grade _____
                                            (poor, fair, good, normal)   (poor, fair, good, normal)

One-handed control: *Right UE* (poor, fair, good, normal)   *Left UE* (poor, fair, good, normal)
                                 Gross-grade _____   Gross-grade _____
                                 Fine-grade _____   Fine-grade _____

Rating values:

1. No comprehension; student is unable to function in this area.
2. Student is unable to perform in this area because of physical limitations.
3. Student exhibits some difficulty with regard to this area, but with assistance task can be completed.
4. Student is able to complete activity independently.

Student is exposed to each activity by spoken directions or demonstrations for a minimum of four times.

Ratings

	Date	Date	Date	Date	Assistive devices	Comments
Cooking activities Blend ingredients by hand						
Stir ingredients by hand						
Scoop						
Clean vegetables with a brush						
Measure dry ingredients using measuring spoons						
Measure dry indredients using measuring cups						
Measure wet ingredients using measuring spoons						
Measure wet ingredients using measuring cups						
Pare or peel vegetables and fruit						
Grate						
Toss						

	Ratings					
	Date	Date	Date	Date	Assistive devices	Comments
Pour cold liquids						
Pour hot liquids						
Pour batter into container						
Sift						
Break eggs						
Slice with knife						
Chop with knife						
Melt						
Simmer						
Boil						
Broil						
Ladle						
Drain using collander or slotted spoon						
Pan fry						
Roll cookie dough or pie crust						
Able to read simple recipe						
Cooking mechanics Turn faucet on and off						
Wash and dry hands						
Apron on and off						
Open and close refrigerator door						
Place and remove items from refrigerator						
Open and close overhead cupboard doors						
Remove and store items in overhead cupboards						
Open and close bottom cupboard doors						
Remove and store items in lower cupboards						
Turn range off and on at proper setting						
Turn oven off and on at proper setting						
Put container in oven						
Take container out and place on counter						
Use toaster						
Use electric mixer						

Continued.

Figure 21-6   Georgia Retardation Center Occupational Therapy Department ADL
in area of food preparation—cont'd

| | Ratings | | | | | |
	Date	Date	Date	Date	Assistive devices	Comments
Cooking mechanics cont'd Open packages						

Open and use wax, plastic
  wrap and aluminum foil
  boxes						

Use can opener						
Open and close bottles and jars						
Knows hot from cold						
Table activities Set table						
Serve the table						
Clear the table						
Clean the table						
Scrape dishes						
Stack dishes						
Wash dishes						
Dry dishes						
Clean up area						
Wipe up spills						
Dispose of garbage						

Recipes used

1.
2.
3.
4.
5.
6.
7.
8.
9.
10.

Figure 21-7 Performance analysis/developmental assessment

Date: _____ Name: _____ Birthdate: _____

Developmental area: Activities of daily living—feeding

Age	Activity and references	Equipment and directions	Scale score							Comments — Information processing and activity analysis
			No 1	Attention 2	Phys. assis. 3	Soc./emot. assis. 4	Verbal assis. 5	Independent 6	Transfer 7	1. Analyze activities considering component parts of each and relationship to: basic senses and function; organization behaviors; cognitive processes and specific concepts; auditory language; gross and fine motor 2. Information processing consider: input; integration; feedback; assimilation; output
3-5 months	5. Anticipation of feeding 2,4,6,11,44,48,50,63 RL-8 AGM-8	Breast or Bottle— Present breast or bottle to child. The child shows signs of recognition without stimulation, for example, quieting, reaching, beginning to suck, puckering or opening mouth.								
	6. Acceptance of pureed solids 2,4,11,44,48	Pureed food, spoon— Observe the child's response when offered pureed food from a spoon. The child opens mouth and removes food from spoon.								
	7. Use of tongue in accepting pureed food 4	Pureed food, spoon— Observe the motion of the child's tongue when accepting pureed food from a spoon. The child moves food around in mouth using tongue to aid swallowing food.								
	8. Swallowing pureed food 4,44,45	Pureed food, spoon— Observe the child's response when accepting pureed food from a spoon. The child swallows food without gagging or choking, and coordinates swallowing with breathing.								

From Vulpe SG: Vulpe Assessment Battery, rev ed, Laurel, Md, 1987, RAMSCO Publishing Co. With permission of the National Institute on Mental Retardation.

22

Children with communicative impairment

FROMA JACOBSON CUMMINGS

COMMUNICATION

Communicative interaction is a basic task of daily living. People who cannot speak or make themselves easily understood by others are frequently assumed to be less competent and less intelligent than others. In the story of Snow White, the nonspeaking seventh dwarf, Dopey, symbolizes society's amused tolerance of its non-articulating members. The assumption that people who cannot talk also cannot think or feel represents an attitude that health professionals and educators must constantly combat in the general public.

One of the best defenses is a system of communication that is tailored to the individual's abilities and disabilities. Each system may include elements of written and oral interactions, gestures, facial expressions, and body language. Occupational therapists, with their commitment to building competence in tasks of daily living and with their skills in activity adaptation and positioning, are among the critical personnel who can help develop communication systems for nonspeaking persons. This chapter introduces the concept of augmentative communication and discusses the occupational therapist's roles and functions in programs for children with motor speech impairment. Methodology for augmenting communication for expressive language and "written" education needs is addressed.

Incidence of oral-motor impairment of speech

It is difficult to establish the number of persons classified as nonoral because of large differences in survey methods and findings. Two 1978 surveys,[5,11] however, suggest that between 200,000 and 1,000,000 persons need some sort of communication augmentation. Similar population statistics were also cited by Montgom-

ery and Hanson in 1984.[10] Nonoral, in this instance, simply means without speech. The population estimate cited is increased by those persons who are temporarily unable to express themselves verbally or in writing because of acute pathological conditions or injuries and persons who are deaf but not otherwise handicapped.

Classrooms for children with special needs include many youngsters who are labeled "unable to test" because of communication impairment associated with physical or developmental disabilities. Diagnoses for these children include but are not limited to mental retardation, cerebral palsy, postcerebral vascular accident, developmental delay, organic brain syndrome, head trauma, spinal cord injury, arthritis, muscular dystrophy, head and neck cancer, developmental language disorders, and autism. Thus, conditions include those that are *congenital* (also profound hearing impairment, developmental apraxia, and developmental aphasia), *acquired* (may include laryngectomy), *progressive* neurological diseases (also multiple sclerosis, amyotrophic lateral sclerosis, AIDS) and *temporary* (including surgery, severe burns, and Reye's syndrome).

Without communication skills, clients must rely on family and professional team members to meet their needs and organize resources to allow achievement of maximal function and independence. This implies that the level of independence achieved will not depend on one's own capacities, but instead will depend on the capabilities of others.

In a study performed in Canada by rehabilitation engineers and reported by LeBlanc,[9] physically handicapped individuals were asked to rank their needs. Communication was accorded the highest priority, with activities, mobility, and ambulation following in order.

Augmentative communication

Imagine sharing information with a colleague, conversing at a party, conducting a transaction at a grocery store, or lecturing to a class. One relies primarily on oral speech for self-expression. However, careful review of these presentations indicates that hands, gestures, body language, eye gaze, pauses, audiovisual equipment, and writing are used to augment the oral messages. These combined components of communication are called *total, adaptive,* or *augmentative communication.* Augmentative communication incorporates all those systems that are used in addition to oral speech to improve understanding of the speaker's message. This can include mechanical systems for nonoral communication that have been designed for persons with physical speech impairment.

The following are examples of children who can be assisted by augmentative communication systems:

1. The child with cerebral palsy whose loss or impairment of motor function includes the inability to reliably produce intelligible expressive speech. Traditional speech therapy may be ineffective. Augmentative communication, including eye gaze, vocalizations, gestures, body language, manual signing, communication boards, and electronic aids, may allow more language development. Functional interaction can then replace frustration.

2. The child with other neurological or developmental deficits makes attempts at speech that range from complete silence to babbling, with varying degrees of word production and comprehension. The prognosis for the development of functional oral speech may be guarded, yet it is desirable that the child have the advantage of communication within physical and cognitive limitations.

3. The child whose speech has been affected by trauma. This child faces additional problems. The child has had speech and is suddenly deprived of it; she may be frustrated in many previously accomplished daily life activities. Loss of control and interaction often disrupts the rehabilitation process. An augmentative communication system in such cases might be temporary, allowing the child to communicate while in the hospital. An alternative system may ultimately be indicated.

4. The severely multi-handicapped child who, on occasion, can very clearly choose and enunciate words and phrases appropriately but whose most typical clinical picture is dominated by anomalies in muscle tone and inability to use expressive verbalization 98% of the time. This "failure" to be able to vocalize clearly may be due to a combination of physical and psychosocial factors. Again, supplemental methods for expressive communication are available when clear speech is not possible.

In the past children with such handicaps have had to rely on "yes-no" indications and "20 questions" routines to make their wishes known. Augmentative systems help these children not only immediately and mechanically but also developmentally. It has been observed clinically that removing the pressure to produce oral speech in fact facilitates its development.

Augmentative communication aids range from very simple ones made in the therapy clinic to the very elaborate, comprehensive systems that are microprocessor or computer controlled. An example of the clinician-made aid is a simple picture board and some type of pointer that is used by the child to indicate the picture showing the desired message.

CLINICIAN-MADE SYSTEMS

Clinician-made systems continue to be quite effective for many children and are recommended in addition to more complex electronic systems. Such aids are reliable and multifunctional. Creativity is employed in developing a communication board that is meaningful to both the speaker and listeners. Objects, miniatures, photographs, pictures, line drawings, symbols, words, letters, and a combination thereof may be used. These representations can be mounted to a vest, belt, apron, pants, or multisurfaced board. Miniboards as well as books can be used.

ELECTRONIC EDUCATIONAL AIDS

Electronic educational aids were introduced in England approximately 25 years ago and allowed even severely physically handicapped children to have appropriate learning experiences. Two examples of these very early electronic systems by POSSUM are the Basic Skill Set and Expanded Keyboard/Scanning Typewriter. The Possum Basic Skill Set* allows children to match items. By hitting a switch, the child moves a light on the board from one selection to another. A correct answer is rewarded with a musical response. The machine gives a negative reinforcement for errors and keeps track of the mistakes. Simple exercises can include object matching, whereas more complex tasks might address such skills as reading comprehension. The manufacturer has also developed an expanded keyboard for adapted direct selection typing. A scanning system for permanent hard copy could be easily accessed by use of input switches.

Many other systems have been developed since this early start, including nonoral communication systems, educational aids, and environmental controls. The technology continues to expand rapidly so that many kinds of aids are available to nonverbal children who are physically handicapped or developmentally delayed. Each system must be selected according to the

---

*From Possum Controls, Ltd, Middlegreen Trading Estate, Middlegreen Rd, Langley, Slough, Berks SL3 6DF; New York office: Twelfth Floor, 105 Madison Ave, New York, NY, 10016.

motor, perceptual, cognitive, receptive, and expressive needs of the child communicator, with consideration of the persons who will be receiving the messages. Psychosocial needs, in relation to self-image and general appropriateness of the system, are always a prime consideration.

Typically, when one envisions a language board, the image is of a piece of cardboard with words arranged in a noun-verb-noun format. This thinking has been expanded to meet the level of the child who uses the system. Again, creativity is the key. Some clinician-made communication boards may be designed in the format of a clear acrylic eye scanner or as shadow boxes, books, folders, flip-top address books, leg chaps, communication handkerchiefs, or vests.

Developmentally, children become familiar with objects long before they are able to read and use the written word. The typical progression of recognition begins with the object itself and proceeds to the miniature, photograph, color picture, line drawing, and, most sophisticated, the word or symbol system. The word should always accompany the item symbol.

SYMBOL SYSTEMS

Some children are not able to read and thus rely on other symbol systems. Three examples of symbolic representation include Bliss, rebus, and Picsyms.

1. *Bliss symbols* were created by Charles Bliss of Australia as a visual graphic system. The symbols are adapted from basic geometric shapes[23] (Figure 22-1, *A*).
2. *Rebus* is the Latin word for thing. Instead of using a spelled word, a meaning can be represented by a thing.[4] Another word for rebus is "pictograph" (Figure 22-1, *B*).
3. *Picsyms** is a picture symbol system and is based on easily recognized line drawings of familiar objects. This system allows nonspeaking preschoolers to "send" messages by choosing a series of symbols (Figure 22-1, *C*).

Additional commonly used pictograph, or rebus, systems may be explored through published picture dictionaries.[6,7,8] For a comprehensive presentation of these systems, see Vanderheiden and Lloyd.[12]

GESTURES AND SIGNING

Pointing, gestures, mime, and any variety of hand systems can be used to complement communication. A significant key to success is the ability of the listener to understand the intent of the speaker. A variety of sign language systems may be employed, but again, for successful communication, it is imperative that the listener understand the signs.

MINSPEAK

Minspeak is a semantic encoding system developed by Baker.[1] It is linguistically based, logically organizes information for easy recall, and is based on five principles: (1) small units of communication do not convey as much information as do full sentences, (2) carefully constructed sets of sentences can fulfill most communication needs, (3) sequences of concepts can summarize most sentences, (4) symbols can represent concepts, and (5) communication speed can be increased by organizing sets of sentences.

Baker developed multimeaning icons to represent concepts and speed communication. Minspeak is a relatively new symbol system that appears increasingly useful.

Classification of aids

An augmentative communication system is designed for the individual according to two main considerations: (1) how the child can best indicate what is to be said and (2) how the message is to be expressed. Therefore aids are commonly classified by (1) the type of input, or selection mode required (direct selection, scanning, or encoding) and (2) the type of display mode (output) that is generated, such as visual display, permanent written copy, synthesized speech, video display, and combinations.

DIRECT SELECTION MODE

Severely handicapped children must have a means of selecting messages that is physically achievable by them. Direct selection, as the name implies, requires

---

*Developed in 1981 by Faith Carlson, Meyer Children's Rehabilitation Unit, Nebraska Medical Center, Omaha.

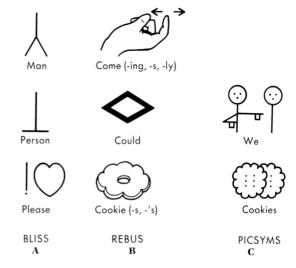

Figure 22-1   A, Bliss. **B,** Rebus. **C,** Picsyms.

the child to specifically select one picture, photograph, object, phrase, word, or letter from an established grouping. Selection is generally accomplished by touching with a finger, fist, hand, elbow, foot, head-stick, light pointer, tongue, eyes, or nose—whatever the child can use most reliably with the best energy efficiency and the least fatigue.

Examples of direct selection modes include the Etran, typewriter keyboard, and picture board. A direct selection mode allows the user to plan and select voluntarily. This mode is relatively fast, simple, and straightforward for those who have appropriate motor control and range of motion. It is easy for the child to learn to use a direct selection mode, and messages are easily understood by the listener.

SCANNING MODE

The display of the scanning mode device looks very similar to the direct selection board, but it is used in a different way. Because a child may not have the necessary skills to use a board independently, the listener points at different options until the desired areas are reached. Possible communications have been arranged in rows or matrices, and the listener assists the client by "narrowing in" on the correct item.

To illustrate, imagine the typewriter keyboard. After establishing the client's ability to indicate a yes-no response, the listener points to two halves of the keyboard and asks, "Is your message in this half or in this half? Is it in this half?" "Yes" or "no" is then indicated by the child using the prearranged response. Through the process of elimination, the listener may then proceed along the rows of keys on the selected half until the desired message is revealed. This method resembles the twenty questions approach, but it is more systematic. Disadvantages of the scanning mode are that messages are limited by the capacity of the system, the methodology is relatively slow, the user must see the display, and the listener is required to be actively involved. However, since minimal motor response is required from the speaker, this mode is more reliable and less fatiguing than others. It is usable by even the most severely involved person. Often external switches are used by the speaker to operate a scanning electronic device.

ENCODING MODE

The encoding mode requires the communicator to use a predetermined code for message selection and the listener to scan down and across a matrix to determine the intended message (Figure 22-2). This presentation mode would be used by a person whose range of motion is too limited to access a larger board, but who has adequate cognitive ability to remember codes. A large board, with the matrix of coded messages, would be placed in an area that is visually convenient to both the speaker and listener. The small coding board would be placed within easy motor access of the communicator. The child may then directly select an area on the horizontal and vertical axes. For example, in the illustration, 1-A would mean "yes." To indicate "I need help," the child would point to 4-A, 7-C, 5-B, 5-B, 4-B, and 6-A.

Encoding is a form of scanning, but it is usually faster than that method. It requires more motor response than scanning and less than direct selection. Therefore it could be less reliable and more fatiguing. It is also more abstract and symbolic than scanning. Other examples of encoding systems are the Morse Code, expansions of abbreviations, and the multimeaning icons of Minspeak.

OUTPUT MODE

With an output mode, the message can be presented by visual display, permanent written copy (paper printout), speech output, video presentation, and a combination of these. This is a matter for individualized choice. Some systems can be incorporated into a lapboard, ranging in size from small and easily transportable to large, cumbersome, and stationary; others cannot.

Elements of visual display output may include lights and a pointing apparatus. It may be large and easy to read, or small and compact. There may be interchangeable overlays for flexibility. Some visual displays have the capacities to chain and remember information.

A simple inexpensive example of visual display that also uses scanning is the clockface communication board (Figure 22-3). These can be clinician made or purchased commercially. Choices are fastened (temporarily) to the clockface and by operating a switch that moves the indicator, the child makes his choices. Varieties of overlays are endless.

One direct selection input aid using visual display is the eye or light selection board—Etran (Figure 22-4). Response choices, either pictures or words, are set onto the board and the speaker responds to queries by looking at his answer or lighting it with special equipment. The board is best made out of a clear material that allows the speaker and listener to see each other. Many clinicians make the boards with a central "look at me" cutout for the same purpose. Any combination of stimuli can be used. In use, it is advisable for the lis-

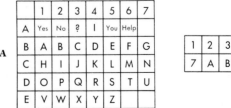
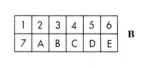

Figure 22-2 Coding matrix and board. **A,** Matrix. **B,** Board.

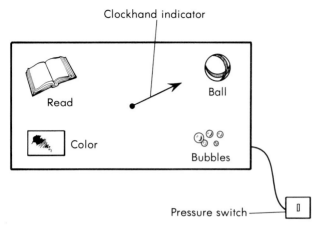

Figure 22-3   Clockface communication board.

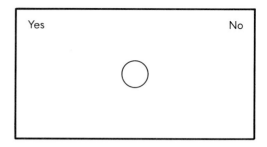

Figure 22-4   Etran light selection board.

tener to repeat the communication to ensure that the user's intent is understood.

Permanent written copy may be produced on strip printers, calculator tape, typing paper, and computer printouts. These systems are most appropriate for academic use, correspondence, permanent copy, or community interaction.

Video/LED display is available with many technical aids. With some there is a short viewing area while others offer a full screen motor. Editing is available.

Aids with speech output produce verbal communications in the form of a recorded voice, synthesized speech, or digitized speech. The client chooses from a variety of stimuli to generate instantaneous speech. Because of the verbal nature of the output, this system can be used most effectively in groups. Memory and capacity of the systems can vary from unit to unit, ranging from words to thousands of sound components.

Portable and stationary microcomputers have become invaluable as communication and education aids. Children with severe motor involvement can use adapted equipment to access the computer and its software.

• • •

As augmentative communication systems become increasingly sophisticated, both in specialization and versatility, one aid can often generate more than one type of output. Computer interfacing is one means by which one system can piggy-back onto another to maximize output. It is also recognized that more than one system may be necessary to meet all the needs of a child in his different functional environments, to provide for communication, education, and environmental control and interaction.

The communication system of a child is more correctly described as a combination of systems. Even the most severely involved child may combine gestures, eye gaze, some eye contact, vocalizations, and facial expres-

sions into his expressive language system. The special-needs child incorporates a variety of efforts of communication to add to the quality or clarity of his "speech."

Therapeutic considerations
FUNCTIONAL COMMUNITY INTERACTION

In contrast to the emphasis of speech and language specialists on language arts, occupational therapists address communication as an activity of daily living. The occupational therapist evaluates communication skills in all life roles and teaches the child to extend these skills beyond the therapy environment to the classroom, play group, Brownie troop, or wherever the child goes. This multienvironment approach generates the term *functional community interaction.* It implies that the individual will be able to interact in all environments of people, both handicapped and able-bodied. Any communication system must be adapted to the child's needs so that the system itself does not limit independence.

Ideally, a specialized communication system should be available to the child for all those postures that are assumed daily, such as prone and supine positions, wheelchair sitting, possibly ambulating, sidelying, and unsupported sitting. Adaptation and flexibility in the choice of systems are important if maximal communication potential is to be reached.

PSYCHOSOCIAL CONCERNS

Therapists will be especially concerned about children's self-images: specifically, how they feel about using the chosen systems. Ideally, children contribute to the decisions concerning the system of choice for them, but lack of speech frequently precludes their making life role decisions. How children accept the devices and how they present themselves to others will affect how others respond to them. This same sensitivity to self-image should be extended to any adaptive aid or position, including splints, headsticks, mobile arm supports, or other devices that are used as interfaces with the communication system.

A closely related issue that is often ignored by professionals is nonverbal communication. What message does the child receive when others:

- "Do for" the child, rather than letting the child perform the task independently?
- Finish a sentence for the child?
- Pretend to understand attempts at oral speech because of limited time?
- Ignore attention-getting efforts to avoid the time-consuming interactions?
- Choose a toy for the child, thereby preventing the development of decision-making processes?
- Pour ketchup on hot dogs and thus presume the child's preference?
- Talk for the child in her presence?

Perhaps the greatest insult is in not asking the child to communicate. Therapists must consider how much this noncommunication affects the child's other developmental processes: gross motor, fine motor, psychosocial, and adaptive. Sensitivity to the feelings of the child nurtures the interpersonal relationships that are crucial to building a communication system and process.

TEAM CONCEPT

Interdisciplinary team involvement is important in the initial choice of systems and in the direct training of children to use the augmentative systems for functional community interaction and ongoing reevaluation process. Team composition is variable but often includes the child, family, certain friends, occupational therapist, physical therapist, educator, speech and language specialist, psychologist, social worker, child advocate, nurse, caretaker, physician, fund-raiser, engineer, computer programmer, vocational counselor, case manager, and adaptive aid specialist. These specialists must know the limitations as well as strengths of their disciplines and personalities and offer interventions ranked by priorities of need to best serve the child. A transdisciplinary approach is essential because of the nature of daily communication needs.

In the emerging field of augmentative communication, the speech and language specialist works with language, using the augmentative system for communication, language development, and syntax. The teacher strengthens the educational program by incorporating newly developed communication skills into classroom activities. The role of the occupational therapist is less well-defined at present, although therapists have traditionally instructed children in typing with and without adaptations.

ROLE OF OCCUPATIONAL THERAPY

The occupational therapist is the key person to bridge the space between the child and the communication system(s). This is done by organizing that space so that the child has access to the system(s) in a consistently reliable manner, by solving problems of position placement, making adaptations, choosing inter-faces, identifying perceptual and motor assets and liabilities, and evaluating reflex patterns. The skills of the occupational therapist can enhance the child's functional access to whatever system(s) the communication specialist deems linguistically appropriate.

Assessment

Occupational therapists evaluate each child to determine:
- Organization of space to make access to equipment easier
- Positions required during the child's typical day
- Visual perception assets and liabilities, including visual tracking, figure-ground discrimination, object performance concepts, spatial relationships, and visual perception of position in space
- Suitable switches and other interfaces, keyboard styles, positioning, placement of switch, and placement of aid
- Most reliable motor responses in a variety of positions
- Adaptations and mounting apparatus
- Potential social, educational, and vocational opportunities that will be made more practical by development of communication skills
- Reaction to types of systems under consideration, including reactions of family members and peer group
- Systems globally appropriate and acceptable to the child's life-style.

The occupational therapist collaborates with the child and the team to select systems that will work for the child. This criterion far surpasses the search for a system that the child can work. As part of the assessment the therapist can also participate with the primary team and the family to gather pertinent information regarding:
- Medical aspects that may affect positioning
- Pending medical procedures
- Adaptive aids presently used, as well as information about aids that were previously used and why they were discarded
- Visual and auditory acuity and perceptualization
- Reliable motor responses used in other activities and with other equipment
- Independence in self-maintenance activities
- Activities performed in a typical day, including participation and positioning
- Child and family goals and priorities

A critical goal within the motor function portion of the evaluation is the identification of an appropriate, reliable, volitional, and controlled movement pattern that will not interfere with the child's concentration on communication. It is advisable to look at all the positions assumed by the child in a typical day, including the optimal and typical, and consider how the typical can be improved.

Some practitioners assert that a child must have a wheelchair that allows optional seating arrangements before a complete assessment for communication systems can be accurate. Others would argue that the need for successful communication is such a strong drive that its blockage can cause severe frustrations reflected in adverse behavior patterns, reflex-dominated postures, spasticity, and inability to relax. The latter group might suggest that by facilitating some form of successful augmentative communication and thus relieving the tension of noncommunication, a more successful mobility system can be fabricated.

Creativity is the key to finding more than one position and movement pattern that will allow access to the system. The reliable motion may be, for example, direct selection with one finger, or oral sucking and puffing, or chin depression or thigh abduction. With an adolescent it may be advisable to look at reflex patterns to consider how these might be used initially to gain access to a system.

During this search many factors must be considered. Important motor components include reflex patterns, overflow, possibility of triggering seizure activity, level of fatigue, range of motion, as well as strength and endurance. Ability to learn new tasks, attention span and attention to the task during the motor response, and probability of success are significant cognitive factors. The need for interfacing adaptive equipment must be considered. And finally, the therapist must focus on such emotional factors as the child's reactions to stress and fatigue, motivation, eye contact during interaction, and, perhaps most important, the child's feelings about using this position and motor response.

In cooperation with the speech and language specialist, who has also evaluated the child and suggested a suitable system, the occupational therapist determines the specific interfaces for that system. The therapist may be able to use a commercially available switch quite well with the child's reliable responses or may need to fabricate a makeshift switch for the evaluation and begin the design for a custom switch. Multisensory feedback, such as tactile, visual, and auditory, must be considered. For the direct selector, the occupational therapist is able to suggest size of menu (number of available items for selection), size of input areas, placement of different areas, and required pressure to obtain an output. To choose a switch for scanning or encoding, the switch placement, pressure for output, need for visual pursuit, and safety precautions must be considered.

Visual perception and cognitive factors must also be evaluated, including figure-ground, position in space and spatial relationships, and visual sequencing ability. Important task components include following directions, making eye contact, taking turns, relating cause and effect, visual memory, visual matching, categorizing information, and visual midline crossing (Figure 22-5).

A final step in the initial occupational therapy assessment is to determine the spatial relationships between the child, interfaces, system, and output modes. These relationships will be different for each position that the child assumes during the day. Options for portable,

---

Figure 22-5 Skills to be assessed when planning augmentative communication systems

MOTOR	*VISUAL PERCEPTION*	
Midline crossing	Spatial relationships	Visual pursuit
Range of motion	Position in space	Visual-auditory discrimination
Eye-hand coordination	Figure-ground	Attention span
Strength	Visual tracking	Attention to task
Speed-accuracy-control	Directionality	Risk taking
Time-energy saving	Ability to follow directions	Information categorization
Reliability of response	Eye contact	Information finding
	Symbol permanence	Visual matching
ACTIVITIES OF DAILY LIVING	Cause-and-effect relationships	Motor planning
Independence using	Timing	
communication	Sequencing	
Communication to enhance	Spelling	
social, education, vocational	Reading	
opportunities	Word recognition	
Communication via phone	Decision making	
Communication for emergency	Problem solving	
Communication for pleasure	Visual-auditory memory	
One-to-one communication		
Group interaction		
Communication to order products		

semiportable, or stationary systems must be considered. Semiportable systems include those that may be lightweight but require several pieces of equipment and interfaces and assistance for assembly and transportation.

The last component of the assessment requires the sensitivity of the entire team. As was discussed previously, severely physically handicapped children have generally not had the opportunities for development that more normal children experience. They have probably never crawled around a kitchen pulling everything out of cabinets, nor knocked over a lamp with a toy. They may never even have been given the chance to choose what they will wear, watch on television, give as a gift, or put on their hot dogs. Family constellations develop, often quite comfortably, wherein the child becomes the recipient of the action, the thing rather than the person. When evaluating children for communication systems, we ask them to make decisions and be involved in a cause-and-effect activity. We respect them as persons who have a lot to say, and we may be preparing them to say what others are not ready to hear. Much more is happening to them than simply spending time with a variety of systems. The first taste of autonomy may be unsettling for both the family and the child. The team must be sensitive to hints from the family and the child's home team. Their suggestions are important to continued successful use of communication systems and skills.

Treatment activities

Successful operation of an augmentative communication system is dependent on many variables. The most obvious are motor access to the equipment and the development of receptive and expressive language skills. The lists in Figure 22-5 suggest other areas to be considered throughout the assessment-training-reassessment process. Activities chosen to facilitate these skills and functional components, individualized to the child and devices, should improve the child's successful operation of the augmentative communication system.

The occupational therapist has traditionally used activities to facilitate functional performance. Figure 22-6 provides a list of recommended activities that will enhance the basic task components of perceptual-motor access to augmentative communication systems. In theory the best response will be obtained through activities such as these, in addition to or instead of drill on the actual system. Obviously this effect is most likely to occur if the selected activities are appropriate to the system and to the skills of the particular child.

Educational component (developmental play)

Motorically challenged and developmentally delayed children differ from their peers even in their very earliest play. Play activities are further complicated for children with sensory limitations and for those who are not able to use oral speech reliably. Although the means are not readily available for developmental growth through play, the needs exist in even greater proportions. Computer technology using hardware, software, and adaptive interfaces can assist these children in their active participation in these developmental activities.

COMPUTER ACCESS TO PLAY—THE PROBLEM

Able-bodied children enjoy four areas of play. These activities are reflected in the variety of experiences provided for special needs children in the classroom and therapy environments. A combination of commercially available hardware, software, and professional creativity can help special needs children achieve more appropriate control and participate in these activities. The input systems, output options, perceptual-motor components, and psychosocial aspects are the same as those discussed in this chapter under the section on augmentative communication.

1. *Early gross motor play,* wherein one learns about oneself in relationship to others, may not have been experienced by the motorically impaired child who has never followed the sequential patterns of rolling, sitting, crawling, creeping, kneeling, and pulling to stand. This affects his ability to understand and manipulate the gross motor spatial propositions. He does not have the background experiences to transfer to a game of cars and trucks, whereby he zooms his cars in front of, around, and in back of each other until they crash in mad collision—only to bring the sirens of the screeching fire engine, ambulance, and police car.
2. *Imaginative play;* make-believe, dress up and playing with makeup are other important skills that help the child learn about self. The severely motorically impaired, functionally nonverbal child may never *choose* which hat to wear or which color nail polish is the most fun. Doing the activity may be great, but choosing, directing, and controlling the activity is even greater!
3. *Explorative play;* young children are tickled to be able to go through mommy's purse and daddy's pockets—playing with the keys, putting on the glasses, examining the wallet, and jingling the coins. These are important growth aspects of role modeling, explorative play, and imaginative play.
4. *Make-believe writing;* children, at a fairly young developmental age, typically begin to take an interest in "writing" with an instrument. A young two-year-old may begin to scribble with a crayon or marker—most appropriately on paper! She "fingerpaints" in her food as she begins to create pictures and images that represent something else. It is not long before she "writes," now making symbols and combining them into "words"—the meanings may not be universal, but they are

Figure 22-6 Activities that facilitate access to augmentative communication systems

SWITCH CONTROL

Battery-operated toys—adapted
Electric trains
Freddy the Frog (Fisher Price)
Oscar the Grouch (Fisher Price)
Monster Dash (Prentke Romich)
Prentke Romich Toy Modifications
Votrax Research Handi Toy
Wall switch for a room light
Remote control television
Garage door opener
Shower
Outside sprinkler system
Garbage disposal
Blue Bird (Fisher Price)
Jumping Jack (Fisher Price)
Molly Moo Cow (Fisher Price)
Ring a Bell bicycle crib toy
Ring a Bell fire engine crib toy
Musical crib toy
Juggler crib toy
Crib aquarium
Surprise boxes
Jack-in-the-box
Pass the nuts
Mattel Tuff-Stuff wordwriter, calculator, letters
Mattel See 'n Say
Battery-operated remote-controlled animals
Push-button telephones
Coleco Good Puppy
Perceptual motor facilitators
Pioneer board
Mechanical pointing boards
Switch-operated cassette player
Switch-operated popcorn popper
Switch-operated blender
Computer activities such as Motor Training Games

CAUSE AND EFFECT

Jack-in-the-Box (variety of)
Surprise box (variety of)
Sesame Street House (Child Guidance)
Push-and-Go toys (Tomy)
Egg timer (Playskool; Fisher Price)
Building blocks (variety of)
Pop beads
Cash register (Fisher Price)
Attention-getting bell

RISK TAKING

Table games
Monster Dash (Prentke Romich)
Candy Land
Chutes and Ladders
Hungry, Hungry Hippos
Possum Basic Skill Set
Old Maid (card game)
Go Fish (card game)
Imitation activities
Pass the Nuts (Tomy)

POINTING

Table games
Push button telephones
Telephone truck (Tonka Toddler)
Operator Telephone (Fisher Price)
Finger painting
Little Maestro (Creative Playthings)
Imitation of postures
Mirror play
Clay
"Show me" activities
Melody Mike (Child Guidance)
Tactile stimulation activities or cards
Little Professor (Texas Instruments)
Speak and Spell (Texas Instruments)
Calculator games
Typing
Bubbles
Active range of motion
Computer games using keyboard or keyboard adaptations

PERCEPTION

Possum Basic Skill Set
Concentration (card game)
Imitation of postures
Gross motor directionality activities
Figure-ground cards or activities
Dot-to-dot games
Puzzles (visual matching, word, symbol)
Two-to-four step sequencing activities
Visual matching cards
Lotto (commercial or clinician-made)
Domino games
Lincoln logs (Playskool)
Peg bus and racing car (Creative Playthings)
Shape sorting toys (variety of)
Systems 80 (Borg-Warner)
Potato head type game
Bristle blocks (Playskool)
Bubbles
Size discrimination activities
Categorization (by color, size, shape, and so on)
Color pegs
Developmental learning materials
Self-care activities
Sequencing cards
Tipsy Tea Cups (Child Guidance)
Blockhead (Saalfield)
"What would you do if?"
Simon (Milton Bradley)

certainly important and meaningful to her. The stages progress through early letter and number formation into a clearly legible form of written communication. The severely physically handicapped child, with spastic upper extremities and reflex domination, may be robbed of these experiences. Thus, the percentage of our population that is motorically and developmentally incapable of functional oral speech may also be limited in written expression.

COMPUTER ACCESS TO PLAY—THE SOLUTION

Computer hardware is commercially available that allows the child (with adaptive interfaces) to access software using direct selection, scanning, and encoding. This technology can also be implemented with the child whose motor limitations preclude success with paper and pencil activities, thus allowing him to produce written communication meaningful to others. He can also use the adaptive systems to enhance his play. A creative clinician is the key to this linkage.

The systems, combining hardware and software, may include a wide-based computer or dedicated system, voice synthesizer or digitized speech, printer, color monitor or display, switch or access mode, and input and other adaptations. Special cards may be used to increase memory and expand adaptability. The following systems are suggested as examples to assist the special needs child in his developmental play and educational growth.

- Switch-operated toys may include any variety of homemade or commercially operated switches used to control battery-operated "toys." Toys may be selected from the toy store (trains, cars, dogs, circus toys) or include cassette players and popcorn poppers.
- Apple compatible computers are available with expanded memory, single disk drive, color monitor, voice synthesizer, adaptive firmware card, Muppets Learning Keys, assorted switches, Unicorn membrane keyboard, printer, and graphics tablet. Software important in early play includes, but is certainly not limited to, the Talking Word Board, Programs for Early Acquisition of Language (PEAL), Motor Training Games, Stickybear games, Face-maker, alphabet games, same/not-same games, and body part activities. This type of system is stationary but yields to maximum flexibility and adaptation. Most preschool software that is commercially available can be driven with adaptations for the motor-impaired child.
- Portable "notebook style" personal computers come equipped with voice synthesizer, LED display, printer, scanning arrays, and expanded keyboards. Activities can be created for customized play, although commercial game disks cannot be used without piggy-backing this system onto another computer. This setup has the advantage of portability and can combine some enjoyable play activities with the user's communication system. Variety is available within the memory constraints of the system.
- Home computers with voice output, color video display, scanning arrays, and adaptations and super computer programmers can accomplish almost anything.
- Dedicated systems may be used alone or to interface computers. Their use is similar to the portable computer.

It is to be emphasized that even without previous computer experience, clinicians can create limitless activities for children.

COMPUTER AS A TEACHING TOOL

In the discussion of technology, reference is made to highly sophisticated units, including computers, for intervention with young, delayed motorically-impaired children. These systems are being used to assist the children in the progression through their developmental milestones; that is, the children are being taught to use the computer not for the sake of using a computer, but for understanding concepts such as cause and effect relationships, using the computer as a modality. It is stressed that using a computer would not be an IEP goal for a young preschooler—the appropriate developmental task continues to be the goal. The goal of effective computer use may be an appropriate goal for an older child in a vocational program.

CREATIVE APPROACHES TO COMPUTER USE IN "TEACHING"

Passive computer "watching" is not as effective as active computer system participation. This section will address the implementation of high technology for the achievement of developmental goals.

1. Switch-operated toys—there are numerous battery-operated toys that can be adapted for remote switch operation. Besides being fun, they can help teach cause and effect relationships, timing, touch and release, and turn taking. They give the child control of his environment. This is also an excellent way to evaluate switch access and choice, position/placement, sustained vs touch-release, pressure, and overflow.
2. Apple compatible computers—combinations for this option are threefold:
   a. Apple, color monitor, voice synthesizer, Adaptive Firmware Card, disk drive, switches, Unicorn keyboard. The firmware card has numerous adaptations to affect commercially available software. A crucial function is the ability to bypass the traditional keyboard to drive commercially available programs, including a range of preschool software. Thus, Facemaker, a preschool favorite, can be played using the expanded keyboard, scanning with switches or encoded choices that use switches.

b. Apple, monitor, single disk drive, voice synthesizer, Adaptive Firmware Card, Unicorn expanded keyboard, Talking Word Board Disk, and keyguard for expanded keyboard (optional). Using this program, an able-bodied person is able to create any variety of activities through overlays. Examples of those used with the children at Upward Foundation's Developmental Achievement Center in Phoenix include choosing colors for art therapy session, makeup, dress up, cooking, holiday songs with activities, paper dolls, grocery store and going to the gas station (Figure 22-7). For the makeup game, the keyboard is divided into eight sections, each with a picture of the makeup and the word underneath. When the child touches the area, the computer says the corresponding phrase, for example, touch the area "I want blue eye shadow," hear "I want blue eye shadow," and help apply blue eye shadow. What fun to see your pretty face in the mirror! Task components in this delightful program include active ROM, spatial memory, figure ground, motor planning, crossing midline, and visual pursuit.

c. Apple, color monitor, voice synthesizer, single disk drive, expanded memory card, Muppet Learning Keys and PEAL software (Programs for Early Acquisition of Language). Using an overlay for the Muppet Learning Keys, the child brings to the screen a color picture—

toys are used with the program to enhance language skills within the play situations. The package includes information for the clinician to assist the child to maximize success in the language development. Popular games are "Baby" and "What's in Mommy's Pocketbook?" Again, the child enjoys the activity while participating in exploratory and representational play (Figure 22-8).

3. Portable computers—the range and design of activities for this type of system is by necessity governed by the expandability of the system. The Epson HX20, with adaptations using Speech Pac or Words + and an expanded keyboard has been used in play activities like those discussed above. Dedicated systems can also be implemented in this manner with possibilities for input including scanning, directed direct selection, direct selection, and encoding.

4. Written communication—a variety of graphic tablets allows the developmentally young child to draw a picture, bring it to the color monitor, save it to disk, and print a permanent copy. Programs allow this to be accomplished using directional keys. This can progress to typing hard copy using: (1) direct selection (could be aided by headpointer, light beam, eye gaze, voice input, expanded keyboard); (2) scanning arrays, using any of numerous switches; and (3) encoding using systems like Morse Code, abbreviation expansions and Minspeak. In the classroom, the child

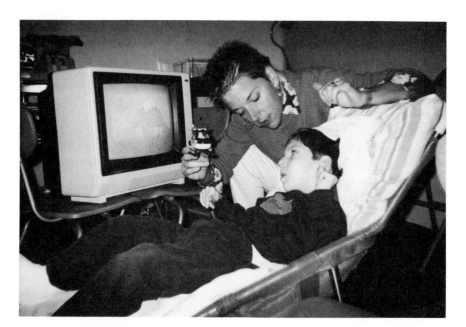

Figure 22-7 Computers allow children to communicate their choices and play otherwise inaccessible games.

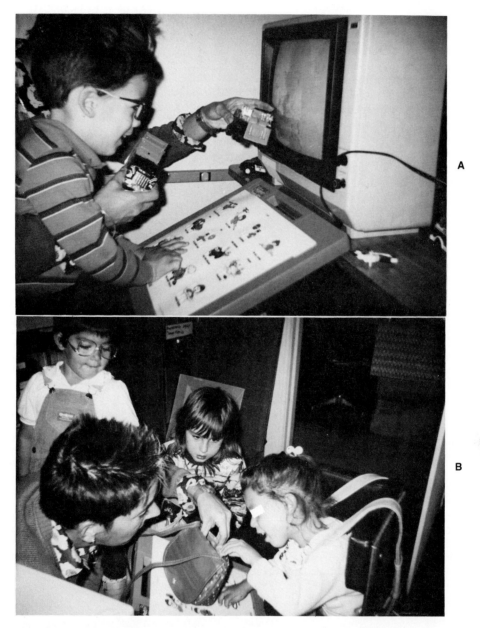

Figure 22-8   Children explore their environments and match their discoveries to board representations. **A,** Toys. **B,** Mommy's pocketbook.

learning to match numerals to a number of objects can have her page of stimuli, count the objects, choose the response from her choices, motorically select, complete the questions, and print her answer sheet. Complex word processing lies at the other end of the spectrum.

It cannot be overemphasized that computers and high technology are being used to supplement and facilitate the child's developmental activities. Thus, in many cases, the software, excellent as it is, need not stand alone.

When playing Stickybear Numbers, it is fun to touch a numeral and watch that corresponding number of objects come onto the screen. This can be enhanced using tactile number cards, feltboard activities, lotto, number charts, bingo, matching games, and listening games. Another popular game, Comparison Kitchen, involves same/not-same activities. This can be enhanced by matching play cookies, cookie dominoes, cookie bingo, cutting out clay cookies, and actually baking cookies!

CASE STUDY

Jane is 4 years, 2 months old. She was brought to Bayshore Rehabilitation Center, an agency offering transdisciplinary evaluation and treatment by specialists in nursing, occupational therapy, physical therapy, and speech therapy.

Medical diagnosis: Cerebral palsy. Evaluation 1 year ago described "severe developmental delays and severe spastic quadriplegia, probably resulting from a hypoxic episode at 3 weeks of age." She has no history of seizures. Additional medical information shows normal hearing in at least one ear with history of chronic ear infections and bilateral myringotomies. She has reduced visual ability because of cortical problems.

Functional status: Jane is dependent in all activities of daily living and self-care:

  Mobility: She is able to roll and crawl on the floor, but is otherwise dependent.

  Dressing: Dependent

  Eating: Manages food in her mouth

  Self-feeding: Dependent, but does indicate food preference by pointing to food choice or verbalizing "more"

  Hygiene: Dependent, but makes motor response to the verbal cue, "Give me your hand."

  Communication: Inconsistent

Previous adaptive equipment: Prone board and Bobath ball. The ball is still used occasionally, but the board was discarded because the mother understood the doctor to say it was no longer needed. Pillow should be used to position her in the standing position.

Present aids: Wheelchair, eyeglasses, corner chair, and mobility aids.

Reliable motor responses: (described by family and transdisciplinary team): Head response yes-no; eye pointing; left and right direct selection is more reliable right of midline area; right joystick; and right rocker switch. Jane's tendency not to cooperate during structured testing situations affected communication and performance to potential during the assessment. She sometimes avoided looking at objects or pictures indicated by therapists.

Reason for referral: It appeared to the transdisciplinary team at Jane's preschool that she exhibits the entry-level readiness skills for enhancement of her present communication modes.

Current communication: Communication methods currently used at home include some verbalization (for example, "sick" and "yeah"), kicking her feet, rolling over to an adult for help, crying, and jabbering. When asked, "Jane, do you want to eat or drink?" she kicks her feet and may verbalize. When responding to a directive, "Are you wet? Come over here," she rolls over to the questioner, crying to express the need to be changed or fed. She has no way to indicate needs. In other environments, including preschool, she interacts by choosing between food or two toys and expresses needs by vocalizing, crying, or smiling.

Spontaneous communications included during the assessment process were occasional word approximations and the perseverative repetition of "ice cream" after she identified a picture of an ice cream cone. She also babbled reduplicated syllables, which also may have been word approximations.

Communication need: Specific needs for Jane include a communication system or combination of systems that will allow her to participate more independently in her educational environment and facilitate and augment her oral speech. Immediate needs include means to make choices and indicate her desires.

Equipment introduced: Zygo 16, joystick, Prentke Romich Training Aid with rocker switch, Apple 2 + computer with disk drive, Echo 2 Voice Synthesizer, video display, Unicorn membrane keyboard, Prentke Romich Lighttalker, Prentke Romich Touchtalker, Speechpac using scanning and direct selection on expanded keyboard, attention-getting bell, and clockface communicator.

Assessment environment: Jane was seen by the transdisciplinary team in multistage assessment at the center. The team members also know Jane through the traditional therapy program at her preschool. The overall atmosphere, therefore, was relaxed and supportive. Jane attempted most tasks and activities asked of her.

Positioning: Jane shows the following movement patterns that may present difficulty in using the special equipment: increased muscle tone in either total flexion or extensor patterns, although Jane has enough control to operate simple switches. Head control is fair and more consistent when she is motivated. No problems with retention of any primitive reflexes. Jane's most functional position is in the corner chair with the lapboard and with switch or board placement at midline. Other recommendations: attach a dowel to her tray for her to hold with her left hand so as to decrease associated movements when she uses her right hand.

Motor response and visual perception: Jane successfully accesses the communication systems while sitting in her corner chair using both scanning and direct selection. For scanning, she used her right arm to approach the joystick and one-way rocker switch. With her head in midline, both the switch and reinforcement are placed in midline to maximize potential for success. Areas on a large membrane keyboard were approached with both the right and left hand, with total access to the interface. When presented with a small keyboard requiring direct selection (3½ inches), Jane exhibited increased tone and drooling. Jane wears corrective eyeglasses and appears to have some visual perception deficits related to the use of augmentative aids. More specifically, she does not appear to cross midline, does not regard materials placed left of midline, has difficulty attending to the task, and shows deficits with visual tracking.

Communication-interaction: Using a membrane keyboard with colored drawings of objects found in a purse, therapists demonstrated naming items in the purse. The keyboard was positioned at midline on the tray of the corner chair in which Jane was sitting. Each item was named by pressing the appropriate picture on the keyboard that activated the computer voice and an identical picture on the video screen. The purse was opened wide, and all items in the purse were visible. As each item was named, it was taken from the purse and given to Jane or placed on the pictured item on the keyboard. She smiled while she watched the demonstration. She did not raise her eyes to look at the video screen, nor did she look toward the pictures on the membrane keyboard. Her gaze moved primarily in the lower quadrant of the board. When encouraged to press pictures to get items in the purse, she pressed mirror and keys, the two pictures closest to her right hand. Some assistance was necessary to help her reach the "keys" picture.

Developmental/Play: Jane shows an interest in her environment and peers, recognizes the cause-effect relationship, appears to engage in some parallel play, is interested in, but limited in color to, paper activities, responds to the "voice" of the computer but not the video display, enjoys music and art, and loves looking in the mirror.

Summary of findings: This child was assessed and showed functional potential to be most effective in her corner chair. Reliable motor responses included scanning, using a rocker switch or joystick approached at the right and placed in midline, and direct selection with bilateral upper extremity access. Visual perception assets and liabilities that could affect success within a program or system are probably related to her motor status and developmental level. These are (1) difficulties with attention to task, (2) midline crossing, (3) regard for the full visual field, and (4) visual tracking.

Important indications of communicative interaction are Jane's ability to indicate choices by touching her choice, her attempts to say words, and head nodding for "yes" and "no." At present she tends to choose items on her right side more frequently than those on her left, her word approximations are often unintelligible, and her head-nodding responses are not reliable. However, Jane is steadily improving in all these areas.

Professional recommendations: Based on these findings the transdisciplinary team made the following recommendations. Because Jane presently responds to objects as stimuli, a progression to photographs seems appropriate. This would encourage her to indicate choices. Direct selection appears to be an appropriate motor response, although a scanning aid might be incorporated into her program to facilitate cause and effect and visual tracking.

Jane's present functional performance and the clinical judgment of this team suggest the probability that she will become a more reliable verbal communicator. Thus efforts should be directed toward the implementation of systems and programs to facilitate her oral speech. Electronic aids would be more directive as educational motivators.

Jane would be more functional in her daily activities if she used systems that encourage verbalization and allow her to participate more independently in her academic readiness program. Clinician-made and commercially available aids that meet these criteria are Zygo 16, using a one-way rocker switch; Communicator, using a one-way rocker switch; Magic Wand Speaking Reader by Texas Instruments; Prentke Romich Training Aid; Systems 80 with five-way rocker switch or scanning interface; Apple 2 + 48K computer with disk drive, color monitor, membrane keyboard; Echo 2 Voice Synthesizer, adaptive firmware cord, Unicorn Keyboard and single switch input; PEAL software with Muppet Learning Keys; Speech Pac with Unicorn Keyboard and developmentally appropriate "games."

Short-term therapy recommendations: Team intervention will be necessary in the development and training of these systems to facilitate more successful interaction. Direct therapy training at the center includes developmental-cognitive and play-work activities, including the communication systems and task components. This will take place in the center within a peer group and, as appropriate, within Jane's community interactions. At the appropriate time, equipment will be made available on a temporary basis to Jane at home. When it has been demonstrated that these systems help Jane to be more functional and assume appropriate life roles, third-party funding will be sought.

Immediate short-term goals for Jane, with assistance from either the therapy team at Jane's preschool or the transdisciplinary team at the center, are as follows:

1. At lunch time Jane will progress from her present stage of pointing to actual food to indicate preference to the stage of pointing to photographs. Long-term goals will expand this to other categories and line drawings.
2. To improve her visual perception, Jane will use the training aid and light scanners.
3. Activities to improve her motor reliability and energy efficiency are recommended.
4. Jane showed interest and success with a joystick. This motor control system might suggest potential for a motorized mobility system.
5. Jane will participate individually and in a small group in language/play activities using the computer. Activities appearing appropriate *at this time* would include songs, PEAL software, make up games, coloring games, dress up games, and turn-taking games.

SUMMARY

Communication is an important activity of daily living, but verbal communication may be beyond the capacity of many children who have physical handicaps, developmental delays, or emotional disorders. Augmentative communication is a skill that is readily used by the typical verbal youngster, but it must be carefully and appropriately integrated into the developmental day and life roles of the nonspeaking child. Technological advances are such that even the most severely physically handicapped child may use an augmentative communication system through knowledgeable choice of motor access, selection mode, and output possibilities.

Multidisciplinary team intervention is indicated for the selection and training of an appropriate system, by use of assessment-training-reassessment model. In efforts to avoid the "dusty device syndrome," careful attention must be directed to positioning, linguistic skills, cognition, motor assets, motivation, expressive and receptive language development, perception, and psychosocial aspects. The occupational therapist is concerned with a traditional evaluation and treatment model directed toward the concept of communication as an activity of daily life. The therapist analyzes the components of related tasks, systems, and program designs and implements an activity program with the child to develop communication skills for functional community interaction.

Believing that "play is the work of the child," then "adapting play is the work of the occupational therapist." Computer and system adaptation, as used for augmentative communication systems, can also be applied to developmental play activities. The therapist's creativity is the key to transforming experiences from real to imaginary and back again for the special needs child.

Indeed, it is through my expressive language as author and your receptive language as reader that I have been able to convey my message to you. I have used an input mode of direct selection on a typewriter and have given you, the reader, permanent, readable, copy (output) in the form of this chapter: a true example of augmentative communication.

STUDY QUESTIONS

1. A primary goal in the implementation of an augmentative communication system is to enhance the child's expressive communication. Describe the role of the occupational therapist in this process.
2. Why would a child need a combination of communication systems?
3. Discuss the phrase "functional community interaction."
4. A primary concern of many parents for their functionally nonverbal children is that the use of an augmentative communication system may interfere with the development of oral language. Discuss this from the OT perspective.
5. Discuss how the creative clinician may help her client choose the facial expression on a jack-o-lantern using a talking computer program.

REFERENCES

1. Baker BA: Whence? Whither? A brief history of Minspeak, Detroit, Mich, Nov 1986, First Annual Minspeak Conference.
2. Bliss CK: Semantography, Sydney, Australia, 1965, Semantography Publications.
3. Bliss CK. and McNaughton S: The book to the film, "Mr. symbol man," Sydney, Australia, 1975, Semantography Publications.
4. Clark CK, Davies CO, and Woodcock RW: Standard rebus glossary, Circle Pines, Minn, 1974, ARS, American Guidance Service, Inc.
5. Firing M: The physically impaired population of the United States, San Francisco, 1978, Firing and Associates.
6. Johnson R, The picture communication symbols, Solano Beach, Calif, 1981, Mayer-Johnson.
7. Johnson R, The picture communication symbols, book II, Solano Beach, Calif, 1985, Mayer-Johnson.
8. Kirstein I, and Bernstein C: Oakland schools picture dictionary, Pontiac, Mich, 1981, Oakland Schools Communication Enhancement Center.
9. LeBlanc M: Personal communication, 1983.
10. Montgomery J, and Hanson R: Augmentative Communication Advocacy 1984, Boston, Mass, 1984, Third International Conference of the International Society for Augmentative and Alternate Communication.
11. Rehabilitation engineering, a plan for continued progress—II, Richmond, Va, 1978, Rehabilitation Engineering Center, University of Virginia.
12. Vanderheiden G, and Lloyd LL: Communication systems and their components. In Blackstone SW, editor: Augmentative communication: an introduction, Rockville, Md, 1986, American Speech Language Hearing Assoc.

SUGGESTED READINGS

Beukelman DR, and Yorkstown KA: Communication system for the severely disarthric speaker with an intact language system, J Speech Hear Disord 42:265, 1977.

Computers and the disabled, Byte: The Small Systems Journal, Sept, 1982.

Copeland K: Aides for the severely handicapped, New York, 1974, Grune & Stratton, Inc.

Fountain Valley School District, Title IV-C ESEA: Nonoral communication, Fountain Valley, Calif, 1980, California State Department of Education.

Hagan C, Porter W, and Brink J: Nonverbal communication: an alternative mode of communication for the child with severe cerebral palsy, J Speech Hear Disord 38:448, 1973.

McDonald ET: Conventional symbols of English, In Vanderheiden G, and Grilley K, editors: Nonvocal communication techniques and aids for the severely physically handicapped, Baltimore, 1976, University Park Press.

Resource Director of Computer and Communication Technology, Except Parent, p. 33, Oct, 1986.

Van Bruns-Connolly S, and Shane HC: Communication boards: help for the child unable to talk, Except Parent, p. F19, April, 1978.

Vanderheiden G: Nonvocal communication resource book, Baltimore, 1978, University Park Press.

Vanderheiden G, and Grilley K: Nonvocal communication techniques and aids for the severely physically handicapped, Baltimore, 1975, University Park Press.

Vanderheiden RC, and Harris-Vanderheiden DH: Communication techniques and aides for the nonvocal severely handicapped. In Lloyd L, editor: Communication assessment and intervention strategies, Baltimore, 1976, University Park Press.

Vickers B: Nonoral communication systems project: 1964-1973, Iowa City, Iowa, 1974, Campus Stores.

23

Sensory integration and children with learning disabilities

FLORENCE CLARK
ZOE MAILLOUX
DIANE PARHAM
JULIE CRITES BISSELL

In the 1940s, a child who had normal measured intelligence but could not learn in a circumscribed area of academics (for example, reading), was simply called an underachiever or, in extreme cases, labeled emotionally disturbed. Sometimes the child as well as the parents were referred for psychotherapy. In the 1950s, a child with this problem was more typically labeled as having minimal brain damage or minimal brain dysfunction, and parents were no longer regarded as contributors to the problem. Educationally handicapped or *learning disabled* are the terms most likely to be used to classify these children today—terms that circumvent the implication of brain damage or dysfunction. Why the periodic changes in the labels attached to these children? Are they merely capricious, or do they reflect some systematic historical trend in how this dysfunction and its origins are viewed? Is it important that the entry-level pediatric occupational therapist be aware of the forces that contributed to these developments?

Today the field of learning disabilities is described as lacking consensus on the basic issues of definition, assessment, and programming.[192] Eminent researchers, Kirk and Kirk,[117] recently called it nebulous and without a unified body of theory and practice. Wiederholt,[204] in a now often cited historical review on the history of the education of children with learning disabilities, identified controversies over definition, territorial rights of respective health and educational professions, and the lack of studies establishing the effectiveness of programs as major problems confronting the field.

Entry-level therapists must understand the history of the learning disabilities field. As they begin their practice in this area, they will be entering a field that has been plagued with uncertainties and controversies.[107] Therapists will be asked to clarify what they mean by a learning disability, to describe what their role is in the remediation of this problem, and to present data that support their practice. The basic assumptions therapists make about the nature of learning disabilities may be challenged by educators or physicians with a different orientation, and therapists must be prepared to address the concerns of such professionals.

This chapter prepares the entry-level-therapist to face and manage such conflict; it is naive to expect to enter this field and avoid the controversies. Facing conflict and managing it requires a broad view of the field and an understanding of the sources of its uncertainties and controversies. Knowledge of the ways in which the disciplines of occupational therapy and education interface with other professions involved in the management of learning disabilities must also be part of the entry-level therapist's preparation. In the first part of this chapter the field of learning disabilities in general is discussed. In the second part the focus is narrowed to occupational therapy intervention with children with learning disabilities. Because sensory integrative procedures are used widely with this group of children, this chapter devotes considerable attention to them. In addition, how the occupational behavior approach might be used with such children is discussed. In the final section of this chapter there is an attempt to sort out the similarities and differences between sensory integrative, perceptual-motor, and sensorimotor approaches to treatment. The intent is that, after reading this chapter, the entry-level therapist will be prepared to communicate, with clarity, to the educators, speech pathologists, physicians, and other professionals about the role of occupational therapy in the treatment of the child with learning disabilities.

A discussion of educational and medical perspectives on learning disabilities should begin with a definition of this condition. Unfortunately, consensus on the definition of this term does not exist within the discipline of special education, much less across disciplines. At this point, much uncertainty exists surrounding the notions on the nature of this disorder. Despite the difficulties inherent in defining the terms, learning disabilities are usually readily recognized,[145] and educators seem to view it as a viable classification.[193] The presentation of the existing, and controversial, definitions of learning disabilities will be deferred until the reader is provided with a historical perspective on the education of these children who seem to defy definition but who are apparently identifiable.

A HISTORICAL PERSPECTIVE ON THE EDUCATION AND IDENTIFICATION OF CHILDREN WITH LEARNING DISABILITIES

The education and identification of some children as learning disabled was spawned by three forces: (1) The results of brain localization studies on adult patients with brain damage; (2) the inference that children with specific learning problems and normal intelligence had brain damage or brain dysfunction that interfered with learning; and (3) the federal legislation in the 1960s and 1970s that mandated educational service delivery to these children. The following analysis of these forces and their effects is based largely on Wiederholt.[204]

Results of brain localization studies: foundation phase

A number of nineteenth century physicians studied the specific effects of circumscribed lesions of the brain. Wiederholt[204] considered these physicians to have laid the foundation for the identification of learning disabilities in children. He called the period in which they worked, from about 1802 to 1933, the foundation phase. These physicians were interested in the disorders of spoken language, written language, and perceptual-motor processes that were the functional correlates of (associated with) specific brain lesions.

In the foundation phase, knowledge about the site of brain lesions and their concomitant effects was acquired through postmortem studies of the brains of patients who had demonstrated specific learning problems. For example, based on autopsy studies, Broca in the 1860s argued that a lesion to the third frontal convolution resulted in aphasia.[175] Later, in 1926, Head[94] extended many of Broca's theories.

Other physicians focused on description of the brain structures implicated in disorders of written, rather than spoken, language.[96,149] Word blindness was defined by Hinshelwood[96] as "a condition in which, with normal vision and therefore seeing the letters and words distinctly, an individual is no longer able to interpret written or printed language." Based on the autopsy of a patient with this condition, Hinshelwood believed the brain's left angular gyrus to be implicated in the condition. He went a step further in that he believed that some children were born with "congenital word blindness," and he suggested a method involving three steps for teaching them to read. Twenty years later Orton[150] questioned many of Hinshelwood's views and presented a theory on alexia (the inability to read) that placed great emphasis on the dominance of one hemisphere over the other for adequacy of reading functions. Orton[151] believed that roughly 10% of school-aged children had reading disabilities because of poorly established dominance.

A third group, made up of psychologists and physicians who conducted research during this period, studied the perceptual-motor disturbances that were associated with brain lesions. Goldstein[86] proposed that, in addition to the specific learning disabilities that seemed to arise from circumscribed areas of brain injury, general manifestations of brain damage were also obvious. He described the behaviors of brain-injured adults as disordered, inattentive, and emotionally explosive. In the 1940s Strauss, a psychiatrist, and Werner, a psychologist, studied the characteristics of brain-injured children who were, in addition, mentally retarded.[184,187,201] In particular, they were interested in determining whether these children would be symptomatically similar to the brain-damaged adults described by Goldstein. Strauss and Lehtinen[186] reported that, like their adult counterparts, brain-injured children had perceptual disturbances, but the children were less able to compensate because they had never possessed intact perceptual abilities. These children with brain damage and retardation were described as uncontrolled, erratic, inhibited, and socially less acceptable than normal children.

Whether they studied disorders of spoken language, disorders of written language, or disorders in perception, the physicians and psychologists who worked during the foundation phase contributed to the overall conceptualization of learning disabilites. First, their studies led to the belief that specific learning disabilities, for example, language or reading problems, were associated with lesions of circumscribed areas of the brain. Second, their studies suggested that more general behavioral problems, such as distractibility, could also be associated with brain damage in both adults and retarded children. Third, they provided descriptions of clinical cases in which the manifestations of brain injuries seemed to be congenitally acquired rather than secondary to a postnatal insult. Finally, they paved the way to educational programs that were based on the assumption that children with learning problems had concomitant brain dysfunction.

Interventions based on inference of brain damage: transition phase

Wiederholt[204] proposed that in the period from around 1930 to 1960 the education of children with handicaps was in a transition phase. In 1955 Strauss and Kephart[185] emphasized the need for professionals to work with the brain-injured child of normal intelligence. Here the conceptual leap was made that children without known brain injury did, nevertheless, possess minimal brain damage. These children were described as having problems in learning, poorly coordinated perceptions, lack of purposeful behavior, distractibility, disinhibition, and perseveration. This cluster of symptoms was called the "Strauss syndrome."[185]

Whereas physicians had been the leaders in the foundation phase, psychologists and educators were the primary contributors to the field during the transition phase. In this phase, programs for educating the child with disorders of spoken language, disorders of written language, and perceptual-motor disturbances were developed. The programs were based on models of brain processing and the assumption that learning disorders were reflections of a dysfunction in, or damage to, the brain. The knowledge of brain function that had been an end product of the earlier autopsy research was now translated into intervention models. It was assumed with these models that by aiming at better efficiency in brain processes, learning disabilities could be remedied. Assessment procedures were developed to identify the dysfunctional brain processes, and corresponding intervention programs were designed to change them. Because the intervention programs focused on changing the processes underlying academic learning, they collectively are referred to as process-oriented approaches.

Models of auditory-language processing were constructed by Osgood[152,153] and Wepman and others[200] and were used to guide the development of the Illinois Test of Psycholinguistic Abilities (ITPA),[118] which today, despite criticism, is widely used in the learning disabilities field.[82] In this test the child is assessed in receptive, associative, and expressive language functions at the automatic and representational levels; both the auditory and visual channels are tested. Educational programs are then developed for teaching these abilities.[140] These process-oriented programs are referred to today as the psycholinguistic approach.

A second approach to developing interventions for children with learning disabilities was also based on the assumption that these children's brains were not processing information adequately. However, this approach presumed, in an additive manner, that the more sensory systems that were called on during a learning activity, the better would be the learning. Called multisensory teaching strategies, they emphasized kinesthetic, auditory, and visual reinforcement during learning tasks.[70,71] For example, a child would be required to say the word *circle* as she drew a circle on the blackboard.

Finally, a third type of intervention was developed in this period and, like those just described, it assumed that learning disabilities were consequent to brain dysfunction. These programs involved an initial assessment on a perceptual-motor test and then training in specific skills,[75,76,110] such as walking a balance beam, making "angels in the snow," or tracing dot-to-dot designs. Although a number of perceptual-motor training programs were developed and subtly differed from one another in some ways, all were based on the assumptions that (1) motor learning provided a foundation for symbolic learning; (2) motor development unfolded hierarchically; (3) unsatisfactory motor development would interfere with academic learning; and (4) remediation of motor deficits should contribute to better coping with traditional academics.[49]

Legislation in the 1960s and 1970s:
INTEGRATION PHASE

The 1960s ushered in what Wiederholt[204] described as an integration phase. Most of the contributions in this period were from the field of education. Educators, motivated by federal mandates and incentives, began to establish educational programs for children with learning disabilities and test the effectiveness of the process-oriented models that had been developed in the transition period.

The federal government was highly instrumental in the 1960s in making services available to children identified as learning disabled. Gearheart[82] provided an excellent review of this legislation. Public Law 89-10, the Elementary and Secondary Education Act of 1965, provided significant monies for local educational programs. Gearheart believes that these programs probably involved children who today would be called learning disabled, since they addressed, in part, children with reading problems and neurological impairment. He qualifies his statement by pointing out that this law did not explicitly fund programs for the child with learning disabilities.

Public Law 91-230, the Education of the Handicapped Act, contained a title (Title VI) that addressed the educational needs of the child with handicaps. Children with learning disabilities were *not* included in the definition of handicapped under this law. However, under Part G, the government was authorized to allocate grants to fund research, training, and model programs for children with learning disabilities. Gearheart singles this out as the first piece of federal legislation that treated learning disabilities as a distinct handicapping condition. In 1969 only 12 states had passed legislation for funding programs for children with learning disabilities. By 1974 all 50 states had programs, although various terms were used to designate this group of children, such as educationally handicapped, neurologically impaired, and learning disabled. Through grants awarded under Public Law 91-230, Education of the Handicapped Act, Title VI, Part 6, Child Service Demonstration Projects (CSDPs) proliferated, and learning disabilities were established as a subcategory of special education.

Finally, in 1975 under Public Law 94-142, the Education for All Handicapped Children Act, funding was provided specifically for the education of children with learning disabilities as well as with other handicapping conditions. Importantly, under this law occupational therapy was mandated as a related service that should be provided to the child with learning disabilities, as well as to children with other handicapping conditions, when this service will improve the child's ability to benefit from special education.

Competition in the 1970s and 1980s:
CONTROVERSY PHASE

Had Wiederholt[204] written about the 1970s and 1980s, he might have called this the controversy phase. This has been a time marked by heated controversy about the nature of learning disabilities and how children with learning disabilities can best be helped.

During the integration phase, many educators began to research the effectiveness of existing programmatic approaches. Studies were conducted on the effectiveness of the educational systems that had been developed during the transition phase.[65,90,134,148,188] In the 1970s this issue came to a head. The perceptual-motor and psycholinguistic approaches were called process-oriented or ability models because the intervention was focused on remediating a particular ability (for example, visual sequencing), rather than on skill development in tasks more directly identifiable as academics. In process-oriented approaches the child typically is given a diagnostic test that identifies the processes in which there is a dysfunction. Remediation is focused on the process, rather than on the area of academic skill in which the child is deficient.

Process-oriented models are contrasted with task analysis models that are aimed directly at acquisition of specific academic tasks. The tasks are analyzed into components based on complexity, and theoretically the child is taught to master simple tasks before more complex ones. The emphasis is on component parts of terminal behaviors. Through incremental gains in academic skills the children are moved from where they are to where they should be.

In 1974, Ysseldyke and Salvia[208] published a study in which they analyzed the predictive efficiency of the most frequently used instruments for measuring abilities. Based on this analysis, they concluded that ability

models essentially were nonvalidated. A few years later, Vellutino and his colleagues[194] provided a lengthy critique of the perceptual-deficit hypothesis of learning disabilities. They argued that data did not support the basic premise that visual perceptual disturbances contributed to reading disabilities and that the effectiveness of perceptual programs had not been established. They then recommended task analysis emphasizing behavioral rather than psychoneurological processes for intervention with children with learning disabilities.

One well-known controversy has surrounded the use of psycholinguistic training based on diagnosis with the Illinois Test of Psycholinguistic Abilities.[118] The controversy began when Hammill and Larsen[90] reviewed 38 studies of psycholinguistic training effectiveness. They reported that a large percentage of the studies did not show positive effects, and therefore the efficacy of psycholinguistic training had not been conclusively demonstrated. In 1978 Lund, Foster, and McCall-Perez[123] countered Hammill and Larsen's conclusions by reevaluating the same group of studies. They argued that, while some of the studies were inconclusive, others yielded strong support for psycholinguistic training. In response, Hammill and Larsen[91] reconfirmed their original position that the training was nonvalidated. Finally, in 1981, Kavale[103] reported on a meta-analysis of 34 psycholinguistic training studies. Meta-analysis is a sophisticated statistical analysis that provides an effect size summarizing the results of a group of experimental studies. An impressive effect of psycholinguistic training on ITPA performance was found, thus substantiating claims of effectiveness of this training.

Perceptual-motor training has also been challenged by some educators.[131] A meta-analysis of 180 efficacy studies of perceptual-motor training indicated that perceptual-motor training is *not* an effective intervention technique.[105] Occupational therapists should be aware that educators are likely to equate sensory integration intervention with perceptual-motor training. However, when sensory integration treatment studies are analyzed separately from perceptual-motor studies, a different picture is revealed. A meta-analysis conducted by Ottenbacher[155] summarized the results of group experimental studies that used only sensory integrative intervention. A very strong positive effect was found, indicating effectiveness of this treatment approach.

Current models of the contributors to learning disabilities

It is misleading to suggest that the entire field of special education rejected psychoneurological approaches in the integration phase. Eminent special educators such as Frostig and Maslow[77] and Cruickshank[60] tenaciously continued to endorse the position that the knowledge of the status of brain functioning is central to remediation for these children. Others argued that neurological considerations are probably relevant for some but not all learning disabilities.[108,132]

In the late 1970s the literature did not reflect a total rejection of the idea that brain dysfunction was implicated in learning disabilities. Papers published in the integration phase did raise questions about the validity of the treatment approaches that had been generated from nineteenth century conceptualizations of brain processes. New explanations of learning disabilities appeared, based on more current ideas on how the brain processes information, matures, or attends to relevant stimuli. Alternative explanations for the presence of learning disabilities emerged as well. A discussion of four of these perspectives follows. Familiarity with these models enables entry-level therapists to bring to their practice a broadened view on current thinking about learning disabilites.

THE ATTENTIONAL DEFICIT HYPOTHESIS

In the attentional deficit hypothesis, learning disabilities are seen as being related to deficient attentional mechanisms. While reading, a child must focus attention on words on the page; during a classroom lecture, the instructor's words must be attended to; working a problem in geometry requires sustained concentration on the task demands. Children who have difficulty directing their attention to relevant stimuli will have problems with learning.

Harris[92] defined attention as "the presence of those behaviors which have become associated with adaptation to classroom environments and yield correct or learned responses to pertinent, task relevant stimuli or stimulus dimensions." Mirsky[141] defined it as "a focusing of consciousness or awareness on some part of the multitude of stimuli from the environment; usually on the basis of learning or training." Kinsbourne and Caplan[115] considered a type of learning disability, called a cognitive-style disorder, to be a problem with attention. These perspectives reflect the current interest in the field of learning disabilities in linking problems with attention to disorders in learning.

The attentional deficit hypothesis of learning disabilities suggests that children with learning disabilities may be unable to filter relevant from irrelevant information. Such impairment may result in problems with selective attention or the ability to attend to only relevant stimuli. In extreme cases the child may appear to be distractible. Selective attention has been found to be age-related.[88,126] With increased age, children become more efficient at blocking out irrelevant stimuli. Research suggests that children with dyslexia acquire selective attention in the same developmental progression as do normal children, but they seem to do so at a slower rate.[190]

Other researchers have linked learning disabilities to problems with attention.[72,102,176] In a particularly interesting study, Shields[177] measured the average evoked responses (AERs) of children with learning disabilities to visual stimuli. In this procedure, as the children looked at the stimuli, very small changes in EEG patterns were recorded and electronically averaged. Results suggested that children with learning disabilities may need to focus more attention on tasks than do children without learning disabilities. Fuller[78] also compared the brain wave activity of children with learning disabilities and normal children. He found that children with learning disabilities, when they were engaged in school-related tasks, showed immature patterns of brain activity. Other studies have suggested that children with learning disabilities spend more time attending to irrelevant stimuli.[63,142]

The studies that support the attentional deficit hypothesis implicate brain dysfunction in learning disabilities. After all, the brain regulates attention. Intervention strategies that have been developed in accord with the position have *not,* however, been similar to the process training systems that were developed in the transition phase. For example, in accepting the position that at least some learning disabilities may result from attentional deficits, Keogh and Margolis[109] suggest that teachers make their task expectations clear and explicit and encourage students to review available responses before acting. These procedures are not reminiscent of either perceptual-motor training or psycholinguistic interventions. They are based on the assumption that some children with learning disabilities act on inappropriate information in the presence of adequate perceptions. Keogh and Margolis[109] believe these children may be responding too quickly or giving insufficient attention to stimuli.

In addition to educational strategies aimed at improving attention problems, medical treatments have also been developed for children with learning disabilities under the assumption that a basic attention deficit exists. The medical diagnosis typically used for such children is *attention deficit disorder,* which is often treated with medication, especially if hyperactivity is a problem. The acronym for this diagnosis is ADD. An attention deficit disorder can exist with or without hyperactivity, according to the *Diagnostic and Statistical Manual of Mental Disorders (DSM III)*[6] of the American Psychiatric Association. When hyperactivity is present, the acronym is ADD-H. The *DSM III* criteria for attention deficit disorder with hyperactivity are as follows: The child displays, for her mental and chronological age, signs of developmentally inappropriate inattention, impulsivity, and hyperactivity. The signs must be reported by adults in the child's environment, such as parents and teachers. Because the symptoms are typically variable, they may not be observed directly by the clinician. When the reports of teachers and parents conflict, primary consideration should be given to the teacher reports because of greater familiarity with age-appropriate norms. Symptoms commonly worsen in situations that require self-application, as in the classroom. Signs of the disorder may be absent when the child is in a new or a one-to-one situation.

The number of symptoms specified is for children between the ages of 8 and 10, the peak age range for referral. In younger children more severe forms of the symptoms and a greater number of symptoms are usually present. The opposite is true of older children.

A. *Inattention.* At least three of the following:
1. Often fails to finish things he or she starts
2. Often doesn't seem to listen
3. Is easily distracted
4. Has difficulty concentrating on school work or other tasks requiring sustained attention
5. Has difficulty sticking to a play activity

B. *Impulsivity.* At least three of the following:
1. Often acts before thinking
2. Shifts excessively from one activity to another
3. Has difficulty organizing work (not due to cognitive impairment)
4. Needs a lot of supervision
5. Frequently calls out in class
6. Has difficulty waiting turn in games or group situations

C. *Hyperactivity.* At least two of the following:
1. Runs about or climbs on things excessively
2. Has difficulty sitting still or fidgets excessively
3. Has difficulty staying seated
4. Moves about excessively during sleep
5. Is always "on the go" or acts as if "driven by a motor"

D. Onset before the age of 7

E. Duration of at least 6 months

F. Not the result of schizophrenia, affective disorder, or severe or profound mental retardation[6] (p. 43).

According to *DSM III,* the criteria for ADD without hyperactivity are the same as those for ADD-H, except that the individual never had signs of hyperactivity (criterion C).[6] Psychotropic drugs are prescribed to more children for hyperactivity than for any other disorder[79] and stimulant drugs are the most effective type and most often used for ADD-H. Ritalin (methylphenidate) is by far the most commonly prescribed, followed by Dexedrine (dextroamphetamine), Cylert (pemoline), and nonstimulant drugs.[79]

There is considerable evidence that these medications are very effective in producing short-term improvements in activity level, behavioral control, and performance on tasks involving vigilant attention and impulse control.[79,156] However, whether they produce improvement in academic achievement has not been conclusively demonstrated.[40,79] It appears that although hyperactive children may settle down and behave more attentively in school when medicated, they may not necessarily learn more than if they had not been medicated. In a meta-analysis of studies of drug treatment of hyperactivity, Ottenbacher and Cooper[156]

found the largest effect size for behavioral and social measures, and the smallest for intellectual and academic achievement measures, thus providing support for the assertion that medication definitely reduces hyperactivity and increases attention span but has a relatively weak effect on improving academic achievement. Follow-up studies of hyperactive children show that medication in childhood does *not* improve long-term outcome in adolescence or adulthood.[198,202]

Given that medication has strong short-term effects in reducing activity level and impulsivity, how does it work? The answer to this question is not known, although there are a number of speculative models attempting to explain medication effects. Most of the models assume that hyperactivity is the result of some abnormality in the arousal function of the central nervous system, and that medication affects arousal through generalized effects on neurotransmitters such as the catecholamines, dopamine, and norepinephrine. Depending on the model, the arousal problem is conceptualized as a brainstem reticular activating system dysfunction, a dysfunction in cortical inhibition, or some combination of brainstem-cortical interaction.[69,167]

Porges[160] has an interesting model in which hyperactivity is viewed as an imbalance between the sympathetic and parasympathetic functions of the autonomic nervous system. He presents physiological evidence that hyperactive children are dominated by the sympathetic component, which is associated with orienting and "fight or flight" reactions. According to his model, the parasympathetic component, which is responsible for sustained attention, is overruled in the child with ADD-H. The child's behavior consequently appears distractible, impulsive, and overactive. Stimulant drugs are believed to improve sustained attention because they increase the action of the cholinergically-mediated parasympathetic nervous system, thus normalizing the autonomic nervous system.

It should be noted that not every child with ADD-H will respond well to medication. For those who do, an optimal dosage is critical in obtaining positive results. If the dosage is inappropriate, the child's attention, cognitive, and behavioral problems may actually become worse.[79] Furthermore, a number of common side effects should be closely monitored in any child taking a stimulant medication. These include insomnia, anorexia, changes in mood and appearance that resemble depression, perseveration in problem-solving tasks, choreoathetoid movements and tics, increased heart rate and blood pressure, and slowing of growth in height and weight.[79,167] Many researchers believe the physical growth and cardiovascular effects are temporary and harmless,[79] but others warn that research in this area is inconclusive.[166] These physiological changes may produce subtle and insidious effects when stimulants are used for long periods of time.[202]

Some researchers[202] have identified important social

effects that emanate from stimulant medication. In particular, the child's self-concept may be affected either positively or negatively. On the one hand, a more positive self-concept may develop if the child had such serious behavior problems that self-concept was already endangered before medication was administered. A negative effect may occur, however, if the child comes to believe that his or her good behavior is solely due to "the pill." Often children refer to their medication as "smart pills" or "good boy pills," as if the pills were the magic solution to their problems. Thus, the child may fail to develop a belief in self as the lovable, competent person who is responsible for the positive changes that occur under medication.[202]

Whalen and Henker[202] suggest that the message adults give about medication influences how the child perceives the situation. They recommend that pills be portrayed as assistive agents that will help boost the child's efforts. Making an analogy may help convey this concept. For example, eyeglasses may help one to read, but will not teach how to read or actually do the reading, just as medication may help a child sustain attention, but will not make him learn or do good things. Another recommendation is that an intervention program such as social skills training be implemented before and concomitantly with the medication. Positive changes are then more likely to be attributed to the child's effort at learning new skills than to "good boy pills." An occupational therapy program focusing on the child's ability to organize his own behavior, as well as to socially interact with others appropriately, therefore could be a critical adjunct to medication.

THE INFORMATION-PROCESSING DEFICIT HYPOTHESIS

The advent of the computer has had its impact on psychology, particularly on how this discipline conceptualizes human information processing. Information-processing models of brain functioning liken the brain to a computer. Farnham-Diggory[68] presented a perspective on learning disabilities that uses an information-processing model. According to Farnham-Diggory, computer models of information-processing mechanisms tend to consist of certain components (Figure 23-1).

Feature detectors register minute pieces of sensory information, feature buffers store the information, and a feature synthesizer integrates it with any information applied to it from a working memory. Programs stored in the system guide how the information will be acted on and what responses will be made. The semantic network consists of memories of interconnected concepts. Information acquires meaning when it is interpreted in relation to the semantic network. The example of reading the word *by* illustrates the functioning of the system: visual feature detectors would register minute visual elements, and a feature synthesizer would enable the child to recognize the letters *b* and *y;* a program

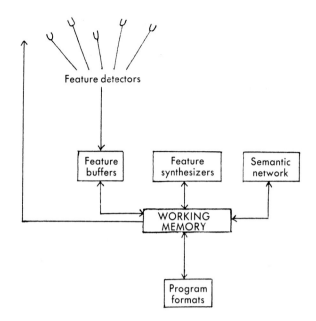

Figure 23-1 A schematic flow chart of the human information-processing system.

From Farnham-Diggory S: Learning disabilities: a psychological perspective, Cambridge, Mass, 1978, Harvard University Press.

directs the child to combine *b* and *y* to form *by;* the child reads *by,* and the meaning she attributes to this word is acquired through reference to her semantic memory. Information-processing models do not describe the actual anatomical areas of the brain that perform these functions, but because the brain is the organ that processes information in humans, the approach implies that information-processing problems may be secondary in some instances to brain dysfunction.

Information-processing models like the one just described generate interesting theoretical explanations for the presence of learning disabilities. Farnham-Diggory[68] suggested that the type of learning disability to emerge may be contingent on the component in the system where breakdown occurs or on the availability of programs. Some children may have perfectly intact components, but they simply never have learned the strategies that enhance learning. Other children may be victims of faulty processing in any one or several of the components. The former group seems less likely to have a brain dysfunction than the latter. The information-processing model, then, suggests that some but not all learning disabilities could be neurologically related.

A number of studies have been conducted to determine at which points, as information flows through the system, a learning disability may emerge. Stanley and Hall[183] suggested that individuals with dyslexia, when compared to normal readers, seemed to retain information in the sensory buffer for longer periods of time and retrieve information less efficiently. Farnham-Diggory[68] interpreted this study to suggest that the feature detector in the individuals with dyslexia was sluggish in clearing itself, and the feature synthesizer was slower in synthesizing information. Individuals with dyslexia appear to retrieve and react to letters more slowly than normal readers; visual images (with the exception of digits) appear to linger for longer periods of time in their memories.[181-183] Farnham-Diggory[68] proposed that, if information persists in the buffer, it may interfere with the registration of new information. She suggested the net effect of this may be a blurring of details. It seems logical to assume that washing away of detail could result in a reading problem.

COGNITIVE STRATEGY DEFICIT HYPOTHESIS

The cognitive strategy deficit hypothesis emerged from information processing theories, and is becoming very popular in learning disabilities research today. Cognitive strategies are analogous to computer programs that organize and integrate information on a higher level than simple detection and storage of sensory data. These strategies are derived from information-processing models that assume that in learning, a person actively generates strategies that impart meaning to the task at hand.[205] For example, when faced with new academic material to learn, a child might relate the new material by familiar knowledge, create mental images, or rehearse the material by silently repeating it. There is some evidence that children with learning disabilities do not spontaneously generate cognitive strategies to the same degree as their normally achieving age-mates.[162,191] Cognitive strategy training, therefore, is beginning to be used by educators to help children with learning disabilities.[1,136]

Metacognition is related to the issue of cognitive strategies. This is defined as the knowledge that one has about one's own cognitive processes.[73] Some examples of behaviors based on metacognition include writing down a phone number to remember it, going to a quiet place to study, and using a mnemonic "trick" such as reciting a poem that provides cues for recalling the cranial nerves in correct order. The person performing each of these behavioral strategies demonstrates an awareness that she will not pay attention or remember unless something special is done. In essence, study skills are metacognitive strategies.[48] Specific metacognitive strategy training is viewed by some as fertile ground for helping children with learning disabilities.[98,122]

One type of intervention designed to improve metacognitive strategies in children with learning disabilities is called cognitive behavior modification.[89,138] Meichenbaum[138] is generally considered the originator of this approach, which employs verbal techniques that emphasize the child's internalized speech as an organizational guide. The child is taught to ask self-questions and answer them in an orderly sequence, such as, "What am I supposed to do? I am supposed to do this and this. Am I doing it? Good, I did it correctly."[121] Although somewhat successful, this kind of training has been questioned regarding its generalization and durability.[1,107,139] The same questions have been raised in relation to other cognitive training techniques. In general, it appears that individual differences among children influence the relative effectiveness of the various cognitive interventions.[108] In other words, what works well for one child may not help another.

THE COGNITIVE DELAY HYPOTHESIS

A group of researchers and theoreticians endorse the position that some so-called learning disabilities are actually nothing more than manifestations of immaturity.[7,58] In this perspective, learning disabilities are explained on the basis of timing. Proponents believe that the vast majority of learning disabilities would be eliminated if educational demands were tailored to the developmental, rather than the chronological, age of the child.[7]

To some extent the cognitive delay hypothesis overlaps with the information-processing and attentional deficit models of learning disabilities. Attentional mechanisms and information-processing strategies are age-dependent and are acquired at a later chronological age in children with alleged learning disabilities.[42,78,88,177,191] Perhaps poor school adjustment is simply a result of the child's unreadiness in her ability to focus attention on relevant stimuli; or it may result from expecting the child to master academic skills for which she has not yet developed sufficient cognitive strategies.

Accepting the position that underachievement is a manifestation of delayed maturity leads to specific guidelines for intervention. Ames[7] recommends that the label *learning disabled* not be used. Instead, she suggests that school officials make a simple adjustment in grade assignment. Placement of the child in a grade with chronologically younger children in which she can meet the task demands eliminates the need for any special program. A counterposition might be to retain the child in a class with children her age, but provide her with a program that might accelerate maturation.

THE NEUROPSYCHOLOGICAL SUBTYPES HYPOTHESIS

The hypothesis that there are different neuropsychological types of learning disabilities is a direct outgrowth of the brain localization studies during the early foundation phase of the field of learning disabilities. In earlier years, researchers treated the concept of "minimal brain dysfunction" as if it were a single disorder responsible for a specific set of symptoms resulting in learning disabilities. Today, however, a more popular view is that there probably are a number of different types of brain dysfunctions that lead to different kinds of learning disabilities. Rather than seeking one basic deficit underlying learning disabilities, researchers now direct their efforts toward identifying the variety of patterns in which learning disabilities may be manifest.[124,133,169,173,175]

Research into neuropsychological subtypes is often referred to as the "subtyping" literature in learning disabilities. Researchers in this area have relied heavily on multivariate statistical techniques, such as factor analysis and cluster analysis, to identify learning disability subtypes.[169] As discussed later in this chapter, this is the same approach that has been used by Ayres and others to identify types of sensory integrative dysfunction.

Much of subtyping research has been conducted on children identified as dyslexic or reading disordered. In a classic study, Mattis, French, and Rapin[133] identified three types of dyslexia: (1) a language disorder in which the children had good visual-motor skills but poor expressive vocabulary and other evidence of linguistic dysfunction; (2) an articulatory and graphomotor disorder, in which subjects had normal linguistic skills but poor articulation and visual-motor skills; and (3) a visuo-spatial perceptual disorder, characterized by visual perceptual impairment, poor visual memory, and relatively good verbal skills. Although subsequent studies have tended to identify more than three subgroups of disabled readers, they have been consistent in distinguishing among disorders that are primarily language-based vs those with more prominent visual-perceptual or visual-motor involvement.[62,124,158,174]

Studies of children more generally identified as learning disabled have revealed similar patterns.[125,137,180] It should be noted that many of the subgroups identified in these studies present a combination of language and visual perceptual deficits rather than purely one or the other. Even so, the distinction between linguistic and visual contributions to academic achievement is intriguing. There is some evidence that different academic skills require varying degrees of language and visual-spatial abilities. Arithmetic, for example, is thought to be heavily reliant on language processing.[168]

The subtyping studies have been linked theoretically to cerebral specialization as a factor in learning disabilities. Evidence is considerable that the left hemisphere of the brain is specialized for verbal functions and tasks requiring sequencing, while the right hemisphere is specialized for visual-spatial and tactile perception.[46,81,114] Some researchers have suggested that learning disabilities may emerge when one cerebral hemisphere is not sufficiently specialized for a function or when, in the presence of adequate specialization, the other hemisphere is dysfunctional.[54] Perhaps the

learning disability subtype characterized by verbal deficits is a result of poor left hemisphere functioning. The visual-spatial type, then, might be due to poor right hemisphere functioning.

Although promising, this area of research has not gone unchallenged. Hiscock and Kinsbourne,[97] for example, state that available evidence indicates that anomalous hemispheric specialization is not associated with cognitive deficit. After reviewing the literature in this area, they found that it was impossible to draw a conclusion about the contribution of cerebral specialization to learning.[116]

ENVIRONMENTAL INTERACTION HYPOTHESIS

In each of the hypotheses about learning disabilities that have been discussed so far, the cause of the problem is assumed to be internal. However, some theorists have argued that environmental variables are critical in whether or not a child becomes labeled "learning disabled."[3,57,104] To ignore the role of situational or experiential factors, then, would lead to false conclusions about the nature of learning disabilities. External factors must be considered if an accurate understanding of learning disabilities is to be acquired.

Kavale and Forness[104] present a model that emphasizes interactions among student attributes, environmental influences, and instructional features. Student attributes include within-child characteristics such as those described in the preceding sections of this chapter, for example, neuropsychological patterns of abilities. Variables that are classed as environmental influences include elements related to general family characteristics and educational environments. Instructional variables are those that relate to teacher behavior, classroom management, instructional processes, and curriculum structure. In this model, learning disabilities occur when a child's special attributes are not compatible with the level of instruction provided in the classroom Kavale and Forness[104] speculate that a mismatch occurs when there is a gap between what is needed by a particular child and what is provided by the teacher. This can lead to motivational problems that compound the problem as the child disengages from the school learning process.

In another model, Adelman and Taylor[3] suggest that learning problems be conceptualized on a continuum with central nervous system (CNS) dysfunction on one end and environmental inadequacies on the other. At the CNS end of the continuum would be those children whose learning problems are *primarily* due to CNS dysfunction; at the opposite end would be children whose problems *primarily* stem from environmentally based problems such as inadequate exposure to challenging experiences and poor teaching. In the middle of the continuum are problems stemming mainly from person-environment interactions. Children who don't learn well in situations that ignore their individual differences or exacerbate their vulnerabilities would be placed here. Adelman and Taylor[3] note that, in keeping with current definitions of learning disability (see following section in this chapter), they reserve the term "learning disabilities" for those children whose learning problems are caused by minor CNS dysfunction. It is important for occupational therapists to realize, however, that many of the children identified by school systems as learning disabled (LD) may not have CNS dysfunction. They may be labeled LD because they need special education to help them achieve in the face of a history of deleterious environmental or personal-environmental interactions.

The definitional quandary: characteristics of the child with learning disabilities

The history of the education of children with learning disabilities has had its impact on the terms used as labels for the condition. Learning disabilities were first identified as concomitants of brain damage. When children without known lesions had the characteristics of persons with brain damage, an inference was made that they too had brain damage, or dysfunction, of a minimal nature. The term minimal brain damage, or dysfunction, was coined and loosely used to classify a variety of children who to one extent or another had learning problems, were hyperactive, had perceptual problems, perseverated, and were clumsy. Generally, children labeled with these terms possessed measured intelligence within the normative range.

Use of the terms minimal brain damage and minimal brain dysfunction, both popular in labeling these children in the 1950s, makes certain assumptions about the precise nature of the condition. The first term, minimal brain damage, implies that a lesion, that is, a site of pathology, exists in the brain. This term might be considered pejorative by both the child and her parents when no hard evidence can be produced indicating anatomic damage to the brain. The term minimal brain dysfunction is more nebulous, softer, and perhaps less offensive. This term does not imply that the child's brain is literally damaged; rather, it suggests that an area of the brain may not be functioning adequately. Although the latter term is less objectionable to parents than the first, it is still unacceptable to some.[82]

In 1963 Dr. Samuel Kirk, at a conference sponsored by the Fund for Perceptually Handicapped Children, argued that the term minimal brain dysfunction was of little use in educational settings because it did not lead to classroom management strategies.[82] He went on to say that he was recently using the term learning disabilities to describe children with disorders in speech, language, reading, and associated communication skills who were neither blind, deaf, nor mentally retarded. He pointed out that this definition had the advantage of avoiding the difficulties inherent in trying to establish with certainty brain dysfunction.

Definitions that have been used at the federal level have, in essence, been in accord with Kirk's ideas. Under Public Law 94-142, specific learning disability is defined as:

A disorder in one or more of the basic psychological processes involved in understanding or in using language, spoken or written, which may manifest itself in an imperfect ability to listen, think, speak, read, write, spell or to do mathematical calculation. The term includes such conditions as perceptual handicaps, brain injury, minimal brain dysfunction, dyslexia, and developmental aphasia. The term does not include children who have learning problems which are primarily the result of visual, hearing, or motor handicaps, or mental retardation, or of environmental, cultural or economic disadvantages.[82]

Gearheart[82] points out that although this definition was accepted on a federal level, it was not accepted without controversy in the field of special education. He suggests that the definition was written into federal law because it was the least unacceptable among several alternatives. Criticisms leveled against the definition have been that it does not sufficiently emphasize the neurophysiological nature of the disorder[59,60] and that it is not sufficiently usable.[204] Standardized tests are not available that reliably differentiate children with learning disabilities from children with emotional disturbance or children who underachieve because of educational deprivation.[204] So much controversy exists regarding an acceptable definition of learning disabilities that the January 1983 issue of the *Journal of Learning Disabilities* featured articles on the topic written by a set of experts.[107,145,172] In addition, data from a survey published in this issue revealed that Child Service Demonstration Centers (the federally funded educational model programs for children with learning disabilities) failed to comply with the federal definition of learning disabilities.[132]

In the Child Service Demonstration Centers, low achievement, language difficulties, perceptual deficits, a discrepancy between ability and achievement, and failure in the mainstream were the most frequently cited criteria for diagnosing children as having learning disabilities.[132] In another study,[66] 14 different operational definitions of learning disabilities (LD) were found in the professional literature. These formulas for classifying children as LD were based on either ability-achievement discrepancy (a difference of 10 or more points between full-scale IQ score and an achievement test score), low achievement (a score of 85 or below on a standardized achievement test), or test score scatter (a discrepancy of 9 or more points between verbal and performance IQ scores).

Despite disagreements over exactly how to identify a particular child as learning disabled, one group of individuals from diverse perspectives was able to agree upon a general definition of learning disabilities. The

National Joint Committee on Learning Disabilities consists of representatives from six professional and parent organizations. Their definition of learning disabilities is cited often:

> Learning disabilities is a generic term that refers to a heterogeneous group of disorders manifested by significant difficulties in the acquisition and use of listening, speaking, reading, writing, reasoning, or mathematical abilities. These disorders are intrinsic to the individual and presumed to be due to central nervous system dysfunction. Even though a learning disability may occur concomitantly with other handicapping conditions (e.g., sensory impairment, mental retardation, social and emotional disturbance) or environmental influences (e.g., cultural differences, insufficient/inappropriate instruction, psychogenic factors), it is not the direct result of those conditions or influences.[147]

Widely used textbooks in the field of learning disabilities reflect the views held by the proverbial average special educator. Gearheart[83] notes a severe discrepancy between academic achievement and ability and learning in a specific area (for example, oral expression and written expression) as being central to identification. He then lists eight other characteristics as shown below.[83] Some of these characteristics are contradictory, but this is reasonable since Gearheart makes the point that not all the symptoms must be present in a single child.

1. *Hyperactivity.* Restlessness; the quality of being unable to sit still. Excessive movement that may interfere with the ability to selectively attend to stimuli. The child is in perpetual motion.

2. *Hypoactivity.* The opposite of hyperactivity; listlessness; sluggishness. Gearheart states that this characteristic is not as common as hyperactivity.

3. *Inattention.* The inability to focus attention on any one task for any sustained length of time.

4. *Overattention.* The inability to break a focus after having been concentrating on an activity for a sustained length of time. Gearheart links overattention to figure-ground ability. Rather than directing the attention to the significant elements in a picture, the child will focus on the background.

5. *Lack of coordination.* The inability to move the muscles in a smooth manner. Gearheart points out that although some children with learning disabilities do not have problems with coordination, many do. At a young age, the signs of poor coordination may be poor or slow achievement of developmental milestones. For example, the child may have difficulty throwing a ball, skipping, or running. The child may be clumsy and trip frequently.

6. *Perceptual disorders.* Gearheart lists problems in visual, auditory, tactile, proprioceptive, and vestibular perception as most common. He states that problems in olfactory and gustatory perception are less likely to be associated with a learning disability, but he does not document his statement. Gearheart points out that visual-spatial problems may interfere with accurate copy-

ing of letters. He suggests that these children may have difficulty distinguishing the ringing of a phone from that of a doorbell. If a sensory acuity deficit is ruled out, perceptual disorders may be present.

7. *Perseveration.* These children may repeat actions persistently in several behavioral domains. Perseveration of verbal responses, but especially in writing and copying, may be noted.

8. *Memory disorders.* Problems may be with either visual or auditory memory or both. The child may be unable to remember a sequence of objects she has just seen or repeat several letters she has just heard. Children with these problems may forget the words in the beginning of a sentence before they read those at the end.

OCCUPATIONAL THERAPY AND THE TREATMENT OF THE CHILD WITH LEARNING DISABILITIES

Children with learning disabilities can be treated in medical, educational, or private practice settings. Each setting has its own sets of constraints and sets of professionals. Chapters 1 and 2 of this text describe these settings and the professional personnel who work within them.

Occupational therapists are concerned with the role performance of the child with learning disabilities. The student role requires competence in learning and in the organization of the customary daily round of activities in which one must engage to foster learning. A learning problem can result when a child's brain is not able to organize sensory input or when the child is inefficient in organizing her behavior and concentrating on learning tasks. A type of neural irregularity may be associated with difficulty in developing habits that support academic achievement, such as automatic use of verbal rehearsal, or the discipline required to do homework and study. The child may be unable to manage daily activities in ways that optimize student role performance.

Most often the occupational therapist has treated the child with learning disabilities with sensory integrative procedures that aim to improve efficiency of neural processing. While research shows that a sensory integrative approach benefits some children with learning disabilities,[20,25,29] it is not appropriate for all. The occupational behavior frame of reference, which can be interpreted to subsume the use of sensory integrative procedures,[127,163] provides a global perspective that expands the focus of occupational therapy from the neurobiological to the sociocultural and environmental dimensions.

Most of this chapter goes into detail on the use of sensory integrative procedures for children with learning disabilities. Initially, however, a brief coverage of the occupational behavior frame of reference in relation to the child who is considered learning disabled is provided. The inclusion of this section reflects the conviction that occupational behavior is a broad conceptual framework that can guide occupational therapy with children with learning disabilities, regardless of whether or not sensory integrative procedures are applied.

The occupational behavior frame of reference and the child with a learning disability

The occupational behavior approach (Chapter 3) has special relevance for the child with learning disabilities. Takata,[189] in the introduction to a series of articles on occupational behavior in pediatrics, states that the movement of pediatric occupational therapy practice from hospitals to schools requires expanding occupational therapy approaches beyond those derived from sensory integrative theory. In the occupational behavior approach, as Takata describes it, the focus is on how effectively the individual occupies particular life roles in the family, in school, and in the community. Children and youth in need of health care are seen not as individuals with categorical disabilities, such as cerebral palsy, or learning disabilities, or mental retardation, but as individuals who are required to meet specific expectations associated with particular roles. This assumption, when applied to the child with learning disabilities, translates into a concern for how well the child is performing in a student role.

ASSESSMENT

When using the occupational behavior frame of reference, the therapist may assess both mother and child and other related individuals using open-ended questions, interviews, and informal observation based on the guiding questions that have already been listed. Standardized assessments may also be used. Mailloux, Knox, Burke, and Clark[130] provide tables that illustrate the assessments that may be used in pediatric occupational therapy when the model of human occupation, a theoretic model in the tradition of occupational behavior, is utilized. Although the case illustrations in this chapter do not focus on learning disability, the general approach does apply to children with learning disabilities. Typically, when the occupational behavior approach is used, the play style and history of the child, the role performance, and the quality of daily engagement in activities is assessed. Florey[74] lists some specific instruments that may be used. In using the occupational behavior approach with the child with learning disability, the therapist might address the following questions:

1. How does the child play? Is play encouraged or discouraged by her parents or by the home environment? Does the child's play support the building of skills that are required to succeed as a student?
2. How is the child proceeding in the occupational choice process? Is she in the fantasy, tentative, or real-

istic stage? Will his or her learning disability render occupational choices unrealistic?[196]
3. How does the child's home environment encourage or discourage success in the student role? Does it contain elements that suggest a valuing of school-related competencies? Is it conducive to an organized approach to studying and mastery of school requirements? What are the family's attitudes toward the skills that support academic achievement and school social adjustment? Will the home environment generate in the child a desire to do well in school?[41]
4. What kind of habits has the child developed? Does he or she effectively organize behavior into routines that are consistent with task requirements, both in the home and in the school setting? To what extent does someone else organize his or her activity?
5. What are the unspoken demands of the home and school environment? Is the child expected to perform beyond current skill levels? What are the requirements of the child's role as student?[41]

These questions were generated from the occupational behavior perspective that was originated by Reilly[163] and that since has been extended in the writing of numerous other therapists. Kielhofner and Burke[111] and Kielhofner, Burke, and Igi[112] have synthesized many of the ideas presented in these papers. In brief, these writers suggest that central to the occupational behavior perspective is the idea that skills are consolidated by the child into habits and internalized roles. Habits are defined as automatic routines that provide consistency in daily life. When habits fail, conscious decision-making (or volition) must be employed. Habits undergo transformations as the child matures. For example, on entry to school, first grade children will apply habits learned at home to the new setting. If they had had the pattern of hanging their coats up when they entered their homes, they would be likely to adapt and use this habit in the new school setting. Similarly, if they had learned to maintain a neat work space during projects at home, it is unlikely they would be messy in task performance in kindergarten.

Internalized roles were defined by Kielhofner and Burke[111] as a personal sense of the complete set of behaviors required in occupying a position in a social group. The role of student encompasses behaviors that support both academic achievement and social adjustment in the classroom. It is conceivable that a child labeled as learning disabled might possess the habits that could support competency in the student role, but is simply oblivious to what is required of him. He may misread the expectations of teachers and peers. For example, he may think that being overattentive is a desirable trait, and enactment of this characteristic might interfere with learning. More commonly, though, the breakdown of role performance of the child with learning disabilities appears to result from insufficient or inappropriate skills and habits that organize behavior, rather than from misconstruing role expectations.

Thus far the discussion of the role dysfunction of the

child with learning disability has focused on the role of student. This focus is consistent with a major tenet of the occupational behavior frame of reference that treats the occupational role as an entity distinct from familial and sexual roles. Occupational roles are defined by Kielhofner and Burke[111] as "the productive roles that determine the bulk of daily routines and thus organize most of the behavior within the system." For the school-aged child, the role of student meets the specifications of this definition. At the same time, it is permissible for the therapist using this approach to address familial and sexual roles, especially in relation to how they influence occupational role performance.

GOALS OF THERAPY

Following assessment of the child with learning disability, a treatment program is developed. Because the aim in this section is simply to provide the reader with a sense of how the occupational behavior perspective could be used with a child with learning disabilities, no attempt is made here to provide specific information on this approach. Instead, a sketch of what form the treatment might take is presented.

The occupational behavior frame of reference holds that skills are learned and mastered within the context of play. If a child with learning disabilities had a specific writing disability, for example, and was clumsy in his or her execution, the occupational therapist might provide a pressure-free environment in which the child could use play experiences to improve coordination. In this arena the child would be free to explore the properties of writing implements and of her own body as the implements are used. The therapist might consult with the child's parents, providing guidance on how play experiences at home could be constructed and encouraged to support writing proficiency.

If the child was found not to have developed sufficient interests to eventually support an optimal occupational choice, and was at the age when this is expected, the therapist might use the therapy situation for exploration of interests. The therapist might involve the child in activities he or she had never engaged in before and encourage the child to appraise how satisfying such an experience was. The therapist additionally might try to familiarize the child with potential occupations with which his or her learning disability would not interfere.

A third goal of therapy might be to make recommendations for how the home environment might be altered to support the child's student role performance. If the child was found to be distractible, a minimally stimulating and isolated area of the house could be designated as a study area for the child. A proper work space could be designed or constructed and supplies could be purchased (presuming the family had sufficient funds); lighting could be assessed and altered if it was found to be less than optimum. The child's daily habits could be addressed. If he or she lacked organiza-

tion, the therapist could work on organization and sequencing of simple daily tasks. If the parents had not provided opportunities for the child to organize his or her own behavior, the therapist could encourage them to do so.

Finally, within the clinic situation the child could be presented with environmental challenges matched to the child's level of skill so that he or she could experience a sense of success. Media such as art, games, and play chosen to be in accord with the child's readiness would be used. While participating in these activities, the therapist could note whether there is improvement in the child's ability to selectively attend to relevant stimuli and improvement in work habits, organization of behavior, risk-taking, and decision-making.

Use of organized games may be a particularly potent means of improving motor performance, cognitive abilities, attention, self-concept, and social interaction.[113] Hurff[99] has described a specific gaming technique that can be applied to teaching strategies of daily living to children with severe learning disabilities. Games differ from play in that they are more systematic and organized and involve goal-oriented interaction with some form of opposition. Although reports of these techniques have been related to individuals with mental retardation, gaming strategies have great promise for use with children with learning disabilities.

The sensory integrative approach
BACKGROUND

Sensory integrative procedures are widely used in occupational therapy practice with children with learning disabilities. Guidelines for the use of these procedures were derived from principles of sensory integrative theory as developed and described by Ayres[21,28,30] (see Chapter 3). For the entry-level therapist to comprehend the place of this approach within the practice of occupational therapy and how it is specifically used with the child with learning disabilities, the knowledge of the forces that contributed to its evolution is essential. The entry-level therapist needs to be provided with an overview of how the applications of sensory integrative theory were developed and underwent change. A perspective is also needed on the current use of these procedures with children with learning disabilities.

Before the development of sensory integrative theory, occupational therapists had traditionally been concerned with the relationship of childhood occupation to disability. Occupations, in this context, refer to the purposeful, culturally defined, and self-directed activities children engage in during their customary daily round of activities.[206] Occupational therapists also had a long history of addressing the disorders of language, movement, and perception that followed brain injury. Sensory integrative procedures, when they emerged, were a logical and natural extension of past practice.

THE TRADITIONAL FOCUS ON CHILDHOOD OCCUPATION

In the 1940s and 1950s pediatric occupational therapy was described by physicians as an essential medically-related profession that contributed to the well-being of the hospitalized child.[44,159,164] Occupational therapists were described as being concerned with the play and daily life activities (occupations) of the child. In this period Allessandrini[4] extolled the virtues of play, arguing that it was a serious undertaking for children, which should not be confused with diversion or ill use of time.

The tradition of using play as a treatment medium has been continued through the development of the occupational behavior frame of reference. However, the idea that culturally defined self-directed and purposeful activity should be used as a treatment medium was also retained in the applications of sensory integrative theory to practice. Treatment in this approach would be directed toward improvement in the organization of behavior through self-directed, purposeful, and pleasurable activity, which in addition was chosen for its organizing effects on the brain.

INTEREST IN DISORDERS OF SYMBOLIC FUNCTION FOLLOWING BRAIN INJURY

Occupational therapists, before the emergence of sensory integrative theory, had had an interest in disorders of symbolic functions following brain injury. Their experience in the area made them a natural choice among the available professions for treating children with learning disabilities. In the early 1950s two papers were published that addressed the relationship of occupational therapy to aphasia.[84,157] Palmer and Berko[157] reviewed the classic works on brain localization and aphasia (for example, studies by Broca) and described Goldstein's ideas on the characteristics of brain-damaged adults. Giden, Eno, and Bosley[84] described how aphasia and other disturbances associated with brain injury affected performance of workshop activities such as weaving. They suggested that with aphasia patients therapists should deemphasize perfection and allow success, and therapists should start with familiar activities and select those that would prepare the patient for future role performance.

McDaniel[135] reiterated many of the ideas originally presented by Giden, Eno, and Bosley. In her paper the aphasia-related disorders were reviewed with descriptions of both the language-related (for example, sensory aphasia and motor aphasia) and the nonlanguage-related disturbances (for example, loss of attention, concentration, perseverance, and poor organizational abilities). McDaniel[135] recommended that occupational therapists provide speech reeducation programs when speech therapists were not available. When they were, she suggested that occupational therapists reinforce speech acquisition within the context of purposeful activity.

The fact that occupational therapists had had a tradition of working with aphasic adults and children before the 1960s when sensory integrative theory was developed probably influenced how that theory would be conceptualized. The publications previously cited[84,135] presented two principles that would be retained in sensory integrative theory. First, they suggested that within the context of occupation (or purposeful activity) language acquisition might be indirectly enhanced. Second, they suggested that engagement in activity could be graded in accord with severity of brain dysfunction.

USE OF SENSORY STIMULATION TO EVOKE COORDINATED MOTOR RESPONSES

Occupational therapists had traditionally practiced in hospital settings with patients who had neuromuscular problems secondary to brain damage (for example, cerebral vascular accident or cerebral palsy). Uncoordinated movement patterns, abnormal muscle tone, and the presence of abnormal reflexes interfered with performance of functional and purposeful activities. It became clear to therapists in the 1950s and 1960s that increased normalization of motor performance was a prerequisite to the achievement of self-care and other skills.

In this period a number of treatment approaches were described in the literature in which neurophysiological principles, emphasizing sensory stimulation, were employed to promote better execution of movement patterns. These approaches are called sensorimotor because all of them emphasized the relationship between sensation and the motor response. Principles of these approaches would be incorporated in sensory integrative theory when it emerged. However, in its concern with occupation, self-directed activity, symbolic functions, and the capacity of the individual to organize his own behavior, sensory integrative theory would depart from these approaches and become a distinct entity.

In the 1950s and 1960s publications by Mysak and Fiorentino,[146] Ayres,[10] and Voss[195] were representative of the sensorimotor approach. Procedures described tended to be specific to particular muscle groups and were based on detailed and precise descriptions of neurophysiological principles derived from laboratory studies on lower animals. Concepts in neurophysiology, such as summation, irradiation, and inhibition, were defined and inferences were made as to how these concepts could be employed in treatment to foster more normal movement patterns in patients with brain lesions. The proprioceptive and tactile base of movement was given strong emphasis.

The sensorimotor approaches armed occupational therapists with numerous techniques based on sound physiological principles for improving patients' neuromuscular responses. The notion that sensory input could improve motor responses would become a major principle of sensory integrative theory.

CONCERN WITH PERCEPTION AND THE ORGANIZATION OF BEHAVIOR

Occupational therapists have had a tradition of being concerned with how brain-damaged and mentally ill patients could learn to better organize their behavior, perceive their environments accurately, and exercise sufficient concentration on a task to complete it successfully. They have been particularly concerned with how occupation could be used to promote these capacities. In 1949 Ayres[8] presented principles of grading activities in accord with organic reactions of the brain to electroshock (a treatment that is used in mental health facilities for depressed patients). She suggested that activities be selected that psychodynamically matched the affective state of the client. Postelectroshock patients were described as having "confused and clouded sensorium"[8] progressive memory loss, impaired coordination, and an inability to perform abstract reasoning or use their imaginations. The ways in which numerous craft activities (occupations) could be adapted to promote organized behavior in these patients were then detailed.

Engagement in purposeful activity required patients to be able to accurately perceive the tools and other objects in their environment, sequence their actions to accomplish a goal and execute the appropriate motor responses. In 1954 Robinault[165] argued that the role of occupational therapy needed to be broadened with the child with cerebral palsy. She suggested it should include the teaching of colors, shapes, and size discrimination. She regarded the focus on the mechanics of grasp and release and on self-care skills as necessary but not sufficient for the rehabilitation of these children.

In the same year Ayres[9] published a paper in which she discussed how principles of ontogeny could be used for developing arm and hand functions. In a paper published in 1958, which was influenced by the ideas of Rood,[166] Hebb,[95] and Strauss and Kephart,[185] Ayres[11] further elaborated on her ideas on the interface between occupational therapy and visual-motor functions, that is, eye-hand coordination. Ayres defined perception as, "the use of sensations, rather than raw sensations in themselves."[11] The perceptual process was defined as being concerned with how the sources of sensation were integrated for use. In contrast to it, Ayres described the motor process as entailing ideation of the task to be performed (ideational motor planning). Principles and procedures for training visual-motor functions involving primarily tabletop activities, such as puzzles and pegboards, were then described.

Occupational therapy's concern with perceptual functions was also reflected in an article by Troyer[192] who presented many ideas on how therapists could use activity to enhance perceptual-motor functions. Troyer maintained that integration of the sensory and motor systems was required for the development of precise, coordinated, active, and perceptive individuals.

The emergence of sensory integrative theory and its research base for practice

Sensory integrative theory has been developed over the course of more than 20 years: 1960 to the present. The theory addresses how humans develop the capacity to organize sensation for the purpose of accomplishing self-directed, meaningful activity. It should be noted that in this chapter, sensory integrative theory is being defined as the concepts presented by Ayres.[21,30,31] We do not consider this theory to be within the same category as the sensorimotor theories of Bobath, Rood, and Voss who have primarily addressed the eliciting of coordinated motor responses, that is, neuromuscular function.[45,166,195] At the same time, we acknowledge, as did Ayres, that some of the principles of the sensorimotor approaches were incorporated into the building of sensory integrative theory. The use of sensory integrative procedures is sometimes referred to as sensory integrative therapy. We discourage the use of this term, because it implies separateness from occupational therapy. Sensory integrative procedures are designed to be used within the context of occupational therapy.

Sensory integrative theory continues to undergo modification. Support for its validity is found in neurobehavioral studies (generally conducted on animals), in studies on child development, and in research on children with learning disabilities, as well as on those with other disabling conditions. In this section, the steps in the research process that Ayres took in developing the theory are reviewed to lessen the potential for misuse of the theory, its procedures, and its instruments. A grasp of the research base of this theory is also essential for those therapists who may be called upon to justify its use in practice, for example, in testifying at an educational placement hearing.

Sensory integrative theory is complex; mastering it requires extensive reading of the neurobiological literature, a solid preparation in neurophysiology and neuroanatomy, and study of Ayres' original writings. We distinguish between the theory, which refers to selected concepts and principles related to central nervous system functioning and development, and the treatment procedures that follow it.

Central to the sensory integrative theory is an explanation of how children develop the capacity to organize their own behavior. Ayres[30] pointed out that the newborn hears, sees, and feels sensations from his or her body, but is unable to judge distances or attach meanings to the sound he or she hears. As the ability to organize sensation and behavior develops, the child may become better able to focus attention on relevant stimuli, remain organized for longer spans of time, and execute a customary daily round of activities in a manner that supports an occupational role. This process of organizing sensory information in the brain to make adaptive responses is what Ayres called sensory integration.[21]

The application of sensory integrative theory practice can be summarized through explication of the following principles that are drawn from Ayres.[21,30,31]

1. *Controlled sensory input can be used to elicit an adaptive response.* Ayres defines an adaptive response as "an appropriate action in which the individual responds successfully to some environmental demand."[30] It implies dealing with the environment in a "creative and useful way."[30] An example of an adaptive response in an infant is observed when she sucks competently. Rocking a hobby horse constitutes an adaptive response in the toddler (in which she must coordinate trunk flexion and extension). For the older child it may be ice skating. Adaptive responses require the child to organize sensation, accurately judge the requirements of the situation, and execute the response competently. Whenever a child experiences the type and amount of sensory stimulation that challenges but does not overwhelm the central nervous system, the evincing of an adaptive response is potentiated (Figure 23-2).

2. *An adaptive response contributes to the development of sensory integration.* Each time a child is able to successfully meet a challenge from the environment, the ability to organize sensory input to meet environmental demands increases. Ayres[21] believes that motor activity is a powerful organizer of sensory input. As adaptive responses are emitted, the nervous system uses its knowledge of the results of past actions to guide the organization of sensory information for future use.

3. *The more inner-directed a child's activities, the greater the potential of the activities for improving neural organization.* This principle assumes that children possess an inborn motivation force toward sensory integration, which Ayres calls "inner drive."[21,30] The child is seen as naturally attracted to activities that require and bring about brain organization of sensory input. For example, it can be speculated that an 18-month-old whose nervous system may be overwhelmed by the vestibular input provided by swinging would shy away from this activity. On the other hand, possibly because of an increased capacity to organize sensation of this type, 3- and 4-year-olds will seek out those activities that incorporate swinging. Therapy that makes use of this inner drive capitalizes on the inherent capacity of the child to seek out those activities that will bring about brain organization (Figure 23-3).

4. *More mature and complex patterns of behavior are composed of consolidations of more primitive behaviors.* Ayres believes that children meld previously learned functions together for the creation of more mature adaptive responses. Emission of increasingly mature adaptive responses is a product of practice of each sensory and motor element. Underlying the changes in behavioral complexity are parallel advances in neural organization. As brain stem processing of sensory input becomes more efficient, higher cortical functions are freed to develop more fully.

5. *Better organization of adaptive responses will enhance the child's general behavioral organization.* While some adaptive responses are simple unitary acts, others require more complex sequencing and timing of motor activities. The child must figure out how to or-

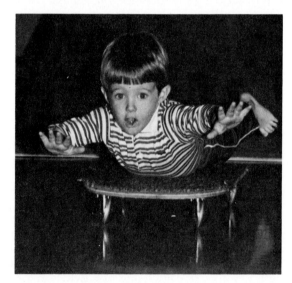

Figure 23-2 Adapted response elicited by linear vestibular stimulation.

Photograph by Dooley Brown.

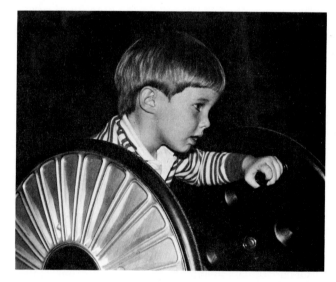

Figure 23-3 This child's expression reflects inner direction, suggesting that this activity requiring motor planning will promote neural organization.

Photograph by Dooley Brown.

der and time a set of motor responses to achieve a goal (Figure 23-4). In essence, the child must program her actions. Ayres reasons that engagement in this process may enhance the child's general programming capacity.[31] For example, an improvement in this general capacity may lead to being better able to organize the usual daily round of activities or the steps required to accomplish a school-related task.

6. *Registration of meaningful sensory input is necessary before an adaptive response can be made.* During the course of a day, individuals notice some but not all of the stimuli in their environments. The stimuli that are noticed influence the motor responses that are made. If a child is oblivious to many of the stimuli in the environment, his or her repertoire of adaptive responses will be limited, and potential for developing more complex behaviors will thus be thwarted. On the other hand, some children seem to register sensory input excessively. These children may be bombarded by input to such a degree that they have a difficulty extracting meaning from sensation or focusing on a goal-directed task.

These principles provide the foundation on which

treatment is based. Discussion of treatment will be deferred until an overview of the steps Ayres took in the construction of the theory is provided.

THE EMPIRICAL BASE OF AN EVOLVING THEORY

Instrument construction. In the late 1950s and early 1960s, based on review of the literature in development, neurobiology, psychology, education, and clinical experience, Ayres formulated hypotheses about which psychoneurological functions might be implicated in learning disabilities. She then constructed the precursors of the 18 tests that were published as the Southern California Sensory Integration Tests (SCSIT).[22] Each test was presumed to be a measure of a psychoneurological process that contributed to the capacity to learn and had set administration and scoring procedures. The tests were given to large groups of normal children, and tables of normative data were prepared. These tables indicated the average performance of children without dysfunction and within specific age groups. The test measured aspects of visual and tactile perception and certain motor functions.

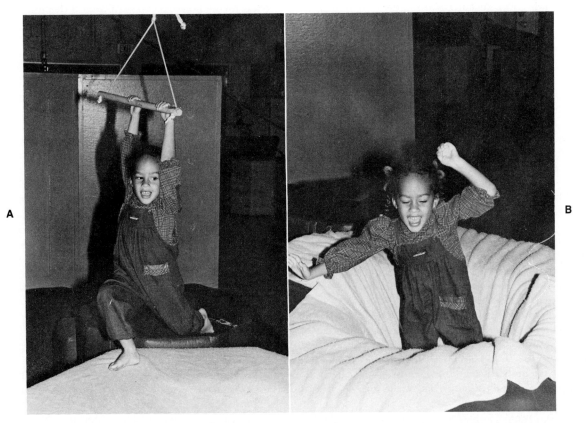

Figure 23-4   Activity requiring sequencing and timing. **A,** Child must push off and grasp the trapeze. **B,** Child then must time the release of her hands and her jump into the blanket.

Photograph by Dooley Brown.

Typology. Ayres was interested in using these tests diagnostically with children who had already been labeled as having learning problems. An assumption she made was that there were probably many different kinds of learning problems, each of which might be associated with dysfunction in a particular neural substrate. Ayres conceived of the Southern California Sensory Integration Tests as tests that would allow for the differential diagnosis of the neural substrates that contributed to learning problems.

Before the Southern California Sensory Integration Tests could be used in this way, a classification system (typology) of neural systems related to learning needed to be constructed. Ayres used a procedure called factor analysis to develop the typology. In this procedure, sets of test scores are grouped according to their associations. Ayres interpreted the clusters that emerged from the factor analytic studies she conducted on children with learning disabilities as being representative of several neural substrates contributing to learning.[21]

The factor analytic studies Ayres has conducted to date are summarized in Table 23-1. In 1965 Ayres[15] administered the precursors of the Southern California Sensory Integration Tests to 100 children suspected of having perceptual-motor handicaps (note that this term was used as a synonym for learning disabled in the 1960s) and to 50 normal children. Ayres was interested in determining whether the neural systems (factors) measured by these tests would differ in the two groups of children. Four of the factors—which she called tactile defensiveness, perceptual dysfunction form position in two-dimensional space, deficit of bilateral integration, and apraxia—emerged only in the dysfunctional group of children. These neural systems were interpreted to represent dysfunction rather than a developmental process. The fifth factor, called figure-ground perception, emerged in both groups and was interpreted as being related to a developmental process.

This study was especially important because it suggested that perceptual-motor problems were associated with neural processes involving integration of input from more than one sensory modality. From the data, the dysfunctional children did not appear to have unimodal sensory disturbances (for example, a discreet problem in visual perception). Each factor (neural system) that emerged was contributed to by at least two sensory systems. It appeared that neural substrates concerned with intersensory integration contributed to learning disabilities. This idea became a major tenet of sensory integrative theory.

In 1966 Ayres[16,17] performed the next two factor analytic studies. In the first of these, the precursors of the Southern California Sensory Integration Tests were given to 92 children, 10% of whom had possible central nervous system dysfunctions. In the second study the tests were given to 64 adopted children, aged 4 to 8, who were within the normative range on the Gesell Developmental Schedules. This study suggested that normal children did not vary in the same way as did dysfunctional children in their performances on the Southern California Sensory Integration Tests. These findings reinforced the idea that the neural systems being measured on the tests in the dysfunctional group were representative of dysfunction rather than a developmental progression. These data found support for the idea that learning disabilities were related to brain dysfunction.

In 1969 Ayres[18] conducted another major factor analytic study. In this study the neural syndromes were further defined by their extent of relationship to auditory-language functions. Ayres gave the 36 children with educational handicaps (another popular term synonymous with the term learning disabled) the Southern California Sensory Integration Tests along with the Illinois Test of Psycholinguistic Abilities. The factor structure (interpreted as neural syndromes) that emerged was relatively consistent with that found in the previous factor analytic study in which dysfunctional children made up the sample. The results suggested that the typology that had emerged could be used for diagnosing types of neural dysfunction in children with learning disabilities.

In 1972 Ayres[23] conducted a factor analysis of scores on 48 tests (including the Southern California Sensory Integration Tests and the Illinois Test of Psycholinguistic Abilities) obtained by 148 educationally handicapped children. Ayres published another paper in which she used statistical procedures (the computation of regression equations) to determine which tests were predictive of the six factors that had been isolated in the study published in 1972.[19] (Note that these two studies seem to have been published out of sequence.) The factors that emerged were labeled form and space perception, auditory-language functions, postural and bilateral integration, praxis, and functions of the left side of the body. These studies found additional support for the notion that the tests were measuring particular neural substrates related to learning that could be used to classify types of dysfunction in learning disabled children.

In 1977 Ayres[26] reported the findings on another major factor analysis. The subjects were 128 educationally handicapped children. Results suggested that Southern California Sensory Integration Tests, along with auditory-language tests, were measuring five major domains: somatosensory processing and motor planning, auditory-language functions, postural ocular responses, eye-hand coordination, and postrotary nystagmus. Importantly, in this study, the results on the Southern California Postrotary Nystagmus Test (SCPNT)[24] were included. This test was a measure of the duration of reflexive and to-and-fro movements of the eyes that are induced by rotation about the body axis. Results of this test were interpreted as an index of the status of some aspects of vestibular function.

Most recently, Ayres and her colleagues[38] have reported results of further analyses to refine our understanding of the precise nature of the sensory integrative dysfunctions that seem to underlie learning and behavior problems. These analyses are similar to those already presented, with two exceptions. First, they used scores on four new praxis tests—Sequencing Praxis, Praxis on Verbal Command, Block Building Test, and Oral Praxis—tests which will, in modified form, become part of the new battery of Sensory Integration and Praxis Tests[34] soon to be published by Western Psychological Services. Second, they incorporated statistical procedures that had not been used in the previous studies. In the study reported by Ayres, Mailloux, and Wendler[38], the major finding was that praxis seems to be a unitary function that is manifest in various tasks. Somatosensory perception was highly related to this factor the authors call a somatopractic function. In the second study, Ayres found once again that tactile and practic scores are related. Short duration postrotary nystagmus was not statistically associated with praxis. Further, inconsistencies between computer-generated clusters over Ayres' subjective categories and those that had been identified through factor analyses elucidated the complexity of practic and tactile functions in the young developing brain.

For the most part, when the Southern California Sensory Integration Tests were given to different samples of children, their factor structure remained fairly consistent. Table 23-2 provides a perspective on which of the factors (neural systems) were isolated most consistently. In the studies through 1977, it can be seen that the apraxia factor emerged in nearly all the studies in which dysfunctional children made up the sample. Deficits in form and space perception were more varied, and the configuration and patterns of the clusters suggested that there were at least two kinds of visual perceptual problems. The first seemed to be related to somatosensory processing, the second to functions associated with the right hemisphere. Deficits in postural and bilateral integration emerged relatively consistently in earlier studies.[15,18] Finally, auditory-language dysfunctions seemed to bifurcate in the same way that visual spatial perception had. One type seemed to be related to the left hemisphere and did not seem to be related to sensory integrative processes. The second type was found in association with vestibular dysfunction and poor bilateral integration. In nearly every study a strong association between tactile defensiveness and hyperactivity was found.

Results across these studies were synthesized, and a typology was adopted for diagnosing types of sensory integrative dysfunction on the basis of the Southern California Sensory Integration Tests and Southern California Postrotary Nystagmus Test scores; results of clinical observations of neuromuscular responses; and information, when available, from auditory-language tests. The following is the typology that has been in use:

1. Vestibular bilateral integration dysfunction
2. Dyspraxia
3. Left hemisphere dysfunction
4. Right hemisphere dysfunction
5. Generalized dysfunction

Detailed descriptions of these neural systems are presented in a subsequent section of this chapter. It should be noted that the factor structure of the tests suggested that the various neural systems were interrelated. It could also be interpreted hierarchically with some factors hypothesized to be substrates for others. The factor structure was found to make sense in relation to neurobiological theory. (See Ayres[21,22] for the interpretation of these factors.) This finding helped to validate that the tests were measuring neurophysiological function. The complexity of the factor structure and its dependence on both scores on standardized tests and on clinical observations suggested that clinical experience, familiarity with tests and measurement theory, and knowledge of sensory integration research and theory were requirements for sound interpretation of the Southern California Sensory Integration Tests. These tests could not be mastered at the undergraduate level.

In recent years, Ayres and her colleagues have been involved in the development and standardization of the Sensory Integration and Praxis Tests (SIPT)[34] which will replace the SCSIT. Standardized on a North American sample of over 2,500 children, validity studies on these tests, not yet reported in the literature, are expected to further refine our understanding of the typology of sensory integrative dysfunctions. Results of these studies should be published by 1989 and will be used for identifying the presence of types of sensory integrative dysfunction in normal children.

Experimentation. The development of the typology enabled experienced therapists proficient in the administration and interpretation of the Southern California Sensory Integration Tests to provisionally and differentially diagnose the type of neural dysfunctions that might be present in children with learning disabilities. However, the ultimate test of the theory's validity rested on whether it could be demonstrated to possess predictive validity. Evidence was needed that, once children were diagnosed as having sensory integrative dysfunction and were then treated in accord with the specific type of dysfunction identified (such as dyspraxia or vestibular bilateral integration dysfunction), the treatment was effective in remediating learning problems. Such studies could provide further evidence that sensory integration was a contributor to some types of learning disabilities and that inferences made to treatment based on the theory were sound.

Ayres[20,29] conducted two studies that addressed

Table 23-1 Purpose, hypotheses, design, results, and contributions of Ayres' factor analytic and regression studies

Year	Purpose	Instruments	Hypothesis	Design	Subjects	Results	Contribution to theory
1965	Identify relationships among sensory perception, motor performance, laterality in normal and children with perceptual problems. Establish construct and discriminant validity	Early versions of the Southern California Sensory Integration Tests, (SCSIT), additional perceptual-motor and laterality tests, also freedom from hyperactivity and tactile defensiveness	Test results would identify factors for children with and without dysfunction. Normal and dysfunctional children will demonstrate different factors	Thirty-three tests Two behavioral parameters Analysis of difference between group means Q- and R-technique factor analysis	N = 100 dysfunctional N = 50 normal Dysfunctional children had learning or behavioral disorders	Tests discriminated between normal and dysfunctional groups Five patterns detected: Apraxia Dysfunction form and space perception Deficit bilateral integration Visual figure-ground perception Tactile defensiveness	Established discriminant validity of early versions of test Most children demonstrated more than one factor, therefore factors related Sensory integration-clusters were not by sensory systems Praxis and tactile functions linked Tactile defensiveness, hyperactivity, distractibility linked Cognitive aspects deemphasized Eye-hand agreement not discriminative Empirical support for syndromes
1966a	Explore perceptual-motor function relationships in a normal sample and compare with prior studies Establish construct validity	Frostig tests, early versions of the SCSIT Also freedom from hyperactivity and tactile defensiveness	That factors would emerge	Seventeen tests Two behavioral parameters R-technique factor analysis (simplified matrix)	N = 92 Formed normal distribution, 10% abnormal, three with mild CP	Praxis accounted for most variance Motor planning, kinesthesia, tactile functions, motor accuracy, bilateral coordination Visual perception factor: Ayres Space Test, Frostig	More support for praxis syndrome Visual component without motor element Perceptual-motor functions correlate as a whole in normative sample Kinesthesia closer to tactile than visual perception as in prior study

1966b	Provide an understanding of whether syndromes represent dysfunction or developmental lag Establish construct validity	Nearly the same as 1966a	That variation in perceptual-motor abilities would be small in a group of normal children	Sixteen tests Two behavioral parameters R-technique factor analysis	N = 64 Adopted, all normal on Gesell	Visual motor ability accounted for most variation Praxis and tactile perception were least variable Hyperactivity, distractibility, tactile defensiveness factor Factors weak because of lack of variance in performance of normal children	Suggested that low scores in praxis and tactile perception represent developmental deviation, not delay Little systematic variation when tests given to normal children Tactile defensiveness-hyperactivity may have a maturational component
1969	To provide an indepth analysis of dysfunctional patterns in children with learning handicaps Establish construct validity	Sixty-four tests and observations: SCSIT, psycholinguistic, intelligence, auditory, postural-ocular reactions, academic achievement	Brain functions involve several levels and will cluster accordingly	Q-technique factor analysis	N = 36 Educationally handicapped children	Five factors identified: Auditory language, sequencing Postural and bilateral integration Right hemisphere dysfunction Apraxia Tactile defensiveness	Hints to left hemisphere dysfunction
1971	To identify predictors of severity of sensory integrative syndromes	Forty-eight tests and observations: SCSIT, psycholinguistic, intelligence, eye-hand usage, postural responses	That predictive equations would emerge	Ten-step regression equations for each syndrome calculated	N = 140 Educationally handicapped	Presence of more than one type of disorder was the norm Prone extension best predictor of postural-bilateral integration Imitation of postures best predictor of praxis	Somatosensory and praxis linked again Elucidated best predictors of syndromes As many children may have apraxia as have postural and bilateral coordination problems

Continued

Table 23-1 Purpose, hypotheses, design, results, and contributions of Ayres' factor analytic and regression studies—cont'd

Year	Purpose	Instruments	Hypothesis	Design	Subjects	Results	Contribution to theory
1972	To further analyze and refine factors Establish construct validity	Same as above	That similar factors as previously would emerge	R-technique factor analysis	N = 148 Educationally handicapped	Six factors identified: Form and space perception Auditory language Postural ocular Motor planning Reading-spelling and IQ Hyperactivity, tactile perception	Further confirmed left hemisphere dysfunction Reconfirmed syndromes found in other samples of learning disabled children
1977	To further analyze interrelationships (add Southern California Postrotary Nystagmus Test [SCPNT]) so that differential diagnosis can be further refined	SCSIT SCPNT, postural-ocular and lateralization measures, dichotic listening, Illinois Test of Psycholinguistic Abilities (ITPA), intelligence, academic achievement Flowers-Costello (auditory)	That clusters would continue to be refined	Series of R-technique factor analyses (not all measures entered each time)	N = 128 Learning disabled	Five major domains identified: Somatosensory-motor planning Auditory-language Postural-ocular Eye-hand coordination Postrotary nystagmus	Further elucidated nature of interhemispheric integration Role of vestibular system clarified

| 1987 | To continue to attempt to differentiate types of sensory integraton dysfunction

New praxis tests as well as many of the tests that had been used in past studies | SCSIT, SCPNT selected ITPA test, Sentence repetition
Clinical observation of praxic extension, supine, flexion, ocular pursuits
Preliminary versions of newly designed praxis tests: sequencing praxis, praxis on verbal command, oral praxis, block building test | Is praxis a unitary function?
Would computer-generated clusters match those that had been identified clinically and through factor analysis? | Screen plot factor analyses, correlation coefficients
Comparison of test profiles of children with diagnoses
Use of computer-generated clusters | N = 182
Learning or behavior disorders | Praxis tests were related with one another
Visual tests correlated with tactile tests
Somato-visual-practic factor identified
Tactile scores and praxis related; short duration postrotary nystagmus; statistical association with praxis | Suggestion of a general somato-practic function
Further verified close association of tactile score and praxis
Computer-generated clusters were not meaningful |

Adapted from Ayres AJ.[13-17,21,24]

Table 23-2 Factors identified in studies by Ayres (1965-1977)

Date of study	Apraxia	Deficit in form and space perception	Deficit in postural and bilateral integration	Deficit in auditory and language functions	Tactile defensiveness	Miscellaneous
1965: 100 dysfunctional, 50 normal	Tactile tests Motor planning (imitation of posture, motor accuracy, MAC, Grommet) Eye pursuits	Frostig tests Kinesthesia Manual form perception Ayres' space test	Right-left discrimination Avoidance crossing midline Rhythmic activities	Not tested	Poor tactile perception Hyperactive-distractible behavior Tactile defensiveness	Figure-ground a separate factor Eye-hand agreement not related to perceptual-motor dysfunction
1966a: Normal distribution of Gesell developmental quotients	Accounted for most variance Motor planning Tactile and kinesthesia Motor accuracy Figure-ground Frostig tests	Figure-ground Frostig spatial relations Ayres' space test		Not tested	Low association of tactile defensiveness with praxis factor	Identified two main factors in normal sample: General perceptual-motor (somatosensory and motor) Visual perception
1966b: Only normal children		Frostig tests Ayres' space test Motor accuracy Figure-ground	Integration two sides of body and tactile perception	Not tested	Tactile defensiveness and hyperactivity—may be a maturational factor involved	Visual-motor ability accounted for most variation in normal children Poor motor planning—tactile perception not seen in normal children
1969: Educationally handicapped children	Tactile Motor planning	Most Southern California Sensory Integration Tests (SCSIT) visual tests not included in analysis Possible right hemisphere dysfunction: eye movement deficits, better right- than left-sided function	Bilateral integration Postural reactions Reading and language problems	Possible left hemisphere dysfunction: Auditory-language Reading achievement Auditory and visual-motor sequencing	Tactile defensiveness and hyperactivity—loaded together but not a separate factor	

1972: Educationally handicapped children	Motor planning Hyperactivity Tactile defensiveness (more emphasis on motor than tactile)	Position in space Illinois Test of Psycholinguistic Abilities visual closure Space visualization Design copying Tactile tests	Poor ocular control Excessive residual primitive postural responses Relatively good left-hand coordination Bilateral integration symptom did not load	Auditory language Intelligence	Hyperactivity-distractibility Tactile perception	Reading-spelling load together Motor accuracy highly associated with all parameters
1977: Learning disabled children	*Analysis 5:* Imitation of postures Composite tactile Kinesthesia	*Analysis 3:* Four SCSIT visual tests Manual form Perception	*Analysis 5:* Prone extension Composite postural Flexion posture Composite tactile Kinesthesia Bilateral integration symptom did not load	*Analysis 5:* Composite language (ITPA) Dichotic listening Flowers-Costello (auditory)	Not measured	Visual tests have strong cognitive component (loaded with IQ on Analysis 2) Space Visualization Contralateral Use (SVCU) score associated with lateralization indices Motor accuracy loaded separately on all

Adapted from Ayres AJ.[13-16,21,24]

these issues. In the first study she tested 148 children with learning disabilities on the Southern California Sensory Integration Tests to identify those in the group who had the type of learning disabilities for which sensory integrative procedures had been designed. The selection process resulted in the constitution of two groups. One group was made up of children judged to have a generalized sensory integrative dysfunction. The second group consisted of 24 subjects considered to have discrete auditory-language problems. In each group one-half of the subjects received sensory integrative procedures along with their usual special education program (the experimental subjects). The remainder received equivalent time in special education (control group). The children in both experimental groups received 25 to 40 minutes of sensory integrative procedures daily over a 5- to 6-month period.

All of the children had been pretested on achievement tests. Following the intervention they were retested on these measures. Results indicated that, within the group with generalized dysfunction, the children who had received the sensory integrative procedures had made greater gains, on the average, in reading and in overall academic achievement than those who had not received therapy. In the group with discrete auditory-language disorders, those who had received the sensory integrative procedures improved more, on the average, than the control group. An additional but important finding was that both experimental groups seemed to make greater gains than their matched control groups in language acquisition.

This study was important because it provided tentative evidence that, for those children who, on the basis of being tested on the Southern California Sensory Integration Tests and on the basis of clinical impressions of an occupational therapist, could be diagnosed as being very good candidates for sensory integrative procedures, the procedures did seem to enhance academic achievement and auditory-language functions. It is essential that therapists be aware that this study did not provide evidence that sensory integrative procedures were appropriate for all learning disabled children. The children who made up the samples were selected from among the general population of children with learning disabilities because they could be diagnosed as having the type of dysfunctions that were thought to be most responsive to sensory integrative procedures. Also, the study did not suggest that perceptual-motor or sensorimotor programs or other facsimiles of these sorts of programs were effective in lessening academic problems. The treatment program that the experimental groups received had the unique features of the sensory approach described by Ayres,[21] and may have borne only a slight resemblance to these other types of programs.

In 1974 Ayres was awarded a grant by the Center for the Study of Sensory Integrative Dysfunction and the Valentine-Kline Foundation for further study of the effects of sensory integrative procedures on learning disabled children. In this study[25,27] she was especially interested in identifying which children with learning disabilities would, and which would not, benefit academically from sensory integrative procedures. (It should be noted that this study had numerous other facets that cannot be covered in an introductory chapter of this kind.) In the one facet of the study that addressed the relationship of sensory integrative procedures to academic achievement, 46 children with learning disabilities received sensory integrative procedures for 6 months. A control group remained in class receiving equivalent time in special education. When the average differences in change in pretest and posttest scores between the groups were compared, no significant differences were found. However, when only the children with depressed nystagmus who had received the sensory integrative procedures were compared with those with depressed nystagmus who had not, significant results emerged. In this analysis it was found that a greater number of children (among those children with learning disabilities with depressed nystagmus) who had received the sensory integrative procedures gained more academically than those who had only been exposed to special education. This study was of much importance because it helped to pinpoint which children with learning disabilities were the best candidates for sensory integrative procedures. The results suggested that not all children with learning disabilities should be provided with the procedures. Children with depressed postrotary nystagmus and other signs of vestibular dysfunction were identified as those most apt to benefit from the procedures.

Carter, Morrison, Sublett, Uemura, and Setrakian[53] reported nonsignificant results on academic outcome measures. Clark and Pierce[56] have pointed out the differences in research design elements that may account for the discrepant findings between this and the previous studies. Such elements include the subject selection criteria and the age of the subjects.

In summary, all but one of these studies suggested that sensory integrative procedures were effective in enhancing academic learning in some children with learning disabilities. They also provided evidence that, because all learning disabled children did not benefit from the procedures, an evaluation process was essential before the recommendation for therapy.

The studies had the net effect of tempering enthusiasm for the approach. Reasonable evidence existed to suggest that the procedures benefited some subgroups of the population with learning disabilities. Because in the studies sensory integrative procedures were provided to children who were also receiving special education, the studies implied that sensory integrative procedures were a supplement to, and not a substitute for, special education.

Several criticisms can be made of the effectiveness studies conducted by Ayres. Perhaps the most obvious one is that the control group children did not appear to receive equal time in individualized attention as did the children in the experimental groups. The argument assumes that within their regular special education program the children were not routinely provided with equivalent individualized attention from classroom, itinerant, or resource room teachers. However, even if the experimental children did receive more individualized attention than the control groups, it is unlikely that the results could be adequately explained on the basis of attention alone. The difficulty in attributing the findings to an effect of attention centers on the fact that some (the children with depressed duration of nystagmus and other signs of vestibular dysfunction) but not all of the children in the experimental group seemed to benefit from the procedures. The possibility that children with attenuated nystagmus are more responsive to individualized attention than other children with learning disabilities is unlikely and strains the argument.

A second criticism that can be made of the studies is that they were conducted by the originator of the theory. Studies of the validity of a theory are more powerful when they are conducted by independent investigators. A number of studies have been conducted by independent investigators on the effectiveness of sensory integrative procedures* but all except two of these were on children without learning disabilities. One of these studies, however, deserves special mention because it was on children who were later identified as having reading failures. White[203] identified 21 children out of 124 when they entered first grade as at-risk for reading failure. Approximately one-half of the children were given the Southern California Sensory Integration Tests and then treated in accord with their diagnoses with the procedures recommended by Ayres[21] (experimental group). Each child received 48 half-hour treatment periods (over a 6-month period). At the end of the year, White reported the experimental group had attained a significantly higher reading level than the control children. Moreover, this difference persisted 1 and 2 years later.

A third type of criticism has been leveled, not against these studies on sensory integrative procedures per se, but against perceptual-motor programs and their facsimiles. The problem is that the writers who take this stand do not distinguish between sensory integrative procedures and the programs that resemble them, and they use the term sensory integration loosely. For example, Kinsbourne and Caplan,[115] a physician and a psychologist, respectively, in providing guidelines for parents on how to choose remedial programs, advise them to avoid "speculative methods." They define speculative methods as "any procedure that relates hypothetically, rather than logically, to educational good." Multisensory approaches and physical

education approaches "purporting to accelerate brain maturation (as opposed to raise morale)" are listed as examples of speculative approaches. Similarly, Reid and Hresko[161] state that "poor performances on perceptual, perceptual-motor, and sensory integrative tasks are characteristics of learning disabled children." But, they maintain, their significance is not clear and their relevance to intervention not validated. These authors make no reference to Ayres' studies or writings because they loosely use the term sensory integration in their statements. Their comments, however, might be inappropriately generalized to sensory integrative procedures. Other authors[47,119,178] have specifically criticized the approach described by Ayres. That is why it is suggested that therapists using the procedures be familiar with these papers. Therapists must "have a handle" on the research base that has both tentatively justified and delineated the use of sensory integrative procedures. They should be able to anticipate criticisms they will need to respond to in practice through familiarity with these publications. Each therapist has a responsibility of being a research consumer who can defend her practice with empirical support.

Inferences for intervention. Sensory integrative procedures have undergone modification throughout the past 20 years they have been in use. In another section of this chapter these procedures are described as they are currently used. As part of this discussion of the empirical base of the use of sensory integrative procedures, an overview of the ways in which the research brought about changes in practice is presented.

As already mentioned, from 1958 through 1960, Ayres recommended perceptual-motor training progressions with a heavy emphasis on the practice of tabletop tasks. The early 1960s were marked by a shift to an emphasis on tactile stimulation and away from cognitive processes. In her Eleanor Clark Slagle Lecture, Ayres[13] described the factors (referred to in this chapter as neural systems or syndromes) that had been isolated in her factor analytic study[15] (discussed in the section on typology).

This study suggested that the factors were related to neural substrates that processed intersensory information. In her Slagle lecture Ayres[13] suggested that tactile functions were especially important to treatment. She also recommended that treatment should focus on sensorimotor behavior, rather than on cognitive processes. The same general line of thought was apparent in a paper Ayres published on body scheme in 1961.[12] In this paper a case study was presented that described therapy procedures that relied heavily on cognitive processes. However, tactile and proprioceptive stimulation to enhance motor planning was also described as part of the program, reflecting Ayres' shifting emphasis on what should constitute therapy.

Just as tactile stimulation had been emphasized in the 1960s, in the 1970s greater attention was given to the vestibular system. The series of factor analytic stud-

---

*References 53, 55, 61, 87, 128, 143, 154, 155, 203.

ies that had been published up through this period had suggested that the neural substrates (factors) could be interpreted hierarchically. For example, the neural systems that seemed to be concerned with vestibular and tactile integration were interpreted as subserving more complex functions such as reading, visual perception, and language. Moreover, because some of the more important structures in the nervous system that were known to integrate sensory information were located in the brain stem, the inference was made that improvement in efficiency of neural processing at this level might enhance higher cortical functions. The result of this line of thought was that in the 1970s treatment relied heavily on procedures thought to enhance brain stem integration of sensory input. Major integrating mechanisms in the brain stem were found to be closely tied to vestibular mechanisms. As a logical development, treatment in this period came to emphasize provision of vestibular stimulation.

In her 1972 text, Ayres[21] listed numerous activities that she hypothesized would improve the efficiency of neural integration at a brain stem level. The procedures incorporated provision of tactile, proprioceptive, and especially vestibular input. Use of the net hammock, platform swing, inner tube, and scooter boards was described and has since become a symbol of the approach, although such equipment is not always used by therapists in accord with the principles of sensory integrative theory.

Therapy was described as relying even less on cognitive processes than it had in the 1960s.[21] Moreover, the concept of self-direction emerged as being critical to the treatment process. Ayres described therapy as providing the child with opportunities to organize her own behavior. The therapist's challenge is to draw out the child's inner drive and to provide a blend of freedom and structure that will promote exploration (Figure 23-5).

In the late 1970s Ayres conducted the major effectiveness study that had implicated the vestibular system in the type of learning disabilities that were responsive to sensory integrative procedures.[28,29] The finding led to even greater emphasis being placed on the provision of many types of vestibular stimulation varying in intensity, directionality, and speed. Concomitant with this evolving focus was a decrease in the emphasis placed on reflex integration and on tactile input, although procedures addressing these were still used intermittently as part of the overall therapy program. Sensory integrative procedures had evolved to the point that they no longer resembled the perceptual-motor systems that had been developed in the 1960s. The procedures required an elaborate array of equipment and overhead beams permitting suspension. They also required highly trained therapists who could tailor the therapy situation so that it drew forth the child's self-direction, yet demanded more complex adaptive responses than the child had previously performed.

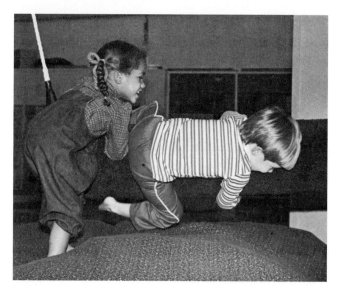

Figure 23-5   This activity, providing potent vestibular stimulation, also taps the children's inner drives.

Photograph by Dooley Brown.

Treating the child with learning disability with a sensory integration dysfunction: current practice

Entry-level therapists should not expect to be able to provide sensory integrative procedures upon graduation. The correct use of these techniques requires a great deal of professional skill and a blend of science and art. Science has generated the knowledge base in neurobehavioral science that provides a foundation for use of the procedures. Science has also furnished the data that tentatively suggest that the procedures are effective in promoting gains in children who have a variety of handicapping conditions.*

However, the provision of sensory integrative procedures also requires considerable artfulness. The therapist must make judgments about whether this approach should be initially recommended for the child. As much as possible, the therapist will use objective data from an evaluation procedure, but some subjectivity may need to enter into this decision. Throughout the treatment sessions the therapist will need to make judgments based on the child's characteristics and history, the equipment available in the treatment setting, relevant theories and facts, and past clinical experience. For each child, and during each moment of the therapy session, procedures are highly individualized in accord with the practical wisdom of the therapist and his or her knowledge of sensory integrative theory.

Although there are limited data to suggest that these

*References 28, 55, 61, 128, 143, 154, 203.

procedures are effective in promoting developmental gains in mentally retarded, autistic, and aphasic children,[36,51,55] this discussion will be confined to their application with learning disabled children. The therapeutic process begins with assessment, with a consequent decision on whether the child should be recommended for therapy. If the child is recommended, treatment is initiated. In this section an overview of the assessment process and guidelines for provision of sensory integrative procedures is presented. The purpose is simply to expose the reader to some of the central considerations that must be addressed in using these procedures. Competence in provision of the sensory integrative procedures is accrued over time through the interplay of advanced study and experience.

ASSESSMENT

An appropriate initial assessment, as well as a means for determining progress, is essential in all areas of clinical practice. Although this process creates a professional challenge for all therapists striving to provide quality care, several unique factors arise when the potential use of sensory integrative procedures is anticipated. Sensory integrative dysfunctions are not directly observable. Their presence is inferred from meaningful clusters of poor performance on a great number of tests and on clinical observations of neuromuscular performance and behavioral organization.

The diagnoses children are given on the basis of this evaluation procedure are not incontrovertible. They represent provisional hypotheses (tentative assumptions) about the nature of the contributors to the child's learning disorder. The correctness of the diagnosis is tested in the therapy situation. If the hypothesis is correct, then the procedures should produce certain predictable effects. The act, then, of arriving at a diagnosis is performed to guide intervention. It is essential that treatment effects (or the correctness of the hypothesis) be carefully documented.

Because sensory integrative theory purports that sensory integrative processes can affect many aspects of the child, in addition to academic performance, evaluation and documentation of change should be multifaceted. No single test can provide information of sufficient magnitude to infer the presence of a sensory integrative disorder—many tests must be used. Change, as a consequence of therapy, may occur in language acquisition, play, self-esteem, self-care, attention to relevant stimuli, or any aspect of the child's role performance. Both the complexity of diagnosis and the wide range of possible treatment effects must be considered in evaluating the child for a sensory integrative dysfunction.

The diagnosis the therapist gives the child will not rest exclusively on the results of the Southern California Sensory Integration Tests (SCSIT) or the Sensory Integration and Praxis Tests (SIPT). Also considered are the child's history and presenting problems, as well as observations of the child's neuromuscular status and behavioral organization. Observations of the following will usually be included: eye pursuits; equilibrium reactions; postural responses; the ability to assume total body patterns, such as prone extension and supine flexion; the presence of choreoathetosis; cocontraction; fine motor coordination; smoothness of movement; eye and hand usage; organization of behavior; spontaneous language; expression and comprehension; clinical motor planning ability; gravitational security; and emotional lability. In some instances the dichotic listening test[27] (see Chapters 9, 10, and 11) is also used to assess cerebral dominance for auditory language functions.

Finally, results of testing conducted by professionals from other disciplines, such as psychology and speech pathology, may be considered in the formulation of an overall diagnosis. In particular, measures of intelligence and auditory-language performance are helpful in rounding out a final impression of what neural processes may be contributing to the child's learning problems.

Documentation of the effects of sensory integrative procedures also requires the use of a variety of tests. Since sensory integrative theory suggests that the purpose of therapy is to enhance the child's capacity to develop and learn through more efficient neural processing,[21] changes are not expected before at least 6 months of intervention. The common expectation of weekly or monthly formal progress reports is often not necessary.

Another consideration in documentation is that the areas in which the child is expected to improve are not the same as those emphasized directly in the activities employed in therapy. Treatment provides a situation in which the child can receive and respond to meaningful sensory input and environmental challenges involving motor planning, ideation, and problem-solving. However, the areas in which parents and teachers initially perceived problems are also those in which changes, as a consequence of therapy, are likely to take place. These areas encompass physical, academic, social, and emotional development. Informal and nonstandardized observations by the child's parents, teachers, and other significant persons outside the therapy environment can buttress the therapist's impressions of the child's progress.

In addition, standardized tests must be used to tease out actual treatment gains from maturational effects. A number of standardized tests are clinically useful for documenting change. The Bruininks-Oseretsky Test of Motor Proficiency[50] is designed for children 4½ years to 14½ years and measures perceptual and motor functioning. It is especially helpful because the areas tested are not specifically addressed in therapy but do seem to depend on efficient sensory processing for performance to meet age expectations. The Development Test of Visual Motor Integration[43] is designed for children 2 years to 15 years and measures visual perception and eye-hand coordination in the form of a design copying test. This test helps provide information on change for the same reason as the above test. An additional test for measuring visual motor integration is the Primary Visual Motor Test by Haworth.[93]

Language scores are especially helpful for documenting change since (1) a large number of children diagnosed as presenting sensory integrative dysfunctions demonstrate speech and language disorders and (2) the language domain may be one of the systems most likely to benefit from the implementation of sensory integrative procedures. Some evaluations that have language items can be administered by the occupational therapist with practice; others should be administered only by qualified speech and language specialists. Tests that are sometimes used include the following: (1) the Peabody Picture Vocabulary Tests,[64] (2) the Expressive One Word Picture Vocabulary Test,[80] (3) the Test for Auditory Comprehension of Language,[51] (4) the Carrow Elicited Language Inventory,[52] (5) the Weiss Comprehensive Articulation Test,[198] and (6) the Sentence Repetition Test.[179]

In addition, academic tests may be useful in measuring the effectiveness of therapy, depending on the child's problems. The Wide Range Achievement Test by Jastak and Jastak[100] or the Woodcock-Johnson Psycho-educational battery[207] may be appropriate. Evaluations of activities of daily living, self-esteem, and student role performance may also be helpful in the assessment of behavioral changes.

PATTERNS OF SENSORY INTEGRATIVE DYSFUNCTION

As was mentioned earlier, there are complexities involved in labeling children as learning disabled. Learning disabled is a catchall term in which children with various characteristics are subsumed. Not all children with learning disabilities will present clinical pictures suggestive of the presence of a sensory integrative dysfunction. Those who do not should not be recommended for the procedures. The evaluation process previously described enables the therapist to generate a hypothesis about the contributors to a child's learning disability. The impressions generated by this process guide the therapist's decisions on what procedures to recommend. Overdiagnosis of children and overenthusiasm for the approach must be counteracted by a sound understanding of the proper use of the tests and knowledge of the data that suggest which types of children with learning disabilities are most apt to benefit from the procedures.

SENSORY INTEGRATIVE DYSFUNCTIONS

Several types of sensory integrative dysfunctions were identified in Ayres' factor analytic studies utilizing the SCSIT (Table 23-2). Preliminary research utilizing the SIPT has contributed to the conceptualization of these disorders and current analyses of SIPT data are expected to expand and refine understanding of sensory integrative dysfunction. The following descriptions of sensory integrative disorders rely heavily on Ayres[21,22,30,31] and Ayres, Mailloux, and Wendler.[38]

Vestibular bilateral integration dysfunction. In Ayres' earlier book,[21] vestibular bilateral integration dysfunction was called postural bilateral integrative dysfunction. Children hypothesized to have this disorder usually are the least affected among the learning disabled. These children may dislike sports and perform poorly in them. They may be poorly coordinated, especially in tasks requiring the hands to work together.[30]

In clinical observations, the therapist may detect that the child's eyes do not seem to be working together properly. A jerk may be noticed as the child's eyes cross their midline. The child may not show a clear preference for one hand, although well beyond the age at which hand dominance should have been established. In the prone position the child may be unable to simultaneously raise his arms, hands, heels, and thighs (in what is called the prone extension posture). On the Southern California Postrotary Nystagmus Test the induced postrotary nystagmus may be depressed in duration relative to that of other children of the same age.[24] This constellation of problems suggests inefficiency in vestibular processing.[30]

It is posited in sensory integrative theory that the vestibular system has a considerable influence on postural tone, ocular pursuits, the coordination of input from the two body sides, the establishment of laterality, language function, and visual perception. Ayres[30] describes the developmental progression of a vestibular-bilateral integrative disorder as follows. In early childhood the child may experience problems mastering directionality (she may turn to the left when asked to turn to the right). In middle childhood she may have difficulty learning to dance (which requires smooth rhythmical movement) or learning to play the piano (which requires the hands to work together with precision). At this age the child may also be identified as having a reading disability.[30]

This cluster of problems is seen in sensory integrative theory as related to inefficiency in vestibular processing.[30] It is thought that these children begin to cognitively compensate for the poorly functioning vestibular systems. For example, to point to the left hand on a command to do so, they will think longer and harder than children normally do. This compensation is then proposed to interfere with adequate establishment of hemispheric dominance for auditory language functions, visual-spatial perception, or both. In other words, both hemispheres may have to deal with the same functions, rather than specializing. Without adequate hemispheric specialization, neither visual-spatial nor auditory-language functions may be performed well. Moreover, activities such as reading, which require both visual perception and auditory language skills, may be impaired because the two hemispheres are thought, when this syndrome is present, to not communicate adequately. Research has suggested that children hypothesized to have this dysfunction are among the best responders to sensory integrative procedures.[25] In therapy these children typically seek out intense and rapid vestibular stimulation.

Developmental dyspraxia

Ayres' study of praxis in recent years has introduced some of the most dynamic conceptualizations of sensory integration disorders. Ayres' view of praxis as a critical link between occupational therapy and sensory integration is evident in the following passage:

Praxis is an uniquely human skill that enables us to interact effectively with the physical world. It is one of the most critical links between brain and behavior. Praxis is to the physical world what speech is to the social worlds. Both enable interactions and transactions[35] (p. 1).

In her earlier writings, Ayres[21-23] used the term *apraxia* to refer to developmental dyspraxia. In more recent work, Ayres[30,35] has stated that the term apraxia is used when the individual (usually an adult) is unable to motor plan. She believes the term *dyspraxia* is better suited for the child who can formulate motor plans but who is slow and inefficient in doing so. Children with learning disabilities who have problems in motor planning almost invariably fall into the latter category.

To understand the way in which developmental dyspraxia may be manifest, Ayres has described three basic practic processes. The first process is referred to as ideation or conceptualization. This aspect of praxis is a cognitive process that allows an individual to form an idea about what to do with an object or how to interact in a given situation. Although cognitive in nature, ideation is thought to depend on efficient sensory processing. Ayres states that children with dyspraxia who have difficulty with ideation are likely to have trouble choosing an activity, using equipment properly, and possibly in organizing themselves for action as in getting ready to go to school.[35]

Planning a course of action is the second practic process described by Ayres. She views planning as "an intermediary process between ideation and action"[35] (p. 23). Planning an action is also a cognitive process in that it requires thinking about actions. Ayres states that the brain must have adequate information from tactile, kinesthetic, vestibular, and visual systems to plan a purposeful act. Planning involves sequencing and timing as well. Ayres gives an example of an activity she frequently uses in therapy that often reveals difficulty in the sequencing and timing aspects of motor planning. In this activity, the child must propel herself with a trapeze off the top of a ramp, swing, and then drop into a pillow. The child must time the release of

the trapeze at the instant she is over the pillow. Early or late releasing may be seen in the child with a poor ability to plan timing and sequencing of actions.

Execution is seen as the final process in praxis. Although executing an action is probably not the main difficulty for children with developmental dyspraxia, it is the only aspect of praxis that can be observed. Ayres differentiates poor execution resulting from inefficient sensory processing from poor muscle control seen in disorders such as cerebral palsy.

Factor analyses utilizing the SCSIT consistently demonstrated a dyspraxia factor emerging in association with tactile and visual perception dysfunction (Table 23-2). The single best indicator of dyspraxia in these studies was the Imitation of Postures Test[19] in which the child is required to quickly snap into a posture the examiner assumes. This test, renamed Postural Praxis, remains an important element of assessing praxis with the SIPT.[34] Other tests that will help assess practic function include Constructional Praxis, Sequencing Praxis, Oral Praxis, and Praxis on Verbal Command. Preliminary research[38] has not revealed a tendency for different types of dyspraxia to emerge but rather supports a notion of praxis as a unitary function. Continuing research with the SIPT will help the occupational therapist delineate presence of dyspraxia in the child with learning disabilities.

Dyspraxia is frequently associated with distractibility and hyperactivity.[23] Children with dyspraxia are considered good responders to sensory integrative procedures.[23] Figure 23-6 depicts an intervention designed to foster constructional praxis.

Generalized dysfunction. Children who, on the basis of results from the Southern California Sensory Integration Tests, are classified as having generalized dysfunction, are thought of as having severe sensory integrative dysfunction. In their cases, academic learning is probably restricted by many factors, only one of which may be related to their sensory integrative dysfunction. When learning problems are a result of a complex interplay of factors, it is doubtful that provision of sensory integrative procedures would appreciably enhance academic learning. These children are not considered prime candidates for sensory integrative procedures. However, a child with generalized dysfunction may benefit from a sensory integrative approach in terms of general adaptive behavior, if a disorder in modulation of sensory input (discussed later) is also present.

CONSIDERATIONS FOR RECOMMENDING OCCUPATIONAL THERAPY BASED ON SENSORY INTEGRATIVE ASSESSMENT

Ayres[32] pointed out that many children in classes for the learning disabled appear to have other nervous system irregularities that could severely interfere with learning. These children, like those hypothesized to have a vestibular bilateral integration dysfunction, are

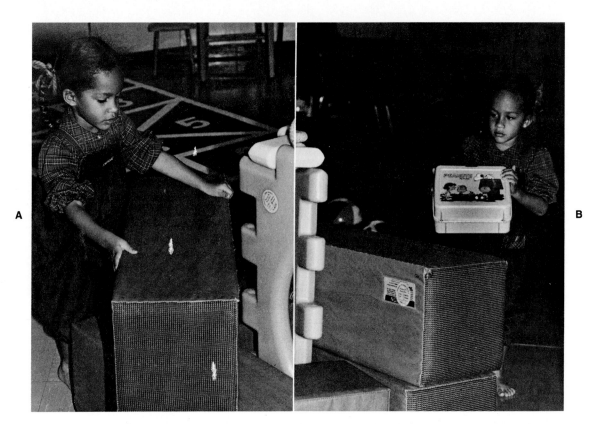

Figure 23-6   Activity requiring constructional praxis. **A,** This child must organize spatial information as she combines objects to build a house. **B,** On completing the activity, the child uses fantasy as she plans to have lunch in the house.

Photograph by Dooley Brown.

likely to score poorly on the Southern California Sensory Integration Tests or the Sensory Integration and Praxis Tests. Because of the type, severity, and complexity of the nervous system disorders, provision of sensory integrative procedures is likely to make little difference in their academic achievement.[32] Therapists who fail to recognize this situation may inappropriately select clients for treatment. They may be overenthusiastic in their recommendations, make unrealistic predictions about the outcomes that are expected from therapy, and generate criticism.

Left hemisphere and right hemisphere dysfunctions were detected by Ayres' factor analytic studies, but experimental data suggested that children with these diagnoses did not benefit academically from sensory integrative procedures.[25] The reader is reminded that occupational behavior concepts may provide a viable basis for occupational therapy treatment.

Left hemisphere dysfunction. As previously mentioned, data exist suggesting that some children with learning disabilities may have a dysfunction in processing information in the left hemisphere.[54] A sensory integrative evaluation can provide tentative evidence of the presence of this kind of dysfunction and assist in the diagnosis. Most right-handed individuals demonstrate left-sided dominance for auditory language function.[27] The diagnosis of left hemisphere dysfunction is suggested when a child demonstrates poor auditory-language skills and a pattern of poorer right-handed performance than left-handed performance in the presence of normal sensory integrative functions. These children do not tend to show hyperactivity, distractibility, or poor postural responses. Postrotary nystagmus is usually prolonged or within normative expectations. It is hypothesized that these children are underachieving because of left hemisphere inefficiency. Data suggest that they do well in traditional special education programs and are not among the best responders to sensory integrative procedures.[29]

Right hemisphere dysfunction. Results of a sensory integrative evaluation may assist in the diagnosis of a right hemisphere dysfunction. Children hypothesized to have this dysfunction may show discrete visual-spatial perceptual problems without other evidence suggestive of a sensory integrative dysfunction. Usually in right-handed persons the right hemisphere specializes in visual-spatial tasks. If this side of the brain is not processing information optimally, visual-spatial perception may be compromised. Children who are hypothesized to have this dysfunction are thought to demonstrate adequate postural responses, unimpaired auditory-language functions, better right- than left-hand performance, and underuse or disregard of the left hand. This dysfunction seems to be one of the less frequently made diagnoses, and only a few children with this diagnosis were included in Ayres' effectiveness studies.[20,25,29] In general, children hypothesized to have this type of dysfunction are not recommended for sensory integrative procedures.

DISORDERS IN MODULATION OF SENSORY INPUT

In addition to the types of dysfunction reviewed earlier, Ayres has described disturbances in modulation of sensory input that may appear along with a sensory integrative dysfunction or in isolation. In contrast to the typology of syndromes, which is quantitatively grounded in test scores, the notion of sensory modulation addresses the more qualitative aspects of sensory processing, which are closely related to the emotions. Specifically, hyperresponsivity to motion and to touch fall within this category.

Two types of hyperreactive vestibular responses are described by Ayres.[30] The first, gravitational insecurity, is defined as intense anxiety and distress in response to movement or to a change in head position. Ayres[30] suggests that the child may experience a sensation of falling when in a stable, but threatening position. Typically, the child prefers to be in secure contact with a firm ground and thus may avoid activities that involve jumping, climbing, swinging, and other forms of active or passive movement. Ambulation tends to be slow and overly cautious. This condition is thought to be associated with inadequate inhibition of vestibular input.[30] The second type of vestibular hyperresponsivity, intolerance to movement, is described as an aversive reaction to rapid spinning and circular movement. For these children, movement is unpleasant but not threatening. They may readily approach movement activities, unlike the gravitationally insecure, but react to vestibular stimulation with excessive nausea and discomfort.

Tactile defensiveness has been associated with vestibular dysfunction as well as with dyspraxia. Defined as an aversive reaction to touch, it was repeatedly linked with hyperactivity and distractibility in Ayres' factor analysis (Table 23-2). Like gravitational insecurity, it is thought to involve oversensitivity to sensory input. The reader is referred to Ayres[14,21] for a lengthy discussion of the hypothesized neural substrates of this disorder and to Royeen[170,171] for a discussion of the manifestations and measurement of tactile defensiveness.

Little research has directly addressed the effects of therapy on tactile defensiveness or gravitational insecurity. Ayres and Tickle[39] found that vestibular and tac-

tile hypersensitivity were among the strongest predictors of a good response to therapy in a group of autistic children. Informal case reports have suggested that significant improvement in adaptive behavior results when sensory integrative procedures are employed with children who are hypersensitive to touch and movement. Further research in this important area is warranted.

OTHER CONSIDERATIONS IN DIAGNOSING THE PRESENCE OF A SENSORY INTEGRATIVE DISORDER

Results of a sensory integration evaluation on some children with learning disabilities do not permit interpretation in accord with the typology presented earlier. Rather than strain to force a diagnosis, it is recommended that the therapist use alternative models for interpretation as presented in the Southern California Sensory Integration Test Manual.[22] Therapists need to be cautious in diagnosing children. As a rule, children with learning disabilities who do not fit the available interpretation models probably should not be recommended for therapy. If the data are suggestive but do not clearly indicate a sensory integrative dysfunction, therapy could be provided on a trial basis with an extensive reevaluation after 6 months. The SIPT will provide a computer-generated basis for interpretation upon which the examiner will need to expand but which will not always allow distinct classification.

Goals and objectives of treatment

The specific objectives of sensory integrative procedures will vary according to the kind of dysfunction that is diagnosed and the individual differences that make each child unique. In short, objectives are individualized for each patient. However, it is possible to list some general goals from which specific objectives can be derived (Figure 23-7). While these goals usually apply to most children involved with sensory integrative procedures, they may not all be appropriate for each child. Furthermore, specific objectives generated toward the same goal may vary substantially from one child to another.

INCREASE IN THE FREQUENCY OR DURATION OF ADAPTIVE RESPONSES TO SENSORY INPUT

Increase in the frequency or duration of adaptive responses to sensory input depends on the therapeutic application of controlled sensory input. During provision of sensory integrative procedures, the therapist constantly monitors the child's responses to be certain that the stimulation is organizing rather than disorganizing, integrating rather than overwhelming. Sensory input is considered optimal when it is neither overstimulating nor understimulating.[30] The therapist "reads" the child's autonomic nervous system response (for example, skin color, breathing rate), as well as

---

Figure 23-7   Goals of therapy using sensory integrative procedures

---

Increase in the frequency or duration of adaptive responses to sensory input.
Development of increasingly more complex adaptive responses.
Increase in self-confidence and self-esteem.
Improvement in cognitive skills, language acquisition, or academic achievement.
Improvement in daily living and personal-social skills.

Adapted from Ayres AJ: Sensory integration and learning disorders, Los Angeles, 1972, Western Psychological Services; Ayres AJ: Sensory integration and the child, Los Angeles, 1979, Western Psychological Services; Ayres AJ: Aspects of the somatomotor adaptive response and praxis. Audiotape, Pasadena, Calif, 1981, Center for the Study of Sensory Integrative Dysfunction.

changes in behavioral organization, and makes judgments about whether the child's responses are adaptive (Figure 23-8). Contingent on this ongoing appraisal is the modification of therapeutic activity. Manipulation of the sensory environment in this way enables the child to produce adaptive responses more frequently and sustain them for longer periods of time than might otherwise be possible.

Stimulation generally is not confined to one sensory modality. The activities that are used provide natural combinations of proprioceptive, vestibular, and tactile stimulation. Sensory integrative procedures, to be appropriate, must provide the right combination of stimulation in accord with the status of the child's nervous system (Figure 23-9). The availability of attractive suspended equipment that can be used for rich provision of vestibular stimulation is essential.

With sensory integrative procedures, active stimulation is usually preferred over passive stimulation, although in some instances passive applications may be used.[30] Passive application of vestibular stimulation, in particular, is more likely to be used in children with severe involvement who appear to have difficulties with sensory registration. Even with these children, active stimulation is encouraged whenever possible, since it is more likely to engage the child's inner drive and lead to more complex adaptive responses. Ayres[31] suggests that sensory registration can be further enhanced in treatment by simplifying the environment so that there are only a few choice pieces of equipment to which the child might attend.

It should be kept in mind that Ayres' definition of an

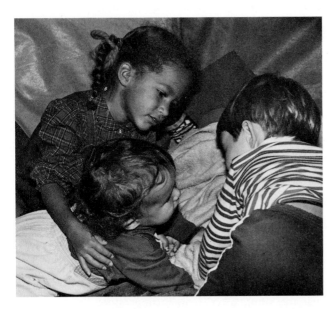

Figure 23-8   The comforting effects of the tactile stimulation these children are receiving are reflected in their facial expressions.

Photograph by Dooley Brown.

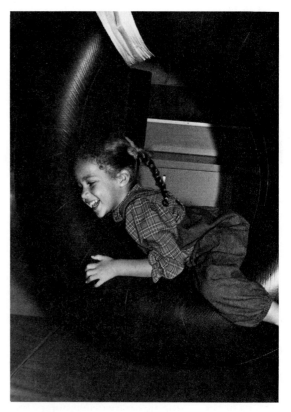

Figure 23-9   Many children place their cheeks on the inner tube, maximizing tactile stimulation (touch-pressure) to the face as they receive vestibular stimulation.

Photograph by Dooley Brown.

adaptive response encompasses a broad range of behaviors. Ayres described it as a purposeful goal-directed response through which motions achieve functional meanings.[21] Recently Ayres coined the term somatomotor adaptive response to mean a motor response that is dependent on integration of vestibular and tactile information.[31] Examples would include equilibrium reactions, protective responses, or lying prone with neck and hips extended to ride successfully on a scooter board. Adaptive responses can vary in complexity, quality, and effectiveness.[31] They may entail sequences of behaviors, such as going down a ramp prone on a scooter board and then knocking down an inflated toy, or single motor patterns, such as sitting on a scooter board and maintaining an upright posture for a sustained period of time[31] (Figure 23-10).

Successful repetition of a new adaptive response provides evidence that the child's nervous system is consolidating new strategies for dealing with sensory information. Similarly, when a child sustains an adaptive response for a longer period of time than ever before, a measure of the internal process of sensory integration is provided. An example is the child who initially was unable to sustain a flexed body position to stay on a swinging suspended bolster for more than a few seconds but who now is able to enjoy a 5-minute ride.

DEVELOPMENT OF INCREASINGLY MORE COMPLEX ADAPTIVE RESPONSES

Not only are adaptive responses expected to occur with greater frequency and duration, they also are expected to become more complex in organization. The goal is based on the assumption that the types of stimulation provided are thought to promote more efficient brain stem organization of multisensory input. It is posited that better neural organization at this level will enhance the child's ability to make judgments about what is in the environment, what can be done with objects, and what specific actions need to be taken to accomplish a goal[31] (Figure 23-11 on p. 492).

Ayres[31] believes that repeating activities is acceptable during the period when the child is perfecting the response; however, development of more complex abilities occurs only when tasks become slightly more challenging than any the child has successfully accomplished before. The therapist uses activity analysis, assessment information, ongoing observations, and knowledge of child development to guide the arrangement of the therapeutic environment so that it will engage the child's inner drive and draw forth more complex interactions with the equipment. For responses to be adaptive, however, they must be successful. Ayres defines therapy as a combination of challenge and success[31] (Figure 23-12 on p. 493).

Minimally involved children are eager to explore sensory integrative equipment and will initiate more complex variations of an activity within a single session. For more involved children, the adaptive responses usually will be less complex, will require more repetition and will advance more slowly. The task of the therapist in such cases is to simplify the challenge so the child can succeed, then gradually change the ac-

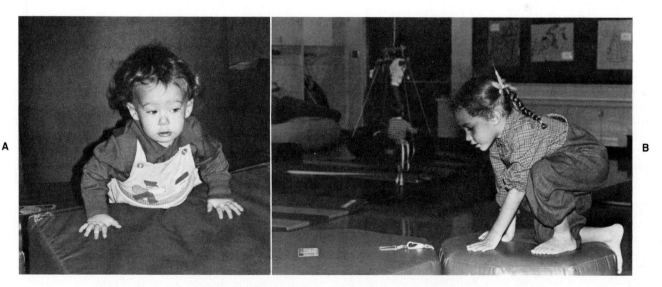

Figure 23-10 Adaptive responses varying in complexity. **A,** Weight-bearing on hands on a stable surface in preparation for climbing, a simple adaptive response. **B,** Weight-bearing on hands on an unstable surface, a more complex adaptive response.

Photograph by Dooley Brown.

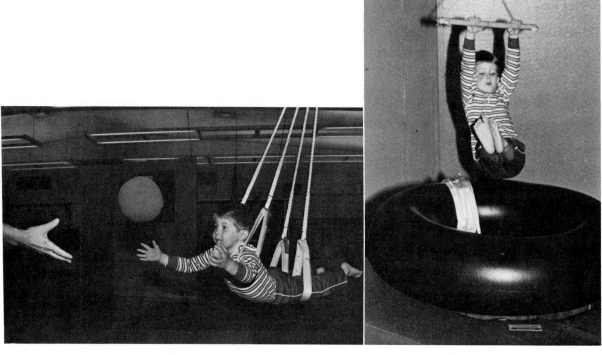

Figure 23-11 This child demonstrates two complex adaptive responses elicited through sensory integrative procedures. **A,** Prone extension pattern as child swings in suspended "helicopter" and attempts to catch a ball. **B,** Hip flexion as child clears his legs in preparation for a jump requiring timing into the inner tube.

Photograph by Dooley Brown.

tivity by altering its components on a fine gradient of complexity. Ayres[31] suggests requiring an adaptive response of only a few parts, rather than the total body, as one means of simplifying the challenge. Ayres also suggests that activities that involve movement patterns that are centrally programmed in the nervous system, such as walking and sitting, and do not require planning will be less demanding than those involving the assumption of unusual positions.[31] A short-term objective for a very gravitationally insecure and dyspraxic child, for example, might be to walk up a large inclined ramp without physical assistance from the therapist.

Other children in the therapy environment can help elicit more complex adaptive responses from a particular child, since they can serve as models of a variety of activity options. It should be noted, however, that sensory integrative procedures are provided dyadically (that is, with a one-to-one child-therapist ratio) in an optimal situation. If other children are present, each should be with her own therapist. When other children are not present, the therapist may model activities.

INCREASE IN SELF-CONFIDENCE AND SELF-ESTEEM

Ayres[30] claims that adaptive responses promote self-actualization by allowing the child to experience accomplishment of a task that previously could not have been mastered. When a child is responding adaptively to demands in the environment, she will appear creative, efficient, and satisfied. Therapy will be fun, and the child will be emotionally involved[30] (Figure 23-13).

From the outset, the therapeutic procedures generally are directed by the child, not the therapist. An assumption of the treatment approach is that children will seek out the stimulation they need to organize their nervous systems.[21] The therapist assists the child in responding adaptively to it. Ayres stated that the adaptive response cannot be imposed on the child by the therapist; it can only be generated within the child. The child wants to accomplish an act and attempts it. The child initiates and emits the response while the therapist helps to ensure success. The child is following an inner drive, while the therapist encourages and

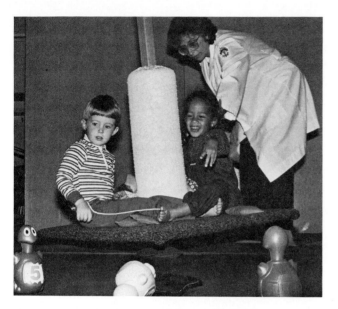

Figure 23-12 After successfully knocking down a turtle with a beanbag while riding the flexor swing, this girl's facial expression shows the characteristic signs of pleasure associated with success.

Photograph by Dooley Brown.

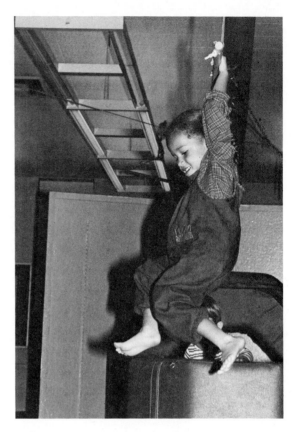

Figure 23-13 Successful accomplishment of adaptive responses are thought to enhance self-confidence and self-esteem.

Photograph by Dooley Brown.

lures the child into pursuing those activities that may enhance nervous system development. Ayres emphasizes that therapy at its best involves a self-directed child.[21]

Therapists can promote self-direction of the child by first structuring the environment so the possible adaptive responses are not beyond the child's capacity and second, by making assistance available so the child will succeed[31] (Figure 23-14). Knowledge of normal development guides the therapist's decision on how to manipulate the environment or offer assistance. Although, in principle, it is suggested that treatment should follow a developmental sequence, Ayres[21] maintains that it is best to allow the child to guide treatment, provided the procedures do not become nontherapeutic. The course of treatment, then, need not invariably follow a strict developmental progression.

The final outcome of therapy that encourages successful self-directed experiences is a child who perceives herself as a competent actor in the world. Therapy entails involvement in challenging activities that are achievable and guided by the child.[31] It is expected that engagement in such activities will promote feelings of mastery and a sense of personal control that resides within the self.[30] The resulting gains in positive self-concept can be critical to the emotional development of children with learning disabilities who often are characterized as having low self-esteem.[129]

Behavioral changes over time can provide an index

of gains in self-confidence and self-esteem. For example, a child whose initial approach to the physical environment was inhibited, constricted, or fearful may demonstrate exploratory and risk-taking behaviors with growing frequency. A child who originally reacted to difficult tasks with destructive actions or self-denigrating remarks may show a decrease in those behaviors along with an increasing willingness to tackle potentially threatening activities.

IMPROVEMENT IN COGNITIVE SKILLS, LANGUAGE ACQUISITION, OR ACADEMIC ACHIEVEMENT

Research discussed earlier in this chapter provides tentative evidence that provision of sensory integrative procedures to some types of children with learning disabilities is associated with enhancement in language and cognitive abilities and increased proficiency in some academic skills.[20,25,29] In treatment, however, the therapeutic techniques do not directly address these functions. Rather, gains in these areas are seen as eventual outcomes of enhancement of sensory registration, sensory integration, and general programming capacity.

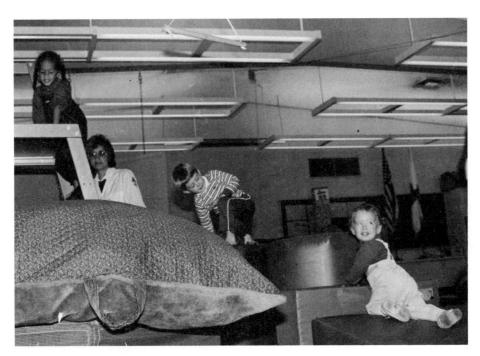

Figure 23-14   Therapists can promote self-direction by structuring the environment in accordance with the child's abilities.

Photograph by Dooley Brown.

Practice of specific visuomotor skills (for example, tabletop activities) or academic tasks are not customarily included in the treatment context.

Recently Ayres[29] speculated that programming of motor actions during sensory integrative procedures may provide a pathway to better programming of language and cognitive functions. She proposed that to accomplish an unfamiliar purposeful activity the child must first generate an idea of what is to be accomplished. Next, a "program" must be formulated for how to accomplish the act. Finally, execution of the task involves sequencing of motor activities.[29]

Specific procedures have been developed by Ayres that are aimed at promoting ideation, sequencing, and programming.[29] Activities requiring these components are a particularly important treatment of a child with dyspraxia. Ayres[29] believes that programming functions can be encouraged through the use of verbal behaviors, such as counting or singing, to regulate motor output (Figure 23-4 on p. 473).

IMPROVEMENT IN DAILY LIVING AND PERSONAL-SOCIAL SKILLS

Sensory integrative procedures encourage the child to organize his or her own activity. The child must generate ideas about what is to be done with a piece of equipment and then program the actions needed to accomplish a goal. In what Ayres calls the "optimum for growth situation,"[21] the child will go on to execute the

acts and experience the consequences of planning. Ayres hypothesizes that, with improvement in programming of action, a general programming ability is enhanced. The outcome of this is a child who is better able to organize behavior, daily routine, and self-care and who is better able to focus attention on relevant tasks that support role demands.[30] As competency develops in life skills, it is usually accompanied by growth in self-esteem. Often the child begins to interact with peers and adults in more effective and enjoyable ways as a function of greater self-confidence and emotional self-control.

Therapy may help the child who is overly sensitive to touch or movement to deal with these sensations in a more adaptive manner. As a result, the child is able to approach the world with greater security. Not only are daily living skills improved, but relationships with others are more likely to be entered with greater physical comfort. The child is better able to enjoy social interaction without the interference of distrust in her own reactions to ongoing sensation (Figure 23-15).

Other treatment considerations
ROLE OF THE THERAPIST

The therapist cannot use a "cookbook approach" in providing sensory integrative procedures. It is inappropriate to enter the therapy situation with a list of activ-

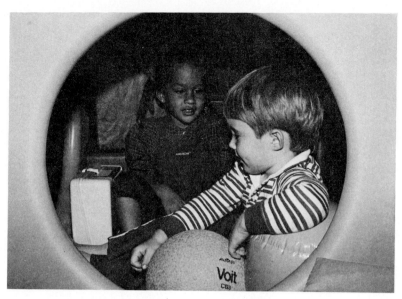

Figure 23-15   After engagement in sensory integrative activities, these children show comfort in peer interaction in a house they constructed.

Photograph by Dooley Brown.

ities the child eventually will be required to do. The therapist's judgments on what should be encouraged in a given treatment session depend on her capacity to imagine what the child is experiencing and the ingenuity to figure out how to help the child accomplish the task successfully.[31] The therapist learns with experience to "read" the child's responses and to anticipate the possible outcomes of the child's behavior. This ability is called artful vigilance by the authors. Within the therapy context, the therapist must learn how to establish rapport with the child and create a sense of safety in the child. A relationship with these characteristics fosters the child's inner urge to explore his environment. The therapist must also decide on a style of interaction with the child. While some children will do better with little and unadorned verbal communication, others may need the therapist to be more verbal, emotive, and enthusiastic.

The central role of the therapist providing sensory integrative procedures is to arrange an environment that is conducive to the child's organization of her own behavior.[31] Ayres believes that preparation of the remedial environment is one of the most demanding requirements of the therapist.[30]

Although, in general, the therapist guides while the child directs the therapy, it should be noted that this is not invariably the case. In instances in which a child shows little or no evidence of an evocable inner drive, the therapist may need to impose a therapeutic procedure.[31]

CHARACTERISTICS OF THE ENVIRONMENT

The availability of a wide range of equipment and a suspension system from which to hang and arrange it is absolutely essential. Just as ultrasound therapy cannot be accomplished without ultrasound equipment, sensory integrative procedures cannot be provided without the appropriate facility and equipment. Ayres[21,30] described the equipment required for sensory integrative procedures.

The clinic setting should provide for accessibility of equipment. It helps if equipment not in use can be hung on pegs within arm's reach of the therapist. Ideally, a number of swivel hooks should be available and secured in the beams that support the ceiling. When it is within the child's capacity, she can assist in rearrangements of the environment during the therapy session.

The treatment area should be designed to allow for subdivisions of space. Movable partitions make possible the blocking off of areas for individualized therapy. This same space can be enlarged by opening the partitions, and it can be used for activities requiring considerable excursion or for tandem therapy in which more than one child, each with her own therapist, receives therapy together.

THE FLOW OF THE THERAPY SESSION

Therapy sessions should have a flow. One activity should follow another in natural succession. Sessions do not consist of the therapist's asking the child to do

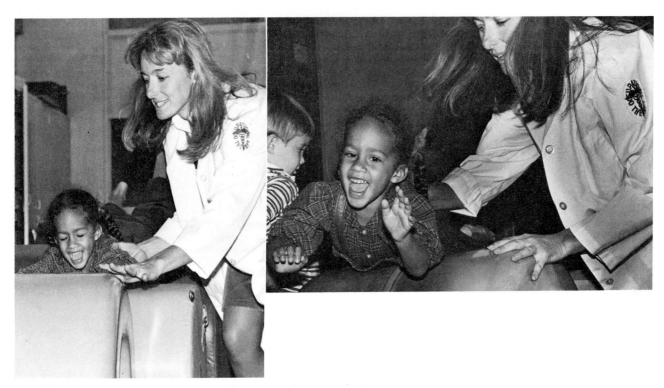

Figure 23-16 The therapist promotes self-direction in the child by making assistance available as the session flows.

Photograph by Dooley Brown.

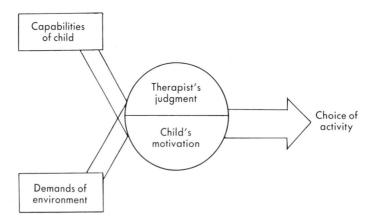

Figure 23-17 The process of activity analysis during sensory integrative procedures.

one and then another preplanned activity. As much as possible, the child should be encouraged to be self-directed. The optimal therapy situation is one in which a balance is achieved between the therapist's structure, and the child's freedom.[21] But the child's self-direction can become chaotic without the structuring provided by the therapist.

The therapist's artful vigilance enables the creation of the balance of structure and freedom that is essential in the therapy environment (Figure 23-16). The therapist attends to the child's behavior, interprets the adaptiveness of her actions, and anticipates the next event, helping the child when necessary. Such help may include adding suspended handles the child can grasp, lowering equipment, or providing a cushion into which the child already swinging can jump.[31]

A well-developed ability to analyze therapeutic activities in relation to individual client needs allows the therapist to create a treatment milieu that falls midway between rigidity and chaos. The flow of the therapy situation is contingent on the proficiency of the therapist in making judgments about when to provide structure vs when to allow the child's self-direction to prevail. The choice of an activity to be used within the therapy context results from interaction of the child with the therapist. The therapist brings to this situation impressions of the child's capabilities, impressions that are formed through the results of formal evaluation and past experience in treating the child. The child similarly brings a conception of his own capabilities. Both therapist and child have some knowledge of the activity options in the environment, although the therapist's knowledge in this area is far more comprehensive and substantive than the child's. Knowledge in these two areas will influence the child's motivation toward particular activities. The therapist, observing the child's self-direction toward a particular activity, makes a decision on whether it is challenging and achievable by the child, with or without the therapist's assistance. If it is, the child's self-direction will determine the choice of activity; if not, another activity may be encouraged by the therapist. A therapy session consists of recurrences of this process, with the choice of each new activity resulting from interaction of child and therapist. A thread of continuity links activities and imbues the session with the qualities of spontaneity and flow (Figure 23-17).

DIFFERENTIAL TREATMENT BASED ON DIAGNOSIS

In general, children diagnosed with a vestibular bilateral integration problem will seek out great amounts of potent vestibular stimulation and will put forth much effort to make responses reflecting increased adaptive capacity. The types of vestibular stimulation they seek may vary in direction, acceleration, and potency. A child may vary her position on a piece of equipment so that a variety of vestibular receptors can be stimulated. Such a child may spend as much as three-fourths of a therapy session involved in the reception of intense vestibular stimulation.

Children with gravitational insecurity or intolerance to movement will not seek out vestibular stimulation. They will want to keep their feet touching the floor. Therapy for these children begins with activities that involve minimal vestibular stimulation while their feet are anchored firmly to the floor. The stimulation is provided in positions in which the head is upright. Security can be furthered by the therapist's holding the child or doing an activity with him. Providing a helmet and bringing attention to the mats and pillows that are under the child may decrease the threat of movement.

A child with dyspraxia typically seeks out vestibular stimulation, but not as much as the child who is diagnosed as having a vestibular bilateral integration dysfunction. Frequently these children are distractible. Providing limited equipment can enhance the flow of the therapy session. There should be more emphasis on ideation and programming of action and on the quality of adaptive responses. For example, a child with dyspraxia may be encouraged to set up an obstacle course and figure out what to do in navigating through it. Because such a child sometimes self-directs toward repetitive activities, she may need to be gently pushed on to new activities. Verbal regulation such as singing or counting can assist such a child in making adaptive responses.[31] Climbing activities may be especially beneficial, as well as activities involving initiating, timing, and sequencing.[31]

Provision of tactile and vibratory stimulation is usually appropriate for children with poor somatosensory processing. It is also central to the treatment of tactile defensiveness. Generally, tactile stimulation is not imposed but is made available to the child through the provision of a variety of brushes, napped fabrics, and other textured objects that can be applied to the skin. Carpeted equipment can effectively provide tactile stimulation in an activity so that attention can be directed to the activity and not to the tactile input, per se. Fuzzy blankets, sheepskins, or cloths with which the therapist can unobtrusively line or pad surfaces are also helpful.

INDIVIDUAL DIFFERENCES

Each child brings to the therapy session unique differences that change over time.[144] Individual differences in children exist in their physical attributes and in their behavior and emotional styles. For example, one child may be emotive while another is apathetic; one may be sociable and another shy. Therapists also have individual differences in their approaches to children. Because sensory integrative procedures are influenced by the individual differences of the child and therapist, a description of the activities that were used in a therapy session is only a partial presentation of the therapeutic process. Indeed, two children may partici-

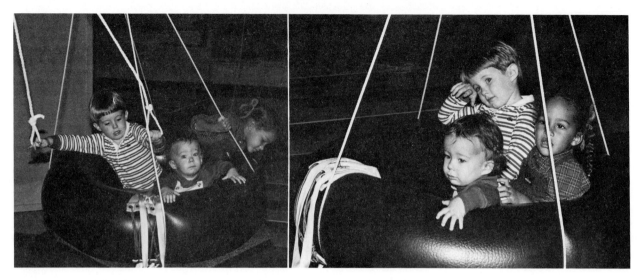

Figure 23-18   The change in affect demonstrated in these children alerts the therapist that the activity is overwhelming.

Photograph by Dooley Brown.

pate in identical activities, but the qualitative aspects of their treatment experience may be diametrically opposed. One child may have experienced success and freedom, the other failure and coercion.

PRECAUTIONS

Sensory integrative procedures should not be administered by occupational therapists with limited clinical experience. Ayres[21] warns that the provision of tactile, and especially vestibular, stimulation can have deleterious effects on the nervous system. There is the danger that the child may experience sensory overload signaled by flushing, blanching, or perspiring. Overinhibition of brain stem mechanisms can result in cyanosis or depressed respiratory functions. Finally, Ayres[21] points out that there is a risk of accident when children who are unskilled and lacking in judgment and accurate perceptions are encouraged to respond to environmental challenges. The provision of sufficient mats, equipment that is kept in a good state of repair, and an artfully vigilant therapist all lessen the risks involved (Figure 23-18).

CASE STUDY

This child demonstrates an excellent response to therapy. Few other children will do as well.

Tammy, an 8-year-old white female, was referred to occupational therapy by an educational psychologist on staff at the public school she was attending. At that time Tammy was having academic difficulties, and her mother reported that she was distractible, frustrated, and often discouraged. In addition, she seemed to be having visual perception problems. An occupational therapist certified in the administration and interpretation of the Southern California Sensory Integration Tests evaluated Tammy on these tests and on a variety of neuromuscular responses considered to be related to learn-

ing to make a decision as to whether Tammy should be recommended for sensory integrative procedures.

The results of the evaluation suggested the presence of a vestibular bilateral integration dysfunction. This impression was supported by the findings of depressed postrotary nystagmus, low muscle tone, inadequate equilibrium reactions, poor balance, difficulty with assumption of the prone extension posture, and irregular eye pursuits. In addition, Tammy demonstrated tactile defensiveness. Scores on the tests measuring visual perception supported Tammy's mother's report of an apparent problem in this domain. The type of vestibular deficit Tammy displayed had been associated with learning disabilities in Ayres' research and was considered a possible contributor to Tammy's academic problems. The processing of vestibular input is proposed to be crucial in sensory integrative theory to many aspects of development because of the numerous neurological associations between this system and other parts of the nervous system. Inefficient processing in the vestibular system was thought to be related to Tammy's distractibility, decreased attention, poor organization of behavior, and difficulty interacting with peers.

Tammy received eight 1-hour sessions of occupational therapy per week for 7 months. Because there was reason to believe that the type of sensory integrative dysfunction Tammy seemed to have would be responsive to sensory integrative procedures, and because the dysfunction seemed to contribute to her underachievement, the school district agreed to finance the therapy. Therapy was aimed at providing Tammy with the opportunity to receive vestibular and tactile input in a manner that allowed her to self-direct the sessions and elicit adaptive responses. Tammy proved to be very self-directed within the nonthreatening milieu of the one-to-one therapy sessions. She demonstrated a strong tendency to seek out the type of stimulation that the therapist had hypothesized had not been efficiently processed by Tammy's nervous system before the intervention (vestibular and tactile input). In general, Tammy selected the activities she would engage in during therapy, while the therapist helped to make the tasks both challenging and achievable.

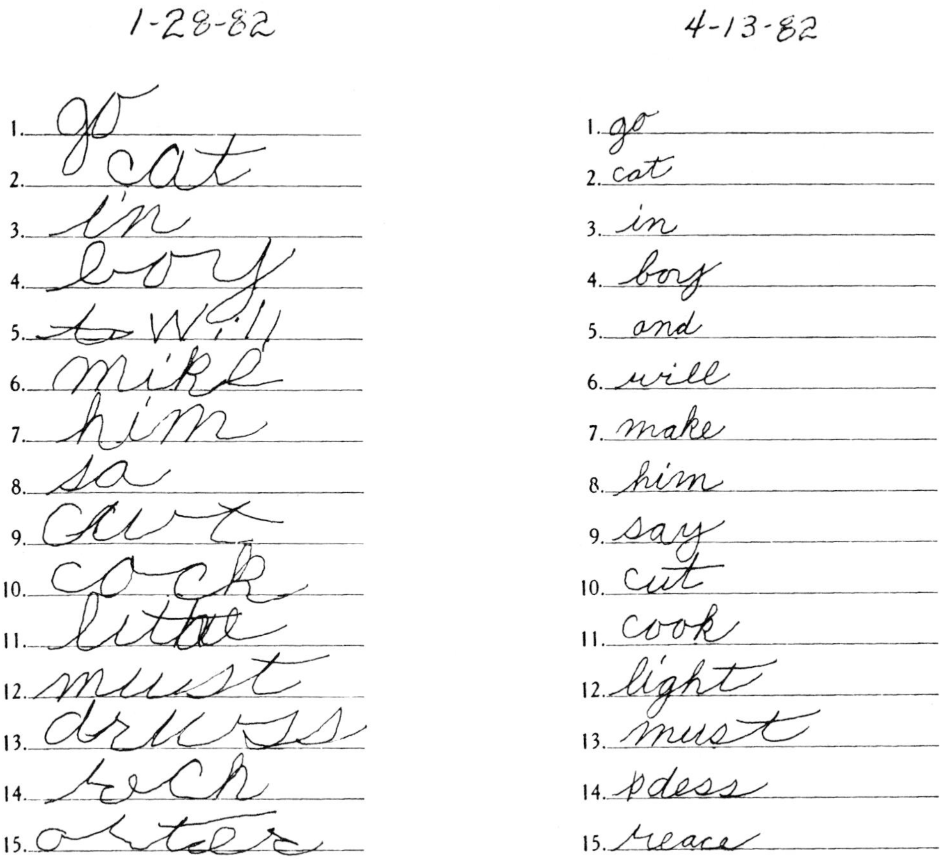

Figure 23-19 Tammy's handwriting samples before and after intervention.

Progress notes recorded during the 8-month period reflected the changes in Tammy that seemed to be a consequence of therapy. In the first month the therapist wrote that Tammy appeared to be "highly motivated but moved without planning," that "she experimented with all the equipment" and seemed to enjoy "self-directed vestibular input," and that she interchanged her right and left hands when throwing objects. Tammy was described as being unable to throw with sufficient force to reach a target. In these instances, the therapist reported, Tammy would become upset.

Four months after therapy had been initiated the progress notes reflected an increase in Tammy's ability to engage in creative play. Improved ability to monitor her own activity was also noted. For example, Tammy was reported to frequently enjoy rolling inside a blue hollow ball, but before rolling she would say, "I need to get organized." Soon after Tammy began to develop better social interactions with other clients who were receiving therapy. A note written at the seventh month of treatment read, "As usual, directs activities pretty much by self," although it should be noted that in the course of time in which sensory integrative procedures were used with Tammy, there were times when she would express boredom. The last note read, "Tammy brought a vase of flowers for the therapists and appeared sad to leave. She did a lot of gymnastic-type tricks using the glider, swing, stacked inner tubes, and trapeze and rings to flip and hang upside down. . . She explored the clinic as though saying farewell. Hugged all therapists—definitely hated to leave."

To assess Tammy's academic and visual-perceptual progress, several standardized tests were administered. These were given in January before intervention, in April (3 months after the initiation of therapy), and in June (5 months after therapy began). The results are in Table 23-3. Samples of Tammy's handwriting before intervention and after are shown in Figure 23-19. It can be seen that considerable progress in this area was made.

Gains made by Tammy in other domains, for example, behaviorally, in peer interaction, and role performance, are difficult to quantify. Comments made by Tammy's mother provide qualitative data that suggest improvements. A year after therapy had been instituted Tammy's mother was interviewed. She stated that "Tammy used to have few friends. She now seems so much happier, interacts very well, and has many friends. What I really notice is how much better her self-concept seems to be and how much more confidence she has." Her mother also said that she was appreciative of an "improvement in the quality of Tammy's life."

Table 23-3 Tammy's test results

Test	January	April	June
Slosson oral reading	3.4 grade	3.7 grade	3.7 grade
Beery visual-motor	6 years, 7 months	6 years, 7 months	8 years, 8 months
Wide Range Achievement Test (WRAT) reading	3.6 grade	4.1 grade	4.2 grade
WRAT spelling	2.6 grade	3.5 grade	3.9 grade
WRAT arithmetic	3.5 grade	3.9 grade	4.1 grade

OTHER APPROACHES TO OCCUPATIONAL THERAPY FOR CHILDREN WITH LEARNING DISABILITIES

Ayres[21] states that "theoretical models, like children, follow a developmental sequence." Although sensory integrative theory and its procedures incorporate some of the principles of perceptual-motor and sensorimotor approaches, in its present state the sensory integrative approach should be treated as a distinct and separate treatment approach not to be confused with the other two types of programs. In the discipline of occupational therapy the terms cognitive perceptual-motor, sensorimotor, sensory-motor-sensory, sensory integration, and multisensory have been used to refer to a variety of neurophysiological approaches to treatment or to processes in the brain.[21,67,85,120] Ayres chose to use the term sensory integration to refer to the theory and procedures she developed, and she provides a sound rationale for doing so. She prefers sensory integration because it emphasizes an organizational process occurring in the brain. Other terms, such as sensorimotor, in contrast focus on the relationship of sensation to specific motor responses. We suggest that sensory integration be used strictly to refer to the theory and treatment that Ayres originated.

Our position may differ from that presented by other therapists. For example, Weeks[197] subsumed the sensory integrative approach developed by Ayres under the general category of sensorimotor integration approaches. Weeks used the term sensorimotor integration in referring to "the multisensory treatment approach, except in discussion of underlying sensory integrative processing or of tests and approaches labeled sensory integration by their developers." However, because Weeks covered the sensory integration approach under the broader category of sensorimotor integration, there is blurring of the distinctions between a variety of approaches.

Farber[67] listed Ayres' approach as one of several sensorimotor integrative treatment approaches. To add to the confusion, the American Occupational Therapy Association[5] listed the term sensory integration under sensorimotor components of occupational therapy treatment and then defined the terms as referring to skill and performance, rather than to neural organization.

In contrast, Ayres' use of the term sensory integration downplays emphasis on the motor response. Instead, it stresses the brain's organization of information (sensory input). In previous sections of this chapter we have stressed that sensory integrative procedures are used to help the child develop a more efficient general organizational capacity. Enhancement of this ability contributes to the development of a child who is more creative and better able to adapt to environmental demands, more proficient in organizing behavior and in performing daily activities, and better able to approach and succeed in academic tasks. The concern is more on how well the child uses his brain to organize information, than on how sensation can be used to produce more normal motor responses.

A distinction should also be made between Ayres' use of the term adaptive response and use of that term by other occupational therapists. Farber,[67] for example, uses adaptive response to refer to a specific neuromuscular reponse that the therapist attempts to bring about in the client through application of a particular hands-on technique. Developmentally appropriate techniques are repeatedly applied until the desired adaptive response is obtained. Ayres,[30] on the other hand, uses adaptive response to refer to a behavioral response that originates in and is controlled by the client in conjunction with therapist manipulation of the environment. The specific adaptive responses that the child will emit often cannot be predicted beforehand, because they arise spontaneously within the child during interaction with the equipment. A therapy session using sensory integrative procedures might elicit adaptive responses at varying levels of complexity, although over many sessions the complexity of overall responses would increase. An adaptive response at a specific developmental level would not be demanded before progression to higher levels is allowed.

Sensorimotor approaches

The treatment approaches that we would choose to classify as sensorimotor are those that are strictly concerned with how sensation and neurophysiological principles can be employed to effect the neuromuscular motor response, per se. The procedures described by Bobath and Bobath,[45] Rood,[166] and Kabat and Knott[101] fall within this category. In their pure form, these approaches are generally used with children and adults suffering from neuromuscular disorders (for example, cerebral palsy or cerebral vascular accidents). They are characterized by hands-on procedures in which the therapist applies pressure or other types of sensation, or otherwise handles the patient so that motor responses reflect more normal movement patterns or tone.

Ayres acknowledges that concepts from the sensorimotor approach have been incorporated into some sensory integrative procedures.[21] The concept of applying sensory stimulation to enhance motor responses originated with Kabat and Knott.[101] Ayres credits Rood[166] with first having elucidated the therapeutic role of tactile and vestibular stimulation. A uniqueness of sensory integrative procedures is that they emphasize potent vestibular stimulation, the type that is provided by swinging in net hammocks and on swings. Sensory integrative procedures also depart from the sensorimotor approaches in that the goals of therapy go well beyond the promoting of a more normal neuromuscular response. Sensory integrative procedures are directed toward the evincing of broadly defined adaptive responses, thereby encouraging the child to organize her own behavior.

Perceptual-motor programs

Another category of neurophysiological approaches is called perceptual-motor programs or systems. As was previously discussed, the characteristics of these programs originated primarily in the field of education. Here the differences between the characteristics of these programs and those of the sensory integrative approach are addressed (Table 23-4).

Perceptual-motor programs are more cognitively oriented than the sensory integration approach. They may ask the child to focus attention on coordinated execution of specific motor acts, often with verbal guidance. For example, they may require the child to practice specific visuomotor activities, such as drawing a circle, while the child or therapist says the word *circle*. With sensory integrative procedures, gross motor activities are heavily used to elicit adaptive responses automatically, and verbalizations are deemphasized.

In perceptual-motor programs the child is required to follow a predetermined sequence of activities. A lesson plan may be used to outline how the session will proceed. The child may be instructed to move on from one activity station to the next and perform certain

Table 23-4 Comparison of perceptual-motor and sensory integrative programs

Perceptual-motor	Sensory integrative
Cognitive orientation	Noncognitive emphasis
Predetermined sequence	Flexible sequence
Repetitive drill	Exploration and creativity
Program-centered	Child-centered
Adult-directed	Adult-guided
Group program	Dyadic interaction
Teach specific skills	Improve brain processing
Suspended equipment optional	Suspended equipment mandatory

skills at each. As was previously illustrated, the choice of activities that will be used in a sensory integration treatment session cannot be predetermined. It results from an ongoing interplay of child self-direction and therapist judgment. The status of the child's nervous system through the course of the therapy session is central in how treatment will flow. The therapeutic situation must be flexible yet simultaneously provide the child with a sense of organization.

Repetitive activity is of value in perceptual programs because, through practice, skills are mastered. In the sensory integrative approach, while repetition may be allowed at times, the emphasis is on exploration and creativity. The child's opportunities to generate ideas about what can be done with a piece of equipment is considered as important as the perfecting of particular skills.

Perceptual-motor programs tend to be more program-centered, while the sensory integration approach is primarily child-centered. In the former a logically developed sequence of activities may be prescribed that makes developmental and neurophysiological sense. The program guidelines determine the lesson plan. In the sensory integrative approach the child is given considerable say in what activities will be done. The therapist assists in making the activities achievable by the child. Knowledge of developmental sequence may guide the therapist in doing this, but a predetermined developmental sequence is not imposed.

The two types of programs also differ in the role of the teacher or therapist. In perceptual-motor programs the teacher may command, expect, or instruct the child to do certain tasks. In the sensory integrative approach the therapist assists the child in organizing her own behaviors.[31] This is accomplished through a variety of techniques, including making available the appropriate equipment, adapting the equipment in accord with the child's needs through activity analysis, asking the child to participate in the arrangement of the equipment, and, of course, allowing the child to choose activities.

Perceptual-motor programs lend themselves to group activity because they clearly map out predetermined sequences of tasks. The use of lesson plans and adult direction makes management of groups feasible. Self-direction of the child, which is so important in a sensory integrative approach, can lead to chaos if permitted in groups. Careful monitoring of autonomic and behavioral responses to sensory stimulation and structuring of the environment to meet individual needs also would be impossible if one therapist were in charge of a group of children. Sensory integrative procedures, then, are best carried out in a one-to-one situation.

Two other characteristics distinguish sensory integrative and perceptual-motor programs. First, an essential feature of sensory integrative procedures is the elaborate array of suspended equipment that can be used to provide potent and varied types of vestibular stimulation. Perceptual-motor programs typically do not involve this. Tabletop activities and gross motor skills involving jumping, balancing, laterality, or coordination are usually described as characteristics of these programs. Second, perceptual-motor programs usually focus on the teaching of specific skills rather than on the enhancement of brain processing.

Classroom consultation

Occupational therapists, especially those working in school settings, are frequently called upon to provide consultation, rather than direct service. As discussed in Chapter 29, consultation to classroom teachers can take a number of forms.

The occupational therapist working in a school system must be able to identify whether or not a sensory processing problem seems to be interfering with the student's ability to benefit from her educational program. In addition, it must be determined if consultation is an appropriate method of intervention. The following case studies are illustrative.

CASE STUDY 1

Patrick is a 5-year, 2-month-old boy in his sixth month of kindergarten who had attended preschool for 2 years before entering kindergarten. His kindergarten teacher observed that he will not touch paste, finger-paint, or certain foods at snack time, and he cries when the teacher attempts to put a painting smock on him. Patrick does not attempt to play on playground equipment during recess, has not made any new friends, and refuses to take his turn during motor activities in the classroom. His teacher reports that because he is reluctant to participate, he is not benefitting from the opportunities provided in her class. An occupational therapist was asked by the school psychologist to provide consultation based upon a teacher's report and observation of the child in the classroom.

Occupational therapist interpretation

Although Patrick is a young kindergartner, he has attended preschool for 2 years. His lack of interaction with school ma-

terials, peers, and playground equipment is not likely to result from limited past experience. Observation revealed that he demonstrated severe reluctance to participate in many classroom activities; this observation, along with the teacher report, suggested a significant sensory processing problem. Expecting the teacher to implement occupational therapy theory for normalizing tactile and vestibular processing is neither realistic nor professional. It may also be detrimental to the child. The occupational therapist in this case may recommend a formal occupational therapy evaluation before making consultation recommendations. It is likely in this case that direct services will be necessary before a classroom consultation program can be effective.

CASE STUDY 2

Jason is a 7-year, 4-month-old boy in his seventh month of first grade. He attended preschool for one year before entering kindergarten. His kindergarten teacher had been concerned because, although Jason had been able to answer challenging questions appropriately, he had had a difficult time following the class routine and rarely finished work on time. Art projects and personal belongings had been very messy and disorganized. Jason's first grade teacher is concerned because Jason is still having difficulty organizing his personal belongings and is having significant trouble with handwriting. His letters, of inconsistent size, are placed without regard to the lines on the paper and spaces are not left between words. Reading comprehension is reported by his teacher to be above average. At recess, Jason typically plays on playground equipment alone or attempts to play chase games which usually end in an argument with a peer. An occupational therapist who was asked to consult with this child's teacher did not observe that Jason sought unusual amounts of sensory stimulation or demonstrated an avoidance of somatosensory or vestibular input. Although Jason had been evaluated by the school psychologist and speech therapist, he did not qualify for special education because no handicapping condition could be certified, such as, an identifiable discrepancy between his academic achievement and his ability.

Occupational therapy interpretation

Jason is one of the older students in his class who had attended both preschool and kindergarten. Thus, problems with finishing his work on time, handwriting, and peer interaction do not appear to result from immaturity or limited experience. The teacher's report and classroom observation suggest that Jason may have motor planning problems related to inefficient processing of somatosensory and visual information. Would consultation be an appropriate method of intervention? In this case, because Jason is participating in classroom activities without reluctance and doing well in some subjects, his sensory processing problem may not be severe enough to eliminate the consideration of consultation. Because Jason does not qualify for special education, he would not qualify for occupational therapy as a related service in the educational system, even if sensory integrative deficits of sufficient severity had been suggested.

An appropriate method of intervention at this time is consultation with this child's teacher. This strategy may prove to be sufficient in lessening the presenting problems. It is possible that this child may qualify at a future date for special education and it is then, according to PL 94-142, that occupational therapy needs as a related service can be addressed through the public school. Still another possibility exists that this child's parents will seek out private occupational therapy in an attempt to prevent a future need for special education. Whatever the future may hold for this child, the following represents the type of action that could be implemented through consultation.

Plan of action

Using a sensory integration frame of reference, an occupational therapist attempts to analyze the sensory and motor factors that may be contributing to the presenting problems. A good rule of thumb in providing consultation for a teacher is never to recommend an activity that is not typically found in childhood play. Sometimes occupational therapists, meaning to be helpful, attempt to train teachers to use therapy equipment such as hammock nets to increase the amount of vestibular stimulation that can be provided in the classroom. This is not an appropriate classroom activity for a group of even five to ten children because the majority of the class cannot participate while one child is in the net. In addition, the intensity of vestibular stimulation could be harmful to the child without ongoing monitoring by a trained therapist. The best consultation action plans emanate from everyday childhood experiences. Through play, the child is challenged and the sensory systems have the opportunity to become better integrated. The goal of the consulting occupational therapist is to bring to a classroom meaningful play experiences for the students while communicating their value to the teacher.

The development of an action plan for classroom consultation begins with a careful activity analysis of the tasks in which the student or the students are having difficulty. Through this process, the teacher can be given general ideas that may benefit not only a specific child but also the entire class. In many situations, an occupational therapist can develop action plans to meet the needs of a few children from which the whole class can benefit. These are usually the easiest for the teacher to implement. Frequently, the ideas center upon motor activities during physical education time or involve art projects. In recommending such activities, process rather than the end product is emphasized with the teacher encouraged to focus on factors such as energy expenditure, coordination, direction following, and social and communication skills. Particularly effective are activities in which the whole class can participate, but which can also be modified to maximize the competency of children with problems.

Action plans may also include specific modifications or physical adaptations that will foster the student role performance of individual students. For example, the therapists may assist the teacher in modifying the paper, tools, desk, chair, schedules, and assignments for a student. In this manner, the teacher and occupational therapist work together to help the child compensate for her problems without lowering classroom expectations or standards. It is sometimes helpful to develop consultation plans that utilize the sensory integration frame of reference by addressing specific sensory systems or processes.

AUDITORY PROCESSING

Difficulty in understanding and interpreting the spoken word can interfere with a child's ability to begin and complete tasks in the classroom. The occupational therapist might check to see if a teacher is scheduling classroom activities with high auditory processing demands at a time when auditory competition outside is at a maximum. It might be recommended that a teacher give one direction at a time and wait a little longer between successive directions to give the child time to analyze the command. Auditory processing can be promoted by classroom teachers through traditional children's games that have songs to coincide with an action.

VISUAL PERCEPTION

Transference of visual spatial notations across two visual planes can make copying from the blackboard difficult. Difficulty with figure-ground perception (identifying objects with a rival background) can contribute to a problem with sorting and organizing personal belongings. Faulty interpretation of the spatial relationships of objects, letters, and words can contribute to reading problems, illegible handwriting, and messy work.

For problems in copying from the chalkboard, an occupational therapist might recommend periodic cleaning of the chalkboard and an effort to keep all notations on it color coded, well-spaced, and uncluttered. These practices may reduce figure-ground problems. Or the therapist may suggest that a teacher reduce her use of the chalkboard by having the children copy from one paper to another with both papers in the same plane. A teacher may be encouraged to try bean bag games in which the targets are placed at approximately the same distance from the child's eyes as is the chalkboard, so that a student can practice focusing and fixating eyes near and far in play. For handwriting spacing problems, the occupational therapist may recommend a decorated tongue depressor to use for spacing words. The possibilities are unlimited.

SOMATOSENSORY PERCEPTION

Hypersensitivity to touch may interfere with peer relationships. Poor discrimination of tactile information may compromise precision in the manipulation of objects of various sizes, shapes, and textures, and with tool control. Inaccurate awareness of where, how, or with what force body parts are moving in relation to objects and people can contribute to torn paper work, broken pencils, an inability to remain in a seat for desk work, and play that is too rough. An occupational therapist might recommend that a teacher designate personal space for each student with masking tape to minimize the threat of inadvertent physical contact. It might be suggested that some students sit or line up in front or back of the line so that the possibility of crowding from both directions is decreased. Tactile discrimination games can be played by finding common objects in a lunch bag without using eyes to help. In the classroom, children can experiment with the correct modulation of force by throwing bean bags into targets at varying distances and pouring liquids and grains into containers without spilling.

VESTIBULAR PROCESSING

Some children need an extra amount of movement before being able to sit still, while other children are easily overstimulated by small amounts of movement. Faulty vestibular processing can interfere with a number of skills needed in the classroom. For example, deficient strength in antigravity muscles (which seems to be related to inefficient vestibular processing) can lower a student's endurance to the point where she expends excess energy just to maintain a seated position. Vestibular-related postural-ocular deficits are thought to make reading and handwriting arduous and frustrating in selected children.

An occupational therapist may recommend that a student who is overstimulated by movement sit in an area where there is limited movement to process in the peripheral visual field. It may be recommended that a student who is having difficulty sitting be encouraged to move through alternate work centers so that she may stand to work, be prone, or sit supported in a bean bag chair. Students with poor ocular control may be provided with a duplicate of blackboard work to reduce the stress of copying. Teachers may be reminded to have the students spend a moment with their eyes closed to rest fatigued musculature between periods of demanding work.

PRAXIS

Motor planning ability is central to success as a student. Almost all classroom activities require that a student have an "idea" of how to interact with objects, tools, and persons in the classroom and be able to develop and successfully implement a motor plan.

There are several ways in which an occupational therapist can stimulate ideation in a classroom. Imaginative games such as a pretend bear hunt or charades can stimulate ideas for movement. Some games encourage each student to come up with a simple movement for the partner to copy, for example, Spinning Statue Freeze.

Some children have adequate ideation; however, they have trouble developing a strategy for the execution of a motor plan. If sequencing appears to be a problem, the occupational therapist can recommend that the teacher write down or illustrate with pictures the sequence of classroom activities. In a classroom, knowing the sequence of events is central to conforming with the classroom routine and making simple transitions from one activity to another. Sometimes problems with constructional praxis result in student completion of messy products through random trial-and-error methods. The occupational therapist may recommend that the teacher either assist the student with thinking about and developing strategies for task execution or provide the students with a prearranged strategy outline on a checklist. If a child appears to have problems with verbal or postural praxis, it might be recommended that the teacher be very careful in how directions are presented. "Simon Says," hand clapping routines, and other games that require a motor or verbal response to words or actions may challenge a child's verbal and postural praxis in the classroom.

SUMMARY

Provision of occupational therapy services for children with learning disabilities was a natural outcome of this profession's previous involvement with patients with brain dysfunction and of trends in special education that identified learning disabilities as one type of handicapping condition. Although a number of exciting hypotheses currently exist to explain learning disabilities, confusion about the definition of the disorder persists. Recent legislation has mandated occupational therapy as a related service in school systems, but occupational therapists also see adults and children with learning disabilities in a wide variety of other settings.

Occupational therapy practice with the child with learning disabilities, using the occupational behavior frame of reference, will focus on play and on maximizing student role performance. Often used in conjunction with the occupational behavior frame of reference, sensory integrative procedures as described by Ayres are widely used with children with learning disabilities. Researched over the last three decades, this approach provides specific guidelines on how children with learning disabilities who also have sensory integrative dysfunctions may be helped to better integrate sensation, become more organized, and perform better at home and in school. The sensory integrative approach can be distinguished from other neurophysiological approaches that may be used with children with learning disabilities. The chapter concluded with a description of how occupational therapy consultation services are provided when direct intervention is not needed.

STUDY QUESTIONS

1. Describe three hypotheses that provide an explanation of learning disabilities.
2. Trace the evolution of sensory integrative theory and practice beginning with its origins in early occupational therapy practice and ending with a description of the current state of the research.

3. Identify six principles or concepts that would be of relevance to the provision of occupational therapy to children with learning disabilities using the occupational behavior frame of reference.
4. List the basic goals and assumptions of sensory integration theory and practice.
5. Describe what Ayres meant by a "pattern of dysfunction." List the characteristics of three such patterns.
6. Compare and contrast two neurophysiologic approaches that are frequently confused with the sensory integrative approach as described by Ayres.
7. Define praxis and describe its essential features.
8. Discuss the differences between consultation and direct service provision to students with learning disabilities in the schools.
9. Describe several ways in which classrooms may be modified to promote the functioning of students with learning disabilities.

REFERENCES

1. Abikoff H: Cognitive training interventions in children: review of a new approach, J Learn Disabil 12(2):65, 1979.
2. Adelman HS, and Taylor L: Learning disabilities in perspective, Glenview, Ill, 1983, Scott, Foresman & Co.
3. Adelman HS, and Taylor L: The problems of definition and differentiation and the need for a classification schema, J Learn Disabil 19:514, 1986.
4. Allessandrini NA: Play—a child's world, Am J Occup Ther 3(1):9, 1949.
5. American Occupational Therapy Association: Uniform terminology for reporting occupational therapy services, Rockville, Md, 1979, American Occupational Therapy Association, Inc.
6. American Psychiatric Association: Diagnostic and statistical manual of mental disorders, ed 3, DSM-III, Washington, DC, 1980.
7. Ames LB: Learning disability: truth or trap, J Learn Disabil 16(1):19, 1983.
8. Ayres AJ: An analysis of crafts in the treatment of electroshock patients, Am J Occup Ther 3(4):195, 1949.
9. Ayres AJ: Ontogenetic principles in the development of arm and hand functions, Am J Occup Ther 8(3):95, 1954.
10. Ayres AJ: Proprioceptive facilitation elicited through the upper extremities. Part 1: background, Am J Occup Ther 9(1):1, 1955.
11. Ayres AJ: The visual-motor function, Am J Occup Ther 12(3):130, 1958.
12. Ayres AJ: Development of body scheme in children, Am J Occup Ther 15(3):99, 1961.
13. Ayres AJ: The Eleanor Clark Slagle Lecture, The development of perceptual-motor abilities: a theoretical basis for treatment of dysfunction, Am J Occup Ther 17(6):221, 1963.
14. Ayres AJ: Tactile functions: their relation to hyperactive and perceptual motor behavior, Am J Occup Ther 18(1):6, 1964.
15. Ayres AJ: Patterns of perceptual-motor dysfunction in children: a factor analytic study, Percept Mot Skills 20:335, 1965.
16. Ayres AJ: Interrelationships among perceptual-motor functions in children, Am J Occup Ther 20(2):68, 1966.
17. Ayres AJ: Interrelations among perceptual-motor abilities in a group of normal children, Am J Occup Ther 20(6):288, 1966.
18. Ayres AJ: Deficits in sensory integration in educationally handicapped children, J Learn Disabil 2(3):44, 1969.
19. Ayres AJ: Characteristics of types of sensory integrative dysfunction, Am J Occup Ther 25(7):329, 1971.
20. Ayres AJ: Improving academic scores through sensory integration, J Learn Disabil 5:338, 1972.
21. Ayres AJ: Sensory integration and learning disorders, Los Angeles, 1972, Western Psychological Services.
22. Ayres AJ: Southern California Sensory Integration Tests, Los Angeles, 1972, Western Psychological Services.
23. Ayres AJ: Types of sensory integrative dysfunction among disabled learners, Am J Occup Ther 26(1):13, 1972.
24. Ayres AJ: Southern California Postrotary Nystagmus Test, Los Angeles, 1975, Western Psychological Services.
25. Ayres AJ: The effect of sensory integrative therapy on learning disabled children: the final report of a research project, Los Angeles, 1976, Center for the Study of Sensory Integrative Dysfunction.
26. Ayres AJ: Cluster analyses of measures of sensory integration, Am J Occup Ther 31(6):362, 1977.
27. Ayres AJ: Dichotic listening performance in learning-disabled children, Am J Occup Ther 31(7):441, 1977.
28. Ayres AJ: Effect of sensory integrative therapy on the coordination of children with choreoathetoid movements, Am J Occup Ther 31(5):291, 1977.
29. Ayres AJ: Learning disabilities and the vestibular system, J Learn Disabil 11(1):18, 1978.
30. Ayres AJ: Sensory integration and the child, Los Angeles, 1979, Western Psychological Services.
31. Ayres AJ: Aspects of the somatomotor adaptive response and praxis, Audiotape, Pasadena, Calif, 1981, Center for the Study of Sensory Integrative Dysfunction.
32. Ayres AJ: Personal communication, Feb 15, 1983.
33. Ayres AJ: Sensory integrative dysfunction: test score constellations. Part II of a final project report, Torrance, Calif, 1986, Sensory Integration International.
34. Ayres AJ: Sensory integration and praxis tests, Los Angeles, In press, Western Psychological Services.
35. Ayres AJ: Developmental dyspraxia and adult-onset apraxia, A lecture prepared for Sensory Integration International, 1985. Published by Sensory Integration International, 1402 Cravens Avenue, Torrance, CA 90501.
36. Ayres AJ, and Mailloux Z: Influence of sensory integration procedures on language development, Am J Occup Ther 35(6):383, 1981.
37. Ayres AJ, Mailloux Z, and McAtee S: An update of the sensory integration and praxis tests, Sensory Integration Special Interest Section Newsletter, p. 1, 1985.
38. Ayres AJ, Mailloux ZK, and Wendler CLW: Developmental apraxia. Is it a unitary function? Occup Ther J Res 7(2):93, 1987.
39. Ayres AJ, and Tickle L: Hyperresponsivity to touch and vestibular stimuli as a predictor of positive response to sensory integration procedures in autistic children, Am J Occup Ther 34:375, 1980.
40. Barkley RA, and Cunningham CE: Do stimulant drugs improve the academic performance of hyperkinetic children? A review of outcome studies, Clin Pediatr 17:85, 1978.
41. Barris R: Environmental interactions: an extension of the model of occupation, Am J Occup Ther 36(10):637, 1982.
42. Bauer RH: Memory processes in children with learning disabilities: evidence for deficient rehearsal, J Exp Child Psychol 24:415, 1977.
43. Beery K: Developmental Test of Visual Motor Integration, Chicago, 1967, Follett Publishing Co.

44. Berko MJ: Mental evaluation of the aphasic child, Am J Occup Ther 5(6):241, 1951.

45. Bobath K, and Bobath B: The facilitation of normal postural reactions and movements in the treatment of cerebral palsy, Physiotherapy 50:246, 1964.

46. Boden JE: The other side of the brain: an appositional. In Ornstein RE, editor: The nature of human consciousness, San Francisco, 1973, WH Freeman and Co, Publishers.

47. Boucher S: Ayres' sensory integration and learning disorders: a question of theory and practice, Aust J Ment Retard 5:41, 1978.

48. Brown AL: Knowing when, where, and how to remember: a problem of metacognition. In Glaser R, editor: Advances in instructional technology, Hillsdale, NJ, 1978, Lawrence Erlbaum.

49. Bruininks RH: Physical and motor development of retarded persons. In Ellis NR, editor: International review of research in mental retardation, vol 7, New York, 1974, Academic Press, Inc.

50. Bruininks R: Bruininks-Oseretsky Test of Motor Proficiency, Circle Pines, Minn, 1978, American Guidance Service.

51. Carrow E: Test for Auditory Comprehension of Language, Austin, Tex, 1973, Learning Concepts.

52. Carrow E: Carrow Elicited Language Inventory, Austin, Tex, 1974, Learning Concepts.

53. Carter E, et al: Sensory integration therapy: a trial of a specific neurodevelopmental therapy for the remediation of learning disabilities, J Devel Behav Ped 5:189, 1984.

54. Clark FA: Right and left hemisphere specialization: implications for the laterality and hemispheric dysfunction hypothesis of learning disabilities. In Tyler NB, editor: Sensory integration topics: faculty reviews, Pasadena, Calif, 1980, The Center for the Study of Sensory Integrative Dysfunction.

55. Clark FA, and others: A comparison of operant and sensory integration methods on vocalizations and other developmental parameters in profoundly retarded adults, Am J Occup Ther 32:86, 1978.

56. Clark FA, and Pierce D: Synopsis of pediatric occupational therapy effectiveness: studies on sensory integrative procedures, controlled vestibular stimulation, and other sensory stimulation approaches and perceptual-motor training, Proceedings of Maternal and Child Health Conference: Occupational Therapy for Maternal and Child Health: Research and Leadership Development, Miramar Sheraton, Santa Monica, Calif, Jan 1986.

57. Coles GA: The learning-disabilities test battery: empirical and social issues. Harv Educ Rev 48:313, 1978.

58. Critchley M: The dyslexic child, ed 2, Springfield, Ill, 1970, Charles C Thomas, Publisher.

59. Cruickshank W: Concepts in learning disabilities, vol 2, Syracuse, NY, 1981, Syracuse University Press.

60. Cruickshank W: Learning disabilities: a neurophysiological dysfunction, J Learn Disabil 16(1):27, 1983.

61. DePauw KP: Enhancing the sensory integration of aphasic students, J Learn Disabil 11(3):142, 1978.

62. Doehring DC, et al: Reading disabilities—the interaction of reading, language, and neuropsychological deficits, New York, 1981 Academic Press.

63. Doyle RB, Anderson RP, and Halcomb CG: Attention deficits and the effects of visual distraction, J Learn Disabil 9:48, 1976.

64. Dunn LM, and Smith JO: The Peabody Picture Vocabulary Tests, Circle Pines, Minn, 1966, American Guidance Service. In Dunn W: Occupational therapy must respond. Occupational Therapy Week, June 18, 1987.

65. Ensminger EE: The effects of a classroom language development program on psycholinguistic abilities and intellectual functioning of slow learning and borderline retarded children, Doctoral dissertation, 1966, University of Kansas.

66. Epps S, Ysseldyke JE, and Algozzine B: Impact of different definitions of learning disabilities on the number of students identified, J Psychoeduc Assess 1:341, 1983.

67. Farber SD: A multisensory approach top neurorehabilitation. In Farber SD, editor: Neurorehabilitation: a multisensory approach, Philadelphia, 1982, WB Saunders Co.

68. Farnham-Diggory S; Learning disabilities: A psychological perspective, Cambridge, Mass, 1978, Harvard University Press.

69. Ferguson HB, and Pappas BA: Evaluation of psychophysiological, neurochemical, and animal models of hyperactivity. In Trites RL, editor: Hyperactivity in children—etiology, measurement, and treatment implications, Baltimore, Md, 1979, University Park Press.

70. Fernald GM: Remedial techniques in basic school subjects, New York, 1943, McGraw-Hill Inc.

71. Fernald GM, and Keller H: One effect of kinesthetic factors in the development of word recognition in the case of nonreaders, J Educ Res 4:355, 1921.

72. Firestone B: Auditory reaction time of reading disabled children on three processing tasks, Doctoral dissertation, 1976, University of Southern California.

73. Flavell JH: Metacognitive aspects of problem solving. In Resnick LB, editor: The nature of intelligence, Hillsdale, NJ, 1976, Lawrence Erlbaum.

74. Florey LL: Studies of play: implications for growth, development, and for clinical practice, Am J Occup Ther 35(8):519, 1981.

75. Frostig M, and Horne D: The Frostig program for the development of visual perception, Chicago, 1964, Follett Publishing Co.

76. Frostig M, Lefever DW, and Whittlesey JRB: A developmental test of visual perception for evaluating normal and neurologically handicapped children, Percept Mot Skills 12:383, 1961.

77. Frostig M, and Maslow P: Neuropsychological contributions to education, J Learn Disabil 12(8):538, 1979.

78. Fuller PW: Attention to the EEG alpha rhythm in learning disabled children, J Learn Disabil 11:303, 1978.

79. Gadow KD: Children on medication, vol 1: Hyperactivity, learning disabilities, and mental retardation, Boston, 1986, College Hill.

80. Gardner M: Expressive One Word Picture Vocabulary Test, Norato, Calif, 1979, Gardner, Morrison Academic Therapy Publications.

81. Gazzaniga MS: The split brain in man, Sci Amer 217:24, 1967.

82. Gearheart B: Learning disabilities educational strategies, ed 2, St Louis, 1977, The CV Mosby Co.

83. Gearheart B: Learning disabilities educational strategies, ed 3, St Louis, 1981, The CV Mosby Co.

84. Giden FM, Eno ML, and Bosley EC: The occupational therapist discusses aphasia, Am J Occup Ther 4(4):160, 1950.

85. Gilfoyle E, and Grady A: Posture and movement. In Hopkins H, and Smith H, editors: Willard and Spackman's occupational therapy, Philadelphia, 1978, JB Lippincott Co.

86. Goldstein K: The organism, New York, 1939, American Book Co.

87. Grimwood LM, and Rutherford EM: Sensory integrative therapy as an intervention procedure with grade one "at risk" readers—a three year study, Except Child 27:52, 1980.

88. Hagen, JW: The effect of distraction on selective attention, Child Dev 38:685, 1967.

89. Hall RJ: Cognitive behavior modification and information-processing skills of exceptional children, Excep Educ Quar 1:9, 1980

90. Hammill DD, and Larsen SC: The efficacy of psycholinguistic training, Except Child 41:5, 1974.

91. Hammill DD, and Larsen SC: The effectiveness of psycholinguistic training: a reaffirmation of position, Except Child 44:402, 1978.

92. Harris LP: Attention and learning disordered children: a review of theory and remediation, J Learn Disabil 9:100, 1976.

93. Haworth M: The Primary Visual Motor Test, New York, 1970, Grune & Stratton Inc.

94. Head H: Aphasia and kindred disorders of speech, vols I, II, London, 1926, Cambridge University Press.

95. Hebb DO: Organization of behavior, New York, 1949, John Wiley & Sons Inc.

96. Hinshelwood J: Congenital word blindness, London, 1917, Lewis Publishers Inc.

97. Hiscock M, and Kinsbourne M: Specialization of the cerebral hemispheres: implications for learning, J Learn Disabil 20:130, 1987.

98. Hresko WP, and Reid DK: Five faces of cognition: theoretical influences on approaches to learning disabilities, Learn Dis Quar 2\4:238, 1981.

99. Hurff JM: Gaming technique: an assessment and training tool for individuals with learning disabilities, Amer J Occup Ther 35:728, 1981.

100. Jastak SR, and Jastak SWB: Wide Range Achievement Test, rev ed, Wilmington, Del, 1976, Guidance Associations of Delaware.

101. Kabat H, and Knott M: Principles of neuromuscular reeducation, Phys Ther Rev 28:107, 1948.

102. Katz P, and Deutsch M: Relation of auditory-visual shifting to regard achievement, Percept Mot Skills 17:327, 1963.

103. Kavale K: Functions of the Illinois test of psycholinguistic abilities (ITPA): are they trainable? Except Child 47:496, 1981.

104. Kavale K, and Forness S: The science of learning disabilities, San Diego, 1985, College-Hill Press.

105. Kavale K, and Mattson PD: One jumped off the balance beam: meta-analysis of perceptual-motor training, J Learn Disabil 16:165, 1983.

106. Keogh BK: Classification, compliance, and confusion, J Learn Disabil 16(1):25, 1983.

107. Koegh BK: Marker variables: a search for compatibility and generalizability in the field of learning disabilities, Learn Disabil Q 3(3):8, 1978.

108. Keogh BK, and Glover AT: The generality and durability of cognitive training effects, Excep Educ Quar 1:75, 1980.

109. Keogh BK, and Margolis J: Learn to labor and to wait: attentional problems of children with learning disorders, J Learn Disabil 9(5):276, 1976.

110. Kephart NC: The slow learner in the classroom, Columbus, Ohio, 1971, Charles E Merrill Publishing Co.

111. Kielhofner G, and Burke J: A model of human occupation. Part 1: conceptual framework and content, Am J Occup Ther 34(9):572, 1980.

112. Kielhofner G, Burke J, and Igi C: A model of human occupation. Part 4: assessment and intervention, Am J Occup Ther 34:777, 1980.

113. Kielhofner G, and Miyake S: The therapeutic use of games with mentally retarded adults, Am J Occup Ther 35:375, 1981.

114. Kimura D: The asymmetry of the human brain, Sci Amer 228:70, 1973.

115. Kinsbourne M, and Caplan PJ: Children's learning and attention problems, Boston, 1979, Little, Brown & Co Inc.

116. Kinsbourne M, and Hiscock M: Cerebral lateralization and cognitive development. In Chall JS, and Mirsky AE, editors: Education and the brain: the seventy-seventh yearbook of the National Society for the Study of Educaton (part 2), Chicago, 1978, University of Chicago Press.

117. Kirk SA, and Kirk WD: On defining learning disabilities, J Learn Disabil 16(1):20, 1983.

118. Kirk SA, McCarthy JJ, and Kirk WD: Examiner's manual: Illinois Test of Psycholinguistic Abilities, rev ed, Urbana, Ill, 1968, University of Illinois Press.

119. Leher RJ: an open letter to an occupational therapist, J Learn Disabil 14:3, 1981.

120. Llorens LA, and others: The effects of cognitive perceptual-motor training approach on children with behavior maladjustment, Am J Occup Ther 23(6):502, 1969.

121. Lloyd J: Academic instruction and cognitive behavior modification: the need for attack strategy training, Excep Educ Quar 1:53, 1980.

122. Loper AB: Metacognitive development: implications for cognitive training, Excep Educ Quar 1:1, 1980.

123. Lund KA, Foster GE, and McCall-Perez FC: The effectiveness of psycholinguistics training, a reevaluation, Except Child 44:310, 1977.

124. Lyon GR: Learning-disabled readers: identification of subgroups. In Mykelbust HR, editor: Progress in learning disabilities, vol 5, New York, 1983, Grune & Stratton Inc.

125. Lyon GR: Identification and remediation of learning disability subtypes: preliminary findings, Learn Dis Focus 1:21, 1985.

126. Maccoby EE: Selective auditory attention in children. In Lippsitt LP, and Spiker CC, editors: Advances in child development and behavior, vol 3, New York, 1967, Academic Press.

127. Mack W, Lindquist J, and Parham D: A synthesis of occupational behavior and sensory integration concepts in theory and practice. Part I: theoretical foundations, Am J Occup Ther 36(7):365, 1982.

128. Magrun WM, and others: Effects of vestibular stimulation on spontaneous use of verbal language in developmentally delayed children, Am J Occup Ther 35:101, 1982.

129. Mailloux Z: The relationship between self-esteem and praxis, visual motor integration and student role performance in learning disabled children, Masters thesis, 1980, University of Southern California.

130. Mailloux Z, and others: Pediatric dysfunction. In Kielhofner G, editor: A model of human occupation: theory and application, Baltimore, Md, 1985, Williams & Wilkins.

131. Mann L: Perceptual training revisited: the training of nothing at all, Rehabil Lit 32:322, 335, 1971.

132. Mann L, and others: LD or not LD, that was the question: a retrospective analysis of child service demonstration centers in compliance with the federal definition of learning disabilities, J Learn Disabil 16(1):14, 1983.

133. Mattis S, French JH, and Rapin I: Dyslexia in children and young adults: three independent neuropsychological syndromes, Dev Med Child Neurol 17:150, 1975.

134. McConnell F, Horton DB, and Smith BR: Sensory-perceptual and language training to prevent school learning disabilities in culturally deprived preschool children, Nashville, Tenn, 1972, the Bill Wilkerson Hearing and Speech Center. Final report, project no 5-0682, grant no OE6-32-52-7900-5025, USOE Bureau of Research.

135. McDaniel M: The role of the occupational therapist in the reeducation of aphasic patients, part III, Am J Occup Ther 8(2):63, 1955.

136. McKinney JD, and Haskins R: Cognitive training and the development of problem-solving strategies, Excep Educ Quar 1:41, 1980.

137. McKinney JD, Short EJ, and Feagans L: Academic consequences of perceptual-linguistic subtypes of learning disabled children, Learn Dis Res 1:6, 1985.

138. Meichenbaum D: Cognitive behavior modification with exceptional children: a promise yet unfulfilled, Excep Educ Quar 1:83, 1980.

139. Meichenbaum D: Cognitive-behavior modification: an integrative approach, New York, 1977, Plenum Publishing Corp.

140. Minskoff E, Wisemann DE, and Minskoff JG: The MWM program for developing language abilities, Ridgefield, NJ, 1972, Educational Associates.

141. Mirsky AF: Attention: a neurophysiological perspective. In Mirsky AF, editor: Education and the brain: the seventy-seventh yearbook of the National Society for the Study of Education, part II, Chicago, 1978, University of Chicago Press.

142. Mondani MS, and Tutko TA: Relationship of academic underachievement to incidental learning, J Consult Clin Psychol 33:558, 1969.

143. Montgomery P, and Richter E: Effect of sensory integrative therapy on the neuromotor development of retarded children, Phys Ther 57:799, 1977.

144. Moore J: Individual differences and the art of therapy, Am J Occup Ther 31(10):663, 1977.

145. Myklebust HR: Toward a science of learning disabilities, J Learn Disabil 16(1):17, 1983.

146. Mysak ED, and Fiorentino MR: Neurophysiological conditions in occupational therapy for the cerebral palsied, Am J Occup Ther 15(3):112, 1961.

147. National Joint Committee on Learning Disabilities: Learning disabilities: issues on definition, J Learn Disabil 20:107, 1987.

148. O'Donnell DA, and Eisenson J: Delacato training for reading achievement and visual-motor integration, J Learn Disabil 2:441, 1969.

149. Orton ST: Word blindness in school children, Arch Neurol Psychiatry 14:581, 1925.

150. Orton ST: Reading, writing and speech problems in children, New York, 1937, WW Norton & Co Inc.

151. Orton ST: A neurological explanation of the reading disability, Educ Rec 20:58, 1939.

152. Osgood CE: Method and theory in experimental psychology, New York, 1953, Oxford University Press, Inc.

153. Osgood CE: Motivational dynamics of language behavior. In Jones MR, editor: Nebraska symposium on motivation, Lincoln, Neb, 1957, University of Nebraska Press.

154. Ottenbacher K: Occupational therapy and special education: some issues and concerns related to Public Law 94-142, Am J Occup Ther 36(2):81, 1982.

155. Ottenbacher K: Sensory integraton therapy: affect or effect, Am J Occup Ther 36(9):571, 1982.

156. Ottenbacher K, and Cooper HM: Drug treatment of hyperactivity in children, Dev Med Child Neurol 25:358, 1983.

157. Palmer MF, and Berko F: The education of the aphasic child, Am J Occup Ther 6(6):241, 1952.

158. Pirozzolo FJ: the neuropsychology of developmental reading disorders, New York, 1979, Praeger.

159. Poncher HG, and Richmond JB: Occupational therapy in pediatrics, Am J Occup Ther 1(5):276, 1947.

160. Porges SW: Individual differences in attention: a possible physiological substrate. In Keogh BK, editor: Advances in special education, vol 2: perspectives on applications, Greenwich, Conn, 1980, JAI Press Inc.

161. Reid DK, and Hresko WP: A cognitive approach to learning disabilities, New York, 1981, McGraw-Hill Inc.

162. Reid DK, Knight-arest, I, and Hresko WP: Cognitive development in learning disabled children. In Gottlieb J, and Strichart SS, editors: Developmental theory and research in learning disabilities, Baltimore, Md, 1981, University Park Press.

163. Reilly M: The educational process, Am J Occup Ther 23(4):299, 1969.

164. Richmond, JB, and Lis EF: Occupational therapy in pediatrics, Am J Occup Ther 3(4):185, 1949.

165. Robinault IP: Perception techniques for the preschool cerebral palsied, Am J Occup Ther 8(1):3, 1954.

166. Rood MS: Neurophysiologic reactions as a basis for physical therapy, Phys Ther Rev 34:444, 1954.

167. Ross DM, and Ross SA: Hyperactivity—current issues, research, and theory, ed 2, New York, 1982, John Wiley & Sons.

168. Rourke BP: Reading, spelling, arithmetic disabilities: a neuropsychologic perspective. In Myklebust HR, editor: Progress in learning disabilities, vol 4, New York, 1978, Grune & Stratton Inc.

169. Rourke BP, editor: Neuropsychology of learning disabilities—essentials of subtype analysis, New York, 1985, Guilford Press.

170. Royeen CB: The development of a touch scale for measuring tactile defensiveness in children, Am J Occup Ther 6(40):414, 1986.

171. Royeen CB: Domain specifications of the construct tactile defensiveness, Amer J Occup Ther 39(9):596, 1985.

172. Sabatino DA: The house that Jack built, J Learn Disabil 16(1):26, 1983.

173. Satz P, and Fletcher JM: Minimal brain dysfunctions: an appraisal of research concepts and methods. In Rie HE, and Rie ED, editors: Handbook of minimal brain dysfunctions—a critical view, New York, 1980, John Wiley & Sons.

174. Satz P, Morris R, and Fletcher JM: Hypotheses, subtypes, and individual differences in dyslexia: some reflections. In Gray D, and Kavanagh J, editors: Biobehavioral measures of dyslexia, Parkton, Md, 1985, York Press.

175. Schuell H, Jenkins JJ, and Jimenez-Pablon E: Aphasia in adults, New York, 1964, Harper & Row, Publishers, Inc.

176. Senf GM, and Feshback S: Development of bisensory memory in culturally deprived, dyslexic, and normal readers, J Educ Psychol 61:461, 1970.

177. Shields DT: Brain responses to stimuli in disorders of information processing, J Learn Disabil 6:501, 1976.

178. Sieben RL: Controversial treatments for learning disorders, Acad Ther 13(2):138, 1977.

179. Spreen O, and Benton A: Sentence Repetition Test, Victoria, Canada, 1977, Neuropsychology Laboratory, University of Victoria.

180. Spreen O, and Haaf RG: Empirically derived learning disability subtypes: a replication attempt and longitudinal patterns over 15 years, J Learn Disabil 19:170, 1986.

181. Stanley G: The processing of digits by children with specific reading disability (dyslexia), Br J Educ Psychol 46:81, 1976.

182. Stanley G, and Hall R: Short-term visual information processing in dyslexics, Child Dev 44:841, 1972.

183. Stanley G, and Hall R: A comparison of dyslexics and normals in recalling letter arrays after brief presentation, Br J Educ Psychol 43:301, 1973.

184. Strauss AA: Diagnosis and education of the cripple-brained, deficient child, Except Child 9:163, 1943.

185. Strauss AA, and Kephart NC: Psychopathology and education of the brain-injured child, New York, 1955, Grune & Stratton Inc.

186. Strauss AA, and Lehtinen LE: Psychopathology and educaton of the brain-injured child, New York, 1947, Grune & Stratton Inc.

187. Strauss AA, and Werner H: Disorders of conceptual thinking in the brain-injured child, J Nerv Ment Dis 96:153, 1942.

188. Sullivan J: The effects of Kephart's perceptual motor training program on a reading clinic sample, J Learn Disabil 5:545, 1972.

189. Takata N: Introduction to a series: occupational behavior research for pediatric practice, Am J Occup Ther 34(1):11, 1980.

190. Tarver SG, and others: The development of visual selective attention and verbal rehearsal in learning disabled boys, J Learn Disabil 8:26, 1977.

191. Torgesen J, and Goldman T: Verbal rehearsal and short term memory in reading-disabled children, Child Dev 48:56, 1977.

192. Troyer BL: Sensorimotor integration: a basis for planning occupational therapy, Am J Occup Ther 15(2):51, 1961.

193. Tucker J, Stevens L, and Ysseldyke JE: Learning disabilities: the experts speak out, J Learn Disabil 16(1):7, 1983.

194. Vellutino F, and others: Has the perceptual deficit hypothesis led us astray? J Learn Disabil 10(6):375, 1977.

195. Voss DE: Proprioceptive neuromuscular facilitation: applications of patterns and techniques in occupational therapy, Am J Occup Ther 13(4):191, 1959.

196. Webster P: Occupational role development in the young adult with mild mental retardation, Am J Occup Ther 34(1):13, 1980.

197. Weeks ZR: Sensorimotor integration theory and the multisensory approach. In Farber SD, editor: Neurorehabilitation: a multisensory approach, Philadelphia, 1982, WB Saunders Co.

198. Weiss C: Weiss Comprehensive Articulation Test, Boston, 1978, Boston Teacher Resources.

199. Weiss G: Long-term outcome: findings, concepts, and practical implications. In Rutter M, editor: Developmental neuropsychiatry, New York, 1983, The Guilford Press.

200. Wepman JM, and others: Studies in aphasia: background and theoretical formulations, J Speech Hear Disord 25:323, 1960

201. Werner H: Comparative psychology of mental development, New York, 1948, International Universities Press.

202. Whalen CK, and Henker B: Hyperactivity and the attention deficit disorders: expanding frontiers, Ped Clin N Amer 31:397, 1984.

203. White M: A first grade intervention program for children "at risk" for reading failure, J Learn Disabil 12:230, 1979.

204. Wiederholt JL: Historical perspectives on the education of the learning disabled. In Mann L, and Sabatino DA, editors: The second review of special education, Philadelphia, 1974, JSE Press.

205. Wittrock MC: The cognitive movement in instruction, Educ Psychol 13:15, 1978.

206. Wolf R, and others: The structure of research in occupational therapy, Unpublished manuscript, 1983, University of Southern California.

207. Woodcock RW, and Johnson MB: Woodcock-Johnson psychoeducational battery, New York, 1978, Teaching Resources.

208. Ysseldyke J, and Salvia J: Diagnostic-prescriptive teaching: two models, Except Child 11:181, 1974.

24

Children with physical and orthopedic disabilities

JANET H. JOHNSON

SCOPE OF THE PROBLEM

This chapter is the result of a sharing of experiences from work with children who have physical and orthopedic disabilities. The disabilities involved are described according to the presenting problem or diagnosis, and they are reviewed and classified according to the difficulties displayed when children perform activities. Assessment procedures, treatment objectives, and intervention techniques are also presented.

We know that learning and development are complicated processes. The mind and the body are not isolated from each other in the acquisition of skills, but depend on the interaction of the various aspects of the whole organism. The inability of one system to function adequately may impede the development of abilities in another area or interfere with the growth process as a whole. Therefore the physically handicapped child often has developmental problems other than those related specifically to his or her physical disability. For example, a child who cannot move about and cannot manage his body to learn how it relates to the space around him may have difficulty with form and space concepts, directionality, and other perceptual concepts. The child with a physical disability may also exhibit learning problems, mental retardation, or emotional or behavioral difficulties that interfere with a full life. It must be noted that this chapter speaks primarily to problems resulting from physical disability. Reference to other chapters and resources is needed to design treatment intervention that incorporates goals related to additional problem areas. The occupational therapist must consider the breadth of skills needed by the child that will enable her to enjoy a satisfying life as a child and as an adult.

Presenting problems or diagnoses of children with physical disabilities

Children with physical disabilities that limit their ability to function normally can often be classified by a diagnosis or a syndrome, and they generally have conditions with a medical orientation. The diagnoses most seen are neurological and orthopedic problems and collagen diseases (Chapter 6). Specific examples are cerebral palsy, myelomeningocele, muscular dystrophies and atrophies, traumatic injuries, orthopedic abnormalities and defects such as absence or loss of limb, dwarfism, arthrogryposis, osteogenesis imperfecta, and rheumatoid diseases. Other less prevalent neuromuscular or orthopedic diseases and syndromes usually exhibit symptoms of weakness, limited joint range of motion, or incoordination, as do the other conditions.

General medical and surgical conditions that limit physical functioning may also be included here (Chapter 6). Examples of this group are children with congenital heart defects, anemias and leukemias, cystic fibrosis, diabetes, and kidney disease. In these cases children are limited in their ability to participate in activities by decreased energy, pain restriction, and certain medications or medical treatments. Occupational therapists may facilitate normalizing growth and development experiences for these children, recommend activities within their energy limitations, or suggest simplification techniques for performing activities.

Although there is some reticence in labeling and categorizing children, a classification such as a diagnosis can simplify communication among those persons working with a child. For example, when discussing a 10-year-old child with muscular dystrophy of the Duchenne type, trained professionals are immediately

510

aware of the common symptoms that this disease exhibits in a child of this age, such as the increasing weakness, the need for braces or a wheelchair, and the tightness seen in certain muscle groups. The time that this knowledge and awareness saves in communication can be significant. However, the danger in categorizing children by diagnosis is the possibility of viewing a child as a medical entity and not perceiving the individual needs and abilities that should be considered in planning and implementing treatment. Such stereotyping should be avoided.

For the purpose of treatment planning and implementation, children with physical disabilities are grouped according to major symptoms that impede function, and not by diagnosis. The causes of the limited function may result from neurological dysfunction, including loss of sensation or musculoskeletal problems. The major symptoms that impede function are:

1. Muscular weakness
2. Limited joint range of motion
3. Incoordination

Other services involved

Children with physical and orthopedic disabilities often have a variety of problems that require intervention beyond that which is provided by the family, through public education, or through routine medical care. For these children to develop into adults, having the freedom to contribute to their own and to society's well-being, the child and his parents may need the services of several kinds of trained professionals, such as physicians, nurses, social workers, dietitians, occupational and physical therapists, teachers, and other special educational personnel. Also included are people not specifically trained but involved in the child's care, such as babysitters, bus drivers, and extended family members.

Each profession brings a specific orientation and frame of reference to serve the child and her family. As unique as each profession is, remarkable similarities are seen in the educational programs and in the development of each specialty service. Because of these similarities, there is much overlap of skills and flexibility in the approach to service delivery. An example of this is the person who teaches the fracture patient how to bathe and dress himself: in one setting the occupational therapist fills this role and in another setting the nurse may do so. This overlap can result in some confusion in role definition, but it can also provide common reference points for child care workers.

Medical and educational services are costly. They are often inaccessible or strained to their limits because of cost, geography, or lack of available trained personnel. Therefore service personnel are increasingly finding it necessary and often desirable to teach the child and the parents to take a greater part in their health care and maintenance. This participation in self-care is evident in prevention, treatment, and habilitation. The health professional must educate clients to be active participants in their health and development. For the child who is not yet able to assume this responsibility, particularly the young child, it is the parent who must do so. The parents or primary caretakers are the most significant coordinators of the child's health care and development. To ignore the parent or caretaker in treatment planning and intervention is to limit the scope of treatment (Chapter 8).

Special characteristics of children with physical and orthopedic problems relevant to occupational therapy
VARIETY OF DIAGNOSES

Children with physical disabilities fall into several diagnostic categories. With the exception of cerebral palsy, myelomeningocele, and possibly muscular dystrophy, the number of children with any one diagnosis that one therapist may treat is small. However, the variety of diagnoses within the patient population is great. For this reason the therapist working with these children continually must refer to published references[6,27] and other professionals and participate in continuing education for information regarding the classical medical picture of those conditions not frequently seen.

PROGNOSIS AND CHANGE

Children with physical and orthopedic disabilities often demonstrate minimal and slow medical change. In many children the symptoms of the condition are present from birth, such as myelomeningocele and orthopedic defects. Others evidence a progressively debilitating condition that does not improve, as in muscular dystrophy or atrophy. Although the occupational therapist can do little to change the medical picture of a child's disease, the therapist can be of great assistance in preventing further disabilities, such as contractures, and in helping the child to compensate for lack of strength, limited joint range of motion, and incoordination. Thus the therapist may enable the child to engage in activities that are useful and meaningful to her.

EQUIPMENT

To perform many activities, children with physical disabilities often need to use adaptive appliances and equipment. Some need braces or splints, wheelchairs, prostheses, personal care equipment, standing tables, feeding equipment, and so on. Equipment may be required to enable a caretaker to care for, transfer, or transport a child. The occupational therapist may fabricate, order, or maintain some of these; the therapist may teach the child or caretaker to use the equipment in some cases as is appropriate to the occupational therapy goals. The therapist must be aware of the equipped artificial and extended parts of the child's body when considering the child's skills and limitations, for the child is often incomplete without them and may incorporate them into his body image.

TYPICAL TREATMENT SETTINGS

Although children with physical disabilities are seen in general hospitals, physician's offices, and home health agencies, the majority are treated by occupational therapists in settings specifically designed for child care and development. Children's hospitals are frequently the center of medical care for these children. Clinics oriented to specific disabilities may follow the child medically. Because of laws that require all children to attend school in the least restrictive setting and because of laws requiring related services to enable this participation, physically handicapped children in this country are seen, treated, and referred to other settings by occupational therapists working in the public schools.

ASSESSMENT PROCEDURES

In any assessment the occupational therapist is attempting to discover what the client can do and how she does it, and what the client cannot do and why she is unable to do so. Once this procedure has been completed, the therapist is more equipped to determine if intervention will help the client accomplish more and what treatment procedures are appropriate to make this happen.

By definition, a child with a physical disability is unable to perform expected or desired activities because of limitations imposed by her body. The occupational therapist determines which activities of self-maintenance, play, and work the child is unable to perform and what limitations her body is imposing. These limitations most often are a result of muscle weakness, lack of functional range of joint motion, or excessive incoordination.

Assessment of task performance

The nature of the physical disability is often expressed in terms of the problems encountered in performing activities. Therefore many occupational therapy assessment procedures used in working with the child with a physical disability are performance oriented. They evaluate or check the child's ability to perform specific tasks. Typical assessments are:

1. Checklists on daily living skills of feeding, dressing, and hygiene
2. Evaluations related to skills needed to function in a particular setting, such as a classroom skills checklist, a prevocational skills checklist, and a homemaking skills checklist
3. Growth and developmental skill evaluations

When the therapist administers these evaluations, or checklists, the child's response in following directions to perform a specific activity is observed. The therapist determines whether the child can perform the activity and how closely the child's response meets the criteria of the test item. For example, when evaluating a child's ability to independently remove his coat, the therapist is not only observing whether the child can take off his coat, but is also observing and judging the quality of the action: Is the coat removed in a reasonable period of time? Does the child use an unusual or adapted method to accomplish the task? Does he need assistance? If so, what kind of help does he need?

Most checklists incorporate some means to record the quality of the child's response. This may be a comments sections that is located by each test item, or following a section or area tested, or at the end of the form. Another method for grading the response is to use a letter or number that represents typical degrees of activity accomplishment. For example, one could use a number from 0 to 3, instead of a checkmark, when recording responses: *zero* could indicate that the child could not accomplish the activity; *one* could indicate difficult accomplishment only with assistance; *two* could indicate task accomplishment without assistance, but with difficulty or taking an excessive amount of time; and *three* could indicate that the child accomplished the activity independently and with ease.

Although information from a recorded history or from interviews can be used to note a child's abilities, the primary method for an occupational therapist to gather assessment information is by observing the child's actual performance of the activity. During the assessment the therapist gains information that goes beyond the specific skills being evaluated. Causes of nonperformance can be observed, solutions to problems can be generated, and methods for treatment may be suggested.

EXAMPLES OF TASK PERFORMANCE ASSESSMENTS

1. *Activities of daily living skills.* Lists of skills needed to perform self-maintenance activities are often compiled in a way to group together the skills needed for one type of self-care. For example, feeding, dressing, and grooming—hygiene are listed separately. The sections of the evaluation may also follow a developmental sequence or a simple-to-complex sequence. The following are examples of checklists of activities of daily living skills:
- Activities of Daily Living[1][*][16]
- Student Check List[33][*]
- "Life Works Tasks"[22]
- Callier-Asuza Scale self-help section[32]
- Learning Accomplishment Profile self-help section[27]
- *Portage Guide to Early Education*—Evaluation of fine motor and self skills[7]

2. *School-related physical skills.* There are certain physical skills that a child needs to function in a school

---

*For further information see Chapters 9 through 11.

setting, aside from the daily living skills previously mentioned. To work with a child, school personnel need to know which of these necessary skills a child can do and which ones must be taught or compensated for in order for the child to take advantage of the educational curriculum. Examples of evaluations of school-related physical skills are as follows:

- Bruininks-Oseretsky Test of Motor Proficiency[8]*
- Fine Motor Skill Evaluation[13]*
- Evaluation of Upper Extremity Function[12]*
- Learning Accomplishment Profile[29] sections on fine and gross motor skills
- Sensory Integration and Praxis Tests[4] information related to motor planning and motor accuracy*

3. *Play skills.* The child uses play as a developmental tool as well as for enjoyment. Physical manipulation of objects is a large part of play. Information regarding these physical skills can be gathered by observing free play, as well as by administering structured evaluation procedures. Examples of assessments of physical skills used in play are as follows:

- Bayley Scales of Infant Development[5]*
- Bruininks-Oseretsky Test of Motor Proficiency[8]*
- Fine Motor Skill Evaluation[13]*
- Denver Developmental Screening Test[14]*
- Learning Accomplishment Profile[29]
- *Portage Guide to Early Education*[7]

Assessment of physical limitations and abilities

In addition to the documentation of specific task performance, there is frequently a need to determine causes for the difficulties encountered by the child or her caretakers. Weakness, limited range of joint motion, and incoordination are the areas most appropriate to assess to determine a measurable level of physical ability or performance. Sensory testing is performed to determine if there is a loss in the tactile or temperature senses, proprioception, or stereognosis.[31] These evaluations give specific information on a particular physical ability, help to focus and set priorities among treatment goals, and give measurable criteria to assess changes in abilities that result from treatment or from the disease process. These changes may not be evident by looking solely at the child's ability to perform a task.

EXAMPLES OF ASSESSMENTS OF PHYSICAL LIMITATIONS

1. *Measurement of muscle strength.* Muscle tests are used to determine the extent and degree of muscular weakness. The results of the tests provide a basis for planning therapeutic intervention, and in conjunction with periodic retesting, they can be used in evaluating the effect of these procedures. Examples of references

related to the measurement of muscle strength are the following:

- Daniels and Worthington's[10] manual muscle tests
- Trombly and Scott's[34] manual muscle tests
- Kellor and others[20] manual muscle tests
- Kendall, Kendall, and Wadsworth's[21] manual muscle tests
- Pedretti's manual muscle tests[27a]
- Hand and pinch strength measurement with a dynamometer[2,17,24,35]*

2. *Measurements of range of joint motion.* Evaluation of the extent of joint range limitation is necessary before treatment. Remeasurement will document the effectiveness following treatment intervention. References related to measuring range of motion are the following:

- Trombly and Scott's[34] goniometric measurement, outline and palm prints, measurement from x-rays, and functional range of motion tests
- Smith's[30] goniometric measurement

3. *Measurements of coordination.* Examples of measurements of coordination are the following:

- Bruininks-Oseretsky Test of Motor Proficiency[8]*
- DeHaven, Mordock, and Loykovich's[11] tests involving speed and smooth movements
- Jebsen's[19] hand function test
- Minnesota Rate of Manipulation Test[25]
- Trombly and Scott's[34] specific tasks for manipulating buttons, scissors, and so on

The more specific the assessment tool, the more specific the information will be regarding areas needing remediation, and the more specifically treatment goals can be stated. Treatment objectives are determined from assessment information, including (1) the reason for referral, (2) information from others about the child, (3) developmental guidelines, and (4) the results of specific assessment procedures.

TREATMENT OBJECTIVES

In the transition from assessment to treatment lies much of the *art* of therapy. The therapist first gathers information about the specific child or children; weighs that information with the classical medical picture of a disability and his or her knowledge of growth and development and what children do in health; balances all this information with a knowledge and feeling about the needs or expectations of the child, the family, the school, or environmental setting; and finally determines a direction for treatment intervention.[3,9] This process is scientifically based in classical occupational therapy theory, but it is determined by sound clinical judgment, experience, and creativity in actuality.

The following points are considered in determining treatment objectives: (1) the child's present level of functioning, which is learned from assessments; (2) the child's expected level of performance according to his

---

*For further information see Chapters 9 through 11.

age or developmental sequence; (3) the environmental expectations or demands from the child's family or school; and (4) the resources available to implement the child's treatment goals.

Objectives for treatment are derived directly from information gathered from assessment results. It is the assessment that describes the areas of strength and the areas needing remediation. Assessments define what limitations a child with a physical disability has and what activities are affected as a result of those limitations. The limitations of a physically disabled child have been identified as weakness, limited range of motion, and excessive incoordination. Typical treatment objectives therefore follow.

Improve or maintain muscle strength and endurance

Muscle weakness may result from the disease process itself, as in muscular dystrophy, or from limited activity because of the difficulties or pain encountered in movement, such as in juvenile rheumatoid arthritis. A medical knowledge of the disease process and prognosis will help determine if it is appropriate to work toward improved muscle strength. Compensation for weakness may be a concurrent or alternative goal. In evaluating a child's ability to perform specific tasks, the therapist may note that the child may have difficulty moving about and using his body to manipulate objects as tools. If assessments show muscle weakness to be a limitation in task performance, improving muscle strength is typically a treatment goal in occupational therapy.

Improve or maintain joint range of motion

Limited range of motion can be observed in task performance. The child may be unable to reach in various directions or to parts of her body and to hold and manipulate objects needed to perform tasks. Assessment of functional range of motion or joint measurement can determine if the joint range is within normal limits.

Range of motion can be affected by muscle weakness or paralysis, as in myelomeningocele. It may be influenced by joint disturbances, as in juvenile rheumatoid arthritis in which range is limited because of pain and changes in the joint structure. Range of motion is also affected by fixed orthopedic disturbances, as in arthrogryposis, or by missing or foreshortened limbs, as seen in phocomelia. In cases where the range is not fixed and where stress on the joint through activity is not contraindicated, the occupational therapist typically may determine that a treatment goal to increase joint range of motion is appropriate. Prevention of contractures, as in splinting a joint, might also be a goal when an increase in range is unlikely and when the limited range could progress to a fixed contracture. For further discussion of splinting, see Chapter 13.

Improve the ability to control movements

Incoordination can result from various neuromuscular disease processes or from trauma. It can also occur in children with sequentially progressive but delayed neuromuscular development, often resulting from a lack of experience in doing activities because they are handicapped. For example, a kindergarten child with a disability, such as osteogenesis imperfecta, may have a great deal of difficulty cutting with scissors. It is common to discover that this may be the first experience for the child in using scissors. It is also common to find an improvement in the child's eye-hand coordination and in his accuracy of scissor use after participating in graded, sequential tasks using scissors. The occupational therapist may design treatment to improve the child's speed and accuracy of movement or to teach compensatory methods for activities affected by incoordination.

Compensate for deficit skills resulting from muscle weakness, limited range of motion, or incoordination

If the therapist finds it inappropriate or unfeasible for the child to strengthen muscles, improve joint range, or improve coordination because of medical contraindications such as pain, sensory loss,[31] or limited prognosis, goals may focus on the child's learning specific skills in a variety of ways that allow him greater participation in activities. These goals are stated in terms of specific behaviors. Some examples of compensatory goal statements follow:
1. The child will improve self-maintenance skills.
   a. The child will feed himself independently (using adapted utensils and dishes as necessary).
   b. The child will remain safely seated when bathed by a caretaker (using a mobile shower chair equipped with a seat and chest strap and wheel locks for transfer and support).
   c. The child will go to the bathroom unassisted (the therapist should note the height of toilet grab bars and type of clothing required for independence).
2. The child will increase her ability to engage in play and leisure time activities.
   a. Using weighted markers, the child will take turns with classmates when playing a board game.
   b. Given three choices of a toy for independent play, the child will make a choice and engage in appropriate play for 10 minutes.
   c. Given a nine-hole pegboard and corresponding pegs in two colors, the child will insert pegs to

play tic-tac-toe with the therapist or another child.
3. The child will perform school-related physical skills.
    a. The child will sit at a desk or table that is positioned to enable performance of classroom assignments.
    b. The child will print legibly using a pencil holder and primary paper secured to the work surface.
    c. Using adapted equipment (head pointer and keymask on a typewriter), the child will copy a short paragraph from the blackboard.

The therapist may determine several treatment goals resulting from observations, history, and formal assessments of the child. These goals and reasons for the goals must be communicated to others. While treatment intervention usually addresses more than one goal statement, there is a limit to the number of goals that can be carried out at any one time. Therefore the therapist must determine treatment priorities by considering the most important skills a child needs to be able to do at a particular time or place. Parents, teachers, physicians, and others may guide the therapist in this determination, and the policies of the setting may set some treatment parameters, but it is the occupational therapist's responsibility to accept or consider these suggestions in view of his or her professional knowledge of what is within the scope of the profession and what is appropriate and important for a particular child.

Within any of these goal areas, the therapist must further define the treatment objectives so that they are workable, measurable, and more easily communicated. The more specifically and clearly the goal is stated, the more clearly it will be understood by the child and others. Specific behaviors are also more clearly measured as to change. Small improvements can be observed, measured, and reported so that child, parent, therapist, and others can see whether treatment is having an effect and its extent.

TREATMENT MODALITIES

Children with physical disabilities are limited by their bodies in their capability to perform activities. As was said previously, some of these activities can be enhanced by improving the body's potential to perform the activity, such as by strengthening muscles, controlling coordination, or increasing range of joint motion. However, if methods designed to increase the physical function of a child are ineffective or inappropriate, adaptive or compensatory methods to achieve a skill are used.

Corrective modalities

Whenever possible, techniques are employed to enhance a child's ability to control and use his body. By so doing, the improved skills can be generalized and used in a variety of activities. For example, increased hand strength can help the child play with Lego blocks, manage buttons, hold a glass and spoon, write a school assignment, model clay, or construct a model airplane. Increasing the child's hand strength is more effective than teaching the child how to perform any one of these skills by compensating for hand weakness.

IMPROVING MUSCLE STRENGTH

During assessment, strength is measured and recorded. This information is necessary to understand the degree of weakness and to determine if there is a change in strength following treatment.

Participation in activities designed to strengthen particular muscles or muscle groups is the key element in the occupational therapy process. In selecting activities to improve muscle strength, two criteria must be considered. One simple consideration is whether the *chosen activity requires the contraction of the muscles* in question and whether substitution by other muscle groups is occurring. A second factor in activity selection is that *the activity should be graded* for resistance, for the length of time, or for the number of repetitions the child does the activity. The activity should be set at a low enough level to ensure muscle contraction, but at a high enough level to allow the upper limits of strength or endurance to be reached or measured within a treatment session. A child can operate a video game with an electronic device that requires pronation and supination of the wrist to activate and direct the video action. Resistance can be added to the electronic switch to require more muscle strength. The time or physical tolerance of operating the switch and the score earned can be measured and increased as the limits of strength of wrist pronation and supination are reached.

Periodically during the course of treatment, muscle strength should be remeasured to determine changes in strength and to note when a plateau or level of no change is reached. At this time it is worth noting any changes in functional abilities that may be occurring during the period of treatment intervention. During periods of reevaluation, determination must be made of whether to continue treatment intervention, to monitor strength levels, or to discontinue therapy.

INCREASING JOINT RANGE OF MOTION

A measurement of the joint range before treatment is essential to provide a baseline against which to judge the effectiveness of treatment and changes in function. Because the cause of limited range of motion can be a result of muscle weakness as well as a result of orthopedic disturbances, it is wise to measure both active and passive range of motion. A discrepancy between the two may indicate muscle weakness, and treatment goals and methods would be determined based on that factor.

Treatment methods for a child having limited joint range of motion fall into three areas: (1) active participation in activities requiring movement to the maximal range possible, (2) splinting a joint in a desired position to prevent contractures and deformities, and (3) administering passive stretching to specified joints.

Participation in activities is the one method that requires the interest and motivation of the child. As such, there is more likelihood for carryover of the responses used in therapy to other tasks throughout the day. Because of these adaptive and assimilated behaviors, activity is the primary method used in maintaining or improving joint range. There are three suggestions in using activities for children with this treatment objective: (1) the activity must require as great a joint movement as possible (lacing a sewing card having a long lace would encourage more movement of elbow and shoulder and therefore greater range than using a short string or lace); (2) the placement of the child or the activity can facilitate maximal joint range by requiring the child to reach (a child removing pegs and placing them in a box in front of her but at a distance requiring maximal elbow extension would be using a wider range in her elbow than if the box receiving the pegs were placed close to the pegboard); and (3) the therapist will need to watch for substitute movement that avoids the desired joint movement (in a reaching activity such as picking up puzzle pieces placed at the extreme range of elbow extension, a child may lean with his trunk to reach the object rather than extend his elbow as therapeutically desired).

When contractures are progressing and activity is unable to counteract the effect, it may be necessary to splint a body part to prevent fixed joint limitations from occurring. Making a splint for a child requires adjusting the splint pattern to fit the child and choosing materials that are as indestructible and washable as possible. The splint may be rigid or movable and may be worn for various lengths of time as determined by the therapist and the child's physician (Chapters 13 and 25).

Occasionally a therapist may find that the only way to keep a joint mobile is through passive range of motion. This can be accomplished through the child's participation in activities such as using a bilateral sander to increase elbow extension or holding a hoop with both hands while being pulled on a wheeled toy such as a scooter board to increase shoulder flexion. Seating a child with her knees extended or standing her with support can help counteract the effect of sitting long periods of time in a wheelchair with her legs flexed. Direct manipulation by the therapist is also employed to maintain or improve joint range. In such cases, the therapist is cautioned to move the joint carefully to, and just beyond, the known passive range, being mindful of the child's diagnosis and its contraindications.

As in all treatment intervention, remeasurement of the joint range at periodic intervals is necessary to see if the range has changed and to what degree. At times of reevaluation, treatment objectives can be altered or eliminated according to the results of reassessment.

IMPROVING COORDINATION

Although children with coordination problems may be treated by being taught compensatory skills, rather than by attempting to change the motor coordination itself, there are some methods that are designed to enable these children to control their excessive or uncontrolled movements. One such method is the *grading of activities to increase the required accuracy of response*. An example is the designing of activities by use of 1-inch, ½-inch, ¼-inch, or ⅛-inch pegs and corresponding pegboards. As the child is able to accurately and relatively quickly insert the 1-inch pegs in the board, activities are designed that use the next smaller size pegs (Figure 24-1). Another example is teaching the child to write by using primary lined paper and progressing to narrow-lined, loose-leaf notebook paper.

Analogous to the increase in accuracy is the *grading of activities to increase the speed of performance*. The child playing the commercial game SIMON can move from level 1 to level 2 or 3 as he responds within the programmed time allotted at each level. Speed can also be graded into activities for the child learning to use the typewriter or the computer in the school setting. Better coordination is thus the increase in speed and accuracy in the performance of activities.

The task of improving coordination does not belong solely to occupational therapy. Indeed, both physical

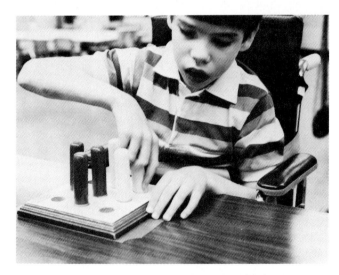

Figure 24-1   Tic-tac-toe is played by inserting 1-inch pegs in a nine-hole pegboard.

Photograph by Darin Derstine.

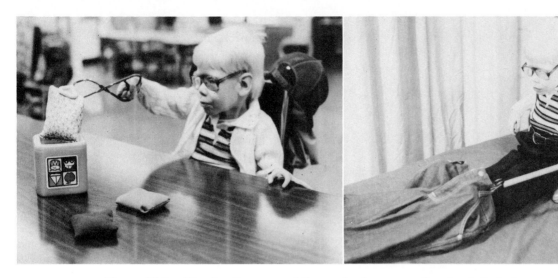

Figure 24-2   "Reachers" can extend the reach when range of motion is limited.

Photograph by Darin Derstine.

education and physical therapy find this is one of the primary objectives within their professions. The occupational therapist can resolve this apparent overlap in roles by focusing on therapeutic efforts and activities in the major areas of childhood performance relevant to occupational therapy: self-maintenance activities, play and leisure time activities, and schoolwork and prevocational activities (Chapters 13 through 17).

Compensatory methods

When attempts to improve muscle strength, joint range of motion, or coordination are unsuccessful or inappropriate, goals may focus instead on the child's learning to perform specific skills in whatever manner allows him to function as independently as possible. In such cases some adaptation or change in the skill is needed. The task is analyzed into its component parts (1) to teach the sequential parts of the skill, (2) to simplify or change the method of performing the skill, or (3) to teach the skill through the use of adaptive equipment or supplies.

There are some key factors to consider in compensatory skill accomplishment. The use of lighter weight objects and energy-saving devices, often electronic, help to compensate for muscle weakness. Devices to improve reach can be used to accomplish a task by compensating for limited range of motion (Figure 24-2). The performance of coordinated movements can be helped by providing stability, for example, using weights, weighted objects, or nonslippery surfaces (Figure 24-3).

When a particular skill cannot be performed by the child following corrective therapeutic procedures or by teaching, simplifying, or adapting the activity itself,

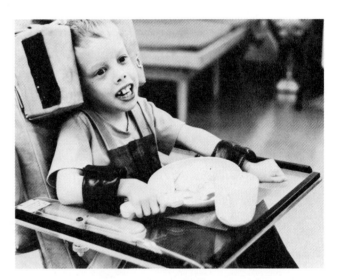

Figure 24-3   Stability to control incoordination is achieved by weights, weighted cup and utensils, and a nonslippery surface.

Photograph by Darin Derstine.

then specific adaptive equipment may be necessary for the most efficient or independent performance of an activity (Figures 24-4 and 24-5). An occupational therapist may teach a child with muscle weakness to write by using an electric typewriter (Figures 24-6 and 24-7), show a child in a full arm cast how to use a card holder to play cards, or teach him how to use a rocker-knife to cut food into bite-size pieces. A splint can serve as a holder or a tool when there is weakness or limited range of motion (Figure 24-7). To make a decision to use a piece of adaptive equipment, the therapist must

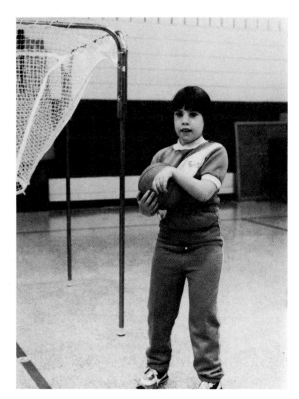

Figure 24-4 Stylish clothing with elastic and Velcro fasteners (see Figure 14-10, *B*) eliminates the need to button, zip, snap, and tie and enables many children to be independent in dressing and toileting.

Photograph by Darin Derstine.

consider the importance of the skill to be enhanced by the equipment (Figure 24-8 on p. 520), the acceptance of the equipment by the child and her family (Figure 24-9 on p. 520), and the cost or effort involved (Figures 24-10 and 24-11 on p. 520).

Techniques and materials

The following suggestions should be considered when working with children with physical and orthopedic disabilities.

LEVEL OF ACTIVITY

Recommended activities should be at a level of complexity that is low enough to allow the child to perform and high enough for the child to improve skill competence. The areas to consider in determining the level of activity are the child's (1) age level, (2) interest level, and (3) physical ability level. An example of an activity used to improve bilateral coordination is stringing beads. A young child in preschool or kindergarten finds random stringing of 1-inch wooden beads to be interesting and within his ability level. A teenage girl is interested in jewelry and has the physical and conceptual ability to string small beads in complex patterns to make a necklace. The interest level can range from stringing one color and shape beads to complex patterns of beading to decorate clothing or make Indian costumes.

SEQUENCE OF ACTIVITY

For the child's abilities to improve, the activities must be sequentially graded to greater levels of diffi-

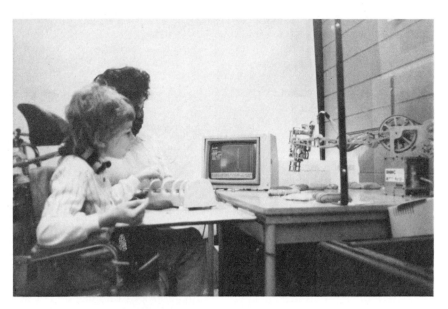

Figure 24-5 The use of a robotic device can enable object manipulation when voluntary grasp and release is limited.[18]

Photograph by Kathy Campbell.

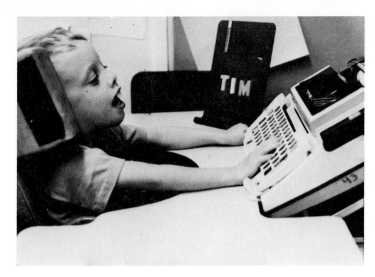

Figure 24-6   This child is learning to type on an electric typewriter with a key mask to help control incoordinated movements. A raised desk stabilizes his arms.

Photograph by Darin Derstine.

culty, requiring increased strength, greater range of motion, or more refined coordination. In the example of stringing beads to improve coordination, certain materials may be selected to make the task physically easier: use beads with large holes; use pipe cleaners or thick, rigid elastic; or extend the length of the rigid tip of the string by dipping it in nail polish or wrapping the string with tape. The materials selected can also require increased coordination for the task: reduce the size of the bead and the size of the bead hole; use a needle and thread instead of a thicker string; or introduce other skill requirements such as twisting a shaped bead to a certain position on a wire or string.

VARIETY AND REPETITION OF ACTIVITIES

Repetition of a skill is necessary to master it; however, a variety of activities is necessary to motivate the child to perform this repetition. Variety is also important to enable the child to generalize the use of the newly developed skill in more than one way. It is a challenge to select a variety of activities that are at the appropriate age, interest, and ability level for a child.

In the bead stringing example, additional examples for activities requiring inserting an object in a defined hole or space are stringing "tribeads" on a pipe cleaner and twisting to form a holiday wreath for a tree decoration; inserting punched notebook paper in a ring notebook; lacing a wallet having prepunched holes with a cord; placing vegetables on skewers for shish kebab; or placing washers and nuts on bolts. As activities become more complicated, additional skill requirements are often needed to perform the activity, such as perceptual skills of sequencing and positioning or conceptual skills related to following directions.

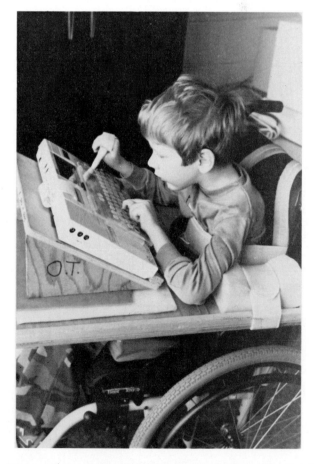

Figure 24-7   Access to a keyboard is possible with a hand splint specifically constructed for that purpose.

Photograph by Kathy Campbell.

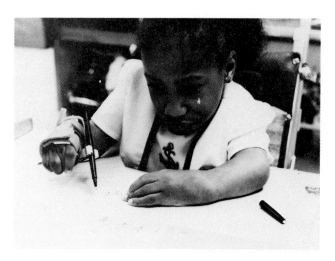

Figure 24-8 By using a splint with a pencil holder, this child who has no grasp is able to write.

Photograph by Darin Derstine.

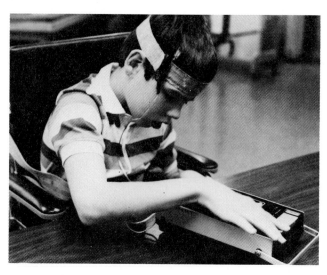

Figure 24-9 A mercury gravity switch is attached to a headband and activates the tape recorder when the child's head is held erect.

Photograph by Darin Derstine.

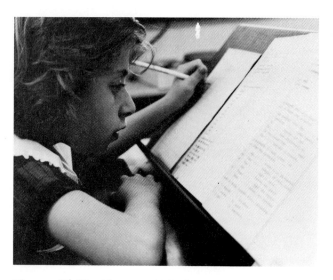

Figure 24-10 After surgical decompression of Arnold-Chiari syndrome, this child benefits from a raised writing surface to avoid stress on the cervical spine.

Photograph by Darin Derstine.

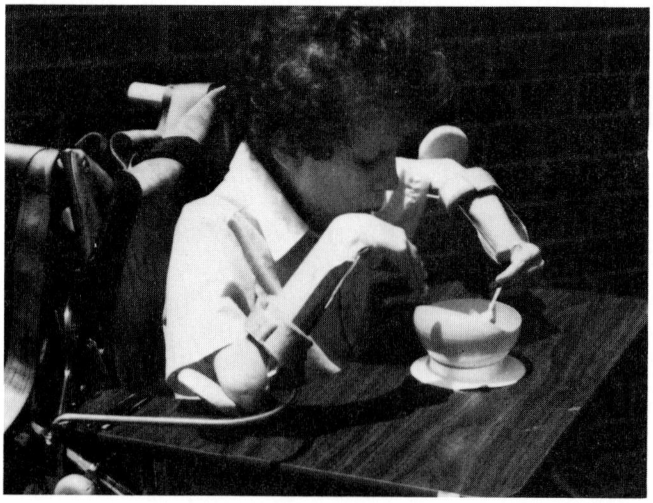

Figure 24-11 A balance forearm orthosis can compensate for weak shoulder and elbow musculature to enable independence in self-feeding.

Photograph by Kathy Campbell.

ADAPTIVE EQUIPMENT

Adaptive equipment may be necessary to perform a skill independently or efficiently. When selecting the most appropriate piece of equipment, the therapist must have a clear understanding of the particular skill that needs to be enhanced and have an awareness of available equipment designed to help perform that skill. If the equipment is not available or cannot be purchased commercially, it may need to be specifically designed and constructed to fit an individual child with a specific skill requirement. It is important for the therapist to have knowledge of available resources in the community, such as medical equipment houses; carpenters or other skilled craftsmen; biomechanical, electrical, and structural engineers; funding sources, both public and private; and other therapists with experience in this area. The reader is referred to Chapters 13 and 17 as well as to companies selling medical equipment and special education supplies and articles in professional journals[15] for examples of adaptive equipment.

COMMUNICATION AND REFERRAL

The multiplicity of problems presented by a child with a physical or orthopedic disability results in a variety of people being involved in his care and development. Therefore much of the therapist's time is spent in efforts with the family and other professionals to help solve the problems a child is experiencing.

Preparation for adulthood

The skills needed to enjoy a satisfying adulthood are many and varied. Social, emotional, and cognitive skills, as well as physical skills, are needed to participate in activities of self-maintenance, leisure, and work. Although the occupational therapist working with children having a physical disability will typically focus treatment on whatever physical skills are needed for maximal independence and satisfaction, goals to enhance social and emotional skills are also considered. Through training, education, and experience the occupational therapist appreciates the breadth of the skills needed in adulthood and reflects this appreciation in treatment, planning, and implementation. Priorities for each child may vary, but goals related to prevocational, sensory-motor, and social-emotional skill development are considered to enable the child to participate as fully as possible as an adult.

CASE STUDY

Billy is a newly enrolled 10-year-old in a class for orthopedically handicapped children. All children in this setting receive occupational therapy services. He has been medically diagnosed as having muscular dystrophy of the Duchenne type.

Planned assessments for Billy include the Activities of Daily Living checklist, the classroom-related skills checklist, and observation and notations regarding play and leisure skills.

Billy ambulates by wheelchair. He can push his wheelchair for short distances, but he fatigues quickly. Although he appears to have good coordination when writing, cutting, or turning the pages of a book, he does not reach for objects and cannot elevate his arm. He cannot lift his school textbooks, carry his school lunch, or open his carton of milk. When he eats, he lowers his head to his hand or to the spoon, rather than lift the spoon to his mouth. He eats very little. Endurance is a problem in all motor activities. Billy talks a lot to classmates and to the teacher. He seems intent or serious when interacting with his classmates. Occasionally during recess a shouting interchange with a classmate is heard. According to bulletin board displays, Billy is one of the best students in the class, having read the most books and reaching the highest rung on the math ladder.

Results of assessments indicate that Billy needs assistance in dressing and hygiene, but he has the ability to feed himself with a spoon or fork once the food is cut and prepared. He is able to write and use scissors to cut paper. His grasp, pinch, and release are functional, but weak. Functional active range is within normal limits in his hands and wrists, but limited in proximal muscle groups of the upper extremities. This limits his reach to perform activities. He appears to have some difficulty interacting with his classmates.

The physical findings correlate with the classical medical picture and demonstrate that the underlying cause of the skill deficits is muscle weakness. To record the present level of strength, the Manual Muscle Test was administered.

Treatment goals

1. Billy will participate in the school curriculum as appropriate to his abilities, using adapted methods or equipment as necessary for functioning.
   a. Billy will sit with his spine as straight as possible, using adaptations to the wheelchair and desk as necessary.
   b. Billy will write classroom assignments with his desk elevated to rest his arms by working short periods of time or using an electric typewriter to reduce fatigue.
   c. Billy will gather materials needed for schoolwork. The therapist will suggest placement and materials to facilitate independence (for example, use of desk organizers to reach materials and lightweight materials when possible).
2. Billy will participate in his self-care as much as possible, using adaptive equipment when necessary.
   a. Billy will use a balance forearm orthosis to enable lifting an eating utensil to his mouth.
   b. When possible, Billy will choose foods that he can manage himself that require no cutting and that have no packages or cartons to open.
   c. Given the appropriate height sink and placement of soap within his reach, Billy will wash his hands independently at school.
   d. Billy will remove a large coat by pulling the cuffs with his opposite hand or with his teeth and shaking out his arm, and will hang the coat on a hook placed within his reach.
3. Billy will participate in play and leisure time activities at school.
   a. Billy will play games within his ability level with classmates (board games, word games), adapting when necessary to participate (for example, scorekeeper, cheerleader).
   b. Billy will participate in individually chosen leisure activities (art, crafts, reading).

4. The therapist will facilitate acceptance of the disease when appropriate.
   a. Refer to agencies or professionals for financial, emotional, or medical assistance, when requested by parents.
   b. Suggest materials and methods to help in Billy's care at home (for example, adaptive clothing or methods of dressing if there are contractures, and leisure time activities for home).
5. The therapist will monitor upper extremity strength by administering muscle tests periodically.

Therapeutic prognosis

Muscular dystrophy is a progressively debilitating disease process evidenced by increasingly weakened muscle strength. The probability of contractures occurring is high, and recurring respiratory problems cause increased threats to life. As Billy becomes weaker, he will benefit from participating in a variety of activities requiring progressively less strength: manipulating objects may need to be replaced by electronically operated equipment for vocational or leisure tasks. Eventually passive activities of viewing and listening at his level of interest will be required. Building interests early and adapting activities to meet these interests in treatment intervention help ensure a full, although short, life. Specific suggestions to enable Billy to participate in activities at his age level, considering his decreasing strength:

1. A power wheelchair will prolong independent mobility.
2. The occupational therapist may consult with physical therapy regarding a ramp at home or lifts for a van to enable Billy to travel from his home to school or the doctor's office, or for shopping or recreation.
3. Using an electric typewriter, a computer with a printer attachment or a word processor may enable Billy to complete school assignments and to play mental games.
4. Providing a desk or wheelchair tray can serve as a work surface, elevating the position of the arms to help maintain the trunk in spinal alignment.
5. Using robotic devices may enable Billy to pick up and place objects for functional use in daily living and classroom activities and for recreational pleasure.
6. Billy could use a speaker phone to eliminate the need to hold the phone to his ear.
7. A wheelchair with reclining back will decrease the gravitational pull of the body into a scoliosis.
8. A mechanical lift may be required to enable a caretaker to transfer Billy in and out of the tub, bed, or wheelchair. Billy's parents and caretakers need to be informed about the disease process and about methods and adaptive equipment to help in Billy's care. They need to be shown how their home treatment programs can delay the effects of the disease, such as the development of contractures, and they need to be informed about programs and assistance available to them (for example, the Muscular Dystrophy Association).

SUMMARY

Children with physical and orthopedic disabilities often have problems of development that are separate from, although stemming from, their physical disability. Therapists must design treatment programs that take the child's developmental status into account as well as the presenting physical problem. Both corrective and compensatory treatment methods were presented in this chapter. Methods of assessment and treatment objectives were also discussed.

STUDY QUESTIONS

1. What are the three major types of symptoms characteristic of children with physical and orthopedic disabilities? Discuss how these problems may differentially affect the daily living skill performance of:
   a. A preschooler with myelomeningocele
   b. An 8-year-old child with juvenile rheumatoid arthritis
   c. A 13-year-old child with muscular dystrophy
   d. A 17-year-old with an above knee sarcoma secondary to osteosarcoma
2. What adaptations might you make for each of the above children that would facilitate his ability to throw a ball one-handed, and, for the older children, to make their beds?
3. What are some of the different compensatory methods that can be used to improve the active range of motion when muscle weakness is present?
4. Using the 1/8-inch pegs, time yourself as you insert 100 pegs into a board under three different conditions:
   a. While using your non-dominant hand with a 5 pound weight on your wrist
   b. While wearing an oversized glove
   c. With your upper arm strapped to your chest so that shoulder movement is eliminated.

What are the differences in time and quality of performance? How can you adapt the activity so that your skill level improves, without removing the handicapping condition?

REFERENCES

1. Activities of daily living, Columbus, Ohio, 1982, Colerain School.
2. Ager C, Olivett BL, and Johnson CL: Grasp and pinch strength in children 5-12 years old, Am J Occup Ther 38:107, 1984.
3. American Occupational Therapy Association: Roles and functions of occupational therapy in early childhood intervention—a position paper. Am J Occup Ther 40:835, 1986.
4. Ayres AJ: Sensory Integration and Praxis Tests, Los Angeles, 1986, Western Psychological Services.
5. Bayley N: Bayley Scales of Infant Development, New York, 1969, Psychological Corp.
6. Bleck EE, and Nagel DA: Physically handicapped children: a medical atlas for teachers, ed 2, New York, 1982, Grune & Stratton, Inc.
7. Bluma SM, and others: Portage guide to early education, Portage, Wisc, 1976, Cooperative Educational Service Agency 12.
8. Bruininks RH: Bruininks-Oseretsky Test of Motor Proficiency, Circle Pines, Minn, 1978, American Guidance Service.
9. Campbell P, McInerney WF, and Cooper MA: Therapeutic programming for students with severe handicaps, Am J Occup Ther 38:594, 1984.
10. Daniels L, and Worthingham C: Muscle testing—techniques of manual examination, ed 4, Philadelphia, 1980, WB Saunders Co.
11. DeHaven EG, Mordock JB, and Loykovich JM: Evaluation of coordination deficits in children with minimal cerebral dysfunction, Phys Ther 49:53, 1969.

12. Evaluation of upper extremity function—occupational therapy, Columbus, Ohio, 1982, Colerain School.

13. Fine motor skill evaluation—occupational therapy, Columbus, Ohio, 1980, Colerain School.

14. Frankenburg WK, and Dobbs JB: The Denver Developmental Screening Test, Denver, 1969, LADOCA Project & Publishing Foundation, Inc.

15. Hall K, and Hammock M: Feeding and toileting devices for a child with arthrogryposis, Am J Occup Ther 33:644, 1979.

16. Hays C, Kassimir J, and Parkin J, Sample forms for occupational therapy, Rockville, Md, AOTA, 1980.

17. Hopkins HL, and Smith, HO, editors: Willard and Spackman's occupational therapy ed 6, Philadelphia, 1983, JB Lippincott Co.

18. Howell R, Damarin SK, Clarke JA, and Lawson J: Design issues in the use of robotic devices as cognitive prosthetic aids with physically handicapped children. In Malick J, and Antonak R, editors: Transitions in mental retardation, Norwood, NJ, Ablex Publishing Corp (in press).

19. Jebsen R: An objective and standardized test of hand function, Arch Phys Med Rehabil 50:311, 1969.

20. Kellor M, and others: Hand strength and dexterity, Am J Occup Ther 25:77, 1971.

21. Kendall HO, Kendall FP, and Wadsworth GE: Muscles testing and function, ed 2, Baltimore, 1971, Williams & Wilkins.

22. Malick M, and Sherry B: Life works tasks. In Hopkins HL, and Smith HD, editors: Willard and Spackman's occupational therapy, ed 5, Philadelphia, 1978, JB Lippincott Co.

23. Mathiowitz V, et al: The Purdue peg board: norms for 14-19 year olds, Am J Occup Ther 3:174, 1986.

24. Mathiowitz V, Weimer D, and Federman S: Grip and pinch strength: norms for 6 to 19 year olds, Am J Occup Ther 10:705, 1986.

25. Minnesota Rate of Manipulation Test, Circle Pines, Minn, 1969, American Guidance Service, Inc.

26. Muscular Dystrophy Association, 810 7th Ave, New York, NY 10019.

27. Nelson WE, and others, editors: Textbook of pediatrics, ed 11, Philadelphia, 1979, WB Saunders Co.

27a. Pedretti LW: Occupational therapy: practice skills for physical dysfunction, ed 2, St Louis, 1985, The CV Mosby Co.

28. Robinault I, editor: Functional aids for the multiply handicapped, Hagerstown, Md, 1973, Harper & Row, Publishers, Inc.

29. Sanford AR: Learning Accomplishment Profile, Chapel Hill, NC, 1974, Chapel Hill Training-Outreach Project.

30. Smith H: Specific evaluation procedures. In Hopkins HL, and Smith HD, editors: Willard and Spackman's occupational therapy, ed 5, Philadelphia, 1978, JB Lippincott Co.

31. Smith H: Sensory testing. In Hopkins HL and Smith HD, editors: Willard and Spackman's occupational therapy, ed 6, Philadelphia, 1983, JB Lippincott Co.

32. Stillman R; Callier-Asuza Scale, Dallas, Tex, 1975, Callier Center for Communication Disorders.

33. Student check list—activities of daily living skills, Columbus, Ohio, 1980, Colerain School.

34. Trombly CA, and Scott AD: Occupational therapy for physical dysfunction, Baltimore, 1977, Williams & Wilkins.

35. Weiss MW, and Flatt AE: A pilot study of 198 normal children: pinch strength and hand size in the growing hand, Am J Occup Ther 25:10, 1971.

25

Children with severe burns

CHRISTINE BOSONETTO DOANE

SCOPE OF THE PROBLEM

"Each year approximately 745,000 children are burned; 40% of these children are burned severely enough to require hospitalization."[17] This is a startling fact when one realizes that in most cases, and even with the best medical help and rehabilitation, the child is left with physical and emotional scars.

Burns in children are usually caused by thermal sources, such as fire or hot water. Certain electrical burns (microstomia) caused by biting an electric cord are also a serious problem. Other causes of burns include sunburn, chemicals, frostbite, and radiation.

On the basis of age, children between 1 and 3 years old are most frequently burned by hot water scald. Children between 3 and 14 years old are most frequently burned by clothing fires. Teenagers are categorized along with adults and are most frequently burned in house or industrial fires.[29]

Burns are life-threatening or major if (1) they cover more than 10% of the total body surface, (2) the child is under age 4, (3) the child has a history of illness or disability, (4) the burns involve the hands, face, or perineum, (5) the child has respiratory or other problems, or (6) the burn is electrical.[1,5,10] A patient with a major burn should be hospitalized where lifesaving efforts can be made.

Skin and burn classification

Recall the anatomy of the skin. The skin is composed of layers of epidermis and dermis; it hosts blood vessels, hair follicles, glands, and nerve cells. Since skin is also the body's largest protective organ, its destruction creates a vulnerability to infection, a loss of body fluids, temperature deregulation, and sensory loss.[3,10]

One of the oldest ways of classifying burns is according to degree. A first degree burn is usually referred to as a minor burn. It can produce redness, slight edema, and soreness; however, blisters do not appear, and it only involves the epidermis.

A second degree burn has blisters and can be superficial or deep with some dermal necrosis. Enough dermis is left, however, to provide for epithelialization. A second degree burn is the most painful, because most of the sensory nerve endings remain effective.

A full thickness burn is also referred to as a third degree burn. Some physicians classify burns further as fourth and fifth degree. Most authors, however, agree that a full thickness burn has the following characteristics: (1) sensation is absent; (2) the burned area is leathery; (3) the color of the burn is usually white or black—if red, it does not blanch with pressure; and (4) the epidermis is completely destroyed, and the dermis is for the most part destroyed. Underlying muscles and tendons can be seriously affected.[1,3,5,10,26]

When the dermis is destroyed, the skin is unable to regenerate; therefore grafting is necessary to cover those body areas that are exposed to infection. Types of skin grafts include (1) autografts, (2) heterografts or xenografts, and (3) homografts. Autografts, which are made of the patient's own skin, are usually grafted from the buttocks or thighs, but can be taken from almost any unburned compatible area. A dermatome is the instrument used to skive the desired thickness of skin from the donor site. Autografts have a high success rate and are considered permanent coverage. Heterografts, or xenografts, are made of pigskin and are used as a temporary cover only. In deep second degree wounds this type of temporary cover allows reepithelialization to take place. Homografts made of cadaver skin are also temporary.[10,12,26]

Whenever full thickness burns occur, the effects of scar tissue must be addressed. Scar tissue is different from normal epithelial tissue, not only in its appearance, but also in the way it grows. Normal skin collagen is laid down in neat organized patterns. After a third degree burn, the collagen becomes more profuse, and the pattern becomes very disorganized; the body loses its ability to reproduce normal skin, and hypertrophic scars result. Scar tissue does not have normal elasticity, but it is contractile. This is thought to be the result of myofibroblasts found in the collagen. Lamberty and Whitaker[18] state,

Fibroblasts contain contractile elements in their cytoplasm similar in appearance to the striations seen in smooth muscle. They also appear to be responsible for, and possibly the main factors in, burn scar contracture.

If patients who have sustained full thickness burns are not appropriately treated, splinted, positioned, and exercised, the unmanaged growth of scar tissue can result in grotesque and serious disfigurement. This deformity in turn causes equally serious limitations in functional performance, including range of motion, strength, dexterity, and activities of daily living.

GENERAL ROLE OF OCCUPATIONAL THERAPY INTERVENTION

The specific professional role of occupational therapy to be demonstrated depends on the policies, the participating physicians, and the history of the institution in which therapy is to be provided. It is important to note that there are slight to significant differences in burn care procedures and methodology. Some general guidelines, however, can be discussed to present the basics of burn care in pediatrics. Hospitals with burn units or beds allocated to burn care would have the greatest opportunity for occupational therapy intervention. However, smaller hospitals that treat less severe burns or see burn patients for joint scar contractures on an outpatient basis have significant need for an occupational therapist as well.

The role of the occupational therapist with the burned child covers the following aspects[14,16,25]

1. To assist in the prevention of deformity, contracture, and hypertrophic scar formation
2. To provide appropriate and carefully selected treatment techniques and therapeutic activities for range of motion, strength, functional coordination, and developmental skills
3. To enable the child to return to as independent a life-style as possible and as is appropriate for the child's age
4. To provide psychosocial therapeutic intervention for the patient's emotional well-being

This role is also translated into services as follows: basic splinting; progressive splinting; exercise through purposeful activities, including educational, avocational, and leisure tasks; activities of daily living, such as hygiene, feeding self, dressing, and playing; provision of adaptive equipment; maintaining developmental abilities as possible; alleviating anxiety; providing opportunities to express underlying emotions and feel-

ings; enhancing self-esteem and self-image; and assisting patients and families with reintegration into society.

Treatment of the burned child presents a very special challenge to the occupational therapist. Most areas of academic learning and practical experience are applied and used daily. Although certain procedures have routine or sequential criteria, it is most usual with burn patients that diversity, creativity, adaptation, and a dynamic challenge are the order of the day. Occupational therapists, therefore, must be prepared to (1) extend themselves beyond the routine and expected, (2) be flexible, (3) be able to deal with significant amounts of human suffering, (4) demonstrate sincerely caring and empathic attitudes, and (5) be willing to attain specialized or additional training to guarantee competence.

Although the team approach is emphasized in most health care areas, it is vitally important to note that burn care *must* be handled by a team.[11,15] The occupational therapist should confer regularly with team members to ensure a unified and consistent progressive treatment methodology with each patient. Burn team members should include the physician, nurse, occupational therapist, physical therapist, and social worker. Additional team members may include the psychologist or psychiatrist, teacher, recreational therapist, vocational counselor for teenagers, and religious leaders.

SPLINTING AND POSITIONING

Splinting, as provided by the occupational therapist, should be a part of the patient's care as early as possible. When the patient is brought to the emergency room, lifesaving efforts are the first priority. However, the occupational therapist may be called to fit the patient with splints in the emergency room or in the intensive care unit.

Malick[21-24] and Willis[35-38] are well-known occupational therapists who are considered respected authorities regarding various aspects of splinting and burn care. Many of the splint designs initially introduced by them remain the most suitable. Both therapists are well-published, and anyone working with burn patients should read their contributions.

The basic splinting rules apply to the burned child. However, extra care must be taken to avoid inappropriate pressure when desensitization is a problem, and infection must be controlled. The general rules of all splint designs include (1) meeting the exact custom needs of the patient, (2) keeping the design simple, (3) providing for easy application and removal, (4) providing for easy cleaning, (5) avoiding any inappropriate pressure, and (6) considering future adjustability.

Most burn specialists agree that splinting a hand with major burns is necessary to prevent contractures and deformities. Positioning the hand is important to maintain a balance between the flexor and extensor tendons. In dorsal third degree burns, permanent damage, including slipping or permanent lesion of the extensor mechanism, is a serious concern. The resulting boutonnière deformity consists of metacarpophalangeal (MP) hyperextension, proximal interphalangeal (PIP) flexion, and distal interphalangeal (DIP) hyperextension.

The burned hand of a child over 4 years old should be splinted in the same position most often used with an adult: wrist neutral to 30 degrees of hyperextension; metacarpophalangeal joints at 45 to 60 degrees of flexion; and proximal interphalangeal and distal interphalangeal joints at 0 degree or full extension (Figure 25-1). Children under 4 years of age may be splinted in a neutral flat pan position. Some therapists prefer to splint the metacarpophalangeal joints at 90 degrees of flexion and the wrist with dorsal burns at 15 degrees of flexion. Other areas splinted early in the course of treatment include the axillas, neck, elbows, knees, and feet.

Axillary splints are used to prevent bands of scars from forming and holding the upper extremity closely adducted to the body (Figure 25-2). Of the splints used, however, axillary splints present the most difficulties. For example, if a patient is not receiving sufficient nutrition, a subclavicular central venous pressure (CVP) line may be inserted for parenteral hyperalimen-

tation. This is the intravenous method of giving high concentrations of nutrient supplements. Placing an upper extremity at 90 degrees or higher with an axillary splint may cut off the flow of the central venous pressure line when it is on the same side of the body. This problem must be worked out with the physician and nursing staff. Hyperalimentation should take priorty over splinting, but often a temporary compromise abducted position of 70 to 80 degrees can be attained.

Axillary splints are also difficult to secure comfortably. Patients seem to complain more about abduction of the shoulder (as a constant position) than any position in which they are placed. One of the reasons may be that it limits their functional ability more than any other position. Hand splints can at least be adapted to hold an eating utensil, but nothing much can be done to assist self-care when both arms are fixed in an over head position. Once patients begin to ambulate, the axillary splint may require additional closures to secure it in the proper position. Because of patient's movement and his size and weight, the splint will have a tendency to slip.

Elbow and knee splints can be made in the simplest form or can be designed to look like a sophisticated brace. The use of a bivalve or two-piece splint is preferred (Figures 25-3 to 25-5). One reason is that using a one-surface splint does not provide sufficient support for an active child. The bivalve splint also provides gentle initial pressure to the anterior surface where scar hypertrophy often creates flexion contractures.

Anterior neck conformers (Figure 25-6) have been described extensively. The most dramatic demonstrations of their ability to prevent and correct deformity are presented by Larson and others[19] and Willis.[37] Neck scars can be so extensive as to eliminate a recognizable neck, creating a triangular shape between the

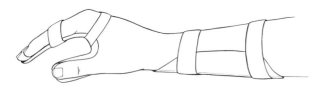

Figure 25-1   Burn hand pan splint.

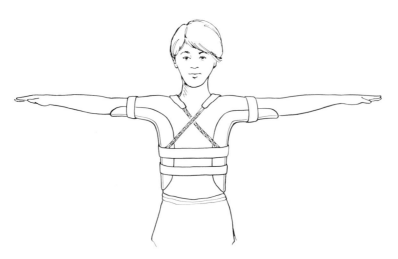

Figure 25-2   Axillary splint.

head and shoulders. Even if the face was not burned, neck scars can create sufficient pull on the facial skin to grossly disfigure the facial features and produce a monsterlike appearance.[9] Standard pillows that increase neck flexion should never be used. However, neck rolls that encourage neck extension are helpful. Precautions must be taken if the patient has any respiratory problems.

Microstomia, or unusually small mouth, frequently results from scarring around the lips and commissures of the mouth.[6,32] Although there are a few variations on the microstomia splint, the prefabricated Microstomia Prevention Appliance (MPA)* has been found to adapt to most patients' needs for a device to stretch the mouth opening and reduce perioral contractures. Both the small and large sizes are adaptable and stretch the mouth between 2.2 and 4 cm. Specially fabricated mouth splints are necessary when an extra large size is needed. This is rare in children.

If patients are left to position themselves, they tend to assume the "position of comfort."[29] This is basically flexion throughout with slight abduction and internal rotation of the shoulders. It becomes obvious, therefore, that splinting is very important to prevent contractures and deformities in those positions. Figure 25-7 provides general guidelines for positioning splints to achieve maximal benefit.

It cannot be emphasized enough that all splints should be worn continuously except for exercise periods, dressing changes, whirlpool treatments, or short-term activity of daily living tasks. Otherwise, splinting benefits are seriously compromised.

The therapist may also be called into surgery to make specific splints following grafting. The purpose of

---

*MPA, Inc, RR 1, Box 176, Iowa City, Iowa 52240.

splinting at that time is to maximize proper positioning immediately and before the patient can become tense or fearful of increased pain. If the therapist is notified ahead of time that a splint must be fabricated in surgery, he or she should make every effort to be totally prepared to avoid any unnecessary time under anesthesia for the patient. The therapist should communicate with the operating room supervisor to have a clear understanding of all operating room dressing and infection control procedures. The operating room supervisor should be made aware of the therapist's needs, for example, an electrical outlet for heat, approved extension, or working surface near the patient. The surgeon who requests that the splint be provided in surgery may prefer that as much of the splint as possible be prefabricated on the patient long before surgery. In this way only final adjustments need to be made in surgery, thereby eliminating extended anesthesia time.

Persons removing or reapplying splints, including physicians, nurses, physical therapists, other occupational therapists, recreational therapists, parents, and sitters, should demonstrate an understanding of appropriate application, positioning, removal, and care of the splints and devices. They should also be provided with careful instruction concerning the hospital's and physi-

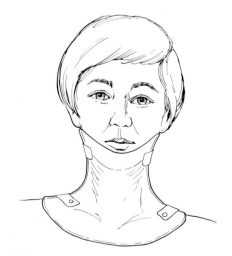

Figure 25-5 Posterior knee splint with padded knee support.

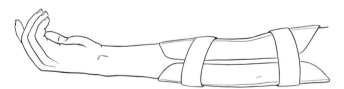

Figure 25-3 Bivalve elbow splint.

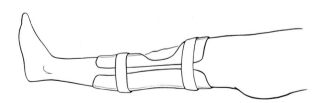

Figure 25-4 Bivalve knee splint with open patella.

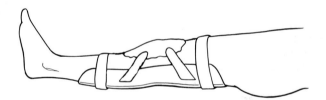

Figure 25-6 Neck conformer.

Figure 25-7 General guidelines for splint positioning

Splints or special devices should provide the following positioning:

Neck: 0 degree or neutral

Shoulders: 90 to 150 degrees of abduction (if possible, include external rotation)

Elbow: Neutral with 5 to 10 degrees of flexion to avoid bony blocks

Wrist: Neutral with 30 degrees of hyperextension

Metacarpophalangeal: 45 to 60 degrees of flexion

Proximal interphalangeal and distal interphalangeal joints: 0 degree or full extension (except with children under 4 years old)

Knees: Neutral, but avoid hyperextension

Ankles: 70 to 90 degrees of dorsiflexion

Figure 25-8 Checklist of points necessary to ensure adequate communication between all persons regarding splints

1. Purpose of the splint
2. Proper application
   a. Exact placement
   b. Closures (straps, gauze, Ace wraps)
3. Amount of time splint should be worn
4. Specific details on proper cleaning procedures per hospital's infection control policies
5. Special precautions
   a. Edema
   b. Pressure areas
   c. Growth factor
   d. Patient's complaints of pain, discomfort, or decreased sensation directly related to the splint or its closures

---

Figure 25-9 Splinting and pressure device supplies

Basic splinting supplies
Orthoplast: plain or perforated
Plastizote: Plain and perforated ¼ and ⅛ inch
Scissors
Heat gun
Method for heating water (stove or electric fry pan)
Velcro regular and self-adhesive hook and pile, 1 and 1½ inches
Velfoam, 2 and 6 inches
Rivets, small, medium, large, and extra large
Hole punch
Hammer
Velcro glue
Carbona
Webbing, 1, 1½, and 2 inches
Reston foam (for nonburned surfaces only)
Stockinette
Gauze
Moleskin
Vinyl
More complete splint supplies and pressure device supplies
K- Splint
Polyfoam
Hexaplast
Uvex
Plaster strips and loose plaster
Alginate material
Drill
Screw drivers
Petroleum jelly
Ultracare sheeting
Files
Sandpaper
Utility knife
Steel wool
Motto tool
D' rings
Elastic for strips
Anvil
Vise and pliers
Wire
Silastic Medical Grade Elastomer (#382)
Dow Corning Medical Fluid (#360)

---

cian's specific infection control policies. See Figure 25-8 for a helpful checklist of important factors to be communicated between all persons involved in the child's care.

Various splinting materials can be used. A few that are easy to use include the Orthoplast, K-splint, Polyform, Aquaplast, Hexaplast, and Plastizote. A list of basic and more complete splinting supplies is provided in Figure 25-9. For complete information on materials and on splinting details, refer to Malick.[21,22]

More complicated methods of positioning that have been successfully used include skeletal suspension, skeletal traction, and surgical procedures involving skeletal pinning or insertion of Kirschner wires. Evans and others[8] give excellent reference with photographs in their article, *Prevention and Correction of Deformity After Severe Burns.*

Patients are positioned by their physicians within the more complex traction techniques. The therapist working with these patients must be sure that any treatment techniques that are used do not disrupt the suspension or traction.

The patient's mobility is significantly deterred by positioning through traction. This in turn creates a need for the therapist to provide the patient with additional self-help aids to enhance independent functioning. Depending on the parts of the body that are immobilized or limited, the therapist can adapt equipment to meet the patient's needs. Ideas to keep in mind include the use of reachers, prism glasses, rocker knives, built-up handles, utility clips on splints, devices for hanging frequently needed items from a traction bar, and mirrors to see around corners or down the hall.

DRESSINGS

Dressings in burn care cover exposed areas to prevent infection and to promote healing. The splint must be congruent in this relationship as well. Splints are usually applied with the dressings, and adequate allowances must be made for required dressing space. If the splint is fabricated before full edema occurs (approximately 24 hours after injury), then the size of the splint should allow for increase in hand and forearm width.

Two commonly used methods of medical treatments involve applying dressings to wound areas that have been debrided of eschar. Eschar is the scablike material or the dead skin that contains bacteria and must be removed. One treatment method requires frequent dressing changes with close infection monitoring, whirlpool treatments, additional debridement, continuous exercise, and opportunities for splint adjustments. The other method involves one surgical debridement, applications of dressing, and possibly splints at that point, followed by application of bulky dressings or a wrap over the extremities. These dressings stay in place for whatever number of days is decided on by the physician unless obvious infection occurs. Skin grafting can also immediately follow surgical debridement.

In both methods it is important that the splints be positioned properly. These are usually held in place with Kerlex or Flexinet. If additional supports or closures are required to hold the splint in place, Velcro straps wrapped in plastic or Ace wrap can be used. Special attention must be given to the possibility of inappropriate pressure in such cases. In the first method the therapist should check the splint fit after each dressing change.

In some hospitals the dressing changes are carried out by occupational therapists, physical therapists, and nurses. In other hospitals each specific area is designated to a professional group, that is, physical therapists will do whirlpools, nurses will apply dressings, and occupational therapists will apply splints.

Innovations in scar reduction

Some of the latest innovations in burn care procedures used by occupational therapists involve the use of specific pressure to avoid or decrease burn scar hypertrophy. Rivers[28,30] is credited with the clear plastic face mask procedure that has been shown to significantly reduce hypertrophy of burn scars. The cellulose acetate butyrate (Uvex) transparent mask is unlike its predecessors made from opaque materials, such as Orthoplast, Polyform, and K-splint. Uvex is totally clear and therefore provides the therapist and physician with visual demonstration of pressure by specific blanching. Although the material is more difficult to work with and requires fabrication of both negative and positive molds, the end result is worth the effort. For specifics on the use of this procedure, refer to Rivers.[28] The procedure has proved helpful in clinical practice. The following is a general overview of the Rivers procedure.

Since the clear plastic Uvex requires a high temperature for fabrication, a mold must be made of the patient's face. Alginate material (a dental impression compound) is used to make an exact impression, or negative mold. This procedure can be difficult with small children who cannot be expected to cooperate. If the child is going to surgery for grafting, the therapist can arrange to make an alginate mold while the child is under anesthesia. The exact steps in taking an impression must be discussed not only with the surgeon but also with the anesthesiologist before making the mold. This is of utmost importance in that the endotracheal tube used for anesthesia and the airway must be protected from becoming dislodged when the impression compound is lifted off. Every effort should be made to take an impression while the child is already under anesthesia for another surgical procedure. If it is determined by the physician that the patient, such as an older teenager, can be cooperative while awake, then straws can be placed in the patient's nose or mouth for an airway, and the procedure can be continued as just described. Care must be taken to reassure an awake patient in order to prevent the fear or panic that can result in aspiration of the alginate material.

Alginate is easily mixed with water until a frosting-like consistency is attained. This is then applied directly to the impression area, which can be prepared with a thin layer of petroleum jelly to provide easy lift off. Once the compound is set, it should be reinforced with plaster strips. When the plaster strips harden, the impression material is removed as a unit with the plaster strips.

The impression is then filled with plaster of paris. After the plaster is set, the alginate is removed. The plaster mold is refined (filed, sanded, wiped, and smoothed down) to remove burrs and approximately ⅛ inch of the plaster that corresponds to the hypertrophic scars. The clear plastic is then heated in a conventional oven and immediately shaped over the plaster mold. Uvex has different properties from those of conventional splinting materials. Therefore the therapist should become familiar with these by practicing with the material before making the first mask for a patient. Once the plastic is molded, typical elastic and Velcro closures can be used to secure the face mask.

Uvex and this procedure can be used on burn scar areas other than the face. Certainly, taking the initial impression becomes an easy task when precautions regarding respiration are not a concern.

Another material that is used more widely than Uvex in providing pressure is Dow Corning's Silastic Medical Elastomer #382. Elastomer is not clear. However, because it is applied in a thick liquid state and hardens to a firm rubbery material, exact specific contact is made with all tissue. Elastomer is easy to use.[24] It can be thinned, reinforced with other materials such as gauze for strength, and used to line splints made with perforated Orthoplast or Plastizote.[2,9] Elastomer hardens quickly after the catalyst has been added, and the patient has a conformer following one fabrication session. Elastomer is most often used in conjunction with Jobst garments. Jobst garments are elastic pressure gradient garments carefully and specifically measured and custom-made to provide 25 mm Hg pressure to burn scar areas.[19] According to Lamberty and Whitaker,[18]

Controlled pressure of greater than 25 mm Hg induces realignment of collagen whorls, increases tissue Pco_2 and decreases tissue 0 vascularity and edema. It is significant that 25 mm Hg is the capillary pressure and it may be that pressure controls the hypertrophic scar by producing a relative ischaemia.

Jobst garments are used internationally with great success. Jobst representatives are available in most major cities and should be contacted for specific information on the appropriate use of their garments.*

Jobst garments stretch over concave areas and therefore cannot provide adequate pressure to these areas (that is, around the clavicles, sides of the nose, chest, and ears). However, by inserting Elastomer conformers, these areas can be provided with appropriate pressure. Malick and Carr[24] give an excellent account of Elastomer uses, fabrication, and results. Although Elastomer is easy to use, the therapist should thoroughly experiment with the material before applying it to a patient. Elastomer must be refabricated during progress made in reduced scar hypertrophy until a totally flat and subtle effect is attained.

Both the Uvex mold and the Silastic Medical Elastomer #382 should be worn continuously (for 20 out of 24 hours per day) until scar growth has been exhausted. They should be removed for brief periods of time (three to four times per day) for cleaning and also to facilitate activities of daily living (that is, the face mask can be removed during meals and at bath time).

SELF-CARE

Basic self-care independence should be started as soon as the physician decides that it is medically safe

to do so. A child who is old enough to eat independently and who is receiving nutrition by mouth should be given every opportunity to succeed in this task with a minimum of physical assistance. The occupational therapist should assess the child's abilities and limitations and provide adaptive techniques and devices immediately, before dependent habits are developed.

Examples of self-help feeding devices for children include built-up handles on utensils; handles and trays covered with Dycem (a nonslip material); large hook-like handles on cups; utensil clips on hand splints, if the patient is not ready for active modified grasp; extra long reusable straws; plate guards; and extra long-handled or curved utensils. *Modified grasp* refers to the ideal position for the burned hand of metacarpophalangeal flexion with proximal interphalangeal and distal interphalangeal extension, with the thumb in opposition.

It is important to note that patients should be encouraged to relinquish devices as soon as possible to maximize their independent behavior and function. Children who are encouraged early to take an active part in their own care display not only less dependent behavior, but also less dependent attitudes overall.

One way to include children in the treatment process is to have them participate in removing their dressings. Their involvement during dressing changes also reduces their anxiety and fear of pain inflicted by others.

With such strong emphasis on early maximal, appropriate independence, the therapist must be very careful not to diminish the child's need for warm human relationships. Providing support, encouragement with positive reinforcement, attention, and companionship should not be confused with assistance. Independence should never result in loneliness.

Often family members and special significant others stay with children receiving specialized burn care. In such situations these individuals can provide the appropriate positive and loving reinforcement for independent behavior, while at the same time providing the physical attention and closeness so often missing. The occupational therapist should be instrumental in educating the family in how to provide the appropriate necessary support.

Independent programs

Independent programs are made up of activities and exercises to be carried out when the therapist is not present. These include both bedside-inhospital programs and postdischarge-home programs. Both are absolutely necessary for the child to derive full benefit from rehabilitation. Burn care is a 24 hour a day procedure. Long after wound closure takes place, burn scars continue to grow. It is mandatory that patients demonstrate their understanding of home programs or independent bedside programs. Written diagrams and

---

*Jobst garments, Box 653, Toledo, Ohio 43694.

posted instructions are very helpful; however, with actual demonstration by the patient, understanding can be documented. This in turn demonstrates quality assurance.

The occupational therapist can be one of the most valuable assets to the patient in planning independent programs. Here the application of activity analysis becomes very important. Hobbies, interests, games, sports, and other leisure activities can be adapted or introduced to make what seems like the never-ending exercises not only bearable but even a little fun.

When the child is ready for discharge, it is very helpful for the parents and responsible persons to have a clearly written out home program to ensure that the patient is receiving all necessary aspects of treatment while reassuring the parents that they are carrying out the program properly.[7]

Such a home program can be developed into a nicely printed or packaged booklet. Some issues that should be covered in home program instructions include skin care, precautions, use of Jobst garments, exercises and positioning, splint care and wear, nutrition, emotional readjustment, and who to call in case of problems or questions, with a list of the burn team and hospital phone numbers.[7]

THERAPEUTIC ACTIVITIES

Therapeutic activities that are intended to increase children's physical function include all the play, developmental, and educational tasks that are used with orthopedically or neurologically involved children. The difference, of course, is in the adaptation of such activities. If the child does not have hand burns, the therapist can use activities with near normal motion for the child. When the hands are involved, the appropriate burn position must be maintained during acute healing. The child should not make a fist until it is determined that the extensor mechanism will not be damaged in the process. One exercise that is frequently used is referred to as "tabletops and curls." This is carried out simply by first assuming metacarpophalangeal flexion with proximal interphalangeal and distal interphalangeal extension. This is the tabletop. Then the patient assumes the opposite position of metacarpophalangeal extension with proximal interphalangeal and distal interphalangeal flexion. This is the curl. In this way all joints are exercised, but a fist is never made.

Active range of motion is most important in burn care. Splints can be removed for these exercises four to five times per day. Needless to say, it is much easier to attain maximal cooperation from children when play is involved, particularly where some discomfort is unavoidable.

DEVELOPMENTAL ASPECTS

It is difficult to accurately assess developmental level when a child is hospitalized for acute burn care.

Initially the child may be too ill, and mobility may be seriously restricted. Also, the therapist can expect anxiety and imposed life-style restrictions to cause a certain amount of regression in the child's level of performance and behavior. This would make standardized testing results invalid in predicting performance outside the hospital environment. Modified, adapted, or partial developmental assessments can, however, be very helpful to the therapist in planning for therapeutic exercise activities that the child needs during the progressive healing stages. The development assessment tools and techniques, and the therapeutic activities that have been presented in all the other chapters of this book, apply to this discussion.

Since the child learns through experiential sensory motor input, including tactile, visual, auditory, proprioceptive, and kinesthetic stimuli, immobilization and confinement can lead to delays in the normal development pattern. The occupational therapist's ability to apply and adapt knowledge of normal neuromotor and psychosocial development to daily living skills and daily exercise tasks will more often result in the patient's being motivated to actively and appropriately participate in, and benefit from, the treatment plan. By using occupational therapy treatment techniques during long hospitalizations, development delays and emotional problems can at least be partially avoided.

PSYCHOLOGICAL ASPECTS

From a psychological standpoint, the burned child experiences feelings that include fear, anxiety, loss and separation, distorted body image, guilt, anger, and depression.[33,34] In a study conducted at the University of Michigan Burn Center, researchers found that the children who were burned before age 11 had the lowest self-esteem. Self-esteem is a long-term treatment problem. Bowden[4] found that patients with low self-esteem spent more days in the hospital and more days in bed after discharge. Occupational therapists have a distinct advantage from training in psychiatry as well as physical disabilities. Providing the child with appropriate channels for self-expression in addition to support and reassurance can begin in the very initial phases of treatment. Passive activities should be initiated early, such as storytelling (bibliotherapy)[33] or specially made talking books that can be played during times when a therapist is not available and the child feels fearful. Subject matter should be carefully selected to provide positive results. Fairy tales with characters such as the Big Bad Wolf can increase the anxiety the small child is already experiencing, whereas stories with positive characters such as popular cartoon characters, or talking dolls and animals can be uplifting and supportive. Talking books and special tape recordings are also useful in special care areas where television sets cannot be operated in conjunction with monitoring equipment.

Relaxation techniques can also be used with children. Children enjoy fantasy, and therefore imagery is easily used both for relaxation and for self-expression. The therapist must be careful to understand the proper use of such techniques to attain positive results.[31]

Often the burned child has other problems. Therefore his history is very important. The therapist should talk to the parents or guardian and establish a workable rapport. The social worker can provide a great deal of assistance with respect to history, family problems, financial concerns, and support systems.

• • •

Children who are developmentally delayed, emotionally disturbed, or physically handicapped present additional challenges to the burn team. During the acute phase these problems may not be apparent without a good history from a responsible party.

In cases of child abuse the parents may not be emotionally able to give an accurate history because of fear or guilt. The burn team members must be aware of specific warning signs of child abuse. Any suspicious cases should be reported to the government agency concerned with child welfare. This is usually the Department of Social Services.

Some of the warning signs include several small burn areas or scars the size of a cigarette tip, unexplained bruises, a history of repeated visits to the emergency room, or a history of accidents or broken bones. Certain burn patterns are indicative of possible abuse as well, for example, burns of the buttocks, feet, and perineum when the backs of knees and anterior hip areas are not burned. This occurs when a child is placed in a tub of hot water. The child reflexes into a protective position by flexing the knees and hips. Burn team members should learn to listen to the child's version of his home life and observe the burned child's behavior.

REINTEGRATION INTO SOCIETY

Part of the therapist's responsibility should include assisting the patient to reenter society. With infants and very small children this of course primarily involves educating parents and significant others in the child's immediate world. With older children this education needs to be taken further to assist the child in making the first difficult transitions.

The occupational therapist may go to the child's school ahead of time with samples of devices, splints, and Jobst garments the burned student will be using and wearing in school. Providing educational information and allowing classmates to try on and experience feeling these garments, splints, or devices can provide an immediate acceptance of the student by peers.

Field trips to shopping centers and public malls can be a part of the occupational therapy treatment plan. The occupational therapist's attitude and presence during the first such excursions can provide reassurance to the child and family and furthermore may mean that such trips will be made much sooner and without anxiety when the child is discharged.[13]

BURN PREVENTION

Since burns are most often accidents caused by human error, educational burn prevention programs are valuable. The participation of the occupational therapist and other burn team members in burn prevention programs is becoming more and more routine. The occupational therapist has an excellent opportunity to help the community by becoming involved in these programs.

The burn team members are seen by people in the community as professionals and experts with a great deal of credibility. This credibility, along with that provided by the fire department, can leave a lasting impression on an audience.

Fire departments have had burn prevention programs for years. They work closely with hospitals that treat burn victims, and they welcome working with the hospital burn team on prevention programs. They voluntarily give speeches at PTA meetings, show burn prevention audiovisual materials to school children, and provide ideas for burn prevention activities to teachers and parents. An excellent resource is *Project Burn Prevention: A Guide to Activities for Children 4 to 7.*[27]

Luther and Price,[20] in *Burns and their Psychological Effects on Children,* present an epidemiological example of appropriate education for the community in burn prevention. They take into account that all three interacting factors—the host (or child), the environment (or kitchen), and the agent (or hot water)—must be dealt with, or the educational process is incomplete.

SUMMARY

It is the occupational therapist's professional responsibility to provide the burned child with every possible benefit that can be derived from occupational therapy intervention. To meet standards of excellence in providing the service, the therapist is usually required to attain additional knowledge and training in this specialty area.

When working with the burned child, particular emphasis is placed on splinting, positioning, special devices for scar reduction, and increased self-help performance. The therapist should also exhibit expertise and versatility in adapting play activities that will incorporate exercise programs. These activities should provide the patient with a psychological outlet, as well as serve as a basis of support.

The therapist's responsibility does not stop when the patient is discharged from inpatient status in the hospital. Burn patients are often followed for years. The outpatient program can be started immediately after discharge with frequent visits for therapy and pressure device follow-up. As the patient progresses, visits become less frequent. The therapist must keep in mind that long-term follow-up is important with children, who will experience changes through growth, both physically and emotionally.

The challenge for the occupational therapist and

other health care specialists increases as more people survive serious burns each year. Approximately 50% more people survive burns than they did 10 years ago. This survival rate refers to the seriously burned population and therefore implies a greater need for health care specialists to work with this population. Medically, scientifically, and practically we are much more knowledgeable with respect to services we can offer to provide burn survivors with a life-style that is significantly more desirable and certainly more normal.

STUDY QUESTIONS

1. Differentiate between full thickness and partial thickness burns. What are the implications of each type in planning occupational therapy intervention with children?
2. What are special considerations in fabricating splints for the burned child?
3. What are the basic methods for treating hypertrophic scar formations?
4. Discuss the social and emotional treatment for the child who has suffered thermal injury.
5. A little boy who is 7 years old has 65% body burn with full thickness burns in the head, neck, chest, left axilla, and left hand; partial thickness burns are scattered along the right arm, hand, trunk, and left upper leg. Using the general problem analysis, develop an intervention plan.

REFERENCES

1. Abston S: Burns in children, Ciba Clin Symp 28:1, 1976.
2. Alston DW, and others: Materials for pressure inserts in the control of hypertrophic scar tissue, J Burn Care Rehabil 2:40, 1981.
3. Bailey W: Pediatric burns, Miami, 1979, Symposia Specialists, Inc.
4. Bowden ML, and others: Self esteem of severely burned patients, Arch Phys Med Rehabil 61:449, 1980.
5. Camacho-Martinez F: Evaluation and complete overview of the burned patient, J Dermatol Surg Oncol 6:10, 1980.
6. Clark WR, and McDade GO: Miscrostomia in burn victims: a new appliance for prevention and treatment and literature review, J Burn Care Rehabil 1:33, 1980.
7. Doane CB, and Fannon MM: Home care guide for burn patients, Atlanta, 1980, St. Joseph's Hospital.
8. Evans EB, and others: Prevention and correction of deformity after severe burns, Surg Clin North Am 50:1361, 1970.
9. Feldman AE, and Mac Millan BG: Burn injury in children: declining need for reconstructive surgery as related to use of neck orthoses, Arch Phys Med Rehabil 61:441, 1980.
10. Feller I, and others: Nursing the burned patient, Ann Arbor, Mich, 1974, Press of Braun–Brumfield, Inc.
11. Feller I, and others: Care of the burned patient: (post graduate course materials), Ann Arbor, Mich, 1976, University of Michigan Burn Center.
12. Gordon M: The burn team and you, Phoenix, 1978, The Burn Treatment Skin Bank.
13. Granite U: Multidisciplinary discharge and rehabilitation planning for burn patients, Qual Rev Bull 5:30, 1979.
14. Hand rehabilitation center procedure manual and teaching syllabus, Loma Linda, Calif, 1980, Department of Occupational Therapy, Loma Linda University.
15. Heimbach D, and Engrov L: Advances in burn care, West J Med 134:274, 1981.
16. Kamil-Miller L: Occupational therapy treatment with burn patients: a learning module, Ann Arbor, Mich, Occupational Therapy Division, University of Michigan Medical Center.
17. Kibbee E: Life after severe burns in children, J Burn Care Rehabil 2:44, 1981.
18. Lamberty BG, and Whitaker J: Prevention and correction of hypertrophic scarring in post-burn deformity, Physio-therapy 67:2, 1981.
19. Larson DL, and others: The prevention and correction of burn scar contracture and hypertrophy, Galveston, 1973, Shriners Burns Institute.
20. Luther SL, and Price JH: Burns and their psychological effects on children, J Sch Health 51:419, 1981.
21. Malick MH: Manual on static hand splinting, Pittsburgh, 1972, Harmarville Rehabilitation Center.
22. Malick MH: Manual on dynamic hand splinting with thermoplastic materials, Pittsburgh, 1974, Harmarville Rehabilitation Center.
23. Malick MH: Management of the severely burned hand, Br J Occup Ther 38:76, 1975.
24. Malick MH, and Carr JA: Flexible elastomer molds in burn scar control, Am J Occup Ther 34:603, 1980.
25. McClellan B: Guidelines for occupational therapy treatment of the patient with upper extremity burns, Masters Thesis, Wayne State University.
26. McDougal WS, and others: Manual of burns, New York, 1978, Springer-Verlag New York, Inc.
27. Project Burn Prevention: A guide to activities for children ages 4-7, Newton, Mass, 1980, Educational Development Center, Inc.
28. Rivers EA, and others: The transparent face mask, Am J Occup Ther 33:108, 1979.
29. Shea P: Notes from lecture materials 1976-1982, Atlanta, Saint Joseph's Hospital.
30. Shons AR, and others: A rigid transparent face mask for control of scar hypertrophy, Ann Plast Surg 6:245, 1981.
31. Trygstad L: Simple new way to help anxious patients, RN 43:28, 1980.
32. Wachtel TL, and others: Management of burns of the head and neck, Head Neck Surg 3:458, 1981.
33. Walker LJS: Psychological treatment of a burned child, J Pediatr Psychol 5:395, 1980.
34. Wernick RL, Brantley PJ, and Malcomb R: Behavioral techniques in the psychological rehabilitation of burn patients, Int J Psychiatry Med 10:2, 1980-81.
35. Willis BA: The use of orthoplast isoprene splints in the treatment of the acutely burned child: preliminary report, Am J Occup Ther 23:1, 1969.
36. Willis BA: The use of orthoplast isoprene in the treatment of the acutely burned child: a follow-up, Am J Occup Ther 24:187, 1970.
37. Willis BA: Burn scar hypertrophy—a treatment method, Galveston, Tex, 1973, Shriners Burns Institute, and Toledo, Ohio, 1973, Jobst Institute.
38. Willis BA: Splinting the burn patient, Galveston, Tex, Medical Communications Department, Shriners Burns Institute.

SUGGESTED READINGS

Corlett RJ: The treatment of deep burns of the hand, Aus NZ J Surg 49:567, 1979.
Davidson TN, and Bowden ML: Social support and post-burn adjustment, Arch Phys Med Rehabil 62:274, 1981.
Denton BG, and Shaw SE: Mouth conformer for prevention and correction of burn scar contractures, Phys Ther 56:683, 1976.

Frist W, Ackroyd F, and Burke J: Long-term functional results of selective treatment of hand burns, Am J Surg 149(4):516, 1985.

Heembach DM, and others: Minor burns, guidelines for successful outpatient management, Postgrad Med 69:22, 1981.

Larson DL, and others: Techniques for decreasing scar formation and contractures in the burned patient, J Trauma 11:807, 1971.

Mangus DJ: A simple sling method for support and aeration of burned legs, Plast Reconstr Surg 68:434, 1981.

Marvin J: Techniques of reaching the public with the burn prevention message, J Burn Care Rehabil 2:50, 1981.

McGourty LK, Givens A, and Fader PB: Am J Occup Ther 39(12):791, 1985.

Newmeyer WL, and Kilgore ES: Management of the burned hand, Phys Ther 57:16, 1977.

Shea PC, and Fannon M: Mayonnaise and hot tar burns, J Med Assoc Ga 70:659, 1981.

Ward JW, Pensier JM, and Parry SW: Pollicization for thumb reconstruction in severe pediatric hand burns, Plast Reconstr Surg 76(6):927, 1985.

Whitaker J, and Lamberty BG: Pressure garments in the treatment of axillary burns contracture, Physiotherapy 67:6, 1981.

26

Children with visual or hearing impairment

BETTY SNOW

Hearing and vision are the distant senses that allow us to understand what is happening in the environment outside our bodies. Those of us with normal sensory function cannot truly understand the total nature of the disability but can be helped by participating in sensory awareness activities. Eating a meal blindfolded to simulate blindness or listening to records that simulate what common songs sound like to an individual with a certain type of hearing loss are examples of sensory awareness activities. They are good exercises, but do not give the total picture. Each person with normal senses has a vast wealth of visual and auditory memories to call on that people with impaired senses do not have. It is important to note that most of the children with sensory loss who are seen in occupational therapy will be congenitally impaired and therefore will have no reservoir of unimpaired information to review.

The *sense organs* (eyes, ears, skin, nose, tongue) are all extensions of the brain. The brain's primary function is to receive information from the world for processing and coding. These sensory stimuli are integrated and associated with past experiences. Since the nature and the intensity of the stimulation to the sense organs vary greatly, one may take precedence over the others, depending on the situation. If a particular sense organ is not working properly, the others do not take over and totally compensate, but another sensation may take precedence.

Ayres[6] developed a *hierarchy of sensory perceptual development* that helps in the understanding of sensory impairments. The senses develop and work in an interactive manner in all everyday activities. They do not perform in isolation, but develop in a building block manner. The *vestibular* system gives information about the body's position in space, movement or lack of movement through space, and direction of move-

ment. The receptors for the vestibular system are located in the inner ear, and it is thought that the auditory system evolved out of the more primitive vestibular system.[5] The vestibular and *tactile* (touch) systems are the foundations of sensation. Visual and auditory sensations are received by the brain against a constant background of tactile stimuli and the body's position in space. It is important to think about the level of alertness required by the brain for auditory and visual perceptual processes to occur. The vestibular system and the *reticular arousal* system have a great influence on this level of alertness. Being either overly alert or not sufficiently alert can obviously have detrimental effects on visual and auditory perceptions.

Vision is the sense we use for understanding the relationships between people and objects. It puts the environment in perspective for us and precedes auditory development by building concepts and perceptual abilities. Children with visual defects often have a diminished verbal language because the relationships and associations between people and objects are not fully grasped. In discussing vision, we have to differentiate between visual acuity, visual awareness, and visual perception. Impairment can occur at any or all levels, and the child has to be assessed accurately.

In addition to its function as the building block for speech, *audition* is the sense that conveys sound. Sound gives information on distance and direction. We can hear a dog bark and without seeing him judge where he is and how far away. Auditory perception is the attachment of meaning to sound patterns. Sound has qualities of tone and pitch that make up auditory acuity. As with vision, impairment can occur at the level of acuity, awareness, or perception. Although language development appears to be the most serious problem for a hearing impaired child, the situation is much more complex, because language is a force in the socialization and development of inner logic of the child.[61] Language is not innate but a product of the child's environment. As the child learns the language, she can exert greater control over her environment.

Piaget[21] discussed development in terms of periods. The first is the sensory motor period and has six stages. The first stage approximates the first month of life and is predominantly reflex behavior. Vision and audition begin to emerge out of reflexive behaviors during the second stage. The infant goes from reflexive visual response to actively following moving objects and will stop crying when he hears a noise, interrupting his activity to listen.

The problems of children with visual or hearing impairments can be enormous. Although deaf and blind children face many shared difficulties, there are also striking differences. For this reason this chapter deals separately with the hearing impaired, the visually impaired, and the multiply impaired. It is important to point out early in the chapter that the occupational therapist is usually not the primary professional for the primary problems of the visually or hearing impaired child, but instead provides critical services for the secondary complications related to the impairments.

The importance of play cannot be overemphasized for these children in particular. Play is the means by which the child learns how to solve problems, to cope with the environment, to face the unknown, and to adapt by changing behaviors.[31,49] For children whose distance senses (and therefore their abilities to perceive the environment) are limited, the development of play skills should be the highest priority.

HEARING IMPAIRMENT
Diagnostic information

It is estimated that 5% of all school-aged children have hearing losses of some degree.[4] Approximately 30% of hearing loss is attributed to prenatal causes, and 70% to postnatal causes.[4] Total deafness is very rare and usually only happens when there is aplasia or failure of the inner ear to develop. A *deaf* person is one whose hearing is so severely impaired that she must depend primarily on visual communication such as writing, lipreading, manual communication, or gestures. A *hard-of-hearing* person is one whose hearing is impaired but not to the extent that he must depend primarily on visual communication.[16,54]

To properly examine the subject of hearing loss, it is important to have a basic understanding of the nature of sound and the anatomy of the ear. Sound sets up a disturbance in the air. Air consists of more than 400 billion particles per cubic inch, and as we speak or make a sound these particles are set in motion, hitting against each other and forming a wave of sound energy. The ear acts as a receiver, amplifier, and transmitter.

The ear is composed of three separate sections (Figure 26-1), and the type of hearing loss that a child has will depend on where the damage is located. The outer ear includes the visible part *(pinna)* and the ear canal extending to the *eardrum (tympanic membrane)*. The function of the outer ear is to collect the sound or acoustic energy and channel it to the eardrum, which vibrates with the sound wave and changes the acoustic energy to mechanical energy. The middle ear consists of the three small bones *(hammer* or *malleus, anvil* or *incus,* and *stirrup* or *stapes)* that conduct vibrations from the eardrum to the inner ear. The stapes is inserted into the *oval window,* beyond which is the fluid-filled vestibule of the middle ear which along with the *semicircular canals* make up the organs of equilibrium. The motions of the bones of the middle ear result in an increase of the mechanical energy of sound so that by the time sound travels from the eardrum to the oval window, it has been intensified many times. The inner ear is composed of the hearing organ, *cochlea,* that coils off the vestibule and the *acoustic nerve* (eighth cranial nerve). The cochlea transforms the mechanical energy of the sound waves into neural energy for reception by the auditory nerve.

There are two types of hearing loss: conductive and sensorineural. In *conductive hearing loss* the problem lies in the sound-transmitting portions, that is, the outer or middle ear. Some common causes of conductive loss are wax buildup, punctured eardrum, or inability of the middle ear bones to move properly. Diagnoses with conductive hearing loss include Treacher Collins' syndrome, a hereditary underdevelopment of the external canal and middle ear, and otosclerosis, a progressive condition occurring as early as late adolescence. We hear by bone conduction as well as by air conduction, and the relationship of these two functions gives diagnostic information about the location of the hearing loss. Fortunately many conductive losses can be corrected by medical-surgical means when detected early. Unfortunately, considerable impairment of the developmental process can occur before the time the child's loss is detected. Poor articulation, delayed speech development, and poor school performance can be caused by conductive hearing loss.

The *sensorineural hearing loss,* or nerve loss, problem occurs in the inner ear with damage to the cochlear hair cells or nerve fibers. A nerve loss is generally not correctable by medical-surgical means, and it requires the use of amplification (a hearing aid). This type of loss often produces problems with loudness and distortion of sound. Sensorineural hearing loss is often associated with meningitis and can be a sequela of ototoxic drugs. Several drugs used especially in early infancy to save lives can have a toxic effect on the hearing organs. Other diagnoses include tumors of the auditory nerve. These are most usually unilateral with the exception of von Recklinghausen's disease, where they are bilateral.

It is common to have a *mixed hearing loss* with

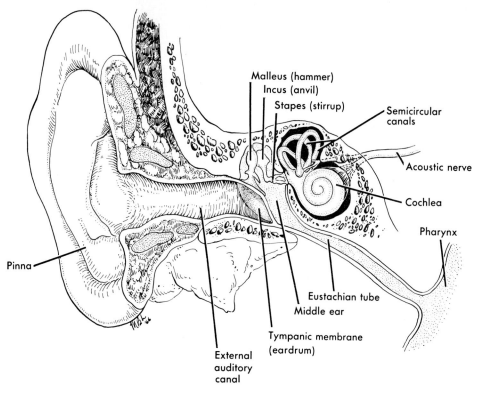

Malleus (hammer)
Incus (anvil)
Stapes (stirrup)
Semicircular canals
Acoustic nerve
Cochlea
Pharynx
Eustachian tube
Middle ear
Tympanic membrane (eardrum)
External auditory canal
Pinna

Figure 26-1   Cross section of the ear.

From Ingalls AJ, and Salerno MC: Maternal and child health nursing, ed 5, St Louis, 1983, The CV Mosby Co.

both conductive and sensorineural loss present. Obviously it is important to medically treat the conductive portion of the loss as efficiently as possible to minimize the total effect. Generally speaking, if a hearing loss is measured in the "marked loss" range, it is likely to include sensorineural components.

The occupational therapist working with the hearing impaired child must have an understanding of the measurement of hearing loss. This includes knowledge of the severity of the loss and its practical meaning to the child. The most common measuring device for hearing loss is the *audiogram* (Figure 26-2). This uses a grid-like score sheet to record the child's response to auditory stimuli. The audiogram has a vertical axis that measures *decibels* (dB). The decibel level is an indication of loudness or intensity of the sound or sound pressure and goes from 0 (the point at which sound is first perceived) to 140 dB (the point or threshold of pain).

The horizontal axis of the audiogram is the *hertz (Hz) level.* This is a measure of the frequency or number of sound vibrations per minute—the pitch or tone of sound. Pitch or frequency ranges from a low of 125 Hz to a high of 12,000 Hz on the audiogram. The range of 500 to 4,000 Hz is the most important because it en-

compasses the majority of speech sounds. On the audiogram the scores are plotted on the graph beginning with the *hearing threshold level* (where the child first begins to hear sounds). On the audiogram of a particular child, the left and right ears are differentiated by use of colors or by the symbol of a circle for right and a cross for left.

Decibel level is related to the distance that a sound moves an air particle and is measured by a particular standard or norm such as the 1969 American National Standards Institute (ANSI). Although it varies slightly with the norm being used, a hearing level from 0 to 25 dB is considered within normal limits. Figure 26-3 details typical loss classifications according to loudness or decibel loss and their respective therapy-education effects.[10] These effects as stated are general in nature and of course will vary somewhat for each individual child and program, but they will give the occupational therapist a general idea of what to expect with a certain level of hearing loss.

Although a person with a mild hearing loss may often use a hearing aid, the greatest benefit is derived when the hearing aid is used with a loss of up to 80 dB. Beyond that point the loss is so severe that only partial help can be obtained from the use of an aid.

Frequency of tones (Hz) lows to highs

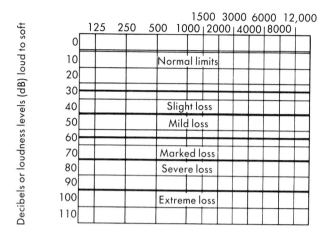

Figure 26-2 Audiogram indicating typical loss classifications.

The hertz level also has to be examined more closely in relationship to the child and her particular hearing loss. The hertz level, or frequency level, is related to the number of times per second the air particle moves and produces tone. In humans the hertz level goes from 20 to 20,000 Hz. Other animals have a much broader range, for example, the porpoise's range is from 150 to 150,000 Hz, and the dog's range is from 15 to 50,000 Hz. A child may have limitation in frequency, and this in turn affects hearing and language development. The hair cells inside the cochlea respond best to varied levels of frequency, depending on location, with the innermost hairs responding best to the low tone frequencies. This means that, depending on the location and extent of damage, there may be high tone loss, low tone loss, or flat loss. Frequency limitations can adversely affect syllable discrimination and understanding of speech.

A *high tone loss* means that the child can hear most of the vowel sounds because they have a lower frequency, but he will miss the consonants. This is serious, because the consonant sounds carry most of the information needed to understand speech. If vowels are removed from a sentence, chances are that its contents will remain clear. However, if the consonants are deleted, understanding will be impossible. With a *low tone loss* the child will miss vowels but will hear many consonants. Voices will sound weak and thin but understandable if the hearing impaired child is close enough to the speaker. A *flat loss* means that all frequencies are evenly affected. Voices will sound far away, and certain strong vowels like the *a* in *ate* will be heard best.

The audiogram will give information on both the decibel and the hertz loss of a particular child, but the therapist should consult with the other professionals

Figure 26-3 Therapy-education implications of typical hearing loss classifications

Slight loss: 25 to 40 dB
May have difficulty hearing faint or distant speech. Needs favorable seating and lighting in therapy or school settings. May need speech therapy, special attention to vocabulary, or aid in some instances.

Mild loss: 40 to 55 dB
Will understand face-to-face conversational speech (at a distance of 3 to 5 feet). May miss as much as 50% of group discussion if voices are low or not in the direct line of vision. May show limited vocabulary and speech anomalies. Will need hearing aid evaluation and training, speech therapy, help in vocabulary and reading, and favorable seating and lighting. May need special class placement or lipreading training.

Marked loss: 55 to 70 dB
Conversation will have to be loud to be understood. Will have increasing difficulty in group discussions. Will show limited vocabulary and is likely to have speech anomalies and be delayed in language use and comprehension. Will need special education services, speech therapy, lipreading instruction, special help with language skills, and hearing aids. Needs to be encouraged in therapy-education settings to pay attention to visual and auditory input at all times.

Severe loss: 70 to 90 dB
May hear loud voices about 1 foot from ear and may be able to identify environmental sounds such as a vacuum cleaner. May have speech difficulties with some ability to discriminate vowels but not all consonants. If loss is present before 1 year of age, the child will not develop spontaneous language. Will need special education services, support services, and hearing aid. Needs a comprehensive program emphasizing language and concept development, speech, and lipreading.

Extreme loss: 90 dB and more
May hear some loud sounds, such as an automobile horn, very close but is aware of vibrations more than tonal patterns. Will have to rely on vision as the primary means of communication, rather than on hearing. Speech will be deficient and will not develop spontaneously, if loss is present before 1 year of age. Will need special education on a comprehensive intensive basis.

involved with the individual child to get an accurate picture of the child's hearing loss.

Other services involved

Although there may be many professionals involved with a particular hearing impaired child, the most common ones are the following:[16,54]

Otolaryngologist A physician who specializes in the anatomy, physiology, and pathology of the head and neck, including the ears, nose, and throat, by using medical and surgical treatment techniques.

Otologist A physician who specializes in the anatomy, physiology, and pathology of the ear, by using medical and surgical treatment techniques.

Audiologist A specialist in the study of hearing who performs various hearing tests and provides rehabilitation and treatment, including hearing aids, for those whose hearing impairment cannot be improved by medical or surgical means.

Audiometrist A technician trained to test and measure hearing ability.

Practice settings

The occupational therapist usually encounters children with hearing impairment in hospitals at the time of diagnosis or later in the school setting. Many will be identified as "suspicious" in the neonatal unit, and others will show up for developmental testing in the clinic. The percentage of deaf children going to state institutions has decreased with the advent of more local programs, although a great number of deaf children (especially those with severe hearing losses or multiple handicaps) still do attend state schools. The occupational therapist has a strategic role in both the local and state school programs in the areas of self-help skills, socialization, fine motor, sensory integration, and perceptual motor development. The increasing number of infant programs also allows for more therapist involvement in the development of the young deaf child and intervention in the all-important mother-child interaction.

Special characteristics relevant to occupational therapy

To the occupational therapist the most important characteristic of the hearing impaired child is the lack of early language development and the profound effect of this on all other areas of the child's development.[26,43,53] What appears at first to be a fairly simple problem becomes quite complicated in consideration of the importance language plays in our society. Language assists in environmental manipulation and gives the child labels for objects and concepts. It plays a critical role in socialization. The infant smiles and quiets with the sight and sounds of his mother. The deaf infant will not respond to his mother's soft voice, unless the mother is in the direct line of sight. Early intervention is imperative, but infantile deafness is often not diagnosed until later. *Babbling* is vocal play, that is, use of the vocal cords and muscles of the mouth, tongue, and larynx, and all children do this. Children who can hear get the stimulus of hearing themselves and their parents' vocalized response. The deaf child, on the other hand, gets insufficient feedback so that the bab-

bling does not continue and progress on to language development. The deaf infant will generally babble normally up until 5 to 6 months,[64] but then, as the normal infant develops a growing repertoire of sounds, the deaf child will not keep up.

Many researchers in the field[42,48] believe that if intervention is delayed until 3 or 4 years of age, the most important formative period of language development is on the decline and permanent damage is done. If the child is denied cortical stimulation by organic means because of impaired auditory stimuli, she will need to conceptualize by other means. Provision of organized alternative stimuli should be one of the main goals of therapy and education for the hearing impaired child.

Occupational therapy assessment procedures with the hearing impaired child

The therapist can use the general scales of child development, such as the Gesell, Denver, and Bayley, with some modification of the language areas and by taking a known hearing loss into account when reporting any score. My bias is to stay away from scores as such, and instead to use the testing results for a description of the individual child's abilities and liabilities and to compare the child against himself at a later point in time. If the child is using a hearing aid, lipreading, or sign language, the therapist should be cognizant of the implications of these specialized techniques. There are some basic suggestions to follow, and these will be covered more in detail in the section on treatment techniques. If the child uses sign language, and the therapist testing the child is unable to give the commands in sign, the test results should include the information that the therapist was unable to speak the language of the child. In some instances a registered interpreter for the deaf is necessary to assure accurate scoring.

Through developmental testing the occupational therapist frequently identifies the child with a mild problem not yet diagnosed. Often a pediatrician will refer a child who is lagging for developmental testing. Part of the problem can be hearing loss. Unfortunately there are no hard and fast rules for development, and each child is an individual. However, certain findings indicate the possibility of hearing loss and suggest referral to appropriate professionals (Figure 26-4).

In most cases the parents are the keenest observers of their infants. Special note should be taken if the mother reports that the infant does not awaken to loud noises, does not respond when called, does not attend to noisy toys, or uses gestures to indicate wants to the exclusion of words. Also notable are the mother's complaints of the child's distractability, inattention to commands, lack of feedback to the mother, or inappropriate responses to verbal stimuli. Obviously all of these

Figure 26-4 Findings that indicate the possibility of hearing loss

Possible hearing impairment must be considered when:
- A newborn does not exhibit a startle (Moro) reflex in response to a sharp clap 3 to 6 feet away
- A 3-month-old has not developed auditory-orienting responses as indicated by not becoming alert to toys that make noise
- An 8- to 12-month-old does not turn to a whispered voice
- An 8- to 12-month-old does not turn to sounds such as a rattle 3 feet to the rear
- A 2-year-old is not using words
- A 2-year-old is unable to identify an object with a verbal clue alone, such as "Show me the ball"
- A 3-year-old has largely unintelligible speech
- A 3-year-old omits beginning consonants
- A 3- year-old does not use two- to three-word sentences
- A 3- year-old uses mostly vowel sounds
- A child of any age speaks in a voice that is too loud, too soft, of poor quality, or of a quality that does not fit his age and sex
- A child always sounds as if he has a cold

difficulties could be attributable to other causes, but hearing impairment should be considered. Also, any child with a history of recurrent ear infections or upper respiratory infections could be a prime candidate for a conductive hearing loss and should be referred to the appropriate professionals.

Other kinds of tests such as prevocational, sensory integration, and activity of daily living checklists can be administered to this population with some adaptation in instructional methods. However, written instructions should be used only if the therapist has in some way made sure that the child has the appropriate level of written comprehension. Writing is language based. We form our sentences in the same way that we form our oral statements. Although research has shown that the deaf have a normal curve on other than language-based instruments, some studies have shown 4 to 7 years lag on other written instruments.[43]

SPECIALIZED ASSESSMENTS

In the area of *psychological testing* several tests are used often with hearing impaired children. The *Hiskey Nebraska Test of Learning Abilities*[3] was developed and standardized on the hearing impaired and covers ages 2 to 17. It consists of 12 subtests selected to cover a broad span of intellectual abilities without lan-

guage. It includes subtests such as bead patterns, picture associations, puzzle blocks, completion of drawings, and memory for digits; it is given in an untimed fashion.[3]

The *Leiter International Performance Scale* is a widely used individual IQ test administered without language with a range from 2 to 16 years. It is a performance test that was developed as a nonverbal counterpart to the Stanford-Binet. It is used with hearing impaired children as well as others, such as those who do not speak English. Directions are pantomimed, and the test is not timed. Administration begins with items below the child's estimated skill level so that the child has an opportunity to become accustomed to the testing procedure. There are numerous subtests divided into three trays for different age levels: tray 1 for 2 to 7 years, tray 2 for 8 to 12 years, and tray 3 for up to 18 years. Pattern strips and blocks are used for subtests such as matching colors, number discrimination, pattern completion, similarities, classification of animals, and spatial relations.[3]

Audiological testing is a complicated and involved process.[54,56] The occupational therapist should consult the professional administering the test on details of testing with the individual child. The most common method of testing requires placement of the child with earphones in a soundproof testing booth. The child indicates when she hears a sound.

There are other forms of testing used with various types and ages of children about which the therapist should be aware. *Behavioral observation audiometry* (BOA) is often used with young children. The mother holds the child in her lap, and the audiologist notes different behavioral responses of the child to sounds at different levels. *Visual reinforcement audiometry* (VRA) teaches the child to orient to a sound source reinforced with light or a visual stimulus. *Tangible reinforcement operant conditioning audiometry* (TROCA) uses a token or candy for reinforcement of sounds identified. In *play audiometry* the child does a certain task, such as putting a cube in a bucket, when the sound is heard. These are all forms of behavioral observations.

There are also some forms of *objective observations* that can be helpful in the diagnosis of hearing impairment. *Evoked response audiometry* (ERA) is often done with infants or unresponsive children. It uses an electro-encephalogram-type machine hooked up to a computer. Earphones are placed on a sedated or quiet child, and a series of clicks are played into the ears. The computer records the brain wave responses to these clicks and supplies information regarding the hearing mechanism response to sound. *Tympanometry* is a procedure to assess eardrum mobility or the presence of fluid in the middle ear. This requires the placement of a probe in the ear canal and can be difficult to perform on an uncooperative child. The *acoustic reflex measurement* is tested with the same instrument as the tympanogram, but measures the response of the two eardrum muscles to the presentation of sound. *Electrocochleography* measures the electrical activity of the inner ear and auditory nerve, while *electroacoustic impedance* testing measures the way sound is conducted by the middle ear to the inner ear. With the advent of newer and more sophisticated technology every day, these types of testing promise much for the future.

Objectives of intervention and treatment modalities

As mentioned earlier, the occupational therapist is usually not the primary therapist with the hearing impaired child. Therapy and educational goals must be coordinated with the special educator, the speech therapist, the audiologist, and others working with the child. Some typical occupational therapy objectives follow. These are by no means all inclusive. Each child should be assessed as an individual by the therapist, and the treatment program should be fitted carefully into the child's total program. Typical goals are the following:

1. *To provide and enhance sensory stimulation.* The hearing impaired child is denied adequate cortical stimulation by auditory channels and must learn to perceive and conceptualize by other means. The functions of the kinesthetic, tactile, and visual systems can be enhanced by the therapist with various activities and techniques. Sensory integrative techniques are useful in developing the kinesthetic system to its fullest. The tactile and proprioceptive systems are very important in the use of sign language. Tactile activities such as having the child locate objects hidden in sand or identify objects behind a shield are among many that can be used. The visual system can be enhanced by tracking exercises, perceptual motor activities, and many games or crafts.

2. *To encourage age-appropriate self-maintenance behaviors.* The occupational therapist can act as a consultant to others for related activities. The parents and others around the child may need consultation regarding what is or what is not appropriate for a certain age. Also, self-maintenance skills involve many concepts that the child should be assisted with in whatever ways possible; for example, the idea of left shoe and right shoe can be shown visually with color coding.

3. *To encourage fine motor and hand coordination skills.* Watch the movements of the hands of a fluent signer and you can easily recognize opposition, finger and thumb flexion and extension, and finger and thumb abduction and adduction. These movements are performed by isolated digits and in total patterns but all in rapid succession and with remarkable coordination. This skill does not come naturally to a deaf child but has to be learned. Occupational therapy's emphasis on hand skills can do much for the deaf child in general and especially for those children who have an identified delay in these skills. Many games and activities can be incorporated in the treatment program.

4. *To encourage socialization.* This part of occupational therapy intervention cannot be done in isolation and is of utmost importance to the hearing impaired child. Socialization can be encouraged by involvement in groups for peer interaction. Developing skills of environmental adaptation and understanding the language-oriented points of behavior can be stressed. Deafness is not an easily visible disability, and therefore a hearing impaired child can be mistaken as being rude if he does not answer questions or respond to social overtures when in fact the child has simply not received the correct stimuli.

SPECIAL TECHNIQUES

The therapist working with the hearing impaired child is intimately involved with the special techniques used with that child. The three most commonly used techniques are lipreading, sign language, and hearing aids.

Total communication is the use of all avenues, such as oral speech, lipreading, sign language, finger spelling, gesture, and body language, simultaneously in communication. Sign language encourages communication and language development.[30,50] There has been a historical battle in the field of deafness between the *oralists* (oral language only through the use of lipreading and speech therapy) and the *sign language users.* The oralists maintain that if taught sign, the child will never learn to talk. The sign language proponents argue that the deaf child needs sign language for early concept development. Fortunately today there seems to be a softening of the lines and a general acceptance of the concept of total communication.

Lipreading would seem easy at first glance. However, consider that only one third of speech sounds are visible to the speech reader.[16] In addition, many of the sounds made in English look alike. For example, *p, m,* and *b* are all made with the same lip movement (lips together). Try looking in the mirror or at a friend and saying *ma, pa,* and *ba* without voice; the problem is readily observed. Another example of look-alike movements would be *f* and *v,* which are both formed with the teeth to the lower lip.

Sign language is not one easily understood entity, but involves many different methods. *Finger spelling* (dactylology) in the United States is done with one hand, each configuration representing a letter in the English alphabet (Figure 26-5). Finger spelling is used by itself or in conjunction with the other forms of sign language. Although it is not too difficult for the hearing person to learn to do, it is very difficult to receive. When receiving or listening, the tendency is to see the individual letter and not the words. With finger spelling it is important that the hand be close enough to the face that the hearing impaired person can see both the lip movements and the finger spelling at the same time.

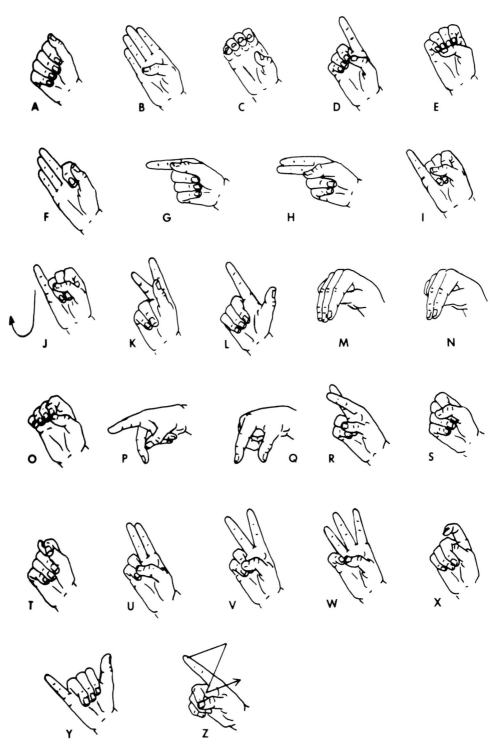

Figure 26-5 American one-hand manual alphabet.

For fluency and readability, the hand has to be held in a comfortable position, not stiffly.

For simplification, sign language can be divided into *Ameslan* (American Sign Language) and *Signing Exact English* (SEE). Ameslan[19,41] is a language in itself and it is not directly translatable to English. Although it is not universal, Ameslan is the primary language of the prelingual deaf in the United States. It has many abbreviations and phrases contained in a single sign and does not conform to the structure of English. Signing Exact English,[32] on the other hand, does conform to the structure and form of the English language and thus is preferred by many educators. There are many arguments for and against both these types and other types of sign. The important thing for the occupational therapist to realize and understand is the philosophy of the particular unit or school that the child is a part of. It is equally important to become as fluent as possible in that particular system. Obviously, for many it will be impossible to learn but a few of the most simple and frequently used words and phrases, but this is important to the therapy of the child. There are many good texts available.[9] However, it is best to attend a class or practice with a friend who knows sign, since it is often difficult to correctly interpret the configuration and movement patterns of the hands.

The occupational therapist can often be involved in the initial stages of learning sign. It is usually best to select the first signs to be taught from those that represent familiar objects, real life situations, and familiar actions. Begin with what is available: things to feel, handle, or do. The parent can be given a likes-dislikes checklist to help the therapist know what is appropriate for the individual child. Often a food item is used first because of its value as a reward. The adult should work at the eye level of the child, obtain eye contact, do the sign, and then physically manipulate the child's hands through the sign. Some basic suggestions for the use of total communication are listed in Figure 26-6. It is hoped that with total communication, the child will demonstrate earlier development of linguistic skills, better interpersonal relationships, and understanding of self and environment.

The occupational therapist also is often involved in the initial stages of *hearing aid use.* Often a history will show that the child had a hearing aid but rejected it. This can sometimes be traced to the lack of professional support for the parents and child during the difficult adjustment period or to the professional's lack of familiarity with the aid. It is regrettable when an instrument that can be of help to the child is not used. One of the problems that occurs is that the aid does not cause the child to hear normally, it only amplifies the sounds in the environment. It does not restore hearing as glasses can restore vision. It does not localize sounds but instead amplifies all sounds in the environment, thus leading to distortion. The therapist can help the parents and child by clarifying realistic expectations of

---

Figure 26-6   Suggestions for the use of total communication

1. Face the child squarely at eye level.
2. Position yourself so that the child can see your face and hands at the same time without strain.
3. Make sure you have the child's attention.
4. Avoid light behind you. If the child has to look into the light, she may be unable to clearly see your lips.
5. Use a normal tone of voice. Do not exaggerate mouth movements, because this practice tends to confuse.
6. Speak the word and give the sign at the same time, rather than in sequence.
7. Use appropriate pauses between words, especially when finger spelling is used.
8. Better results will be obtained when you sit close to the child, rather than across the room.
9. Keep instructions simple and to the point.
10. Be consistent, especially with the young child.
11. Above all, *talk* to the child. She needs to receive the same amount of input as a hearing child, although the method may be altered.

---

the aid and what it can and cannot do for the child.

One of the main problems found in children with new aids is *tactile defensiveness.* The therapist can work on this with the parents and the child. The head is often the most sensitive portion of the body. The child must learn to think of the aid as a piece of clothing that is put on automatically in the morning along with shoes and socks. The earlier an aid is fitted to a child and put into use, the better the chances for language development.[56] The young infant learns much about language as he watches his mother's face while being held in her arms. The major need is to get used to the feel of the aid initially. It is usually best to begin wearing the aid during a quiet activity that involves the speech of just one person. The maximal benefit from an aid is obtained in relatively quiet settings. Because the aid does not localize sounds, the following situations will present difficulties: a place with a lot of background noise; a group with three to four people speaking at once; listening to reamplification such as with a television or tape recorder; and distance listening.

The hearing aid is a sensitive piece of equipment with several parts and can often be out of order. Everyone involved with the child should be aware of some of the common problems, since an improperly working aid is useless to the child. Some of the common problems are (1) dead batteries, (2) squeal—check for looseness of the cord or earmold, (3) batteries improperly placed or corroded, and (4) opening of earmold impacted with wax.

The type of hearing aid prescribed for a particular child depends on the degree and configuration of the loss.[34] There are three major types. The *in the ear* aid is used only for very mild losses and has no external wires. The *behind the ear* aid is usually for mild to severe losses and can be built into eyeglasses. It is a small unit made up of a microphone, amplifier, and receiver located together behind the ear and connected with a short tube to an earmold. The *body aid* is by far the type most commonly used with children. It is usually prescribed for marked to extreme losses. The microphone, amplifier, and power supply are together in a case carried in a pocket or harness worn by the child. The case is connected by small wires or earmolds seated directly in the ear. A monaural aid signifies just one aid, while binaural refers to the use of two separate aids. The parts of the body aid (Figure 26-7) are as follows:

1. *Microphone* picks up the sound waves and converts them to electrical signals. It is usually behind a protective grill. The aid should always be worn with the microphone facing away from the body.
2. *Amplifier* increases the strength of the signal and is located inside the case.
3. *Battery* provides the energy source.
4. *Receiver cord* extends from the case to the ear and is the most vulnerable part of the aid.
5. *Receiver* changes the electrical signals back to sound waves and is attached to the earmold.
6. *Earmold* is custom-formed of plastic to the shape of the individual's ear.

PREPARATION FOR ADULTHOOD

The hearing impaired adolescent must try to blend into a hearing world. Although this task is difficult, there have been many advances in social acceptance of individuals with hearing impairment. The growing technology of communication has improved future prospects. One of the important tasks of most adolescents is learning to drive a car. Most schools for the deaf have special driving training available. All students are taught by driving instructors to constantly scan the environment visually. To the deaf student this is of utmost importance.

Another important aspect of blending into the hearing world is the use of the telephone, a daily communication device often taken for granted. The telephone companies have various forms of amplification devices available. Some hearing aids have a telephone setting. If amplification alone is not sufficient to understand conversation, the Telephone Typewriter (TTY) is available. The Telephone Typewriter is a communication device that uses the telphone lines with a typewriter keyboard to "talk" and a printout device to "listen" or receive the conversation. The telephone ring is replaced with a flashing light or a fan that moves back and forth to indicate an incoming call. The obvious disadvantage is that both ends of the line need to be equipped with this system for it to work. Today technology is, however, making the system cheaper, easier to use, and more portable.

Television provides another aspect of daily life. The frequency of closed-captioned programs has increased, and in 1976 the FTC authorized the Public Broadcasting Service to develop more special programs for the deaf. The deaf use a decoding device, a "black box," to view the same programs as the regular audience but with the addition of captions. Another approach is the use of a sign language interpreter in a cameo spot, but the disadvantage is that this is difficult to read on smaller television screens.

One medical problem of deaf adolescents is of such magnitude that it should be mentioned: *Usher's syn-*

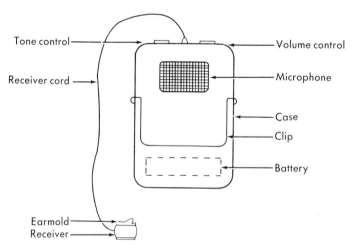

Figure 26-7   Diagram of a body aid.

drome. This is a genetic disease that affects 3% to 6% of all congenitally deaf. It is marked by the progressive blindness of *retinitis pigmentosa,* a degeneration of the retina that progresses from impaired night vision, to gradual constriction of the visual field with loss of peripheral vision, to blindness, usually by 20 to 30 years of age. There is much emphasis on early screening for this problem because of the obvious changes it would make in the education and vocational choice of the deaf adolescent.

Occupational choice has always been difficult for the deaf. Schein and Delk[63] stated that the average deaf worker earns 25% less than the average hearing worker and is usually employed in skilled manual labor. Gallaudet College in Washington, D.C. was for a long time the only place available to a deaf student for higher education. There are now many programs available where deaf students are integrated with the hearing students because of the availability of special services such as interpreters and notetakers. California State University at Northridge and New York University have well-established model programs.

In addition to the obvious communication problem, there are three factors that adversely affect occupational choice for the deaf[63]: (1) psychological perception differences that affect self-perception and perception of reality, (2) restricted life space that adversely affects knowledge of areas outside of the immediate social or geographical area, and (3) limited sociocultural understanding. Although no one can make the deaf child hear normally, the occupational therapist and other professional workers can help alleviate these three blocks to fuller participation in occupation. For resources for additional study and information on hearing impairment, see the reference section of this chapter.

CASE STUDY 1

Ed is 2 years, 3 months old. He had meningitis during the neonatal period with resultant hearing loss of a severe degree. Ed is the first and only child to date of a young couple. Both parents are employed. Ed attends a local day program for children younger than 3 with handicaps of all types. He has been assessed by use of the Gesell Developmental Scale and by subjective observation. Ed performed as follows:

Motor area: Ed passed all items at the 24- month level except the cube tower of six to seven where he functioned at the 21-month level. Although he passed items such as walking up and down stairs alone, it should be noted that he often stumbled and appeared uncoordinated. However, on subjective observation, a great deal of this could be attributed to his "looking everywhere," that is, searching for visual output.

Adaptive area: Again Ed passed all items except for the cube tower and adaptation of form board. The item that requires repetition of three to four syllables was deleted from the testing. Distractability was noted.

Language area: Ed passed none of the items suitable for 24 months. He had vowel sounds and receptive total communication vocabulary of five words and no expressive vocabulary to date. He attempted to form words verbally and with sign language.

Personal- social area: Ed passed all items at the 24-month level except toileting items, communication items, and the play item of parallel play. He demonstrated domestic mimicry and would pull a person to show (21-month level).

As noted, Ed attends a day program with a teacher as the primary professional and with speech therapy, audiology, and occupational therapy as supportive services. Occupational and speech therapies are available on a half-time basis, and the audiologist is employed on a consulting basis.

Treatment program

1. *Tactile desensitization* of the head and face area to promote acceptance of the hearing aid: activities such as rubbing different textures; touching different parts of face on therapist, self, dolls, and felt board (this activity also promotes body identification and sign skills); and playing dress up with different hats.

2. *Improvement of fine motor coordination* through activities and games such as busy box, geometric form ball, putting items in containers, stacking toys, and picking up small pieces of food.

3. *Improvement of attention to activities* through activities such as mimicry games, vestibular stimulation activities such as self-regulated swinging in net and using rocker board, and use of "look" sign in gross motor playground activities.

4. *Consultation regarding toileting* to both school and home and establishment of schedule.

VISUAL IMPAIRMENT
Diagnostic information

It is estimated that 12.5% of all school-aged children have some degree of visual defect.[4] However, less than 10% of these children can be diagnosed as legally blind. Total blindness is found in only a very few children and is often a result of *anophthalmos* (absence of the eyeball). Hereditary causes account for approximately one half of all childhood blindness. Numerous low incidence syndromes with eye and associated deformities are seen. *Retrolental fibroplasia*[40,67] was a disease that surfaced shortly after World War II when oxygen was used liberally to save the lives of premature infants. In the middle 1950s, it was discovered that because the blood vessels of the eyes of premature infants are not fully developed, they are especially sensitive to oxygen. Raised oxygen levels cause hemorrhaging, followed by retinal detachment and the formation of a membrane behind the lens. Today, even with controlled oxygen use, *retinopathy of prematurity*[60] occurs due to the immaturity of the eye in 25% to 30% of infants who weigh 1500 g or less at birth. Once the condition has been identified, it is difficult to determine whether the process will continue and become a major problem. It is estimated to cause an average of 550 cases of blindness yearly. The neurological damage from *maternal substance abuse* can also cause visual deficits.

The legal definition of blindness is important to understand. In the United States it is defined as:

Central visual acuity of 20/200 or less in the better eye after correction, or visual acuity of more than 20/200 if there is a field deficit in which the widest diameter of the visual field subtends to an angle distance no greater than 20 degrees.[37]

To put it more clearly for our understanding, this means that the legally blind child can see an object clearly at 20 feet that a normally sighted child can see at 200 feet. *Acuity* refers to central vision. The *peripheral vision,* or second part of the definition, means that the child can only see in a field of 20 degrees where a normally sighted child can see in a field of over 180 degrees. This peripheral vision is most important in mobility and general observation of the environment. There are some generally accepted gradations of acuity with correction (Figure 26-8). Acuity is not the only factor, and two children with equal acuity can have different visual functions. Of course with many children it will be difficult to know where and how a child sees. Spotty or irregular visual loss may occur in both the central and peripheral areas. The young child may use postural accommodation or head tilt to position herself to a focus point, or where she sees best.

As with the ear, it is important for the occupational therapist to have a basic understanding of the anatomy and physiology of the eye to understand visual impairment. The eye (Figure 26-9) functions to transmit light to the retina. It focuses images of the environment on the retina. The eye is shaped to refract the rays of light so that the most sensitive part of the retina receives rays at one convergent point. The *cornea* is at the front of the eye and is part of the outermost layer of the eyeball. It plays a large part in focusing or bending the rays

---

Figure 26-8 Gradations of acuity with correction

20/20 to 20/70	= Normal to slightly defective vision
20/70 to 20/100	= Mild visual limitation or good partial vision
20/100 to 20/200	= Moderate visual impairment or fair partial vision
20/200 to 20/1,000	= Legally blind with severe impairment
Over 20/1,000	= 1. Finger counting ability
	2. Form perception
	3. Hand movement
	4. Light perception (sees light and can tell where it is)
	5. Light perception (sees light but cannot locate it)

---

of light. Behind the cornea is the *aqueous humor,* which is a clear fluid. The pressure of this fluid helps maintain the shape of the cornea and helps in focusing the rays. The colored part of the eye, or *iris,* with its center hole, the *pupil,* is directly in back of the cornea. The iris governs the amount of light entering the eye by increasing or decreasing the size of the pupil. The light then progresses through the crystalline *lens,* which does the fine focusing for near or far vision, and through the jellylike substance called the *vitreous humor.* The eye has three layers: the *sclera* is fibrous and elastic, helping to hold the rest of the eye structure in place; the *choroid* is primarily blood vessels that supply the eye; and the *retina* is the innermost layer. The retina layer is composed of the nerve cells that contain a chemical that is activated by light. The *fovea centralis* (located on the retina) is the point of sharpest and clearest vision. It is most responsive to daylight and must receive a certain quantity of light before it will transmit the signal to the optic nerve. The retina has three types of receptor cells:

1. *Cones:* Used for color perception and visual acuity
2. *Rods:* Used for night and peripheral vision
3. *Pupillary:* Controls opening (dilation) and closing (constriction) of the pupil

The *optic nerve* (second cranial nerve) transmits the visual sensory messages to the brain for processing.

Visual impairment can occur within the structures of the eyeball, at the retina, along the nerve pathway to the brain, and in the brain itself. *Refractive errors* occur when there is deviation in the course of the light rays as they pass through the eye, preventing sharp focus on the retina. The most common are the following:[60]

1. *Myopia, or nearsightedness.* This child sees most clearly at close range and much less efficiently at a distance. The eyeball is too long or refractive power is too strong so that the focus point is in front of the retina; the child has blurred vision, possibly external strabismus when looking at a distance, and often holds printed material close to his eyes.

2. *Hyperopia,* or *farsightedness.* This child has blurred vision and may have headaches when trying to focus. The eyeball is too short and underdeveloped, the refractive power too weak, and the focus point is behind the retina. This child sees most clearly at a distance, and with constant effort to focus at close range, will become fatigued.

These refractive errors can usually be corrected with lenses but can have a devastating effect on the development of the child in all areas if left undiagnosed or untreated during early school years.

Cataracts are often a congenital problem that give rise to poor vision. A cataract occurs when the lens of the eye changes from clear to cloudy or opaque. After removal of the lens, the child will have to wear correc-

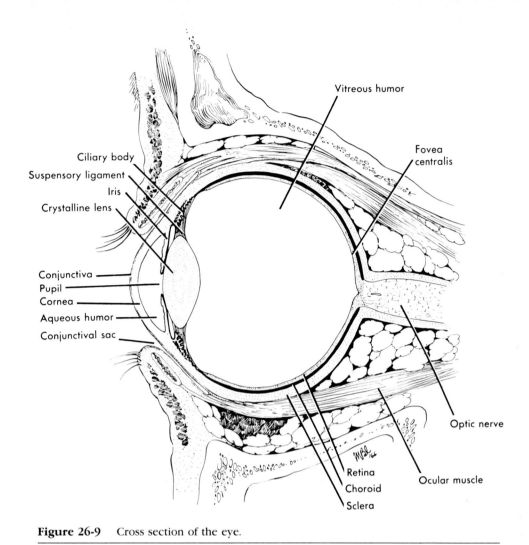

Figure 26-9   Cross section of the eye.

From Ingalls AJ, and Salerno MC: Maternal and child health nursing, ed 5, St Louis, 1983, The CV Mosby Co.

tive lenses. Although often the result of heredity, childhood cataracts have other common causes:

1. *Juvenile diabetes,* or other metabolic disease: Cataracts can occur as early as 3 years of age
2. *Down syndrome:* Approximately 60% of these children develop cataracts from 8 to 17 years of age
3. *Rubella, or German measles:* Approximately 75% of infants whose mothers contracted the disease within the first trimester will have cataracts at birth

Glaucoma is another visual problem that can occur in childhood. Glaucoma is an increase in the intraocular pressure of the eyeball resulting in hardening of the eye and damage to the cornea. The congenital type occurs in the first year of life, and the infantile type occurs between 6 and 12 years of age. It may be secondary to ocular inflammation or neurological diseases.

There are many *other eye conditions* the occupational therapist may encounter. Some of the most important of these are listed here along with common optical terms.[37,55]

Accommodation The power of altering the size of the lens to adjust the focus of the eye.

Optic atrophy Degeneration of the optic nerve fibers.

Patching Covering one eye temporarily to promote use of the other eye.

Nystagmus Rapid involuntary movement of the eyes. May be hereditary, and results in inability to fixate accurately and constantly. The movement is repetitive and may be lateral, vertical, rotary, or mixed.

Strabismus Squint or cross-eyes. Failure of the eyes to converge properly on an image, or both eyes not directed at the same point. This condition is often caused by muscle imbalance and often results in double vision. In esotropia the eye turns inward; in exotropia the eye turns outward; in vertical strabismus the eye turns up or down.

Amblyopia A condition of diminished visual acuity that usually cannot be relieved by lenses. The child may have depth perception problems and may tilt her head. Sometimes called lazy eye.

Astigmatism Unequal curvature of the refractive surfaces of the eye. This may result in focusing problems, because light is not sharply focused on the retina but spread over a more or less diffused area. Distorted images may result.

Cortical blindness The ocular structures are intact, but the child is functionally blind because of severe insult to the visual cortex of the brain. Occurs as a result of near drowning or prolonged shock, for example.

Ptosis Drooping eyelid resulting from weak or absent muscle and usually does not interfere with vision.

Retinoblastoma Malignant tumor of the retina and eye orbit, either unilateral or more often bilateral.

Toxoplasmosis Parasitic disease that can be congenital or acquired from household pets; causes scarring, usually on retina and choroid.

Coloboma Congenital defect of the eye due to its failure to complete growth in the part affected (usually iris, choroid, or ciliary body).

Micropthalmos An abnormally small eyeball.

Cytomegalovirus A herpes virus transmitted transplacentally to the fetus that can cause chorioretinitis, microcephaly with retardation, and other conditions.

Visual acuity is most often tested with the use of the *Snellen chart.* This tests central visual acuity with letters, numbers, or symbols in graded sizes drawn to Snellen measurements. Each size is labeled with the distance it can be seen by the normal eye. The child stands 20 feet from the chart and indicates to the examiner what he sees line by line. Eye report terms include *OD,* which refers to the right eye, *OS* to the left eye, and *OU* to both eyes.

Other services

Visually impaired children often have a number of other professionals involved in their treatment. The most common are the following:

Ophthalmologist A physician who specializes in the diagnosis and treatment of defects and diseases of the eye, performing surgery when necessary and prescribing other types of treatment, including corrective lenses.

Optometrist A licensed specialist in vision (OD) who is trained in the art and science of vision care. Specializes in the examination of the eyes and the preservation and restoration of vision by optometric means; measures refractive errors and eye muscle disorders.

Optician A person who grinds lenses, fits them into frames, and adjusts frames to the wearer.

Orientation and mobility specialist An individual specializing in orientation and mobility training of the visually impaired. *Orientation* is the process of using the remaining senses to establish one's position and relationship to all other significant objects in one's environment. *Mobility* is the ability to move safely and

efficiently from one point to another in the environment. This specialty began with the war blind of World War II. Today specialists in this field come primarily from graduate programs such as that started in 1960 at Boston College, although some programs are available at the undergraduate level.

Practice settings

The visually impaired child is more likely to be identified earlier in life than the hearing impaired child. The occupational therapist will encounter these children in the neonatal and acute units of the hospital. Visually impaired children will often be referred by pediatricians to outpatient clinics for developmental testing and treatment, because the effects of visual impairment on development are more medically evident than those of auditory impairment. The number of blind children going to state schools has been drastically reduced in recent years with the advent of more local programs. The therapist will be involved in both local and state school settings.

Special characteristics relevant to occupational therapy

There are many developmental deviations found among visually impaired children. Blind children have to learn about the world with their hands. Normally sighted children will develop eye-hand coordination early in life, but blind children will have to wait for ear-hand coordination to come at a later stage in development. They need good tactile system performance for exploration and concept development.[45] These children have to pick up a ball and feel it to tell if it is round: there is no other way to develop that concept and know what *round* means. Yet, because of their blindness these children will often exhibit tactile defensiveness. They also need to learn to move their bodies to understand how they move and that there is space (environment) for their bodies to move into. Blindness itself often results in fear of movement. The blind child will have difficulty progressing through the developmental sequence of random-to-purposeful movements.

Lowenfeld[44] talked about three major restrictions imposed by blindness:

1. *Restriction in range and variety of experiences with people and the environment.* Problems of physical accessibility, size, and danger impede the child's ability to interact.

2. *Restriction in ability to get about.* The child needs assurance from others to know what is out there and how to get to it, around it, or away from it.

3. *Restriction in control of the environment and self in relationship to the environment.* The child lacks information from distance sense as to form, size,

position, and general orientation and is unable to read people and determine nonverbal communication.

Behavior deviations can occur, and many authors trace these to early sensory deprivation.[38,23] Blind children are deprived of adequate visual stimuli and are often secondarily deprived of tactile, vestibular, kinesthetic, and proprioceptive stimuli because of the lack of mobility. Further, due to the lack of stimuli, these children are often extremely resistant to change, setting up a cycle reinforcing resistance to new stimuli. Fraiberg[23] stated that it is not uncommon for these infants to sleep or lie untouched for 14 to 18 hours a day. Also, as toddlers they walk late and are not as mobile as sighted children. Studies of animal deprivation[38] clearly show that sensory deprivation during the formative periods can result in the failure of the deprived system ever to achieve maximal development. Multisensory deprivation has an even more pronounced effect.

"Blindisms" may also develop. These include eye poking and flicking hands. Such actions appeal to children because they break up light and change what little they are able to see. However, blindisms make it impossible for them to try to use residual vision for purposeful activity. Blindisms need to be limited and activity diverted to other more productive avenues.[33,71]

Hendrickson[35] discussed some of the implications of blindness for concept development. Vision is normally used to identify the position of things in space, to recognize shapes without feeling them, and to know the length of a room without pacing it. These concepts and many more have to be acquired by the blind child by alternate means.

Occupational therapy assessment procedures with the visually impaired child

Developmental differences characteristic of children with visual impairment are important for the therapist to note. The usual developmental scales can be used with notation as to the child's impairment. Every area of development will be affected, but it should still be kept in mind that generalizations may not apply.

The sighted infant takes hold of her world with her eyes long before she learns to use her hands.[27,29] The infant has monocular fixation at first, but by the eighth week binocular vision is dominant. The infant has sustained fixation on a nearby object (that is, mother's face) during the first week and on more distant objects by the end of the first month. All of this visual grasping is a prelude to hand grasp and use. By 20 weeks the normal infant will usually pick up the pellet on the Gesell test and by 44 weeks has a neat pincer grasp. This performance contrasts sharply with the visually impaired infant who develops ear-hand coordination (the ability to locate and reach for sound), but not until almost the end of the first year. This *ear-hand coordination* begins at about the 10- to 12-month level,[23,33] but does not reach proficiency until the first year of life.

The normal child learns to associate visual experiences with symbolism, and although vision always retains a concrete core, the child learns to associate visual experiences with words. The absence of the association of words with visual experiences explains why, although the blind child receives the same auditory stimuli, *language development* will be affected. Pronouns can be especially difficult for the young blind child to understand. The blind child often will learn to use language for reassurance or as an attention-getting device.

Gross motor development will also be greatly affected by visual limitation. The blind infant will mold to her mother's shoulder like the sighted infant, but she will not spontaneously turn her head as will the sighted child.[1] The prone position without sight is not particularly interesting or comfortable. A fixed supine position is definitely preferred. The blind child will learn to creep, if at all, only after the development of ear-hand coordination. Often the child will prefer to scoot on his back to move around. The blind child will demonstrate a delay in crawling of approximately 6 months.[2] Sitting will usually develop within sighted norms, because it is a static position, but the blind child will have to be positioned in sitting and will have difficulty with fluid movement to and from sitting. Also, time spent in this position will be limited because of the lack of the visual stimulation that motivates the child's attention. Standing is also a static position and will occur roughly within the normal age range. However, walking is a dynamic movement and may be delayed by approximately 7 months.[1] Walking involves a self-initiated movement, and the blind child will need to learn the hazards and layout of the environment. Stair climbing will also be delayed and will require a great deal of guidance. The typical climbing and exploring of the 18- to 24-month old does not take place spontaneously.

Fine motor development is strongly affected by the delay in ear-hand coordination. The blind child will sit and manipulate toys within reach, but once out of reach, the toy disappears. The sound of a familiar noise toy is not spontaneously connected with the feel of the toy. The child develops age-appropriate object transfer and hand play at midline, but manipulation of objects may well be delayed.

In the *social-emotional area* a delay in the development of play may be anticipated. A doll or a toy truck will initially have no meaning. As miniatures of visual objects, these will be difficult to perceive. Parallel play and mimicry are difficult to learn without the opportunity to see and imitate others.

Development of peer relationships can be difficult because the child cannot see the smile or the frown of playmates. The visually impaired child may find it difficult to accurately read the feelings of others without the clues of body language and facial expressions.

Feeding may well be delayed by parental apprehension about the mess and by the child's initial difficulty in coordinating the hand-to-mouth pattern. Also, many blind children have difficulty weaning away from familiar and comforting routines such as the use of the bottle. Feeding problems involve tactile sensitivity and the blind child's natural resistance to change. Difficulty in introducing new foods, storing food in cheeks, spitting out different textures, and finding and sorting out lumps are all common feeding behaviors.

There will be lags in *adaptive skill development.* Discrimination of shape and space, which normally appears from 12 to 18 months, does not occur in the blind child until 24 to 36 months.[58] Concept development is problematic. The blind child will have difficulty learning that one word signifies many different tactile experiences. For example, a chair can have many different shapes, sizes, and textures, but all related forms are identified by that one word.

Figure 26-10 lists some observations that an occupational therapist will most likely make about a blind child. These are based on some possible problem areas.[15,75] The list is not all inclusive and would have to fit the particular situation and the child's developmental level.

The therapist may wish to administer portions of the Sensory Integration and Praxis Test to the child. Several parts of the test do not require sight and others can be adapted. The scores should not be strictly interpreted, because the test has not been standardized for the blind. However, test results can give important information on the child's spatial awareness or orientation, proprioception, and tactile awareness or orientation. Parts of the test that can be administered most readily include finger identification, graphesthesia, localization of tactile stimuli, standing balance, kinesthesia, praxis on verbal command, and the second half of the manual forms. Any interpretation of postrotary nystagmus responses would be difficult, because blind children often have ocular nystagmus as part of their visual deficit.

SPECIALIZED ASSESSMENTS

There are several tests especially adapted or devised for use with the blind. One of special interest to therapists and psychologists is the *Maxfield-Buchholz Social Maturity Scale for Blind Pre-School Children.*[46] It is an adapted version of the Vineland Social Maturity Scale and helps to obtain an accurate developmental picture of an individual child. Previously known as the Maxfield-Fjeld Adaptation, its development was initiated in 1936 shortly after Dr. Edgar Doll published the Vineland Social Maturity Scale. The Maxfield-Buchholz scale covers seven areas of the Vineland scale: self-help

---

Figure 26-10 Observation of the visually impaired child

Posture: Is the child's head up and held at midline? Often the head is down or the child displays unusual posturing. This needs to be noted because of its relation to the prevention of back problems and the promotion of social acceptance. Caution must be taken in interpreting unusual postures or head tilts as these may be natural ways for the child to try to see most effectively.

Balance and stability: Can the child maintain a position well? How good is her balance on one foot? This is important for mobility training.

Ambulation and gait: Is the gait stiff? Are the steps normal in size? How does the child manage on stairs or uneven surfaces?

Strength and tone: Is the child's tone normal, and is his strength adequate for his age? Such children often have low tone because of the lack of movement.

Endurance: Can the child pursue a gross or fine motor task for an appropriate length of time?

Coordination: The dexterity of visually impaired children can be subjectively assessed on tests, such as the Minnesota Rate of Manipulation Test (MRMT). The MRMT in particular has norms for the blind.

Identification of body planes and body parts: Does the child know front from back? Can she identify body parts at an age-appropriate level? The visually impaired child needs to know "boundaries of self."

Laterality: Can the child identify right and left on himself and others and locate objects placed to either side? This is necessary in exploring the environment.

Directionality: Can the child tell which direction to go to reach an object or person, moving or stationary?

Controlled isolated body movements: Are extraneous movements present? Control is important for work and school skills, as well as social acceptance.

Tactile discrimination: Can the child use her hands and body to their fullest to explore?

Auditory discrimination: Can the child discriminate distances of sound and types of sound and identify different people by voice?

Spatial orientation: Is the child able to judge distances? This is important in mobility.

---

general, self-help dressing, self-help eating, communication, socialization, locomotion, and occupation. The Maxfield-Buchholz scale is designed for preschoolers to children of the 5- to 6-year level. Of the 95 items on the Maxfield-Buchholz scale, 44 are from the Vineland scale. The Maxfield-Buchholz items were all standardized with blind children and give the examiner information about how a blind child compares to other blind children. It is administered exactly as the original Vineland: the parent or parent figure gives information about the usual performance of the child.

Another test of interest is the *Reynell-Zinkin Developmental Scales for Young Visually Handicapped Children.*[57] Similar to the Bayley Scales, the Reynell-Zinkin has two parts—one covering mental development and one assessing motor development. The mental scales include sections on social adaptation, sensorimotor understanding, exploration of the environment, response to sound and verbal comprehension, expressive language and communication. The motor scales cover hand function, locomotion, and reflexes. They utilize a profile-type of scoring with no attempt to standardize due to the lack of a "standard" blind population. Age equivalents are given, however, for up to 5 years for sighted, partially sighted, and blind populations.

The *Oregon Project Developmental Checklist*[11] has also been developed for assessing the visually impaired child up to 6 years of age and for writing educational and treatment objectives. It covers the areas of socialization, self-help, fine motor, cognition, language, and gross motor. This checklist also takes into account the fact that there is a vast difference in the degree of visual impairment by indicating items that are acquired at a later age by totally blind and those that may not be appropriate at all for the totally blind child. Several intelligence tests have also been adapted for use with the visually impaired, including the Binet and the Wechsler. Other oral tests are easily adaptable. The American Foundation for the Blind publishes a comprehensive listing[65] of psychological, vocational, and educational tests appropriate for use with the visually impaired.

Visual testing has had many subjective and objective aspects. As with audiological testing, it is becoming more sophisticated with increased technology. In addition to the Snellen-type acuity examinations, there are others developed to test young children and retarded children. Sheridan[66] published a series of vision tests including such items as matching distant pictures to objects on a table. Observation of the young child's functional vision is important; her use of objects and toys often provides the skilled observer with more information than the actual physical examination. The subjective description of functional vision from the mother, teacher, or therapist can add greatly to the physician's assessment. Physicians use an ophthalmoscope to view the internal structure of the eye. Electroretinography (ERG) can be done under sedation for a thorough examination of the retina and fundus. A visual evoked response (VER) test may be done with the use of an electroencephalogram to assess cortical response to light stimulation. Good results indicate that there is no gross defect in the eye, optic nerve, or visual cortex.

The *Erhardt Developmental Vision Assessment*[18] (EDVA) developed by Rhoda Priest Erhardt in 1986 measures development of vision from birth to 6 months at which time maturity of visual development is essentially achieved. This assessment is divided into a section on primarily involuntary visual patterns (eyelid reflexes, pupillary reactions, and doll's eye responses) and a section on voluntary patterns (fixation, localization, ocular pursuit, and gaze shift). It can be very helpful to the therapist in determining the visually impaired child's developmental level and functional abilities.

Objectives of intervention and treatment modalities

The occupational therapist may be the primary therapist for a visually impaired child, but most often works with a team that includes the special educator, the physical therapist, and the orientation and mobility specialist. Other professionals are involved as the child's needs indicate. The treatment plan is based on the individual assessment of the child. The following are some typical intervention goals for this group:

1. *To discourage blindisms and divert the child to more productive behaviors.* Blindisms are persistent stereotyped mannerisms that can seem similar to those exhibited by autistic or retarded children. However, these mannerisms in the visually impaired child are not tied to some psychological or retardation level but to the degree of blindness. As the sensory deficit increases, the need for substitute self-stimulation increases. Eye rubbing or eye poking, for example, causes excitation of the neural portion of the eye and generates impulses in the retina and through the optic nerve.[71] (People who have sight experience this in an unpleasant fashion when they poke their eyes and "see stars.") Blindisms interfere with the development of other more useful behaviors and are socially not well accepted in the sighted world. Substitution with other types of more productive stimulation seems to be the most effective therapy intervention.

2. *To encourage movement in space.* The infant's position must be changed often early in life to counteract the resistance to movement and change. Prone positions should be encouraged. The underdevelopment of dynamic movements, such as crawling and walking, cannot be totally eliminated, but much can be done in the therapy setting to help compensate for these. Crawling over different surfaces and movements on bolsters, therapy balls, and other objects are helpful activities. A chair or wagon can be pushed to develop security in walking. Balance activities are helpful to decrease fear of movement.

3. *To encourage sensory integration.* The blind child needs considerable vestibular stimulation from

tilt boards, swings, scooters, and so on. Sensory feedback in blind children is interrupted and can cause distortion of movement.[17] It is important, however, that safety be maintained in the use of equipment and that the child be allowed to control the movement. Excessive fear of falling, poor grasp of room layout, and inability to organize or cross midline are all indications of difficulty in sensory integration.[73] Van Benschoter[73] outlined a successful summer camp experience for blind children that stressed sensory integrative programming. Children at the camp aged 6 to 21 were given a sensory integration treatment program that had a positive effect on the movement skills of the children involved. Baker-Nobles and Bink[7] studied three adults who, after six months of sensory integration treatment, improved in areas of mobility, activities of daily living, handwriting, and behavior.

4. *To provide parental counseling.* The parents and the family of the blind child should be encouraged to handle the child as they would a normal infant and not leave the child in the crib. They need to talk to the child and explain the environment, allowing the child to do as much tactile exploration as possible. Early intervention is a must for this population.

5. *To decrease tactile defensiveness.* The blind child does not see the approach of people and objects and can exhibit a very defensive reaction to touch. Use of a firm touch is better than a light touch, which can be interpreted as being aversive, as a tickle. Allowing the child to touch textures and to play in such media as sand, water, and clay constitutes good therapy techniques.

6. *To encourage use of hands for manipulation.* At first the world has to come to the blind child. Toys should be maintained within reach, tied to the crib, walker, or tabletop. Later the child can be taught to search for and locate lost objects using a constantly expanding circle.

7. *To encourage socially acceptable behaviors.* The child should be encouraged to look at people when they speak, to smile appropriately, to keep her head up in midline, and to avoid posturing.[36] She must learn how others are reacting based on voices rather than gestures, facial expressions, or body language. Hill[36] in her article on intervention with blind preschoolers, stressed the area of parental and professional encouragement of socially acceptable behaviors in the visually impaired child.

8. *To maximize residual vision.* The therapist should always use whatever vision the child has in the treatment program activities. The more a child uses visual pathways, the better his vision develops.[8] Visual awareness and discrimination activities are important, such as color or shape recognition and matching.

9. *To encourage language and concept development.* The blind child must consciously be taught to develop cognitive schemes that the sighted child picks up in a relatively casual manner. This is done with verbalization and the use of the remaining senses. Those things that cannot be touched or heard, such as clouds, need to be explained in particular.

10. *To develop self-maintenance skills at age-appropriate times.* The therapist can consult with those who work with the child about the developmental sequence of self-maintenance skills. Eating and dressing activities should be "motored through," that is, the therapist physically manipulates the child through the performance of the activity. If abnormal eating patterns develop and are not corrected, they usually do not get better. Good supportive seating is important to the self-feeding process. For dressing, differential tabs can be sewn on clothing to indicate front and back. The child will need a lot of practice time with buttons and zippers. Toilet training can be facilitated by (1) a consistent schedule, (2) an established route to the bathroom, (3) the familiar sounds and smells of the room, (4) consistent use of one or two words for toileting, and (5) establishing an association between changing wet clothes and going to the bathroom.

11. *To develop maximal tactile perceptual abilities.* The blind child obviously needs to maximize tactile abilities to learn about her environment and eventually braille, if she will need it. Activities such as finger painting, finding and identifying objects hidden in sand or beans, and identifying gradations of textures and puzzles are among those that increase tactile awareness.

12. *To develop maximal auditory perceptual abilities.* The blind child has to learn to identify sounds and their meanings and react to them appropriately. Sounds come from three basic sources: toys, speech, and the environment. Active rather than passive listening should be emphasized. Activities such as locating a squeak toy, identifying sounds such as cars and trains, and following directions from persons and recordings are helpful.

13. *To encourage knowledge of parts of the body and body planes.* The child has to know his own body before understanding how it moves and fits into the environment. Body image is important to mobility and social function.[15] Obstacle courses can teach the child how large his body is in relation to other objects. Touching body parts on others is helpful. Life-size dolls can also be used.

14. *To encourage laterality and directionality.* Especially for mobility skills, a blind child must know the concepts of right-left, up-down, in-out. The child must develop the awareness that things outside the body have sides and must be able to measure distance and direction.

15. *To strengthen cognitive skills such as object permanence, cause and effect, object recognition, and ability to match and sort.* Games and many simple craft activities can easily be used to accomplish these

goals. The blind child needs these skills to progress intellectually and academically.

SPECIAL TECHNIQUES

Children with severe visual handicaps will usually have to rely on braille and talking books for their education. For the person who will eventually use braille in school, the importance of early tactile perceptual training cannot be overemphasized. Braille is a system of six raised dots arranged in a cell (Figure 26-11). These dots are arranged in various configurations to form the letters of the alphabet, numbers, and words.[59] Braille can be written in three levels or grades, depending on the degree of contraction used. It is read left to right with one or two hands. Usually the index finger is used with a light touch. As for the child with cerebral palsy who is eating, positioning is critical to the blind child's performance with braille reading. Braille was developed by a young blind French student, Louis Braille, in 1824 and was found to be more efficient than attempting to read the raised Roman alphabet. Speeds do vary, but 104 words per minute is the average, which makes it quite useful in the educational setting. Braille is produced on a special slate or machine called a braillewriter.

Talking books are also available for almost any subject at any age level. The young blind child can be tuned in to listening with short storytelling sessions. The adult should carefully monitor the child's attention to promote good listening skills. Scratch-and-sniff books and tactile books are also available to help in early storytelling. Large print books may be used by those who can discriminate a large typeface.

There are various types of lenses available for the visually impaired, from the relatively common ones used to correct refractive errors to telescopic and microscopic lenses that are used as low vision aids with certain types of blindness. There are also projection devices and magnifying devices such as the opticon, which converts inkprint into a readable vibrating tactile form.

In *mobility training* such techniques as using the Seeing Eye dog, sighted guides, and long canes are taught.[39,76] The techniques of echo detection, trailing, and body protection are also important. Seeing Eye dogs are specially selected and expertly trained. Sighted guides usually walk a half-step in front of the blind person, who holds the guide's arm just above the elbow with fingers inside (next to guide's body) and the thumb outside. A small child may do better holding the guide's wrist. With this use of the sighted guide, body movement on uneven surfaces and changes of direction can best be perceived. Should the blind person need to change sides the guide gives a verbal clue and the blind person slides over, tracing a finger along the guide's waist in back of the guide, switching hands to the guide's opposite elbow. In going through a narrow passage the guide puts his elbow behind his waist as a clue and the blind person falls back to a full step behind the guide with elbow straight and more directly in back rather than to the side. For stairs, the sighted guide gives a verbal indication of stairs ahead, whether they are up or down, as well as information on rail availability and placement. One technique is for the guide to pause and turn at a right angle to the blind person and they go down one step at a time in a foot to step fashion with the guide one step ahead of the blind person. Another technique involves using the rail, if available, the guide goes down or up, without turning, one step ahead of the blind person. Cane technique is also a very specialized procedure that requires the training skills of a professional in the field.

Although as a rule the orientation and mobility specialist is the one who teaches trailing and body protection, there are certain basic principles that the occupational therapist should know. Trailing is the use of a wall as a guide for walking. The hand closest to the wall is extended at hip level until the outside of the little finger touches the wall, then the back of the fingertips are used to guide the person in walking. In the protection technique the upper arm is held at shoulder height and parallel to the floor with the palm facing out

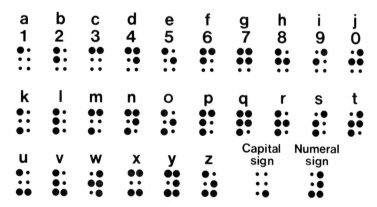

Figure 26-11   The braille alphabet and numbers.

to meet any obstacle before the body does. The lower arm is extended downward and forward with the palm facing out. Another protection technique is to extend the arm palm out in front of the head while bending down to retrieve a dropped object. The blind child can search for a lost object by touching the ground to establish a beginning point and then searching in an ever widening concentric circle pattern. A technique for exploring a room is to search the parameters of the room first, then mentally divide it into grids to be methodically searched. This is extremely helpful in introducing the blind child to a new classroom or new home setup. The use of landmarks and clues such as the grass edge of the sidewalk are important for independent travel as is the idea of "squaring off" or using one point of reference to locate another. Chairs can be approached from the side and checked with hands prior to sitting.

Low vision training is another specialized technique.[8,22] Some educational personnel will specialize in this method. The basic premise is that the child can be taught to use vision. Visual acuity is by itself not really the most important part of visual ability. Through planned stimulation, visual efficiency can be increased. Often light is used initially to increase focusing ability. Once fixation is achieved, the child can learn to discriminate global aspects of the image. When this happens, the child can move on to analyze discrete elements of the image and finally to identify form, outline, and other aspects. Obviously this method does not work with all visually impaired children, but it does have good results with others, especially when combined with a good overall program to heighten the child's levels of perception.

High technology with increasing use of sophisticated electronics and miniature computers will continue to result in positive results for training the visually impaired. Schaefer and Specht[62] discuss the use of one such device in occupational therapy—a light sensor that enables the blind to detect variable light intensities and that may be adapted to various industrial uses in rehabilitation training.

PREPARATION FOR ADULTHOOD

The most obvious challenge for the blind adolescent is the choice of an appropriate occupation. Options are even more limited than for the deaf adolescent, but the situation has improved with more colleges and training programs offering special services for the blind student. Almost all textbooks are available in braille or talking books. The job is to fit the personality and talent areas of the adolescent to the occupational choices. Lack of exposure to many vocational options can be a problem that the occupational therapist can address through community orientation and various activities to give the child more prevocational experiences.

There are certain mannerisms that should be discussed, because these behaviors often interfere with optimal social interaction. Again, these are things that the therapist and all the other professionals involved with the child should work to eliminate:

1. Standing too close to others
2. Rocking the body
3. Blinking, rubbing, or rolling the eyes
4. Stamping or shuffling the feet
5. Not looking at a person when speaking
6. Feeling whatever is bumped into

Daily living skills such as cooking, cleaning, and recreation become increasingly important as the child reaches adolescence. The American Foundation for the Blind puts out a comprehensive list[2] of aids and appliances. For the kitchen there are such devices as a sugar meter that dispenses one half a teaspoon of sugar at a time and an elbow-length oven mitt to prevent accidental burning. A canned goods marking kit is available, as well as self-threading needles and tools with marking gauges. For recreational activities there are braille cards and low vision cards, as well as table games such as Scrabble and Monopoly with braille markings.

Self-care can be facilitated by careful organization of the wardrobe and tactile clues for color of clothing. Handling money and shopping can be difficult tasks and require much training and assistance.

Leisure time activities are important for well-rounded adulthood. Exercise groups, weight lifting, dance classes, and bowling are all excellent physical activities that should be encouraged, since many blind adults lead very sedentary lives. Blind persons can play ball sports with sound balls and can run or jog with minimal track guidance aids. For resources for additional study and information on visual impairment, see the reference section of this chapter.

CASE STUDY 2

Bonnie is 7 years, 4 months old. She had congenital cataracts removed during her first year of life. Her resultant condition is legal blindness with form perception. Bonnie is the third and last child of a couple who have divorced since her birth. The mother works while Bonnie attends a local grammar school where she is mainstreamed into a regular second grade class. She has been assessed informally by the therapist, and parts of the Southern California Sensory Integration Tests have been administered. Bonnie performs as follows:

Motor area: Bonnie can trail in familiar settings such as home and school but needs a sighted guide for unfamiliar areas. Her gait is shuffling and hesitant, and she fears falling. Balance activities are difficult, and she can only stand on one foot momentarily. She has difficulty with motor planning. Her coordination skills, grasp, and pinch are age-appropriate.

Language area: On the school testing she is 1 to 2 years behind in vocabulary. She enjoys music and talking books. Her attention span is variable and auditory discrimination poor for sound location.

Personal-social area: Bonnie was in an infant stimulation program before school placement and has acquired some play skills but remains shy and withdrawn especially in playground activities and physical education. She feeds herself, but her mother has a great deal of difficulty getting her to dress herself. The mother attributes this in part to her own inability to "let go."

As noted, Bonnie is in a regular second grade class. She receives occupational therapy on an itinerant basis, as well as visually handicapped special education services three times a week. She attends regular physical education with some adaptation of requirements.

Treatment program

1. *To increase balance, motor planning, and equilibrium skills.* Use of swing, bolster, tilt board, and scooter activities. Counseling with the teacher and the physical education instructor to provide tactile input for planning motor activities.

2. *To increase dressing skills.* Provide counseling to the mother regarding age-appropriate dressing skills. Refer mother to social worker for counseling related to "letting go" and coping with single parenthood of a handicapped girl. Practice with the child on manipulation of fasteners and use of tactile strips for clothing identification. Home visits to observe and assist in arranging clothing for ease of identification.

3. *To increase social skills.* Have the child plan and participate in group activities with small groups of her classmates. Cooking or craft projects might be used.

IEP objectives for present school year

1. Will be able to stand and balance on one foot for 10 seconds.

2. Will be able to manipulate buttons, snaps, and zippers 100% of the time.

3. Will plan with therapist four group activities during the school year.

MULTIPLE SENSORY IMPAIRMENT (DEAF-BLIND AND MULTIPLY IMPAIRED)
Diagnostic information

There is one important concept to understand regarding any multiple involvement, whether it is deaf-bindness, deaf-retarded, blind-cerebral palsy, or any combination of handicapping conditions: The result is not just a simple addition of the results of the handicaps, but rather a *multiplication of disability.* This combination of sensory losses with each other and with other problems presents the most devastating results, and the interaction of the problems has to be considered.

A common challenge for the occupational therapist is the child whose primary problem is a physical handicap or mental retardation and who additionally has visual or hearing deficits. Cerebral palsy and mental retardation are discussed fully in preceding chapters, but it is important to realize that whenever there is brain damage to a developing brain (such as in cerebral palsy) the chances of additional handicaps are great. For instance, 50% of children with cerebral palsy have some visual deficit and 13% have some form of auditory problem; the percentages of visual and auditory deficits are also high for children with mental retarda-

tion. With both of these diagnoses, accurate assessment of acuity, awareness, and perception is often difficult because these children cannot give reliable feedback to the examiner. The examiner has the additional burden of trying to ascertain the child's true developmental level despite the multiplicity of the handicapping conditions. The asymmetrical tonic neck reflex (ATNR) pattern of the young cerebral palsy child can be reinforced by the pattern of the young blind child preferring the supine position. Thus, in the blind-cerebral palsy child, the examiner must determine how much of the ATNR is reflex patterning and how much is volitional patterning. The combination of sensory deficits added to mental retardation or cerebral palsy creates a true challenge to the therapist. Further adaptations and activity analysis must be added to the treatment techniques described earlier in Chapters 20 and 21.

Another special problem encountered in the therapy setting is deaf-blindness, most often caused by congenital rubella. With rubella, also known as the 3 day or German measles, a fairly mild infection in the mother causes serious damage to the developing embryo. Almost every system of the body can be affected, but the most common triad is congenital cataracts, sensorineural hearing loss, and congenital heart defects. These children are often small for their age, hypotonic, and have abnormal electroencephalographic patterns. The worst damage to the eyes and heart is done during weeks 2 to 6 of pregnancy, but inner ear and hearing damage continue until the last half of pregnancy.[14] A major rubella epidemic during 1963 to 1965 in the United States affected approximately 50,000 women, resulting in 20,000 stillbirths or miscarriages and 30,000 children born with handicaps. Of these children, approximately 5000 had the double handicaps of deafness and blindness.[14] Rubella incidence is reduced today by the live vaccine developed in 1960 and by an active ongoing antibody testing program. However, cases of congenital rubella are still reported, especially among the children of young adolescent mothers who contract the disease early in pregnancy and may not know they are pregnant at the time or may not have consulted a physician.

The rubella epidemic of the 1960s brought attention to the plight of the deaf-blind. Before that time few programs were available to educate or treat these children. The Perkins School was an exception. It is a residential facility in Massachusetts for the blind that has had many deaf-blind pupils, the most famous being Helen Keller.[20] A young instructor, Annie Sullivan, was sent, in 1887, to Alabama where the 6-year-old Helen Keller lived. Helen had been deaf-blind since 19 months of age and was unable to communicate in any rational way. The instruction was difficult at first, but eventually the two returned to Perkins School where Helen continued her education. Today, due mostly to increased knowledge stemming from the rubella epidemic, there is a wealth of educational and therapeutic information about the implications of deaf-blindness and its treatment.

Rubella is not the only disease that causes a combination of visual and hearing deficits. Embryological studies show that there is much similarity in the timetable of development of the eye and the ear.[69] Therefore, many diagnoses involve both systems such as cytomegalovirus infections, toxoplasmosis, congenital syphilis, Hurler's syndrome, Waardenburg's syndrome, and Goldenhar's syndrome. Meningitis is the leading cause of noncongenital deaf-blindness in children.

Other services

An extraordinary number of professionals may be involved with the multiply handicapped. Orthopedists, neurologists, and cardiologists are a few medical specialists whose expertise is often needed. As the severity of the child's disability increases so does the chance that the occupational therapist will become involved. The occupational therapist may be a major team member, especially with the physically involved child who has visual deficits or with the deaf-blind child. Very often the occupational therapist's first contact with visual or hearing impairment is through a multiply involved child.

Practice settings

The number of children with multiple sensory handicaps is often too small to establish an effective local program. The number of residential placements tends to rise with the level of impairment. Also, as children grow older they need more specialized programming. Although most professionals would favor local programs that allow children to live at home, there are very definite advantages to residential programs as the child matures. These are:
1. No long summer or holiday breaks to lose skills
2. Continuity of program and skills training
3. Twenty-four-hour care and supervision
4. Transition for those who will always need assistance

Special characteristics relevant to occupational therapy

There are some behaviors characteristic of rubella deaf-blind children.[13] Typically they show extreme tactile defensiveness. They do not like anything new or different, and changes of any type are not well accepted. There is a great deal of oral defensiveness, and the change from smooth to textured foods is quite difficult. Rubella children are usually hypotonic early in life. There is hypermobility of the joints, unless the child suffered additional brain damage from hypoxia, thereby incurring spasticity. Such children will usually learn to walk but will be delayed and cautious about giving up support. They can go from walking holding onto a wooden stick, then a smaller stick, then a piece of rope, then a piece of yarn, then a thread and still immediately fall if the thread is taken away. They often have had difficult infancy periods, setting up a cycle of negative reactions to parental handling that led to less and less parental handling. They can be "too deaf to be deaf," that is, not responding at any level. This seems to evolve because the stimuli do not make sense to the deaf-blind children, so they choose to block them out.[47] They can have many primitive withdrawal reactions and can seem autistic. Blindisms such as eye poking, eye rubbing, flicking hands in front of eyes, head bumping, hair twirling, and rocking are often present and can become self-abusive. Perseverative behaviors are common, as are teeth grinding and masturbation. Certainly, every child is different and may manifest these behaviors to different degrees.

With the visually or auditorily impaired child who is also physically or mentally handicapped many of the above characteristics will also be noted, such as autistic-like behaviors, tactile defensiveness, and resistance to change. One of the important characteristics for the occupational therapist to keep in mind is that these children will need consistent repetition to learn skills. Progress can be made but will often be extremely slow. A simple task, such as learning the hand-to-mouth pattern necessary for self-feeding, may well take years of hand over hand practice with multiple clues and much consistency. Therefore, the therapist, in addition to being the direct service provider, must take on the role of consultant or monitor. Campbell, McInerney and Cooper[12] found that more normal patterns of movement were achieved at faster rates when multiply handicapped children were able to practice the desired movement patterns more frequently; therefore, specific techniques were taught to school staff and parents. The therapist has to be able to assess the child and identify very specific tasks or movements to be worked on, to determine the appropriate intervention strategies, and to instruct others to carry out the tasks or movements with accuracy. Training caretakers and school staff becomes extremely important. It is important for the occupational therapist to remember that parents of a handicapped child have had experience only with their own multiply involved child. The caretaking/school staff may see many of these children over their careers but are not approaching them from the unique and distinct point of view of the therapist. Often the caretaking/school staffs change frequently and with the changes certain programs get "lost in the shuffle." Skills like using hand over hand guidance to have the child feed herself rather than having the adult spoon feed the child can be lost. All too often skills are learned only to be neglected and forgotten due to changes in caretakers or the environment. The occupational therapist can make a conscious effort to check the developmental history fully and to keep in mind the child's occupational behaviors and tasks and the future consequences of not fully attaining occupational skills. A prime example is in the area of activities of daily living skills where the occupational therapist may be able to set up and monitor a toilet scheduling program to have the child become toilet trained. It may take many years and much classroom and home time, but this is basic to the child's acceptance in society. The role of consultant or monitor is difficult, although a superficial impression is that this type of therapy takes less time and effort than direct service. In reality, if done correctly, it may take more time, because it is done on an irregular basis as opposed to the regularity of direct treatment. The therapist will have to develop a rapport with the persons doing the training and develop the ability to encourage and reward others to keep them following the program correctly. As a "combination cheerleader and policeman" the therapist will have to do repeated inservice training to assure that techniques are carried out accurately. In many cases written programs with diagrams or pictures will be used, and the directions will need to be clear and simple without confusing medical jargon. Monitoring entails not just watching others do a program but doing it oneself on occasion to get the feel of the child and her performance. Direct service based on specific goals is also given, but the pervasive characteristic of the handicaps in the multiply involved child neccesitates involvement of all personnel in attaining developmental skills.

Occupational therapy assessment procedures with the multiply impaired

Developmental scales can be used for assessment and treatment planning of the deaf-blind. Of special interest are the prehension and tactile abilities, since almost everything will have to be taught in a "hand over hand" manner. The Callier-Asuza Scale[70] is a checklist for use with this population. It has five areas of subscales: motor development, daily living skills, language development, perceptual abilities, and socialization. It covers developmental skills up to approximately the age of 7 and is based on observations of spontaneous behaviors in structured and unstructured situations. Each subscale is further divided; for example, the daily living skills subscale consists of dressing and undressing, personal hygiene, development of feeding skills, and toileting. The directions specify that it should be administered by an individual familiar with the child. The teacher or therapist should spend a substantial period of time (at least 2 weeks) working directly with the child before attempting to use the checklist. It is also suggested that aides, parents, and others be consulted about their observations of the child to obtain the most accurate picture.

A complete descriptive assessment of levels in all areas of development must be done for children who have physical or mental handicaps in addition to visual and auditory impairment. The therapist must pay special attention to play and social skills, activities of daily living, arm and hand skills, and prevocational skills. According to the child's diagnosis testing may include assessments of developmental age levels, range of motion, reflexes, tone, and noting the presence of any deformities or behaviors that interfere with function. The child should be observed in structured and unstructured settings and significant others should be consulted about the child's skills. The therapist will sort out what part each of the contributing factors plays in the total picture of the child's difficulties.

SPECIALIZED ASSESSMENTS

Psychological testing of the child with multiple sensory handicaps is challenging and must be done on an individual basis with subjective observation, rather than by standardized testing. This is also true of visual and auditory assessment, although the new technology of the evoked response testing shows much promise with these children.

Objectives of intervention and treatment modalities

Although the goals of treatment will depend on the individual assessment of the child and identified levels of functioning, some typical treatment goals follow:

1. *To minimize tactile defensiveness.* Since very little can be done with these children until they are able to accept touch, this is usually a basic goal. The child should be gradually introduced to a large variety of tactile stimulation activities and encouraged to reach out and explore independently.

2. *To provide early parental intervention.* If possible, the child and mother should be involved in an intervention program from the moment of diagnosis.[52] The cycle of diminished or negative responses from the child leading to decreased stimuli from the mother must be stopped as soon as possible. The child needs to be out of the crib and placed in the room where activity is taking place and given much gentle but firm stimulation.

3. *To provide adequate positioning.* The multiply involved child often cannot or will not, because of fear, move by herself. Adequate positioning of the child to take advantage of the environment and to prevent contractures and deformities is extremely important. Reflex patterns, behavioral patterns, and tonal problems that interfere with development should be counteracted in the positioning process. Functional positioning, so that the child can take advantage of any residual senses available, is the aim of much treatment. For those children not moving by themselves, teaching the caretakers and school staff different positions and encouraging them to change these positions often is important.

4. *To provide maximal adaptation.* With these children it is necessary to take techniques found in many other diagnostic areas and adapt them with the visual or auditory handicap in mind. For example, the lap tray for a blind-cerebral palsy child should have raised edges so the child can easily explore a defined area without pushing objects off the tray and thus out of reach. The resourcefulness of the occupational therapist can be put to maximum use devising equipment that fits the child's unique pattern of disability.

5. *To maximize movement.* The child at first needs to be moved, and later encouraged, if able, to move by himself. For the child with reflex or tone problems, much effort has to be made to provide movement so that the cycle of lack of movement, contractures, and deformities is interrupted. Practice time should be allowed and new items introduced gradually. Activities with tilt boards, swings, and bolsters are useful, but most important is movement with another person, such as walking (holding on) or rocking together. The child will need much help in letting go of the supportive surface.[33] Moersch[51] detailed a treatment program that strongly emphasizes the use of meaningful activity, play, and movement in treating the multiply involved child.

6. *To improve feeding skills.* Feeding is often a problem for multiply involved children. Often they have had stormy neonatal periods with long periods of tube feedings. Therapy intervention with the neonate should focus on obtaining good sucking skills (good rhythm and appropriate strength) and decreasing facial tactile defensiveness. Later, problems such as tongue thrusting, taking too long to feed, and poor coordination of mouth movements occur. Learning to accept textured foods and chewing will usually require intervention. Physically moving the child through the movements of chewing and cup placement is often necessary. Tactile defensiveness and resistance to change are two major difficulties that can be intensified with the presence of increased tone and reflex patterns.

7. *To improve self-maintenance skills.* As much independence as possible should be the goal for each individual child. Toileting is often a problem because of resistance to the potty chair and difficulty in understanding what is required. For the child who is physically handicapped in addition to visually or auditorily impaired, the use of toilet scheduling techniques may be needed. The adult should place the child on the toilet at scheduled times and note the results to determine if the child has a pattern that can be used to allow her to stay continent without actually being able to place herself on the commode. Often the next step is the establishment of some type of indicator (verbalization, sign or gesture, or body language) that indicates that the child needs to void. Dressing and hygiene skills are also often difficult, requiring adaptation and hand over hand guidance.

8. *To develop cause-and-effect relationships.* The child needs to learn to make things happen outside herself. Play activities such as jack-in-the-box or busy box are useful.

9. *To develop productive behaviors.* Not only must the perseverative, nonproductive behaviors be stopped, but more productive behaviors must be substituted. Otherwise, equally undesirable behaviors will be established. The child will need consistency and continuity. If tactile signs are used, they should be simple initially and consistent from one person to the next. The development of interpersonal and play skills is crucial.

SPECIAL TECHNIQUES

Many of the specialized techniques used with these children deal with the development of some form of communication. *Clueing* is a system that was developed primarily by the mother of a rubella child in England.[25] It is a signal-type of language (one-way communication) between the mother and child. In this technique the daily activities of the child must be analyzed for clues or signals that can be picked up by the child. These signals tell the child what is happening or about to happen and form the beginning of communication. For example, the mother might rub the child's arms with a warm wet cloth before putting him into the bath.

TADOMA is a method of teaching speech and speech reading by placing the child's hand on the speaker's face and throat and thereby having the child pick up the vibrations that are made by sound. Children usually place the thumb on the speaker's lips and spread the fingers over cheek and neck.

Coactive movement is a system developed by Dr. J. Van Dijk in Holland.[74] He began the system with what he called the "resonance phenomenon": the therapist goes with the child's action, rocking or crawling, or whatever it is. This is to develop a rapport at the child's level. In the next stage of coactive movements, the therapist moves with the child in a prearranged sequence. This leads to nonrepresentational reference with such activities as identifying body parts on self and others, and then to imitation. *Imitation* uses body movements or positions and leads to natural gesture, a system that describes the object according to what is done with it; for example, a toothbrush would be identified by making toothbrushing movements with the hand. This system is developed for very low functioning children and is based on the premise that the rubella child will not naturally explore and that the world outside himself does not exist.

There are other more sophisticated communication techniques that are often used by people who developed the double handicap later in life, such as the blind child who has lost her hearing, the meningitis child with the double handicap, or the deaf adolescent with Usher's syndrome. These are methods such as the following:

1. Printing in the palm. The block letters of the alphabet are traced in the palm of the person's hand.
2. Alphabet glove. A thin glove with the letters of the alphabet placed on different parts of the hand is worn by the deaf-blind person; the interpreter simply spells out the words.
3. Tellatouch machine. The interpreter uses a machine with a standard typewriter keyboard on one side and a space for the deaf-blind person's index finger on the other side. As the keys are hit on the typewriter, the letters pop up in braille under the index finger of the deaf-blind person.

With multiply involved children and their slower pace of development, task analysis and breaking a task down into its smallest component parts can be very useful in setting realistic goals for therapy and in establishing steps for the team to work on. Task analysis can be especially useful in activities of daily living and vocational skills. The total task, such as buttering a piece of bread, is broken down into its smallest components, and then backward or forward chaining of steps is used. In forward chaining the object is to teach the first step until it is mastered, then the second, and so on. In backward chaining the last step is taught until mastered, then the next to last, and so on. It is important to fade out assistance, but still give as much as needed. Each time a repeated error is corrected, enough information to correct the error should be provided, but not as much as before.[28]

Another useful technique with the multiply involved is *behavior modification*. This is a systematic approach to alter the child's behavior through environmental programming. Reinforcement is often used, and detailed records of the child's responses are kept. Often a positive trait needs to be reinforced, such as urinating when placed on the potty, or a negative trait such as eye poking needs to be extinguished. These behaviors are charted, and positive reinforcement is given for the desired behavior. Although being ignored can be a good behavioral conditioner for many children, deaf-blind and multiply involved children are often quite happy to be left alone. Therefore, this technique may not have the desired effect.

For the severely physically and mentally involved multiply impaired child, the therapist may decide to teach splinter skills. These may often be related to survival or self-care skills that the child will benefit from even if learned in a rote manner and only carried over into one setting. Carryover should be sought if possible, but after weighing all factors, therapeutic judgment may support concentrating on certain splinter skills.

PREPARATION FOR ADULTHOOD

The multiply handicapped child is usually prepared for sheltered employment rather than for independent living. Approximately 75% of the rubella children will need sheltered living and employment.[68] There are four levels of independence to consider:

1. Custodial care—sheltered living: Not capable of taking care of own needs, although may have some self-help skills and may participate in recreation programs.
2. Sheltered employment—sheltered living: Capable of working with close supervision and living in group home situation with supervision and assistance in some tasks.
3. Sheltered employment—semisheltered living: Capable of working in sheltered workshop and living with some support services available.
4. Self-sufficient: Employed and competent in daily living skills.

Some of the behaviors that the adolescent will have to develop for more self-sufficient living are (1) communication of at least basic emergency/survival words such as stop, eat, more, no, and finish; (2) social skills; (3) self-care skills; (4) telling time; (5) cooking and shopping skills; (6) home management; (7) travel and mobility; and (8) housekeeping. Workshop activities are manipulative for the most part and can include folding, stamping, collating, counting, gluing, bending, sorting, assembling, wrapping, stuffing, filing, measuring, stapling, and clipping.

If the child has remained at home with the family unit through school, adolescence is often the time when a move must be made to a residential facility. Both the family members and the child must be prepared for this.[72] Also, the emerging sexuality of the child has to be dealt with at the level of the child's understanding. For resources for additional study and information on multiple sensory impairment, see the reference section of this chapter.

CASE STUDY 3

Mary is 17 years, 3 months old. She had congenital rubella syndrome with cataracts, with resultant severe hearing loss and markedly delayed development. Mary is presently in a state residential facility for the blind that has a deaf-blind treatment unit. She is gradually being transferred from the school program into the sheltered workshop program. She has been at the state facility since the age of 10 when her parents could no longer maintain her at home because of self-abusive behaviors and the need for constant supervision. Since her placement, she has been placed on a behavior modification program that has markedly reduced her self-abusive behaviors. She was assessed with the Gesell scale and a self-help skills checklist used by the school. She has difficulty with cup placement in eating, with fasteners in dressing, and with rigidity in walking. She understands and uses some tactile sign language and is functioning overall on a level of about a 3- to 4-year-old.

Treatment goals

1. *To increase coordination and manipulative skills for workshop experience.* Include activities such as sorting nails by size and shape, folding letters, and stamping envelopes.
2. *To improve eating skills.* Reinforce techniques to lo-

cate tabletop and to place cup upright with gradually fading physical assistance.

3. *To improve dressing skills.* Practice fasteners on self, practice boards, and dolls.

4. *To decrease rigidity in walking.* Movement through space activities such as trampoline, swimming, tilt board, and scooter board.

SUMMARY

This chapter has provided an overview of occupational therapy intervention with the child with visual or hearing impairment. Degrees of impairment have been investigated, as well as typical causes of impairment. Eye and ear anatomy has been reviewed to give information on the dynamics of a sensory loss. Emphasis in occupational therapy assessment has been placed on the interruption in the developmental process caused by the loss of one or both of these distance senses. General treatment goals have been given, stressing provision of activities and experiences to allow the child to develop adaptive behaviors and to develop to her fullest potential. Brief explanations have been given regarding specialized techniques used with these children, including the use of hearing aids, sign language, braille, and low vision aids. It is my hope that the profession of occupational therapy will become increasingly involved with these children because of its emphases on adaptation, activity analysis, and developmental sequence.

STUDY QUESTIONS

1. Sean is 6 years old with mild mental retardation and left hemiparesis. He is completely blind in his right eye and legally blind in his left. He has been referred to occupational therapy for improvement in postural stability, gross motor skills, fine motor skills, and self-care skills. He is also receiving services from a mobility instructor. Using the general problem analysis, plan an intervention program.
2. Children with hearing impairment may use one of four basic methods to improve communication skills. How would use of each method affect occupational therapy intervention?
3. What are common problems of children with visual impairment that would suggest the need for referral to occupational therapy? How can the occupational therapist help them with each of these problems?
4. Imagine that Helen Keller had been born in the 1980s instead of the 1880s and she was referred to you for occupational therapy. What would you do, and why?
5. You have a 10-year-old child with spastic quadriparesis who is severely mentally retarded. She was referred to you for assistance with oral motor control and feeding techniques. You learn that she is also cortically blind. What would you recommend to her teacher?

REFERENCES

1. Adelson E, and Fraiberg S: Gross motor development in infants blind from birth, Child Dev 45:114, 1974.
2. Aids and appliances for the blind and visually impaired, New York, 1970, The American Foundation for the Blind.
3. Anastasi A: Psychological testing, London, 1982, Macmillan Publishing Co.
4. Arena JM: Davison's compleat pediatrician, Philadelphia, 1969, Lea & Febiger.
5. Ayres AJ: The influence of the vestibular system on the auditory and sensory systems, new techniques for working with deaf blind children, Denver, 1973, Mountain Plains Regional Center.
6. Ayres AJ: Sensory integration and learning disorders, Los Angeles, 1973, Western Psychological Services.
7. Baker-Nobles L, and Bink MP: Sensory integration in the rehabilitation of blind adults, Am J Occup Ther 33:559, 1979.
8. Barraga N: Impaired visual behavior in low vision children, New York, 1964, The American Foundation for the Blind.
9. Basic pre-school signed English, Washington, DC, 1973, Gallaudet University Press.
10. Bernero RJ, and Bothwell H: Relationship of hearing impairment to educational needs, Springfield, Ill, 1966, Illinois Department of Public Health and Office of the Superintendent of Public Instruction.
11. Brown D, Simmons V, and Mathvin J: The Oregon project for visually impaired and blind preschool children, Medford, Oregon, 1984, Jackson County Education Service District.
12. Campbell PH, McInerney WF, and Cooper MA: Therapeutic programming for students with severe handicaps, Am J Occup Ther 38:594, 1984.
13. Chess S: Behavioral study of children with congenital rubella, New York, 1967, New York University Rubella Project.
14. Cooper LZ: Congenital rubella in the United States in infections of the fetus and newborn infant, New York, 1975, AA Gershon.
15. Cratty BJ: Movement and spatial awareness in blind youth, Springfield, Ill, 1971, Charles C Thomas, Publisher.
16. Davis H, and Silverman SR: Hearing and deafness, New York, 1970, Holt, Rinehart & Winston Inc.
17. deQuiros J: Neuropsychological fundamentals in learning disorders, San Rafael, Calif, 1976, Academic Therapy Publications.
18. Erhardt RP: Sequential levels in the visual-motor development of a child with cerebral palsy, Am J Occup Ther 41:43, 1987.
19. Fant LJ: Ameslan—an introduction to American sign language, Silver Springs, Md, 1971, The National Association for the Deaf.
20. Fish AG: Perkins Institute and its deaf-blind pupils, Watertown, Mass, 1934, Perkins School for the Blind.
21. Flavell JH: The developmental psychology of Jean Piaget, New York, 1963, Van Nostrand Reinhold Co Inc.
22. Fonda G: Management of the patient with subnormal vision, ed 2, St Louis, 1970, The CV Mosby Co.
23. Fraiberg S: Insights from the blind: comparative studies of blind and sighted infants, New York, 1977, Basic Books Inc, Publishers.
24. Fraser BA, Hensinger RN, and Phelps JA: Physical management of multiple handicaps, Baltimore, Md, 1984, Paul H Brookes Publishing Co.
25. Freeman P: Parent's guide to early care of a deaf-blind child, London, 1966, The National Association for Deaf-Blind and Rubella Children.
26. Furth HG: Deafness and learning: a psychological approach, Belmont, Calif, 1973, Wadsworth Inc.
27. Gesell A, Ilg FL, and Bullis GE: Vision: its development in infant and child, New York, 1967, Hafner Publishing, Inc.
28. Gold M: Try another way, Washington, DC, 1977, The National Children's Center.
29. Gregory RL: Eye and brain—the psychology of seeing, New York, 1972, McGraw-Hill Inc.
30. Grinnel MF, Dentamore KL, and Lippke BA: Sign it successful—manual English encourages expressive communication, Teach Except Child, p 123, 1976, Spring Publications Inc.

31. Gunn SL: Play as occupation—implications for the handicapped, Am J Occup Ther 25:285, 1971.

32. Gustafson G, Pfetzing D, and Zawalkow E: Signing exact English, Silver Springs, Md, 1975, Modern Sign Press.

33. Halliday C: The visually impaired child: growth, learning, development—infancy to school age, Louisville, Ky, 1970, The American Printing House for the Blind.

34. Hearing aids for children, Lansing, Mich, 1966, Michigan Department of Public Health.

35. Hendrickson H. In Orem RC: Montessori and the special child, New York, 1969, The Putnam Publishing Group Inc.

36. Hill L: Working with blind pre-schoolers, Am J Occup Ther 31;417, 1977.

37. Illinois Society for the Prevention of Blindness: Definition of words relating to vision, Springfield, Ill, 1964, The Society.

38. Jastrzembska ZS: The effects of blindness and other impairments on early development, New York, 1976, The American Foundation for the Blind.

39. Kaarela R, and Widerberg L: Basic components of orientation and movement techniques, Kalamazoo, Mich, 1970, Western Michigan University.

40. Kinsey E: Retrolental fibroplasia—cooperative study of the use of oxygen and RLF, Arch Ophthalmol 56:481, 1956.

41. Klima ES, and Bellugi U: The signs of language, Cambridge, Mass, 1978, Harvard University Press.

42. Leenenberg EH: Biological foundation of language, New York, 1967, John Wiley & Sons Inc.

43. Liben LS: Deaf children: developmental perspectives, New York, 1978, Academic Press Inc.

44. Lowenfeld B: Our blind children, Springfield, Ill, 1969, Charles C Thomas, Publisher.

45. Lydon WT, and McGraw LM: Concept development for the visually handicapped child, New York, 1973, The American Foundation for the Blind.

46. Maxfield KE, and Buchholz S: A social maturity scale for blind pre-school children, New York, 1957, The American Foundation for the Blind.

47. McInnes JM, and Teffry JA: Deaf-blind infants and children, Toronto, Canada, 1982, University of Toronto Press.

48. Meadow PM: Deafness and child development, Berkeley, Calif, 1980, University of California Press.

49. Michelman S: The importance of creative play, Am J Occup Ther 25:285, 1971.

50. Mindel ED, and Vernon M: They grow in silence-the deaf child and his family, Silver Springs, Md, 1971, The National Association for the Deaf.

51. Moersch M: Training the deaf-blind child, Am J Occup Ther 31:425, 1977.

52. Moucka S: The deaf-blind infant in the family, parent counseling and infant stimulation, Denver, 1973, Mountain Plains Regional Center.

53. Myklebust HR: The psychology of deafness: sensory deprivation, learning and adjustment, New York, 1964, Grune & Stratton, Inc.

54. Newby H: Audiology, New York, 1972, Appleton-Century-Crofts.

55. Perera CA: May's diseases of the eye, Baltimore, Md, 1957, Williams & Wilkins.

56. Pollack D: Educational audiology for the limited hearing infant, Springfield, Ill, 1970, Charles C Thomas, Publisher.

57. Reynell J, and Zinkin P: Reynell-Zinkin Developmental Scales for Young Visually Handicapped Children, Windsor, England, 1979, NFER Publishing Company, Ltd.

58. Robbins N: Educational beginnings with deaf-blind children, 1960, Perkins School for the Blind.

59. Rugers CT: Understanding braille, New York, 1969, The American Foundation for the Blind.

60. Ryan SJ, Dawson AK, and Little HL: Retinal diseases, Orlando, Fla, 1985, Grune & Stratton, Inc.

61. Sapir R: Culture, language and personality, Los Angeles, 1966, University of California Press.

62. Schaefer KJ, and Specht MA: A light probe adapted for use in training the blind, Am J Occup Ther 33:640, 1979.

63. Schein JD, and Delk MT: The deaf population of the United States, Silver Springs, Md, 1975, The National Association for the Deaf.

64. Schlesinger HS, and Meadow KP: Sound and sign: childhood deafness and mental health, Berkeley, Calif, 1972, University of California Press.

65. School G, and Schaun R: Measurement of psychological, vocational, and educational functioning in the blind and visually handicapped, New York, 1976, The American Foundation for the Blind.

66. Sheridan MD: Manual for the STYCAR Vision Tests (Screening Tests for Young Children and Retardates), Berks, England, 1969, NFER Publishing Company, Ltd.

67. Silverman WA: Retrolental fibroplasia: a modern parable, New York, 1980, Grune & Stratton, Inc.

68. Smith B: Potentials of rubella deaf-blind children, 1980 is now: a conference on the future of deaf-blind children, Sacramento, Calif, 1974, John Tracy Clinic and Southwestern Regional Center.

69. Smith DW: Recognizable patterns of human malformations, Philadelphia, 1982, WB Saunders Co.

70. Stillman RD: The Callier-Asuza Scale, Dallas, 1973, Callier Speech and Hearing Center.

71. Thurnell RJ, and Rice DFG: Eye rubbing in blind children: application of a sensory deprivation model, Except Child 36:325, 1970.

72. Tretaloff M: Counseling parents of handicapped children, Ment Retard p 7231, 1969.

73. Van Benschoter R: A sensory integration program for blind campers, Am J Occup Ther 29:617, 1975.

74. Van Dijk J: The non-verbal deaf-blind child and his word: his outgrowth towards the world of symbols, St Michielsgestel, Holland, 1965, Insituut Voor Doven.

75. Warner DH: Blindness and early childhood development, New York, 1984, The American Foundation for the Blind.

76. Welsh RL, and Blasch BB: Foundations of orientation and mobility, New York, 1980, The American Foundation for the Blind.

RESOURCES FOR ADDITIONAL STUDY AND INFORMATION ON HEARING IMPAIRMENT

Alexander Graham Bell Association for the Deaf, 3417 Volta Place, NW, Washington, DC 20007. (Publishes *The Volta Review.*)

American Speech and Hearing Association, 19801 Rockville Pike, Rockville, Md 20852. (Information on deafness, audiology, and speech therapy.)

California State University, Northridge, National Center on Deafness, 18111 Nordhoff, Northridge, Calif 91324.

Conference of American Instructors of the Deaf, 5034 Wisconsin Ave, NW, Washington, DC 20016. (Publishes *American Annals of the Deaf.*)

Deafness Research and Training Center, New York University, 80 Washington Square East, New York, NY 10003.

Gallaudet College, 7th and Florida Ave, NE, Washington, DC 20910.

John Tracy Clinic, 806 West Adams Blvd, Los Angeles, Calif 90007. (Correspondence course for parents of deaf preschoolers.)

National Association for the Deaf, 814 Thayer Ave, Silver Springs, Md 20910. (Publishes *The Deaf American,* clearing house of information.)

National Captioning Institute, PO Box 57064, Washington, DC 20037. (Information on tv and film captioning.)

National Hearing Aid Society, 24261 Grand River, Detroit, Mich 48219. (Information on hearing aids and dealers.)

National Technical Institute for the Deaf, 1 Lomb Memorial Dr, Rochester, NY 14623.

Professional Rehabilitation Workers of the Deaf, 814 Thayer Ave, Silver Springs, Md 20910. (Publishes *Journal of Rehabilitation of the Deaf.*)

RESOURCES FOR ADDITIONAL STUDY AND INFORMATION ON VISUAL IMPAIRMENT

American Academy of Ophthalmology and Otolaryngology, 15 Second St SW, Rochester, Minn 55901. (Information on low vision aids and ophthalmology.)

American Academy of Optometry, 1506-1508 Forshey Towers, Minneapolis, Minn 55402. (Information on low vision aids and optometry.)

American Association for the Blind, 15 West 65th St, New York, NY 10011. (Publishes *Journal of Visual Impairment and Blindness.*)

American Foundation for the Blind, 15 West 16th St, New York, NY 10011. (Disseminates information, research, films, publications. Publishes *New Outlook for the Blind.*)

American Printing House for the Blind, 1839 Frankfort Ave, Louisville, Ky 40206. (Publications, talking books, large print and braille publications.)

Association for the Education of Visually Handicapped, 919 Walnut St, 4th Floor, Philadelphia, Pa 19107. (Publishes *Education of the Visually Handicapped.*)

Division for the Blind and Physically Handicapped, Library of Congress, 1291 Taylor St NW, Washington, DC 20542. (Regional libraries of large print, braille, and talking books.)

Howe Press, Perkins School for the Blind, Watertown, Mass 02172. (Games, writing, and educational aids publications.)

National Association of the Visually Handicapped, 305 East 24th St, New York, NY 10010. (Large print publications and information.)

National Society for the Prevention of Blindness, Inc, 79 Madison Ave, New York, NY 10016. (Studies the causes of blindness, clearing house of information.)

Recording for Blind, Inc, 215 East 58th St, New York, NY 10022. (Taped and recorded educational material.)

RESOURCES FOR ADDITIONAL STUDY AND INFORMATION ON MULTIPLE SENSORY IMPAIRMENT (DEAF-BLIND)

Centers and Services for Deaf-Blind, Special Services Branch, Bureau of Education for the Handicapped, US Office of Education, Donohue Bldg Rm 4046, 400 Maryland Ave SW, Washington, DC 20202. (List of regional centers and state educational agencies working with the deaf-blind.)

Helen Keller National Center for Deaf-Blind Youths and Adults, 111 Middle Neck Rd, Sands Point, NY 11051. (Information on the deaf-blind, especially vocational training.)

John Tracy Clinic, 806 West Adams Blvd, Los Angeles, Calif 90007. (Correspondence learning program for parents of preschool deaf-blind children.)

27

Children with emotional or behavioral disorders

ANNE F. CRONIN
WITH CONTRIBUTIONS BY DIANA P. BURNELL

Mental or emotional health has been defined as "the degree of freedom an individual has in choosing from among alternative types of behavior"[22] (p. 128), with emotional disturbance inferred from inflexible behavior patterns. This concept is complicated by the fact that many behaviors considered "maladaptive" in adults are recognized as normal at some earlier stage of child development.[16,22,30] Consequently, literature on identification and diagnosis of emotionally disturbed children is often ambiguous and occasionally contradictory.

Incidence of emotional disturbance in children is also difficult to determine. Although less than one in every thousand school-aged children is hospitalized annually for mental illness, about four children per thousand are seen for outpatient psychiatric care; this is twice the rate for adults. Recent statistics indicate that the general prevalence of psychiatric disorders among school-aged children is between 6% and 7%.[38] Children with chronic organic disorders have a much higher incidence of emotional disturbance, ranging from 12% to 58%, according to the specific organic problem.[31,38]

With these issues in mind, this chapter presents occupational therapy for children with emotional and behavioral disorders, both as primary and secondary problems. Discussion begins with a brief historical review of occupational therapy intervention, which is supplemented later with citations from the literature that illustrate different theoretical approaches to treatment. A review of diagnostic information (see Chapter 6) and typical practice settings is included. Discussion

of theoretical approaches, assessment procedures, and treatment modalities is followed by presentation of a sequence of case studies.

HISTORICAL PERSPECTIVE

The treatment of emotional and behavioral disorders of children and adolescents is considered a complex and highly specialized area of pediatric occupational therapy. In the last 50 years many psychological approaches have been used successfully. Between 1930 and 1954 the psychoanalytic approach guided most of the treatment of psychotic children. Adolescents with conduct disorders who were institutionalized in correctional facilities were treated by use of an unstructured behavioral approach. During the 1950s and 1960s psychoanalytic theories still regulated most of the goals and treatment modalities used in occupational therapy. However, the developmental approach was used to justify tutoring, skill development, and work programs. From the 1960s, with the development of psychotropic drugs, the biophysical approach was included with other current approaches in a therapeutic milieu environment. Vestibular and sensory stimulation were used to improve cognitive-perceptual-motor functions. Some programs were reported to have used several theories for establishing goals. The behavioral approach began to replace the psychoanalytic model as the guide for occupational therapy with disturbed children and adolescents in the 1970s. A sociocultural approach derived from systems theorists, influenced the design of therapeutic community programs for adolescents with drug and alcohol abuse problems. In the 1980s a renewed interest in the treatment of autism

The contributions of Dr. Burnell to sections on history and classification systems are gratefully acknowledged.

brought forth the recommendation that occupational therapists working in this area look for answers to treatment in the neurobiological literature. Occupational therapists in this specialty area use all the general psychological approaches as a means of assessing, planning, and documenting treatment intervention with children and adolescents. Knowledge of these approaches is necessary for the understanding of past treatment, communication with other professionals, and future practice.

CURRENT THEORETICAL MODELS OF CHILDHOOD PSYCHOPATHOLOGY

The etiologies of most emotional disorders involve a complex interaction of neurological, family, environmental, intrapsychic, and specific precipitating causes. Researchers and clinicians in child psychopathology have organized these factors according to four general conceptual models.[16] These models are intended to both systematize and direct the clinician's thinking and the progression of therapy. The knowledge of and use of such models is particularly important in mental health because of the complexity of the disorders and the need for consistency among all service providers to the child.

The four major theoretical models presented here are: psychoanalytic, social learning and behavioral, systems analytic, and developmental.[16] Each of these models is presented briefly with specific focus on issues relevant to occupational therapy.

Psychoanalytic

The psychoanalytic theories of behavioral disturbances in children focus on deviations from the developmental process that result in maladaptive function, fixation, or regression.[16,37] Although psychoanalytic approaches in adulthood stress elaborate defense mechanisms and unconscious projections, the clinician who works with children must incorporate a more developmental orientation. As described by Kaplan and Sadock, ". . . the maladaptive defensive functioning is directed against conflicts between impulses that are characteristics of a specific developmental phase and environmental influences"[16] (p. 951).

Two psychic operations that were originally described by Freud are of particular importance in the psychoanalytic view of childhood and childhood emotional disturbance. These are fixation and regression—common responses to conflict that are believed to be consistent with the lack of sophisticated cognition processing in children through the latency period of development (approximately 7 to 11 years).

Fixation refers to an overinvestment in a particular stage of development as a result of some pathological experience. Excessive use of this mechanism is believed to lead to inhibition or aberration of the child's emotional development.[14,37] Fixation is typically demonstrated when the child is not emotionally prepared to cope with a novel situation, so that he in fact resists growing up. In contrast, *regression* refers to the child's tendency to revert to an earlier, successful pattern of adapting behaviorally. As described by Simon and Pardes, ". . . this might happen particularly in the face of a current threat or if the individual has great difficulty mastering a new developmental task"[37] (p. 512). An example is the child who becomes angry and insists on riding her tricycle after she has fallen off her new bicycle several times.

Overall, the psychoanalytic model focuses on difficulty in achieving or resolving the developmental tasks necessary for continued psychic growth and adaptation. Intervention tends to emphasize free expression of thoughts and feelings, use of guided play and play environments to enhance emotional expression (traditionally known as "play therapy"[1]), and encouraging the substitution of new adaptive mechanisms. Although the use of projective techniques (see Chapter 10) is widely associated with psychoanalysis, it is generally held that this method is less effective with most prepubescent children, who do not have mature abstract thinking capacity. However, projective techniques may be used to encourage social expression.[21,25]

Social learning and behaviorism

Intervention derived from these theories is based on the concept that all behavior is a consequence of a basic process of acquisition and maintenance.[16] This approach has evolved from the work of Watson and Pavlov, and emphasizes the concepts of conditioning, behavioral antecedents, consequences, reinforcers, and modeling.[16,37] Issues of psychic development, motivation, and emotional expression are not a focus of the behavioral model, which instead emphasizes observable, objective actions and events. Behaviors may be learned and unlearned, and what renders any specific behavior (or class of behaviors) maladaptive is the social significance of those actions. In their presentation of the behavioral model, Kaplan and Sadock[16] described two types of abnormal behavior: deficits that result from a failure to learn, and deficits that are a consequence of inappropriate learning.

Clinicians who use the behavioral model generally plan intervention through the controlled application of reinforcement, with an emphasis on rewarding previously unnoticed or undernoticed good behavior.[16,26] Because of the objective scientific method used by adherants of this approach, it tends to be more widely researched and documented than the other models presented. Strengths of the approach include the speed with which it can eliminate specific dangerous or self-destructive behaviors. In addition, it has the advantage of not implying parental guilt and it offers specific techniques to elicit change.

Systems analysis

The *family systems* and *transactional analysis* approaches share a common foundation in their application of general systems theory to mental health intervention. Both approaches see the family as ". . . a self-regulating open system that possesses its own unique history and structure. Its structure is constantly evolving as a consequence of dynamic interactions . . ."[16] (p. 952). These approaches direct intervention to the family system rather than exclusively with the child, and tend to focus on family development life cycles, functions, roles, values, goals, and structure. The transactional analysis approach also defines specific roles and functions of the individual and attempts to identify and analyze all of the possible interactions that will occur between two or more people, with variations according to individual ego states.[1,7]

Family systems therapies generally use counseling and are less activity oriented than the other approaches mentioned. The specific counseling techniques that are used require specialized training and are not commonly used in pediatric occupational therapy. However, familiarity with the techniques can be an asset when negotiating occupational therapy goals with family needs and expectations. Transactional analysis has been more widely used by occupational therapists and reportedly was used successfully with school-aged children to enhance communication skills and parent-child interactions.[15]

Developmental

The developmental model incorporates the works of Gesell, Piaget, Erikson, and others, and includes the recent growing field of developmental neuropsychology. The primary assumption of this model is ". . . that in the absence of unusual interferences, children mature in basically orderly predictable ways. . . "[16] (p. 952). Emotional crises, physical limitations, learning disabilities, or chronic illness may interfere with adaptation to such a degree that cognitive and emotional development are challenged.[11,17,31]

Developmental intervention focuses on facilitating skills acquisition and encouraging expression of emotions through socially acceptable means. Task mastery and social competence are emphasized, and programs are generally delivered through a play or activity format.[13,16,25] Activities are designed to carefully elicit social, interpersonal, and emotional adaptive skills through control of the environment and personal interactions.

DIFFERENTIAL DIAGNOSIS AND CLASSIFICATIONS
Classification systems

There are two compatible resources that may be used to recognize and describe emotional and behavioral disorders arising in infancy, childhood, and adolescence: the *International Classification of Diseases,* ed 9, published in 1977 by the World Health Organization (ICD-9),[44,45] and the *Diagnostic and Statistical Manual of Mental Disorders,* ed 3, published by the American Psychiatric Association in 1980 (DSM-IIIR).[43]

The ICD-9 is a statistical classification of all diseases, injuries, and causes of death. It was designed for use in gathering worldwide data and for indexing and retrieval of medical records. After the ICD-9 was published, psychiatrists in the United States complained that the classification system was not specific. Therefore a revised version was developed, the ICD-9-CM. This classification system includes all mental disorders found in the DSM-III, as well as many other codes and terms; however, the DSM-III is generally employed as the resource for coding diagnosis in most mental health facilities.

The DSM-III uses a multiaxial organization and description of mental disorders. This means that each individual is assessed through different categories of information called axes. There are five axes in the DSM-III assessment classification. Axes I and II include all classifications of mental disorders. Mental disorders are generally thought to be patterns or syndromes associated with behavioral, *psychological, or biological* dysfunction. A clear boundary between the various syndromes is not believed to exist. It is important to understand that the term *mental disorder* in the DSM-III is used to classify behavior patterns observed in the individual, not the person himself.

Axis I: Applies to clinical syndromes or focus of treatment
Axis II: Records personality or developmental disorders
Axis III: Provides the clinician with a category to define any physical disorders that may accompany the mental disorder
Axis IV: Describes the severity of psychosocial stressors that may have caused the mental disorder
Axis V: Codes the highest level of adaptive functioning manifested during the past year

The last two axes are especially important for occupational therapists. It is in these areas that the therapist's expertise may be best used by the treatment team.

The following two examples are provided to illustrate how this classification system is used with emotional disorders in children and adolescents.

A 5-year-old child who has been accepted into a program for autistic children might have the following DSM-III diagnoses and their respective codes:

Axis I: 313.89 Reactive attachment; 299.00 Disorder of infancy with autistic features
Axis II: 315.90 Atypical specific developmental disorder
Axis III: Rule out neurological dysfunction

Axis IV: 4-5 Moderate to severe psychosocial stressors

Axis V: 4-5 Fair to poor adaptive development

An adolescent admitted to an acute psychiatric hospital might have the following DSM-III diagnoses:

Axis I: 309.00 Separation anxiety disorder with mixed emotional features; 305.30 Substance abuse, hallucinogens; drug-induced psychosis

Axis II: Deferred

Axis III: Mild physical symptoms

Axis IV: Fair psychosocial stressors

Sometimes the psychiatrist will code one syndrome, or several, on an axis; while at other times the coding will be deferred until further information is available on the patient. It is not unusual to find in a long case history one or two additional DSM-III diagnoses that reflect either an update of the patient's condition or a difference of opinion between clinicians. Occupational therapists should regard the most recent diagnosis for planning treatment.

Major classifications

It should be remembered that psychopathology is less clearly differentiated in childhood than in adulthood.[38] Childhood disorders are seldom discrete and classifications are inconsistent. The diagnostic categories presented in this chapter are intended to reflect patterns of dysfunction most commonly seen by occupational therapists, but this content is not all inclusive of any possible childhood psychiatric disorders.

PERVASIVE DEVELOPMENTAL DISORDERS OF CHILDHOOD

The group of disorders represented under this classification share two features: a widespread disruption to development in several areas simultaneously, and deviations or aberrations in personality organization that are qualitatively abnormal at any stage of development.[16,26] The pervasive developmental disorders are considered the most severe forms of childhood psychopathology[16] and include infantile autism.

Clinical manifestations of autism include extreme social isolation, mutism or atypical language, and bizarre responses to the environment. Associated features are labile mood, aberrant sensory responses, and rigidly stereotyped play behavior and body movements.[16,26,38] Autism is described in depth in Chapter 6. The prognosis for intervention with these children is mixed and is an arena of continuing research.

CONDUCT DISORDERS

Conduct disorders include repetitive and persistent patterns of antisocial behavior that violate the rights of others.[16] For diagnostic purposes, it must be established that the child's behavior is severe and repetitive enough to distinguish it from ordinary negative behav-

iors that are common to children and adolescents.

Conduct disorders are very common, particularly among boys. Parental attitudes and family socioeconomic status appear to be major correlational factors.[16] In addition, research has demonstrated links between conduct disorders and learning disabilities, attention deficit disorders, and organic brain disease.[19,33,38] Prognosis appears to be biased by the individual's social responsiveness. The more socialized child demonstrates a relatively favorable prognosis, whereas undersocialized children and adolescents tend to have more persistent patterns and less favorable outcome.[16]

ANXIETY DISORDERS OF CHILDHOOD AND ADOLESCENCE

Anxiety disorders of childhood and adolescence manifest themselves differently that adult anxiety disorders, thus warranting a separate diagnostic category. Children have less developed and less symbolic reactions to anxiety, and patterns are not as persistent as those exhibited by adults. A wide variety of symptoms may be demonstrated, including irritability, lack of energy or hyperactivity, intrusiveness, excessive demands for attention, and generally "whiny" unhappiness.[16] Anxiety disorders are usually reactions to real or perceived stress; they develop increasing complexity with the age of onset. Prognosis is good if the stressor can be identified and appropriate intervention implemented.

EATING DISORDERS

Eating disorders include any conspicuous disturbance in eating behaviors. These disorders are primarily seen in adolescence, or in combination with mental retardation or pervasive developmental disorder.[16,26] Bulimia and pica are typical examples.

The most common eating disorder is *anorexia nervosa,* which occurs primarily in females and often results in hospitalization. This condition is characterized by an intense focus on weight loss, an unrealistic fear of becoming fat, and peculiar patterns of handling food.[16,40] Although anorexia is believed to be psychogenic in origin, it may lead to serious metabolic and other physical problems. Anorexics have been described as demonstrating increased motor activity and distorted body image, but neither symptom is wholly supported by research.[43] Other characteristics that have been described but not supported by research findings include fear of failure, overperfectionism, and poor self-concept. Anorexia nervosa is generally considered episodic, and the short-term response to hospitalization is good. Prognosis is less favorable with later ages of onset.

ORGANIC MENTAL DISORDERS

Organic mental disorders include mental and behavior impairment secondary to cortical damage. These disorders may be caused by closed head injuries, systemic diseases, or poorly developed central nervous system (CNS) organization. Of these, the problems seen in children following head injury have probably received the greatest attention recently. Substance-induced dementias are included in this classification. Although no single set of symptoms is specifically manifest by any of these disorders, because of the variability of brain lesion sites, Kaplan and Sadock[16] present the following list of common characteristics:

1. Memory impairment, especially in short-term recall
2. Impaired abstract thinking, generalization, logical reasoning, conceptualization, problem-solving
3. Impaired ability to learn and perform novel tasks
4. Impaired ability to attend to salient features of tasks or information
5. Impaired judgment, with decreased sensitivity to and awareness of behavioral consequences
6. Impaired orientation to time and space
7. Distorted perception of one's body and one's environment

The incidence of mental illness increases greatly in the presence of organic disorder. In a 1970 study conducted by Rutter et al that was reported by Spreen and others,[38] among a general population of 3300 Welsh school-aged children, the incidence of psychopathology was 6% to 7%. In dramatic contrast, children with lesions above the brain stem without epilepsy had a 37.5% incidence and those children who had both above brain stem lesions and epilepsy or other seizure disorder had a rate of 58.3%.

In a study of behavioral sequelae of closed head injury,[38] the most prominent disturbance reported was a state of disinhibition. The investigators noted that socially inappropriate behavior, insensitive and embarrassing actions or verbalizations, and inability or failure to follow social norms were typical. Other patterns of behavior observed included excessive talking, poor hygiene, and poor impulse control. Little information is available on long-term prognosis of the psychiatric sequelae of closed head injury, but clinically the outcome appears to be directly related to the degree of brain damage.

AFFECTIVE DISORDERS

Childhood affective disorders have the same clinical feature as the adult disorders and therefore are not differentiated in DSM III.[45] The common feature of this classification is a disturbance in mood accompanied by cognitive, psychomotor, and interpersonal difficulties.[16] Affective disorders in children are often diagnosed in conjunction with adjustment disorders, thus classifying them as secondary affective disorders. Depression, whether related to another psychiatric disorder or associated with a medical disease, is the most commonly reported affective disorder in children. Pless and Pinkerton,[31] in their discussion of psycho-

logical maladjustment in children with chronic illness, reported disturbances in self-esteem, motivation, and interpersonal relationships. This is consistent with the description of depression presented by Kaplan and Sadock,[16] including a pervasive loss of interest or pleasure, psychomotor agitation, or suicidal thoughts. Prognosis of affective disorders is generally good when the causative factors can be identified and treated. Disorders that are secondary to chronic physical dysfunction or illness may be more difficult to ameliorate.[31]

OTHER DISORDERS

Other psychosocial disorders listed by DSM III[45] as first evident in infancy, childhood, or adolescence are described elsewhere in this text. These include mental retardation (Chapters 6 and 21) and attention deficit disorders (Chapters 6 and 23).

ADJUSTMENTS AND IDENTITY DISORDERS OF ADOLESCENCE

According to the literature, the main cause of adjustment conflicts is found in the failure to adequately process challenges, resulting in developmental lags. Kaplan and Sadock[16] described these as ". . . acute regressive states manifest by anxiety, depression, eating and sleeping disorders, clinging to peers or parents, psychosomatic disorders or impulsive acting out" (p. 947). This pattern seems to be based on an exaggerated focus on developmental issues of independence and expectations for adult role behavior. These disorders are generally acute and have a good prognosis.

SUBSTANCE ABUSE

Statistics indicate a surprisingly high rate of substance abuse among school-aged and adolescent children. Adolescents seem particularly vulnerable, because of their need for peer acceptance, engagement in "adult" activities, and need to reduce the stress and demands associated with their age. The range of substances commonly associated with adolescent abuse is broad, including alcohol, nicotine, marijuana, LSD, cocaine, amphetamines, barbiturates, and heroin.[30] In a 1980 study conducted by the National Institute of Drug Abuse,[30] 65% of high school seniors said that they had used some illegal drugs during their lives.

The impairments in social and occupational function associated with substance abuse have been described in the DSM-III-R as disturbed social relations, erratic and impulsive behavior, and inappropriate expression of aggressive feelings.[45] Many adolescents with substance abuse problems also demonstrate conduct disorders or adolescent adjustment reactions. Occupational therapy intervention with youths who are substance abusers will therefore vary according to the individual's history of single or recurrent episodes, secondary diagnoses, and family patterns.

PRACTICE SETTINGS, SERVICES, AND RELATIONSHIPS
Typical settings and service delivery systems

INPATIENT CHILDREN'S MENTAL HEALTH CENTERS

Although many inpatient programs are specialized for treatment of specific populations, very few are designed exclusively for children. In an informal survey of local mental health centers conducted by this author, about 30% had a children's unit, and 70% of the children's units employed occupational therapists. Inpatient, residential units for children tend to deal with more severely impaired children, including autistic and developmentally delayed children. This is consistent with the view of residential programs presented in Chapter 1.

OUTPATIENT MENTAL HEALTH CLINICS

Larrington[19] described services in an outpatient mental health clinic, stating that occupational therapy services were established to deal with a number of children whose problems were loosely identified as "organic" and who were not considered appropriate candidates for treatment using the program's psychoanalytic frame of reference. The organicity observed was described as hyperactivity and learning disability. The children were seen twice weekly for 50-minute sessions, and the general program approach was sensory integrative. This outpatient model seems to be the most widely used for children with emotional problems who are seen by occupational therapists outside of the school system. Some therapists may provide similar services through private practice as well.

INPATIENT ADOLESCENT MENTAL HEALTH CENTERS

Whereas few younger children are seen in residential programs, many facilities have inpatient programs for adolescents. As described by Lordi, "Hospitalization is a mark that the family system cannot maintain, sustain, or repair the adolescent's problem"[28] (p. 248). Most residential treatment programs utilize a model of intermediate care, meaning that the average hospitalization is between 9 and 24 months. These programs frequently employ occupational therapists, who often see adolescents in groups with therapy emphasis on self-esteem, communication, and improving role and skill development. As the incidence of suicide attempts and substance abuse among teenagers is on the rise, these are the most common problems.

DAY TREATMENT CENTERS AND PARTIAL HOSPITALIZATION PROGRAMS

Day treatment programs are being used increasingly for children and adolescents to maintain family relationships and reduce costs of residential care. Typically, the child participates in an intensive program with multiple therapies during the day and goes home at night. Because the public schools now meet most service needs of older children with emotional or behavior disorders, most day treatment programs provide services mainly to preschool children. The types of problems that are commonly seen include the pervasive childhood disorders. Partial hospitalization programs, with weekends or variable evenings at home, are increasingly used to assist with the transition of children and adolescents coming from residential programs.

SCHOOL SERVICES

The bulk of current occupational therapy services to emotionally disturbed children are delivered in an academic setting. Many children seen in schools carry no psychiatric diagnosis, but have been identified because of their inability to conform to the behavioral constraints of the classroom.[22] Children may thus be classified as emotionally handicapped or behaviorally disturbed. The specific behaviors that become the focus of special education include an inability to learn, unsatisfactory interpersonal relationships, inappropriate behavior, and general unhappiness. Occupational therapists in these settings work to support the child's educational goals, as described in Chapters 1 and 29. Many of the children that occupational therapists serve in school systems demonstrate the concept of "organicity" described by Larrington, and treatment models parallel those described for outpatient programs.

ACUTE CARE HOSPITALS

Increasingly, children are referred to occupational therapy services for treatment of emotional problems that are secondary to medical illness and hospitalization. Among children who require long-term, high technology treatments, such as those with cancer or renal disease, mental health problems are well-documented.[4,42] Disorders in interests, motivation, and play behavior have also been observed.[18] Watson[41] stated that "It is the occupational therapist's role to promote, through use of functional activities, performance and explore with the patient the meaning of his or her illness or disability" (p. 339). It is also important to enhance developmental progression and provide an environment of developmental relevance to the child.[4,41]

Others involved in mental health service delivery

In the hospital or other clinical settings, occupational therapists serve as part of the medical team. Other personnel typically include physicians, psychologists, nurses, social workers, and child life specialists.

The occupational therapist must be able to articulate therapy goals and work within the treatment model that is supported by the team and facility.

In all of these settings, the occupational therapist interfaces with family members and teachers. Family intervention has been detailed in Chapter 8 and is explored further in this chapter as it relates to the child with emotional or behavioral disturbances. Even in medically oriented and residential settings, a teacher is available to maintain children's academic skills at grade level. Occupational therapy goals tend to strengthen and enhance educational goals when program planning is collaborative.

OCCUPATIONAL THERAPY INTERVENTION APPROACHES

Treatment theories are used to explain the basis for problems observed and to guide intervention. In collaboration with other team members, therapists may apply approaches like the psychoanalytic or behavior management. In addition, several treatment theories have been developed by and for occupational therapists. These include the works of Reilly, Kielhofner, Ayres, Nelson, and Llorens, and their colleagues—the focus of the following discussion. It is important to see the holistic scope covered by the theories described, as well as their focus on the dynamic interaction between the child, therapist, environment, and activities. Each theoretical approach has its own organization, but all share an emphasis on the use of activities to facilitate change.

Reilly: an explanation of play

Mary Reilly formulated a theoretical explanation of play, presented in this text in Chapter 3. To summarize, Reilly's theory proposed that play has an organizing effect on behavior and that play in childhood is a critical precursor to adult competence and achievement.[32] This concept is supported by others who have recognized play as a means of developing skills in communication, expression of emotion, and motor competencies, as well as a foundation of the individual's self-esteem.[1,5,14] Reilly's work used a systems approach to the analysis of play, seeing the child as an open system in dynamic interaction with the human and non-human environment. Through a progression of play behavior that is guided by the therapist through interactions, activity selection, and environmental manipulation, the child may attain a sense of competence and achievement. Reilly proposed that as the child develops competence through play, self-esteem and a sense of efficacy are also realized. At the achievement level of play, the child acquires a sense of mastery and mature motivation.[32] Incorporating this approach into therapy, developing the child's play behaviors, through engagement in arts, games, role-playing, puppetry, and dance, is used to enhance progression through the exploratory, competency, and achievement continuum. It is important to remember that Reilly's focus on play behavior is different from the more psychoanalytically oriented "play therapy," which uses play as a modality to promote emotional expression.[1]

Kielhofner: a model of human occupation

This model of occupational therapy intervention was originally derived from, but expands considerably on, Reilly's occupational behavior theory, so many similarities in concepts and language may be noted. The human occupation approach, presented by Kielhofner, Burke, Barris, Neville, and others[17] builds on the open systems concepts proposed by Reilly. The authors describe persons with psychosocial dysfunction as sharing ". . . the general characteristics of maladaptive output, either a cessation of occupational behavior or

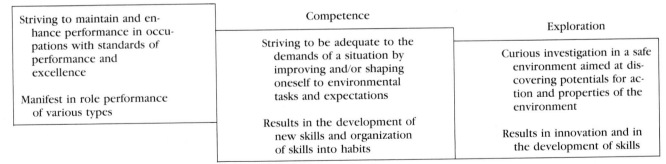

Achievement

| Striving to maintain and enhance performance in occupations with standards of performance and excellence

Manifest in role performance of various types |

Competence

Striving to be adequate to the demands of a situation by improving and/or shaping oneself to environmental tasks and expectations

Results in the development of new skills and organization of skills into habits

Exploration

Curious investigation in a safe environment aimed at discovering potentials for action and properties of the environment

Results in innovation and in the development of skills

Figure 27-1   Three levels of occupational function.

Reproduced with permission from Kielhofner GS: Model of human occupation, Baltimore, Md, 1985, Williams & Wilkins.

engagement in activities that hold no meaning for them"[17] (p. 248). Kielhofner[17] described levels, characteristics, and outcome of occupational function as exploration, competence, and achievement (see Figure 27-1) and contrasting levels of dysfunction as helplessness, incompetence, and inefficacy.

The proponents of this approach believe that intervention is directed at the maladaptive cycle of behavior that results from dysfunction. Therapy goals of this approach may include specific work on performance skills and habits through a variety of activities. Therapy should promote a positive sense of personal causation and develop the individual's values and interests.[17,20]

Ayres: sensory integration

The theory of sensory integration, as developed by Ayres[2] and others, is widely used by occupational therapists in the treatment of emotionally disturbed children. This approach, described in detail in Chapters 3 and 23, requires assessment of children for specific sensory integrative deficits. Both the occupational therapy and neuropsychology literature indicate that there are much higher incidences of learning disability and sensory integration problems among the emotionally disturbed population.[19,31,33,38]

Children who can participate in standardized testing are treated according to the model presented in Chapter 23. However, many children with severe emotional disturbance are not formally testable. Ayres[3] also utilized the sensory integration approach with autistic children. She postulated that many such children have sensory processing disorders and stated that ". . . when autistic children are able to cooperate well enough to take a standard test for sensory integrative function, their scores are usually similar to those of dyspraxic children"[3] (p. 123). Her studies identified three aspects of poor sensory processing that are common to autistic children. These include inadequate sensory registration, poor modulation of sensory input, and difficulty integrating sensations to form a clear perception of space. These three areas of dysfunction particularly affect motor planning, initiation of activity, and motivation.[3]

Therapy goals for the autistic child that are based on sensory integration theory emphasize attaching meaning to sensation through activity, careful sensory stimulation, and helping the child experience sensations in a positively motivating fashion. A key difference in the treatment is that, unlike the learning disabled child, the autistic child rarely engages in self-directed activity.[3]

Nelson: structured activities as therapy

Nelson[26] studied concepts from the work of occupational therapists and other professionals to develop his approach of structured activities as therapy. He identified and described two major approaches regarding activity therapy as directive and non-directive and differentiated the uses, strengths, and weakness of each approach with developmentally delayed children.[26]

The *directive* approach requires a highly structured environment, clearly defined expectations, and ensured success. This approach draws from the behavioral model in that it does not allow the child to escape from planned activity, is therapist controlled, and uses physical prompts with immediate consequences. The *non-directive* approach is also highly structured, ensures success, and has clearly defined expectations. However, it draws more from sensory motor theories as the child is encouraged to direct the activity, with the therapist acting as a catalyst. The environment of a non-directive approach is designed to elicit desired responses, rather than present a structured task, and the materials used are inherently reinforcing.[26]

Nelson offered the following guidelines for appropriate selection and application of the two activity approaches. The directive approach works faster to reduce negative behavior and to improve performance of specific tasks related to school, work, and daily living skills. In contrast, the non-directive approach is more suited to work with the unhappy (compulsively joyless) child and to developing play and social interaction skills.[26]

Llorens: developmental application of performance skills

Llorens' work represents a developmental approach; her general theory was presented in Chapter 3. When the approach is applied with emotionally disturbed children, Llorens and Rubin[21] stated that "attention is paid to developing both the physical and adaptive skills as well as social competence, with the implicit recognition that the increase in his capacity to cope successfully with the demands of the environment will allow the child to enjoy more meaningful social interaction" (p. 14). Specific treatment utilizing this approach incorporates the use of media that are meaningful to the child and allow practice of the appropriate developmental skills. Additional information about Llorens' practice theory is included in Chapters 3 and 15.

OCCUPATIONAL THERAPY INTERVENTION
Assessment

Assessment of the child with emotional or behavioral dysfunction follows the same general sequence presented in Chapter 7. However, as with any specialized population, the occupational therapist emphasizes specific information. This includes data about:

1. *Behavior patterns:* past and present, including the type, frequency, and location of maladaptive behavior incidents

2. *Environmental influences:* differential patterns of behavior noted at home, at school, with adults, or peers
3. *Play history:* using the format developed by Takata[39] and shown in Chapter 9
4. *Temperament:* including general levels of dependence and independence, typical affect, motivational patterns, and approach to novelty and personal interactions
5. *Family dynamics:* including parent-child interactions, appearance, attitudes, and concerns

Many of the instruments and procedures discussed in Chapters 9 through 11 are appropriately used for assessment of the child or adolescent with psychopathology. Assessment tools selected for this chapter are those that have been used in mental health settings. Of particular importance are interviews with the child and caretakers; these provide critical objective and subjective information about many of the factors listed above.

SENSORY- MOTOR FUNCTION AND SKILL PERFORMANCE

Since performance deficits commonly occur in emotionally disturbed children, the level of skill development must be determined. Although many motor skill tests may be used successfully, the Bruininks Oseretsky is particularly useful for children aged 4 through 14 because of its correlation with the motor aspects of the Southern California Sensory Integration Tests (SCSIT).[46] (See further discussion of this study in Chapter 10.) The SCSIT and the Sensory Integration and Praxis Tests (SIPT) and clinical observations are also appropriate when used by clinicians who are trained in their administration and interpretation with this population. For younger children, the Gesell Developmental Scale, Early Intervention Developmental Profile, and the Play Skills Inventory (all presented in Chapter 11) provide useful information.

COGNITIVE AND EMOTIONAL FUNCTION

Of the instruments presented earlier in this text, the most useful for assessment of cognitive and emotional function include the Goodenough-Harris Drawing Test, the Piers-Harris Children's Self-Concept Scale, the Pre-School Play Scale, the Adolescent Role Assessment, and Burk's Behavior Rating Scales (Chapters 10 and 11). It should be noted that although the Goodenough-Harris Drawing Test was designed as a quick test of intelligence, it is often clinically used by occupational therapists as a projective tool. However, there are no reliability or validity studies of its projective applications.

Other tests that have proven clinically useful in mental health assessment of children and adolescents include the following:

1. *Kinetic Family Drawing (KFD):* In this test the child is asked to draw any family member engaged in an activity. Objective scoring of the drawings was described by Burns and Kaufman.[5]

2. *Personal Reaction Inventory:* This instrument, developed by Nowicki and Strickland[29] was designed to indicate the school-aged child's degree of internal and external orientation and locus of control. The inventory can be administered in interview format or as a pencil and paper test.
3. *Expectancy Questionnaire:* This assessment tool is a structured interview designed by Farnham-Diggory.[8] The child is asked to respond to open-ended questions like "What do you expect to be doing a year from now?" The test provides information about locus of control, interests, values, and motivation. Interpretation is basically subjective and no reliability and validity data are available.
4. *Interest Checklist:* This widely used and much modified instrument was originally reported by Matsutsuyu,[23] as used with adolescents and adults to determine activity interests. A modified version by Neville and Kielhofner[27] includes a historical perspective on participation in activities as well as identifying interests.
5. *Occupational Role History:* Florey and Michelman[9] reported on the modification of the original format developed by Moorhead.[24] The modified version is used as a screening tool to collect data on life-style and experiences, as well as the individual's strengths and weaknesses.

EVALUATION THROUGH ACTIVITY SYNTHESIS

Many of the more severely disturbed children, such as those with pervasive developmental disorders, are unable to attend to or complete a formal test. The most common means of assessing behavior and function of such children is known as "activity synthesis." Mosey[25] defined this method as the process of selecting or creating an activity for the purpose of eliciting a desired response. Through this method activities can be created to identify the unique interests and abilities of the child, as well as to test the therapist's hypotheses about the underlying causes of dysfunction. The effective use of activity synthesis requires good clinical judgment and observational skills, and will vary with the therapist's knowledge of child development, functions, and treatment theories.

Priorities for treatment

As discussed in Chapter 12, goal setting and program planning complete the assessment process. As the therapist becomes more familiar with the individual child, goals may be adjusted to more accurately reflect the child's needs.

It is generally accepted in the mental health literature that some goals will have more immediate priority, particularly when the child's problems are severe. Schopler, Reichler, and Lansing[36] suggested the following sequence for determining goal priority, with goals related to #1 demanding the most immediate attention:

1. Problems that risk the child's life, such as running into a busy street or self-destructive behavior
2. Problems that threaten the child's future with the family, such as aggressive or destructive behavior in the home environment
3. Problems that threaten the professional intervention process, such as noncompliance with programs
4. Problems that prevent adaptation in the broader community outside of the home and school

This system seems quite pertinent to occupational therapy intervention.

Setting goals and objectives

The determination of specific goals is guided by the therapist's choice of treatment theory. With this in mind, the therapist who uses a behavioral approach may identify specific maladaptive behaviors to change, whereas a therapist who chooses the sensory integrative approach may adopt a strategy to carefully elicit sensory processing and thereby enhance adaptive function. For the same child, therapy goals would be expected to differ markedly between approaches, although long-term expectations related to occupational performance would be similar.

The choice of treatment approach should be based on knowledge of each theory or model and its relative strengths and weaknesses in comparison to the needs of the child. Because of the holistic natures of both emotional disturbances in childhood and occupational therapy practice in general, the therapist must carefully study and effectively use assessment information.

The art of therapy

Another important concept in mental health intervention is the therapist's conscious use of self in selecting and directing the therapy approach. Many of the occupational therapy theorists presented in this chapter make special reference to the "art of therapy." Ayres[2] emphasized that it is the child who must change herself, and the therapist should be available to promote and guide. She urged therapists to be sensitive to the child and to change the activity or environment as required to better meet the child's needs. In his discussion of establishing a therapeutic environment, Nelson[26] emphasized the need for the therapist to be skilled at more than one approach and to select an approach that is based on the needs of the child rather than on the bias of the therapist.

Treatment approaches may differ in how they identify problems and choose intervention strategies, but it seems clear that to be effective, the therapist must develop and employ a wide range of treatment skills. The art of therapy relies on a host of variables. These include the therapist's skill in integrating information about treatment approaches, the values of the treatment team, space and equipment available, and the competence of the treating therapist in applying an approach.

Treatment modalities
PLAY THERAPY

Play therapy is a widely used method for treatment of emotionally disturbed children. Many other professionals also use this form of play treatment. Play therapy originally evolved from the psychoanalytic treatment model,[1] but has been adapted and integrated into all of the major psychosocial approaches.[35] The wide acceptance of play therapy lies in the concept that "play is to the child what verbalization is to the adult"[35] (p. 200). This means that play may be utilized as a medium for expressing feelings, describing important experiences, and practicing new skills and roles.

Occupational therapists in acute hospital settings often use play therapy as the primary mode of intervention for children with emotional problems. The use of puppets to act out hospital experiences and to maintain a sense of personal control has been beneficial in assisting the child's overall adjustment to hospitalization.[4,13,20,34,35] Research literature shows that children hospitalized for serious chronic illness have low self-esteem and a sense of being punished for some real or imagined wrongdoing. Play therapy allows such children to act out their anxiety, anger, and frustration. The research on long-term treatment of children with cancer states that there are measurable cognitive changes in children who receive radiation therapy, and their knowledge that they have a life-threatening illness creates a need for what Rosenfeld described as "islands of comfort"[34] (p. 384). She stated that activities should be intrinsically motivating, focus on areas of interest to the child, and allow for the expression of feelings.

BEHAVIOR MANAGEMENT

Unlike play therapy, which emphasizes emotional expression, behavior management programs aim to structure the environment so that the child can learn adaptive, acceptable behavior patterns. This method is based on positive learning experiences and can be applied to a wide variety of therapy tasks. Therapists who use this method will identify a few observable and measurable behaviors, and take baseline data before instituting the treatment program. Changes in the child are effected through judicious application of behavioral consequences, including positive and negative reinforcement. Nelson[26] described several techniques that are used to reduce maladaptive behavior. One example is "Differential Reinforcement of Other Behavior" (DRO). This strategy involves reinforcing appropriate behaviors that are physically incompatible with the negative target behavior. For example, the distractible child who does not remain seated to complete classroom activities is rewarded for performance of activities that require in-seat behavior. Behavior management is widely used in school settings because it works quickly on specific problems and lends itself well to documentation and measurement.

SENSORIMOTOR AND SENSORY INTEGRATIVE TREATMENT

These neurodevelopmentally-based programs are designed to remediate the underlying sensory processing or neuromotor causes of behavioral deficits, rather than targeting specific behaviors. There is little difference in application of treatment techniques between working with learning disabled and emotionally disturbed children, so that guidelines from Chapter 23 are pertinent. However, as mentioned previously, application of sensory integrative therapy requires specialized training, particularly with this population, who may require more direction than learning disabled children.

ACTIVITY GROUP PROGRAMS

As presented by Llorens and Rubin[21] activity groups are designed to develop physical and social interaction skills, and to improve adaptive behavior, feelings of adequacy, and self-esteem. Another focus of group programs is the enhancement of more positive interpersonal relationships. Activity groups are usually graded to develop children's personal responsibility in activity selection, clean-up, and completion. Groups may also be structured to incorporate role-playing, with a focus on leadership and authority issues.[21]

VALUES CLARIFICATION GROUPS

These program methods have derived from the systems analysis approaches. Values clarification groups are frequently used in residential treatment for adolescents and are designed to stimulate thinking about values, improve problem-solving capacities, and establish valued priorities. Additional goals include increasing self-awareness and learning to accept individuals with other sets of values. Groups usually center around some shared task that involves forced choices or ranking of values. For example, the participants may answer and discuss the following questions: Are you more of a spender or a saver? Are you more like a daisy or a rose?

THE THERAPIST'S USE OF SELF

This component of intervention, which has been described by many authors, applies to the choices therapists make about their own behavior throughout a given therapy session and across treatment modalities. These choices include when and how to intervene in activity performance, when to establish rules, and when to encourage independence. As stated by Nelson,[26] the therapist must ". . . analyze his or her own actions. Inadvertent actions might negatively influence the child" (p. 161). Being sensitive to one's impact on individual and group dynamics is imperative in maintaining a therapeutic environment.

Preparation for adulthood
GENERALIZATION TO NATURAL ENVIRONMENTS

In his discussion of therapy progressions, Nelson[26] emphasized that therapists should adapt treatment to build advanced skills. He argued that skills developed in highly structured environments, such as an occupational therapy clinic, need to be sequenced to enable the child to function in his or her own natural environments.

Accordingly, Nelson[26] outlined a series of 17 abilities that relate to the generalization of adaptive behavior skills in the broader community. These may be summarized as follows:

1. Perseverance and delay of gratification
2. Determining when to generalize and when to differentiate
3. Problem-solving through self-correction, trial and error, and rule use
4. Learning and planning from past mistakes
5. Identifying and accepting alternative ways to accomplish tasks
6. Weighing and making choices from different alternatives
7. Planning and preparing
8. Planning one's time
9. Dealing with novelty and unexpected events
10. Coping successfully with ambiguity and uncertainty
11. Recognizing one's feelings about a situation
12. Choosing actions appropriate to situations regardless of personal feelings
13. Being assertive about one's likes and dislikes
14. Adapting to social norms and roles
15. Being empathetic with others
16. Identifying with others and their feelings
17. Engaging in activities with industry and creativity

This list of abilities is consistent with developmental research in cognitive and moral development through early adolescence.[6,28,30] In the early teens, individuals begin to crystallize their ideas about future vocations. Problems that are common to emotionally disturbed children, such as low self-esteem, strongly externalized locus of control, low frustration tolerance, and poor communication skills, can significantly affect vocational development and the transition to adult roles.

These findings are also consistent with the literature related to long-term adjustment to chronic illness. In a discussion of adolescents with cerebral palsy, Freeman[11] described a number of changes in adolescence that exacerbate existing emotional weakness. These included the need to curtail fantasies about the possibility of a cure, greater sensitivity to the attitudes of peers, the heightened importance of sexual attractiveness, and other problems associated with psychosexual maturation. Freeman also described the increased incidence of academic problems and poor goal orientation often seen in these adolescents.[11]

Often individuals with chronic illness have poorly defined values and interests and difficulty making plans for the future. Gorski and Miyake[12] noted the ". . . lack of connectedness adolescents felt from their school experience and their upcoming adult roles" (p. 40). It is clear that all adolescents, and particularly those with emotional disturbance, need to build skills to prepare them for productive "worker" roles and they need to believe that they have access to these roles.[6,10,26]

OCCUPATIONAL THERAPY IN ADOLESCENT LIFE/WORK PLANNING

Many authors have focused on the occupational therapist's role in facilitating the transition to adulthood. This topic is addressed in detail in Chapter 16 and throughout this text. The model of human occupation would appear to lend itself well to organizing therapy services related to adult role transition. Of particular relevance to treatment of youth with emotional or behavioral disorders was a report by Gorski and Miyake.[12] They described a preventive approach intended to alleviate problems before the development of maladaptive patterns. The program was organized in a classroom format with the occupational therapist acting as facilitator and teacher of new skills. The program was divided into the following five stages:

1. Learning about oneself, and focusing on expression of interests and values
2. Learning about the world of work, including information about categories of jobs, job site visits, and role playing
3. Goal planning, including individual identification of long- and short-term goals
4. Maximizing one's potential through encouragement, support, and practice in skill development to address specific problems and concerns
5. Closure, to review strategies learned

This model was designed for a community based program, but could easily be adapted to other settings. By taking a positive approach through identification of interests, values, and skills, the tasks of vocational exploration and implementation are more likely to be perceived as achievable goals and aid the transition to adulthood.

CASE EXAMPLES

This chapter concludes with a series of case examples from the literature and clinical practice. The examples illustrate use of different treatment approaches within a range of service settings. A variety of ages and clinical diagnoses are represented.

Sensory integrative intervention in a pediatric mental health clinic

This program was reported by Larrington,[19] a member of the faculty for the Center for the Study of Sensory Integrative Dysfunction. Between 1971 and 1983, the program provided occupational therapy services to children aged 5 to 21 years. Children were referred from two sources: the mental health outpatient program and from physicians in the community. All children were evaluated with standardized sensory integration tests. Over the course of time, Larrington noted that children demonstrated dysfunctional patterns that tended to be differentiated by the referral source. Those children who were referred through the mental health clinic were, as mentioned previously, loosely defined in referrals as having organic deficits manifest through learning disabilities or hyperactivity. Since clinical signs of neurological impairment were minimal, it had been previously assumed that problems were behavioral, and thus their entrance into the system was through the mental health program. In contrast, children who were referred for outpatient treatment through community medical resources tended to have more strongly manifest signs of neuromotor deficit, including cerebral palsy. As the results of testing accumulated, Larrington found that those children referred through the mental health program typically demonstrated disorders in vestibular and bilateral integration (VBI). In contrast, children who had been referred by physicians tended to demonstrate apraxia or speech and language problems. The balance of this summary of her report deals with the children who demonstrated VBI deficits. Larrington reported also that family relationships for this group tended to be strained, secondary to stress about the presumed behavioral etiology of the children's problems.[19]

Although specific treatment goals were not stated in Larrington's report, the treatment that was instituted emphasized child-directed sensory integrative play experiences, with equipment and materials that provided vestibular, tactile, and proprioceptive stimulation. Treatment was initiated on a one-to-one basis, and generally lasted for 1 to 1½ years. Children were seen twice a week for 50-minute sessions. After some time, therapy was implemented through small groups, as the one-to-one adult/child ratio was maintained through the assistance of parents and aides.[19]

Larrington noted that dramatic behavior changes often occurred within 6 weeks, and that these changes tended to follow a pattern. Children began to assert themselves, becoming bossy and opinionated during play in treatment. They demonstrated new levels of physical interaction with their surroundings, becoming more forceful and propulsive during motor play. She stated that they often "threw themselves through the air for a full-body landing in the sand table"[19] (p. 185). Although the children still looked like "motor disasters" during this period, and their safety during the forceful activities was a concern, none of the children hurt themselves.[19]

At the same time, children were demonstrating improved independence and assertiveness at home. Independent performance of self-care activities increased and improved. Parents were assisted by the therapist to cope with their children's new behaviors, and experience showed that the children tended to settle within a month. In addition, family relationships became less strained as the parent's guilt related to the previously assumed behavioral problems decreased. Continued treatment led to more positive and appropriate interactions, improvement in spatial orientation, organization, and self-esteem.[19]

Play therapy intervention in an acute hospital setting

Shannon was referred to occupational therapy for activities to maintain mental alertness and enhance developmental play. She was 6 years old and was hospitalized for a bone marrow transplant. Her family was actively involved.

ASSESSMENT

Shannon was first seen by the occupational therapist in her hospital room. Because of the need to maintain a sterile environment, she could only play with toys that could be permanently issued to her or could be easily disinfected. The therapist used the Denver Developmental Screening Test as a guideline for parent interview, to determine Shannon's levels of function both before the onset of cancer and before this hospitalization. A play history that assessed prehospitalization and current patterns of interactions was also completed.

Following the parent interview, the therapist utilized the Preschool Play Scale to describe and analyze Shannon's skills during a free play period. Problems observed were low self-esteem, depression, decreased attention, and fatigue. The child evidenced little interest or motivation regarding play activities and generally remained a passive participant, often clinging to her mother. More formal testing was not attempted because of the need to maintain the sterile environment and avoid fatigue.

Goals and priorities were as follows:
1. Develop a trusting relationship to enhance socialization and self-expression
2. Create an environment that encouraged initiation of activity
3. Improve self-esteem and sense of control through play activities
4. Increase endurance in activity level as medically feasible

OCCUPATIONAL THERAPY PROGRAM

Games and puzzles were selected for initial intervention because of their portability and ease of disinfection. Shannon gradually accepted and began to look forward to her daily visits from the occupational therapist. As this indicated that the first program goal had been met, the therapist began to direct Shannon toward activities that involved more creative expression. Through the use of magazine picture collages, Shannon began to talk about her loneliness, about missing first grade, and about her fears that her illness was hurting her parents. As her health improved, Shannon's parents were involved in therapy when they were available. The therapist discussed adaptations with them so that Shannon could play with familiar, preferred activities in spite of her problems of strength and endurance. By the time of discharge, Shannon demonstrated a positive, outgoing affect and was performing most activities at a developmentally appropriate level.

Behavioral intervention in elementary school

Nick was an active, distractible, developmentally delayed 9-year-old in a special education class for children with behavior disorders. He could not get along with classmates in the room or on the playground. The maladaptive behaviors described in his Individualized Education Plan (IEP) included insufficient visual attention to the task or teacher, irrelevant activity that interfered with task completion, frequent out-of-seat behaviors, making audible sounds while working, and occasional disruptive behaviors involving contact with other students.

OCCUPATIONAL THERAPY ASSESSMENT

Formal assessment through standardized testing was impossible on initial evaluation due to Nick's poor ability to follow directions and attend to task. Items from the preschool version of the Early Intervention Developmental Profile were administered in a non-standard form, and performance was analyzed using observation and activity synthesis. Problems were noted in the following areas:

Motor control: Included impaired postural control, decreased bilateral motor coordination, and poor rhythm and timing of movements.

Sensory processing: Difficulty screening environmental stimuli.

Perceptual and fine motor skills: Poor pencil grasp and difficulty manipulating scissors, inconsistent stereognosis.

Cognitive function: Unable to independently seriate more than three items consistently; poor awareness of time and topographical orientation.

Self-care skills: No initiation of self-care tasks; unable to spatially orient clothing; unable to identify and correct errors.

Clinical observation indicated that Nick was affectionate and cooperative with familiar persons in a structured setting, but that he generally became impulsive and disruptive in more natural environments. Nick was verbal and able to express himself in short sentences, although he frequently relied on one and two word answers.

GOALS AND PRIORITIES

Because Nick's abilities varied greatly in dyadic and classroom settings, the IEP team agreed that he should be seen individually by the occupational therapist once weekly, to work on specific self-care and school-related tasks. In addition, the therapist would be available in the classroom once weekly to assist in developing and monitoring behavioral strategies in a group work setting. Specific IEP goals were to:

1. Promote positive work and attending behaviors by reinforcing behaviors incompatible with the maladaptive behaviors (using DRO).
2. Structure the classroom environment to reduce distractors and enhance success at task completion.
3. Clearly identify and implement specific consequences for both desirable and undesirable behaviors.

Because of the number of maladaptive behaviors that had been consistently demonstrated by Nick, the teacher, psychologist, and occupational therapist developed a priority list of behaviors to be changed. The primary focus was to increase attending behavior and reduce disruptive behaviors involving contact with other students. The classroom program was designed with input from the entire team and the individual occupational therapy program was planned to be consistent with the team approach.

OCCUPATIONAL THERAPY PROGRAM

The individual and monitoring services that were implemented dealt with environmental adaptations, increasing attention and task completion, and reducing out of seat behavior as follows:

1. Nick's classroom work station was moved to a corner of the room. He was separated from the next child using a screen. It was found that Nick remained less agitated and required fewer reprimands when he was able to work in a standing position. He was therefore provided with an appropriate height work surface and a stool to use when tired of standing. With this intervention, Nick developed a clear concept of "his" work area and reduced his negative interactions with the teacher.
2. It was determined that Nick worked well for token reinforcement. Assignments for both classroom and individual work were selected to be achievable in length and difficulty. Task completion was rewarded with a token. As tokens were earned, social praise was added to strengthen the value of natural reinforcement. Occupational therapy tasks focused primarily on sensory motor

and self-care skills, to complement the cognitive, social, and perceptual-motor goals.
3. The use of standing working station eliminated the immediate problem of out-of-seat behavior in the classroom. However, this problem was the focus of all one-to-one intervention in occupational therapy. The therapist collected baseline on in-seat behavior and found that Nick left his seat without permission 29 times in a 50-minute period. It was also observed that he greatly enjoyed vestibular activities.

Accordingly, the 30-minute treatment session was divided into a 20-minute task-focused period, followed by a 10-minute child-directed vestibular activity. Nick was told that he would receive the 10-minute "free play" period if he did not leave his seat, and that 1 minute would be deducted from his free play period each time he left his seat without permission.

With this program, Nick improved rapidly in attention and task completion. Although improvement was also noted in balance and postural control, Nick continued to prefer to do classroom assignments in standing position. To advance his progress, the screen was removed from Nick's work area and he began to participate in a small group gross motor activity program in occupational therapy. Goals were expanded to improve peer interaction, incorporating games to enhance his awareness of rules and social roles.

By the end of the school year, Nick was no longer disruptive in the classroom, although he occasionally had difficulty in unstructured or novel environments. His parents reported improved affect and self-confidence, as well as overall behavior at home. Shortly before the end of the first school year, Nick's work station was lowered for sitting. He continued to have difficulty sitting on a static surface for long periods, but was able to maintain sitting adequately on a large therapy ball. The IEP goals for the following year were to emphasize continued progress on behavioral goals and developing Nick's skills in a more natural school work environment.

Developmental intervention in an adolescent intermediate care facility

Cathy, aged 18, was a voluntary admission to the adolescent treatment program. Her problems on admission included substance abuse and depression, with history of psychiatric intervention related to sexual abuse by her stepfather.

In this inpatient program, hospitalization generally lasted from 4 to 6 months. The program was divided into levels, with the actual in-hospital behavior of the individual determining the first level of placement. Accordingly, Cathy was admitted to Level One. She spent her first few days with no shoes or street clothes, and was limited to highly controlled activities on the living unit. No visitors or gifts were allowed.

With acceptable behavior, Cathy progressed to Level Two. Street clothes were permitted, and Cathy was allowed to leave the living area to attend the school program. The art, physical education, and music classes were run by the activity therapy department. After transfer to Level Three, Cathy began to participate in activity therapies, which included occupational, music, dance, and art therapies. The occupational therapy assessment included use of Kinetic Figure Drawings, a modified Interest Checklist, and an interview using Black's Adolescent Role Assessment.

Cathy was initially resistant to all activities, saying that she always failed at or broke anything she ever cared about. The therapist guided her to color in preprinted designs as an easy, success-oriented project. The positive feedback and confidence in her ability projected by the therapist led Cathy to gradually choose more complex and demanding projects. Since the occupational therapy sessions were generally held in small groups, Cathy began to demonstrate some confidence with her peers, and became a more active participant in recreational programs. Additionally, Cathy's ability to initiate, direct, and organize tasks was observed in the activity program.

Because she was performing adequately in both school and therapy programs, an increased focus was placed on interpersonal relationships. When Cathy was able to spontaneously confide in one peer and in one staff person, she progressed to Level Four. The occupational therapist had identified "high status" activities and made engagement in these level-dependent to provide incentive and future orientation in treatment. Cathy was allowed to select activities, with a focus on:

1. Developing personal goals and attainable steps in meeting those goals
2. Developing more mature positive interpersonal skills
3. Continuing to improve confidence and self-esteem
4. Developing time management strategies to balance school, work, self-maintenance, and leisure time.

Cathy expressed interest in cooking and the horticulture program. Although she saw both of these as leading to adult roles, when she talked about her future expectations, she had no clear vocational path. The increased emphasis in occupational therapy on planning for her future and a discussion with the high school vocational counselor led Cathy to begin to think more realistically. She began to demonstrate more productive use of her time.

These interests and concerns were new to Cathy and she was supported by her therapy sessions. She became quite invested in the horticulture program and on several occasions was nearly dropped back a level because of her difficulty assimilating failures or coping with unexpected developments. The therapist helped Cathy to deal with these frustrations by identifying and modifying unrealistic personal goals and expressing underlying feelings. Within this context, Cathy began to express her concerns about impressing her mother, feeling pressured to please her stepfather, and the subsequent alienation of both parents.

At Level Five before her discharge, Cathy took on a supervisory role in horticulture, teaching both staff and peers about the work expectations of the program. Activities were focused on growing house plants and selling them to local florists. Cathy began to develop a bookkeeping system to plan and monitor schedules for seeding the various plants.

After 5 months, Cathy was discharged during days to the public high school, with continued occupational therapy services after school through a partial hospitalization program. In school, Cathy was able to maintain adequate grades. She discussed the frustrations and temptations of her new school environment with the occupational therapist as she continued in her horticulture work program. The therapist assisted her to continue to focus her interests and values, and Cathy progressed further. About 3 months after her return to public school, Cathy obtained a part-time job with a local florist and was discharged from occupational therapy.

SUMMARY

The treatment of emotional and behavioral disturbances in children and adolescents crosses diagnostic categories that include primary psychopathology and secondary problems resulting from chronic or neurological illness. Occupational therapy is therefore often provided in settings other than traditional mental health facilities. The primary approaches to mental health intervention include psychoanalytic, social learning and behavior, systems analysis, and developmental. Through studies of these approaches, in conjunction with a focus on the role of activity, occupational therapy theories for mental health have been developed by Reilly, Kielhofner, Ayres, Nelson, Llorens, and their associates. Careful consideration of these theories, combined with effective application of their use in practice, is critical to appropriate selection of a theoretical approach to meet a child's needs. Occupational therapy assessment of children with emotional or behavior disorders uses a range of familiar instruments and procedures, but the emphasis of data collection is on patterns of behavior, expression of emotions, and interpersonal interactions. The structured use of children's and adolescents' activities through play therapy, behavior management, groups, and other methods was presented in this chapter. Finally, a series of case studies provided examples of the integration of theoretical approaches with assessment, goals, and program in different settings for children with different clusters

578

of problems. To reiterate, this chapter is considered introductory to a highly specialized area of occupational therapy, and additional study of the primary resources is warranted.

STUDY QUESTIONS

1. Consider the case example that presents Larrington's sensory integration program. How might goals and program activities have been different if a structured activity group approach had been used? What might be similar?
2. Review the case example of Nick. How would his goals and program have been different if a sensory integrative approach were used? As you review his case, what elements do you notice that are consistent with other approaches?
3. Review the case example of Cathy. Consider what her goals and program might have been if she had been hospitalized in a facility that utilized a behavior management approach.
4. A 10-year-old girl in fifth grade was in an auto accident 2 months ago and sustained closed head injury involving the right frontal and temporal lobes. She was comatose for about 2 weeks after, and then received early treatment in an acute hospital. What types of psychopathology might you expect to see when she is referred for occupational therapy in an inpatient physical rehabilitation unit? Discuss how two different approaches to treatment might be used to deal with her residual emotional, behavioral, and cognitive deficits.

REFERENCES

1. Axline VM: Play therapy, revised edition. New York, 1969, Ballantine/Del Rey/Fawcett Books.
2. Ayres AJ: Sensory integration and learning disorders, Los Angeles, 1972, Western Psychological Services.
3. Ayres AJ: Sensory integration and the child, Los Angeles, 1983, Western Psychological Services.
4. Brunquell D, and Hall MD: Issues in the psychological care of pediatric oncology patients, Annual Progress in Child Psychiatry and Child Dev Part IV, number 27:430, 1983.
5. Burns R, and Kaufman H: Actions, styles, and symbols in kinetic figure drawing K.F.D., New York, 1972, Brunner/Mazel, Inc.
6. Cotton NS: Childhood play as an analog to adult capacity to work, Child Psychiatry and Human Dev 14:135, 1984.
7. Cromwell FS: Occupational therapy for adolescents with disability, New York, 1985, The Haworth Press Inc.
8. Farnham-Diggory S: Self, future, and time: A developmental study of the concepts of psychotic, brain damaged, and normal children, Monographs by the Society for Research in Child Development, vol 31 (1, serial no. 103).
9. Florey L, and Michelman S: Occupational role history: a screening tool for psychiatric occupational therapy, Am J Occup Ther 32:301, 1978.
10. Freedman BJ, and others: A social-behavioral analysis of skill deficits in delinquent and non-delinquent adolescent boys, J Consult Clin Psy 46:1448, 1978.
11. Freeman RD: Psychiatric problems in adolescents with cerebral palsy, Dev Med and Child Neurol 12:64, 1970.
12. Gorski G, and Miyake S: The adolescent life/work planning group: a prevention model. In Cromwell F, editor: Occupational therapy for adolescents with disability, New York, 1985, The Haworth Press, Inc, p. 139.

13. Hindmarsh WA: Play diagnosis and play therapy, Am J Occup Ther 33:770, 1979.
14. Hinsie C: Psychiatric dictionary, ed 3 New York, 1960, Oxford University Press Inc.
15. James M, and others: Techniques in transactional analysis, Reading, Mass, 1977, Addison-Wesley Publishing Co.
16. Kaplan HI, and Sadock BJ: Modern synopsis of psychiatry IV, Baltimore, 1985, Williams & Wilkins.
17. Kielhofner GS, editor: A model of human occupation, Baltimore, Md, 1985, Williams & Wilkins.
18. Kielhofner GS, and others: a comparison of play behavior in hospitalized and non-hospitalized children, Am J Occup Ther 37:305, 1983.
19. Larrington G: Sensory integrative intervention in a pediatric mental health clinic. In: Occupational therapy in practice, Rockville, Md, 1985, American Occupational Therapy Association, Inc, p. 184.
20. Lederer JM, Kielhofner G, and Watts JH: Values, personal causation and skills of delinquents and non-delinquents, Occup Ther in Mental Health 5:59, 1985.
21. Llorens LA, and Rubin E: Developing ego functions in disturbed children, Detroit, 1967, Lafayette Clinic Handbooks in Psychiatry.
22. Long NJ, Morse WC, and Newman RG: Conflict in the classroom: the education of emotionally disturbed children, Belmont, Calif, 1965, Wadsworth, Inc.
23. Matsutsuyu J: The interest checklist, Am J Occup Ther 23:323, 1969.
24. Moorhead L: The occupational history, Am J Occup Ther 23:326, 1969.
25. Mosey AC: A model for occupational therapy, Occup Ther in Mental Health 1:11, 1980.
26. Nelson DL: Children with autism and other pervasive disorders of development and behavior: therapy through activities. Thorofare, NJ, 1984, Slack, Inc.
27. Neville A, and Kielhofner G: Modified interest checklist, 1983 (unpublished workbook, National Institutes of Health).
28. Novello JR: The short course in adolescent psychiatry, New York, 1979, Brunner/Mazel Inc.
29. Nowicki S, and Strickland B: A locus of control scale for children, Journal of Consulting and Clinical Psychology 40:148, 1983.
30. Papilia DE, and Olds SW: A child's world: infancy through adolescence, ed 3 New York, 1982, McGraw-Hill Inc.
31. Pless IB, and Pinkerton P: Chronic childhood disorder: promoting patterns of adjustment, London, 1975, Year Book Medical Publishers, Inc.
32. Reilly M: Play as exploratory learning: studies in curiosity behavior, Beverly Hills, Calif 1974, Sage Publications Inc.
33. Rider B: Perceptual-motor dysfunction in emotionally disturbed children, Am J Occup Ther 27:316, 1973.
34. Rosenfeld MS: Crisis intervention: the nuclear task approach, Am J Occup Ther 38:382, 1984.
35. Schaefer CE, and O'Conner KJ: Handbook of play therapy, New York, 1983, John Wiley & Sons Inc.
36. Schopler E, Reichler J, and Lansing M: Individualized assessment and treatment for autistic and developmentally delayed children, Baltimore, Md, 1980, University Park Press.
37. Simons RC, and Pardes H: Understanding human behavior in health and illness, Baltimore, Md, 1977, Waverly Press, Inc.
38. Spreen O, and others: Human developmental neuropsychology, New York, 1984, Oxford University Press.
39. Takata N: The play history, Am J Occup Ther 23:314, 1969.
40. Van Deusen J, and Allen L: Is perceptual motor dysfunction a

problem in anorexia nervosa?, Phys and Occup Ther in Pediatrics 5:51, Winter 85-86.

41. Watson LJ: Psychiatric consultation-liaison in the acute physical disabilities setting, Am J Occup Ther 40:338, 1986.

42. Whitley SB, Branscomb BV, and Moreno H: Identification and management of psychosocial and environmental problems of children with cancer, Am J Occup Ther 33:711, 1979.

43. Williams JBW, editor: Diagnostic and statistical manual of mental disorders, ed 3, Washington, D.C., 1980, The American Psychiatric Association.

44. World Health Organization: Manual of the international statistical classification of diseases, injuries, and causes of death, vol I and II, 9th revision, Geneva, 1977, The World Health Organization.

45. World Health Organization: Mental disorders: glossary and guide to their classification in accordance with the ninth revision of the international classification of diseases, Geneva, 1978, The World Health Organization.

46. Ziviani J, Poulsen A, and O'Brien A: Correlation of the Bruininks-Oseretsky Test of Motor Proficiency with the SCSITs, Am J Occup Ther 36:519, 1982.

28

The dying child

PEGGY BARNSTORFF

On a pediatric ward in a large medical center, I met two people who challenged me to learn more about death, especially children's perceptions of death.

Jan was an 11-year-old girl with a distorting facial malignancy that had been in progress for over 2 years. She had been seen periodically in various outpatient clinics, interspersed with hospital stays both in her hometown and in the regional medical center. The treatment she received, as well as the disease process, was extremely painful.

Finally, when Jan was dying in the medical center, she was in a private room that was darkened at all times. Her contacts with the outside world were few. The medical staff rarely visited her room, except to administer medications or during rounds.

Donna, a nursing student, was Jan's only meaningful contact with the outside world. Jan looked for Donna's visits, asked for her when she was not there, and allowed only Donna to spend extended periods of time with her. It was a relationship full of meaning for both, and it sparked my interest in the problems of dying children.

THE SCOPE OF THE PROBLEM

One hundred years ago, childhood deaths were very common, and many families had to learn to accept the loss of a child. Today, children's deaths are more unusual and often unexpected, even though a child may have a terminal disease. Our beliefs in the medical system and its ability to cure us leave us unprepared for death. Therefore children's deaths grievously affect all of those around the child: the family, the medical staff, and the community of friends and professionals.

In the United States it is expected that tens of thousands of children will die annually. The most prevalent cause of childhood deaths is accidents; however, neoplastic disease is the second major cause of death. These chronic neoplastic diseases include leukemia; solid tumors such as lymphomas, neuroblastomas, Wilms' tumor, rhabdomyosarcomas; tumors of the-

brain, bone, and eye; and soon to be in the forefront is acquired immunodeficiency syndrome (AIDS) in children.[23]

When a child is terminally ill, with an acute or chronic situation, there are various people who will care for that child: the medical staff, consisting of the child's primary care physician and the many specialists who work together to provide diagnosis and treatment; and the nursing staff, dealing with the dying child on a daily basis, taking care of the child, administering the medications, charting the course of the disease, and providing opportunities for the child to use daily living skills. Allied health personnel also may be involved in the child's care and include the social worker, the physical therapist, the occupational therapist, the dietitian, and the medical technician.

Children who are dying also have the concern of parents, grandparents, aunts and uncles, siblings and cousins, as well as members of the community, such as teachers and family friends. All of these individuals are affected by, and may be involved in the care of, the dying child.

It is typical for a child who is an accident victim to die in the hospital. However, children with terminal illnesses are now more often involved in home care programs, hospice, or respite care programs, such as the Ronald McDonald Houses attached to hospitals in major cities.[5,24,32] Here they are followed by nurses, physical therapists, occupational therapists, aides, and hospice volunteers. Other agencies that work with these children and their families include those that grant children's wishes, such as the "Make a Wish Foundation" and the "Sunshine Foundation," as well as those that provide familial bereavement counseling, such as the "Compassionate Friends" in Illinois or "the Candlelighters" in Washington, DC.[36]

Children with more chronic diseases are seen in outpatient clinics until they become too ill. Then they

580

are admitted to the hospital and wait for a remission so that they may be released to go home. In the last 10 years a trend has developed to allow the child for whom treatment fails to have the option to die at home, rather than in a hospital. This has been fostered through programs such as the hospice and individually developed programs at various medical centers.[19]

CHILDREN'S PERCEPTIONS OF DEATH

Depending on one's frame of reference for understanding children, there are either three or four stages in the development of a child's understanding of death. Nagy,[20] one of the earliest individuals to study this topic, suggested three stages: (1) from birth to 5 years the child believes that death is a reversible process in which life activities such as growing, hearing, and feeling can take place, (2) from the ages of 5 to 9 years the child personifies death as a distinct personality, and (3) from the age of 9, onward, death is understood to be a cessation of corporeal life and is a universal phenomenon.

Kane[10] and Koocher[12,13] related the development of a child's perception of death to Piaget's stages of development during the preoperational, concrete operations, and formal operations states. Their research suggested that as a child's mind matures, the cognitive stages will be reflected in the child's understanding of death.

Childers and Wimmer[3] studied children's perceptions of death, and their results indicated that differential awareness of death is a universal function of age. Among the subjects of their study, the understanding of death as being irrevocable was not demonstrated systematically until age 10.

Meliar[18] suggested that there are four stages to the development of the concept of death: (1) the majority of 3- and 4-year-olds demonstrate a relative ignorance of the meaning of death, (2) among 4- to 7-year-olds death is seen as a temporary state, (3) 5- to 10-year-olds appear to function in a transitional state: these children believe that death is final, but that the dead function biologically, (4) to most older children death is a cessation of all biological functioning.

Infants

As a child matures from infancy to adulthood, his or her concepts of self, life, and eventual death parallel Erikson's and Piaget's developmental theories. The postpartum infant facing death reacts only physiologically, using all of his strength to continue living. As the child reaches the end of the period of bonding at around 6 months of age, he reacts to the physical process of the disease symptoms and the resulting treatment procedures. At this age the infant is capable of recognizing that he disturbs people, especially his parents. The infant equates this with being bad. The infant

may respond to treatment with anxiety and fear, which is further aggravated by separation anxiety. These reactions continue throughout the ages of 2 and 3. It is also during this period that the child learns the word *death,* but the word has little or no meaning for the toddler.

Preschool children

Egocentricity diminishes as the child is introduced to a world larger than the one known during the toddler years. At 4 years of age the child is beginning to conceptualize himself or herself as an individual; however, this conception is accompanied by that of "not me" as well. Feelings of being and not being must be dealt with by a preschooler. The thought of not being is very anxiety-producing, because if one is no longer being, that means separation from family and also loss of all the independence that has so far been acquired. The child focuses on the single dimension of comparing objects at a given time. Therefore the child focuses on life, which means being with others on earth as compared to death, which means separation from loved ones. Death also means that one becomes immobile, unable to move.[26] Thus thoughts of dying suggest dependency and loss of the self-control that a child of this age has just begun to acquire. Disease then threatens a child's very psychosocial existence.

Although children of 4 and 5 approach death with fantasy reasoning and magical thinking,[12,34] they can begin to appreciate the meaning of a diagnosis, and this greatly influences their reactions to the world around them. Television, radio, magazines, books, and communications with others disclose many ideas. They hear words, view the responding emotions, and develop associations that can· be applied to later experiences. Children begin this application process as they come to identify with others. Concurrently they develop an increased curiosity about burial, dead animals and flowers, and the accidental features of death.

For 3- to 5-year-olds death means absence or going away and is a temporary, impermanent state.[18] Death is seen as a continuation of life, but in a different place. Preschool children are not capable of cognitively understanding the process as being irreversible; such a concept is indicative of the ability to abstract thought. This is also true of retarded children who function cognitively at the preoperational level. Neither are these children realistic about the permanence or timing of death.[31] The most painful aspect of dying is the realization of separation. Denial is processed to overcome feelings of helplessness and the sense of loss. Narcissism develops with the threat to life and the recognition of the reality of the situation.[4]

School children

Children of school age come to realize that death is irreversible, it is the cessation of bodily functions as we know them, and it is universal to the species.[27]

The prognosis and its significance are understandable to children of 5 to 7 years of age. Although children may realize that death is imminent, thoughts about this are seldom vocalized. They perceive absence and death with a sense of impending tragedy. By this time the concept of time has been mastered. School children can think of an object as a whole, as well as consider its parts. With the vivid imagination that is also present at this time, the physical change and deterioration that occurs with death can be visualized. Death is specific and concrete and has both internal and external causes.[26] The prognosis becomes absolute and creates such anxiety that the child can no longer cope. As increasing age brings increased emotional and intellectual capability, it also brings greater meaning to a child's own death. This leads to needing more help in coping.

Going to school full time adds to the child's continually changing social role and relationships within it. A 6- or 7-year-old realizes that with death there comes a change in previously established relationships. Again, death symbolizes separation from loved ones. This breeds anxiety. The child now understands that separation cannot be avoided, and because of this knowledge he learns to be a "good patient": death is not mentioned and feelings of pain and emotions are repressed. The rules of life are learned. At this time there is an emotional shift from anxiety to fear of physical injury and mutilation, operations, body intrusions, and needles.[29] Often these children die lonely, pretending they will not die, even though all others around them are aware of this. They rarely ask questions related to their disease or treatment, and they tend to avoid the topic of death, as if to protect their families from their approaching demise.[9]

From ages 5 to 9, death is personified and thought of as a contingency. Death as a personality is usually invisible, either having no form or going through the night so that it cannot be seen.[4] This is the time of life when children may have difficulty going to bed at night in the dark for fear that they may not wake the next morning. There is much talk at this age about the boogeyman. Death is remote, it exists outside of one's self, and through careful living it can be kept at a distance. This is also a period of interest in animate and inanimate things, which evolves into a transition period of superstitions and rituals around death, being uncertain as to whether death is funny or fearful—"Don't step on the crack, it will break your mother's back."

It is not until children become 8 or 9 that play and verbal expressions come to terms with each other. Weininger[35] found that previous to this age, when children were told that a doll was sick and going to die, they tended to talk about the doll's death as being permanent, but continued on in the play situation to have the doll return to life, recovering.

Egocentricity is decreased in the 9- and 10-year-old, while mature concepts of time, space, quantity, and causality are emerging. These children appreciate living and begin to understand death as the physical finality of living. Anxiety about death is characteristic in preadolescents and serves as a lead-in to adolescence.[33]

Adolescents

Adolescence is the bridge from childhood to adulthood; it is a period of transition. These transitions occur not only in the physiological, but also in the cognitive, psychodynamic, and sociocultural aspects of development. Cognitively adolescents move into the world of abstract thought. They learn to speculate on possibilities beyond reality and what might occur, as well as what does occur.[26] In this exploration adolescents will delve into the limits of life and the meaning of death.

Adolescents appreciate the reality of death.[22] However, personal death is not accepted.[17] The adolescent tends to assume the attitude of "Everyone else but me can die." Adolescence is a period of intense present, with the immediate life situation being important, and past and future being pallid. More structure is given to the past than to the future, but the past represents a period of confusion. Attitudes toward the future are subjective and distinctly negative. Often the future is viewed as being risky and devoid of any positive values.[4] Even if imminent, death is thought of as remote, because it distorts the importance of the present.

Adolescence represents the drive for complete independence and self-sufficiency. It is a time of group identity with peers and the development of personal ideas and behavior, usually through the peer group relationships. Guilt and vague feelings of badness are felt during rejection of parental control. This rejection bothers the adolescent. As most deaths in this age group occur secondarily to trauma or accidents (frequently resulting from the breaking of rules), death becomes a confirmation of badness and is perceived as punishment that is meted out by the unforgiving parent. This idea leads to fear of the authority figure and eventual bitterness and resentment, deepening the adolescent's guilt and accentuating his or her depression.[6]

Death also means rejection by the gang, as it emphasizes the vulnerability of the individual, as well as the difference between individuals. The rejection cannot be tolerated by an emerging independent individual. Death then becomes a function of dependency in isolation.

As the child gets older, there is an increase in expressed death anxiety in relation to illness. Before the age of 9 this anxiety is expressed in terms of separation or mutilation fears. After 9 it is expressed in the younger patients as anxiety demonstrated through symbolization and physiological expression. Older boys tend to act out, while older girls are prone to depression.[4] This expression appears to be directly related to our society's role models and the inability on the part of men to actively express emotion. Anxiety may also appear as regression to an earlier stage of development.

It may be concluded that children at any age perceive their own death according to their developmental level and through the catalyst of some crisis event, such as a catastrophic illness (Table 28-1).

THE IMPACT OF HOSPITALIZATION

At some time a dying child will be hospitalized for medical intervention. Even to the most carefully briefed child, the hospital represents something fearful, simply by virtue of its difference and newness in a child's repertoire of experiences.

The *toddler* views home as the seat of security, safety, and guidance. When hospitalized, the toddler experiences separation anxiety, separated from his familiar surroundings, routine, and family. Compounding the strangeness of the hospital setting, the treatment personnel cause the child pain and discomfort. The child, in turn, reacts to the physical pain and his perceptions of his parents' discomfort rather than to any understanding of the end of his own existence.[6]

Erikson pointed out that with increasing age, increasing independence develops. The preschool child does not separate thinking from concrete reality. Thus hospitalization is thought of as punishment for bad thoughts.[6] The child reacts with guilt and noncomprehension of the treatment. He is angry with the hospitalization process, and the treatment he receives he views as a form of punishment. Anger is usually directed toward the treatment team or other patients. In addition to anger and guilt such a child also must deal with loneliness.

The awareness of self increases as children develop. They begin to think in terms of "me" and "mine" versus "not me" and "not mine." The thought of not being

---

Table 28-1   Developmental stages: children's perception of death compared with Erikson's psychosocial and Piaget's cognitive stages

Erikson's psychosocial stages	*Piaget's cognitive stages*	*Perception of death*
1. *Trust vs mistrust* (birth to 1 year) Development of the sense of trust through the pairing of the infant's actions with pleasant events.	1. *Sensorimotor period* (birth to 2 years) Based on the formation of action schemas for skilled movement, language, visual perception, and object permanence.	1. *Birth to 1 year* Reacts physiologically. Without bonding there is little desire to live (failure to thrive).
2. *Autonomy vs doubt, shame* (1 to 3 years) The terrible twos. Beginning development of control over one's body, self, and environment.	2. *Preoperational period* (birth to 7 years) The ability to symbolize through language, thought, drawing, and play. Egocentricity. Asks questions and *why?* Is more able to employ past events and to consider more than one aspect of an event at a time.	2. *One to four years* Responds with fear and anxiety to treatment. Death has little or no meaning. 3. *Four to six years* Has the concept of "me" and "not me." Fantasy reasoning with an increased curiosity about dead animals, flowers, burial, and so on. Death is temporary.
3. *Initiative vs guilt* (3 to 5 years) Beginning exploration of the physical environment through senses and the social, physical worlds through language.	3. *Concrete operations* (7 to 11 years) Time of real, concrete thought. Orders, counts, and thinks in terms of cause and effect. Beginning to compare own views and ideas.	4. *Six to eight years* Death means being separated from loved ones and causes anxiety. The child learns to be a good patient. Superstitions about death predominate.
4. *Industry vs inferiority* (5 to adolescence) Begins to be a worker. Wants to please. Learns the meaning of rules and uses them.	4. *Formal operations* Beginning of abstract thought and reasoning. Ability to form hypotheses and test them.	5. *Eight to eleven years* Death is realized to be permanent.
5. *Identity vs role diffusion* Merging of past identity with future expectations (bodily, societal, and one's own).		6. *Adolescence* Speculates about what occurs after death. Death is perceived in terms of loss of independence and identity.

produces anxiety, thus children react through the process of denial. Denial allows them to deal with more tolerable and productive subjects that will ultimately lessen the anxiety. These children avoid speaking of death. Often their play behavior centers around accidents and disasters as they attempt to prove to themselves that existence can be controlled just as toys are controlled.[6] Frequently hospitalized children of this age also show less maturity in the level of their play, as well as less playfulness when compared to nonhospitalized children.[11]

The *grade-school child* is busy learning rules and is expected to exert some self-control and cooperation. Intellectually the child of this age is able to solve problems through thoughts, as well as by action. The child develops increased self-awareness, leading to independence from parents. Meanwhile, parental beliefs are internalized. By late grade school, the child has developed special friends, and the children teach and help each other.

Studies suggest that children in this stage are aware of the seriousness of their disease, even though they may not be capable of speaking about it,[30] and even though no one has told them how ill they are.[29]

Smallness, vulnerability, and inadequacy characterize the grade-school child. Such a child deals with these feelings through the use of denial and reaction formation.[6] For example, he or she may try to act fearless.

Grade-school children are also aware of their own identity. This allows them to think beyond self boundaries and to imagine. They understand about past and future concepts and fantasize about death and the idea of their own deaths. Thus they develop an alternative to death, seen in such forms as heaven, paradise, and hell.[6] Children want their existence to continue. Through learning rules, they pattern themselves after other individuals, leading to the realization that their parents are not perfect. Children therefore seek alternative heroes, groping for something to believe in and worship. These beliefs allow them to organize their worlds methodically, including a cause and purpose behind every action. This is then followed by a reward or punishment. Death being perceived as a punishment causes religious guilt.[16] Secondary to this perception of punishment, dying children may reject the idea of heaven, which then represents only separation from family. Understanding of death increases throughout this stage, but these children tend to think that death comes suddenly and quickly. They may blot out feelings of death and in turn rely on parental authority (God, physicians, or teacher) for final protection from death.

Hospitalization involves various degrees of separation from family and friends. The grade-school child is lonely, scared, and sad, as well as fearful of the unknown. A study by Spielberger and others[28] indicated strong support for the hypothesis that terminally ill children show greater awareness of their hospital experience than do children who are chronically ill. These same children also expressed more hospital and nonhospital-related anxiety. Homesickness, anger, frustration, and anxiety are usually expressed to the treatment staff in the form of refusing to cooperate.[6] Some children might withdraw and become obviously depressed; however, the usual course of behavior is one of regression. They learn quickly from others and become sensitive to the feelings of the team. When involved with the hospital through the use of activities, children may become happier, and their self-image tends to improve. As death approaches, they may become sad and bitter, not wanting to leave. They feel lonely from the realization that this is one trip that must be made alone. Thus comfort and security are sought.

In dealing with death the *adolescent* progresses through the stages outlined by Dr. Elisabeth Kübler-Ross[15]: (1) denial, (2) anger, (3) bargaining, (4) depression, and (5) acceptance. Emotions in adolescents are more likely to be expressed than in younger children. Death is representative of loneliness and passivity. Hospitalized adolescents fear being returned to the dependent role and may overtax their strength through continued independence. Although they long for warmth and caring, they reject support and thus force people to withdraw from them, even while dreading loss of control. With approaching death, they become weakened and allow themselves to be loved and cared for. At this point they rationalize that control will be regained as strength is. The adolescent wants to live, but at the same time may be fascinated with the concept of death.[6]

Death in the middle teens defeats the newly developed self-control, self-confidence, and self-direction that all led to the enjoyment of self. Older grade-school children and adolescents who know they are dying and accept death's finality prepare their families for the event. They gradually withdraw their expectations from the family and seemingly reject them. It is as if they are trying to comfort their families and ease them through the final phase of death with as little pain as possible.

On the whole, then, most children recognize the severity of their own illness whether or not they have been presented with the diagnosis.[30] They react according to their stage of development, as well as their sociocultural expectations. For the most part a terminal illness and the resulting thoughts of death are recognized by the children as the removal of independence. This and the intense feelings of separation affect their response to their own deaths.

ASSESSING THE CHILD'S UNDERSTANDING OF DEATH

Assessing the child's understanding of death is important when working with a terminally ill child. This process helps the therapist to know how to deal with the child's understanding of what is happening to him or her. Therefore it is helpful to assess what stage of Piaget's cognitive and Erikson's psychosocial development the child evidences (Table 28-1). This gives a fairly accurate assessment of the child's understanding of death. It is also easier than trying to get a child to talk about death, since most children tend to avoid this subject with someone they have just met.

A second consideration in assessing the child's understanding is to record the parents' understanding of death and any relevant sociocultural ideas they have. These sociocultural aspects will color a child's perception of death and may differ from the occupational therapist's. When working with terminally ill children, one should also ask what expectations the parents have, whether they are willing to have their child told that he or she is terminally ill, and what approach they are using with the child.

OBJECTIVES FOR OCCUPATIONAL THERAPY INTERVENTION

Determining objectives for the terminally ill child is often very difficult for the staff. The staff members realize this is a child who will not get well and who is different from the usual pediatric patient for whom they can set goals and develop long-term expectations. Therefore their objectives are mainly psychological in nature, emphasizing quality of life, with less emphasis on physical aspects. The focus is not only on the child, but also on family members and their ability to develop adaptive responses. They are to:

1. Understand the origin and intensity of the child's anxiety
2. Allow thoughts or reactions to death to come into the open
3. Encourage expression of grief
4. Provide support
5. Facilitate and maintain independence
6. Facilitate and maintain participation in activities of daily living
7. Facilitate age-appropriate play skills
8. Facilitate adaptive child-family relationships

TREATMENT MODALITIES

The underlying principle when providing occupational therapy care for terminally ill children is to add quality to their remaining days. Two modalities are available to occupational therapists for terminally ill children: play activities and activities of daily living.

Until the age of 5, children learn exclusively about their world through play. They learn and practice activities before incorporating them into practical application. Once they go to school, play and teaching help them learn. The more playful and interesting the subject, the more likely they are to learn. Therefore the use of play is encouraged when dealing with terminally ill children.

Activities that are appropriate for the child's developmental level, physical level (including endurance and tolerance), intellectual level, and emotional state should be chosen. Play will allow the child to work through some of the feelings that he either has no words for, or cannot express. It also will allow the child to focus his interests on something other than himself, something in the world around him. The occupational therapist can also suggest activities appropriate for the family.

The second treatment modality that is useful in treating terminally ill children is activities of daily living. Too often adults take away the independence that a sick child has acquired. Parents and staff often jump to perform an activity such as bedmaking, dressing, or eating to save the child's strength. However, by doing so they take away the vestiges of independence that remain for the child and imply that there are no more decisions the child can make. Encouraging the continuation of routine activities of daily living allows a child to look forward to consistency and to know and have some control over what is coming. As the child becomes weaker, energy conservation methods can be taught to parents and introduced to children, allowing them to continue functioning independently. These modifications can be as simple as changing from metal to plastic utensils, using Velcro fastenings on clothing, and using pushcarts so that the child does not have to carry objects as weakness progresses. These modifications allow the child to continue functioning and to feel useful, rather than force the child to spend numerous hours on the sofa or bed watching countless television programs. The focus is not only on the child, but also on family members and their ability to develop adaptive responses.

WORKING WITH THE FAMILY OF THE DYING CHILD

Parents must deal with the loss of their child throughout the process of the illness. They must also deal with the idea that they will continue to survive after their child's death.

Parents often suspect the severity of the child's illness and anticipate the news.[21] Their reaction on hearing the diagnosis may range from loss of control to outward calm. Those who display a lack of affective response do so as a defense mechanism to allow themselves to deal realistically with the problems at hand. Clinical observers, as well as parents, report that it takes several days or weeks for the realization of the diagnosis to sink in. Typically both parents are eager to hospitalize the child once it is suggested, as this renews their hope that the diagnosis is faulty and that treatment will cure their child.

With the realization of the diagnosis and the major

decisions made as to treatment, the parents are then free to react to the situation. Initially the reaction appears as shock or denial contaminated by guilt.[21] This guilt takes the form of the parents' thinking either that they are the cause of the illness or that they had not paid enough attention to the child. This, combined with questioning of the medical staff, represents an attempt to search for meaning or understanding of the situation. A problem occurs, however, if feelings of guilt become prolonged in nature and lead to overindulgence or to lack of discipline.

Denial is seen as the underlying reason for seeking other opinions,[7] representing the hope that the diagnosis is wrong and that the physician and medical staff have been in error. Binger and others[2] studied 23 families of terminally ill children and found this reaction is not usually shown by the immediate family, but rather by the grandparents and friends of the family.

Intellectualization also occurs. Parents seek information about the disease and cures, especially from other parents on the hospital ward and in support groups. This behavior is healthy up to a point. It gives the family an intellectual understanding of the disease to help them deal with the situation and the decisions that surround the treatment. However, the increasing numbers of questions usually indicate increasing anxiety and guilt, which are not resolved by more information and should be dealt with realistically.

Throughout the course of the child's illness, hostility and anger are expressed by parents. Initially this reaction appears as a fight to reverse the diagnosis. Next, parents often feel resentment that they should suffer in such a manner. This may be complicated by guilt over their feelings of resentment. Resentment is usually channeled outward, often directed toward the treatment team. Third, anxiety of the unknown produces feelings of anger and hostility. Further, in the course of an illness, sick children often do not act sick, which reinforces the parents' denial.[6]

Parents often want to stay with their child during the course of his or her hospitalization. Urging the parents to return home may add to feelings of distress and guilt. Often other children at home are neglected, thus increasing sibling rivalry and resentment toward the sick child. Seeking to cheer a child is a constant need felt by the parents. However, this does not acknowledge a child's true feelings. Hospitalization promotes feelings of separation and anxiety on the part of the parent and the child. The parents are eager to hospitalize the child, but are fearful to let the child go. Hospitalization represents a loss of control. No longer is the parent in charge; the authority is transferred to the medical personnel, and eventually the parents come to depend on the strength and support of the hospital.

Resentment is increased if the physician is unable to provide a curative treatment. This is complicated by the child's feelings. The child expects his parents to ease the pain and make him well. The parents are unable to do this, and the child becomes angry. This leaves the parents confused with feelings of failure.

A remission is anticipated eagerly until the child is allowed to return home. The child's parents then realize that they are in sole care of the child, and this increases their anxieties. Overprotective behavior displayed by the parents leads to resentment by others and affects all family matters.[21]

A relapse confronts the parents with the cold reality of the situation. They may react as if they had just learned of the diagnosis. A relapse causes great stress, and effective coping behavior is needed. There is a dynamic balance of emotional states, and transient episodes of ineffective coping are not uncommon. Successful coping behavior protects the parents from being overwhelmed by environmental and psychological stress while they continue to function in the medical and psychological care of their child.

Anticipatory grief is the gradual occurrence of mourning behavior, precipitated by the first acute critical phase of a terminal illness.[4] It is typically characterized by somatic symptoms: apathy, weakness, preoccupation with thoughts of the ill child, sighing, occasional crying at night, and appearing depressed. At other times, there is increased motor behavior and increased talk about the child. These symptoms help to reintegrate the feelings with the gradual redirection of external energies.[8]

Physical complaints are gradually replaced by resignation and the desire to have it over with. Parents turn their energies to other matters. Visits become a duty; the parents seem detached from their own child and more interested in the remaining children on the ward.[4] This is indicative of acceptance. Mourning energies are being converted to more constructive means.

Exhaustion of treatment options accelerates the grieving. The child's parents may experience decreasing understanding and become more prone to anger.

In chronic terminal cases the parents have had time to rehearse how they will act. They usually control their expressions of grief, taking death calmly. However, if the parents have expressed denial continually throughout the course of their child's illness, death will be a shock, an experience of immediate loss. The parents will often need many months before they can speak about the child without distress.

Finally, death is experienced with relief, and guilt is tinged with remorse.[16] Mourning may deepen feelings of self-value through thoughts of death. Also, the love and warmth felt for the dead child may lead to a greater sense of self-worth. Three to six days after the child's death, the parents' mourning becomes less pronounced. However, there tends to be a continued interaction with the hospital through such things as gifts, initiation of research foundations, and library donations. After the child's death there is a tendency of the parents to reverbalize the guilt, which is bound up with the feelings of relief.

Binger and others[2] found that in half of the 23 families they studied, one or more members required psychiatric help after a child's death, although none had required it before. Mulhern et al found, in the families they worked with, 50% of the bereaved families had at least one member who had sought psychiatric/psychological care, 70% reported serious marital discord following the child's death, and 25% to 50% of the surviving siblings experienced significant emotional, behavioral, or academic difficulties.[19] This finding makes it important to understand the three types of unhealthy family protective maneuvers that can occur. The first is the *conspiracy of guilt* that occurs when the parents feel the death was preventable. Communication about the lost child is shrouded and evasive to protect the living members of the family. This tends to support the idea that if the parents had acted differently, the child would still be alive. Therefore guilt is maintained, and there is no chance for the exploration of the event for fear that someone will be blamed.[14] Surviving children in such a family live in a world of distrust and in constant fear of what may be in store, and they are hesitant to ask for clarification. A second unhealthy coping mechanism is the *preciousness of the survivor.* This leads to overprotection and shielding of the surviving children with fantasied attributes and expectations placed on them. This may lead to implications of specialness and good fortune placed on the survivors. Survivors may be filled with feelings of omnipotence and the desire to test fate, which limits their ability to develop practical coping mechanisms.[14] The last type of unhealthy coping is the *substitution for the lost child* in one of the survivors or a new child. The chosen child is likely to be vulnerable and forced to live a dual life: one of his own, and one of the dead sibling's. Because of this, the child is not likely to develop a secure sense of identity.[14] Unhealthy coping strategies used by families require outside intervention from mental health professionals. Even in the healthier families, as evidenced by their more adaptive coping patterns, one finds persisting guilt, sadness, and health fears that continue to be problematic after a child's death.[19]

After their experiences, families of dying children have made the following suggestions to health professionals. Listening seems to be the most valuable asset of a medical staff.[21] This is followed in importance only by offering reassurance, which often calms a parent's guilt feelings. Knowledge presented at the parents' level of understanding is calming. Questions should be answered patiently, kindly, and realistically. Families may be grateful, as well as angry. These angry feelings are dealt with best if the treatment team does not react to them as a personal insult or attack, and if the anger can be channeled productively. If information is available on support groups, the staff members should make it known to parents.

General components of good management include the following:[1]

1. Competence of staff
2. Availability of staff
3. Continuity of care
4. Personalized care
5. Well prepared procedures
6. Active treatment role for the child
7. Questions encouraged
8. Supportive actions and discussions

After a child's death, the family also experiences difficulty relinquishing the ties with the health care personnel who have been involved with their child's treatment. Increasing numbers of agencies and facilities offer bereavement counseling to aid the family through the first year after the child's death. This is thought to be the average length of time for family grief to be resolved.[36]

WORKING WITH PERSONNEL CLOSE TO THE DYING CHILD

Among the personnel who treat the dying child and counsel the family, there may be a feeling of ambivalence in which compassion struggles against repulsion inherent in the threat of death. The degree of success in resolving this conflict determines the degree of success of the health care worker. Therapists should be aware of this ambivalence in their colleagues and in themselves as well.

Since the primary goal of a health care worker is to help the sick child get well, a dying child prevents reaching this goal, thus causing feelings of frustration and anger. However, one cannot get angry with a sick child, so instead this situation often leads to feelings of guilt and even greater anger toward the one causing the guilt. This emotional state may become cyclic. Sack et al, studying medical residents, found that the physicians used the following coping strategies to deal with a child's death: (1) they had a tendency to try to master anxiety-provoking situations; (2) they tended to want to change the environment and not themselves; and (3) they habitually used intellect to master their anxieties. These patterns benefit neither the child, the family, nor the health care team involved with the child.[25]

Reactions of the personnel toward the child are influenced by previous experiences with death. The health care personnel may take the approach of being overprotective toward the child. This overprotectiveness often leads to overt or covert reactions of anger by the child. On the other hand, the staff members may be overindulgent, and thereby put an added burden of guilt on the child; after all, what has the child done to deserve this special treatment? When both types of behaviors are shown by the staff, there is inconsistency and confusion within the child, who then may not know how to behave.

When treatment fails, workers may accuse each other of failure, thus redirecting toward each other the anger, frustration, and irritation they feel because they were unable to help.

One staff member reacted to a dying child by hopping into his sports car and racing the highways until he had worked through his distressed feelings. This is one method of coping; however, in this case it produced anxiety in the rest of the staff until he returned. More constructive methods can channel anger and irritation into productive actions, whether oriented to motor release or to talking. Some of the methods currently used by staff members to deal with a child's death include individual counseling, team support group meetings, and case conferences where a child's course of treatment and eventual death are discussed.

Although a child's death is painful to all, it can also be a time of learning about life, love, and the appreciation of others. The best advice is often the hardest to take. Parents recommend trying to live each day as it comes, and with each day enjoying one's child.[2] Occupational therapists are able to provide aid and support to these very special children and their families.

CASE STUDY

When Jan, the 11-year-old girl described at the beginning of this chapter, first had treatment, her facial cancer was hardly noticeable. She often came down to the playroom. In the playroom, occupational therapists worked with the children, allowing them to express their feelings about the medical procedures through the use of play, for example, playing nurse and doctor with a doll and actual nonharmful medical items, and encouraging the children to play with age-appropriate toys.

After several admissions and subsequent surgery, Jan began to withdraw to her room. The staff initially tried to get her to come out, but eventually obeyed her wishes and went to her in her room. By this time, Jan preferred quieter activities, such as painting, drawing, sewing, and crafts. These activities offered recognizable end products and allowed her to feel purposeful, able to accomplish a task from the beginning to the end. As she became weaker because of the disease and the treatment for it, the activities often consisted only of talking and reading. Now Jan was being bathed primarily by the nursing staff, although she was encouraged to perform at least part of the routine. She could still feed herself most of her meals, although her intake was supplemented with intravenous feedings. She continued to refuse to leave her room. At the same time she began to draw away from the majority of the staff, as well as her parents—as if to spare them the pain of death. She allowed only a few within her realm, thus adding to her life an element of control respected by the staff. It was during this time that Donna, the nursing student, became important to her. Donna and Jan talked together as Jan grew weaker and lost her ability to perform activities. Treatment eventually failed to produce a response, and Jan grew weaker and died.

CASE STUDY

Suzi was an 11-year-old who initially was seen in the pediatric neurology clinic. Throughout her grade-school years, she had been an "A" student. Recently though her grades had begun to slip, and it was recommended that she have a thorough neurological workup to try and pinpoint the cause of her academic difficulties. Suzi, a pretty, bright sixth grader,

was admitted to the hospital. Two weeks later, after an extensive medical workup, including psychological testing and an occupational therapy evaluation, Suzi was diagnosed as having SSPE (subacute sclerosing panencephalitis), a deteriorating neurological condition associated with the measles virus. She was still up and able to get around, although she had periods of memory lapses and found it difficult to learn new material. Her parents' grief began.

Suzi was followed as an outpatient in the clinic. One month later she was readmitted. At this time, she complained of weakness in her legs, had poor endurance, and was unable to walk. The neurologic exam showed increased muscle tone and deteriorating balance. Occupational therapists explored hobby ideas with Suzi and her parents, focusing on previously acquired skills, since she found new learning so difficult. Her parents were encouraged to allow Suzi to be as independent as possible in areas such as eating and dressing, but they were taught how to help with transfer techniques for toileting and travelling. At the same time, occupational therapists discussed desirable alterations in Suzi's home. Suzi's parents were also referred to a home health care agency.

Several months later, Suzi was admitted on an emergency basis to the hospital. She was comatose, her posture was decorticate, she was unable to swallow, and her temperature regulation mechanism had failed. Although medically stable, Suzi needed to have a gastric tube surgically placed into her stomach for nourishment. A thermoregulating blanket helped to control her temperature fluctuations. At this time, occupational therapy services were provided to the parents to teach them to provide maintenance range of motion and stimulation, as well as to allow them to express some of their anger toward the medical staff.

When Suzi's parents decided to take her home, they were taught the care of a comatose patient, including routine medical monitoring and feeding and hygiene techniques. Services with the home health agency were renewed. Several months later, after several outpatient visits to the clinic to monitor her deteriorating condition, Suzi died quietly at home.

SUMMARY

In working with dying children, occupational therapists must be aware of developmental differences in the way children view death. These differences, added to the impact of hospitalization, affect children's responses to treatment and to surrounding people. Therapists can be effective with play activities and activities of daily living. It is important to understand the positive and negative emotions affecting parents, staff, and self.

STUDY QUESTIONS

1. Write down your feelings about working with children who are dying. How do you think these feelings are going to influence your ability to work professionally with dying children?
2. Children's understanding of death varies from age to age. How would this affect occupational therapy intervention with a preschool child, a grade-school child, and an adolescent?
3. What is the major role of the occupational therapist with the family of the dying child?

4. How does the therapist's own view of death affect his or her interactions with the family?

REFERENCES

1. Bergman AB: Psychosocial aspects in the care of children with cancer, Pediatrics 40(3):492, 1967.
2. Binger CM, et al: Childhood leukemia: emotional impact on patients and family, N Engl J Med 280:414, 1969.
3. Childers P, and Wimmer M: The concept of death in early childhood, Child Dev 42:1299, 1971.
4. Cook SS, et al: Children and dying: an exploration and a selected bibliography, New York, 1973, Health Sciences Publishing Corp.
5. Dominica F: The dying child, Lancet 1(8333):1107, May 14, 1983.
6. Eason WM: The dying child: the management of the child or adolescent who is dying, Springfield, Ill, 1970, Charles C Thomas, Publisher.
7. Evans PR, et al: The management of fatal illness in childhood, Proc R Soc Med 62:549, 1969.
8. Friedman SB: Care of the family of the child with cancer, Pediatrics 40:498, 1967.
9. Jeffrey P, et al: The role of the special school in the care of the dying child, Dev Med Child Neurol 24(5):693, 1982.
10. Kane B: Children's concepts of death, J Gen Psychol 134:141, 1979.
11. Kielhofner G, et al: A comparison of play behavior in non-hospitalized children and hospitalized children, Am J Occup Ther 37(5):305, 1983.
12. Koocher GP: Childhood, death, and cognitive development, Dev Psychol 9(3):369, 1973.
13. Koocher GP: Talking with children about death, Am J Orthopsychiatry 44:404, 1974.
14. Krell R, and Rabkin L: The effects of sibling death on the surviving child: a family perspective, Fam Process 18(4):471, 1979.
15. Kubler-Ross E: On death and dying, New York, 1969, Macmillan Publishing Co.
16. Lewis M, and Lewis DO: The crisis of death: a child dies, Curr Probl Pediatr 3:1, 1973.
17. McDonald RT, and Carroll JD: Appropriate death: college students' preferences vs actuarial projections, J Clin Pychol 37(1):28, 1981.
18. Meliar JD: Children's conception of death, J Gen Psychiatry 123:359, 1973.
19. Mulhern RK: Death of a child at home or in the hospital: subsequent psychological adjustment of the family, Pediatrics 71(5):743, 1983.
20. Nagy M: The child's view of death. In Feifel WH, editor: The meaning of death, New York, 1959, McGraw-Hill Inc.
21. Noland RL: Counseling parents of the ill and the handicapped, Springfield, Ill, 1971, Charles C Thomas, Publisher.
22. O'Brien CR, et al: Death education: what students want and need, Adolescence 13(52):729, 1978.
23. Oleske J, et al: Immune deficiency syndrome in children, JAMA 249:2345, 1983.
24. Pizzi M: Occupational therapy in hospice care, Am J Occup Ther 38(4):252, 1984.
25. Sack WH, et al: Death and the pediatric house officer revisited, Pediatrics 73(5):676, 1984.
26. Salladay SA, and Royal ME: Children and death: guidelines for grief work, Child Psychiatry Hum Dev 11(4):203, 1981.
27. Speece MW, et al: Children's understanding of death, Child Dev 55(5):1671, 1984.
28. Spielberger CD, et al: Children's state-trait anxiety inventory, Palo Alto, Calif, 1972, Consulting Psychologist's Press.
29. Spinetta JJ: The dying child's awareness of death: a review, Psychol Bull 81(4):256, 1974.
30. Spinetta JJ, et al: Anxiety in the dying child, Pediatrics 52(6):841, 1973.
31. Sternlicht M: The concept of death in preoperational retarded children, J Gen Psychol 137(2):157, 1980.
32. Tigges KN, et al: The treatment of the hospice patient: from occupational history to occupational role, Am J Occup Ther 37(4):235, 1983.
33. Toews J, et al: Death anxiety: the prelude to adolescence, Adolesc Psychiatry 12:134, 1985.
34. Von Hug-Hellmuth H: The child's concept of death, Psychoanal Q 34:499, 1965.
35. Weininger O: Young children's concepts of dying and dead, Psychol Rep 44:395, 1979.
36. Wessel MA: The primary physician and the death of a child in a specialized hospital setting, Pediatrics 71(3):443, 1983.

ADDITIONAL READINGS

Kubler-Ross E: On children and death, New York, 1983, Macmillan Publishing Co.
Oremland EK, and Oremland JD: The effects of hospitalization on children, Springfield, Ill, 1973, Charles C Thomas, Publisher.
Picard HB, and Magno JB: The role of occupational therapy in hospice care, Am J Occup Ther 36(9):597, 1982.

PART VII

SERVICE DESIGN AND MANAGEMENT

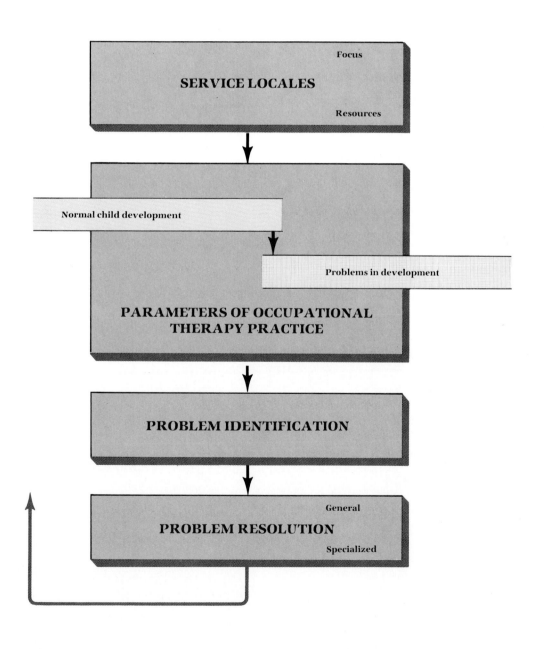

29

Occupational therapy in the school system

LINDA C. STEPHENS

All children are required to spend considerable time in an educational setting in preparation for adult roles in life. Education has been defined as "a continuous process by which individuals learn to cope with their environments" (p. 1257).[17] The occupational therapist who works in a school setting has the unique opportunity to help students become more functional in their own environments. This chapter discusses the educational environment as it relates to the occupational therapist, as well as the therapist's roles and functions in this setting.

LEGISLATION

The Education of All Handicapped Children Act of 1975 (PL 94-142) and Section 504 of the Rehabilitation Act of 1973 dramatically changed the focus and availability of education for handicapped children in the United States. Before the enactment of this federal legislation many handicapped children were excluded from public schools, received education in private schools (at their parents' expense), were institutionalized, or remained at home. In 1975, when the Education of All Handicapped Children Act was enacted, approximately 1.75 million handicapped children in the United States were receiving no education at all, and 2.5 million were receiving inadequate services.[18]

The Education of All Handicapped Children Act[4,p.42474] and its regulations have four main purposes:

1. To ensure that all handicapped children have available to them a free appropriate public education;
2. To ensure that the rights of handicapped children and their parents are protected;
3. To assist states and localities to provide for the education of handicapped children;

4. To assess and ensure the effectiveness of efforts to educate such handicapped children.

Section 504 of the Rehabilitation Act of 1973 was enacted to prohibit discrimination against handicapped persons in programs or activities receiving federal funds. This act states that "no otherwise qualified handicapped individual . . . shall, solely by reason of his handicap, be excluded from the participation in, be denied the benefits of, or be subjected to discrimination under any program or activity receiving federal financial assistance" (p. 22676).[16] This legislation also provides for a free appropriate education for handicapped children and requires that nonacademic services and extracurricular activities be available to handicapped students on the same basis as nonhandicapped students.

Federal legislation provides for the use of certain "developmental, corrective, and other supportive services as are required to assist a handicapped child to benefit from special education" (para. 121a.13).[4] Occupational therapy is identified as one of these related services. As a result, greater numbers of occupational therapists are being employed by school systems to provide this related service to children in special education. Public schools are mandated to develop programs to provide adequate education for all handicapped children. Consequently, a significant portion of the practice of occupational therapy has shifted from medical settings to public schools.

THE EDUCATIONAL ENVIRONMENT
Systems theory

The educational environment can be analyzed and understood in terms of systems theory. A *system* is a functional unit that consists of a structuring of events or happenings rather than physical parts; it describes a pattern of relationships. Every system is made up of a number of *subsystems* and is also part of larger interacting *suprasystems*. All systems have definite boundaries, or limits, and are interdependent with surrounding systems.

The occupational therapist can be considered a subsystem interacting with other subsystems within larger systems and suprasystems. Figure 29-1 shows some of these interactions. In this example, the occupational therapist interacts with other subsystems, such as special education, speech therapy, physical therapy, and the student. As various schools have contact with one another, they represent interacting systems within the larger suprasystem—the educational organization and school administration. The suprasystem has an infinite number of contacts and interactions with other suprasystems, such as the State Board of Education, the community, and the state, local, and federal governments.

Many occupational therapists working in school settings are itinerant; they are expected to travel among several schools to provide services to handicapped children. It is important for these therapists to realize that they are moving from one system to another within the same suprasystem. Each system and subsystem has "its own distinctive function, develops its own norms and values, and is characterized by its own dynamics" (p. 99).[11] The effective itinerant therapist is one who recognizes the differences between systems and adapts to each unique environment.

Each occupational therapist, as an individual, can be considered a unique subsystem with different combinations of background, training, professional experience, personality, race, values, perceptions, and childhood experiences. Figure 29-2 illustrates the components of the individual as a subsystem and the interactions with other subsystems. These components are sometimes taken for granted when an individual interacts with individuals from similar backgrounds. When there are substantial differences, these must be examined so that interpersonal relationships can be developed for the therapist to be effective on a professional level. Some examples are the white middle-class therapist working in an inner-city black school, or an urban therapist working in a rural area.

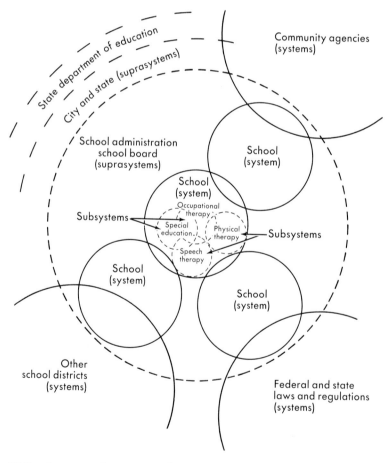

Figure 29-1   Systems, subsystems, and suprasystems in the schools.

A public school is a system made up of elements from the community reflecting the culture, traditions, and values of that community. It is a relatively open system, accepting any child within its geographical boundaries and usually encouraging participation from families and other community members. The system itself develops its own values and traditions, establishes channels of communication, and bestows power on certain individuals. As a system of interacting elements with a purpose of education, the school sometimes becomes inflexible and resistant to change.

Regan[19] described the characteristics of a rural school system and its suprasystems. Rural areas often have a high incidence of poverty, resulting in substandard housing, poor nutrition, and inadequate medical care. The rural schools are likely to have fewer funds and less modern equipment than urban schools. Rural persons often have more conservative religious and moral values and live in more homogeneous communities than do urban persons. Regan[19] stated that "not until the population's needs and resources, as well as the school administrative structure are understood can therapists deliver their services with the cooperation and support of the community and the administrative hierarchy" (p. 88).

Medical and educational models

The occupational therapist typically receives training and experience in a system referred to as the medical model. In this model, dysfunction or disease is identified, and strategies are developed to increase function and to alleviate disease and dysfunction. The occupational therapist, as a subsystem working within the medical model, interacts closely with other medical subsystems (nurses, physical therapists, and so on) under the direction of the physician. Treatment may end once the patient is considered cured or has reached a "maintenance" level. The patient enters the system voluntarily at any point in time, receives services, and then leaves the system.

The educational system is concerned primarily with the "normal" child who is expected to gain increasing skill, knowledge, and competency in moving through the system. Although educators are increasingly working in interdisciplinary teams, there is no one recognized leader, and the close interaction found in the medical model is not required (for example, the educational planning team does not have the same type of interdependence and need for a leader that a surgical team has). The consumer in the educational model is the student who enters the system at a predetermined time (typically age 5 or 6) and remains within the system for a set length of time (usually 12 or 13 years). A comparison between the hospital and school, as examples of the medical and educational systems, is found in Table 29-1.

Role conflict

The occupational therapist, as a member of a health profession working in an educational setting, may experience role conflict. Role conflict occurs when there is an inability to reconcile inconsistencies between two or more simultaneous sets of expected role behaviors. The therapist, trained in a medical model, might have a perception of the occupational therapist's role that is different from the educator's perception of that role. "Providing services that are medically and behaviorally oriented to programs that are designed to enhance students' learning may cause further confusion in the occupational therapists' perception of their roles and functions as a related service" (p. 6).[5]

As an example, an occupational therapist received referrals for students in a class for the severely mentally handicapped. The therapist, after assessing the students, determined that the students needed maintenance programs that could be carried out by the teacher and the aide. The occupational therapist perceived her role as an indirect one, instructing the teacher and the aide and returning periodically to check the students' progress. The teacher's perception of the occupational therapist's role was different. The teacher thought that the therapist should take the students out of class for a half hour twice each week and give them therapy. These differences in role perceptions resulted in confusion and friction. The teacher thought that the therapist was "not doing her job," and the therapist thought the teacher was "uncooperative."

Another source of role conflict is derived from the nature of the occupational therapist's role in an educational environment. The occupational therapist deals with students with problems and frequently must be

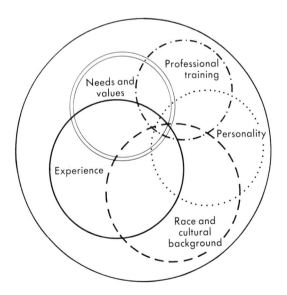

Figure 29-2 The occupational therapist as a subsystem.

Table 29-1 Comparison of medical and educational systems

	Hospital	*School*
Function	Saving lives, caring for the sick, curing or healing the injured	Instruction and development, preparation for life
Type of system	Relatively closed; must have credentials to participate; restricted areas; may be located at a distance from consumer; must pay fee or make appointment to enter	Relatively open; public has general knowledge and experience; building open to all; part of community; records accessible; parents and others urged to participate
Contact with system	Intermittent; contact when problem arises; consumer chooses when and where to enter system	Constant; continues through age 16 + ; admittance and attendance required by law
Barriers to consumer/provider interaction	Medical mystique; lack of understanding of terminology, clothing (nametags, uniforms, patient's gowns); inaccessible records; accessible only through receptionist or answering service	Teachers' lounge; teachers' dining area
Delivery of services	Cooperative team headed by physician; consumer usually not part of team	Individual professionals or collaborative and consensual decision-making by team; consumer (parent) is team member
Administration	Appointed board members (prestigious citizens); board meetings usually closed with little consumer input	Board members elected by public (members of community); board meetings open with frequent consumer input
Funding	Private pay; insurance; federal funds; grants; taxes; fee for service; salaries usually not public	Property taxes; state and federal funds; indirect pay for service; salaries public knowledge

creative in finding solutions to those problems. The educational organization is often a bureaucracy that resists change and does not know how to handle the unusual situation. The system that has no difficulty in purchasing hundreds of desks for students may be stymied by a request to build an adapted desk for one handicapped student. "The degree to which a given role demands innovative activity is associated significantly and positively with both the degree of role conflict and the amount of tension the role occupant experiences on the job" (p. 127).[11]

Role conflict for the occupational therapist also occurs when the therapist is in a position requiring a liaison or boundary-spanning function. The occupational therapist working in a school setting may perform this function between the educational and medical systems with different role expectations from both systems.

There are several strategies the occupational therapist can employ to deal with role conflict to reduce tension and frustration. First, the therapist should expect role conflict to be a part of the job. It is unrealistic to expect all persons in an educational setting to have an accurate perception of the functions of an occupational therapist. Demands for innovative solutions to problems and for liaison functions are necessary parts of the occupational therapist's role, but they tend to increase role conflict. A second strategy is to develop support systems with other occupational therapists in neighboring

school systems or in professional organizations. Third, the presence of role conflict can be considered an opportunity to develop innovative ideas and to act as a change agent in the resolution of conflicts. This gives the occupational therapist an opportunity to be creative and to derive satisfaction from successful problem solving.

ROLES OF THE OCCUPATIONAL THERAPIST
Description of roles

What does an occupational therapist do in the school system? The occupational therapist is concerned with improving functional skills and developing coping behavior through the use of purposeful activity. The basis of occupational therapy intervention is a functional inability to perform.[23] Occupational tasks for the student in an educational setting are those tasks necessary for adequate performance in the classroom. It is the occupational therapist's role to provide intervention to enable the student to overcome or compensate for his or her functional inability in order to benefit from special education.

Five major roles identified by Gilfoyle and Farace[7] have been officially adopted by the American Occupational Therapy Association (AOTA):

1. Evaluation: The identification of the student's def-

icits and needs in order to plan an occupational therapy program

2. Program planning: The determination of an appropriate occupational therapy program that is coordinated with the student's total education program

3. Program delivery: The implementation of an occupational therapy program designed to enhance the student's functioning and to enable the student to benefit from special education

4. Consultation: To provide training and information for school personnel and parents, which enables them to be more effective with the student

5. Management and supervision: To plan, supervise, and direct others as needed to implement occupational therapy services for the school or school system

The AOTA has developed standards for occupational therapists in school systems[22] and has adopted official guidelines for the provision of occupational therapy services in this setting.[8]

Occupational therapy as a related service

Occupational therapy, as defined by the regulations of PL 94-142, is a related service that can be provided to a handicapped student to enable him to benefit from special education.[4] Occupational therapists who are funded with federal monies must adhere to these guidelines by providing therapy only when the student needs it to benefit from special education. It is possible that a student may need occupational therapy in the clinic setting (medical model) but would not be eligible for services in the educational setting. "Every pediatric occupational therapist must recognize that school-based therapy services are not simply clinic therapy services delivered under the school building's roof" (p. 20).[15] Therapy provided within the school setting is designed to enhance the student's abilities to participate in the educational process.

Those students whose handicapping conditions do not interfere with the student's ability to benefit from special education are ineligible for school-based occupational therapy. If a student is able to participate in regular education and is not eligible for special education services, then that student is usually not eligible for related services, despite the presence of a handicap. Temporary handicapping conditions (for example, a fractured bone) usually do not make a student eligible for school-based therapy, although the student may need occupational therapy in a medical setting.

A very bright first-grader had a mild left hemiparesis from cerebral palsy. This student participated in all aspects of the educational program, including physical education, with few adaptations. The disability did not interfere with the student's educational program; therefore, she was not eligible for occupational therapy in school despite the fact that she did not have full use of her left hand. In another case, a teenager suffered traumatic amputation of the left arm in an automobile accident. He returned to his high school classes and was able to participate in everything except typing class. The occupational therapist consulted with the typing teacher and gave her material on one-handed typing, but did not have any contact with the student. The student continued to receive occupational therapy services on an outpatient basis at a rehabilitation center.

To determine eligibility for a student to receive occupational therapy as a related service, the therapist must determine if the student's handicap interferes with specially designed instruction and if occupational therapy could enable the student to benefit from that instruction. This is usually done by a process of screening and evaluation. Eligibility criteria vary so state and local guidelines need to be consulted.

Assessment role and evaluation procedures
SCREENING

The first step in developing or implementing occupational therapy services in an educational setting is to identify those children who need occupational therapy services. The occupational therapist needs to be involved in screening programs to accomplish this. Screening involves setting certain criteria for a particular population and identifying those children who do not meet the criteria and who therefore need further evaluation. A determination of the need for occupational therapy services is not made in the screening process, only the determination that further evaluation is needed.

There are several ways in which an occupational therapist can be involved in the screening process in a school. Many school systems have established educational or health screenings of certain age groups, especially of children who are entering school for the first time in kindergarten or first grade. It is appropriate for the occupational therapist to become involved as a member of the educational team charged with the responsibility to identify children who deviate from the norm.

The occupational therapist might choose to screen certain populations of children, such as classes for the mentally handicapped, physically handicapped, or learning disabled. The teachers of such classes are valuable sources of information for identifying those children who have problems or whose performance deviates from that of other children in the class. Information can be obtained through record review, teacher checklist, teacher interview, and observation.

According to AOTA guidelines,[8] the systematic screening of a certain group of students to identify those who need in-depth evaluation is termed "Type 1 screening." An individual student may also be screened following referral for special education. The purpose of this screening is to determine the need for occupational therapy referral and is usually accomplished through record review, interviews, and observation of performance. According to the guidelines, this is "Type 2 screening."

Screening instruments need to be chosen that are "appropriate to the chronological, educational and functional level of the student and shall not be racially or culturally discriminatory" (p. 900).[22] It is appropriate for the school-based occupational therapist to screen in one or more of the following areas: self-care, occupational tasks (school, leisure, play, or home), prevocational or vocational skills, developmental levels, neuromuscular functioning, and psychosocial functioning. By using information obtained through the screening process, the therapist can determine if a referral for a full evaluation is appropriate (Chapter 9).

REFERRAL

The referral for an occupational therapy evaluation is usually the initial step in obtaining occupational therapy services for a student. This is step 1 of the flowchart found in Figure 29-3. The referral should follow guidelines established by the American Occupational Therapy Association Statement on Referral.[8]

The student who is initially identified as possibly needing special education placement is usually referred by a teacher or principal to an educational evaluation team or educational planning committee. This team determines which educational or related service evaluations are needed and makes appropriate referrals. If an occupational therapy evaluation is requested, the occupational therapist contributes data to the educational team to help determine a student's special education placement and need for related services.

In the case of a student already placed in a special education setting, referrals may come from a variety of sources. Screening programs may identify students who need occupational therapy evaluations; parents and teachers might have concerns about problems that interfere with the child's ability to function in the special education setting; or requests might come from physicians or community agencies. When a problem is suspected or a request made, the referral for occupational therapy evaluation should be generated through the educational planning team that follows procedures established by the local school system for referrals to related services. A sample referral checklist appears on p. 167.

Usually the major criterion for referral to occupational therapy is the functional inability to perform, which interferes with the child's ability to benefit from special education. The functional inability may relate to occupational performance (self-care activities, home-school-work activities, play-leisure activities, prevocational activities) or to dysfunction in neuromuscular development, sensory-integrative development, emotional development, social development, or cognitive development. However, some children might have a dysfunction in one of these areas which does not interfere with their ability to benefit from special education. For example, a mentally handicapped child might have a developmental age of 3 years, which is significantly below the chronological age. In the areas of social development, cognitive development, and self-care activities the child may perform consistently on a 3-year-old level. In the absence of any neuromuscular or sensory-integrative impairment, the child may not be eligible for related services. In this case the child's dysfunction does not interfere with the ability to benefit from special education, which is geared to the child's developmental level.

Licensure laws in some states or policies established by some local education agencies may require a physician's referral before occupational therapy services are initiated. Every school-based occupational therapist must be cognizant of local laws and regulations. Even when a physician's referral is not required, it is the occupational therapist's professional responsibility to seek medical information and management when indicated. The occupational therapist should work with the educational planning committee to counsel the parent or guardian regarding the need for medical services.

EVALUATION

Step 2 in the flowchart (Figure 29-3) is to obtain parental consent for evaluation. The parents or guardian of a child have a right to be informed of any special evaluations or procedures given to their child at school, and they also have a right to give or withhold permission for evaluations. Parental permission for evaluation must be in writing and becomes part of the confidential records maintained by the school.

Step 3 is the occupational therapy evaluation. The evaluation process consists of data gathered from several sources. Examples are educational and medical records, interviews with teacher and parents, observation of the student, and administration of standardized and nonstandardized tests. The occupational therapist should choose tests and evaluation instruments that are appropriate for the chronological and functional levels of the student, and should take care that they are administered in a manner that is not culturally or racially discriminatory. The therapist should use test results and clinical judgment in assessing the student's abilities and dysfunction (Chapters 10 and 11).

Once the evaluation is complete, the therapist must communicate results and make recommendations to parents, teachers, and other involved persons (step 4). Often this reporting is done orally in a parent or teacher conference or in the educational planning meeting. Results also must be documented in writing in the occupational therapy evaluation report (Figure 29-4). At this time the occupational therapist deter-

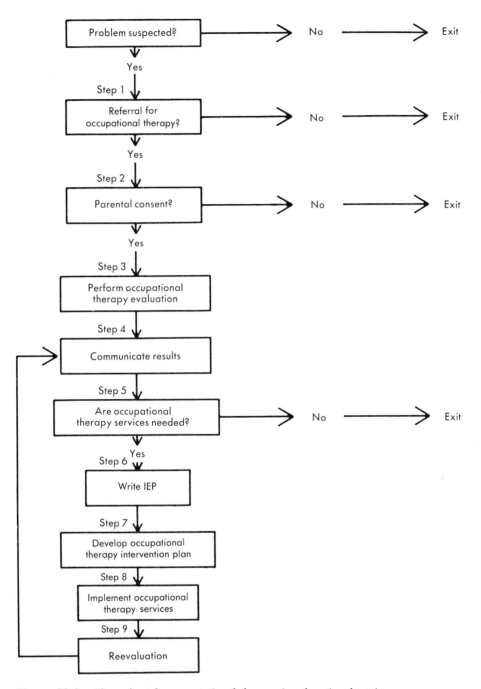

Figure 29-3   Flow chart for occupational therapy in educational settings.

mines if the student or family needs additional services in the community (rehabilitation, medical, vocational, counseling) and makes appropriate recommendations. A determination is then made as to the student's eligibility for occupational therapy services in the school setting (step 5).

Program planning

The second role identified for occupational therapists in the school system is concerned with program planning. The occupational therapist, using results of the occupational therapy evaluation, determines expected outcomes following intervention and estab-

Figure 29-4 Outline for evaluation report for school-based occupational therapist

1. General information
   a. Relating to student: name, age, school, birthdate, educational placement, summary of developmental-medical history
   b. Relating to referral: Referral source, presenting problems, diagnosis
   c. Relating to evaluation: Date of evaluation, tests administered, other sources of data
2. Psychosocial skills
   a. Relationships: Peer relationships, dyadic interaction, family relationships
   b. Behavior: Coping skills in classroom, behavior during evaluation, self-expression, self-control
   c. Self-concept—self-identity
   d. Play and leisure interests; extracurricular activities
3. Developmental skills
   a. Performance levels for physical-emotional-social components
   b. Manipulative hand skills
4. Daily living skills
   a. Daily personal care: Grooming, hygiene, feeding-eating, dressing, functional communication, use of adapted equipment
   b. Prevocational skills: Work process skills and performance, work product quality
   c. Use of environment: Functional mobility, restrictions imposed by environmental barriers
5. Sensorimotor skills
   a. Neuromuscular: Reflex integration, range of motion, gross and fine motor coordination, strength and endurance
   b. Sensory integration: Sensory awareness, visual-spatial awareness, body integration
6. Cognitive skills: Orientation, concentration, attention span, memory, generalization, problem solving
7. Preventive measures taken or needed: Energy conservation, joint protection, body mechanics, positioning
8. Conclusions: Summary of student's functional levels, including strengths and weaknesses; identification of areas of dysfunction needing intervention
9. Recommendations: Need for other services; need for occupational therapy intervention, including type of intervention, service delivery model, frequency, duration, and goals
10. Name and signature of occupational therapist

lishes educationally relevant long-term and short-term goals. These goals are coordinated with goals from special education and other educational or related services the student receives and are included in the student's Individualized Education Program (IEP). Detailed planning is done by the occupational therapist by outlining methods and activities to be used to reach goals.

INDIVIDUALIZED EDUCATION PROGRAM (IEP)

The Individualized Education Program is a written plan for a handicapped child required by federal regulations. It must be written and in effect before special education and related services are provided to a student. It is usually developed at a staffing or Individualized Education Program meeting by a team made up of a supervisory person, the child's parents, the child (where appropriate), and other individuals involved with the child. The latter could include an occupational therapist who has evaluated or provided services to the child.

According to federal regulations for Public Law 94-142, the Individualized Education Program must include the following[4]:

1. Present levels of functioning
2. Goals and short-term objectives
3. Special education and related services to be provided
4. Dates for initiation and duration of services
5. Criteria for evaluating the achievement of goals and objectives (para. 121a.346)

EDUCATIONAL PLANNING TEAM

The IEP is the vehicle by which interdisciplinary team planning is accomplished to meet the individualized needs of the handicapped child. The occupational therapist, as a member of this team, contributes to the description of present levels of performance and to the development of overall goals and objectives for the student (Step 6, Figure 29-3). Ideally, the IEP is comprised of consensus goals that "should not represent the perspective of any one profession, but rather the overall needs of one student" (p. 17).[8]

Occupational therapy goals, which may be in team consensus goals, must relate to the student's educational outcomes. These goals are reviewed annually and are revised or rewritten as needed. In this way the occupational therapist shows how occupational therapy intervention can improve the child's functional abilities in the classroom to enhance his or her ability to benefit from special education.

WRITING GOALS

A statement of present levels of performance describes a child's function at a particular time in a particular setting. When used as a reason for referral or as data gathered from an interview or observation, it is compared to the expected level of performance for a child of similar chronological or developmental age. When the described level of performance does not meet the expected level of performance, then a functional inability to perform exists. It is this functional inability to perform occupational tasks that provides the basis for occupational therapy intervention.

Long-term goals are generally broad and may take an extended length of time to accomplish. These may be determined by the entire team as consensus goals and reflect expectations of the student's eventual functioning. It may require the coordinated efforts of more than one discipline to work toward the same goal. Short-term goals, on the other hand, are specific and measurable. Many school systems require goals to be written in behavioral terms so that outcomes can be measured. To be measurable the goal must have at least three components: a *condition* statement, a *behavioral* statement, and a *performance* criterion (see p. 223). The following is an example of occupational therapy goals in an educational setting.

CASE STUDY

Present level of performance: Mary slumps over her desk, rests her head on her arm, and tilts her head when writing. She frequently turns sideways in her chair or sits half off the chair when doing seat work.

Long-term goal: Mary will remain in an appropriate position when doing seat work in class.

Short-term goal 1: When doing written work at her desk in the classroom (condition), Mary will demonstrate the ability to cross the midline of her body by writing from left to right, maintaining an erect posture (behavior), turning sideways in her chair no more than one time in 15 minutes (criterion).

Short-term goal 2: When doing written work at her desk in the classroom (condition), Mary will demonstrate greater postural stability by maintaining an erect posture, with feet on floor, left hand holding paper (behavior), slumping over the desk no more than one time in 15 minutes (criterion).

OCCUPATIONAL THERAPY INTERVENTION PLAN

The occupational therapist, in working toward goals generated by the team, develops an occupational therapy intervention plan (step 7, Figure 29-3). This plan, unlike the IEP, specifically details the methods and activities the therapist plans to use in working toward identified goals. The occupational therapist draws on his or her knowledge of normal and abnormal functioning, along with various theoretical frameworks for ameliorating the inability to function, to devise a plan of intervention and to predict its effect. This reflects the unique role of the occupational therapist's contribution to the improvement of the student's overall functioning. The intervention plan is not part of the IEP but remains in records maintained by the therapist. The following is an example of an occupational therapy intervention plan using the previously cited case.

CASE STUDY

Functional inability to perform: Mary does not maintain acceptable posture at her desk. Her writing is messy and slow; she does not finish her work.

Causes of functional inability: Lack of integration of righting reaction causes entire body to follow when head turns; inability to maintain prone extension pattern indicative of hypotonic postural muscles; lack of integration of two sides of body; poor eye tracking (tendency to use one eye only); inability to inhibit or screen out inappropriate auditory or visual stimuli (involuntarily turns toward noise or movement in the classroom); poor eye-hand coordination aggravated by postural instability.

Methods of occupational therapy intervention: Sensory integrative treatment emphasizing vestibular and tactile input and adapted responses to enhance postural stability, integration of the two sides of the body, and normal movement patterns.

Occupational therapy program objectives: (1) Normalize response to vestibular and tactile stimuli, (2) develop ability to maintain prone extension position for 10 seconds, (3) demonstrate ability to cross midline of the body, (4) demonstrate integration of neck on body righting reaction when tested by the arm extension test, (5) maintain sitting position without external support.

Occupational therapy program activities: Spinning in net hammock (seated and prone); riding scooter board down ramp (prone); wheelbarrow-walking across room; reaching for beanbags while gliding on scooter board; rolling across rug with one arm up and one arm down; throwing Velcro darts across midline while sitting on T-stool.

Program delivery

IMPLEMENTATION OF THE OCCUPATIONAL THERAPY PROGRAM

The third role identified for school-based occupational therapists is that of implementing an intervention program (step 8, Figure 29-3). There are several aspects to consider in the implementation of occupational therapy services: (1) determining the appropriate service delivery model, (2) balancing the needs of the student with available resources, (3) determining the maximum and minimal frequency of service, and (4) determining the duration of the program, including the appropriate time to discontinue.

Service delivery models. The two major models for service delivery are those of direct service and monitoring. According to Gilfoyle,[20] *direct services* are "those related services within a student's educational program for which the occupational therapist has the primary responsibility" (p. 2). Direct service can be conducted on an individual or a group basis, but it must be implemented personally by the therapist or assistant. Weekly contact is usually considered the minimal frequency of intervention.

Monitoring programs are planned by a therapist but administered by another person. This could be a parent, teacher, or aide who is trained and supervised by the therapist for specific activities. Appropriate activities to be monitored are those specified for a particular student that *do not require the presence of a qualified therapist to be carried out in a safe and effective manner.* Regular and periodic contact is necessary to update programs and supervise the manner in which programs are implemented. Examples of activities that could be monitored are handling, positioning, use of equipment, and techniques used to adhere to medical precautions.

Methods of providing services. Either of the service delivery models can be implemented on a centralized or a decentralized basis. The centralized system can be compared to the occupational therapy clinic in a hospital or rehabilitation center in which all clients are physically located in one building and are transported to the occupational therapist in a space established primarily for that purpose. Some advantages of this system include more efficient use of the therapist's time, greater flexibility in scheduling and grouping, permanent establishment of equipment, easy accessibility to stored supplies, and greater accessibility of the occupational therapist to students and staff.

In the decentralized system the occupational therapist is itinerant, traveling to the students' locations. It can be compared to the home health model of providing occupational therapy services. Often it is necessary for the occupational therapist to carry equipment and supplies from place to place and to set up temporary therapy areas for providing services. While this system is less efficient for the therapist, it has definite advantages for the student. Students may be able to attend their neighborhood schools and attend some classes with nonhandicapped peers (mainstreamed), thus giving them greater opportunity for normal life-styles than if they were transported to a special school that housed only handicapped students. Even severely mentally and physically handicapped children can benefit from the stimulation of contact with nonhandicapped children in the school.

In one city several classes for severely mentally handicapped children were located within an urban elementary school. Even though these children were not capable of participating in classes with nonhandicapped children they did attend assemblies and other special school functions. The children enjoyed the music and activities on these occasions and benefited by the change from their classroom routine. In turn, the nonhandicapped children became accustomed to the sight of children in wheelchairs or children whose behavior deviated from the norm. Some of the nonhandicapped children made a habit of stopping to speak to or touch a hand of a handicapped child and enjoyed the handicapped child's delight at this special attention.

The trends toward mainstreaming handicapped children and providing itinerant therapy pose challenging problems for the therapist, especially in rural areas. Some school systems have equipped special therapy vans as mobile therapy rooms. One project in New York made use of a converted bus to provide transdisciplinary services to children in rural areas.[14]

TERMINATION OF SERVICES

It is sometimes difficult to determine the appropriate duration of occupational therapy intervention for the handicapped student in school. It is the responsibility of the occupational therapist to make decisions regarding termination of services according to several criteria. If occupational therapy is no longer necessary for the student to benefit from special education or if the student no longer requires special education, then the student ceases to be eligible for school-based occupational therapy. It may be appropriate, however, for that student to receive occupational therapy in another setting, such as an outpatient clinic.

In general, it is appropriate to discontinue occupational therapy when the student has met established goals or no longer makes progress even after a variety of intervention strategies have been tried. Discharge plans for these students should reflect any need the student may have for continuing support services within the school system or the community. The educational planning committee needs to be involved when termination of services is considered so that smooth transitions can be made. In some cases it may be appropriate for the occupational therapist to discontinue services for a period of time, then resume services when the student reaches a new developmental level or must cope with new environmental demands. For example, a student with cerebral palsy functioned very adequately in an elementary school environment and occupational therapy services were terminated. However, physical growth, adolescent issues, and the stresses of a middle school environment made it necessary for the student to resume occupational therapy to cope with disability in a new environment.

ADAPTED EQUIPMENT IN THE CLASSROOM

The occupational therapist can make a valuable contribution to the educational process by providing or fabricating adapted equipment needed by the student to function in the classroom. This includes equipment needed for seating or other positions in the classroom, as well as adapted equipment for managing classroom materials, writing, eating, dressing, and toileting.

The ambulatory, physically handicapped child may lack adequate labyrinthine or optical righting reactions to maintain a seated position without external support. This is the case with the children pictured in Figure 29-5. Obviously when a child must exert a great deal of effort to remain in his seat, he will lack the proximal stability necessary for control of distal musculature necessary for writing. When an occupational therapist developed adapted seating to provide external support for one child, the child's writing improved dramatically (Figure 29-6).

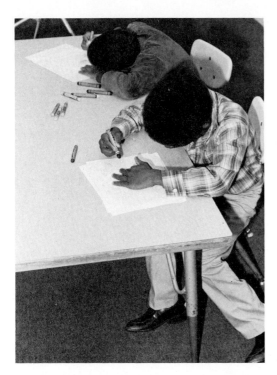

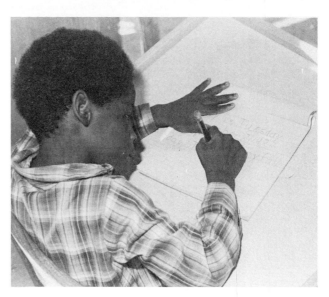

Figure 29-6   The use of a cutout table tilted to 45 degrees provides the support this child needed for writing.

Courtesy Atlanta Public Schools, Atlanta, Ga.

Figure 29-5   Although initially seated correctly, these children make increasing use of the table to provide trunk support as they become absorbed in the activity. Note position of the child's legs.

Courtesy Atlanta Public Schools, Atlanta, Ga.

The nonambulatory child may need wheelchair adaptations or special adapted seating to increase functional abilities. Such adaptations should aid in normalizing body alignment, neutralize primitive reflexes, facilitate appropriate motor behavior, and provide comfort and security[6] (Figure 29-7).

Some therapists have used thick corrugated cardboard (Tri-wall) for fabricating adapted seating for physically handicapped children. This material is lightweight and less expensive than plywood, yet adequately meets the adapted seating needs of the young child whose rapid growth makes frequent changes necessary.

Devising functional positioning for the severely involved physically handicapped child may require some ingenuity on the therapist's part. One therapist made a seat by cutting out portions of a plastic kitchen garbage can, adding padding and supports where needed.[8] This therapist also devised a sidelying positioner from a cardboard box.

Adapted equipment, such as prone standers, corner chairs, bolster chairs, and sidelying positioners, is commercially available from a number of sources. It is the occupational therapist's responsibility to choose or make equipment to meet each child's needs, based on the occupational therapy evaluation.

The physically handicapped child who is capable of performing academic work in a regular classroom may challenge the therapist's problem-solving abilities and creativity. An adapted device (Figures 29-8 and 29-9) must meet at least three criteria to be satisfactory:

1. It must increase the child's functional abilities for the intended task. If the child can do just as well without the device, leave it off.
2. It must be accepted by the child, other students in the classroom, and the teacher.
3. It must be simple. Elaborate adapted devices often require too much effort to set up and need frequent adjustment or repair.

It must be kept in mind that the occupational therapist's role in the school setting is to enable the student to benefit from special education. Any adapted devices must be for that purpose and become the property of the school system, not the student. It may be advisable to devise adapted classroom seating rather than extensive wheelchair modifications. The occupational therapist can, however, consult with the family regarding wheelchair adaptations and other adapted equipment for the home and guide the family to available resources for obtaining needed equipment.

REEVALUATION

The ninth, and final, step in the flowchart in Figure 29-3 is reevaluation. This can be done whenever the therapist determines it is appropriate, but should be

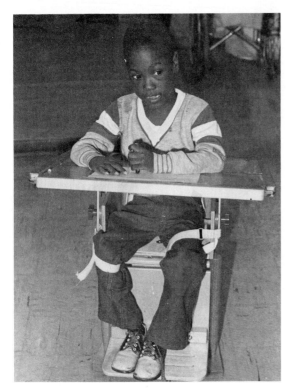

Figure 29-7 The use of an adapted classroom chair with tilted lap tray and adequate foot-leg support helps this child inhibit abnormal reflexes to maintain a functional position.

Courtesy Atlanta Public Schools, Atlanta, Ga.

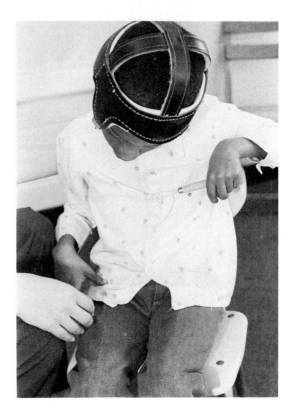

Figure 29-8 This child learned to use a button aid to increase independence in dressing.

Courtesy Atlanta Public Schools, Atlanta, Ga.

done at least once a year. When reevaluating a student, the therapist determines if goals have been met and if there is a further need for occupational therapy services. Reevaluation results are communicated to the parent and teacher (step 4) and are documented. If occupational therapy services continue to be needed, goals are revised or rewritten, the Individualized Education Program is reviewed and revised, and appropriate intervention is given.

In most states comprehensive reassessment of all students who receive special education is required every 3 years. This could include students in institutions or residential school settings or other students who are not in local schools. The occupational therapist may be involved as part of an assessment team to determine such students' educational needs. If occupational therapy is needed the student is referred to the appropriate sources.

Consultation
CONSULTANT ROLE IN THE SCHOOLS

The fourth role identified for occupational therapists in the school setting is to consult with school personnel and parents regarding occupational therapy for the student. According to the Standards of Practice of Occupational Therapy Services in Schools[22] "consultation is a service in which the occupational therapist's expertise is used to help the educational system achieve its goals and objectives . . ." (p 12). There are three major types of consultation in the school setting: case, colleague, and system.[8]

Case consultation. Case consultation involves a specific student, usually with short-term needs. An example might be devising special adaptations or seating arrangements to enable the student to function in the classroom. This type of consultation might be appropriate to help the student adjust to a change from a self-contained classroom to a regular class. In some states (for example, New York) this type of consultation is known as "transition-support services."[15]

Colleague consultation. Colleague consultation is used to provide resources and assistance to other professionals in the educational setting or to help them with specific problems or to increase their skills and knowledge. In an example given earlier in this chapter (p. 599) the occupational therapist gave colleague consultation when she provided instructional materials for one-handed typing to a teacher who had a student with an upper extremity amputation.

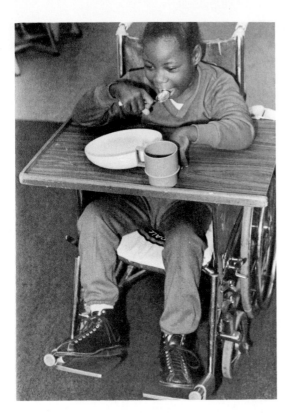

Figure 29-9 The use of an offset spoon and scoop dish enable this child to feed herself independently.

Courtesy Atlanta Public Schools, Atlanta, Ga.

In-service training, in which an organized presentation of material is given in a group setting, is often an effective method of providing colleague consultation. Teaching methods might include lecture, discussion, demonstration, role-playing, and use of audio-visual aids. Lemerand[13] listed four kinds of in-service programs: (1) concept exploration, (2) skill demonstration, (3) material adaptation, and (4) case study analysis.

Topics for in-service training should be planned to meet the needs of the group receiving the training. Some appropriate topics for teachers and aides include lifting and handling techniques for physically handicapped students; techniques for teaching self-help skills to mentally handicapped students; feeding techniques for children with oral-motor problems; and how sensory integrative problems of learning disabled children affect their performance in the classroom. (See Chapter 21 for additional information on in-service training.)

System consultation. System consultation is used to address the needs of the organization rather than an individual. Examples are giving recommendations for eliminating architectural barriers, acting as a liaison to community health agencies, or providing parent training classes.

CONSIDERATIONS FOR EFFECTIVENESS

Gilfoyle[3] described a consultant as "a person who has expertise in a profession and can communicate this expertise to help others achieve identified goals and objectives" (p. 19). According to West,[24] a consultant is an individual who is "a change agent, a catalyst in decision-making, an enabler and a helper/adviser" (p. 51). The consultant and the consultee are involved in an unusual problem-solving relationship in which there is no obligation for the consultee to accept the help, suggestions, or recommendations offered. To be effective, the consultative relationship should be based on mutual trust and respect.

The effective consultant is one who listens to the needs, concerns, and problems of the clients and guides them in developing skills to meet those needs or solve their problems. The ineffective consultant tries to apply solutions or give advice without developing a helping relationship or taking the time to understand the client's real concerns.

There are a number of barriers to effective consultation. A major barrier is difficulty in communication resulting from the lack of mutual trust and respect. Establishing rapport is especially difficult if there are cultural differences between consultant and client, or if the consultant is much younger or less experienced than the client. To be effective, the consultant must have respect for the client's expertise and experience and have some understanding of that person's needs, values, and perceptions. Communication takes place only after two persons have developed some common or shared expectations and attach similar meanings to messages exchanged.[1]

An example of the difficulty in developing shared meaning might be the difficulties encountered by a therapist from a large northern city who is employed by a rural mountain southern school system. The therapist, seeking to consult with families of handicapped children, might find real differences in perceptions and values based on cultural differences in life-styles, traditions, and religion that result in lack of understanding and communication. There may also exist a distrust of the "outsider," regardless of how well-meaning the therapist might be. The therapist will need to develop communication and shared meaning on a personal level before it will be possible to develop a helping relationship on a professional level. This often takes time to develop—months or even years.

Other barriers to effective consultation may be attitudinal ones. Here are some examples:

1. Hostility: "Don't try to show me anything!"
2. Anger: "I don't want to be here."
3. Dependency: "You do it for me."
4. Apathy: "Who cares?"
5. Indifference: "Why change?"
6. Frustration: "Whenever I want to try something new, I can't get supplies."
7. Discouragement: "We tried that before, and it didn't work."

8. Denial: "Everything is fine; we don't have any problems."
9. Passive aggression: Verbally accepts suggestions, but later finds reasons not to carry them out.
10. Defensiveness: Gives excuses; excessive need to explain action or lack of action.

Administration and management

The fifth, and final, role of the occupational therapist in a school-based program is managing and supervising the occupational therapy program. This role includes developing and maintaining the occupational therapy program, managing occupational therapy personnel, documentation, and time management.

DEVELOPING THE OCCUPATIONAL THERAPY PROGRAM

The occupational therapist charged with the responsibility of developing an occupational therapy program in a school system uses exactly the same process as the occupational therapist charged with the responsibility of providing occupational therapy service to an individual child. This process includes needs assessment, program planning, implementation, and reevaluation.

The needs assessment, or evaluation phase, includes data collection and identification of needs, problems, and priorities. The therapist will find it helpful to collect data regarding the number of schools in the district, the number of handicapped students, the types of handicaps, the geographical locations of schools with handicapped children, and other related services available to students. In performing a needs assessment, the occupational therapist considers the occupational therapy needs of the school system. Have some children already been identified as needing therapy? What are high priority needs identified by school administrators for inservice training, consultation, and direct service? What needs have been identified by special education teachers? What are the expectations of parents regarding occupational therapy services? Are there particular problems to be addressed by the occupational therapist?

Once needs and priorities have been identified, the occupational therapist can design an occupational therapy program to meet these needs. Timelines should be established as guides for implementing the program. The program plan should include screening programs, service delivery models, types of therapy needs, recommendations for staff, anticipated caseloads, and budget for equipment and supplies.

The implementation phase includes the process of carrying out the established program plan. The occupational therapist evaluates, plans, and carries out intervention for individual students, as well as performs consultative and administration functions.

Reevaluation is concerned with assessing the effectiveness of the occupational therapy program. Goals and objectives of the program are reviewed along with the criteria for judging the effectiveness and efficiency of the program. Peer review or record review could be used in assessing the quality of occupational therapy services provided to individual children. As a result of the reevaluation process and quality review, weaknesses can be identified, and new needs may emerge. The circular process continues with additional program planning, implementation, and reevaluation (see also Chapter 31).

PERSONNEL

The occupational therapist in the school system is required to maintain certification and state licensure, if applicable. Some states also require teacher certification for therapists employed in school systems. The occupational therapist has a professional responsibility to maintain competency with current professional knowledge and skills. Some states require continuing education units as a part of licensure or teacher certification requirements.

Occupational therapists in the school system may have the responsibility for supervising other personnel, such as paraprofessionals (aides) or volunteers. This responsibility may include informal or formal training, assigning duties, overseeing the performance of these duties, and evaluating employee performance.

Certified occupational therapy assistants (COTAs) can make valuable contributions to the provision of occupational therapy services in the schools. It is appropriate for the COTA to implement occupational therapy services for certain students under guidelines established by the supervising occupational therapist. As the assistant demonstrates competency in the use of each procedure or treatment technique the need for close supervision decreases. Appropriate for the COTA are maintenance or repetitive treatments, those that can be defined without the need for ongoing professional judgment or interpretation, and some data gathering. The American Occupational Therapy Association has detailed roles of both levels of personnel in the school setting and set guidelines for supervision.[21]

DOCUMENTATION

Even though paperwork may appear to be a time-consuming burden, it is necessary to keep careful records for legal and professional reasons. Documentation is necessary for communication with team members, physicians, parents, and others. It is needed for careful and responsible planning, and is essential if a case is taken to court. A therapist may be required to prove that a child received adequate services or he may need to use documented evidence for defense against a charge of malpractice.

A therapist may keep personal records apart from the official files. These records may include written observations, personal anecdotal notes, and other recorded information maintained solely for personal use.

Test protocols also fall into this category, but the written report and interpretation are part of the official record.

In general, the following types of records should be kept:

1. General information
   a. Caseload date: Names, ages, and educational placement
   b. Number of times each student received occupational therapy and type of intervention (direct, monitoring, or consultation)
   c. Colleague consultation given, including in-service education
   d. Number and names of schools served by the itinerant occupational therapist
   e. Use of therapist's time for direct service, travel, supervision, monitoring, consultation, and meetings
2. Individual student information
   a. Referral, parental consent for evaluation, and assessment report
   b. Medical information and physician's referral, if indicated
   c. Individualized Education Program including occupational therapy goals and objectives, frequency, service delivery model, and duration of service
   d. Occupational therapy intervention plan
   e. Mid-year and/or end-of-year progress reports
   f. Case consultation reports for each contact
   g. Occupational therapy discharge report

CASELOADS AND TIME MANAGEMENT

Determination of an appropriate caseload and allocation of the therapist's time are subject to many variables: frequency of services needed by the child based on the therapist's evaluation, number of schools in which children are located, geographical distribution of schools, and time required for travel. Other variables are the amount of time required for meetings and staffings, amount of consultation requested, need for community contacts, time required for documentation, number of requests for in-service programming, and availability of paraprofessionals.

The School Systems Task Force of the American Occupational Therapy Association developed a formula to determine appropriate caseload numbers (Figure 29-10). By using this formula, an occupational therapist can account for the variables that influence time available for intervention and can also take into consideration the types of service delivery used.

The therapist first figures the actual amount of time available each week for direct service and monitoring. This is done by taking the total number of working hours and subtracting time used for other duties: assessments (including documentation), IEP and other meetings, consultation, research, travel between schools and supervision of aides. The time remaining is

Figure 29-10 Caseload Formula

$$ITA = 25 - T - S$$
ITA is *Intervention Time Available*
T is *Travel*
S is *Supervision*
$$ITA = 1.25\,DI + 0.625\,DG + 0.625\,M$$
DI is *Direct, individual*
30 minutes, twice a week
DG is *Direct, group*
2 per group, 30 minutes, twice a week or
4 per group, 1 hour, twice a week
M is *Monitoring*
30 minutes per week

Intervention Time Available (ITA) for direct service, monitoring, and documentation.

It is important to allot adequate time for documentation. In the formula, one quarter hour of documentation time is provided for every hour of student contact. The amount of time needed for a given number of students is calculated according to the service delivery model: individual, group, or monitoring.

Example: A therapist works a total of 35 hours per week in a local school system. He usually assesses one student per week, which includes one hour with the student, one hour writing the report, and ½ hour for other data collection. An average of 3 hours per week is spent in IEP and faculty meetings, and 2 hours per week are spent in colleague consultation. He spends an additional 2½ hours per week on a research project. Total time is figured as follows:

Assessment	2.5 hr
Meetings	3.0 hr
Consultation	2.0 hr
Research	2.5 hr
TOTAL	10.0 hr

When this figure is subtracted from 35 working hours this leaves 25 hours per week for direct contact, monitoring, and travel between schools. How many students should be on this therapist's caseload?

The therapist has been assigned to four schools. To visit each school at least twice a week requires that he spend a total of 2 hours travel time. Therefore the intervention time available (ITA) is 25 minus 2, or 23 hours per week. By substituting in the formula in Figure 29-10, the therapist has the following:

$$23 = 1.25\,DI + 0.625\,DG + 0.625\,M$$

At this point the therapist looks at his assigned caseload and planned intervention. He has 8 students for individual therapy twice a week and 10 students in groups of 2 twice a week. Each therapy session is ½ hour. The therapist needs to figure the number of additional students he can monitor. This is done by substituting in the formula:

$$23 = 1.25(8) + 0.625(10) + 0.625\,M$$
$$23 = 10 + 6.25 + 0.625M$$
$$23 = 16.25 + 0.625M$$
$$23 - 16.25 = 0.625M$$
$$6.75 = 0.625M$$
$$\frac{6.75}{0.625} = M$$
$$M = 10.8$$

Therefore, this therapist can handle ten more students for monitoring. Total caseload is 28 students.

CASE STUDY

Initiation of special education

Parent request. Brian, aged 5 years, 6 months, entered kindergarten in an urban elementary school in January of the school year after having attended a private nursery school. Brian's mother requested a staffing to explore the need for special education, and she obtained reports of recent evaluations for the in-school team to review.

Record review. Psychological, medical, occupational therapy, and physical therapy evaluations had been completed on an outpatient basis at a local hospital. According to the psychological reports, Brian had a low normal IQ, showed low self-esteem, was easily frustrated (especially with motor tasks), displayed acting-out and aggressive behaviors, and was depressed. The therapists reported these problems: crossing the midline of the body, equilibrium, fine and gross motor planning, graphic skills, prehension, and visual perception. It was reported that Brian was considerably delayed in language development and that his speech was difficult to understand. Medical reports indicated a normal physical examination with a history of ear infections and allergy. Hearing and vision were within normal limits. In addition to the services received from the hospital, the family participated in counseling sessions with a local agency.

Initial staffing. The in-school team, made up of the classroom teacher, speech therapist, occupational therapist, resource teachers for behavior disorders and learning disabilities, school psychologist, and parent, met on Brian's second day of school. The purpose of the meeting was to recommend evaluations and to decide on a 30-day interim placement while those evaluations were being completed. As a result of this meeting, Brian was placed in a regular kindergarten class with daily resource help from the behavior disorders teacher. Referrals were made for speech, occupational therapy, learning disabilities, and behavior disorder evaluations. Based on reports of previous evaluations and classroom observations, some goals were developed for the 30-day period. These were concerned with developing appropriate classroom behaviors and decreasing aggressiveness and fighting.

Occupational therapy assessment

Preevaluation data collection. The data collection for the occupational therapy assessment began with a review of the records, especially those of the previous occupational ther-

apy evaluation. After consulting with the occupational therapist who had worked with Brian previously, the present therapist decided to use the following in assessing Brian: parent and teacher interviews, informal observation, the Southern California Sensory Integration Tests, clinical observations, and informal assessment of play and developmental skills.

An interview was conducted with Brian's mother by use of a questionnaire of developmental and sensory behaviors. Responses to the questionnaire revealed a possible tactile problem. Brian had a habit of touching everything in sight; he frequently withdrew from touch, bumped and pushed other children, and wore a coat when not needed. Brian's mother also described coordination problems, possible auditory perception problems, and slowness in reaching developmental milestones. Brian turned over at 7 months, was slow talking, and, according to the mother, had trouble walking.

Brian's kindergarten teacher described an active, talkative child who pushed and hit other children and had difficulty attending to class activities. He lagged behind his classmates in readiness skills for reading and writing. Classroom observation during show-and-tell revealed that Brian sometimes watched and listened, but more often played with a toy car or wandered around the room.

Occupational therapy evaluation

Psychosocial skills: In the one-to-one testing environment Brian was lively and restless, sometimes refusing to attempt tasks presented to him. Although his behavior was often stubborn and manipulative, he appeared to have a desire to gain approval from adults. He responded well to a reward system that used a brightly colored sticker for appropriate behavior. However, in an unstructured group situation Brian had difficulty following rules, disobeyed adults, and antagonized his peers. When observed with his mother, Brian seemed rebellious and hostile.

Although Brian appeared aggressive and rebellious, he may have been using these behaviors to hide a low self-esteem and feelings of insecurity. His refusal to attempt tasks could be a defense mechanism to avoid failure. Brian refused to draw a boy, but did finish a drawing of an incomplete man. The therapist talked to Brian about this drawing, asking, "How does he feel inside?" Brian's only response was to scribble vigorously on the stomach of the man in the drawing. When asked, "Is he happy or sad?" Brian replied, "He's angry, angry at you!"

Brian enjoyed playing with small cars and trucks and toy guns, but avoided drawing and coloring, as well as toys that required fine motor skills. His play was often destructive in nature. He made pretend bombs, destroyed towns made of blocks, or had cars and trucks engage in massive wrecks. Brian's play was usually solitary; he had not yet developed interpersonal skills needed to play cooperatively with other children.

Developmental skills. Gross motor skills that did not require a great deal of balance, such as jumping, hopping, and skipping, were developmentally on age level. The abilities to balance on one foot and to walk heel-to-toe were 1 to 2 years below his chronological age. Upper extremity gross motor planning, as measured by the Imitation of Postures Test, was above the norm.

Brian's ability to manipulate small objects was on age level, although he would not remain on task for more than a few minutes. Eye-hand coordination, as measured by the Motor Accuracy Test, was above the norm for the right hand but significantly below the norm for the left. Brian is right-handed, but his left eye is dominant for sighting. He tended to use each hand on its own side of space, rather than crossing the midline of his body. Visual-motor integration, as indicated by the Design Copying Test, was significantly above the norm.

Although Brian's behaviors seem extreme, they must be viewed in light of normal emotional development. The 5½- to 6-year-old child is typically emotional, with aggressiveness and a false sense of self-confidence.[10] Brian's emotional difficulties appear to magnify and intensify the negative aspects of normal 6-year-old behavior.

Daily living skills. Brian was independent in age-appropriate feeding, dressing, and grooming skills, although his mother described his eating as sloppy. Occupational skills needed for the classroom were on the whole adequate. Brian could manipulate scissors to cut straight lines; he made jerky circular cuts when cutting a circle. He was learning to print letters of his name and displayed immature, but adequate, prehension patterns with pencils and crayons. Visual perceptual tests showed average functioning.

Sensorimotor skills. Sitting balance was poor with a dependence on external support. Brian was hypotonic and was unable to assume the prone extension position or maintain the flexed supine position. Brian was very unstable in a quadriped position and objected to having the therapist put her hands on his head to test for reflexes. He giggled and pulled away when he was touched and did not want his sleeves rolled up. There were indications of residuals of the symmetrical tonic neck reflex and lack of integration of righting reactions.

In addition to the clinical manifestations of tactile defensiveness, Brian scored poorly on tests for graphesthesia and localizing tactile stimuli. There were irregularities in diadochokinesia, rapid thumb to finger movement, and eye tracking. He was observed to avoid crossing the midline of the body in hand activities and in eye tracking. He also showed deficiencies in coordinating the two sides of his body.

The occupational therapist suspected vestibular problems because of Brian's low muscle tone, lack of postural stability, eye tracking problems, and difficulty with bilateral integration. However, Brian could not maintain a sitting position on a moving nystagmus board, and overhead hanging equipment for a net hammock was not available at his school. Therefore duration of nystagmus was not measured.

Evaluation summary. The occupational therapy evaluation indicated that Brian had a sensory integrative dysfunction in the areas of bilateral and postural integration, which could be a result of ineffective processing of the tactile system and possibly the vestibular system. There was also a disorder in psychosocial functioning in that the child displayed maladaptive methods of coping with his environment and in developing relationships both with adults and peers.

The following summary was written for the in-school team: This evaluation shows moderate sensory integrative dysfunction primarily in the areas of tactile functioning and bilateral motor integration. Significant findings are evidence of tactile defensiveness (avoidance of touch), difficulty in coordinating the two sides of the body (including avoidance of the midline and poor performance of nondominant hand), and unstable gross motor movement patterns.

The presence of tactile defensiveness has been linked with behavioral problems in some children who display aggressiveness and hyperactivity. Brian's tendency to overreact to tactile stimuli (fight-or-flight pattern) may account for some of his behavioral problems in the classroom.

Brian's inability to stabilize large postural muscles makes his movements appear clumsy and uncoordinated. When he is seated in a chair, his motor planning with his arms is adequate, but when he is seated in a cross-legged position on the mat, he can be pushed over easily. It is very important for Brian to have a chair of the proper size in the classroom so that his feet can be firmly on the floor. Round tables are not recommended, as they do not give enough surface for arm support.

Placement staffing

Review of evaluation data. The in-school team reconvened after the 30-day evaluation period to write goals and determine placement for Brian. Evaluation results were discussed. The speech therapist found no language deficits, but indicated that there were some articulation errors that interfered with the intelligibility of Brian's speech. Speech therapy was recommended twice a week. Testing in the area of learning disabilities showed that Brian did not meet the state requirements for this exceptionality and therefore would not need help from the learning disabilities teacher. The behavior disorders teacher found significant deficiencies in accepting authority from adults, relating to peers, and in developing acceptable behavior patterns. The occupational therapist reported on the results of the occupational therapy assessment and recommended occupational therapy on an individual basis two times a week.

Development of the Individualized Education Program. All of the evaluation results were used in developing statements of present levels of performance for the Individualized Education Program. These were in the following areas: academic achievement, social-emotional adjustment, communication skills, psychomotor skills, career-vocational areas, self-help skills, and physical-medical considerations. Next, goals were written for each of the identified deficit areas needing intervention from special education and support services. The occupational therapy goals were as follows:

Annual goal: To improve sensory integration and postural stability.

Objectives:

1. When working on a pencil-and-paper task at the table, Brian will remain in his chair and cross the midline of his body 80% of the time without verbal reminders.
2. When touched on the arm, leg, or face without visual cues, Brian will locate the touch accurately without withdrawing four out of five times.
3. Brian will play a game requiring him to balance on three extremities without falling 70% of the time.

Special education placement. Based on the information gathered and the needs that had been identified, the team agreed that Brian's primary exceptionality was behavior disorders. The next task was to decide on the most appropriate and least restrictive educational placement for Brian. The team agreed that Brian's needs could be met with placement in a regular kindergarten class with a resource class for behavior disorders 2 hours daily and itinerant services from the speech therapist and occupational therapist. All of these services were available at the present school, so no change in school placement was needed. Brian's mother agreed to this placement.

Occupational therapy intervention

Frequency of service. Brian was considered to have high priority for occupational therapy services. However, when Brian entered school in January, the therapist already had more than the maximum number of children on her caseload. Consequently Brian received occupational therapy only one time a week.

Occupational therapy activities. A sensory integrative approach was used, with an emphasis on tactile and vestibular input. Brian participated eagerly and responded positively to the tasks presented, but sometimes continued his manipulative behaviors. As a result, it was necessary to provide therapy sessions that were structured, yet included opportunity for movement exploration and experimentation.

Therapy activities included numerous scooter board activities and games that challenged balance in quadruped and sitting positions. Tactile input was given by rubbing the extremities with various textures and by rolling up in a rug. Brian especially enjoyed the latter, which probably indicated a need for the moving touch-pressure stimulus it provided. Spinning was used cautiously, as Brian sometimes complained of nausea or headache following this stimulation. Proprioceptive input was given with activities such as the wheelbarrow walk.

Review staffing

In June of the school year the in-school team met again to review goals and objectives in the Individualized Education Program and to write a program for the next school year. The team agreed that Brian had made tremendous progress during the year. Some of the goals for improving behavior and interpersonal skills had been met, and his kindergarten teacher felt he was ready for first grade. The occupational therapist's progress report read in part:

> "Brian has shown a great deal of improvement in the short time he has received occupational therapy. He is better able to tolerate tactile (touch) stimuli and has much better control of large muscle movements. Although Brian sometimes acted in a manipulative, demanding, or stubborn manner, he always responded to firm limits and completed the task. He appeared to enjoy the sessions, and on a one-to-one situation, his behavior was controllable. However, on at least one occasion he verbalized hostile, destructive feelings toward the school and adults, saying, 'I'm going to put bombs in the school,' and 'I want to shoot arrows in all the teachers.' "

The occupational therapist recommended continuation of occupational therapy for the next school year in a group of two or three children. Previous goals for occupational therapy had not yet been achieved, so they were carried over to the next year's Individualized Education Program. In addition, the occupational therapist and behavior disorders teacher agreed to work jointly to develop appropriate group behavior and classroom coping skills. The following goals were added:

Annual goal: To improve classroom behavior and coping skills.

Objectives:

1. When working on an activity in a group of three children, Brian will remain in his place and allow the other children to participate in the activity without interruption 70% of the time.
2. Brian will take turns while playing a game with another child without adult direction 80% of the time.
3. When frustrated with a task, Brian will ask for assistance without destroying materials four out of five times.

A new Individualized Education Program was completed with goals for behavior disorders, speech therapy, and occupational therapy. It is anticipated that Brian will continue to improve with these services so that eventually he can participate fully in a regular educational environment.

SUMMARY

This chapter described occupational therapy in the school system and the roles of the occupational therapist within that setting. These roles are evaluating, program planning, implementing services, consulting, managing, and supervising. The occupational therapist, in carrying out these roles, provides occupational therapy services in nine steps: (1) obtain referral, (2) obtain parental consent, (3) perform evaluation, (4) communicate results of the evaluation, (5) determine need for services, (6) write IEP with Educational Planning Team, (7) develop intervention plan, (8) implement intervention, and (9) reevaluate students.

The function of the occupational therapist in the school system is to provide related services to students with impairments in functional abilities in the classroom. The purpose of occupational therapy intervention is to increase functional levels of students so that they are able to benefit from special education.

STUDY QUESTIONS

1. How do the differences in medical and educational models contribute to role conflict for the occupational therapist in a school setting?
2. What are some reasons why a child who receives occupational therapy in a medical clinic might not be eligible for occupational therapy at school?
3. Name some appropriate ways of screening students for occupational therapy in the school setting.
4. What are the purposes and functions of the educational planning team?
5. How does the occupational therapy intervention plan differ from the IEP?
6. What are team consensus goals?
7. How does the school-based occcupational therapist determine when to terminate services to a student?
8. Name the three types of consultation. How do they differ?
9. Discuss the role of the certified occupational therapist assistant in the school system.
10. How many students can a therapist schedule for individual sessions if she has 20 hours available for intervention (after travel has been deducted) and already has 16 students in group sessions? She has no students for monitoring.

REFERENCES

1. Baskin OW, and Aronoff C: Interpersonal communication in organizations, Santa Monica, Calif, 1980, Goodyear Publishing Co, Inc.
2. Binder-Macleod C, and Walden G: Adaptive equipment construction with Tri-wall cardboard. In Occupational therapy in practice, vol 1, Rockville, Md, 1983, The American Occupational Association, Inc.
3. Consultation. In Gilfoyle E, editor: Training: occupational therapy educational management in schools, vol 3, module 5, Rockville, Md, 1980, American Occupational Therapy Association, Inc.
4. Education of handicapped children: implementation of part B of the Education of the Handicapped Act, Fed Reg 42:163, 1977.
5. Educational/medical models and occupational therapy as a related service. In Gilfoyle E, editor: Training: occupational therapy educational management in schools, vol 4, module 8, Rockville, Md, 1980, American Occupational Therapy Association, Inc.
6. Farber SD: Neurorehabilitation: a multisensory approach, Philadelphia, 1982, WB Saunders Co.
7. Gilfoyle E, and Farace J: The role of occupational therapy as an education-related service, Am J Occup Ther 35:811, 1981.
8. Guidelines for Occupational Therapy Services in School Systems, Rockville, Md, 1987, American Occupational Therapy Association, Inc.
9. Houston J: Inexpensive adaptive positioning equipment for a multiply handicapped child, Occupational Therapy in Practice, vol 1, Rockville, Md, 1983, American Occupational Therapy Association, Inc.
10. Ilg FL, and Ames LB: The Gesell Institute's child behavior, New York, 1981, Harper & Row, Publishers, Inc.
11. Kahn RF, and others: Organizational stress: studies in role conflict and ambiguity, New York, 1964, John Wiley & Sons, Inc.
12. Katz D, and Kahn R: Social psychology of organizations, New York, 1966, John Wiley & Sons, Inc.
13. Lemerand P: Inservice training packet. In Gilfoyle E, editor: Training: occupational therapy educational management in schools, vol 4, module 7, Rockville, Md, 1980, American Occupational Therapy Association, Inc.
14. Magrum WM, and Tigges KN: A transdisciplinary mobile intervention program for rural areas, Am J Occup Ther 36:90, 1982.
15. Muhlenhaupt M: Occupational therapy in New York public schools, Northport, NY, 1985, The Press Room at TMC.
16. Nondiscrimination on basis of handicap: programs and activities receiving or benefiting from federal financial assistance, Fed Reg 42:86, 1977.
17. *PARC vs Commonwealth of Pennsylvania,* 344 F Supp 1257, 1971.
18. Rebell MA: Implementation of court mandates concerning special education: the problems and the potential, J Law Educ 10:335, 1981.
19. Regan NN: The implementation of occupational therapy services in rural school systems, Am J Occup Ther 36:85, 1982.
20. Service delivery. In Gilfoyle E, editor: Training: occupational therapy educational management in schools, vol 3, module 5, Rockville, Md, 1980, American Occupational Therapy Association, Inc.
21. Roles of Occupational Therapists and Occupational Therapy Assistants. In: Guidelines for occupational therapy services in school systems, Rockville, Md, 1987, The American Occupational Therapy Association, Inc.
22. Standards of practice for occupational therapy services in schools. In: Guidelines for occupational therapy services in school systems, Rockville, Md, 1987, The American Occupational Therapy Association, Inc.
23. Task force on target populations, Am J Occup Ther 28:158, 1974.
24. West WF: The principles and process of consultation. In Llorens LA, editor: Consultation in the community: occupational therapy in child health, Dubuque, Iowa 1973, Kendall/Hunt Publishing Co.

SUGGESTED READINGS

Creighton C: The school therapist and vocational education, Am J Occup Ther 33:373, 1979.

Gilfoyle E, editor: Training: occupational therapy educational management in schools, vols 1-4, Rockville, Md, 1980, American Occupational Therapy Association, Inc (Supported by Grant #G007801499, US Dept of Education, Office of Special Education and Rehabilitative Services.)

Gilfoyle E, and Hays C: Occupational therapy roles and functions in the education of the school-based handicapped student, Am J Occup Ther 33:565, 1979.

Kinnealey M, and Morse AB: Educational mainstreaming of physically handicapped children, Am J Occup Ther 33:365, 1979.

McCormick L, and Lee C: PL 94-142: mandated partnerships, Am J Occup Ther 33:586, 1979.

Mitchell MM: Occupational therapy and special education, Children 18:183, 1971.

Mitchell MM, and Lindsey D: A model for establishing occupational therapy and physical therapy services in public schools, Am J Occup Ther 33:361, 1979.

Ottenbacher K: Occupational therapy and special education: some issues and concerns related to PL 94-142, Am J Occup Ther 36:81, 1982.

Punwar A, and Wendt E: Certification of occupational therapists in the public schools: The Wisconsin experience, Am J Occup Ther 34:727, 1980.

30

Private practice in pediatric occupational therapy

JANICE POSATERY BURKE

In recent years dramatic changes in the health care delivery and financing industry have occurred. Increased consumer involvement and decentralized, noninstitutional health care models have provided for "an unprecedented expansion and innovation in an industry that appeared tradition bound and impervious to the forces of supply and demand."[4] These changes have created greater opportunities for entrepreneurial efforts in providing care to acutely and chronically ill individuals.

Occupational therapists have been part of the new health care movement, having owned and participated in private practices for many years. Within the last 10 years, many more pediatric occupational therapists have entered private practice. The 1986 American Occupational Therapists Association (AOTA) Member Data Survey[1] reported 6% of all occupational therapists to be in private practice, as contrasted to 1.3% in 1973. This rising number of therapists in private practice is greatly a result of Public Law 94-142, which mandated education in public schools for all handicapped children. Opportunities immediately arose for entrepreneurial occupational therapists to sell services under various privately administered formats to the public school system.

Many health care agencies have become more interested in attracting private practice occupational therapists for many reasons. Economically speaking, many facilities cannot afford full-time occupational therapy services. There are also "people power" reasons. Institutions may be unable to attract full-time occupational therapy services because of locale, salary scale, character of facility, degree of professional isolation, or legal and economic agendas. Facilities may need to come into compliance with federal and state regulations and accreditation. In some cases, facilities have been unaware of occupational therapy. Along with these institutional based needs for private practice, demand for direct, non-institutional, private therapy has grown.[9]

"Occupational therapy is fast becoming known as a friend to a growing society of smart patients and health care personnel who want delivery on their own terms."[4] Occupational therapists in private practice are no longer unknown community resources and are finding many advantages in private practice. They are reaching more people as they offer tailor made services to address individual patient needs.[5] Their ability to provide these services is enhanced when they are released from the constraints of hospital or clinic policy. Therapists in private practice are able to offer services following hospital discharge. They can schedule appointments for times that best serve client goals. Appointments can be made during dinner time to work on feeding skills, or during bath time to help with self-care skills. A private practice allows a great deal of flexibility with program development and implementation. There are few bureaucratic procedures for initiating a new program. In a private practice, the therapist identifies a need, develops the program, identifies the patients, and offers the services.

On the other hand, the private practitioner must develop competence in two very different areas: one, as the professional therapist with a specific set of knowledge and skills; and two, as the business person, able to organize and administer a business and make timely and key financial decisions.

☐ The author wishes to express her appreciation to Erna Blanche, Tamera Lynch, and Bonnie Nakasuji, her associates in practice at Therapy West in Culver City, California.

612

CURRENT MODELS OF PRIVATE PRACTICE

In a private practice, the therapist has the opportunity to select the kind of practice that reflects individual skill and style as well as community need. For example, a therapist living in a rural area may have a practice that is primarily oriented to consultation—seeing individuals for evaluation and recommending a course of treatment to be carried out by someone else; another therapist in a more urban area may choose to specialize in treating only children or only a specific diagnostic group. The style selected depends on the population served, their needs, funding sources, and the clinician's personal goals.

The world of private practice increases the number and variety of individuals with whom one does business. Landlords, insurance agents, accountants, builders and carpenters, office equipment and medical equipment sales representatives—all are business contacts with whom the private practitioner enters into contract negotiations, lease agreements, and financial arrangements. Private practitioners have great control over their individual practices. As in any small business where the owners set their own hours, they often work extremely hard at first. In time, the owners of new businesses establish their individual pace and define the specific areas of interest where they enjoy success in doing what they most want to do.

Sole practitioner

Working alone, the sole practitioner offers services directly to patients on a fee-for-service basis. In this type of practice, the therapist works by and for herself, other than during vacations or other temporary periods of absence (such as maternity leave, short-term consulting out-of-town, disability, or an increase in other service-related demands).

A major benefit to being a sole practitioner is autonomy and independence in everyday work. The sole practitioner establishes policy for office procedures, makes decisions about the shape and form of the practice, and solves problems that are met along the way. These policies include the kinds of services to be provided and the fee and payment schedules. Initially, the owner may have empty client hours to fill while setting up the practice and may contract with other agencies to fill out her work week. For example, she may provide 8 hours of evaluation and consultation for a nearby preschool for children with disabilities.[5]

Contracting individual clients as a sole practitioner is the basis for generating paid patient contact hours. The description of the services provided form the details of the agreement between the service provider and the client being served. The product of the sole practitioner is the individual work that she does herself or hires others to perform. The private practitioner in some cases may hire other therapists (both registered and assistant) to provide for treatment and evaluation. This is known as subcontracting.

When the individual service provider meets parents who are interested in having their child evaluated and treated by a therapist, the service provider must demonstrate self-confidence, competence, and an understanding of what specific services the child needs. Both the background and experience of the private practitioner contribute to her ability to communicate information directly to the parents. Parents are looking for help. They want to match the personality and skill of the practitioner to their child's needs, as they perceive them.

A private practice includes a collage of professional roles and positions. A private practitioner may choose to define her practice as oriented in a specific area such as evaluation and treatment, education, writing, or special workshops. Some practitioners act as vendors for the equipment that they provide to patients. Some practitioners combine small research grants into their practices. The choice is an individual one that reflects the specific desires of the individual practitioner.

Group practitioner

Alternatives to being a sole practitioner include the combining of two or more sole practitioners into an association, joint venture, or partnership. As an associate, one may continue to maintain one's private practice with sole responsibility for it, but work with, hire, or subcontract parts of the business to other occupational therapists, speech therapists, nutritionists, or physical therapists.

Two or more therapists may form an associate relationship to meet a specific need; for example, to share space and equipment. Other associate relationships may include professionals from other disciplines who collaborate on specific cases, providing consultation and services to complement specific patient needs.

The associate relationship must be based on a written agreement that is legally binding. This agreement must outline the roles and responsibilities of each associate. The nature of the relationship, financial considerations, rights and duties of individuals, terms of termination, and other similar issues are spelled out in this document.

Registry services

Sometimes the focus of a practice shifts to matching the needs of agencies and individual patients to other therapists. This business might take the form of an occupational therapy registry or a clinic where the owner provides sales, marketing, and managerial skills, and hires therapists to provide services to individuals and health agencies. There are many ways to assemble administrative and therapeutic skills to meet the needs of agencies and individual clients. Enterprising therapists can design and benefit from many models of business organization, under the rubric of private practice.

CHARACTERISTICS NEEDED IN PRIVATE PRACTICE

When thinking about establishing a private practice, it is important to seek first hand knowledge by spending time with other individuals engaged in the kind of practice you want to have. This may include other occupational therapists who are doing the specific activities you want to do as well as other health care professionals who have the kind of private practice desired. After spending time with various private practitioners (occupational therapists, psychologists, nutritionists, physicians), a sense of the kind of qualities or skills that are common denominators emerges: idea-oriented vision, capacity for risk-taking, persistence and energy, public relations skills, and money management skills.

Idea-oriented vision. Occupational therapists in private practice must have ideas for new areas of practice that are generally different from offerings in established clinics and schools. Visions for uncommon and innovative treatment strategies are often the foundation of a successful private practice.

Capacity for risk-taking. Starting new programs and developing a new business means stepping off into the unknown. This situation demands coping with great levels of uncertainty. Risk-takers[10] view this as a challenge rather than a stress.

Persistence and energy. Reaching the goal of establishing and developing a private practice is directly related to the energy and persistence applied to it. Being organized with identified support systems and resource people to call on for specific issues will permit energy to be focused on what must be done. It is important to find support among other professionals who can provide knowledge in unfamiliar areas (such as accountants, special equipment manufacturers and suppliers) and those who can provide collegial support as peers.

Public relations skills. Generally, a small business owner who deals directly with the public must have good person-to-person skills. He must be able to communicate, hearing a client's concerns, fears, and goals, and be able to present himself, his skills, and his position on an issue in an organized and professional way. Private practitioners must be able to generate confidence in their services and their profession. In addition, it is necessary to communicate with a wide range of persons, not only health professionals and parents, but other business people as well. Effective communication contributes dramatically to the stature of the practitioner within the health and the business communities.

For example, many offices and businesses share parking lots, and available disabled parking spaces are often used indiscriminately. Because this affects patients, the therapist must approach the other businesses and enlist their cooperation in keeping the space clear for patients. The therapist's attitude about the patients she serves directly influences her business neighbors.

Money management skills. It takes time to turn the corner on any business and begin to make money rather than spend it. One should be prepared financially to decrease present earning levels while developing the business that can eventually increase financial opportunities. Both income and expenses must be managed so that times of decreased earnings and low census do not present a fiscal emergency. The books must be kept in an orderly and timely fashion. Patients must be asked to pay and be reminded when they do not fulfill their obligations.

Experience. An occupational therapist who wants to work in private practice must ask himself: Do I have enough background and experience to effectively handle the variety of complex health care issues and treatment demands that will face me? Would I be better off seeking additional training and work experience first? Would I be better off working in a group with more experienced therapists? Although there are no formal guidelines concerning how much clinical experience a therapist needs before working as a sole practitioner, there is no doubt that it is not a work situation for the recent graduate. A sole practitioner must have expertise, maturity, and advanced reasoning skills.

DEVELOPMENT AND ORGANIZATION OF THE PEDIATRIC PRIVATE PRACTICE

The first and most important step in developing a private practice is to envision services as a business and to develop a business plan. The business plan is a detailed description of the proposed private practice. A wide range of resources on starting businesses are available at libraries and bookstores. In addition, business courses are offered in community colleges, adult education programs, and through the Small Business Administration of the federal government. The components of a business plan are:

- Defining the service
- Determining the existing market
- Determining sources of income
- Estimating start-up and operation costs
- Projecting income
- Setting a realistic time table

Defining the service one intends to offer and the population one intends to serve is the first step. From this information, goals are set and strategies to meet them are determined. The therapist should take an inventory of her own skills (what she does well) and her level of motivation (what she most likes to do) and then determine:

- What population she wants to serve
- What needs of this population are unmet

- What services she would enjoy providing
- Where the patients are geographically located
- What economic condition prevails in the area
- How the projected population will pay for service
- What competition exists

Determining the existing market requires a careful and realistic appraisal of the need for the service and the kind of work that is required to get the service into operation.[6,11] In pre-practice discussions one may approach various potential referral sources, asking them to estimate how many patients they may be able to refer, in what time frame, and the kinds of problems those individuals may have. From this kind of raw data fruitful contacts may be identified and numbers of patients estimated. Also, in discussions with other private practitioners, one can begin to estimate how many "potentials" turn into "real" fee-generating work.

Determining sources of income, other than patient fees, then budgeting time and effort for them is important. Initially there is much expenditure of time and money with less than adequate pay-off, or so it appears. With careful attention you will be able to determine which ones will be investments in the future of the practice.

At this point, thinking becomes concrete. How many patients will be seen for evaluation, treatment, and consultation in a given month? How many patients will be seen regularly? Occasionally? How many total hours will be spent in treatment and evaluation, with estimations of indirect costs? Indirect cost of time and money should include non-service activity such as writing reports and telephone time.

Estimating start-up costs requires the therapist to clarify on paper exactly what will be needed to begin serving patients (Figure 30-1). If treatment space is rented, rental costs must be estimated for the time it will take before enough money is earned to pay expenses. One-time expenses, such as a logo or the design work necessary for your practice, the occasional costs such as printing business cards and stationery, and costs for such regular needs as accounting and cleaning must also be included.

In addition, the cost of both office and treatment equipment and any structural changes necessary to make the space safe and durable must be included in intitial cost figures. Additional costs are those such as making the bathroom accessible, installing the beam necessary for suspended equipment, making the lighting adequate, and installing suitable flooring.

Other costs to consider are phone service installation, deposit, and phone equipment; answering machine and service fees; first and last months' rent and security; large treatment equipment; and postage.

Net income is projected by subtracting expenses from gross income. At this point, it is necessary to be realistic about what actual income is necessary to make ends meet. The target income should be established by calculating how many patients must be seen in a week

---

Figure 30-1 Expenses

ONE TIME EXPENSES

Structural changes to office space such as: overhead beam installation and flooring
Fabrication of hook system
Telephone system
Therapy equipment
Lease-related expenses (first and last months' rent, security deposits)
Artwork/graphics for letterhead, cards, brochures
Computer and related equipment
Office furniture

OCCASIONAL EXPENSES

Printing stationery, cards, brochures
Special mailings
Therapy materials/supplies
Repairs
Accounting and legal fees
Business license, permits
Taxes
Insurance premiums (professional and general liability, health, disability)
Educational expenses
Professional organization fees, Chamber of Commerce fees

REGULAR EXPENSES

Phone
Rent (office, equipment)
Postage
Copying
Outreach
Expenses related to billing, bookkeeping
Employee salaries and benefits
Offices and routine therapy supplies
Cleaning expenses

---

and the number of hours that must be worked to achieve it.

Any realistic plan must also build in room for unforeseen change. Agencies that initially were considered "good" possibilities may close, may change their policy, or decide to hire a full-time therapist. Underestimations and overestimations are possible and plans must be flexible.

Establishing a bank account is part of opening a business; the account becomes an important record for accurately tracking gross income (what comes in) and net income (what is left after expenses). Talking with bank personnel will identify the range of financial services available and the convenience of those services; all will require careful records of time spent with patients, in consultation, and in administrative tasks.

Consultation with an accountant will help clarify the need for financial services.[9] Client account records are merely logs of the actual transactions of the practice. In addition to setting these up, an accountant is knowledgeable about small businesses, can provide advice regarding leasing or subleasing, and can help determine the amount of capital necessary to support business start-up and how far funds can and should be stretched.

After each step of the business plan is written, a *realistic time-table must be set* for each task and a realistic time frame developed for the growth of the business. Certain business tasks precede the establishment of any business: obtaining a business license and establishing a record system. Employee records are required by law. These and other records such as tax, interest, and purchasing are useful for accurately understanding the financial aspects of the business and answering financial questions—is it making or losing money? Is financing adequate for day-to-day operation?

Records allow the estimation of tax payments and establish the worth of the business for future ventures such as taking in a partner or selling the practice.

Finding suitable space. Space needs are defined by the kind of practice and will vary for consultant in-home and office-based services. Will service be provided in the therapist's home or the patient's? How is equipment to be stored or transported? What office space is required? Among the considerations for clinic space (known as studio space to realtors) will be the kind of treatment to be given, the number of patients to be seen at any given time, and the interval between treatments. Consider logistics such as whether children will arrive with rain and snow gear that must be stowed, and whether siblings and extended family will accompany patients to treatments regularly and require a waiting room.

What age children will the practice serve? A wide range in ages and needs necessitates different kinds of treatment areas—an infant evaluation area, an area for visual motor activities, appropriate space for sensory integration treatment. Are separate testing areas and meeting space needed? Project how the practice should be operating in 6 months, 1 year, 3 years. For example, one plan might be to subcontract services out to other therapists within 9 to 12 months of starting, which would require as many as three therapists to use the office during a given treatment hour. Is space adequate to accommodate that number of children, caretakers, and siblings? Natural lighting, accessibility and convenience, parking, noise generated within office and treatment areas are additional factors to consider when leasing or subleasing an office.

Another option is to establish the practice out of the therapist's home, using space there for phone and desk work and doing all of the treatments in patients' homes. There are many benefits to such an in-home based practice. Financially, there is less risk because of no investment in office space. Expenses are primarily in special equipment (such as a portable sensory integration system), evaluation and assessment tools, and treatment materials (toys, toys, toys). Freedom from rent payments and other overhead makes starting up such a practice much less stressful. There are, however, hidden costs and expenses such as car maintenance and repair, gasoline, and weather factors. There are problems inherent in storing and transporting treatment equipment and materials and finding adequate space in each home to perform treatments. In addition, time and distance between patient contacts must be considered. If it takes 1 hour to get from child to child, then contact hours will be reduced by 50%. In turn, earnings will be down by one half.

An in-the-child's home practice may be a necessity for the target population. Children who are ventilator-dependent or oxygen-dependent, older children who are more physically involved and more difficult to transport, and children who are residents of a skilled nursing facility or other extended care home would be likely candidates for this model of practice.

A significant advantage of testing children in their own homes is the valuable opportunity it provides to look at the child's ability to adapt to everyday life situations. What happens to the child who has a moderate motor disability when her big sisters and friends come around? How does she keep up? Is she included in part of their play? Is she able to cope? What are the demands on the caregivers? Is it realistic to ask the mother to work on feeding skills with her child at dinner time when in reality she has two other small children to feed along with other evening responsibilities?

Starting the business. Establishing therapy policy is a way of ensuring that professional standards are maintained throughout the practice.[8] Policies are related to a philosophy and principles of practice. When in private practice, one must have internalized standards that reflect what occupational therapy is and how it should be practiced. Treatment policy must be clearly defined in written form if the practice includes hired employees. In this case, a handbook that explains in detail the requirements and responsibilities of personnel in the practice is useful. Such a document may include a general description of the practice (goals and objectives), job descriptions for personnel, referral, evaluation, and treatment procedures, billing specifications, a statement regarding standards of practice, note-writing guides, and any pertinent therapy procedures. Insurance and legal issues include the need for *comprehensive general liability insurance* to protect the practice against non-professional claims such as accidents to clients, families, or personnel that may occur during business operations. Additionally, treatment that is performed in another facility (for example, an extended care facility) must also be covered by insurance. Many insurance companies provide general liability plans.

The second type of essential insurance is *professional liability insurance.* This insurance protects the therapist against claims arising from real or alleged malpractice errors or negligence in the course of professional duties. *Health and disability insurance* are an integral part of the overall insurance package. All self-employed persons, and this includes professional practitioners, must establish these traditional benefit packages for themselves. The therapist must seek out insurance and benefit packages that suit the needs of the specific private practice organization. Local insurance agents are appropriate sources of direct and indirect assistance. Ongoing evaluation will be necessary to determine if the purchased packages will fully satisfy the needs of the practice.

Generating referrals will require that the population that is right for the therapist's service be identified and the service made known to the population. One strategy may be to offer free screenings in preschools or elementary schools that will show whether in-depth occupational therapy evaluations should be undertaken. Provided as a service to parents and referral agencies, these screenings build visibility for the practice and yield referrals for treatment.[12] (See Marketing, page 619.)

A private practice has its own cycles of high and low census or "seasonal effects."[7] Patterns of high referral, low absences, or more frequent cancellations appear regularly. With children some periods of evaluation and treatment cycles are predictable. For example, a new school year may bring more referrals; holiday and winter time bring more absences. Summer vacations bring new treatment schedules and possibilities for group, camp, or other special program offerings.[7]

Among the specific skills that assist in establishing a caseload are the interdisciplinary skills for communicating with other professionals who may refer patients, and family communication skills for interacting with the patient and family. Specifically, the therapist needs to be able to develop skills in (1) giving and receiving information; (2) understanding cues and clues from parents; (3) establishing rapport—nothing happens until everything that can possibly get in the way gets out of the way; (4) setting pace and rhythm of a family interview; (5) judging comfort and mood; (6) establishing an empathic identification with a parent—be who they are, see as they do; (7) being able to give information, using examples and checking that it has been accurately received; (8) reinforcing changes parent and child make; and (9) confronting difficult behavior.

The therapist's practice is a reflection of oneself. All of the subtle details (where it it located, how it is maintained, how the practitioner presents himself through dress and other particulars) will give parents and colleagues an idea or feeling about the practitioner's competence. Therefore, attention must be paid to specific details to create an environment that conveys the desired message. As an example, cards and stationery should be carefully chosen. A card with printed credentials is an introduction of one's professional status. It also gives colleagues and potential clients the information they need about location and telephone number. Whether to develop a logo or business identification design is a personal decision. The choice of such design will depend on the kind of persons to be attracted and the image to be conveyed. For example, one pediatric dentist had his card printed on paper that represented a school blackboard. The lettering was printed to resemble a child's printing, complete with several reverse letters. A nutritionist who counsels young women has a pink card. Other images conveyed through paper and lettering include sophistication, technical skill, humor, gender-related characteristics, a feeling of caring, stability, healing, or affluence.

ADMINISTRATION AND MANAGEMENT OF PEDIATRIC PRIVATE PRACTICE

In managing a private practice, primary consideration must be given to the kinds of contracts available, the kinds of records to be kept, and marketing efforts.

Contractual practices

Independent contractors set up the terms of service obligations to a particular agency in constrast to the full-time paid employee who fills a previously established terms of service contract in return for a regular salary along with a benefit package and supervised, regular work. Independent contractors construct their own terms for providing the necessary work, based on their professional judgment and standards of practice (Figure 30-2).

In both the consultative and service contract, the therapist and administrator spell out the specific details of their relationship in a formal, written agreement. This contract outlines the service to be provided, the term of the agreement, the fees for service, and the details regarding liability, equipment, space, and other specifics of the obligation. Timetables for renegotiation and termination should be spelled out.

Contracts are best negotiatied by the person defining the service, that is, the therapist. Her ability to give accurate and complete information, clarify communications, and answer concerns in a confident and thoughtful way will lend credence to her professional image and is essential to establishing a fruitful working relationship with an administrator. Renegotiating a previous contract provides the opportunity to change things that did not work the first time around.

Any contract negotiation requires a clear idea of what is needed to provide the quality and quantity of service requested. A contracting therapist assumes a wide range of risks. The number of evaluations and treatments to be delivered varies and there are no traditional employee benefits such as sick time, vacation time, and health insurance. An independent contrac-

Figure 30-2   Employee status vs private practitioner status

EMPLOYEE	PRIVATE PRACTITIONER
Fixed, regular income	Pay negotiable with each individual patient, contract, or other service rendered
Minimal wage-related record keeping	Detailed record keeping required
Minimal administrative burden	Maximum administrative responsibilities
Benefits built into salary	Carry and pay insurance coverage, no paid sick leave, vacation time
Facilities/equipment provided by employer	Rent/own office, purchase/rent equipment
Facility sets work schedule	Establish own work patterns
Taxes withheld routinely	Quarterly tax payment made
Identification with an organization	Establish own identity in health community
Continuing education/travel expenses provided	Pay own continuing education/travel expenses
Fit into allotted work space within facility	Select and design work space
Support services provided (xerox, typing)	Provide own support services
Patient billing services provided	Handle billing to third party payors, private individuals, and/or contract agencies
Access to other professionals within facility	Must seek out other professionals for advice, case consulation, collaborative endeavors
Development decisions made for you	Plan and develop practice based on own ideas and efforts
Job and income security	Less secure income

tor's rate for reimbursement should be higher than that of a regular employee because of the assumption of these risks.

Clinical and administrative records

There are two kinds of records to be kept—patient records and business records. Patient records include all patient-related data such as intake forms (Figure 30-3), reports, evaluations, histories, progress notes, attendance records, videotapes, and still pictures. Business records include all documents that relate to business transactions such as accounting records, bank statements, invoices and receipts for supplies and equipment, insurance policies, rental agreements, inventories of equipment and supplies, and contracts.

In both cases, the ability to keep organized and systematic records is important to the practice. For example, all intake information on patients should be kept in the same way, noting important details such as the referral source, initial evaluation dates, and fee and payment plans. By devising forms and procedures and establishing files, one can collect and maintain professional and business data so that it is useful and easily accessible.

Organized records and a computer are valuable aids for analyzing certain aspects of business: where referrals are coming from, what type of outreach and advertising efforts have paid off, or how many patients are seen in an average month. Such organization also assists in maintaining the kind of practice planned for,

with letters and requests answered routinely, referrals acknowledged promptly, and billings and receipts handled in a timely way.

Other procedures for handling records and information such as daily charting are established in accordance with professional and legal requirements. Along with formats for evaluations, reports, and charting, a set format for routine writing tasks saves time and energy. In all cases, it is critical to develop writing skills. Insurance carriers, contracting agencies, and other professionals all prefer information that is brief, concise, and coherent.

In general, paperwork is a time-consuming aspect of any work situation. Because time is directly linked to income and work is directly linked to credibility, it may be helpful to establish some routines to help keep things in place: using the same block of time each week to take care of scoring evaluations and writing reports, using another for answering and initiating correspondence. In both cases, it is critical to build time into the daily schedule for such tasks.

Issues associated with setting and collecting fees are often emotionally and professionally charged for private practitioners. Establishing a fee that reflects the therapist's personal sense of worth along with her comfort is the first step in conquering this new territory. Fees are based on a serious and careful review of target income less expenses. It is helpful to determine what other professionals such as inpatient, outpatient, and home health providers are paid for comparable services. It is important to develop skill in verbally han-

---

Figure 30-3   Sample intake form

PATIENT INFORMATION

Today's date   Referral source:

Child's name:
Birthdate:
Parents:
Address:
Phone numbers: (home)
                          (Work-mother)
                          (Work-father)
                          (Daycare)
Payment:
Insurance carrier:
Child's pediatrician:
Other physicians, psychologists, therapists (including
    agencies) involved with child:
Other agency information:
    Case manager
School information:
    School
    Grade
    Teacher
Plan:

Figure 30-4   Sample release form

I hereby authorize _____ *(name)*
                        _____ *(address)*
                        _____
to release all medical, educational, psychosocial,
    developmental, _____ *(other)*
information regarding _____ *(name)*
                        _____ *(birthdate)*
to: Janice P. Burke, MA, OTR
    101 Any Street
    Hometown, USA 00007
                        Signed: _____
                        Relationship: _____
                        Date: _____

---

dling questions about fees. One of the best ways to do this is to practice by creating imaginary situations or anticipating potential issues before a particular meeting or contract negotiation. Practitioners should feel comfortable and confident with the fees they establish.

Billing forms should include diagnostic codes that reflect the patient diagnosis, evaluation, and treatment codes for the service rendered. Relative value scales (RVS) are established within each state by the medical association. These coded listings are a method of providing uniform information for insurance and government agencies. The RVS manual is available for purchase through the state medical association.

The process that an insurance or medicare claim is subject to is complex. The claim is received and processed by non-medical personnel who essentially "enter" the data from the form into a computer system for sorting and determining whether the service is eligible under a certain policy. Since the person entering that information may have no knowledge of occupational therapy, they may have difficulty determining even what to enter as the treatment. Standardized codes for the services offered and specific treatments given ensure that the information will be entered accurately. Insurance carriers want claims that are "simple, brief, easily comprehensible statement[s]" (p. 44).[7]

It is important to choose words and phrases describing treatment and progress very carefully, as they affect approval for third party reimbursement. Like the RVS

codes, certain key words and phrases are part of the insurance system and are recognized and accepted. Discussions with other private practitioners and insurance representatives help clarify the terminology that should be used.

Consent forms give permission to receive information from other professionals about their work with a child and family and release forms (Figure 30-4) give permission to release information to others. This applies to written reports and evaluations. When pictures (either videotape or film) are taken of a patient, signed permission is necessary, both to take the picture and to show it to other professionals, for educational or other purposes. Each purpose must be fully spelled out in the release form and must be signed and dated by the parent or legal guardian.

Outreach activities and marketing

Expanding the practice and increasing occupational therapy's recognition in the community is an exciting and rewarding activity, yet there frequently is little time or energy for such outreach. However, this activity benefits a professional reputation and gains recognition for the practice as a valuable commodity.[6,11] It should, therefore, be included in monthly time planning. One should plan to take part in a wide range of civic and community activities such as sponsoring an entrant in a walkathon, placing an ad in a special events publication, providing a free screening, buying a raffle ticket for a police or firefighter function, or donating time to a local drug prevention program.[12]

The most consistent and powerful source for marketing the practice is the therapist. His ability to present himself as competent, articulate, and professional is the most effective form of salesmanship. In establishing a private practice, the early identification of facilities and agencies that do not offer occupational therapy is important. The administrators of these agencies should be sent proposals that outline the kinds of occupational therapy services provided by the new practice. Included in such a plan, in addition to an explanation of the kinds of services offered, is a description of the types of patients who may most benefit from such services.

All written communications will reflect on the writer and the profession. A clear, well written report to another professional who is working with the child is an excellent introduction to services. The next time that professional sees a child with a similar problem, she will remember where the child was helped. It is not uncommon to receive a phone call from someone who received a copy of a report, asking about the services you provide and suggesting a conference. So, too, a poorly written report will be remembered by another professional as too long and detailed, or in some other way unprofessional. These negative incidents unfortunately affect the profession of occupational therapy more powerfully than the well received work.

Meetings, special workshops and topical lecture series and courses are opportunities to meet other professionals and market services to them. Professional associates have regular meetings to discuss specific cases and other issues. These meetings are excellent opportunities for educating oneself and others. Other sources of marketing contacts may be found in specialized groups such as women in health networks, alumni groups, and local professional organizations.

Another opportunity for marketing is presenting programs for individuals in special settings such as in-service programs in hospitals and schools (especially preschools), gyms and recreation programs, pediatric medical practices, or in parenting series offered at local hospitals, adult education, or the YMCA.

Mailings and brochures are obvious ways to transmit the practice's message. There is certainly value in developing mailings to announce the opening of a business, expansion in service, relocation, or other major changes. Other useful strategies to advertise available services are sponsoring a parent/child lecture series, bringing in guest professionals to address key issues in parenting, and advertising these by mail.

A brochure that describes in words and pictures the kinds of services that are available through the therapist's practice may prove to be a valuable marketing tool; this is especially useful in reaching large numbers of professionals who may have limited knowledge of occupational therapy. Pictures of therapists performing evaluations and providing treatment with patients in a variety of situations and with a range of modalities are highly informative, illustrating perceptual motor, sensory integration, group, and individual treatment sessions, as well as prosthesis fitting and adaptive equipment for feeding.

It is highly desirable to meet other professionals who may be ultimate referral sources; this should be considered among the first responsibilities of the practice. Many networks are available of professionals who provide various types of care to children. Pediatricians and pediatric nurse practitioners, educators (especially in early education centers), prevention coordinators in health centers who are involved in early identification of children at risk—all these may provide good information about other referral and contact sources.[12] The degree to which this happens depends on the therapist's ability to explain what kind of services this new practice provides (Figure 30-5).

Word of mouth is one of the most beneficial indirect marketing tools for any practice. Satisfied parents are the best publicity available. They communicate with other parents and begin sharing ideas and information on the kinds of people, places and things that have most helped their child. A parent who speaks highly of a therapist's skills and abilities essentially sells that therapist to other parents.

Writing, consulting, and teaching are other ways the therapist can market the practice. Writing a column in a local paper about toys, identifying the need for and developing the means of procuring play equipment that encourages children with disabilities to interact on a public playground are two activities that are interest-

---

Figure 30-5   Potential referral sources

Pediatricians, neurologists, orthopedists, disability specialists, developmental pediatricians
Teachers (for special populations and general population)
Preschool personnel
Gyms and sports programs for children
Speech therapists
Physical therapists
Psychologists
Nutritionists
Special schools/private schools/public schools
Social workers
Friends and neighbors
Clergy
Occupational therapists in acute care hospitals, rehabilitation centers
Specialists from blind children's centers/programs
State funded advocacy and support agencies
Screening program
Attorneys
Community colleges (child care training programs)
Well baby programs
Home health agencies, Visiting Nurses Association
Health Maintenance Organizations, pre-paid health plans

ing, worthwhile, and good exposure for the practice. Writing in professional newsletters for teachers, parent network newsletters, school nurse publications, and local papers are other examples.

Other occupational therapists in the community should also be contacted. Therapists in traditional facilities may be unaware of new services. Through state newsletters, presentations at local occupational therapy association meetings, and conferences, other occupational therapists can learn about new services that augment their own, such as home visits, discharge follow-up, school visits, or continued outpatient treatment sessions. Children with chronic illnesses or disabilities are often more appropriately treated within their own local communities. This type of treatment offers the obvious benefit of being close to home. It also is functionally oriented, with the child seen as an active member of his everyday community, not segregated in the hospital environment.

Small business persons in general believe that one never really knows where the next source of business may come from. For this reason, it is worthwhile to be able to communicate at various levels of complexity about occupational therapy. Develop a set of explanations and try them out on friends and relatives, other occupational therapists and therapy professionals, physicians, and "on-line" health care personnel. As these explanations of occupational therapy practice develop, the therapist will acquire a sense of how much information to give an inquiry without overwhelming, and how to guide interactions with others to facilitate understanding.

SUMMARY

The shape and form of a private practice is a reflection of the practitioner and patients who make up the practice. It is interesting to contrast the different models that therapists have constructed to meet the unique qualities in themselves, the patients and families they work with, and the health care community they are placed in. Additionally, therapists are influenced by the broad state, national, and international perspectives regarding children and their families as well as the professional and associated professional groups that work with similar issues.

Away from the traditional settings a private practice offers new opportunities in occupational therapy and business. Private practice gives the therapist an increased sense of confidence, competence, personal power, and fulfillment.

This chapter has described the difference between solo and group practice and discussed developing a business. Space needs, insurance and legal issues, developing the caseload and therapeutic policies are vital to any plan. There are differences between clinical and business records, both in use and purpose, and exam-

ples of each were given. Finally, marketing services is essential—directly, indirectly, and as outreach.

STUDY QUESTIONS

1. Make a line down the center of a piece of paper. On the left side of the line title the column "assets"; on the right side of the line title the column "liabilities." Begin to list all of the assets and liabilities you feel you have to consider about yourself and the health community where you live to make an accurate decision about your potential to have a successful private practice. Your work habits, business experience (or access to an individual with business expertise), your professional experience and reputation, financial and emotional resources should all be considered.

2. To realistically cover your expenses and make a profit (salary) you must establish your expenses and determine a fee for service. Compile two lists, one that will target the number of hours you will need to be involved in revenue-generating activity (direct patient care, employing a therapist, assistant, or aide to fulfill a contract), and a second one that will reflect a realistic expectation of your expenses. Ask yourself, "What is the minimum number of hours needed to 'make ends meet?' How many hours will be needed for me to begin to realize a profit? To generate the kind of income I would like to have? How long will it take me to achieve these different levels of income generation?"

3. Compile a list of the various services you intend to offer as part of your private practice. Services may include screening, testing, consultation to family, to a facility, to a physician, lecturing, and so forth. For each service indicate two potential referral sources that you would contact to solicit work. Establish a fee for each of the services you intend to offer.

REFERENCES

1. AOTA 1986 Member Data Survey, Research Information and Evaluation Division, American Occupational Therapy Association, Rockville, Md, 1986, AOTA, Inc.
2. Epstein C: Consultation: communicating and facilitating. In Bair J, and Gray M, editors: The occupational therapy manager, Rockville, Md, 1985, American Occupational Therapy Association.
3. Frazian B: Establishing and administrating a private practice in a hospital setting, Am J Occup Ther 32:296, 1978.
4. Frazian B: Tidal surge and private practice: the historic eighties, Occup Ther Health Care 2:7, 1985.
5. Goldenberg K, and Quinn B: Community occupational therapy associates: a model of private practice for community occupational therapy, Occup Ther Health Care 2:15, 1985.
6. Kautzmann L: Marketing occupational therapy services, Occup Ther Health Care 2:91, 1985.
7. Knickerbocker B: One person's experience in private practice, Occup Ther Health Care 2:37, 1985.
8. Koeltz C: Private practice in nursing, Maryland, 1979, Aspen Systems Corp.
9. McFadden S: Private practice in mental health settings: a therapist's experience. MHSIS Newsltr.
10. McFadden S, and Hanschu B: Risk taking in occupational therapy, Occup Ther Health Care 2:3, 1985.
11. Olsen T: Marketing. In Bair J, and Gray M, editors: The occupa-

tional therapy manager, Rockville, Md, 1985, American Occupational Therapy Association.

12. Shuer J, and Weiner L: Developing pediatric programming in a private occupational therapy practice, Occup Ther Health Care 2:53, 1985.

ADDITIONAL READINGS

Bair J, and Gray M: The occupational therapy manager, Rockville, Md, 1985, American Occupational Therapy Association.

Cauldwell-Klein E: O.T.s in private practice. Physical Disabilities Specialty Section Newsletter 2:1, 1979, Rockville, Md, American Occupational Therapy Association.

Cromwell F: Private practice in occupational therapy. Occupational Therapy in Health Care, New York, 1985, Haworth Press.

Hall K, and Hickman L: Establishing a private practice. Sensory Integration Specialty Section Newsletter 3:1, 1980, Rockville, Md, American Occupation Therapy Association.

Small Business Administration: Management Aids Series, St Louis, Mo.

31

Evaluation research and pediatric occupational therapy

CHARLOTTE BRASIC ROYEEN

"Research consciousness" is increasing within the occupational therapy profession; the discipline may be considered to be undergoing a "scholarly rite of passage"[20] (p. 3). However, the research emphasis of the field has been focusing on traditional research methods. The interests of the profession may be better served, in part, by including and fostering the more recently evolved types of investigation that collectively comprise evaluation research. This chapter is devoted to consideration of evaluation research as specifically applied to pediatric occupational therapy.

Gillette[12] stated that "the issue is the ability and willingness of the profession of occupational therapy to document the value of its services through research and quality assurance" (p. 499). The climate of accountability, fiscal conservatism, and competition between professions has created a situation in which occupational therapists must accept responsibility for evaluation research of occupational therapy programs. If they do not, professionals from other disciplines will design and carry out the evaluation process, without fully understanding and delineating the substance of occupational therapy programs. Thus it is in the best interests of the profession, as well as the interests of the children it serves, to conduct evaluation research in pediatric occupational therapy.

This chapter introduces evaluation research for programs in pediatric occupational therapy in the following manner: Evaluation research is defined and differentiated from client evaluation and what is more commonly thought of as research. Purposes, categories, and

levels of evaluation research are presented, as well as a brief historical review of the development of this type of investigation. The process of evaluation research is delineated and specific applications in pediatric occupational therapy discussed. Finally, the most common design categories of evaluation research are described and examples of each given.

Definition

Evaluation research is comprised of designing and executing planned, rigorous strategies to appropriately gather specific data or information on specific programs or components thereof, for use by designated individuals or groups. Simply stated, these strategies consist of measurement or description, data analysis, generation of formal reports, and dissemination of results.[25] Cooley and Lohnes[8] summarized evaluation research as follows:

An evaluation is a process by which relevant data are collected and transformed into information for decision-making. Evaluation is defined as a process rather than a product. Evaluation research transcends research and extends into decision-making (p. 3).

The four main functions of evaluation research as identified by Suarez[28] are:

1. Determining if program objectives are met
2. Acquiring information necessary for policy makers or administrators
3. Determining the effectiveness of the program
4. Judging the value or worth of the program

The final analysis of most evaluation research concerns the fourth function, the generation of a judgment regarding value of a given program or program

□ Dr. Royeen is affiliated with the Office of Special Education Programs, U.S. Department of Education. The U.S. Department of Education does not endorse this chapter as a social policy nor should it be inferred as such.

623

Table 31-1   Important differences between research and evaluation research

Characteristic	Research	Evaluation Research	Reference
Purpose	Develop or test theory Prediction Understanding	Product delivery Mission accomplishment	Yerxa[31]
Function	Determination of truth	Determination of value	Popham[25]
Outcomes	Conclusions	Decisions	Popham[25]
End Products	Discovery of new knowledge	Determination of goal achievement	Yerxa[31]
Application to Other Persons and Places	High	Low	

component.[15,25] Thus there is an inherent political nature to evaluation research[17] that must be recognized; it is discussed in detail later in this chapter.

Evaluation research compared to client evaluation and traditional research

Evaluation research is quite different from client evaluation. The word "evaluation" has different meanings in each process. To illustrate, in Chapter 7, assessment of an individual client is defined as ". . . an evaluative process based on facts (data collected through different formal and informal objective measures of children's functions and performance) and sound clinical judgment" (p. 128). Thus, in the case of client evaluation, one is assessing an individual. In contrast, evaluation research seeks to assess one or more programs of service delivery or components thereof.

In addition, evaluation research should be clearly differentiated from what is commonly thought of as "research." In a discussion of concepts developed by Neighbor and Schulberg[19], Royeen[27] stated that:

Evaluation is related to research, but differs with regard to values, purposes and resources. Whereas clinical research questions center on the search for "truth," evaluation research focuses on program effectiveness, efficiency, and responsiveness (p. 812).

Another distinction that has traditionally been made between research and evaluation research is in regard to their respective relationships to theory. Research typically is designed to develop or test theory, whereas evaluation research is not necessarily related to any theory.[31] Research and evaluation research also differ on other key points, as summarized in Table 31-1.

Categories of evaluation research

Evaluation research may be categorized by purpose and by time frame. The purpose categories are *program and project evaluation* and the time-related forms are *formative* and *summative.*

The first basic level of evaluation research is program evaluation. Such investigations are designed to describe what the program does and how objectives

Table 31-2   Differentiation of levels of evaluation research

Type of Evaluation Research	Category	Level	Function
Program evaluation	Basic	First	Describe roles and functions of pediatric occupational therapy services within a given setting
Project evaluation	Advanced	Second	Evaluate how well or effectively such services are delivered

are accomplished.[29] Examples of questions that might be addressed in program evaluation research include:

- What mechanism is used to determine who receives pediatric occupational therapy services?
- What are the roles and functions of pediatric occupational therapists in this program?
- How do the roles and functions of the pediatric occupational therapist differ from those of other professionals in the program?
- How are pediatric occupational therapy services delivered—direct service, consultation, or monitoring?
- In what settings are pediatric occupational therapy services delivered—home, school, hospital, outpatient clinic?

Program evaluation research in pediatric occupational therapy, therefore, consists of a description and analysis of the roles and functions of pediatric occupational therapy within a given program or setting.

Somewhat differently, project evaluation may be considered a more advanced, second level of evaluation research. Such investigations determine quality and effectiveness of service delivery.[29] In pediatric occupational therapy, project evaluation investigates how well or effectively the identified roles and functions are operationalized within a given setting. Table 31-2 summarizes these two levels of evaluation research.

Table 31-3 Differences between formative and summative evaluation

Characteristic	Formative Evaluation	Summative Evaluation	Reference
Purpose	Assist in program development	Assist in evaluation of program that has been delivered	Morocco[18]
Goal	Improve program	Demonstrate value or worth of program	Suarez[28]
User of results	Program developer	Decision maker/Consumer	Popham[25]
Associated methodologies	Descriptive phenomenological	Empirical hypothesis based	Morocco[18]
Associated processes	Inductive	Deductive	

It is important for program evaluation to precede project evaluation. A solid base of clearly identified roles and functions is needed before the effectiveness of service delivery via those roles and functions can be evaluated. Indeed, pediatric occupational therapy needs to expand the data base regarding roles and functions of therapists before advancing to project level research.

Popham[25] stated that *formative evaluation* occurs while a program is still in operation, so that findings can be used by program developers to change or modify the program. In contrast, *summative* evaluation is conducted after services are delivered, to measure the effectiveness of the program. Therefore, formative evaluation can be summarized as relating to program development,[18] whereas summative evaluation determines the merits and worth of a completed program.[25] A summary of characteristics of formative and summative evaluation is provided in Table 31-3.

History of evaluation research

Historically, evaluation research is associated with the development of the "Great Society" during the Johnson administration of the 1960s. During that time, the increase in number and scope of federal programs necessitated the development of mechanisms to evaluate use of funds, and the process of evaluation research began to evolve.[5] Methodologies for executing evaluation research have followed what Guba and Lincoln[14] called a four-generational model. That is, the conceptualization and execution of evaluation research has evolved through four stages. These were characterized by Guba and Lincoln as follows:

Stage 1: Evaluator served as technician for measurement of performance

Stage 2: Evaluator measured performance and described strengths and weaknesses.

Stage 3: Evaluator took on stronger role in judgment of value and worth of program

Stage 4: Evaluator assumed role of facilitator and elicits judgments based on values of interested parties for "stakeholders"

The current trend is to increase the relatedness of

the process of evaluation research on a given program or project to the theoretical approach espoused by a particular program.[6] This is an interesting development, but may create a paradoxical situation in which it is more difficult to differentiate between traditional and evaluation research in clinical settings.

Other trends in evaluation research include use of multiple methods in controlled inquiry (qualitative and quantitative) and the development of "user focused" techniques.[23] The use of both qualitative and quantitative strategies can allow for a better understanding of individuals and the meaning of their behaviors.[30] Of particular note among the more qualitatively oriented evaluation technologies is the "naturalistic" approach of Guba[13] and the case study method of Yin.[32]

User focused evaluation research is designed and executed with the consumer of the findings in mind. For example, the pediatric occupational therapist might determine what kind of information interests teachers, principals, administrators, parents, or student advocacy groups, and then develop program evaluation strategies to extract this particular data.

The overall purpose of evaluation research as it is currently practiced is multi-faceted. Phillips[24] explained it well: "Evaluation studies serve other purposes than information purposes. They legitimate. They advocate. They explain" (p. 23). Thus, evaluation research can potentially serve the field of pediatric occupational therapy well by describing, advocating, and legitimizing services.

The process of evaluation research

The process of evaluation research should be based on a detailed plan. Suarez[28] stated that "a plan for evaluation is a detailed formulation of the procedures and actions by which an evaluation is to be conducted" (p. 193). Plans for evaluation of programs in pediatric occupational therapy should address the questions posed in Figure 31-1. Each of the questions is discussed further to provide a conceptual framework for the process of evaluation research.

Question 1. Why is the evaluation being conducted?

Typically, evaluation research is conducted in re-

Figure 31-1   Questions to be addressed in the plan for the evaluation

ITEM QUESTION
 1. Why is the evaluation conducted?
 2. What is the mission of the home institution/organization?
 3. What are the roles and functions of the pediatric occupational therapy program?
 4. How is the mission statement of the home institution/organization the same as or different from the roles and functions of the pediatric occupational therapy services?
 5. What is the theoretical base for delivery of the pediatric occupational therapy services?
 6. What are key components of the program?
 7. Who are key "stakeholders" regarding findings from the evaluation?
 8. What are the proposed questions to be answered by the evaluation?
 9. Why were those specific questions addressed?
 10. What data are necessary to answer each proposed question?
 11. What is an appropriate strategy or research design for the evaluation?
 12. How will data be organized and verified?
 13. What are the criteria for interpretation of the data?
 14. How were the criteria determined?
 15. What are considerations regarding communication with key "stakeholders?"

sponse to an administrative, agency, or third party request. However, for each evaluation, the "why" may be somewhat different, so it is imperative that an evaluator clearly establish the impetus for any specific investigation.

Question 2. What is the mission of the host institution/organization?

It is also important to establish the context in which the pediatric occupational therapy program exists. Therefore, the goals and objectives of the institution or organization within which the occupational therapy service operates should be clearly identified. This can be accomplished by reviewing mission statements, interviewing staff, and talking with those served by the agency.

Question 3. What are the roles and functions of the pediatric occupational therapy program?

The purpose of providing occupational therapy services must be precisely determined. This description should include clear delineation of services and how such services are delivered. Both the formally and informally recognized roles and functions of the occupational therapist should be specified.

Question 4. How is the mission of the host institution/organization the same as or different from the roles and functions of the pediatric occupational therapy services?

Comparing these two aspects serves to identify conflicts and inconsistencies. Identification of any such inconsistencies serves to alert responsible individuals to the need for action to remedy the situation by reevaluating goals and priorities.

Question 5. What is the theoretical base for delivery of the pediatric occupational therapy services?

As mentioned by various authors throughout this text, occupational therapists frequently use an eclectic approach to intervention with children. However, it is still essential to clearly identify the overall conceptual model or theory base from which the actions and clinical reasoning of the staff are generated.[28] Typically, there is one primary theory that "drives" the program,[6] such as sensory integration, neurodevelopmental treatment, or occupational behavior.

Question 6. What are the key components of the program?

The description of the program must include breakdown of key components such as age and type of client populations served, settings in which services are delivered, staffing patterns, and funding sources and constraints.

Question 7. Who are the key "stakeholders" regarding findings from the evaluation?

In evaluation research, the term "stakeholder" refers to those individuals or groups who have a "stake" or vested interest in the findings or outcome of a study. Stakeholders should be identified, if possible, before the evaluation process is planned, and ideally should participate in the design and execution of the evaluation research project. At the very least, the evaluators should attempt to initiate and maintain communication with the stakeholders throughout the course of the research.

Question 8. What are the proposed questions to be answered by the evaluation?

Chadwick et al[5] suggested that there are no fixed evaluation questions. Indeed, the particular questions that are to be addressed in any given evaluation need to be generated specifically for that time, situation, and setting. As mentioned previously, evaluation questions are best generated by including stakeholders in the process of identifying and refining the areas to be investigated. Question development is a crucial step in the process of evaluation research since each item has implications regarding the type of data and research strategies that will be needed.

Question 9. Why were those specific questions addressed?

It is equally important to understand the motivation behind the selection of specific questions. For example, it may be that a particular question was included because it will provide information mandated by a legislative body. Another question might seek to compare results of different theoretical approaches to treatment because the therapists need to know what is most effective in their particular setting. Or, third party payors might need to know the cost implications of including pediatric occupational therapy services in their coverage. The reasons for each of these examples are different and each has slightly different political implications. It is critical for the evaluator to be aware of these political implications as the motivation behind question selection is determined.

Question 10. What data are necessary to answer each proposed question?

Given that one or more evaluation questions have been posed, the investigator must determine what data are needed to provide the required information. For example, if the question is, "Has the pediatric occupational therapy program had a successful impact on community preschools serving handicapped children?", then the evaluator knows that information from preschools will be necessary. Another question could be: "Within this pediatric occupational therapy program, which intervention strategy—one based on sensory integration or one based on neurodevelopmental treatment—is more effective with infants who have a congenital defect of the cleft palate?" To answer this question, data will be needed regarding a variety of developmental and maturational levels of children who have cleft palate.

Table 31-4 lists data collection procedures commonly used in evaluations of pediatric programs.

Question 11. What is an appropriate strategy or research design for the evaluation?

There are also no standard or perfect evaluation strategies.[10] Rather, there are categories of research design strategies from which a particular format can be adopted and adapted for a given situation. Within this context, the four most common types of evaluation research design are presented.

Criterion- or objectives-based evaluation is commonly used for program evaluation.[28] Simply stated, the research design consists of identifying the objectives of the program and then determining whether they have been met. For example, many chapters in this book recommend program goals and objectives. A therapist might adopt a set of goals and objectives, implement the author's program modalities and recommendations, and then determine if the program goals and objectives have been met.

Cost-effectiveness evaluations were defined by Andrieu[2] as:

. . . the application of economics for determining the efficient use of resources in all sections of the economy. Its main objective is to identify and quantify program effects as "benefits" and compare them to program costs. Overall, if benefits exceed the costs, the well being of the community is expected to increase as a result of the program (p. 219).

Although it is relatively simple to calculate program expenses, cost-oriented evaluations require very difficult judgments to determine the financial worth of seemingly non-quantifiable entities such as benefits to the broad community. For example, in a cost-effectiveness study of preschool programs, Barnett[3] had to esti-

Table 31-4 Data collection procedures commonly used in evaluation research

Assessment Area	Types of Data Collected
Child development	Standardized tests Observations Parent or teacher reports Anecdotal records
Interactions between child and others	Observations Sociometric devices Critical incidence techniques
Parental attitudes, knowledge, and skills	Tests Questionnaires Rating scales Observations Interviews
Environments	Observations Anecdotal records Unobtrusive measures
Placement	Agency records Parent interviews
Staff attitudes, knowledge, and skills	Tests Questionnaires Rating scales Observations Interviews
Cost effectiveness	Outcome measures Program costs record

Adapted from TM Suarez[28] (p. 203).

mate the reduction in welfare costs for and increased potential earning power of those students who had participated in the preschool experience.

The final analysis of cost-effectiveness studies is to determine if the cost of program services is a profitable social investment.[3] Reports of this type of study are rare in occupational therapy, although a micro-costing analysis by Mansfield[16] is a promising beginning.

Most evaluation research within pediatric occupational therapy has been executed using the strategy of *single subject or multiple baseline designs.* These may be considered as project evaluation, and are employed to determine the efficacy of intervention services.[21]

However, across all disciplines, the vast majority of evaluation research has utilized what may be considered *quasi-experimental designs.* Generally, such designs attempt to measure change of one or more groups of subjects who receive intervention. The typical design may be represented as:

$$C = X2 - X1$$

where:
C = Change score
$X1$ = Subject performance before intervention
$X2$ = Subject performance after intervention

It is typical for such investigations to use ANOVA, t-tests, ANCOVA, or equivalent nonparametric procedures for data analysis.[26] Such quasi-experimental designs for evaluation research present the same potential confounds that undermine traditional research through threats to internal validity.[4] Superficially, the measurement of change is simple. But, as Fortune and Hutson[10] pointed out, in reality it is difficult and problematic for the following reasons:

1. Measurement errors will occur since no instrument or test is 100% reliable
2. A correlation between pre-test and post-test scores may exist and confound the difference scores
3. There may be problems in how subjects were assigned to groups
4. The phenomenon known as "regression to the mean" may occur and confound the difference scores

Table 31-5 categorizes selected articles from occupational therapy and related literature that provide examples of strategies employed for design of evaluation research.

Question 12. How will the data be organized and verified?

Given that a particular strategy has been selected, procedures and mechanisms for data organization and verification need to be planned and organized. For example, who will check on completeness of all scoring sheets? Who will be responsible for seeing that all data have been properly coded and entered into the computer? This is a crucial step that is frequently overlooked in the planning stages.

Question 13. What are the criteria for interpretation of data?

Basically, the answer to this question identifies what will be considered a successful program result.[5] The investigator needs to decide, before conducting the evaluation, what guidelines or predetermined standards will be used to guide interpretation of results. What constitutes success? What constitutes lack of success?

The criterion may be a level of significance on some statistical test (usually a probability value of alpha = 0.05 or less), or a practical measure of performance (such as the ability of a child to eat independently). Sometimes, a sequence of data is required to provide a logical argument that the program outcomes constitute success. In other instances, "expert" testimony or literary references are used to set criteria for evaluation of findings.

Question 14. How were criteria determined?

The evaluator should specify how the criteria were set. This allows the consumer of the evaluation research to better understand the meaning of the project results.

Question 15. What are considerations regarding communication with key stakeholders?

As Patton[23] stated: "Utilization is not something to become suddenly concerned about at the end of an evaluation" (p. 83). Since ". . . one primary purpose of evaluation research is to advocate interests . . . the sharing of information pertaining to evaluation findings is a legitimate mechanism to use in the competition for funding" (p. 23). Therefore, the evaluator determines not only who the stakeholders are, but also who may be the audience for evaluation findings. Suarez[28] stated that these may be program staff, funding and administrative agency staff, parents, staffs of similar programs, policy makers, the general public, members of the press and media, related professionals, and professional program sponsors, adoptees, and advocates.

Potential users of the evaluation findings should be contacted before the evaluation begins to establish rapport and communication.[1] Furthermore, as part of the evaluation plan, the investigator should establish a time

---

Table 31-5 Examples of design categories of evaluation research related to pediatric occupational therapy

Design Foundation of Evaluation Study	Article/Example	Authors
Criterion- or objectives-based evaluation	Starting a level I fieldwork program	M.B. Cole[7]
Cost effectiveness-based evaluation	Micro-costing analysis: a measure of accountability	M. Mansfield[16]
	Benefit-cost analyses of the Perry preschool program and its policy implications	W.S. Barnett[3]
Single subject and multiple baseline	Oral sensorimotor therapy in the developmentally disabled: a multiple baseline study	K. Ottenbacher, J. Hicks, A. Roark, and J. Swinea[22]
Quasi-experimental	A program for improving energy conservation behaviors in adults with rheumatoid arthritis	G.P. Furst, L.H. Gerber, C.C. Smith, S. Fisher, and B. Shulman[11]
	A program for parents of children with sensory integrative dysfunction	B. Friedman[9]

frame and procedures for continuing communication with these audience members throughout the course of the project.

To draw an analogy, just as one can use manual facilitation techniques to bias muscle tone in a hemiplegic person prior to cued intentional movement, one can use rapport and community support to influence the political climate prior to the reporting of evaluation research findings[27] (p. 812).

SUMMARY

This chapter has been designed to introduce the reader to important concepts and characteristics of evaluation research as applied to programs in pediatric occupational therapy. At this point in its development, the discipline and its clients can be well served by pediatric clinicians' participation in the basic level of evaluation research: descriptions of roles and functions. As this information is refined, those with special interests, ability, and resources can further legitimize and advocate the need for pediatric occupational therapy services through conduct of the second level, advanced evaluation research that measures the efficacy of how roles and functions are operationalized.

STUDY QUESTIONS

1. Define and differentiate research as it is traditionally considered and evaluation research as presented in this chapter.
2. Explain how evaluation research can be used in pediatric occupational therapy.
3. Differentiate clinical evaluation and evaluation research. How might evaluation research affect the process and content of clinical evaluation of a child?
4. Define and differentiate between formative and summative evaluation. Suppose that you were the first occupational therapist to provide services in a rural school system. How might you use each of these during your first year to assist you with program development and to determine the need for additional therapy services and staff during the second year of operation?
5. This chapter has summarized the evaluation research process via a 15 question format. Given the hypothetical situation in study question #4 above, what resources could you use to answer the 15 process questions?
6. Define and differentiate between basic, first level evaluation research and advanced, second level research. For the hypothetical situation in study question #4, prepare three research questions that might be addressed by a basic level study. How might these same evaluation topics be rephrased for an advanced, second level study?

REFERENCES

1. Aiken MC, and Daillak RH: A study of evaluation utilization, Educational Evaluation and Policy Analysis 1(4):41, 1979.
2. Andrieu M: Benefit cost evaluation. In Rutman L, editor: Evaluation research methods: a basic guide, Beverly Hills, Calif, 1977, Sage Publications Inc.
3. Barnett WS: Benefit-cost analysis of the Perry preschool program and its policy implication, Educational Evaluation and Policy Analysis 7(4):333, 1985.
4. Campbell DT, and Stanley J: Experimental and quasi-experimental designs for research, Chicago, 1966, Rand Publishing Co.
5. Chadwick BA, and others: Evaluation research. In Social science research methods, Englewood, NJ, 1984, Prentice-Hall Inc.
6. Chen H, and Rossi PH: Evaluation with sense: the theory driven approach, Evaluation Review 7(3):283, 1983.
7. Cole MB: Starting level I fieldwork programs, Am J Occup Ther 38(9):584, 1985.
8. Cooley WW, and Lohnes PR: Evaluation research in education, New York, 1976, John Wiley and Sons.
9. Friedman B: A program for parents of children with sensory integrative dysfunction, Am J Occup Ther 36(9):586, 1982.
10. Fortune JC, and Hutson BA: Selecting models for measuring change when true experimental conditions do not exist, J Educ Res 77(4):197, 1984.
11. Furst GP, and others: A program for improving energy conservation behaviors in adults with rheumatoid arthritis, Am J Occup Ther 41(2):102, 1987.
12. Gillette NP: A data base for occupational therapy: documentation through research, Am J Occup Ther 36(8):499, 1982.
13. Guba EB: Toward a method of naturalistic inquiry in educational evaluation, Los Angeles, 1978, Center for the Study of Evaluation.
14. Guba EB, and Lincoln YS: The countenance of fourth-generation evaluation: description, judgment and negotiation, Evaluation Studies Review Annual 11:70, 1986.
15. Hamilton JL, and Swan WW: Measurement references in the assessment of preschool handicapped children, HECSE 1(2):41, 1981.
16. Mansfield M: Micro-costing analysis: a measure of accountability, Am J Occup Ther 37(4):239, 1983.
17. McLemore JR, and Neumann JE: The inherently political nature of program evaluators and evaluation research, Evaluation Program and Policy Analysis 10:83, 1987.
18. Morocco CC: The role of formative evaluation in developing and assessing educational programs, Curriculum Inquiry 9(2):137, 1979.
19. Neighbor WD, and Schulberg, HC: Evaluating the outcomes of human services programs: a reassessment, Evaluation Review 6(6):731, 1982.
20. Ottenbacher K: A scholarly rite of passage, Occup Ther J Res 7(1):3, 1987.
21. Ottenbacher K, and York J: Strategies for evaluating clinical change: implications for practice and research, Am J Occup Ther 38(10):647, 1984.
22. Ottenbacher K, and others: Oral sensorimotor therapy in the developmentally delayed: a multiple baseline study, Am J Occup Ther 37(8):541, 1983.
23. Patton MQ: Creative evaluation, Beverly Hills, Calif, 1981, Sage Publishing Co.
24. Phillips LA: Evaluation program results. In Radsey-Rusch, editor: Conference proceedings from the project directors' annual meeting, November 4-6. Washington, DC, 1985, United States Department of Education, Office of Special Education Programs.
25. Popham WJ: Educational evaluation, Englewood Cliffs, NJ, 1975, Prentice-Hall, Inc.
26. Porgis SW: Ontogenetic comparisons, International J of Psych 11(3):203, 1976.
27. Royeen CB: Evaluation of school-based occupational therapy programs: need, strategy, and dissemination, Am J Occup Ther 40(1):811, 1987.
28. Suarez TM: Planning evaluation of programs for high risk and handicapped infants. In Ramey CT, and Trohanis PL, editors:

Finding and educating high-risk and handicapped infants, Baltimore, Md, 1982, University Park Press.

29. Wholey JS, and others: Federal evaluation policy: analyzing the effects of public programs, Washington, DC, 1971, The Urban Institute.

30. Williams DD: Naturalistic evaluation: potential conflicts between evaluation standards and criteria for conducting naturalistic inquiry, Educational Evaluation and Policy Analysis 8(1):87, 1986.

31. Yerxa EJ: Evaluation versus research: outcomes or knowledge? Am J Occup Ther 38(6):407, 1984.

32. Yin RK: Case study research: design and methods, Beverly Hills, Calif, 1984, Sage Publications Inc.

Appendix

Children's Hospital at Stanford occupational therapy time—oriented record activities of daily living assessment

CHILDREN'S HOSPITAL AT STANFORD

ACTIVITIES OF DAILY LIVING ASSESSMENT*

Name of patient _____ Hospital no. _____

Diagnosis _____ Onset _____

Birth date _____

Sex: M   F   Handedness: R   L

               Assessor's signature   **Date**

1. _____

2. _____

3. _____

4. _____

5. _____

6. _____

7. _____

8. _____

Subtests utilized:

Basic ADL	Communication	Adolescent self-care	Transfers
Wheelchair	Household activities	Equipment list	

*From Bleck, E. E., and Nagel, D. A., editors: Physically handicapped children: a medical atlas for teachers, New York, 1975, Grune & Stratton, Inc. By permission.

Reprinted with permission from Coley IL, Pediatric assessment of self-care activities, St Louis, 1978, The CV Mosby Co.

<table>
<tr><td colspan="2"></td><td colspan="2" align="center">CHILDREN'S HOSPITAL AT STANFORD
OCCUPATIONAL THERAPY</td></tr>
<tr><td colspan="2" align="center">addressograph stamp</td><td colspan="2" align="center">TIME-ORIENTED RECORD

ACTIVITIES OF DAILY LIVING ASSESSMENT</td></tr>
</table>

Key to scoring: 4 . . . Independent
3 . . . Independent with equipment and/or adaptive technique
2 . . . Completes but cannot accomplish in practical time
1 . . . Attempts but requires assistance or supervision to complete
0 . . . Dependent—cannot attempt activity
— . . . Nonapplicable

The **Year-Month** vertical column represents the | Order of developmental sequence | or approximate age when the child accomplishes the activity; the horizontal column represents the chronological age of the child being assessed.

Visit number		1		2		3		4		5		6		7		8	
Julian date																	
	Yr. Mo.																
BED	Order of dev. seq.	R.	L.	R.	L.	R.	L.	R.	L.	R.	L.	R.	L.	R.	L.	R.	L.
1 Supine position	Birth																
2 Prone position	Birth																
3 Roll to side	1-4 wk.																
4 Roll prone to supine	0.6																
5 Roll supine to prone	0.7																
6 Sit up	0.10																
7 Propped sitting	0.6																
8 Sitting/hands props	0.7																
9 Sitting unsupported	0.10-0.12																
Reaching																	
10 To midline	0.5																
11 To mouth and face	0.6																
12 Above head	—																
13 Behind head	—																
14 Behind back	—																
15 To toes	1.3																
FEEDING																	
16 Swallow (liquids)	Birth																
17 Drooling under control	1.0																
18 Suck and use straw	2.0																
19 Chew (semisolids, solids)	1.6																
20 Finger foods	0.10																

ACTIVITIES OF DAILY LIVING

Continued.

CHILDREN'S HOSPITAL AT STANFORD
OCCUPATIONAL THERAPY

TIME-ORIENTED RECORD

ACTIVITIES OF DAILY LIVING ASSESSMENT

Key to scoring: 4 . . . Independent

3 . . . Independent with equipment and/or adaptive technique

2 . . . Completes but cannot accomplish in practical time

1 . . . Attempts but requires assistance or supervision to complete

0 . . . Dependent—cannot attempt activity

— . . . Nonapplicable

The **Year-Month** vertical column represents the | Order of developmental sequence | or approximate age when the child accomplishes the activity; the horizontal column represents the chronological age of the child being assessed.

	Visit number	Yr. Mo. Order of dev. seq.	1 R.	L.	2 R.	L.	3 R.	L.	4 R.	L.	5 R.	L.	6 R.	L.	7 R.	L.	8 R.	L.
	FEEDING—cont'd																	
	Utensils																	
21	Bottle	0.10																
22	Spoon	3.0																
23	Cup	1.6																
24	Glass	2.0																
25	Fork	3.0																
26	Knife	6.0-7.0																
	TOILETING																	
27	Bowel control	1.6																
28	Bladder control	2.0																
29	Sit on toilet	2.9																
30	Arrange clothing	4.0																
31	Cleanse self	5.0																
32	Flush toilet	3.3-5.0																
	HYGIENE																	
33	Turn faucets on/off	3.0																
34	Wash/dry hands/face	4.9																
35	Wash ears	8.0																
36	Bathing	8.0																
37	Deodorant	12.0-																
38	Care for teeth	4.9																
39	Care for nose	6.0																

	CHILDREN'S HOSPITAL AT STANFORD
	OCCUPATIONAL THERAPY
	TIME-ORIENTED RECORD
	ACTIVITIES OF DAILY LIVING ASSESSMENT

Key to scoring: 4 . . . Independent
3 . . . Independent with equipment and/or adaptive technique
2 . . . Completes but cannot accomplish in practical time
1 . . . Attempts but requires assistance or supervision to complete
0 . . . Dependent—cannot attempt activity
— . . . Nonapplicable

The **Year-Month** vertical column represents the [Order of developmental sequence] or approximate age when the child accomplishes the activity; the horizontal column represents the chronological age of the child being assessed.

Visit number			1		2		3		4		5		6		7		8	
		Yr. Mo.																
		Order of dev. seq.	R.	L.	R.	L.	R.	L.	R.	L.	R.	L.	R.	L.	R.	L.	R.	L.
	HYGIENE—cont'd																	
40	Care for hair	7.6																
41	Care for nails	8.0																
42	Feminine hygiene	Puberty																
	UNDRESSING																	
	Lower body																	
43	Untie shoe bow	2.0-3.0																
44	Remove shoes	2.0-3.0																
45	Remove socks	1.6																
46	Remove pull-down garment	2.6																
	Upper body																	
47	Remove pull-over garment	4.0																
	DRESSING																	
	Lower body																	
48	Put on socks	4.0																
49	Put on pull-down garment	4.0																
50	Put on shoe	4.0																
51	Lace shoe	4.0-5.0																
52	Tie bow	6.0																
	Upper body																	
53	Put on pull-over garment	5.0																

ACTIVITIES OF DAILY LIVING

Continued.

<table>
<tr><td colspan="2"></td><td colspan="9">CHILDREN'S HOSPITAL AT STANFORD
OCCUPATIONAL THERAPY

TIME-ORIENTED RECORD

ACTIVITIES OF DAILY LIVING ASSESSMENT</td></tr>
</table>

Key to scoring:
- 4 . . . Independent
- 3 . . . Independent with equipment and/or adaptive technique
- 2 . . . Completes but cannot accomplish in practical time
- 1 . . . Attempts but requires assistance or supervision to complete
- 0 . . . Dependent—cannot attempt activity
- — . . . Nonapplicable

The **Year-Month** vertical column represents the | Order of developmental sequence | or approximate age when the child accomplishes the activity; the horizontal column represents the chronological age of the child being assessed.

Visit number			1	2	3	4	5	6	7	8
		Yr. Mo.								
	FASTENERS	Order of dev. seq.								
	Unfastening									
54	Button: front	3.0								
55	side	3.0								
56	back	5.6								
57	Zipper: front	3.3								
58	separating front	3.6								
59	back	4.9								
60	Buckle: belt	3.9								
61	shoe	3.9								
62	Tie: back sash	5.0								
	Fasten									
63	Button: large front	2.6								
64	series	3.6								
65	back	6.3								
66	Zipper: front, lock tab	4.0								
67	separating	4.6								
68	back	5.6								
69	Buckle: belt	4.0								
70	shoe	4.0								
71	insert belt in loops	4.6								
72	Tie: front	6.0								
73	back	8.0								
74	necktie	10.0								
75	Snaps: front	3.0								
76	back	6.0								
	Assessor's initials:									

ACTIVITIES OF DAILY LIVING

addressograph stamp	CHILDREN'S HOSPITAL AT STANFORD OCCUPATIONAL THERAPY TIME-ORIENTED RECORD ACTIVITIES OF DAILY LIVING ASSESSMENT

Key to scoring: 4 . . . Independent
3 . . . Independent with equipment and/or adaptive technique
2 . . . Completes but cannot accomplish in practical time
1 . . . Attempts but requires assistance or supervision to complete
0 . . . Dependent—cannot attempt activity
— . . . Nonapplicable

Visit number	1		2		3		4		5		6		7		8	
Julian date																
COMMUNICATION	R.	L.	R.	L.	R.	L.	R.	L.	R.	L.	R.	L.	R.	L.	R.	L.
Writing																
1 Sharpen pencil																
2 Print																
3 Write																
4 Erase																
Typing																
5 Insert paper																
6 Press space bar																
7 Press key																
8 Turn carriage																
9 Remove paper																
Telephone																
10 Remove receiver																
11 Hold receiver																
12 Dial																
13 Speak																
14 Replace receiver																
15 Take message																
16 Use telephone book																

ACTIVITIES OF DAILY LIVING

	CHILDREN'S HOSPITAL AT STANFORD
	OCCUPATIONAL THERAPY
	TIME-ORIENTED RECORD
addressograph stamp	ACTIVITIES OF DAILY LIVING ASSESSMENT

Key to scoring: 4 . . . Independent
3 . . . Independent with equipment and/or adaptive technique
2 . . . Completes but cannot accomplish in practical time
1 . . . Attempts but requires assistance or supervision to complete
0 . . . Dependent—cannot attempt activity
— . . . Nonapplicable

	Visit number	1		2		3		4		5		6		7		8	
	Julian date																
	ADOLESCENT SELF-CARE	R.	L.	R.	L.	R.	L.	R.	L.	R.	L.	R.	L.	R.	L.	R.	L.
	UNDRESSING																
1	Remove nylons/panty hose																
2	Remove girdle/garter belt																
3	Remove brassiere																
4	Remove necktie																
	DRESSING																
5	Put on nylons/panty hose																
6	Put on girdle/garter belt																
7	Put on brassiere																
8	Put on necktie																
	AIDS																
9	Put on eyeglasses																
10	Remove eyeglasses																
11	Put on hearing aid																
12	Remove hearing aid																
	HYGIENE																
13	Shampoo hair																
14	Set hair																
15	Shave face																
16	Shave underarms																
17	Shave legs																
18	Apply deodorant																
19	Apply makeup																
20	Groom fingernails																
21	Groom toenails																

ACTIVITIES OF DAILY LIVING

addressograph stamp	**CHILDREN'S HOSPITAL AT STANFORD** **OCCUPATIONAL THERAPY** **TIME-ORIENTED RECORD** **ACTIVITIES OF DAILY LIVING ASSESSMENT**	

Key to scoring: 4 . . . Independent
                 3 . . . Independent with equipment and/or adaptive technique
                 2 . . . Completes but cannot accomplish in practical time
                 1 . . . Attempts but requires assistance or supervision to complete
                 0 . . . Dependent—cannot attempt activity
                 — . . . Nonapplicable

	Visit number	1	2	3	4	5	6	7	8
	Julian date								
	TRANSFERS								
	Specify: ambulatory								
	with crutches								
	with wheelchair								
1	To bed								
2	From bed								
3	To toilet								
4	From toilet								
5	To bathtub								
6	From bathtub								
7	To shower								
8	From shower								
9	To regular chair								
10	From regular chair								
11	To car								
12	From car								
13	To bus								
14	From bus								

ACTIVITIES OF DAILY LIVING

<table>
<tr><td colspan="2" rowspan="2"></td><td colspan="17">CHILDREN'S HOSPITAL AT STANFORD
OCCUPATIONAL THERAPY

TIME-ORIENTED RECORD

ACTIVITIES OF DAILY LIVING ASSESSMENT</td></tr>
<tr></tr>
</table>

addressograph stamp

Key to scoring:
- 4 . . . Independent
- 3 . . . Independent with equipment and/or adaptive technique
- 2 . . . Completes but cannot accomplish in practical time
- 1 . . . Attempts but requires assistance or supervision to complete
- 0 . . . Dependent—cannot attempt activity
- — . . . Nonapplicable

	Visit number	1		2		3		4		5		6		7		8	
	Julian date																
	WHEELCHAIR SKILLS	R.	L.	R.	L.	R.	L.	R.	L.	R.	L.	R.	L.	R.	L.	R.	L.
1	Sitting balance																
2	Fasten belt																
3	Unfasten belt																
4	Lock brakes																
5	Unlock brakes																
6	Propel forward																
7	Propel backward																
8	Propel corners																
9	Open doors																
10	Close doors																
11	Go up ramp																
12	Go down ramp																
13	Raise footrests																
14	Lower footrests																
15	Swing footrests to side																
16	Remove arms																
17	Replace arms																
18	Pick up object from floor																
19	Sitting push-ups (10)																
20	Adjust position																
21	Reach crutches, holder																
22	Place crutches, holder																

ACTIVITIES OF DAILY LIVING

<table>
<tr><td colspan="2" rowspan="3">addressograph stamp</td><td colspan="9">**CHILDREN'S HOSPITAL AT STANFORD**
OCCUPATIONAL THERAPY

TIME-ORIENTED RECORD

ACTIVITIES OF DAILY LIVING ASSESSMENT</td></tr>
</table>

Key to scoring: 4 . . . Independent
3 . . . Independent with equipment and/or adaptive technique
2 . . . Completes but cannot accomplish in practical time
1 . . . Attempts but requires assistance or supervision to complete
0 . . . Dependent—cannot attempt activity
— . . . Nonapplicable

Visit number	1	2	3	4	5	6	7	8
Julian date								
HOUSEHOLD ACTIVITIES								
Food preparation								
1 Open: milk								
2 packaged food								
3 bottles, capped								
4 screw lids								
5 Pour: liquids								
6 dry ingredients								
7 Mix: with spoon								
8 egg beater, manual								
9 electric mixer								
10 Sift flour								
11 Break egg								
12 Peel vegetables/fruit								
13 Cut vegetables/fruit								
14 Use: measuring spoons								
15 cups								
16 can opener								
17 rolling pin								
Range								
18 Operate: burner controls								
19 oven controls								
20 Place pans on range								
21 Remove hot pans from range								

ACTIVITIES OF DAILY LIVING

Continued.

	CHILDREN'S HOSPITAL AT STANFORD OCCUPATIONAL THERAPY TIME-ORIENTED RECORD ACTIVITIES OF DAILY LIVING ASSESSMENT

Key to scoring: 4 . . . Independent
3 . . . Independent with equipment and/or adaptive technique
2 . . . Completes but cannot accomplish in practical time
1 . . . Attempts but requires assistance or supervision to complete
0 . . . Dependent—cannot attempt activity
— . . . Nonapplicable

	Visit number	1	2	3	4	5	6	7	8
	Julian date								
	Range—cont'd								
22	Oven: open								
23	place pans (2-4 lb.)								
24	remove pans (2-4 lb.)								
25	Broiler: in								
26	out								
27	Storage areas: open								
28	close								
	Refrigerator								
29	Open								
30	Close								
31	Food: in								
32	out								
33	Handle ice trays								
	Sink								
34	Dishes, utensils: wash								
35	dry								
36	store								
37	Faucets: reach								
38	turn on/off								
39	Wash sink								

ACTIVITIES OF DAILY LIVING

	CHILDREN'S HOSPITAL AT STANFORD OCCUPATIONAL THERAPY TIME-ORIENTED RECORD ACTIVITIES OF DAILY LIVING ASSESSMENT

Key to scoring:
4 . . . Independent
3 . . . Independent with equipment and/or adaptive technique
2 . . . Completes but cannot accomplish in practical time
1 . . . Attempts but requires assistance or supervision to complete
0 . . . Dependent—cannot attempt activity
— . . . Nonapplicable

	Visit number	1	2	3	4	5	6	7	8
	Julian date								
	Table								
40	Set								
41	Clear								
42	Serve food								
	Shopping								
43	Make list								
44	Travel to store								
45	Carry parcels								
46	Handle money								
47	Store purchases								
	Cleaning								
48	Use: dust cloth								
49	dust mop								
50	broom								
51	dust pan								
52	Clean: stove								
53	wash bowl								
54	toilet								
55	Empty waste basket								
56	Floors: wash								
57	polish								
58	vacuum								

ACTIVITIES OF DAILY LIVING

Continued.

		CHILDREN'S HOSPITAL AT STANFORD **OCCUPATIONAL THERAPY** **TIME-ORIENTED RECORD** **ACTIVITIES OF DAILY LIVING ASSESSMENT**

Key to scoring: 4 . . . Independent
3 . . . Independent with equipment and/or adaptive technique
2 . . . Completes but cannot accomplish in practical time
1 . . . Attempts but requires assistance or supervision to complete
0 . . . Dependent—cannot attempt activity
— . . . Nonapplicable

	Visit number	1	2	3	4	5	6	7	8
	Julian date								
	Cleaning—cont'd								
59	Furniture: polish								
60	vacuum								
61	Bed: change								
62	make up								
	Laundry								
63	Clothes: wash								
64	hang								
65	dry								
66	fold								
67	Ironing: dampen								
68	set up board								
69	set up iron								
70	put away clothes								
	Sewing								
71	Thread needle								
72	Tie knot								
73	Use straight pins								
74	Use scissors								
75	Sew button								
76	Mend								
77	Use sewing machine								

ACTIVITIES OF DAILY LIVING

CHILDREN'S HOSPITAL AT STANFORD **OCCUPATIONAL THERAPY** **TIME-ORIENTED RECORD** **ACTIVITIES OF DAILY LIVING ASSESSMENT**									

Key to scoring: 4 . . . Independent

3 . . . Independent with equipment and/or adaptive technique

2 . . . Completes but cannot accomplish in practical time

1 . . . Attempts but requires assistance or supervision to complete

0 . . . Dependent—cannot attempt activity

— . . . Nonapplicable

Visit number	1	2	3	4	5	6	7	8
Julian date								
Child care								
78 Bathe								
79 Dress								
80 Undress								
81 Feed								

ACTIVITIES OF DAILY LIVING

Index